To Dr. Jordan Katz
and
To Sherrie, Benjamin, Sarah, Mom, and Dad

Contributors

TAMESHWAR AMMAR, M.D.
Assistant Professor of Anesthesiology, Mt. Sinai School of Medicine, New York, New York
Uncommon Cardiac Diseases

ALLEN W. BURTON, M.D.
Assistant Professor, Department of Anesthesiology, University of Texas Medical Branch, Galveston, Texas
Renal Disease

JOHN V. DONLON, M.D.
Associate Clinical Professor Anesthesia, Harvard Medical School; Chief, Department of Anesthesia, Massachusetts Eye and Ear Infirmary, Boston, Massachusetts
Eye, Ear, Nose, and Throat Diseases

C. J. EAGLE, M.D.
Professor of Anaesthesia, University of Calgary; Director, Department of Anaesthesia, Foothills Hospital, Calgary, Alberta, Canada
Hepatic Diseases

JOHN H. EISELE, JR., M.D.
Professor and Chairman, Department of Anesthesiology, University of California Davis, Davis, California
Connective Tissue Diseases

MARK EZEKIEL, M.D.
Assistant Clinical Professor, Department of Anesthesiology, University of California at Irvine, Orange, California
Gastrointestinal and Nutritional Disorders

DAVID D. FRANKVILLE, M.D.
Associate Clinical Professor of Anesthesiology, Department of Anesthesiology, University of California San Diego; Director, Pediatric Anesthesia Services, University of California San Diego Medical Center, San Diego, California
Uncommon Malformation Syndromes of Infants and Pediatric Patients

DAVID R. GAMBLING, M.B., B.S.
Associate Clinical Professor of Anesthesiology, University of California San
Diego; Co-Director, Obstetric Anesthesia, University of California San Diego
Medical Center, San Diego, California
The Pregnant Patient and the Uncommon Disorders of Pregnancy

AHMED F. GHOURI, M.D.
Assistant Clinical Professor, Department of Anesthesiology, University of
California Irvine, Orange, California
Gastrointestinal and Nutritional Disorders

RANDALL GOSKOWICZ, M.D.
Assistant Clinical Professor, Department of Anesthesiology, University of
California San Diego School of Medicine; Director of Anesthesia for Liver
Transplantation, University of California San Diego Medical Center, San Diego,
California
Uncommon Poisoning, Envenomation, and Intoxication

JAN CHARLES HORROW, M.D.
Professor and Vice Chair, Department of Anesthesiology, Allegheny University
of the Health Sciences; Chief of Service, Anesthesia, Allegheny University
Hospitals–Hahnemann Division, Philadelphia, Pennsylvania
Hematologic Diseases

JOEL A. KAPLAN, M.D.
Horace W. Goldsmith Professor and Chairman, Department of Anesthesiology,
Mt. Sinai School of Medicine; Senior Vice President of Clinical Affairs, Mt.
Sinai Medical Center, New York, New York
Uncommon Cardiac Diseases

JOHN P. McCARREN, M.D.
Associate Clinical Professor, Department of Anesthesiology, University of
California San Diego; Chief, Anesthesia Services, Thornton Hospital, La Jolla,
California
Respiratory Diseases

DOUGLAS G. MARTZ, Jr., M.D.
Assistant Professor of Anesthesiology, University of Maryland School of
Medicine; Director of Clinical Quality Management, Department of
Anesthesiology, University of Maryland Medical System, Baltimore, Maryland
Neurologic Diseases

M. JANE MATJASKO, M.D.
Martin Helrich Professor and Chairman, Department of Anesthesiology,
University of Maryland School of Medicine, Baltimore, Maryland
Neurologic Diseases

RICHARD I. MAZZE, M.D.
Professor of Anesthesiology, Stanford University; Chief of Staff, Veterans
Administration Palo Alto Health Care System, Palo Alto, California
Renal Disease

JORDAN D. MILLER, M.D.
Associate Professor, Department of Anesthesiology, University of California Los Angeles School of Medicine, Los Angeles, California
Muscle Diseases

JONATHAN L. PARMET, M.D.
Associate Professor, Department of Anesthesiology, Allegheny University of the Health Sciences; Anesthesiologist, Allegheny University Hospitals–Hahnemann Division, Philadelphia, Pennsylvana
Hematologic Diseases

BRIAN L. PARTRIDGE, M.D.
Adjunct Assistant Clinical Professor, Department of Anesthesiology, University of California San Diego School of Medicine; Anesthesiologist, Anesthesia Services Medical Group, San Diego, California
Skin and Bone Disorders

DONALD S. PROUGH, M.D.
Professor and Chairman, Department of Anesthesiology, the University of Texas Medical Branch, Galveston, Texas
Renal Disease

DAVID L. REICH, M.D.
Associate Professor of Anesthesiology, Mt. Sinai School of Medicine; Co-Director of Cardiothoracic Anesthesia, Mt. Sinai Medical Center, New York, New York
Uncommon Cardiac Diseases

LAURENCE S. REISNER, M.D.
Professor of Anesthesiology and Reproductive Medicine, University of California San Diego; Acting Chair, Department of Anesthesiology, and Co-Director, Obstetric Anesthesia, University of California San Diego Medical Center, San Diego, California
The Pregnant Patient and the Uncommon Disorders of Pregnancy

MICHAEL F. ROIZEN, M.D.
Professor and Chairman, Department of Anesthesia and Critical Care, and Professor, Department of Medicine, University of Chicago Division of Biological Sciences, Pritzker School of Medicine, Chicago, Illinois
Diseases of the Endocrine System

HARVEY ROSENBAUM, M.D.
Clinical Associate Professor, Department of Anesthesiology, University of California Los Angeles School of Medicine, Los Angeles, California
Muscle Diseases

DAVID L. SCHREIBMAN, M.D.
Assistant Professor of Anesthesiology and Surgery, University of Maryland School of Medicine, Baltimore, Maryland
Neurologic Diseases

LEO STRUNIN, M.D.
Boc Professor of Anaesthesia and Director, Anaesthetics Unit, St.
Bartholomew's and the Royal London School of Medicine and Dentistry, Queen
Mary and Westfield College, University of London; The Royal London
Hospital, London, England
Hepatic Diseases

D. EDWARD SUPKIS, Jr., M.D.
Assistant Professor of Anesthesiology, Department of Anesthesiology, The
University of Texas M.D. Anderson Cancer Center; Medical Director of
Respiratory Care and Chairman, Capital Equipment Technology Committee,
Associate Professor, M.D. Anderson Cancer Center, Houston, Texas
Uncommon Problems Related to Cancer

JOSEPH VARON, M.D.
Assistant Professor of Anesthesiology, Critical Care and Medicine, The
University of Texas M.D. Anderson Cancer Center; Director, Surgical Intensive
Care Unit, and Assistant Director, Respiratory Care Services, M.D. Anderson
Cancer Center, Houston, Texas
Uncommon Problems Related to Cancer

WILLIAM C. WILSON, M.D.
Assistant Clinical Professor of Anesthesiology and Critical Care Medicine,
University of San Diego Medical Center; Associate Director, Surgical Intensive
Care Unit, University of California San Diego Medical Center, San Diego,
California
Uncommon Poisoning, Envenomation, and Intoxication

Preface

The fourth edition of *Anesthesia and Uncommon Diseases* is dedicated to Dr. Jordan Katz because his original concept, the raison d'être for the book, remains the same: i.e., to bring vital, yet widely scattered, clinical information to the practicing anesthesiologist and nurse anesthetist. In order to do this as best as possible the fourth edition of *Anesthesia and Uncommon Diseases* has been significantly revised and restructured. The overriding goal of this revision has been to retain the best of the past while ensuring that all material is current, concise, and clinically meaningful. From an editorial point of view, the current economics of medicine in the United States has made this task more difficult.

The book has been reorganized into sections consisting of uncommon diseases of specific organs and systems, uncommon diseases and problems by type of patient, and uncommon multisystemic diseases and anesthetic problems. Two important new chapters have been added: one on uncommon anesthesia problems related to cancer and one on problems related to poisoning and intoxications. In addition, a host of talented, well-respected authors have added fresh perspective to many challenging topics. The basic approach of first presenting the pathophysiology of the uncommon disease, and then the anesthetic management, has been largely retained. The intent of this unique mixture of old and new is to reach the full potential of Dr. Jordan Katz's original concept and teaching contribution.

JONATHAN L. BENUMOF

Contents

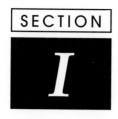

SECTION

I

Uncommon Diseases of Specific Organs and Systems

Neurologic Diseases

Douglas G. Martz, Jr., M.D.,
David L. Schreibman, M.D.,
and M. Jane Matjasko, M.D.

I. BASAL GANGLIA DISORDERS

The entities to be considered next include Parkinson's disease, Huntington's chorea, Sydenham's chorea, torsion dystonia, and spasmodic torticollis. All have similar symptoms of chorea, athetosis, and dystonia. These symptoms may also occur because of cerebrovascular insufficiency or during drug therapy (most notably phenothiazines and butyrophenones), or as a result of hypoxic encephalopathy or central nervous system (CNS) trauma. Because the functional deficiency in all these entities is in the basal ganglia, the anesthetic considerations are similar.

A. NEUROANATOMIC AND NEUROPHYSIOLOGIC CONSIDERATIONS

The basal ganglia (extrapyramidal system) subserve motor functions that are distinct from those attributable to the corticospinal tracts (pyramidal system). The major nuclei are the caudate and the putamen (which together are called the *striatum*), the internal and external segments of the globus pallidus, the subthalamic nucleus, and the substantia nigra (Fig. 1–1). There are many neural connections between these nuclei, each contributing excitatory and inhibitory impulses. These impulses, channeled through the globus pallidus to the thalamus and then to the cerebral cortex, along with some modifications from the cerebellum, determine motor function controlled by the corticospinal tracts. If one or more of the supporting nuclei are damaged, the sum of the impulses to the globus pallidus changes and mobility is disordered.

The most important neurotransmitter substances in terms of basal ganglionic function are acetylcholine (ACh), dopamine, and γ-aminobutyric acid (GABA), although serotonin, substance P, somatostatin, and enkephalin exert some neuromodulatory effects. ACh, which is most concentrated in the striatum, exerts an excitatory effect on striatal neurons, whereas dopamine, which is concentrated in the substantia nigra, exerts an inhibitory effect. GABA is also thought to act as an inhibitory neurotransmitter and is very concentrated in the substantia nigra, striatum, and globus pallidus.

B. CLINICAL MANIFESTATIONS

The symptoms of extrapyramidal diseases can be divided into primary functional deficits (negative symptoms due to loss of connectivity) and secondary release effects (positive symptoms of excessive activity). *Akinesia,* which can be prominent in Parkinson's disease, refers to inability of the patient to initiate changes in activity and to perform volitional movements rapidly. *Bradykinesia* and *hypokinesia* describe lesser degrees of impairment.

Muscle tone is defined as the amount of resistance encountered when a relaxed limb is moved passively. In *rigidity,* the muscles are in continuous contraction and resistance to passive movement is constant. This tends to be more prominent in flexor muscle groups. *Cogwheel rigidity* occurs when a hypertonic muscle is stretched passively and the resistance is jerky, as though controlled by a ratchet; it is a common manifestation of Parkinson's disease. *Chorea* refers to a widespread arrhythmic, jerky, restless type of movement. It is often constant and may affect any part of the body. Generalized chorea is the predominant manifestation of Huntington's and Sydenham's choreas. *Athetosis* is characterized by inability to sustain a muscle group in one position; it occurs most often in the hands, although it can be generalized. Athetotic movements are slower than those associated with chorea. Athetosis is usually seen in torsion dystonia and cerebral palsy. *Dystonia* refers to abnormally increased muscle tone that causes fixed abnormal postures, although some patients exhibit shifting postures. It generally involves trunk muscles, as opposed to extremities, and is increased during volitional motor activity and stress, as in torsion dystonia. Focal dystonias—more common than torsion dystonia—include such dis-

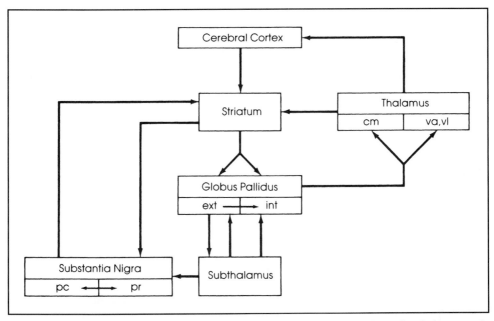

FIGURE 1–1. Schematic diagram of the major neuronal connections between the basal ganglia, thalamus, and cerebral cortex. The projection from the internal segment of the globus pallidus constitutes the principal efferent pathway from the basal ganglia. Key: ext, external; int, internal; pc, pars compacta; pr, pars reticulata; cm, centromedian; va, ventroanterior; vl, ventrolateral. (From Growden JH, Young RR: Paralysis and other disorders of movement. In Braunwald E, et al (eds): Harrison's Principles of Internal Medicine, ed 11. New York, McGraw-Hill, 1987, pp. 79–91.)

orders as spasmodic torticollis and writer's cramp. *Hemiballismus* is a hyperkinetic movement disorder characterized by violent, flinging arm motions; it occurs in a number of extrapyramidal disorders.

C. SYDENHAM'S CHOREA

Sydenham's chorea occurs primarily in children, most often in females, usually as a consequence of β-hemolytic streptococcal infection. It is rarely fatal but recurs within a year in as many as 30 to 35 per cent of children. Particularly important is its association with endocarditis (20 per cent) and the high incidence of electrocardiographic (ECG) abnormalities in asymptomatic siblings. Irritability and emotional lability are frequently seen, although more severe mental symptoms can occur. Pathologically, scattered areas of cell degeneration are found in the cerebral cortex, basal ganglia, substantia nigra, and cerebellum, as is arteritis with hyalinization of small vessels.

The onset of symptoms is often insidious, but the diagnosis is not difficult when one observes choreiform movements in a child. These movements are most prevalent in the upper extremities and stop during sleep.

They may also be diminished by phenothiazines and barbiturates, which are the principal drugs for treatment, although some patients are treated successfully with corticosteroids and levodopa.

There is no reported anesthetic experience with Sydenham's chorea. Preoperative assessment should include careful evaluation of cardiac status, particularly ECG abnormalities, and appropriate antibiotic prophylaxis for rheumatic heart disease. Premedication with barbiturates is appropriate. The anesthetic plan must consider potential interactions with the patient's current drug therapy (see the section on Parkinson's Disease).

D. HUNTINGTON'S CHOREA

Huntington's chorea, also termed *chronic progressive chorea* and *adult chorea*, is a genetic disease transmitted in an autosomal dominant pattern with an incidence of 4 to 5 per million. Pathologically, there is marked atrophy of the caudate nucleus with some atrophy of the putamen and globus pallidus. Neurochemical studies of the basal ganglia show decreased levels of GABA and its synthesizing enzyme and increased amounts of somatostatin. The onset of the disease occurs at age 35 to 40 years; clinical manifestations include chorea, ataxia, and dysarthria. As a general rule, dementia increases as the motor disorder worsens. Although no form of treatment exists to halt the relentless progression of the disease, phenothiazines and butyrophenones are somewhat effective in alleviating symptoms.

Reported anesthetic experience consists of a small number of case reports and letters. One case of delayed recovery from thiopental may have been dose related and has not been substantiated in other reports.[1–4] Propofol has been used successfully as an induction agent and for anesthetic maintenance.[5, 6] Interestingly, the incidence of decreased pseudocholinesterase activity is substantially higher in Huntington's chorea patients than in the normal population; this may explain the single report of prolonged response to succinylcholine.[7] Thus it appears that no anesthetic agent or muscle relaxant is contraindicated, although succinylcholine may have prolonged effect.[8, 9] The use of muscle relaxants not metabolized by pseudocholinesterase certainly may be warranted. Use of butyrophenones and/or phenothiazines in the anesthetic regimen may help to control choreiform movement perioperatively. Glycopyrrolate may be the preferred anticholinergic agent since central anticholinergic effects may exacerbate choreiform movements. Other concerns regarding the anesthetic management are determined by the level of physiologic debilitation in the individual patient.

E. SPASMODIC TORTICOLLIS

Spasmodic torticollis and other craniocervical spasms are intermittent, arrhythmic, brief, or prolonged contractile spasms of the facial, jaw, lingual, sternocleidomastoid, trapezius, and other neck muscles. Other diseases in this group include blepharospasm (Meige's syndrome), oromandibular dystonia, and spasmodic dysphonia.

Spasmodic torticollis usually begins in early to middle adulthood and is manifested by rotation and partial extension of the head. Although the most prominently affected muscles are the sternocleidomastoid and the trapezius, electromyographic (EMG) studies show sustained activity in the posterior cervical muscles as well. The pathogenesis is not known, although hyperactivity of the dopamine system in the striatum has been postulated. Surgical interruption of the spinal accessory nerve and the first three cervical motor roots bilaterally has been the most successful therapy. There is a risk of transient or permanent paralysis of the diaphragm secondary to inadvertent phrenic nerve damage. Postoperatively, swallowing may be difficult if the patient cannot reflexly lift the chin. There are no reported adverse anesthetic reactions; spasms are relieved with muscle relaxants, and, interestingly, nitrous oxide at analgesic concentrations ameliorates the dystonic movements.[10]

F. TORSION DYSTONIA

Torsion dystonia (dystonia musculorum deformans, Oppenheim's disease) is a genetic disease that can have its onset in adulthood (the autosomal dominant form) or childhood (autosomal recessive or autosomal dominant with variable penetrance). Clinical onset is gradual; involuntary writhing movements and torsion spasms are characteristic symptoms. The spasms commonly involve the vertebral column; lordosis and scoliosis are seen when the disease is of long duration. Adults may have a fixed cervical spine, and an awake intubation may be indicated in these cases. There are no reported adverse effects of anesthetic agents. Heavy premedication may relieve spasms because symptoms are absent during sleep.[11]

Other rare disorders that affect the basal ganglia and lead to extrapyramidal symptoms include status marmoratus (double athetosis); Hallervorden-Spatz syndrome (pigmentary degeneration of the globus pallidus); Creutzfeldt-Jakob disease, a slow virus disease; and Wilson's disease, an inherited defect of copper transport and storage associated with the absence of ceruloplasmin, a copper-binding globulin. There are no reports of anesthetic experience with these syndromes, but Creutzfeldt-Jakob and other slow virus infections require strict operating room technique to avoid transmission to personnel during brain biopsy.

G. PARKINSON'S DISEASE

Parkinson's syndrome can follow (1) long-term administration of drugs such as reserpine, phenothiazines, and butyrophenones; (2) carbon monoxide or manganese poisoning; (3) encephalitis (such as encephalitis lethargica); and (4) CNS trauma following repeated blows to the head (common in boxers). Most often, however, the cause of Parkinson's syndrome is not known, and it is this entity that is referred to as *Parkinson's disease* (paralysis agitans). The disease begins most often between 40 and 70 years of age (peak onset in the sixth decade). In the United States about 1 per cent of the population older than age 50 are affected.

Although the pathophysiology of Parkinson's disease is unclear, it is due to a relative deficiency of dopamine in the caudate nucleus and putamen, which creates an imbalance between inhibitory (dopamine) and excitatory (ACh) control of the basal ganglia. A decrease in basal ganglia dopamine is found with experimental ablation of the substantia nigra, and, indeed, in Parkinson's disease the most consistent pathologic findings are loss of pigmented cells in the substantia nigra and the presence of Lewy bodies (eosinophilic cytoplasmic inclusions) in the remaining pigmented nuclei. Experimental and illicit use of the neurotoxin MPTP causes irreversible parkinsonian symptoms. It is postulated that the degradation of MPTP by the enzyme monoamine oxidase-B (MAO-B) causes destruction of the substantia nigra. Inhibition of MAO-B has shown some clinical benefit.

Diagnosis is made on clinical grounds. Initial symptoms are usually mild and unilateral but, if untreated, often progress to a debilitating level. In its fully developed form, clinical manifestations include stooped posture, stiffness and slowness of movement, mask-like facies, rhythmic tremor of the extremities that subsides with active, willed movement or complete relaxation, shifting, unsteady gait, and monotone voice. Approximately one third of all patients have some degree of dementia—and often depression.

The goal of treatment in Parkinson's disease is to balance striatal activity by reducing cholinergic activity or enhancement of dopaminergic function. Drugs used include levodopa, selegiline, anticholinergics, amantadine, and bromocriptine. Levodopa (L-dopa), unlike dopamine, crosses the blood–brain barrier and is converted to dopamine in the CNS by the enzyme dopa-decarboxylase. Dopa-decarboxylase is present in the systemic circulation and tissue, and therapy with L-dopa increases systemic dopamine levels as well. The concurrent administration of a decarboxylase inhibitor, carbidopa, allows the total dose of L-dopa to be decreased, thus reducing the dose-related side effects.

Side effects from chronically increased serum dopamine concentrations include nausea and vomiting (prominent during early phases of therapy), myocardial irritability, and reduced activity of the renin-angiotensin system leading to decreased intravascular volume and orthostatic hypotension. Other side effects of long-term L-dopa administration include CNS effects such as confusion, depression, agitation, on-off syndrome (in which, in a matter of minutes or from one hour to the next, the patient may shift from a state of relative mobility to one of complete or nearly complete immobility), and dyskinesia, which invariably occurs in every patient and is the limiting factor in the use of L-dopa.

Dyskinesia is treated by reducing the L-dopa dose or concurrently administering anticholinergics; the most common of the latter are trihexyphenidyl (Artane), benztropine mesylate (Cogentin), and amantadine, an antiviral agent. Amantadine acts by releasing stored dopamine from presynaptic terminals. Amantadine and anticholinergic drugs are especially effective against tremor in the early stages of the disease. Bromocriptine, a dopamine agonist, is most effective in the treatment of Parkinson's disease in the early stages or when used in combination with L-dopa. Selegiline, an MAO-B inhibitor, exerts its effect by blocking dopamine catabolism. Treatment in the early course of the disease has delayed progression to disability and the need to initiate L-dopa therapy.[12, 13]

Although not common today owing to the success of drug therapy, stereotactic obliteration of the globus pallidus or ventrolateral thalamus is still performed occasionally in young, healthy patients with severe unilateral tremor. Implantation of fetal adrenal medullary tissue into the caudate nucleus has had modest preliminary success in improving motor function.[13]

H. ANESTHETIC CONSIDERATIONS

Patients with Parkinson's disease most often require surgery for urologic, ophthalmic, and orthopedic procedures.[14] Preoperatively, pharmacologic therapy should be maintained up to and through the morning of surgery. Drugs that potentially cause or exacerbate extrapyramidal symptoms, such as phenothiazines, butyrophenone derivatives (droperidol), and metoclopramide (Reglan), should be withheld. Anesthetic agents (such as halothane) that sensitize the heart to arrhythmias from catecholamines should be excluded, owing to the potential for arrhythmias with L-dopa.[15, 16] Selegiline is an MAO-B inhibitor and theoretically should not cause the exaggerated sympathetic response associated with other MAO inhibitors. There are no reports of selegiline and perioperative reactions. Vasopressor therapy should be planned accordingly.

Although ketamine has been used successfully in patients taking L-dopa, its use has been questioned, since it may precipitate an exaggerated hypertensive response.[17] Opioids, especially in large doses, have been implicated in precipitating rigidity; however, opioids in analgesic concentrations have not been reported to increase symptoms of the disease.[18] Inhalation anesthetics have been implicated in exacerbating rigidity in the postoperative period. In one case report a patient showed classic signs of parkinsonism on emergence from general anesthesia. His condition returned to baseline, but he was diagnosed with Parkinson's disease 18 months later.[19] Propofol has been reported to abolish parkinsonian tremors perioperatively. The mechanism of this effect is not known.[20] There are no absolute contraindications to regional anesthesia. There is a case report of exacerbation of parkinsonism intraoperatively during spinal anesthesia, but this was most likely due to low levels of the patient's medication regimen. Interestingly, intraoperative tremors can mimic ventricular arrhythmias during continuous ECG monitoring.[21] There is one reported case of a hyperkalemic response after succinylcholine administration, but it is unclear whether the patient had intercurrent peripheral denervation.[22] From other series it appears that the response to succinylcholine is normal in Parkinson's disease.[23] The response to the nondepolarizing muscle relaxants is normal.

Preoperative hypotension is likely because there may be relative hypovolemia, norepinephrine depletion, and varying degrees of autonomic dysfunction. If vasopressors are needed, a dilute direct-acting agent such as phenylephrine hydrochloride (Neo-Synephrine) is indicated. Diphenhydramine (Benadryl), an H_1 receptor–blocking antihistamine that has central anticholinergic activity, has been reported to be an excellent drug for sedation and control of mild tremor in the awake patient undergoing surgery with local anesthesia.[24] Postoperatively, it is advantageous to resume drug therapy as soon as possible, to avoid recurrent extrapyramidal symptoms. If the drugs have been discontinued for prolonged periods, gradually increasing dosage schedules should be used when therapy resumes, to minimize side effects.

II. MOTOR NEURON DEGENERATION

The motor neuron degenerative diseases (Table 1–1) share the clinical findings of muscle weakness and wasting with intact sensory pathways. The anesthetic management is similar for each of these diseases, the most common of which is amyotrophic lateral sclerosis (ALS).

TABLE 1–1

Degenerative Motor Neuron Diseases

Amyotrophic lateral sclerosis (ALS)
   Progressive muscular atrophy
   Primary lateral sclerosis
   Pseudobulbar palsy
Inherited motor neuron diseases
   Autosomal-recessive spinal muscular atrophy
      Type I: Werdnig-Hoffmann, acute
      Type II: Werdnig-Hoffmann, chronic
      Type III: Kugelberg-Welander
      Type IV: Adult-onset disease
   Familial ALS
   Familial ALS with dementia or Parkinson's disease (Guam)
   Other
      Arthrogryposis multiplex congenita
      Progressive juvenile bulbar palsy (Fazio-Londe)
      Neuroaxonal dystrophy
Associated with other degenerative disorders
   Olivopontocerebellar atrophies
   Peroneal muscle atrophy
Friedreich's ataxia
Guillain-Barré syndrome
   Baló's disease
Acute disseminated encephalomyelitis following measles, chickenpox, smallpox, and (rarely) mumps, rubella, or influenza
Acute and subacute necrotizing hemorrhagic encephalitis
   Acute encephalopathic form (Hurst's disease)
   Subacute necrotic myelopathy
   Acute brain purpura

A. AMYOTROPHIC LATERAL SCLEROSIS

ALS is a degenerative disease of motor cells throughout the CNS; males are affected more often than females. When the degenerative process is limited to the motor cortex and the efferent pathways, the syndrome of primary lateral sclerosis occurs; when the disease involves the brain stem nuclei it is termed *pseudobulbar palsy*; and when limited to the anterior horn cells of the spinal cord it is called *progressive muscular atrophy*. A remarkable feature of the disease is the selectivity of neuronal cell death. The entire sensory apparatus, the regulatory mechanisms for the control and coordination of movements, and the intellect remain intact. There is also some selectivity in motor involvement, since the extraocular muscles and the sacral parasympathetic neurons that innervate the sphincters for bowel and bladder control are spared.

The disorder has its peak incidence between ages 40 and 50 years. Although it is uncommon, well-documented instances of familial genetically patterned disease occur, and family histories have been traced for both a dominant and a recessive pattern of inheritance. These genetically linked cases tend to occur at a younger age, usually in the late teens.

The incidence of ALS in the Chamorro natives of Guam and the Mariana Islands is 100 times that in other countries. In addition, there is frequent association of a Parkinson's-dementia complex with ALS in Guam.[25] Diagnosis is made by clinical observation and EMG studies, which show a reduction in the number of motor units and an increase in the size of individual muscle action potentials.

Both upper and lower motor neuron degenerative processes are almost invariably identifiable when the disease is well established, although one or the other may predominate in the early phases of the disease. ALS begins with atrophy, weakness, and fasciculations, very often involving one of the limbs, but most muscles are involved within 1 to 2 years. Occasionally the first symptoms may be related to spasticity and associated spastic weakness, especially in the lower extremities. As the disease progresses, both spasticity and atrophy may be evident in many muscles.[26]

In some persons the early signs are prominent in bulbar-innervated striated muscle. Early bulbar symptoms are commonly those that affect precision of speech. Swallowing abnormalities are particularly troublesome, owing to the increased risk of regurgitation and aspiration. In addition, inability to control emotional responses is present. It appears that affect and feelings may be quite normal, but when confronted with a stimulus that evokes sadness or laughter patients may burst into uncontrollable facial spasms.

The characteristic fasciculations are simultaneous contractions of bundles of contiguous muscle fibers, which are often visible through the skin. They are more evident with fatigue and exercise.

The usual course of the disease is relentless progression, without periods of improvement or stabilization of symptoms. Most often death is due to pulmonary infection. There is no effective treatment that influences the pathologic process. Modern rehabilitative measures, including mechanical aids of various kinds, help patients to overcome the effects of their disabilities; respiratory support can prolong survival. Thyrotropin-releasing hormone (TRH) infusions have been observed to cause transitory (not long-term) improvement of motor function.[26] ALS is associated with malignant tumors, but not nearly as often as the myasthenic syndrome (for example, Eaton-Lambert disease) that accompanies certain neoplastic diseases.

B. SPINAL MUSCULAR ATROPHY

In spinal muscular atrophy (SMA), peripheral motor neurons are affected without involvement of the upper motor neurons. SMA generally affects a much younger age group and tends to be hereditary (usually autosomal recessive).

Werdnig-Hoffmann disease (SMA type I) is a rapidly progressive disease of infancy that can even be apparent in utero because of decreased fetal movement. Affected infants are alert but weak and hypotonic. Death usually occurs within the first year of life. SMA type II is clinically similar to type I, except that the evolution of the disease is considerably slower and patients survive into adolescence or even young adulthood. Kugelberg-Welander disease (SMA type III) manifests itself during late childhood and has a slow, indolent course. Typically, muscles of the trunk and proximal limbs are most severely involved. SMA type IV is a slowly evolving adult form of SMA. Other very rare motor neuron diseases not discussed here are listed in Table 14–1.

1. Anesthetic Management

Because the cause of poor neuromuscular transmission in motor neuron degenerative diseases is not clear, a major concern of anesthetic management is the use of muscle relaxants. A reduction in the enzyme choline acetyltransferase, which is involved in the synthesis of ACh, probably occurs secondary to degeneration of anterior horn cells.[27] The resultant decreased levels of ACh would increase the patient's sensitivity to nondepolarizing muscle relaxants.[28]

The clinical implications are more troublesome when the respiratory muscles are affected by the disease, since residual neuromuscular block may contribute to postoperative respiratory difficulties. If nondepolarizing muscle relaxants are indicated, the dose should be titrated and neuromuscular blockade continuously monitored. Succinylcholine should not be given to persons with motor neuron degenerative diseases, owing to its association with a hyperkalemic response and myotonia-like contractures.[29, 30]

There is no evidence that any specific anesthetic technique or drug is deleterious to those with motor neuron degenerative disease. If regional anesthesia is planned, the anesthetic level should not compromise accessory respiratory muscle function. Neuraxial narcotics for postoperative analgesia have been administered—with good results.[31] Risk of pulmonary aspiration is increased in patients with bulbar involvement.

During general anesthesia, assisted or controlled ventilation is recommended; postoperatively, residual anesthetic or the location of the surgical wound may cause respiratory compromise. Postoperative ventilatory support, especially in Werdnig-Hoffmann disease, may be required.

C. FRIEDREICH'S ATAXIA

Friedreich's ataxia is the prototype for all forms of progressive ataxia. It is distinguished from them by the involvement of the spinal cord; other forms of progressive ataxia are caused by cerebellar lesions (familial cortical cerebellar atrophy) and brainstem lesions (familial olivopontocerebellar and spinocere-bellar degeneration and olivopontocerebellar atrophy).

Friedreich's ataxia occurs between 10 and 30 years of age and is usually inherited in an autosomal-recessive manner, although an autosomal-dominant subset exists. It is characterized by degeneration of long ascending and descending fibers in the spinal cord, including the spinocerebellar tracts, with concomitant dorsal root ganglion atrophy. It is therefore a mixed upper and lower motor neuron disease, with cerebellar signs predominating. Clinical manifestations include ataxia, dysarthria, and nystagmus combined with weakness, spasticity, and atrophy. Pes cavus and kyphoscoliosis are common associated abnormalities; a hypertrophy-like cardiomyopathy is present in about half of the cases. ECG monitoring may demonstrate sinus tachycardia and a variety of arrhythmias. Many patients die as a result of their arrhythmias or from complications of congestive heart failure.

Anesthetic management in progressive ataxia is similar to that described for the motor neuron degenerative diseases. With Friedreich's ataxia appropriate measures should be taken if during the preoperative assessment restrictive pulmonary disease or a cardiomyopathy is discovered. Onset and recovery from nondepolarizing muscle relaxants appear to be normal.[32, 33] Use of regional anesthesia has been reported without exacerbation of neurologic symptoms.[32, 34]

D. GUILLAIN-BARRÉ SYNDROME

The cause of Guillain-Barré syndrome (acute idiopathic polyneuritis) is unknown, but evidence suggests that the clinical manifestations of the disorder are the result of a cell-mediated immune response of the peripheral nerves. A mild respiratory or gastrointestinal infection precedes the neurologic symptoms by 1 to 3 weeks in 60 to 70 per cent of patients. Other preceding events include surgical procedures, viral exanthems and other viral illnesses, certain vaccinations, and lymphomatous disease.

The major clinical manifestation is weakness that evolves more or less symmetrically over several days. Proximal as well as distal limb muscles are involved, usually lower extremities first with ascending spread; 50 per cent of patients have bulbar involvement. The disease can vary from paresis of the legs alone to total motor paralysis. Paresthesias are frequent; muscle pain occurs in about one third of cases. Disturbances of autonomic function are common; symptoms include fluctuating hypertension and hypotension, sinus tachycardia, diaphoresis, and orthostatic hypotension.

The diagnosis is made by clinical findings confirmed by increased cerebrospinal fluid (CSF) protein (presumably due to inflammation of nerve roots) with a normal cell count, although 10 per cent of patients show CSF lymphopleocytosis. The essence of treatment is symptomatic care. Ventilatory support should be implemented if pharyngeal and respiratory involvement impairs the ability to protect the airway or to adequately maintain ventilation and oxygenation.[35] Some guidelines for mechanical ventilatory assistance include an alveoarterial oxygen tension gradient greater than 300 mm Hg with an inspired oxygen fraction of 1.0, arterial PCO_2 greater than 50 mm Hg, maximum static inspiratory and expiratory pressure less than 30 cm H_2O, and vital capacity less than 14 mL/kg.[36]

Frequently, treatment of hypertension and hypotension from autonomic dysfunction is necessary. A therapeutic trial of prednisone can be beneficial in some cases, but if a definite response does not occur within a few days it should be discontinued. Plasmapheresis, if implemented within 2 weeks of onset of symptoms, has been shown to significantly reduce the time to recovery. The majority of patients recover spontaneously and completely. In an intensive care environment mortality is about 2 per cent.

Considerations in anesthetic management of the Guillain-Barré patient focus on the severity of disease, in terms of respiratory status and autonomic dysfunction. Succinylcholine-induced hyperkalemia and increased sensitivity to nondepolarizing muscle relaxants are present, as in motor neuron degeneration.[41] Because of the possibility of significant variations in blood pressure, continuous intraarterial pressure monitoring should be implemented before anesthetic induction. Treatment of autonomic dysfunction is the same as for congenital dysautonomia (see the section on Dysautonomia). No abnormal responses to anesthetic agents are reported, but residual respiratory effects from anesthetic agents and muscle relaxants may necessitate postoperative ventilation. The use of regional anesthesia is controversial; two case reports have cited no ill effects from regional anesthe-

sia, but one article has implicated regional anesthesia as a cause of the disease. Clinical experience suggests that patients are sensitive to local anesthetics, and thus doses should be titrated to effect.[35, 41-45]

In a parturient with Guillain-Barré syndrome, a regional anesthetic for labor would be beneficial, because autonomic dysfunction may trigger an exaggerated hemodynamic response to pain. Epidural anesthesia for abdominal delivery has been reported.[43] For patients with respiratory compromise the risk-benefit ratio of regional anesthesia versus general anesthesia should be individualized.[46]

III. GENETICALLY DETERMINED POLYNEUROPATHIES

Polyneuropathies in association with systemic disease (e.g., diabetes mellitus, uremia, sarcoidosis, metastatic cancer) or a substance (e.g., isoniazid, vincristine, chronic alcoholism, vitamin B_{12} deficiency) are well described in various medical textbooks. However, three groups of genetically determined polyneuropathies can be identified according to their main clinical features—a pure motor type, a predominantly sensory type, and a mixed sensorimotor-autonomic type. A few representative polyneuropathies are described.

Charcot-Marie-Tooth disease (peroneal muscular atrophy) is inherited in an autosomal dominant mode. Its onset is usually in the second decade, and it generally affects the distal leg musculature, although later in life atrophy of the hand and forearm muscles occurs. High pedal arches and clubfeet are common; the most common clinical manifestation is foot drop. Diagnosis is based on abnormal nerve conduction velocities and sural nerve biopsy.[1] The main disability difficulty is walking, owing to a combination of weakness and sensory ataxia. Treatment includes foot bracing and surgical ankle fusion.

Déjérine-Sottas disease (progressive hypertrophic neuropathy) follows an autosomal recessive pattern. It begins in childhood and is slowly progressive. Pain and paresthesias in the feet occur early and are followed by development of symmetric weakness and wasting of the distal limbs. Roussy-Lévy syndrome (hereditary areflexic dysstasia) is probably an autosomal recessive disorder. It presents in infancy and is characterized by sensory and motor deficits affecting mainly the lower legs and eventually the hands. Kyphoscoliosis is a commonly associated finding.

The anesthetic experience for hereditary polyneuropathies consists of a few case reports and a retrospective review of patients with Charcot-Marie-Tooth disease.[37-40] Preoperative assessment should include evaluation for restrictive pulmonary disease if phrenic nerve involvement is suspected. Patients with significant motor and sensory deficits are sensitive to thiopental.[40] Successful use of succinylcholine has been reported; however, it seems appropriate to avoid succinylcholine when there is even a suspicion of muscular denervation, to avoid a hyperkalemic response. Onset of and recovery from nondepolarizing muscle relaxants appears to be normal. There are no reports of malignant hyperthermia episodes. No other anesthetic agents appear to be contraindicated. Anesthetic management should be tailored to accommodate any concomitant systemic abnormalities.

IV. ABNORMALITIES OF CEREBROSPINAL FLUID PATHWAYS

A. CEREBROSPINAL FLUID PHYSIOLOGY

The intracranial contents consist of 86 per cent brain tissue, 10 per cent CSF, and 4 per cent blood. The CSF spaces, by virtue of their larger volume and compressibility, are the best buffers against increasing intracranial pressure. The total CSF volume—130 to 200 mL—is divided equally between the intracranial compartment (25 to 50 mL in the ventricles) and the spinal subarachnoid space. CSF pressure in the lumbar subarachnoid space is approximately 100 mm H_2O when a subject lies supine and 300 mm H_2O when sitting. CSF is formed in the choroid plexus lining the ventricles at a rate of 500 to 600 mL per day.[47] The majority of CSF production is by Na/K-ATPase–mediated active transport and the remainder by passive filtration that is dependent on capillary hydrostatic pressure. CSF is isotonic to, but not an ultrafiltrate of, plasma.

Factors that affect CSF formation include choroidal blood flow, temperature, serum ventricular osmolarity, intraventricular hydrostatic pressure, hypocapnia, intrathoracic venous pressure, and sympathetic innervation. Many drugs inhibit CSF formation, including acetazolamide, digoxin, corticosteroids, spironolactone, furosemide, and ethacrynic acid. Maximum inhibition of only 70 per cent is obtained, despite using a combination of inhibitors. Aminophylline increases CSF production by increasing Na/K-ATPase.

CSF circulates from its site of formation in the two lateral ventricles in the cerebral hemispheres through the paired foramina of Monro to enter the midline third ventricle. The third ventricle is connected to the fourth ventricle through the aqueduct of Sylvius. Communication between the fourth ventricle and the cisterna magna (cerebellomedullary cistern) is via the paired lateral foramina of Luschka and the single midline foramen of Magendie. From there, the CSF circulates in the intracranial and spinal subarachnoid spaces. Spinal subarachnoid space CSF flow is sluggish, as compared with intracranial flow, and there is essentially no circulation in the central spinal canal.

Absorption of CSF occurs principally at the arachnoid villi located along the sagittal sinus. The mechanism of absorption is a bulk flow phenomenon utilizing a combination of transepithelial channels and pinocytosis. The major factor affecting CSF absorption is hydrostatic pressure, which is determined by CSF and venous pressure. Absorption begins when CSF pressure exceeds venous pressure.[48, 49] The rate of absorption equals the rate of formation of CSF. The balance between absorption and formation produces a CSF volume that determines intracranial pressure.

Anesthetic agents may affect the balance between the formation and absorption of CSF (Table 1–2).[50] The magnitude of the effect that anesthetic agents have on CSF dynamics is minimal but may become relevant when intracranial compliance is reduced. Thiopental, propofol, narcotics, isoflurane, and nitrous oxide have little effect on the balance between CSF formation and absorption.[51] Mannitol, an osmotic diuretic used to decrease intracranial pressure, probably works by multiple mechanisms, including by decreasing CSF formation, brain water content, and cerebral blood volume.[52]

B. HYDROCEPHALUS

Hydrocephalus is a pathologic process characterized by accumulation of excess CSF.

TABLE 1–2

Effects of Anesthetic Agents on Cerebrospinal Fluid Formation and Absorption

Agent	Formation	Absorption
Inhalation		
Halothane	Decreased	Decreased
Enflurane	Increased	Decreased
Isoflurane	No change	Increased*
Desflurane	No change	No change
Sevoflurane	Decreased	Decreased
Nitrous oxide	No change	No change
Intravenous		
Alfentanil	No change	Decreased*
Etomidate*	No change	No change
Fentanyl	Decreased	Increased*
Ketamine	No change	Decreased
Midazolam*		
Low dose	No change	Decreased
Int dose	No change	No change
High dose	Decreased	Decreased
Ermediate		
Propofol	No change	No change
Sufentanyl	No change	Increased*
Thiopental*		
Low dose	No change	No change
High dose	Decreased	Increased

*Effect is dose dependent.
Adapted from Artru AA: New concepts concerning anesthetic effects on intracranial dynamics: Cerebrospinal fluid volume and cerebral blood volume. American Society of Anesthesiologists, 38th Annual Refresher Course Lecture (Lecture 133), 1987.

The most common pathogenesis is an obstruction of CSF pathways, but overproduction (as in choroid plexus papilloma) or inadequate absorption of CSF may also cause hydrocephalus. The distinction between communicating and noncommunicating hydrocephalus rests on whether a portion of the ventricular system is isolated from the CSF circulation.

Hydrocephalus may be classified as either congenital (incidence 3 in 1000 live births) or acquired. It is associated with the following congenital syndromes: aqueductal stenosis, myelomeningocele, Arnold-Chiari malformation, and Dandy-Walker cyst. Intracranial lesions such as neoplasms, arachnoid cysts, and vascular malformations also cause congenital hydrocephalus. Acquired hydrocephalus occurs in the pediatric population from fibrosis of the leptomeninges caused by meningitis or intraventricular hemorrhage. Adults develop hydrocephalus from neoplastic disease or after trauma, meningitis, or subarachnoid hemorrhage.

Signs and symptoms of hydrocephalus depend on the age of the patient and the rapidity of its onset. In infants, hydrocephalus leads to increased head circumference, split sutures, and tense fontanelles, even in the upright position. The child exhibits irritability, nausea, vomiting, lethargy, abducens nerve palsy, paralysis of upward gaze, difficulty swallowing secondary to brain stem traction, and seizures if the process is allowed to progress untreated. In children, slow onset of hydrocephalus can cause headaches, mental retardation, behavior and gait disturbances, visual changes (due to papilledema and subsequent optic nerve atrophy), or endocrine abnormalities.

In adults acute hydrocephalus initially causes headaches, nausea, vomiting, lethargy, confusion, and papilledema. Progression leads to transtentorial herniation and brainstem compromise. Patients may have an irregular respiratory pattern, decerebrate or decorticate posturing, ECG abnormalities, bradycardia, and hypertension. Chronic hydrocephalus, with its slow onset, may cause headaches and nausea only.

The diagnosis of hydrocephalus is made by computed tomography (CT) or magnetic resonance imaging (MRI), which may show ventricular dilatation, obstructive masses, midline shifts, and vascular abnormalities. Ventricular dilatation and failure to visualize the fourth ventricle suggest the diagnosis of aqueductal stenosis.

Acute deterioration in a patient with hydrocephalus may require immediate decompression with an intraventricular catheter. Definitive management of hydrocephalus requires surgical correction—that is, placement of a pressure-regulated CSF shunt or removal of obstructing lesions. Nonsurgical therapy has not been shown to be effective. The ventriculoperitoneal (VP) shunt is the preferred procedure because of its benign nature and ease of revision. Alternative sites include ventriculoatrial (VA), lumboperitoneal (LP), ventriculopleural, ventriculocholedochal, and ventriculovesicular shunts. The most common complications of shunt placement are disruption of shunt integrity (obstruction, disconnection, migration, or extrusion of the catheter), infection, and headache from intracranial hypotension. Complications unique to VA shunts include air embolus during placement, vascular perforation, thrombosis of the internal jugular vein or superior vena cava, and nephritis from chronic bacteremia. Surgical procedures may also be required for removal, replacement, or revision of an existing shunt.

The major anesthetic consideration is the maintenance of adequate cerebral perfusion pressure. Premedication that leads to oversedation, hypoxia, hypercarbia, and increased cerebral blood volume should be avoided. Smooth induction with an intravenous agent, mild hyperventilation, propofol or low-dose inhalation agents (with or without narcotic supplementation), and a short-acting nondepolarizing neuromuscular blocking agent provide anesthesia for these short procedures. Pediatric patients may benefit from premedication with oral midazolam, rectal midazolam or methohexital under direct observation, or an inhalation induction that may minimize increased intracranial pressure associated with crying and struggling.[53] Intravenous access can then be secured and intubation accomplished with a short-acting nondepolarizing neuromuscular blocking agent. If the child is lethargic or irritable or has tense fontanelles, intravenous induction should be seriously considered.[54]

Overzealous decompression of large ventricles can lead to upward herniation of the brain stem, resulting in hypotension, bradycardia, arrhythmias, and altered respiratory pattern. Too rapid decompression of the ventricular system can also cause tearing of bridging veins between the dura and brain, resulting in a subdural hematoma.

C. NORMAL-PRESSURE HYDROCEPHALUS

Normal-pressure hydrocephalus (NPH) consists of the classic triad of memory difficulty, gait apraxia, and urinary incontinence.[55] The mental deficit associated with NPH is more of a subcortical frontal nature: forgetfulness, inattentiveness, slowness in processing complex information, and impaired ability to manipulate acquired knowledge.[56] NPH has been described in pediatric patients with preexisting neurologic disease after the onset of new deficits.[57] Diagnosis of NPH is made by CT evidence of ventriculomegaly that is out of proportion to cerebral atrophy accompanied by normal or low CSF pressure as measured by lumbar puncture. The clinical syndrome is thought to be due to periventricular hypoperfusion related to hydrocephalic compression and stretching of periventricular vascular and neural structures.[56] Fewer than 50

per cent of patients chosen for surgery benefit from surgical shunting procedures.[58] The predictive value of CSF shunting success has been attempted by using CSF tap test (40 to 50 mL), continuous external lumbar drainage for 4 or 5 days, positron emission tomography (PET), and single-photon emission CT (SPECT) studies.[59] Anesthetic management is identical to that of patients with hydrocephalus. Of note is that NPH is associated with a higher incidence of cardiac and arteriosclerotic disease, particularly arterial hypertension.[60]

D. PSEUDOTUMOR CEREBRI

Pseudotumor cerebri (benign intracranial hypertension, idiopathic intracranial hypertension) is a clinical entity characterized by (1) elevated intracranial pressure (greater than 200 mm H_2O and as high as 600 mm H_2O) that is not related to a pathologic process, (2) normal CSF composition, and (3) no alteration in consciousness. There are two distinct patient populations—adults and infants. The adult form occurs predominantly in obese women, who exhibit headache, nausea, vomiting, and dizziness or blurred vision without other signs of cerebral dysfunction. Headache, the most common symptom, is generalized, throbbing, and episodic. Typically, the headaches are worse in the morning and are exacerbated by head movement and Valsalva maneuver. The visual disturbances begin as an enlargement of a blind spot and inferonasal field deficit but at presentation the complaint may be diplopia, blurred vision, or blindness. Pseudotumor is often self-limited, although as many as 10 per cent of adult patients may have residual visual impairment from prolonged papilledema. Clinical symptoms can vary with weight, menstrual cycle, pregnancy, or use of oral contraceptives. Physical findings are usually unremarkable except for papilledema. CT may reveal normal or small lateral ventricles with slit third ventricles and effaced cerebral sulci.[61]

The infantile form of pseudotumor does not show a female preponderance. Patients exhibit rapid head growth, split sutures, and tense fontanelles while they normally achieve developmental milestones. CT shows enlarged ventricles and fluid spaces over the brain.

The cause of pseudotumor varies (Table 1–3), and a single cause is not usually identified. Many mechanisms have been proposed to ex-

TABLE 1–3

Causes Associated with Pseudotumor Cerebri

Endocrine
　Addison's disease, menarche, pregnancy, hypo/
　　hyperthyroid, hypoparathyroidism,
　　pseudohypoparathyroidism, empty sella
　　syndrome
Dietary
　Obesity, hypo-/hypervitaminosis A, vitamin D
　　deficiency, malnutrition
Drugs
　Steroid withdrawal, estrogen, oral
　　contraceptives, lithium, tetracycline,
　　trimethoprim-sulfamethoxazole, nitrofurantoin,
　　nalidixic acid, thyroid supplements, danazol
Impaired cerebral venous drainage
　Otitis media, mastoiditis, idiopathic cerebral
　　venous/dural sinus thrombosis, superior vena
　　cava syndrome, arteriovenous malformation,
　　right heart failure, jugular vein ligation,
　　subclavian vein, thrombosis
Others
　AIDS, systemic lupus erythrematosus, polyarteritis
　　nodosa, polycythemia vera, anemia
　　(pernicious, iron deficiency), Guillain-Barré
　　syndrome, thrombocytopenia

plain the pathophysiology of pseudotumor, but it appears that venous pressure is increased, probably because extracellular edema and the resultant increased brain volume compress cerebral venous sinuses.[62] The elevated intracranial venous pressure leads to resistance to CSF absorption. CSF and intracranial pressures increase to restore the required pressure gradient for CSF absorption into the venous system.[63]

Therapy is directed at treatment of any intercurrent medical process and discontinuation of any potentially inciting or aggravating medication. Patients should be encouraged to lose weight. In general, symptoms respond to medical therapy, including furosemide, acetazolamide, and dexamethasone. Serial lumbar punctures and removal of 30 mL of CSF, or a 50 per cent reduction of the opening pressure, have been recommended to alleviate symptoms.[64]

Surgery is reserved for patients whom medical management fails and whose visual symptoms progress (by visual field testing). CSF diversion procedures, particularly lumboperitoneal shunts, exhibit a failure or complication rate approaching 50 per cent. Some 64 per cent of all shunts required reoperation less than 6 months after insertion, owing to shunt malfunction or low-pressure headaches.[65] For patients with visual dysfunction,

optic nerve sheath decompression can reverse or stabilize progressive vision loss and may lead to the resolution of headaches.[66] Optic nerve decompression is accompanied by a 32 per cent failure rate that may occur any time after surgery and, so, requires long-term follow-up.[67]

Anesthetic management differs from that for patients with hydrocephalus in that epidural and subarachnoid anesthesia are not contraindicated. Lumbar puncture is safe and beneficial, and isolated reports have not noted variations in the dermatomal spread of anesthesia from the normal population. In the patient with an LP shunt, regional anesthesia may damage the shunt device or deposited anesthetic may be lost via the shunt.[68]

E. SYRINGOMYELIA AND SYRINGOBULBIA

Syringomyelia is the progressive formation of an enlarged, CSF-filled intramedullary cavity surrounded by reactive gliosis without associated inflammation or vascular compromise. Communicating or congenital syringomyelia is most often associated with a Chiari malformation. Noncommunicating syringomyelia, filled with proteinaceous CSF, is caused by spinal cord tumor, trauma, or arachnoiditis. Hydromyelia is the dilatation of the central canal. Syringobulbia is the pathologic cavitation of the brain stem.

Many mechanisms have been postulated for the pathogenesis of syrinx formation and growth. Most theories involve the dissociation of intracranial and intraspinal pressures transmitted by arterial or venous pulsations related to hindbrain herniation[69] or impaired CSF circulation.

Syringomyelia is characterized by slow, progressive dysfunction over many years. The most common presentation, especially of a traumatic syrinx, is pain originating at the site of the syrinx radiating to the neck and upper extremities. Signs and symptoms of syringomyelia include asymmetric loss of pain and temperature of the upper extremities due to destruction of crossing spinothalamic tract fibers, with preservation of touch and position sensation. Lower motor neuron destruction causes hyporeflexia and atrophy of the affected extremity. The loss of deep tendon reflexes antedates the discovery of the syrinx.[70] Weakness of the paraspinal musculature leads to thoracic scoliosis.

The most common presenting symptom of

syringobulbia is a pounding occipital headache. Other clinical features involve dysfunction of the involved lower cranial nerves.[71] This can lead to paralysis of the tongue, palate, and vocal cords and the loss of facial sensation. Valsalva maneuver and coughing may exacerbate neurologic findings.

Diagnosis of syringomyelia is made by subarachnoid contrast-enhanced immediate and delayed CTs, which may display reflux of contrast material into the cystic cavity and enlargement of the involved spinal cord. The advent of high-resolution MRI may make invasive CT obsolete for determining the extent of involvement. Ultrasound has been utilized to detect congenital syringomyelia in neonates and may become useful in adults through a transesophageal technique.[72]

Surgical therapy for communicating syringomyelia involves craniocervical decompression. For noncommunicating syringomyelia, decompression of the syrinx is recommended, with the establishment of a communication between the syrinx and the subarachnoid space. Procedures include percutaneous aspiration, laminectomy and syringostomy, or a shunting procedure to the peritoneal or pleural cavity.

The anesthetic considerations for patients with syringomyelia often include many of the problems involved in patients with spinal cord injury (SCI): sympathetic areflexia, autonomic hyperreflexia, respiratory insufficiency, and poikilothermia. Significant muscle wasting may lead to a hyperkalemic response to succinylcholine, contraindicating its use.[73] There may be an exaggerated response to nondepolarizing neuromuscular blocking agents; therefore, careful titration and monitoring of the neuromuscular blockade are recommended. Thoracic scoliosis can lead to cardiorespiratory complications, especially in the postoperative period. The presence of syringobulbia may lead to diminution of protective airway reflexes that can complicate intubation and extubation. Some of these surgical procedures may be done with the patient in the sitting position, requiring appropriate preparation and monitoring.

V. SPINAL CORD INJURY

A. ACUTE SPINAL CORD INJURY

In the acute phase of SCI, anesthesiologists provide emergency cardiovascular and respi-

ratory management, general anesthesia for surgery involving an associated injury, and anesthesia for stabilization or decompression laminectomy.[74] The annual incidence of traumatic SCI ranges from 11.5 to 53.4 per million population.[74] SCI commonly occurs in males between ages 15 and 25 years; the majority are related to motor vehicle accidents and involve the cervical spine.[75] The most frequent level of cervical spine injury is C5–6, the fulcrum of cervical spinal cord mobility, whereas the most frequent site of thoracolumbar transection is at T12–L1. The fatality rate for SCI is 48 per cent, mortality being greatest in patients younger than 15 or older than 75.[76–78]

Spinal cord injuries are accompanied by other associated trauma in 25 to 65 per cent of cases. The most common associated injuries involve the head; that is, intracranial hemorrhage and skull or facial fracture, producing rhinorrhagia or otorrhea.[79] The presence of a skull or facial fracture is not associated with a higher risk of a cervical spine injury.[80] The soft tissue injuries most often overlooked are located in the thorax, such as rib fractures, hemothorax, and pneumothorax.[81] Coexisting intra-abdominal injuries are rare and should be suspected when there is persistent hemodynamic instability or evidence of adjacent major trauma.[82] Vertebral artery injury may occur in association with a cervical spine injury and should be suspected in patients who display brain stem or cerebellar dysfunction.[83]

Spinal cord blood flow (SCBF) autoregulation is similar to the cerebral circulation; that is, normal blood flow is maintained between mean arterial pressures of 50 and 150 mm Hg. Arterial CO_2 tension influences SCBF, which remains constant from 40 to 50 mm Hg $Paco_2$, increases linearly from 50 to 90 mm Hg and decreases with hyperventilation.[84] When arterial oxygen tension is less than 60 mm Hg, there is a sharp increase in SCBF.[85] Endogenous endorphins indirectly decrease SCBF by causing hypotension and hypoventilation.

The pathophysiology of SCI initially involves the gray matter. Small gray matter blood vessels are disrupted, with endothelial breakdown and subsequent hemorrhage and edema.[86] This rapid decrease in gray matter SCBF is followed by hypoperfusion in the white matter. As the injury progresses, there is a loss of local antoregulation, decreased tissue oxygen tension, increased lactic acid production and the resultant spinal cord ischemia, with the potential for caudal and cranial extension. A biochemical cascade leads to the release of potent vasoconstrictors, causing further ischemia, generation of free radicals leading to lipid peroxidation, and necrosis of neuronal tissue. By 24 hours, the central gray and adjacent white matter are necrotic.[87] Early effective therapy—within 8 hours, in theory—may spare adjacent white matter and limit the degree of functional impairment. The only clinically effective therapy for SCI at present is large doses of corticosteroids. A regimen of methylprednisolone, a loading dose of 30 mg/kg followed by an infusion of 5.4 mg/kg per hour for the next 23 hours, produced both sensory and motor improvement.[88] Many other therapeutic modalities have been proposed, but experimental results are not encouraging following use of naloxone, thyrotropin-releasing hormone, local hypothermia, hyperbaric oxygen, catecholamine antagonists, dimethyl sulfoxide, gangliosides, diuretics, and calcium channel antagonists.

All comatose patients and polytrauma patients are considered to have an SCI until it is proven otherwise.[74] The vertebral column must be immobilized at the scene in the neutral position to prevent further embarrassment of a potentially injured spinal cord. If these patients require airway support, experienced personnel should ventilate or intubate while the patient's head and neck are held in the neutral position, manually or with skeletal traction, as necessary. Patients with lesions above C4 require assisted ventilation; lesions below this level should not cause respiratory impairment unless complicated by another injury. To ensure optimal neuronal survival, PaO_2 should be greater than 100 mm Hg and $PaCO_2$ less than 45 mm Hg. Indications for intubation include PaO_2 less than 100 mm Hg; $PaCO_2$ greater than 45 mm Hg; maximum inspiratory force less than 20 cm H_2O; vital capacity less than 15 mL/kg; PaO_2–FiO_2 ratio less than 250; and an abnormal chest roentgenogram revealing atelectasis, pulmonary edema, or pulmonary infiltrate.[77, 89]

Pulmonary edema is a common cause of mortality from acute SCI: the prevalence is greater than 40 per cent in some series. The edema may be due to overzealous fluid repletion or a neurogenic response. Neurogenic pulmonary edema is related to a transient, centrally mediated sympathetic discharge (predominantly α-adrenergic), leading to a shift of blood from the high-resistance peripheral vascular beds to the low-resistance pulmonary bed. After the initial phase, pulmonary and systemic pressures become normal. The high protein content of the edema fluid and evident frank hemorrhage seem to indicate a vascular injury, leading to an alteration in capillary permeability.[77, 90, 91]

Acute SCI above T5 is characterized by autonomic hypo- and hyperactivity. Initially there is an immediate but transient hypertensive response associated with increased systemic vascular resistance (SVR), increased myocardial contractility, and dysrhythmias.[77] Within minutes, interruption of the spinal sympathetic tracts leads to hypotension from the pooling of blood in the dilated peripheral vascular beds, bradycardia due to lack of competitive inhibition of the now dominant parasympathetic nervous system, and loss of cardiac accelerator nerve fibers located from T1–4. Even if intravascular volume is adequate, patients with SCI may be unable to maintain adequate cardiac output without the compensatory sympathetic-induced constriction of venous capacitance vessels and arterioles.[77, 85]

Spinal shock is characterized by complete loss of somatic and visceral sensation, flaccid paralysis, absent deep tendon and abdominal reflexes and plantar responses, and retention of urine and feces. Blood pressure is decreased owing to loss of sympathetic vascular tone or of cardioaccelerator fibers, depending on the level of the lesions. The end of spinal shock is indicated by the return of elicited spinal cord reflex arcs such as abnormal cutaneospinal reflexes or exaggerated muscle spindle reflex arcs in a caudocraniad manner.[92] Spinal shock may last 3 days to 6 weeks.

Hemodynamic stability and appropriate intravascular volume repletion must be established to maintain perfusion pressure of the spinal cord and other organs. A pulmonary artery catheter is recommended for optimal management of these patients, because there is often a discrepancy between pulmonary artery and central venous pressures. Intravenous fluids—not inotropic agents—are used to maintain blood pressure and ensure tissue perfusion. Judicious fluid challenges can be used to produce individualized ventricular function curves. If cardiac filling pressures are maintained, spinal cord perfusion is optimized and the risk of pulmonary edema minimized.[78, 90, 91, 93]

Atropine has been advocated for acute therapy of SCI when the patient is hypotensive and bradycardic and exhibits poor tissue perfusion. The pure chronotropic effect has been shown to increase mean arterial pressure and cardiac index.[94] Inotropic therapy is warranted when poor tissue perfusion persists despite adequate fluid administration. Isoproterenol is a β-adrenergic agonist whose positive inotropic and chronotropic actions make it an ideal agent for bradycardia patients.[77] Dopamine is preferred for patients with ischemic heart disease or stenotic valvular lesions because of its less chronotropic properties. Vasopressors such as phenylephrine may be used in the emergency setting but should be avoided because they counteract the increased cardiac output provided by the low systemic vascular resistance.

Pulmonary complications are the most common cause of death in the first 3 months for quadriplegics.[77] The combination of a high cervical injury (C7 or above) and inadequate ventilation leads to ventilation-perfusion inequalities, increased dead space, hypoxia, hypercarbia, pulmonary vasoconstriction, retention of secretions, atelectasis, pneumonia, and respiratory failure.[74] An injury above C5 leads to complete loss of diaphragmatic innervation (C3–5) and demands ventilatory support. Paralysis of the intercostal muscles, which elevate the thoracic cage on inspiration, causes decreased alveolar ventilation, paradoxical respiration, and an ineffective cough, leading to retention of secretions and inadequate gas exchange. Abdominal muscles, innervated by the lower six thoracic segments and L1, function predominantly in forced expiration and provide abdominal wall tone.[95–97]

Quadriplegics' ventilatory parameters are optimal in the supine or 20° Trendelenburg position rather than a sitting position. In the latter, the flaccid abdominal musculature protrudes and the abdominal contents fall toward the pelvis, leading to a short diaphragmatic descent on inspiration and no abdominal rebound during expiration. In the supine position, diaphragmatic descent is accompanied by compression of the abdominal contents and forward protrusion of the abdominal wall, which causes elastic recoil of the wall and more cephalad movement of the diaphragm on expiration.[77, 95]

After acute SCI, pulmonary function testing reveals decreases in vital capacity, tidal volume, total lung capacity, expiratory reserve volume, forced expiratory volume in one second (FEV_1), forced vital capacity (FVC), expiratory flow rates, and functional residual capacity, and an increase in residual volume. The FEV_1–FVC ratio is normal, indicating a restrictive defect.[95] Hypoxemia may be present, often without hypoventilation, probably owing to microatelectasis. Alveolar hypoventilation may be more pronounced during sleep in the first week after injury. Pulmonary function improves when intercostal and abdominal muscle spasticity occurs, which leads to increased abdominal wall elastic recoil and a decreased end-expiratory volume. Serial testing is recommended for monitoring respiratory function.

Gastric atony, paralytic ileus, and the resulting abdominal distention—common during the first 2 weeks—cause further respiratory embarrassment, limited diaphragmatic excursion, and increased risk of aspiration. Further deterioration of respiratory function in the first 48 hours may be due to rostrad extension of the spinal cord lesion.[95–98]

The use of prophylactic chest physiotherapy (including postural drainage, chest wall percussion, breathing exercises, and tracheal suctioning) has been shown to decrease the incidence of pulmonary complications in mechanically ventilated and spontaneously ventilating patients.[77, 95] Tracheal suctioning of quadriplegics has been associated with bradycardia and cardiac arrest secondary to an unopposed vasovagal reflex, especially when accompanied by hypoxia. Preoxygenation and atropine pretreatment are beneficial.[89] Patients may exhibit bronchial hyperresponsiveness after cervical SCI owing to unopposed cholinergic bronchoconstrictor tone.[99] The use of β_2-adrenergic agonist nebulizer therapy during spinal shock may be associated with hypotension, owing to a further decrease in systemic vascular resistance.[100]

Surgical management is indicated in SCI to achieve alignment when nonsurgical manipulation has failed, to decompress an injured spinal cord, to stabilize persistent subluxation, and to treat any accompanying injuries.

1. Preoperative Evaluation

The preoperative evaluation of a patient with acute cervical SCI undergoing a surgical procedure must include a careful assessment of the respiratory and hemodynamic status. Because of the high incidence of associated injuries, a careful physical examination is imperative. Hemorrhagic shock may be present despite a pulse rate of less than 60. The respiratory analysis includes an arterial blood gas determination, pulmonary function tests (at minimum, bedside spirometry), and chest radiography. Hemodynamic evaluation includes the placement of a pulmonary artery catheter to assess cardiac reserve and intravascular volume status. ECG is of value in identifying posttraumatic myocardial ischemia or myocardial contusion. Routine electrolytes, especially sodium and calcium, are important to evaluate preoperatively. Hyponatremia occurs in patients with cervical and chronic SCI, for a variety of reasons.[101] After 10 days, patients with SCI may have hypercalcemia, owing to the mobilization of calcium from bone, which predisposes to intraoperative arrhythmias. Prolonged immobilization can cause venous thrombosis and pulmonary embolism, requiring autoregulation therapy; these must be corrected before surgery.

Premedication with sedatives or narcotics, if necessary, should be titrated to effect in the operating room to prevent hypoventilation and depression during the neurologic examination. Atropine is a valuable premedicant for a patient whose pulse rate is less than 70 since it may counteract the vagal effects of some anesthetic agents.

2. Intraoperative Management

Monitoring required for surgery for acute SCI includes an arterial line, ECG, and a pulmonary artery catheter to assess pulmonary artery pressure, cardiac output, and mixed venous blood gases. Intracranial pressure monitoring may be indicated in patients with an intercurrent head injury. Somatosensory-evoked potential (SSEP) monitoring of posterior column function may be indicated during stabilization and decompression procedures in patients who are neurologically intact. Intraoperative awakening has been used to evaluate patients during lumbar decompression and stabilization.

The patient with an acute SCI is considered to have a full stomach and to be at increased risk for passive regurgitation of gastric contents. Factors that make regurgitation more probable include gastric atony, supine position, a nasogastric tube, paralyzed abdominal musculature, and preintubation positive-pressure ventilation. Cricoid pressure must be applied cautiously to a patient with a cervical cord injury.

The method of intubation depends on the patient's condition, the extent of neurologic injury, the time elapsed since injury, and the preference and experience of the anesthesiologist. An awake intubation, after appropriate topical anesthesia and sedation, is preferable, because it permits neurologic assessment before and after intubation. Nasotracheal or orotracheal intubation can be performed blind or with the aid of a fiberoptic bronchoscope without moving the neck. "Topicalization" of the nasopharynx and oropharynx, superior laryngeal nerve blocks, and transtracheal administration of local anesthetic may be used to minimize discomfort to the patient. Difficult airways may be secured by retrograde intubation using a Tuohy needle and a wire passed through the cricothyroid membrane into the oropharynx or transtracheal jet ventilation through a needle cricothyroidotomy. Tracheostomy or cricothyroidotomy should be avoided unless direct tracheal injury, severe facial trauma, or technically difficult intubation makes them unavoidable, because they may interfere with future surgical access to the neck.[89] Neck stability is maintained throughout intubation by longitudinal axial traction.

The use of succinylcholine is contraindicated for SCI patients, especially with the advent of new nondepolarizing neuromuscular blockers. The hyperkalemic response produced by succinylcholine (as high as 14.7 mEq/L) is due to proliferation of cholinergic receptors in extrajunctional areas of the muscle, which occurs within a day and lasts up to 9 months after injury. The amount of potassium released is proportional to the degree of muscle involvement, not to the succinylcholine dose. Defasciculating doses of nondepolarizing neuromuscular blockers do not necessarily attenuate the hyperkalemic response. Pancuronium is a good choice for muscle relaxation because of its chronotropic effects.

Positioning must be done with extreme care, to avoid exacerbating the spinal cord injury. Positioning the patient awake allows a neurologic examination to be done after positioning and before the induction of anesthesia. Precipitous moving and tilting of patients with a lesion above T1 can have disastrous hemodynamic consequences, owing to the absence of compensatory vasoconstrictor reflexes that usually maintain venous return and cardiac output. Placing the patient rapidly into a head-up position can lead to hypotension and even cardiac arrest, whereas the head-down position can lead to ventricular failure and pulmonary edema. Hemodynamic status of patients with SCI without sympathetic compensatory reflex activity may be further depressed during anesthesia by anesthetic agents that have myocardial depressant and vasodilating effects, hypoxia, positive-pressure ventilation, hemorrhagic shock, positioning, and suctioning. Slow, careful induction is recommended.[78, 102, 103] Postoperative neurologic deterioration may be caused by direct intraoperative trauma to the spinal cord, bony malalignment, postoperative hematoma, or edema. Emergent reoperation may be indicated, with or without radiologic confirmation. The anesthetic technique should permit timely neurologic examination at the conclusion of surgery.

Lesions above T1 impair thermoregulation because sympathetic fibers carrying temperature sensation to hypothalamic thermoregulatory centers are disrupted. Affected patients are essentially poikilothermic and require attention to temperature maintenance in the operating room.

3. Postoperative Care

Respiratory support may be necessary postoperatively, despite adequate preinduction respiratory status, owing to the residual effects of anesthesia.[80, 104] Weaning and extubation are likely to be successful when the patient meets extubation criteria, has no associated chest or head injury, and has no difficulty with secretions. Intense respiratory physiotherapy should be continued in the postoperative period as necessary.

4. Pediatric and Elderly Patients

Patients at the extremes of life who have an SCI exhibit unique features. Pediatric SCIs account for fewer than 10% of all SCIs.[105] The type and distribution of pediatric SCIs vary according to the age of the patient. Children younger than 8 years have a higher incidence of injury to the upper cervical spine and craniovertebral junction, a higher incidence of SCI without radiographic abnormality (SCIWORA), and a higher incidence of complete SCI.[106, 107]

Many anatomic and biomechanical factors combine to produce this unique pattern of injury. The immature spine is protected by its physiologic elasticity secondary to lax ligaments, underdeveloped neck and paraspinous muscles, incompletely ossified wedge-shaped vertebrae, and the shallow horizontal orientation of the upper cervical facet joints.[108] The large size of the infant's head in relation to the torso leads to the large number of atlantooccipital injuries.[108] Fractures that do occur involve the cartilaginous vertebral endplate and injure growth zones.[107] By age 8 years, roentgenographically, the spinal column assumes an adult configuration, producing the mature pattern of SCI.[109]

SCIWORA is defined as objective signs of traumatic myelopathy without evidence of vertebral column injury on plain spine films and CT.[110] These children belatedly develop a neurologic deficit: their condition either deteriorates slowly after a latent period[105] or recurs after a trivial, yet similar injury.[110] The mechanism for the delayed appearance is an ischemic event initiated by the trauma[111] or an incipient instability that occurs with the initial trauma and is reactivated by a trivial yet similar mechanism of injury.[110] SCIWORA has been associated with a high incidence of complete myelopathy.[107] In the setting of SCIWORA, MRI has been advocated because of its ability to detect soft tissue and spinal cord lesions.[112]

The only significant determinant of outcome after pediatric SCI is the neurologic status of the patient at the time of admission.[106] The prognosis for a full recovery is excellent, except with a complete injury. Most patients can be managed conservatively, utilizing external immobilization.[108] Methylprednisolone has also been advocated for use in the pediatric population if administered within 8 hours of injury.[107] The basic tenets of resuscitative and anesthetic management of the pediatric SCI are similar to those for adults. The adequacy of ventilation, oxygenation, and spinal cord perfusion must be ensured.

Adolescents with a chronic SCI should be considered at high risk for development of a latex allergy because of their extensive exposure to products containing latex.[113]

Elders are more often injured by falls and tend to suffer a hyperflexion or extension injury and exhibit a central cord syndrome.[114] Central cord syndrome characteristically presents with disproportionate weakness of the arms, as compared with the legs, urinary retention, and variable sensory loss below the level of injury. Elderly patients with narrowing of the spinal canal, particularly ossification of the posterior longitudinal ligament or ankylosing spondylitis, may suffer exaggerated SCI with even trivial trauma.[115] An index of suspicion is required, as their symptoms may be delayed and they can present with SCIWORA. Elderly patients have a smaller chance of neurologic recovery and higher mortality rates than other age groups owing to preexisting medical conditions and intolerance of prolonged immobilization.

B. CHRONIC SPINAL CORD INJURY

The life expectancy of the patient with an SCI is increasing, owing to improved management of the myriad special conditions with which they present.[116] Patients with chronic SCI present most commonly for urologic, plastic, or orthopedic surgery. The level of SCI determines the extent of cardiovascular reflexes. Lesions above T4 cause varying degrees of postural hypotension, depending on the degree of adaptation that has occurred. After several months there is often an increase in renin-angiotensin system activity and capacitance vessel tone. A decrease in cerebrovascular resistance allows cerebral perfusion at lower blood pressure. A quadriplegic patient's complete interruption of the sympathetic nervous system causes the loss of compensatory cardiovascular reflexes and autonomic hyperreflexia.[78] These patients present with a slower basal heart rate than their paraplegic counterparts, owing to their unopposed vagal tone.[117]

Respiratory function may improve by 6 months after injury, as evidenced by improvement in pulmonary function tests (vital capacity, FEV_1, and maximal inspiratory force). Arterial blood gas evaluation often reveals hypoxemia with a normal $Paco_2$. Spontaneously breathing quadriplegics have optimal respiratory function in the supine or Trendelenburg position.

Renal failure is the principal cause of death in patients with chronic SCI. Chronic urinary tract infections lead to calculus formation, hypoproteinemia, hypocalcemia, and renal failure. Anemia is caused by renal insufficiency and gastrointestinal bleeding from nonsteroidal antiinflammatory drugs. Poor wound healing may occur. Ninety per cent of paraplegics—especially those with cauda equina lesions—present with pain syndromes. Many of these patients have drug dependency problems.[118]

Transferring and positioning must be done carefully. Rapid and precipitous movements can trigger orthostatic hypotension, owing to the lack of compensatory cardiovascular reflexes. Osteoporosis can lead to pathologic fractures despite extreme care. Skin breakdown may occur in less than 2 hours, particularly if too little attention is paid to pressure point padding. Patients who are febrile or anemic are more prone to form decubiti. Kyphoscoliosis may be present in patients with asymmetric spinal cord lesions because of the imbalance of muscle tone.[118]

Poikilothermia is still a problem, and conscientious heat conservation during the operative period must be continued. Muscle denervation hypersensitivity leading to hyperkalemia contraindicates use of succinylcholine, especially in patients with concurrent renal insufficiency; however, newer neuromuscular blocking agents have made this controversy obsolete.

C. AUTONOMIC HYPERREFLEXIA

Autonomic hyperreflexia is characterized by acute generalized autonomic overactivity in response to cutaneous or visceral stimuli below the spinal cord lesion. Stimuli capable of inducing the response include bladder, bowel, or intestinal distension, skin stimulation, pyelonephritis, muscle spasm, uterine contractions, and surgery. Autonomic hyperreflexia occurs in 65 to 85 per cent of patients with SCI above T7 but is unlikely with injuries below T10. The mechanism involves absence of the supraspinal inhibitory influence on thoracolumbar sympathetic outflow. Sympathetic spinal reflex activity results in a nonspecific response (mass spinal reflex) proportional to the stimulus' intensity. Signs and symptoms of autonomic hyperreflexia include hypertension, bradycardia, dysrhythmias, headache, nasal congestion, blurred vision, sweating, vasoconstriction, piloerection below the spinal cord lesion, vasodilatation above the lesion, hyperreflexia, convulsions, cerebral hemorrhage, pulmonary edema, and even death.[119, 120]

During surgery, sufficient anesthetic depth provided by general, regional, or adequate local anesthesia can prevent autonomic hyperreflexia, whereas topical anesthesia, sedation, or lack of anesthesia has led to hypertension in these patients. Topical anesthesia advocated for cystoscopy does not block bladder muscle stretch receptors. Regional anesthesia, particularly spinal or epidural, provides protection by blocking afferent pathways. Difficulties in administering regional anesthesia include inexact determination of the anesthetic level, hypotension (prevented by previous volume loading), and technical difficulties due to bone deformities, osteoporosis, and problems in positioning. Autonomic hyperreflexia may also follow anesthesia (for example, in the recovery room).[80]

Primary therapy of autonomic hyperreflexia requires the elimination of the precipitating stimulus. General anesthesia must be deepened or the regional anesthetic level raised. Pharmacologic therapy has involved the use of ganglionic blockade (trimethaphan, pentolinium), α-adrenergic antagonists (phentolamine, phenoxybenzamine), calcium channel blockade (nifedipine), and direct vasodilatation (nitroprusside, hydralazine). Alpha-adrenergic blockade has not been consistently effective in stopping an autonomic hyperreflexic crisis, as it is more effective against circulating cholecholamines than at displacing norepinephrine from receptor sites.[121] Sublingual nifedipine has been shown to abate the hypertension of autonomic hyperreflexia.[122] Drugs that lower blood pressure by a central action (clonidine, methyldopa) are not effective in treating autonomic hyperreflexia. Dysrhythmias may be treated with β-sympathetic antagonists,[4, 30] although β-blockade alone may aggravate the hypertension because of unopposed α-adrenergic activity.

VI. DEMYELINATING DISEASE

The accepted pathologic criteria for demyelinating disease include destruction of the myelin sheaths of the nerve fibers, relative sparing of the other elements of nerve tissue, infiltration of inflammatory cells in a perivascular distribution, a particular distribution of lesions (often perivenous and primarily in white matter), and relative lack of wallerian or secondary degeneration of fiber tracts. A classification of the demyelinating diseases is shown in Table 1–4.

Multiple sclerosis (MS), the most common demyelinating disease, is the only one for which anesthetic experience has been docu-

TABLE 1–4

Demyelinating Disease

Multiple sclerosis (disseminated or insular sclerosis)
  Chronic relapsing encephalomyelopathic form
  Acute multiple sclerosis
  Neuromyelitis optica
Diffuse cerebral sclerosis
  Schilder's disease

mented. In addition, there is a group of dysmyelinating diseases that includes the leukodystrophies and Krabbe's disease. These affect newborns, the primary defect being a genetically determined enzyme deficiency that causes defective myelin formation.

A. MULTIPLE SCLEROSIS

The incidence of MS varies with geographic latitude, from less than 1 in 100,000 in equatorial regions to 6 to 14 in 100,000 in the southern United States and southern Europe and 30 to 80 in 100,000 in Canada, northern Europe, and the northern United States. Epidemiologic studies have shown that MS is associated with particular regions rather than with a particular ethnic group in those regions, thus enhancing the importance of environmental factors in the genesis of the disease. A 5- to 14-fold increase of the incidence of MS in first-degree relatives and the more frequent association of HLA antigens B7 and Dw2 suggest a genetic contribution. An increase in CSF immunoglobulin G (IgG) and serum viral antibodies in some patients suggests a role of autoimmune factors as well. About two thirds of cases of MS have their onset between age 20 and 40 years, approximately one third occurring between 45 and 60 years.

The clinical course of MS is characterized by periods of exacerbation and remission at unpredictable intervals. Onset of symptoms varies, some evolving in minutes and hours and others evolving insidiously over years. Typically, symptoms develop over the course of a few days and improve over a few weeks or months. Signs and symptoms reflect the specific area in the CNS where demyelination is present and thus can encompass a multitude of neurologic findings. Common clinical manifestations include optic neuritis, decreased visual acuity, diplopia, nystagmus, weakness, paresthesias, spasticity in one or more limbs, ataxia, and bladder dysfunction.

Factors such as emotional upset, infections, pregnancy, trauma, and stress (including the perioperative stress of surgery and anesthesia) are implicated in exacerbation of symptoms and conversion of subclinical lesions into overt clinical expression. A higher probability of exacerbation in the postpartum period may be related to emotional or physical exhaustion or to hormonal fluctuation. Body temperature elevation, even as little as 0.5° F, can aggravate symptoms. It has been shown that a rise in temperature can block conduction in marginally functioning demyelinated axons.[123] In one series, 75% of MS patients showed temporary exacerbation of symptoms with a standardized increase in body temperature.[124]

The diagnosis of MS is made on the basis of clinical findings and the support of various laboratory tests and imaging. The most useful of these include MRI, in which "plaques" are prominent in the proton-density images; abnormal visual, somatosensory, and auditory evoked potential responses; and elevated CSF IgG and myelin basic protein.

There is no definitive drug therapy for MS. Therapeutic interventions are directed toward amelioration of acute exacerbations, prevention of relapses, and relief of symptoms. In some patients adrenocorticotropic hormone (ACTH) and prednisone have proved to have a beneficial effect on recovery from, and reduction of, acute relapses, especially of optic neuritis. Immunosuppressive agents such as azathioprine, cyclophosphamide, and cytosine arabinoside (ara-C) have shown some benefit in reducing relapses. Other experimental therapeutic regimens include hyperbaric oxygen, linoleate diet supplementation, plasmapheresis, and interferon. Antispasmodics are used for relief of bladder dysfunction and muscle spasticity in severe cases.

1. Anesthetic Management

Because of the variable course of MS, it is important to discuss the effects that the perioperative period may have on the symptom complex. Surgery and anesthesia have been implicated in the exacerbation of MS, owing to stress; however, there is no evidence that the perioperative period increases the incidence of exacerbation, except when associated with postoperative fever.[125]

General anesthetic agents have no adverse effects on MS. Theoretically, it may be advisable to avoid agents with anticholinergic properties, to decrease the possibility of a rise in body temperature.[126] Early reports of deleterious effects of thiopental[127] have not been supported in more recent publications.[25, 128, 129] Patients who are severely debilitated from their disease and have associated neurologic deficits and muscle atrophy, have the potential for a succinylcholine-induced hyperkalemic response; for a patient in remission or with mild symptoms, however, succinylcholine can safely be used. There are no reports of abnormal responses to nondepolarizing muscle relaxants.

The use of regional anesthesia in MS patients is controversial. In one large study, Schapira and colleagues demonstrated that diagnostic lumbar puncture alone did not induce relapses.[130] The blood–brain barrier may be more permeable to local anesthetics, and thus the toxic dose may be lower than for normal healthy patients.[131] It is theorized that demyelinization of neural tissue in MS predisposes the spinal cord to local anesthetic histotoxicity. It is suggested that epidural anesthesia may be less of a risk than spinal anesthesia because the concentration of local anesthetic in the spinal cord white matter is lower.[132] This advantage may diminish with repeated or continuous epidural administration of local anesthetic that may occur during management of labor and delivery. The patient should be well-informed about the possibility of exacerbation of symptoms before regional anesthesia is initiated. A number of case reports and series found no increase in exacerbation of MS symptoms after epidural or spinal anesthesia. These authors postulate that exacerbation of symptoms after regional anesthesia is no more than the usual incidence of relapse.[133–137] The use of lower concentrations of local anesthetics during epidural anesthesia for labor analgesia is recommended, because multiple "top-ups" theoretically increase the CSF concentration of local anesthetic.[136] Neuraxial narcotics for postoperative analgesia have been used without exacerbation of symptoms.[133, 137]

Additional considerations in the anesthetic management of MS include careful attention to perioperative temperature control, with particular attention to prevention and treatment of even a mild hyperthermic response. MS patients receiving chronic steroid therapy should have their drug supplemented in the perioperative period. Finally, a postoperative neurologic examination should be performed to document new or exacerbated symptoms for appropriate follow-up.

VII. NEUROECTODERMAL DISORDERS

The group of neuroectodermal disorders that includes neurofibromatosis (von Recklinghausen's disease), von Hippel-Lindau disease, Sturge-Weber disease, and tuberous sclerosis is of particular importance to the anesthesiologist because of the unusual location of the neuroanatomic deformities and their association with other diseases.

A. NEUROFIBROMATOSIS

The incidence of neurofibromatosis is 1 in 3000 and is consistent with an autosomal-dominant mode of inheritance. Café au lait spots are common, and six or more spots greater than 1.5 cm in diameter is considered diagnostic. A neurofibroma may occur in any area of tissue that arises from the embryonic neural crest; this accounts for some of the unusual presentations of the disease. Neurofibromas can involve the skin, peripheral nerves and nerve roots, and the viscera and blood vessels, owing to their autonomic innervation. Reported sites of lesions include pharyngeal, intraoral, and intratracheal ones, which may present as unexpected airway obstruction during anesthetic induction.[138–140] There is a 5 per cent incidence of intracranial tumors associated with neurofibromatosis; these include astrocytomas, acoustic neuromas (often bilateral), meningiomas, and primary neurofibromas. Cranial nerve involvement may impair the swallowing mechanism or eliminate gag reflexes. Spinal cord tumors are rare; most spinal cord dysfunction is due to compression of the dorsal nerve roots or spinal cord by fibromas. Skeletal disorders occur in 50 per cent of cases and include scoliosis, mandibular or maxillary deformities, congenital pseudoarthroses, and asymptomatic cervical spine abnormalities involving both alignment and structure.[141]

Other associated disorders include (1) fibrosing pulmonary alveolitis with obliteration of alveoli and blood vessels, leading to pulmonary hypertension, and (2) tumor-related vascular stenosis, which may cause re-

nal hypertension, right ventricular outflow obstruction, or coarctation of the aorta.[135, 142]

Neurofibromatosis is part of the multiple endocrine neoplasia type III syndrome, which includes pheochromocytoma and medullary carcinoma of the thyroid. The incidence of seizures is 20 times higher than in the general population. Last, some degree of intellectual impairment is common but usually is not profound. Any suspected abnormalities should be investigated preoperatively and anesthetic management tailored accordingly.

There are no reported adverse effects of anesthetic agents in neurofibromatosis, although there are some reports of a variable response to succinylcholine and increased sensitivity to nondepolarizing agents.[143–145] A retrospective review of 114 general anesthetics showed normal response to depolarizing and nondepolarizing muscle relaxants.[146] Monitoring of neuromuscular blockade with incremental doses of muscle relaxants is recommended. Regional anesthesia has been used successfully in patients with neurofibromatosis; however, when intracranial fibromas or spinal cord compression is suspected, the increased risks of regional anesthesia should be weighed.[147]

B. VON HIPPEL-LINDAU DISEASE

Von Hippel-Lindau disease is a rare autosomal dominant disease with incomplete penetrance and variable expression. The characteristic lesion is the capillary hemangioblastoma of the retina (60 to 70 per cent of patients) or of the CNS (30 to 50 per cent of patients). The majority of the CNS lesions are located in the cerebellum. Renal and pancreatic cysts, hypernephroma, erythrocytosis, and pheochromocytoma (often bilateral) are also associated with the disease.

There are three reported cases of anesthetic management in von Hippel-Lindau disease. One describes the successful use of epidural anesthesia for elective cesarean section in a patient who had previously undergone resection of a cerebellar hemangioblastoma. The second describes the complications encountered during resection of a cerebellar hemangioblastoma in a patient who also had an active pheochromocytoma. A third describes the anesthetic management of a caesarean delivery followed by a pheochromocytoma resection under general anesthesia.[148–150] Despite the rare association of pheochromocytoma with von Hippel-Lindau disease, it seems prudent to exclude the diagnosis preoperatively, owing to the stated 25 to 50 per cent perioperative mortality rate for undiagnosed pheochromocytoma. No specific anesthetic agents are contraindicated in von Hippel-Lindau disease, and anesthetic management should be tailored according to associated findings (such as pheochromocytoma or intracranial mass lesions). The high incidence of asymptomatic spinal cord hemangioblastomas found during autopsy should be considered when contemplating regional anesthesia.[151]

C. STURGE-WEBER DISEASE AND TUBEROUS SCLEROSIS

Sturge-Weber disease presents as unilateral angiomatous lesions of the leptomeninges and upper face, linear cerebral calcifications, contralateral hemiparesis, seizure disorders, and mental retardation. The incidence of Sturge-Weber disease is not known, although in institutionalized persons it is 1 in 1000. There have been no reports of anesthetic experiences in these patients.

Tuberous sclerosis (Bourneville's disease) is an autosomal dominant disease with an incidence of 1 in 30,000. Patients have a classic triad of adenoma sebaceum, epilepsy, and mental retardation. The adenomatous lesions are most common on the skin but may occur in the heart, lungs, or kidneys. Fifty per cent of cardiac rhabdomyomas are due to tuberous sclerosis. When infiltration of the heart occurs, ectopic beats may be evident. The earliest diagnostic feature is a depigmented ash leaf–shaped area on the trunk of the infant. There is a 75 per cent mortality rate before adulthood, although this may improve with better anticonvulsant therapy. Reports exist in the neurosurgical literature of craniotomies for excision of epileptigenic foci; presumably no unusual anesthetic experiences occurred. There are two case reports that show no unusual reactions to the general anesthetics employed. Antiepileptic medications should be continued in the perioperative period.[152, 153]

VIII. MUCOPOLYSACCHARIDOSES

The mucopolysaccharidoses are hereditary enzyme deficiency disorders characterized by abnormal metabolism of the polysaccharides (heparan sulfate, dermatan sulfate, and keratan sulfate). The result is a abnormal deposition of mucopolysaccharides in body tissues, which leads to serious functional and structural disorders, especially in cartilage and bone tissue. All the subtypes are inherited in an autosomal recessive pattern except for Hunter's disease, which is an X-linked trait. A well-defined classification system for the mucopolysaccharidoses is shown in Table 1–5, along with a summary of clinical features.[154] The majority of these patients die of cardiac or pulmonary complications, although in Morquio's syndrome mortality from cervical cord injury is increased.

The stated anesthetic morbidity and mortality for the mucopolysaccharidoses is 20 to 30 per cent. Morbidity is almost always related to ventilatory difficulties. It is difficult to establish and maintain an airway because of a variety of upper airway abnormalities, including micrognathia, macroglossia, patulous lips, hypertrophic tonsils, restricted motion of the temporomandibular joints, friable tissues, and the presence of copious viscous secretions. In addition, a short neck, an anterior and narrow larynx, and thickened, friable pharyngeal tissue lead to an increased incidence of difficult or failed intubations.[155] Tracheotomy can also be technically difficult and in one case report was impossible even post mortem.[156] Cervical instability, potential spinal cord damage, and severe thoracic and lumbar skeletal abnormalities make positioning and intubation difficult.[157] Intraoperative positioning must be a primary concern and can be facilitated by tailoring a plaster mold to optimize intraoperative position.[158]

Cardiac disease is common in the mucopolysaccharidoses. Both clinical and histologic studies of the cardiovascular system show progressive involvement of the coronary arteries, heart valves, and myocardium. The lumina of the coronary arteries are narrowed, owing to deposition of collagen and mucopolysaccharides in the intima. As children with these diseases grow older, the incidence of valvular disease and cardiomyopathy increases. Both pulmonary and systemic hypertension are common. Two reported intraoperative deaths due to cardiac events occurred in patients who had undergone extensive preoperative cardiac testing.[159]

Respiratory compromise is a frequent clinical finding. Thoracic skeletal abnormalities lead to restrictive pulmonary disease associ-

TABLE 1–5

Classification of Mucopolysaccharidoses

Syndrome	MPS Type	Incidence	Clinical Features
Hurler	IH	1/100,000	Severe involvement of heart, liver, skeleton, airway. Dwarfism, corneal opacities, gargoyle facies, macroglossia. Progressive mental retardation. Conductive deafness.
Scheie	IS	1/500,000	Milder than IH. Slowly progressive skeletal, airway involvement. Cardiac valvular disease common. Corneal opacities. Normal stature and intelligence.
Hurler-Scheie	IH/IS	1/115,000	Intermediate between IH and IS. Mental retardation. Micrognathia common.
Hunter	II	1/70,000–1/150,000	Mild to severe forms. More slowly progressive than IH. Mild mental retardation. Cardiac involvement common.
Sanfilippo	III	May be as high as 1/30,000	Progressive severe mental retardation. Mild progressive somatic involvement.
Morquio	IV	Very rare	Prominent skeletal involvement. Aortic valve disease common. High incidence of odontoid hypoplasia/cervical myelopathy. Normal intelligence.
	V		No longer used. Same as Scheie syndrome.
Maroteaux-Lamy	VI	Very rare	Variable severity of somatic involvement. Normal intelligence. Severe skeletal deformities.
Sly	VII	Very rare	Moderate skeletal abnormalities. Mild mental retardation.

ated with recurrent bouts of pneumonia. Hepatosplenomegaly can result from accumulation of mucopolysaccharides or right-sided heart failure; however, functional impairment of these organs seldom occurs.

Although the mucopolysaccharidoses are rare, the patients tend to come to surgery frequently, the majority for ear, nose, and throat procedures or hernia repair. Thorough preoperative evaluation of cardiac, pulmonary, and neurologic function with appropriate work-up is indicated. It is important to establish which type of disease is involved.[160] Types I and II carry a higher incidence of cervical myelopathy. Age and degree of mental retardation are important considerations in choosing a method of anesthesia. A review of past anesthetic experiences, good inspection of the oropharynx, and radiologic examination of the trachea may warn of possible airway difficulties.[161] One should be cautioned that airway abnormalities can worsen with time: a previously "easy airway" can become a difficult one. Premedication with benzodiazepines may be beneficial with an uncooperative mentally retarded patient but otherwise is best omitted. An antisialagogue should be administered to diminish secretions. Glycopyrrolate and scopolamine may be preferred for patients with heart disease, owing to their less pronounced chronotropic effect as compared with atropine.

Most of the reported anesthetic management difficulties involve airway or positioning problems and concern about preservation of spinal cord function.[162–165] It seems prudent to perform regional anesthesia, if warranted for the surgical procedure and if patient cooperation permits. Airway control for a general anesthetic may require topicalization of the airway and awake intubation by direct laryngoscopy or with the aid of the fiberoptic bronchoscope. The "reverse guidewire" technique, following appropriate sedation, is also possible.

If general anesthesia is to be induced before an airway is secured, inhalation induction may be preferred with maintenance of spontaneous ventilation.[159, 166] Some authors prefer intravenous induction for severely mentally retarded patients who are less willing to accept inhalation induction.[159, 161, 166, 164] Regardless of what technique is employed, intravenous access should be established before anesthetic administration. "Difficult airway" equipment should be immediately available. Nasotracheal intubation is not recommended, owing to difficulties with anatomically constricted nasal passages and potential hemorrhage from soft tissue trauma. Ketamine has been used successfully as the sole anesthetic in these diseases.[167] Preoperatively, airway obstructive symptoms appear to increase the incidence of airway obstruction in the immediate postoperative period.[159] Once an airway is established, careful consideration should be given to positioning and to concomitant cardiac disease. Withdrawal of airway support should be carefully planned and followed by an appropriate monitoring period, because these patients have an increased incidence of atelectasis and airway obstruction secondary to traumatic tissue edema. There are no reported abnormal responses to anesthetic agents or muscle relaxants. Interestingly enough, patients who undergo successful bone marrow transplantation exhibit reversal of preimmunosuppression, airway obstruction, and intracranial hypertension.[159]

IX. DYSAUTONOMIA

Dysautonomia may be congenital, idiopathic, or secondary to a systemic disease. Congenital dysautonomia is present at birth; the idiopathic type usually appears between age 40 and 60 years.[168] If there are central neurologic signs and symptoms, the condition is referred to as the Shy-Drager syndrome. Autonomic dysfunction due to systemic diseases such as diabetes, alcoholism, and nutritional disorders is not discussed, as they are addressed in most basic medical texts.

A. CONGENITAL DYSAUTONOMIA

Congenital or familial dysautonomia (Riley-Day syndrome) is an autosomal-recessive disorder that typically affects Jewish children. The primary genetic defect is not known, although certain pathologic and biochemical markers have been observed. Peripheral nerve biopsy reveals a decrease in the number of small myelinated and unmyelinated fibers; post-mortem examination of sympathetic, parasympathetic, and dorsal root ganglion cells demonstrates reduced numbers of cell bodies. Associated—and potentially related—biochemical changes are reported, including significant decreases in serum dopamine β-hydroxylase (the enzyme that converts dopamine to norepinephrine), urinary vanillylmandelic acid (VMA), and elevation of urinary homovanillic acid (HVA). VMA originates from the degradation of epinephrine and norepinephrine, whereas HVA originates from their precursors. This suggests that dysautonomic patients have a deficiency related to an enzyme defect and an excess of catecholamine precursors.

The disease affects CNS development and manifests clinically as autonomic nervous system dysfunction, generalized decreased sensation, and emotional lability (Table 1–6). Of particular concern is the dysautonomic crisis that is commonly triggered by stress and is characterized by intractable vomiting, hypertension, tachycardia, erythematous skin blotching, and diaphoresis.[169] Elevated serum dopamine levels have been observed during crisis. Diazepam, which increases GABA, is effective in alleviating a crisis by suppressing central dopamine release.[170, 171]

The anesthetic management of familial dysautonomia is both complex and challenging. Decreased autonomic innervation of blood vessels and organs and variable baroreceptor sensitivity to circulating catecholamines lead to blood pressure lability.[168, 169, 172, 173] Baseline systemic vascular resistance is low. Cardiac output responds poorly to increased demand and is very dependent on preload, owing to a relatively fixed inotropy and chronotropy. Patients are extremely sensitive to direct-act-

TABLE 1–6

Signs and Symptoms of Familial Dysautonomia

Diminished pain perception
Erratic temperature control
Labile blood pressure
Postural hypotension
Recurrent pneumonias
Aspiration/bronchiectasis
Cyclical vomiting
Dysphagia
Decreased gastrointestinal motility
Increased salivation
Muscle weakness/incoordination
Scoliosis
Retarded growth
Emotional lability
Defective lacrimation
Smooth tongue

ing vasopressors and have erratic responses to indirect-acting sympathomimetics, owing to diminished sympathetic innervation.

Respiratory function is often compromised by aspiration pneumonia. Poor respiratory muscle function and varying degrees of scoliosis contribute to the restrictive lung disease. In addition, the centrally and peripherally mediated responses to hypoxia and hypercarbia are diminished, a finding that implies greater sensitivity to CNS depressants.

1. Anesthetic Management

Preoperatively, the major goals are to optimize respiratory function, ensure adequate hydration, and reduce patient anxiety.[169, 174] Since chronic dehydration is common, hydration with intravenous crystalloid should be undertaken to achieve a euvolemic state before induction of anesthesia. Preoperative medication with benzodiazepine is recommended because it is the treatment for dysautonomic crisis. Narcotic administration should be minimal or omitted, owing to the increased sensitivity manifested by dysautonomic patients. Antisialagogues should not be administered routinely, to avoid inspissated secretions. Before surgery, chest physiotherapy and prophylactic antibiotics should be given, as necessary. Acid aspiration prophylaxis should be utilized in this patient group at risk.

Severe hypotension has been reported to follow administration of thiopental and inhalational anesthetics to familial dysautonomia patients.[175–178] However, adequate preoperative hydration can prevent significant hypotension with thiopental, narcotic, or volatile anesthetic administration.[169] Dysautonomic patients require smaller doses of anesthetic drugs, perhaps owing to decreased pain sensation or an inability to release catecholamines in response to painful stimuli.[168] Continuous appropriate monitoring should be instituted before induction. Because of the gastrointestinal effects of the disease, rapid-sequence induction should be considered. Controlled ventilation via an endotracheal tube should be maintained during surgery, owing to a tendency for atelectasis in these patients.

There have been no reported adverse or prolonged responses to succinylcholine or nondepolarizing muscle relaxants, whereas the response to muscle relaxant reversal agents is unpredictable. Atropine is effective in the treatment of bradycardia. If hypotension is unresponsive to fluid challenge, small, incremental doses of direct-acting α-adrenergic agents are indicated. Theoretically, regional anesthetic techniques should be tolerated well for the appropriate surgical procedure. Temperature should be monitored during the perioperative period owing to poikilothermic tendencies in dysautonomia.

Postoperatively, the goals are to maintain adequate ventilation, control pain and reactive blood pressure responses, and prevent aspiration. Postoperative pain, if present, should be treated to avoid provoking a dysautonomic crisis. Mechanical ventilation is advised until narcotics are discontinued. Vigorous pulmonary toilet and prophylactic antibiotics should be administered appropriately.

B. SHY-DRAGER SYNDROME AND IDIOPATHIC AUTONOMIC DYSFUNCTION

Shy-Drager syndrome and idiopathic autonomic dysfunction (IAD) are degenerative diseases of middle to late adulthood that result in autonomic dysfunction. IAD involves abnormalities of postganglionic sympathetic neurons; the parasympathetic system is relatively spared. The Shy-Drager syndrome is a central abnormality involving preganglionic neurons, the cerebellum, and the basal ganglia; the patient has extrapyramidal and cerebellar symptoms as well as autonomic dysfunction. The most common signs and symptoms are orthostatic hypotension, anhidrosis, impotence, and urinary and bowel incontinence, although patients may have all of the signs and symptoms of familial dysautonomia listed in Table 1–6.[179] They do not develop dysautonomic crisis.

Anesthetic considerations are similar to those for familial dysautonomia. It is important to note that, in the Shy-Drager syndrome, in which the defect is central, response to indirect-acting sympathomimetics is unpredictable and the response to direct-acting sympathomimetics is still exaggerated, owing to denervation hypersensitivity.[180]

Case reports of anesthetic management in IAD and Shy-Drager syndrome underscore the importance of meticulous cardiovascular and respiratory monitoring and maintenance of adequate preload, both of which are more important than the choice of anesthetic.[168,]

[173, 181] Although ketamine has been used without apparent difficulty in Shy-Drager syndrome, the potential for an unpredictable blood pressure response should obviate its use.[182]

X. KLIPPEL-FEIL SYNDROME

Klippel-Feil syndrome—congenital fusion of the cervical vertebrae—is characterized by a short neck with limited range of motion and a low posterior hairline. Two types are described: type I involves fusion of all cervical vertebrae and varying numbers of upper thoracic vertebrae with occasional fusion with the occiput; type II involves fusion of the C2 and C3 vertebral bodies and spina bifida in all cervical and some upper thoracic vertebrae. Type II is the more common presentation and is often associated with upward displacement of the scapulas (Sprengel's deformity), cleft palate, maxillomandibular deformities, and significant kyphoscoliosis.[183] Skull asymmetry, basilar impression (where the occipital bone is flattened and pushed upward by the upper cervical spine), brachycephaly, and a number of other organ system anomalies have been reported. Clinical manifestations are secondary to compression of the cervical spinal cord, pons, and/or medulla and stretching of cranial nerves. Syncopal episodes may be precipitated by sudden rotary movements of the neck that cause basilar artery insufficiency.

The anesthetic management of Klippel-Feil syndrome includes a complete preoperative evaluation of associated skeletal and organ system anomalies and delineation of any neurologic deficits. The decision on intubation asleep versus awake depends on the neurologic stability of the patient; spontaneous ventilation should be maintained until intubation is performed, owing to the greater likelihood of difficult intubation. The neck should be maintained along a neutral axis during laryngoscopy and positioning, to avoid neurologic sequelae.[184] Muscle relaxation should be maintained with nondepolarizers if neurologic deficits are present. There are no contraindications to any anesthetic agents for Klippel-Feil patients. Case experience with both a general anesthetic after awake fiberoptic intubation and a continuous spinal anesthetic for caesarean section have been reported.[185, 186]

XI. ARNOLD-CHIARI MALFORMATION

The Arnold-Chiari malformation (ACM) is a group of congenital hindbrain anomalies of downward displacement of the cerebellar tonsills through the foramen magnum (and possibly into the cervical spinal canal) and downward displacement of the lower pons and medulla. There are four types of malformation, of which types I and II constitute the vast majority.

Type II ACM, which presents in infancy, is associated with myelomeningocele. Although the initial problem is progressive hydrocephalus, symptoms secondary to cranial nerve, cerebellar, or brain stem dysfunction become more prominent with age. The most common clinical manifestations include inspiratory stridor (representing tenth nerve palsy), episodic apnea, a depressed or absent gag reflex, nystagmus, fixed retrocollis, weak or absent cry, and spastic upper extremity weakness. During myelomeningocele repair in type II ACM, a ventriculoperitoneal shunt is often placed to treat hydrocephalus. Type I ACM, which presents in adulthood, has symptoms secondary to those of the primary defect or associated syringomyelia. The most common clinical manifestations include ataxia; pain in the neck, shoulders, or arms; upper extremity and hand atrophy; spastic paraparesis; headache; nystagmus; vertigo; and, eventually, bulbar symptoms with tongue fasciculations and atrophy, dysphagia, or respiratory embarrassment. Type III ACM involves caudad displacement of the cerebellum and brain stem into a high cervical meningocele, and type IV consists of cerebellar hypoplasia without herniation.

Once the diagnosis is confirmed, surgical intervention is the recommended therapy for progressively symptomatic lesions. This is most often a posterior fossa exploration, including a suboccipital craniectomy, a C1, C2 laminectomy to decompress the caudally displaced cerebellum and brainstem, lysis of subarachnoid adhesions, incision of dural bands, and a duroplasty. In most instances, associated syringomyelia resolves spontaneously after the decompression procedure. Preoperative anesthetic considerations include assessing neural function, especially as it affects upper airway control, protecting from aspiration, and gas exchange; determining if symptoms occur or are exacerbated during flexion-extension of the neck; and determining the presence or absence of increased intracranial pressure.[188, 189]

Intraoperative anesthetic considerations include avoiding extremes of flexion and extension of the neck, owing to possible compression of neural structures, following anesthetic principles for increased intracranial pressure if appropriate, and preparing for possible hemorrhage and air embolism when the procedure is done with the patient seated. In the infant a diffuse venous sinus, which eventually coalesces into the occipital sinus, is normally present in the area of the foramen magnum. In types I and II ACM, the transverse and the torcular sinuses are displaced caudad with the cerebellum and brain stem. Violation of these structures during dural incision can cause massive hemorrhage and air embolism when the patient is sitting or lying prone. Intraoperative monitoring should include continuous arterial pressure and somatosensory evoked potentials. Postoperatively the most common problem is cranial nerve damage leading to upper airway dysfunction with increased risk of aspiration and ventilatory difficulties.[187]

XII. NEUROLOGIC MANIFESTATIONS OF HUMAN IMMUNODEFICIENCY VIRUS INFECTION

Neurologic disease is a frequent complication of human immunodeficiency virus (HIV) infection. Clinically evident neurologic disease occurs in approximately 50 per cent of all HIV-infected persons. As established by the Centers for Disease Control and Prevention the presence of neurologic disease is sufficient to change a diagnosis from HIV infection to acquired immunodeficiency syndrome (AIDS).

The most frequent interactions of anesthesiology personnel and HIV patients with neurologic disease is during the perioperative care of patients for diagnostic stereotactic biopsy, therapeutic stereotactic drainage of brain abscesses, and spinal column laminectomy or drainage of epidural abscesses.[190] Before stereotactic biopsy many patients are started on a 2- to 3-week empiric course of antibiotics that cover the opportunistic organisms that commonly infect the CNS, especially *Toxoplasma*. Stereotactic biopsy is considered for patients who show no improvement after antibiotic therapy, manifest neurologic deterioration, or have a solitary brain lesion discovered by brain imaging. The most common diagnoses from biopsy include primary brain lymphomas, progressive multifocal leukoencephalopathy, and *Toxoplasma* encephalitis.[191] Most stereotactic biopsies can be performed with local anesthesia and monitored anesthesia care and intravenous sedation as needed. General anesthesia may be necessary if the patient's cooperation is impaired (e.g., by AIDS-related dementia).

Anesthetic considerations for epidural abscess drainage should include assessment of associated debilitating conditions and cervical and lumbar spine stability. Attention should be given to preventing increasing neurologic injury secondary to intubation and positioning. As in any procedure, strict adherence to universal precautions is mandatory. The risk of contracting HIV from contaminated percutaneous injuries is extremely low but has been reported. The majority of percutaneous injuries are caused by needles attached to syringes, intravenous or arterial catheter needle-stylets, suture needles, and needles used for secondary intravenous infusions.[192]

XIII. UNUSUAL CEREBROVASCULAR DISEASES

A. INTRACRANIAL ANEURYSMS

Subarachnoid hemorrhage (SAH) from intracranial aneurysms occurs in approximately 28,000 patients a year in North America. Mortality related to massive bleeding, rebleeding, misdiagnosis, late referral, vasospasm, and surgery approaches 66 per cent. Because surgical mortality is 5 to 7 per cent in most reported series, the overall mortality indicates the severity of the nonsurgical complications associated with SAH. Elective surgery for asymptomatic, unruptured intracranial aneurysms is associated with low morbidity (4.1 per cent) and mortality (1 per cent).[193] Educational efforts are necessary to improve recognition of signs of an expanding aneurysm (oculomotor nerve palsy) or of a warning leak (headache, meningismus), so that risks of morbidity and mortality can be reduced for many patients whose diagnosis and therapy would otherwise be delayed. Early surgery (in the first 24 to 48 hours) in grade 0 or 1 lesion patients does not increase mortality or decrease the incidence of vasospasm, and morbidity may be higher than after late surgery; however, with the neck of the aneurysm secured with a clip, vasospasm therapy (intravascular volume expansion, increased blood pressure) can proceed without the risk of rebleeding.[194] Early surgery may also reduce the incidence of medical complications related to prolonged bed rest and hospitalization, such as pulmonary, thomboembolic, and metabolic problems.[195, 196]

The risk of rebleeding is greatest within the first 24 hours after the initial SAH. Recurrent hemorrhage is responsible for major neurologic morbidity and mortality; therefore, efforts are directed at reducing rebleeding by early aneurysm clipping, preventing clot lysis with antifibrinolytic agents, and controlling the transmural pressure across the aneurysm (*transmural pressure* equals *mean arterial pressure* minus *intracranial pressure*) at the lowest level commensurate with adequate cerebral perfusion. Since the specific cause of vasospasm is unknown, prevention and treatment strategies vary. It is clear that maintaining cerebral perfusion pressure (CPP) in the presence of vasospasm can improve outcome.

The perioperative management of an SAH patient from the anesthesiologist's viewpoint is discussed in most current textbooks and will not be repeated here. This section is devoted to the management of uncommon aneurysms, which present interesting and challenging therapeutic considerations.

1. Multiple Aneurysms

After SAH, patients require four-vessel cerebral angiography to detect (single or multiple) aneurysms, which may be above or below the tentorium and ipsilateral or contralateral. Many surgical dilemmas are evident in the presence of multiple aneurysms. Which aneurysm bled? Can multiple clip placements be accomplished during the same craniotomy? Are all of the aneurysms amenable to clip placement? The aneurysm responsible for the SAH may be identified by physical signs (oculomotor nerve palsy) or radiographic criteria such as localized vasospasm on angiography, size of aneurysm, or location of subarachnoid blood on CT. None of these is foolproof; at times the surgeon is forced to choose to clip one aneurysm while leaving others

unsecured for some time. The anesthesiologist must be prepared to carefully control MAP during emergence and in the postoperative period to reduce the likelihood of hemorrhage from the unclipped aneurysm(s). For subsequent craniotomy, brain volume is much easier to optimize if the aneurysm is incidental or SAH occurred in the distant past.

2. Giant Aneurysms

The surgical goal is to clip-ligate the necks of these aneurysms, which may be quite difficult if the dome of the aneurysm totally obscures the parent vessel and access to it. Frequently it is possible to ligate temporarily the parent vessel to permit aneurysmotomy and ligation or suture of the neck. Because the problems and their solutions depend on the anatomy of the aneurysm and feeding vessels, the surgeon and anesthesiologist must plan intraoperative care case by case. A number of options may arise; for example, if sacrifice of the parent vessel is likely, an extracranial-intracranial (EC-IC) bypass may be indicated 3 to 4 days before aneurysm clipping. The EC-IC bypass may not remain patent for long if normal cerebral flow is present; therefore, surgery on the aneurysm is not delayed beyond 3 to 4 days. If a giant basilar aneurysm exists, the team may consider hypothermia or hypothermic cardiac arrest with cardiopulmonary bypass. Barbiturate or etomidate suppression of cerebral metabolism may be sufficient and efficacious in certain circumstances when administered prior to temporary clip occlusion of a major intracranial vessel. Electroencephalographic (EEG) monitoring is indicated to document the therapeutic end point (for example, burst suppression) of maximal cerebral metabolic depression. Simultaneous somatosensory evoked potential monitoring of appropriate cortical areas (since they are resistant to barbiturates) can indicate improper clip placement.

3. Vein of Galen Aneurysms

The vein of Galen is a single midline structure formed by the convergence of the internal cerebral veins and the basal veins of Rosenthal posterior to the splenium of the corpus callosum. It continues posteriorly to join the straight sinus. During embryonic development, cerebral arteries and veins cross close to one another; fistulous connections may occur, because only a few cell layers separate them. Fistulas persist because of the arterial-venous pressure gradient. The size and number of AV fistulas determine the size of a vein of Galen aneurysm and thus the amount of shunt, the presence (or absence) and degree of high-output congestive heart failure (CHF), the severity of compression of the aqueduct of Sylvius (obstructive hydrocephalus), and the viability of local and hemispheric brain tissue exposed to direct pressure or "steal" phenomena. Fistulas that are symptomatic in the neonatal period are very large: as much as 80 per cent of the cardiac output may be shunted. This tremendous volume load leads to cardiomegaly and eventually to high-output cardiac failure that is refractory to medical therapy. Older infants and adults are more likely to develop mild cardiomegaly and failure, hydrocephalus, or symptoms of cerebral ischemia or an intracranial mass lesion.

Arteriovenous malformations (AVM) of the vein of Galen presenting in the neonatal period are often fatal, owing to severe refractory CHF in utero or postnatally, ischemic brain damage, other congenital anomalies, failure to make the diagnosis, or complications of surgery. Clearly, the neonate with this condition is at great risk, with or without surgical intervention. Current anesthetic and surgical techniques and skills may permit survival even if the fistulous connections are only partially ligated. Indeed, this approach may reduce myocardial stress and, when combined with treatment for the obstructive hydrocephalus, may permit survival, growth, and normal neurologic development. In an older, healthier child, additional surgery may be necessary to totally obliterate the AVM.

The causes of death of neonates with this condition are (1) intractable cardiac failure associated with subendocardial ischemia or transmural myocardial infarction, (2) acute circulatory overload after feeding vessel ligation, (3) intraventricular hemorrhage, (4) cerebral infarction secondary to the "steal" phenomenon or to thrombosis of the aneurysm, (5) status epilepticus, or (6) irreversible shock due to intraoperative hemorrhage.

With intraoperative bleeding, the wide pulse pressure may be aggravated so that diastolic filling of the coronary vessels is severely compromised; myocardial ischemia may occur, heralded by intractable hypoten-

sion, bradycardia, or ventricular arrhythmias. Deliberate hypotension is therefore not recommended intraoperatively. Volume replacement must be optimal for cerebral and myocardial perfusion.[197]

Ligation of the feeding vessels may suddenly raise systemic vascular resistance and cause acute volume overload and exacerbation of the heart failure; too vigorous afterload reduction with peripheral vasodilators may compromise coronary perfusion. With abrupt ligation of the feeding vessels to the AVM, flow to vessels supplying the brain in proximity to the malformation may suddenly increase. Normal-pressure perfusion breakthrough may lead to massive brain swelling.

A solution to the dilemma posed by the presence of CHF in a neonate with a potentially surgically correctable AVM may be to slowly obliterate the feeders with temporary—and then permanent—clips and to stage the cranial procedure. This approach allows medical therapy for the CHF to be effective, and eventually unnecessary; it also eliminates the potentially fatal intraoperative hemodynamic changes produced by the more extensive surgery required to completely obliterate the AVM. Control of the CHF and hydrocephalus may permit normal growth and development.

B. CAROTID CAVERNOUS FISTULAS

Carotid cavernous fistulas may result from head or facial trauma or from intracavernous rupture of an aneurysm. Patients present with pulsating exophthalmos, blindness due to prolonged ocular venous pressure elevation, and an ocular bruit audible to the patient and to the examiner with a stethoscope. Treatment techniques have included common carotid compression or ligation; ligation of the cervical internal carotid artery; intracranial ligation of the internal carotid artery before it bifurcates into anterior and middle cerebral arteries, with or without intracranial occlusion of the ophthalmic artery (the trapping operation); the trapping operation plus muscle embolization; hypothermia, with or without hypotension and common carotid occlusion; direct attack on the carotid artery within the cavernous sinus during hypothermia and cardiac arrest; injection of acrylic into the intracavernous portion of the internal carotid artery at the site of the fistula; Gelfoam embolization; and occlusion of the fistula with a balloon-tipped catheter.

It is obvious from this array of suggested procedures that no ideal treatment modality has been found. Each fistula is anatomically different and may have flow characteristics beyond angiographic analysis or significant collaterals that may increase with the age of the fistula.

The ocular bruit is the clinical sign commonly monitored to document obliteration of the fistula; however, stethoscopic appraisal of the disappearance of the bruit can be technically unsatisfactory and objectively difficult in the operating room. A Doppler ultrasonic flow detector placed over the involved eye may be a more reliable method, since it affords continuous monitoring intraoperatively.[198] Regardless of what surgical technique is used, adequate preoperative angiography and intraoperative documentation of the disappearance of the ocular bruit have proved to be necessary for satisfactory treatment of the fistulas.

The appropriate anesthetic technique relates to the mode of therapy for the carotid cavernous fistula chosen by the surgeon and is not different from basic neuroanesthesia principles. EEG and/or somatosensory evoked potential monitoring may permit the diagnosis of unintentional intraoperative occlusion of major cerebral vessels.

RELATED READING

Adams RD, Victor M, (eds): Principles of Neurology, ed 5. New York, McGraw-Hill, 1993.

Azar I: The response of patients with neuromuscular disorders to muscle relaxants: A review. Anesthesiology 61:173–187, 1984.

Braunwald E, Isselbacher KJ, Petersdorf RG, et al., (eds): Harrison's Principles of Internal Medicine, ed 13. New York, McGraw-Hill, 1994.

REFERENCES

1. Davies D: Abnormal response to anaesthesia in a case of Huntington's chorea. A case report. Br J Anaesth 38:490–491, 1966.
2. Blanloeil Y, Bigot A, Dixneuf B: Anaesthesia in Huntington's chorea. Anaesthesia 37:695–696, 1982.
3. Farina J, Rauscher L: Anaesthesia and Huntington's chorea. A report of two cases. Br J Anaesth 49:1167, 1977.
4. Browne M: Anaesthesia in Huntington's chorea. Anaesthesia 38:65, 1982.
5. Gaubatz CL, Wehner RJ: Anesthetic Considerations for the patient with Huntington's disease. AANA 60:40–44, 1992.
6. Soar J, Matheson KH: A safe anaesthetic in Huntington's disease? Anaesthesia 48:743–744, 1993.
7. Giulandi W, Bonfanati G: A case of prolonged apnea in Huntington's chorea. Acta Anaesthesiol 19:235, 1968.
8. Costarino A, Gross J: Patients with Huntington's chorea may respond normally to succinylcholine. Anesthesiology 63:570, 1985.
9. Johnson K, Heggie N: Huntington's chorea. A role of the newer anaesthetic agents. Br J Anaesth 57:235, 1985.
10. Gillman MA, Sandyk R: Nitrous oxide ameliorates spasmodic torticollis. Eur Neurol 24:292–293, 1985.
11. Steen SN: Anesthetic management for basal ganglia surgery in patients with movement disorders. Anesth Analg 44:66–69, 1965.
12. The Parkinson Study Group: Effect of deprenyl on the progression of disability in early Parkinson's disease. N Engl J Med 321:1364–1371, 1989.
13. Spencer DD, Robbins RJ, Naftolin F, et al.: Unilateral tranplantation of human fetal mesencephalic tissue into the caudate nucleus of patients with Parkinson's disease. N Engl J Med 327:1541–1548, 1992.
14. Brindle GF: Anesthesia in the patient with parkinsonism. J Primary Care 4:513–528, 1977.
15. Bevan DR, Monks PS, Calne DB: Cardiovascular reactions to anaesthesia during treatment with levodopa. Anaesthesia 28:29–31, 1973.
16. Shipton EA, Roelofse JA: Anaesthesia in a patient with Parkinson's disease. S Afr Med J 65:304–305, 1984.
17. Ngai SH: Parkinsonism, levodopa and anesthesia. Anesthesiology 3:344–349, 1972.
18. Severn AM: Parkinsonism and the anaesthetist. Br J Anaesth 61:761–770, 1988.
19. Muravchick S, Smith DS: Parkinsonian symptoms during emergence from general anesthesia. Anesthesiology 82:305–307, 1995.
20. Anderson BJ, Marks PV, Futter ME: Propofol—contrasting effects in movement disorders. Br J Neurosurg 8:387–388, 1994.
21. Reed AP, Han DA: Intraoperative exacerbation of Parkinson's disease. Anesth Analg 75:850–853, 1992.
22. Gravelee GP: Succinylcholine-induced hyperkalemia in a patient with Parkinson's disease. Anesth Analg 59:444–446, 1980.
23. Cooperman LH: Succinylcholine-induced hyperkalemia in neuromuscular disease. JAMA 213:1867–1871, 1970.
24. Stone DJ, DiFazio CA: Sedation for patients with Parkinson's disease undergoing ophthalmologic surgery. Anesthesiology 68:821, 1988.
25. Tandon R, Bradley WA: Amyotrophic lateral sclerosis: Part 2. Etiopathogenesis. Ann Neurol 18:419–431, 1985.
26. Tandon R, Bradley WA: Amyotrophic lateral sclerosis: Part 1. Clinical features, pathology and ethical issues in management. Ann Neurol 18:271–283, 1985.
27. Mulder DW, Lambert EM, Eaton LM: Myasthenic syndrome in patients with amyotrophic lateral sclerosis. Neurology 9:627–631, 1959.
28. Rosenbaum KJ, Neigh JT, Strobel GE: Sensitivity to nondepolarizing muscle relaxants in amyotrophic lateral sclerosis: Report of two cases. Anesthesiology 35:638–641, 1971.
29. Gronert GA, Lambert EM, Theye RA: The response

of denervated skeletal muscle to succinylcholine. Anesthesiology 39:13–22, 1973.

30. Beuch TP, Stone WA, Hamelberg W: Circulatory collapse following succinylcholine: Report of a patient with diffuse lower motor neuron disease. Anesth Analg 50:431–437, 1971.

31. Kochi T, Oka T, Mizuguchi T: Epidural anesthesia for patients with amyotrophic lateral sclerosis. Anesth Analg 68:410–412, 1989.

32. Bell CF, Kelly JM, Jones RS: Anaesthesia for Friedreich's ataxia. Anaesthesia 41:296–301, 1986.

33. Campbell AM, Finley GA: Anaesthesia for a patient with Friedreich's ataxia and cardiomyopathy. Can J Anaesth 36:89–93, 1989.

34. Kubal K, Pasricha SK, Bhargava M: Spinal anesthesia in a patient with Friedreich's ataxia. Anesth Analg 72:257–258, 1991.

35. Massan M, Jones RS: Ventilatory failure in Guillain-Barré syndrome. Thorax 35:557–558, 1980.

36. Gracey DR, McMichan JC, Divertie MB, Howard FM: Respiratory failure in Guillain-Barré syndrome. Mayo Clin Proc 57:742–746, 1982.

37. Brian JE, Boyles GD, Quirk JG, Clark RB: Anesthetic management for cesarean section of a patient with Charcot-Marie-Tooth disease. Anesthesiology 66:410–412, 1987.

38. Roelofse JA, Shipton EA: Anaesthesia for abdominal hysterectomy in Charcot-Marie-Tooth disease. S Afr Med J 67:605–606, 1985.

39. Antognini JF: Anaesthesia for Charcot-Marie-Tooth disease: A review of 86 cases. Can J Anaesth 39:398–400, 1992.

40. Kotani NK, Hirota K, Anzawa N, et al: Motor and sensory disability has a strong relationship to induction dose of thiopental in patients with the hypertrophic variety of Charcot-Marie-Tooth syndrome. Anesth Analg 82:182–186, 1996.

41. Feldman JM: Cardiac arrest after succinylcholine administration in a pregnant patient recovered from Guillain-Barré syndrome. Anesthesiology 72:942–944, 1990.

42. Crawford JS, James FM, Nolte H, et al: Regional analgesia for patients with chronic neurological disease and similar conditions. Anaesthesia 36:821–822, 1981.

43. McGrady EM: Management of labour and delivery in a patient with Guillain-Barre syndrome. Anaesthesia 42:899–900, 1987.

44. Steiner I, Agrov Z, Cahan C, Abramsky O: Guillain-Barré syndrome after epidural anesthesia: Direct nerve root damage may trigger disease. Neurology 25:1473–1475, 1985.

45. Plaugher ME: Emergent exploratory laparatomy for a patient with recent Guillain-Barré recurrence: A case report. AANA 62:437–440, 1994.

46. Hughes S: Anesthesia for the pregnant patient with neuromuscular disease. *In* Shnider S, Levinson G (eds): Anesthesia for Obstetrics. Baltimore, Williams & Wilkins, 1987, pp. 420–421.

47. Carpenter MB: Human Neuroanatomy, ed 7. Baltimore, Williams & Wilkins, 1976, pp. 1–20.

48. Segal MB, Pollay M: The secretion of cerebrospinal fluid. Exp Eye Res (Suppl) 25:127–148, 1977.

49. Domer FR: Basic physiology of cerebrospinal outflow. Exp Eye Res (Suppl) 25:323–332, 1977.

50. Artru AA: New concepts concerning anesthetic effects on intracranial dynamics: Cerebrospinal fluid volume and cerebral blood volume. American Society of Anesthesiologists, 38th Annual Refresher Course Lecture (Lecture 133), 1987.

51. Artru AA: Relationship between cerebral blood volume and CSF pressure during anesthesia with isoflurane or fentanyl in dogs. Anesthesiology 60:575–579, 1984.

52. Donato T, Shapira Y, Artru A, Powers K: Effect of mannitol on cerebrospinal fluid dynamics and brain tissue edema. Anesth Analg 78:58–66, 1994.

53. Rockoff MD: Pediatric neurosurgical anesthesia. *In* Ryan JF (ed): A Practice of Anesthesia for Infants and Children. Orlando, Grune & Stratton, 1986, pp. 209–220.

54. Hollinger I: Pediatric neuroanesthesia. Anesthesiol Clin North Am 5:553–556, 1987.

55. Adams RD, Fisher CM, Hakim S, et al: Symptomatic occult hydrocephalus with "normal" cerebrospinal fluid pressure. N Engl J Med 273:117–126, 1965.

56. Vanneste J: Three decades of normal pressure hydrocephalus: Are we wiser now? J Neurol Neurosurg Psychiatry 57:1021–1025, 1994.

57. Barnett GH, Hahn JF, Palmer J: Normal pressure hydrocephalus in children and young adults. Neurosurgery 20:904–907, 1987.

58. Black PM: Idiopathic normal pressure hydrocephalus: Results of shunting in 62 patients. J Neurosurg 52:371–377, 1980.

59. Kristensen B, Malm J, Fagerlund M, et al: Regional cerebral blood flow, white matter abnormalities, and cerebrospinal fluid hydrodynamics in patients with idiopathic adult hydrocephalus syndrome. J Neurol Neurosurg Psychiatry 60:282–288, 1996.

60. Krauss JK, Regel JP, Vach W, et al: Vascular risk factors and arteriosclerotic disease in idiopathic normal-pressure hydrocephalus of the elderly. Stroke 27:24–29, 1996.

61. Rothwell PM, Gibson RJ, Sellar RJ: Computed tomographic evidence of cerebral swelling in benign intracranial hypertension. J Neurol Neurosurg Psychiatry 57:1407–1409, 1994.

62. Malm J, Kristensen B, Markgren P, Ekstedt et al: CSF hydrodynamics in idiopathic intracranial hypertension: Long-term study. Neurology 42:851–858, 1992.

63. Karahalios DG, Rekate HL, Khayata MH, Apostolides PJ: Elevated intracranial venous pressure as a universal mechanism in pseudotumor cerebri of varying etiologies. Neurology 46:198–202, 1996.

64. Jain N, Rosner F: Idiopathic intracranial hypertension: Report of seven cases. Am J Med 93:391–395, 1992.

65. Rosenberg ML, Corbett JJ, Smith C, et al: Cerebrospinal diversion procedures in pseudotumor cerebri. Neurology 43:1071–1072, 1993.

66. Kelman SE, Heaps R, Wolf A, Elman MJ: Optic nerve decompression surgery improves visual function in patients with pseudotumor cerebri. Neurosurgery 30:391–395, 1992.

67. Spoor TC, McHenry JG: Long-term effectiveness of optic nerve sheath decompression for pseudotumor cerebri. Arch Ophthalmol 111:632–635, 1993.

68. Abouleish E, Ali V, Tang RA: Benign intracranial hypertension and anesthesia for cesarean section. Anesthesiology 63:705–706, 1985.

69. Old Field EH, Murazko K, Shawker TH, Patronas NJ: Pathophysiology of syringomyelia associated with Chiari I malformation of the cerebellar tonsils and implications for diagnosis and treatment. J Neurosurg 80:3–15, 1994.

70. Biyam A, El Masry WS: Posttraumatic syringomyelia: A review of the literature. Paraplegia 32:723–731, 1994.

71. Morgan D, Williams B: Syringobulbia: A surgical appraisal. J Neurosurg Psychiatry 55:1132–1134, 1992.
72. Haubitz B, Daniel W, Mügge A, et al: First experiences with syringomyelia imaging using a transoesophageal ultrasound technique. Acta Neurochir 123:157–225, 1993.
73. Roelofse JA, Shipton EA, Nell AC: Anaesthesia for cesarean section in a patient with syringomyelia. A case report. S Afr Med J 65:736–737, 1984.
74. Tator CH, Duncan EG, Edmunds VE, et al: Changes in epiemiology of acute spinal cord injury. Surg Neurol 40:207–215, 1993.
75. Burney RE, Maioe RF, Maynard F, Karvnas R: Incidence of spinal cord injury at trauma centers in North America. Arch Surg 128:596–599, 1992.
76. Kraus JF, Franti CE, Riggins RS, et al: Incidence of traumatic spinal cord lesions. J Chronic Dis 28:471–492, 1975.
77. Mackenzie CF, Ducker TB: Cervical spinal cord injury. In Matjasko J, Katz J (eds): Neuroanesthesia and Neurosurgery. Orlando, Grune & Stratton, 1986, pp. 77–134.
78. Frase A, Edmunds-Seal J: Spinal cord injuries. Anaesthesia 37:1084–1098, 1982.
79. Meinecke FW: Frequency and distribution of associated injuries in traumatic paraplegia and tetraplegia. Paraplegia 5:196–209, 1967.
80. Oller DW, Meredith JW, Rutledge R, et al: The relationship between face or skull fractures and cervical spine and spinal cord injuries: A review of 13,834 patients. Accident Anal Prev 24:187–192, 1992.
81. Ryan M, Klein S, Bongard F: Missed injuries associated with spinal cord trauma. Am Surgeon 59:371–374, 1993.
82. Albuquerque F, Wolf A, Dunham CM, et al: Frequency of intra-abdominal injury in cases of blunt trauma to the cervical spinal cord. J Spinal Disorders 5:476–480, 1992.
83. Deen HJ, McGirr SJ: Vertebral artery injury associated with cervical spine fracture. Spine 17:230–234, 1992.
84. Kobrine AL, Doyle TF, Martins AN: Autoregulation of spinal cord blood flow. Clin Neurosurg 22:573–581, 1975.
85. Bendo AA, Giffen JP, Cottrell JE: Anesthetic and surgical management of acute and chronic spinal cord injury. In Cottrell JE (ed): Anesthesia and Neurosurgery. St. Louis, CV Mosby, 1986, pp. 393–405.
86. Osterholm JL: The pathophysiological response to spinal cord injury. J Neurosurg 40:5–33, 1974.
87. Hall ED, Wolf DL: A pharmacological analysis of the pathophysiological mechanisms of posttraumatic spinal cord ischemia. J Neurosurg 64:951–961, 1986.
88. Bracken MB, Shepherd MJ, Collins WF, et al: A randomized, controlled trial of methylprednisolone or naloxone in the treatment of acute spinal cord injury. N Engl J Med 322:1405–1411, 1990.
89. Green BA, Eismont FJ, O'Heir JT: Spinal cord injury—a systems approach: Prevention, emergency medical services, and emergency room management. Crit Care Clin 3:471–493, 1987.
90. Troll GF, Dohrmann GJ: Anaesthesia for the spinal cord injured patient: Cardiovascular problems and their management. Paraplegia 13:162–171, 1975.
91. Theodore J, Robin ED: Speculation on neurogenic pulmonary edema. Am Rev Respir Dis 113:405–411, 1976.
92. Atkinson PP, Atkinson JLD: Spinal shock. Mayo Clin Proc 71:384–389, 1996.
93. Mackenzie CF, Shin B, Krishnaprasad D, et al: Assessment of cardiac and respiratory function during surgery on patients with acute quadriplegia. J Neurosurg 62:843–849, 1985.
94. Mackenzie CF, Shin B: Cardiac effects of atropine in bradycardic quadriplegics during spinal shock. Crit Care Med 9:150, 1981.
95. McMichan JC, Michel L, Westbrook PR: Pulmonary function following traumatic quadriplegia. JAMA 243:528–531, 1980.
96. Quimby CW, Williams RN, Greifenstein FE: Anesthetic problems of the acute quadriplegic patient. Anesth Analg 52:333–340, 1973.
97. Ohry A, Mocho M, Rozin R: Alterations in pulmonary function in spinal cord injured patients. Paraplegia 13:101–108, 1975.
98. Ledsome JR, Sharp JM: Pulmonary function in acute cervical cord injury. Am Rev Respir Dis 124:41–44, 1981.
99. Dicpinigaitis PV, Spungen AM, Bauman WA, et al: Bronchial hyperresponsiveness after cervical spinal cord injury. Chest 105:1073–1076, 1994.
100. Soni BM, Vaidyanathan S, Fraser MH, et al: Acute hypotension associated with terbutaline nebulizer therapy in a traumatic tetraplegic patient during spinal shock phase. Case report. Paraplegia 33:300–301, 1995.
101. Petrozzi WT, Shapiro BA, Meyer PR, et al: Care Med 22:252–258, 1994.
102. Giffen JP: Anesthesia for acute and chronic spinal cord injuries. Am Soc Anesthesiol Refresher Courses in Anesthesiology 13:69–80, 1985.
103. Denken YK, White RJ, et al: Anaesthesia for laminectomy and localized cord cooling in acute cervical spine injury. Br J Anaesth 43:973–979, 1971.
104. Poe RH, Reisman JL, Rodenhouse TG: Pulmonary edema in cervical spinal cord injury. J Trauma 18:71–73, A78, 1978.
105. Pollack IF, Pang D, Sclabassi R: Recurrent spinal cord injury without radiographic abnormalities in children. J Neurosurg 69:177–182, 1988.
106. Hamilton MG, Myles ST: Pediatric spinal injury: Review of 774 hospital admissions. J Neurosurg 77:700–704, 1992.
107. Osenbach RK, Menezes AH: Pediatric spinal cord and vertebral column injury. Neurosurgery 30:385–390, 1992.
108. Hadley MN, Zabramski JM, Browner CM, et al: Pediatric spinal trauma: Review of 122 cases of spinal cord and vertebral column injuries. J Neurosurg 68:18–24, 1988.
109. Ruge JR, Sinson GP, McLone DG, Cerullo LJ: Pediatric spinal injury: the very young. J Neurosurg 68:25–30, 1988.
110. Pang D, Wilberger JE: Spinal cord injury without radiographic abnormalities in children. J Neurosurg 57:114–129, 1982.
111. Choi J, Hoffman HJ, Hendrick EB, et al: Traumatic infarction of the spinal cord in children. J Neurosurg 65:608–610, 1986.
112. Felsberg GJ, Tien RD, Osom AK, Cardenas CA: Utility of MR imaging in pediatric spinal cord injury. Pediatr Radiol 25:131–135, 1995.
113. Vogel LC, Schrader T, Lubicky JP: Latex allergy in children and adolescents with spinal cord injuries. J Pediatr Orthop 15:517–520, 1995.
114. Johnston RA: Management of old people with neck trauma. Br Med J 299:633–634, 1989.

115. Katoh S, Ikata T, Hirai N, et al: Influence of minor trauma to the neck on neurological outcome in patients with ossification of the posterior longitudinal ligament (OPLL) of the cervical spine. Paraplegia 33:330–333, 1995.
116. Geisler WD, Jousse AT, Wynne-Jones M, Breithaupt D: Survival in traumatic spinal cord injury. Paraplegia 21:364–373, 1983.
117. Leaf DA, Bahl RA, Adkins RH: Risk of cardiac dysrhythmias in chronic spinal cord injury patients. Paraplegia 31:571–575, 1993.
118. Desmond J: Paraplegia: Problems confronting the anaesthesiologist. Can Anaesth Soc J 17:435–451, 1970.
119. Lambert DH, Deane RS, Mazuzan JE: Anesthesia and the control of blood pressure in patients with spinal cord injury. Anesth Analg 61:344–348, 1982.
120. Schonwald G, Fish KJ, Perkash I: Cardiovascular complications during anesthesia in chronic spinal cord injured patients. Anesthesiology 55:550–558, 1981.
121. Chancellor MB, Erhard MJ, Hirsch IH, Stass WE: Prospective evaluation of terazosin for treatment of autonomic dysreflexia. J Urol 151:111–113, 1994.
122. Dykstra DD, Sidi AA, Anderson LC: The effect of nifedipine on cystoscopy-induced autonomic hyperreflexia in patients with high spinal cord injuries. J Urol 138:1155–1157, 1987.
123. Davis FA, Michael JA, Neer D: Serial hyperthermia testing in multiple sclerosis: A method for monitoring subclinical fluctuations. Acta Neurol Scand 49:63–70, 1973.
124. Edmund J, Fog T: Visual and motor instability in multiple sclerosis. Arch Neurol Psychiatry 73:316–320, 1955.
125. Siemkowicz E: Multiple sclerosis and surgery. Anaesthesia 31:1211–1216, 1976.
126. Jones R, Healy T: Anaesthesia and demyelinating disease. Anaesthesia 35:879–884, 1980.
127. Baskett PJ, Armstrong R: Anaesthetic problems in multiple sclerosis. Anaesthesia 25:397–401, 1970.
128. Bamford C, Sibley W, Laguna J: Anesthesia in multiple sclerosis. J Can Sci Neurol 5:41–44, 1978.
129. Kytta J, Rosenberg P: Anaesthesia for patients with multiple sclerosis. Ann Chir Gynaecol 73:299–303, 1984.
130. Schapira K, Poskanzer DC, Miller H: Familial and conjugal multiple sclerosis. Brain 86:315–320, 1963.
131. Eickhoff K, Wikstrom J: Protein profile of cerebrospinal fluid in multiple sclerosis with special reference to the function of the blood-brain barrier. J Neurol 214:207–215, 1977.
132. Warren T, Datta S, Ostheimer G: Lumbar epidural anesthesia in a patient with multiple sclerosis. Anesth Analg 61:1022–1023, 1982.
133. Berger J, Ontell R: Intrathecal morphine in conjunction with a combined spinal and general anesthetic in a patient with multiple sclerosis. Anesthesiology 66:400–402, 1987.
134. Crawford JS: Regional analgesia for patients with chronic neurological disease and similar conditions. Anaesthesia 36:821–822, 1981.
135. Abouleish E: Neurological diseases. In James FM, Wheeler AS (eds): Obstetric Anesthesia: The Complicated Patient. Philadelphia, FA Davis, 1988, pp. 110–111.
136. Bader AM, Hunt CO, Datta S, et al: Anesthesia for the obstetric patient with multiple sclerosis. J Clin Anesth 1:21–24, 1988.
137. Leigh J, Fearnley SJ, Lupprian KG: Intrathecal diamorphine during laparotomy in a patient with advanced multiple sclerosis. Anaesthesia 43:640–642, 1990.
138. Fisher M: Anaesthetic difficulties in neurofibromatosis. Anaesthesia 30:648–650, 1975.
139. Crozier W: Upper airway obstruction in neurofibromatosis. Anaesthesia 42:1209–1211, 1987.
140. Dodge TL, Mahaffey J, Thomas J: The anesthetic management of a patient with an obstructing intratracheal mass: A case report. Anesth Analg 56:295–298, 1977.
141. Yong-Hing K, Kalamchi A, MacEwen D: Cervical spine abnormalities in neuro-fibromatosis. J Bone Joint Surg 61:695–699, 1979.
142. Krishna G: Neurofibromatosis, renal hypertension, and cardiac dysrhythmias. Anesth Analg 54:542–544, 1975.
143. Mauser J: Abnormal responses in von Recklinghausen's disease. Br J Anaesth 42:183, 1970.
144. Magbagbeola JAO: Abnormal responses to muscle relaxants in a patient with von Recklinghausen's disease. Br J Anaesth 42:710, 1970.
145. Baraka A: Myasthenic response to muscle relaxants in von Recklinghausen's disease. Br J Anaesth 46:70, 1974.
146. Richardson MG, Gurudatt KS, Rawood SA: Responses to nondepolarizing neuromuscular blockers and succinylcholine in von Recklinghausen neurofibromatosis. Anesth Analg 82:382–385, 1996.
147. Dounas M, Mercier FJ, Lhuissier C, Benhamou D: Epidural analgesia for labour in a parturient with neurofibromatosis. Can J Anaesth 42:420–424, 1995.
148. Matthews AJ, Halshaw J: Epidural anaesthesia in von Hippel-Lindau disease. Anaesthesia 41:853–855, 1986.
149. Tempelhoff R, Modica P: Anesthetic management of a patient with multiple posterior fossa tumors and an active pheochromocytoma. Anesth Rev 25:13–20, 1988.
150. Joffe D, Robbins R, Benjamin A: Caesarean section and phaeochromocytoma resection in a patient with Von Hippel-Lindau disease. Can J Anaesth 40:870–874, 1993.
151. Otenasek FJ, Silver ML: Spinal hemangiomas (hemangioblastoma) in Lindau's disease. J Neurosurg 18:295–300, 1961.
152. Lee JJ, Imrie M, Taylor V: Anaesthesia and tuberous sclerosis. Br J Anaesth 73:421–425, 1994.
153. Tsukui A, Noguchi R, Honda T, et al: Aortic aneurysm in a four-year-old child with tuberous sclerosis. Pediatr Anaesth 5:67–70, 1995.
154. McKusick VA: Heritable Disorders of Connective Tissue, ed 4. St. Louis, CV Mosby, 1972.
155. Walker RW, Darowski M, Morris P, Wraith JE: Anaesthesia and mucopolysaccharidoses. A review of airway of problems in children. Anaesthesia 49:1078–1084, 1994.
156. Hopkins R, Watson J, Jones J, Walker M: Two cases of Hunter's syndrome. The anaesthetic and operative difficulties in oral surgery. Br J Oral Surg 10:286–289, 1973.
157. Beighton P, Craig J: Atlantoaxial subluxation in the Morquio syndrome. J Bone Joint Surg 55:478–481, 1973.
158. Birkinshaw K: Anaesthesia in a patient with an unstable neck. Morquio's syndrome. Anaesthesia 30:46–49, 1975.
159. Belani KG, Krivit W, Carpenter LM, et al: Children

with mucopolysaccaridoses: Perioperative care, morbidity, mortality and new findings. J Pediatr Surg 28:403–410, 1993.

160. Baines D, Keneally J: Anaesthetic implications of the mucopolysaccharidoses: A fifteen year experience in a children's hospital. Anaesth Intensive Care 11:198–202, 1983.

161. Herrick I, Rhine E: The mucopolysaccharidoses and anaesthesia: A report of clinical experience. Can J Anaesth 35:67–73, 1988.

162. Sjogren P, Pedersen T: Anaesthetic problems in Hurler-Scheie syndrome. Report of two cases. Acta Anaesthesiol Scand 30:484–486, 1986.

163. King D, Jones R, Barnett M: Anaesthetic considerations in the mucopolysaccharidoses. Anaesthesia 39:126–131, 1984.

164. Kempthorne P, Brown T: Anaesthesia and the mucopolysaccharidoses: A survey of techniques and problems. Anaesth Intensive Care 11:203–207, 1983.

165. Linstedt U, Maier C, Joehnk H, Stephani U: Threatening spinal cord compression during anesthesia in a child with mucopolysaccharidosis VI. Anesthesiology 80:227–229, 1994.

166. Diaz JH, Belani KG: Perioperative management of children with mucopolysaccharidoses. Anesth Analg 77:1261–1270, 1993.

167. Sjogren P, Pedersen T, Steinmetz H: Mucopolysaccharidoses and anaesthetic risks. Acta Anaesthesiol Scand 31:214–218, 1987.

168. Sweeney BP, Jones S, Langford RM: Anaesthesia in dysautonomia: Further complications. Anaesthesia 40:783–786, 1985.

169. Axelrod FB, Donenfeld RF, Danzier F, Turndorf H: Anesthesia in familial dysautonomia. Anesthesiology 68:631–635, 1988.

170. Axelrod FB: Familial dysautonomia. In Gellis S, Kagan B (eds): Current Pediatric Therapy. Philadelphia, WB Saunders, 1986, pp. 92–95.

171. Pearson J: Familial dysautonomia (a brief review). J Auton Nerv System 1:119–126, 1979.

172. Smith AA, Dancis J: Exaggerated response to infused norepinephrine in familial dysautonomia. N Engl J Med 270:704–707, 1964.

173. Malan MD, Crago RR: Anaesthetic considerations in idiopathic orthostatic hypotension and the Shy-Drager syndrome. Can Anaesth Soc J 26:322–326, 1979.

174. Beilin B, Maayan CH, Vatashsky E, et al: Fentanyl anesthesia in familial dysautonomia. Anesth Analg 64:72–76, 1985.

175. Stenquist O, Sigurdsson J: The anaesthetic management of a patient with familial dysautonomia. Anaesthesia 37:929–932, 1982.

176. Meridy MW, Creighton RE: General anaesthesia in eight patients with familial dysautonomia. Can Anaesth Soc J 18:568–569, 1971.

177. Kritchman MM, Schwartz M, Papper EM: Experiences with general anesthesia in patients with familial dysautonomia. JAMA 170:529–533, 1971.

178. Inlester JS: Anaesthesia for a patient suffering from familial dysautonomia. Br J Anaesth 43:509–512, 1971.

179. Bevan DR: Shy-Drager syndrome. A review and a description of the anaesthetic management. Anaesthesia 34:866–873, 1979.

180. Stirt JA, Frantz RA, Gunz EF, Conolly ME: Anesthesia, catecholamines, and hemodynamics in autonomic dysfunction. Anesth Analg 61:701–704, 1982.

181. Cohen C: Anesthetic management of a patient with the Shy-Drager syndrome. Anesthesiology 35:95–97, 1971.

182. Saarnivaara L, Kautto UM, Teravainen M: Ketamine anaesthesia for a patient with the Shy-Drager syndrome. Acta Anaesthesiol Scand 27:123–125, 1983.

183. Nagib MG, Maxwell RE, Chou SN: Identification and management of high-risk patients with Klippel-Feil syndrome. J Neurosurg 61:523–530, 1984.

184. Naguib MG, Heram F, Wahab A: Anaesthetic considerations in Klippel-Feil syndrome. Can Anaesth Soc J 33:66–70, 1986.

185. Dresner MR, MacLean AR: Anaesthesia for Caesarian section in a patient with Klippel-Feil syndrome. The use of a microspinal catheter. Anaesthesia 50:807–809, 1995.

186. Burns AM, Dorje P, Lawes EG, Nielson MS: Anaesthetic management of Caesarean section for a mother with pre-eclampsia, the Klippel-Feil syndrome and congenital hydrocephalus. Br J Anaesth 61:350–354, 1988.

187. Hoffman MJ, Hendrick EB, Humphreys RP: Manifestations and management of Arnold-Chiari malformation in patients with myelomeningocele. Childs Brain 1:255–259, 1975.

188. McLeod ME, Creighton RE: Anesthesia for pediatric neurological and neuromuscular diseases. J Child Neurol 1:189–197, 1986.

189. Bell WO, Charney EB, Bruce DA: Symptomatic Arnold-Chiari malformation: Review of experience with 22 cases. J Neurosurg 66:812–816, 1987.

190. Levy RM, Berger JR: Neurosurgical aspects of human immunodeficiency virus infection. Neurosurg Clin North Am 3:443–469, 1992.

191. Luzzati R, Ferrari S, Nicolato A, et al: Stereotactic brain biopsies in human immunodeficiency virus–infected patients. Arch Intern Med 156:565–568, 1996.

192. Greene ES, Berry AJ, Arnold WP, Jugger J: Percutaneous injuries in anesthesia personnel. Anesth Analg 83:273–278, 1996.

193. King JT, Berlin JA, Flamm E: Morbidity and mortality from elective surgery for asymptomatic, unruptured, intracranial aneurysms: A meta-analysis. J Neurosurg 81:837–842, 1994.

194. McGrath BJ, Guy J, Boul CO, et al: Perioperative management of aneurysmal subarachnoid hemorrhage: Part 2. Postoperative management. Anesth Analg 81:1295–1302, 1995.

195. Gelb AW, Newfield P: Intracranial aneurysm. In Matjasko J, Katz J (eds): Clinical Controversies in Neuroanesthesia and Neurosurgery. Orlando, Grune & Stratton, 1986, pp. 233–256.

196. Kassell NF, Boarini DJ, Adams HP, et al: Overall management of ruptured aneurysm: Comparison of early and late operation. Neurosurgery 9:120–128, 1981.

197. Matjasko J, Robinson W, Eudaily D: Successful surgical and anesthetic management of vein of Galen aneurysm in a neonate in congestive heart failure. Neurosurgery 22:908–910, 1988.

198. Matjasko J, Williams JP, Fontanilla M: Intraoperative use of Doppler to detect successful obliteration of carotid-cavernous fistulae. J Neurosurg 53:634–635, 1975.

Eye, Ear, Nose, and Throat Diseases

John V. Donlon

For many patients presenting for ophthalmic or ear, nose, and throat (ENT) surgery, the surgical problem is merely one aspect of a systemic disease complex. Although the surgeon may be able to focus on that one aspect of the patient's condition, the anesthesiologist must consider the whole patient and his or her disease. In this chapter I discuss many eye and ENT diseases that are uncommon; many of them are also reviewed in detail elsewhere in this book.

I. EYE DISEASES: GENERAL CONSIDERATIONS

A. CATARACTS AND SYSTEMIC DISEASE

Cataracts can be associated with metabolic diseases, exogenous substances, infections, skin diseases, genetic diseases, and hematologic problems.[1]

Metabolic diseases include diabetes mellitus, galactosemia, hypoparathyroidism, hypothyroidism, hepatolenticular degeneration (Wilson's disease), phenylketonuria, Refsum's disease, Fabry's disease, and xanthomatosis.

Exogenous substances that can cause cataracts include steroids, phenothiazines, naphthalene, ergot, and parachlorobenzene.

Infections such as rubella, mumps, herpes, influenza, and toxoplasmosis have been associated with cataracts.

Congenital causes of cataracts include Turner's, Down's, Patau's, Conradi's, Pierre Robin, and Sjögren's syndromes. Lowe's (oculocerebrorenal) syndrome is associated with cataracts and glaucoma.[2] The syndrome includes mental retardation, hypotonia, renal acidosis, osteoporosis, and vitamin D deficiency. Anesthetic considerations include attention to acid-base balance, serum calcium levels, brittle bones, and renal dysfunction.[3]

B. ECTOPIC LENS

Spontaneous lens dislocation is associated with Marfan's syndrome, Crouzon's syndrome, and Ehlers-Danlos syndrome and with homocystinuria.

C. RETINAL COMPLICATIONS OF SYSTEMIC DISEASES

Most commonly, retinal problems such as vitreal hemorrhage and detached retina are associated with hypertension and diabetes mellitus. The presence of central retinal artery occlusion indicates severe generalized arteriosclerotic disease. Most collagen diseases, such as systemic lupus erythematosus, scleroderma, and polyarteritis nodosa, can cause vitreal hemorrhages, edema, or retinal detachment.[4] Retinal problems are also associated with Marfan's syndrome, sickle cell anemia, the Wegner-Stickler syndrome, macroglobulinemia, Tay-Sachs disease, Niemann-Pick disease and hyperlipidemia.

D. CORNEAL PROBLEMS ASSOCIATED WITH SYSTEMIC DISEASES

Inflammatory diseases, such as rheumatoid arthritis, Reiter's syndrome, Behçet's syndrome, and sarcoidosis, can cause pathologic conditions of the cornea. The connective tissue disorders of Wegener's granulomatosis, scleroderma, Sjögren's syndrome, and ankylosing spondylosis have been associated with corneal problems.[5] Skin diseases such as pemphigus and erythema multiforme, Marfan's syndrome, and Ehlers-Danlos syndrome have corneal manifestations.

Other causes of corneal lesions include metabolic disease secondary to enzyme deficiencies, such as disorders of carbohydrate metabolism, Wilson's syndrome, hyperlipidemia, cystinosis, and gout. Chronic renal failure, leprosy, tuberculosis, and Graves' hyperthyroid disease all can have corneal features. Finally, mandibulooculofacial dyscephaly (Hallermann-Streiff syndrome) is of particular interest to anesthesiologists because of the likelihood of difficult intubation.[6]

The eye lesion that brings a patient to ophthalmic surgery is often merely one manifestation of a systemic disease that may have consequences for safe anesthesia. Cataracts, a detached retina, a dislocated lens, and eye muscle abnormalities are all eye problems associated with general systemic disease.[7]

II. EYE DISEASES: SPECIFIC CONSIDERATIONS

A. MARFAN'S SYNDROME

Marfan's syndrome is a disorder of connective tissue that involves primarily the cardiovascular, skeletal, and ocular systems. It is inherited as a dominant trait with variable expression, occurring in 1.5 in 100,000 population. The patients are tall with long, thin extremities and fingers. Loose joint ligaments lead to frequent dislocations of the hips and mandible. Pectus excavatum and a high-arched palate can also be present.[8]

Cardiovascular manifestations include dilation of the ascending aorta and aortic insufficiency. The loss of elastic fibers in the media can also account for dilatation of the pulmonary artery and mitral insuffiency resulting from extended chordae tendineae. Heart failure and dissecting aortic aneurysm are not uncommonly associated with Marfan's syndrome.

The ocular manifestations of Marfan's syndrome include severe myopia, spontaneous retinal detachments, displaced lenses, and glaucoma.

Early manifestations of Marfan's syndrome can be subtle, so the diagnosis may not yet have been made when the patient comes to surgery. The anesthesiologist should be suspicious when a tall, young patient with a heart murmur presents for repair of a spontaneously detached retina. These young patients should have chest x-ray studies and an electrocardiogram—and possibly even an echocardiogram—before surgery.

Intubation may be difficult because of an elongated larynx; a high-arched, narrow palate; and possible subluxation of the temporomandibular joint. Severe pectus excavatum and kyphoscoliosis can compromise both respiratory and cardiac function. The tendency for these patients to dislocate joints requires careful attention to positioning and movement on the operating room table.

Significant aortic insufficiency warrants concern for proper blood pressure maintenance; the blood pressure should be high enough (especially the diastolic pressure) to provide good coronary blood flow but not so high as to risk dissection of the aorta. As a rule, the patient's normal blood pressure should be a guide. Concurrent mitral insufficiency and prolonged heart disease can leave the patient with minimal cardiac reserve and, thus, more susceptible to the depressive effects of anesthetic agents. These valve problems may require antibiotic prophylaxis for bacterial endocarditis.

An anesthetic regimen using nitrous oxide, a narcotic (fentanyl 3 to 5 μg/kg or an equivalent), a muscle relaxant technique, and suffi-cient isoflurane to control blood pressure usually works well.

B. GRAVES' DISEASE

Graves' ophthalmopathy includes proptosis, corneal ulcerations, and severe exophthalmos. Infiltrative ophthalmic problems are present in 10 to 20 per cent of patients with Graves' disease, and 3 per cent of them have severe exophthalmos. The cause of exophthalmos is unclear. When medical management (usually steroids) fails, these patients require surgery. Lateral (Krönlein's) or supraorbital (Naffziger's) decompression is performed.[9]

Graves' syndrome includes hyperthyroidism, goiter, exophthalmos, and pretibial myxedema and is associated with the production of excess thyroid hormone. It occurs in about 3 in 10,000 adults (usually women) between 30 and 50 years of age. Graves' disease is felt to be an autoimmune disease directed against thyroid antigens and possibly exacerbated by emotional stress. There is a strong hereditary factor in Graves' disease.

Symptoms, which can be subtle, include weakness, fatigue, weight loss, tremulousness, and increased tolerance to cold. Eye prominence, double or blurred vision, and decreased visual acuity can occur. Cardiac symptoms include a hyperactive heart, atrial fibrillation, palpitations, tachycardia, and dyspnea on exertion.

The pathologic eye condition associated with Graves' disease is due to infiltration of retroorbital tissue and extraocular muscles by lymphocytes, plasma cells, and mucoproteins. The extraocular muscles are often swollen to five to ten times their normal size. Infiltrative ophthalmopathy usually develops in association with hyperthyroidism and responds to medical treatment. If proptosis is severe and muscle function or visual acuity deteriorates, steroid therapy (prednisone 20 to 40 mg/day) is indicated, especially when retrobulbar neuritis develops. Disease resistant to steroid therapy requires surgical intervention.

The three main concerns of the anesthesiologist in these cases relate to steroids, thyroid storm, and tracheal deviation secondary to a large neck mass. These patients usually take large doses of steroids that must be maintained (or increased) during the stress of surgery. Although Graves' disease has usually been diagnosed and controlled before surgery, attention to the level of thyroid function is important.[10] Sudden thyroid storm secondary to stress or infection is always possible. Sudden severe hyperkinesis, tachycardia, hyperpyrexia, vomiting, and dehydration can quickly progress to shock and coma.[11] Therefore the preoperative evaluation must assess the effectiveness of thyroid therapy, documenting triiodothyronine (T_3) and thyroxine (T_4) plasma levels, heart rate, and absence of symptoms.

Finally, an enlarged thyroid gland may cause tracheal pressure or deviation and make intubation difficult. If there is concern about the airway for this reason, x-ray studies of the trachea should be consulted.

C. INCONTINENTIA PIGMENTI

Incontinentia pigmenti is a rare autosomal-dominant disease that occurs mainly in females or as a lethal X-linked trait in males.[12] It is usually present at birth and is first manifested as inflammatory linear skin vesicles or bullae that progress to verrucous papillomata and eventually to skin pigmentation.[13] Other ectodermal abnormalities exist in 60 per cent of patients.

The eyes, teeth, central nervous system, extremities, and heart can be affected. Ocular problems include strabismus, detached retina, exudative chorioretinitis, optic atrophy, and a retrolental membrane.[14] Neurologic problems can include seizures, spastic paralysis, mental retardation, and microcephaly.

The anesthetic management of these patients should focus on the fact that the obvious external ectodermal changes may be harbingers of hidden ectodermal abnormalities in the heart or central nervous system.

D. HOMOCYSTINURIA

Homocystinuria is a rare biochemical abnormality caused by one of several genetic disorders, usually cystathionine β-synthase deficiency, which is inherited as an autosomal recessive trait.[15] Disease occurs in the homozygote, but the heterozygote is without risk. There is an apparent frequency of 1 in 200,000 population.

The most consistent finding is ectopia lentis occurring during early childhood. Since many of the manifestations of homocystinuria are related to abnormal connective tissue, outwardly these patients may appear to have marfanoid characteristics.

Kyphosis and osteoporosis involving the spine may eventually develop. Mental retardation, seizures, and pectus excavatum can be present.

The major life-threatening complication of cystathionine β-synthase deficiency is thromboembolism. Vascular occlusions can occur at any age and involve cerebral, cardiac, renal, or pulmonary emboli, especially after surgery. The pathogenesis of the thrombotic tendency is not clear, but it could be related to increased platelet adhesiveness or aggregation, Hageman factor activation, or increased platelet consumption secondary to endothelial damage. The number and severity of clinical complications vary widely. The diagnosis is suggested by ectopia lentis and thromboembolic events and may be confirmed by specific urine tests for homocystine.

The major anesthetic problem in these patients at any age is the risk of thromboembolism in a major organ system (brain, heart, kidneys, lungs) causing significant damage or death.[16] Low-flow, hypotensive states must be avoided. It is essential that these patients be kept well-hydrated and well-perfused and that hypotension is avoided.[17] Early postoperative vascular support stockings prevent stasis thrombi in leg veins. The platelet function and bleeding parameters should be checked before surgery, and consideration should be given to using aspirin or dipyridamole to decrease platelet adhesiveness or increase platelet survival.

Another concern in the perioperative period is hypoglycemia. Hypermethioninemia can trigger hypoglycemia secondary to hyperinsulinemia.[20] Blood glucose levels must be monitored, and intravenous solutions should contain glucose.

E. HEMOGLOBIN DISEASES

Hemoglobin diseases are inherited disorders of hemoglobin synthesis that reflect structural abnormalities of globin polypeptides or, as in thalassemia, impaired synthesis of globin chains. In hemoglobin S (Hb S), a single amino acid (valine) substitution in the beta chain has no influence on oxygen affinity or molecular stability, but it causes an intermolecular reaction, forming insoluble structures within the erythrocyte, leading to sickling.[21] Low oxygen tension and acid pH are critical determinants of the degree of sickling.

Sickle cell anemia (homozygous for Hb S) is a serious disease characterized by hemolytic anemia, recurrent pain and fever, and organ system involvement. About 8 per cent of American blacks are heterozygous carriers of Hb S; thus, about 0.5 per cent of blacks are homozygous for Hb S disease. A crisis episode of sickling can be precipitated by cold, infection, or hypoxia or during conditions that cause increased vascular stasis.

Bone and bone marrow infarctions, spinal osteoporosis, leg ulcers, jaundice, and recurrent episodes of pneumonia tend to occur. The heart may be enlarged, and congestive heart failure may develop with age.

Although ocular abnormalities such as proliferative retinopathy can occur in all types of sickling diseases, they are more common in adults with Hb SC or Hb S thalassemia (60 per cent) than in those with Hb SS (10 per cent). The proliferative retinopathy seen during the third or fourth decade of life is due to vascular occlusion.

Fortunately, patients with Hb SC, Hb S thalassemia, or Hb SA (sickle trait) have less severe symptoms than patients with Hb SS, and usually present with only mild anemia and splenomegaly.

The vascular occlusion of retinal vessels leads to ischemia, neovascularization, vitreous hemorrhage, fibrosis, traction, and retinal detachment or atrophy.[22]

Conditions that precipitate sickling crisis in patients with Hb SS must be avoided.[23] They include hypoxia, cold, acidosis, and vascular stasis. Therefore, these patients must be kept well-oxygenated and monitored with a pulse oximeter well into emergence in the recovery room. A 40 per cent oxygen face mask supplement must be used during awakening. Good hydration, avoiding hypotension and hypothermia, and encouraging early ambulation with elastic support stockings prevent vascular stasis. An alkaline buffer intravenous solution may be appropriate, and controlled ventilation monitoring of end-tidal carbon dioxide at 35 to 40 mm Hg helps prevent intraoperative respiratory acidosis. Airway obstruction, either at induction or during emergence can lead to hypoxic, acidotic episodes, and care must be taken to ensure adequate oxygenation during these periods. Preoperative evaluation should focus on eliminating any infectious process and ensuring good functioning of the lungs and a stable blood count. Postoperative pneumonia can lead to a sickling crisis and can be fatal in these patients. Any anesthetic technique that supports the preceding caveats will be useful in patients with homozygous sickle cell anemia (Hb SS).

F. RETINOPATHY OF PREMATURITY

Retinopathy of prematurity (ROP) is usually associated with low–birth weight preterm neonates who require oxygen therapy. The theory is that hyperoxia causes vessel constriction in the developing retina, creating areas of peripheral ischemia, poor vascularization, and proliferation of an abnormal retinal vessel network (neovascularization), which causes hemorrhages, scarring, fibrosis, and retinal detachment.[24]

The incidence of ROP is once again increasing as neonatal medicine improves the survival rate (65 per cent) of very low–birth weight neonates. The assumption that ROP may be caused only by excess oxygen in this population seems unwarranted in sight of a recent reexamination of data.[25] ROP is of multifactorial origin in these very immature infants.[26]

The infants undergo prolonged care in the intensive care unit after birth and are subject to a wide range of medical problems. ROP may develop in 40 to 75 per cent of premature infants who weigh less than 1000 g. There is an inverse relation between birth weight and the incidence of ROP.

These premature infants usually have problems with episodes of apnea and bradycardia, neonatal jaundice, patent ductus arteriosus, bronchopleural dysplasia, intraventricular hemorrhage, delayed mental development, and seizures.

Since the American Academy of Pediatrics has stated that there is no association between short-term hyperoxia and ROP, these patients should receive unrestricted oxygen, as required, during surgery.[27] When oxygen was restricted in these patients, the incidence of respiratory complications was high.

Elective surgery should be postponed until after 44 weeks' gestational age. Cryotherapy to ablate the avascular retina and prevent neovascularization is a new approach performed in newborns just weeks after birth. More conventional ophthalmic surgery for ROP occurs at 4 to 12 months of age and removes membranes or corrects retinal detachments. Although by age 4 months many of these neonates who weighed less than 1000 g seem to be thriving, the anesthesiologist must still be concerned about poor lung function, recurrent apnea, a propensity for bradycardia, and sudden hypoxic periods.[28]

These patients should be monitored for apnea and bradycardia, perioperatively and continuously for at least 24 hours postoperatively.[29] Treatment with caffeine or theophylline may be necessary to decrease the number of episodes of apnea. Patients taking theophyllin may be more likely to have arrythmias during halothane anesthesia. Since these patients depend on heart rate to maintain cardiac output, bradycardia must be avoided. Premedication with atropine is indicated.

Oxygen saturation should be monitored with a pulse oximeter or transcutaneous oxygen monitor and should be kept at 95 to 98 per cent for safety.

The usual anesthetic management principles for neonates apply. The child should be kept warm, and end-tidal carbon dioxide and fluids should be monitored closely. Preoperative evaluation of pulmonary function, heart function, and seizure control should be satisfactory before anesthesia begins.

G. RETINITIS PIGMENTOSA

Electroretinography (ERG) is a stimulated reflex response study performed to evaluate a patient for retinitis pigmentosa and visual function. When this test is performed in small children, the ophthalmologist may request general anesthesia to ensure their full cooperation. Although retinitis pigmentosa per se does not pose a problem for anesthetic care, the conditions of the test and the influence of anesthetics on the results are of interest.

These tests are performed in a dark, Faraday cage room with a flashing light source placed over the patient's face. The anesthesiologist may find himself or herself working in cramped quarters, without the usual operating room lighting or equipment readily handy and with a young, uncooperative patient whose face will be partially obscured by ophthalmologic equipment.

Anesthesia equipment must include a suctioning apparatus and an instant light source, if necessary. Monitoring equipment includes an automatic blood pressure cuff, an electrocardiograph, a pulse oximeter, and an end-tidal carbon dioxide capnogram. The patient should be intubated.

The choice of anesthetic agents is interesting. Although ERG is only a simple rod-cone reflex response study, anesthetic agents may affect both the amplitude and latency of the ERG responses, distorting the interpretation.

Although ketamine, a phencyclidine derivative, is known to cause nystagmus and increased electroencephalogram (EEG) activity, it is felt that it does not alter ERG responses significantly in rabbits.[30] Since vomiting, aspiration, and laryngospasm have been associated with ketamine, its use in ERG studies is dangerous unless the patient is intubated.

Isoflurane has been shown to decrease the amplitude and increase the latency of visual evoked potential in a dose-dependent fashion.[31, 32] Enflurane, which can produce seizurelike activity in the EEG, increases the amplitude of visual evoked potentials. Neuroleptanalgesia with fentanyl and droperidol had no effect on visual evoked potential amplitude but did increase latency.[32] No consistent influence of nitrous oxide on visual evoked potential has been demonstrated.[31]

Studies have not been done on the effects of volatile agents on ERG responses, but in general cortical evoked potentials are more sensitive to anesthetics than are subcortical evoked potentials, such as ERG responses.

H. EYE TRAUMA

Eye trauma requires some special anesthetic considerations. Such trauma may be penetrating or blunt. Open-eye injuries requiring surgical repair may vary from a small corneal leak to a totally disrupted globe and contents. Tissue damage may involve the cornea, iris, and lens, and the loss of vitreous gel, choroidal vessel hemorrhage, scleral laceration, and a detached retina.

The open-eye injury must be managed carefully to prevent sudden increases in intraocular pressure (IOP) that could damage further the eye by extrusion of vitreal contents.[33] Increased IOP can occur from active squeezing by extraocular muscles, direct external pressure (face mask), and increased venous pressure caused by coughing, straining, bucking, obstructive breathing, or Valsalva's maneuver. The IOP will also be increased by succinylcholine and endotracheal intubation (especially when it is difficult or prolonged).[34]

In general, sedatives, narcotics, nondepolarizing muscle relaxants, barbiturates, and volatile general anesthetics lower IOP.

Choroidal hemorrhage is more likely in open-eye situations when hypertension and increased venous pressure are also present.

Direct pressure on the eye from a face mask should be avoided. Rapid-sequence intubation is in order for a patient who has an open-eye injury and a full stomach. Succinylcholine increases IOP transiently. The mechanism is unclear. Preventing fasciculations by pretreating with a small dose of a nondepolarizing muscle relaxant can attenuate the IOP response to succinylcholine. This method has been used clinically without causing obvious eye damage.[35]

The increase in IOP after laryngoscopy and intubation may be attenuated by pretreatment with intravenous lidocaine, 1.5 mg/kg.[36] Pretreatment with clonidine,[37] beta-blockers, and high-dose short-acting narcotics[38] has also been shown to minimize this IOP response to intubation.

If a nondepolarizing muscle relaxant such as vecuronium, 0.15 mg/kg intravenously, is chosen for the intubation relaxant, at least 90 seconds must elapse and four monitors must indicate full relaxation before laryngoscopy and intubation are attempted.[39]

Intraoperative management suggests documented muscle paralysis to prevent bucking, controlled ventilation to prevent hypercarbia, and use of an antiemetic for postoperative emergence. Extubation of "full-stomach, open-eye cases" should be performed after nasogastric tube drainage of the stomach and with intravenous lidocaine and a narcotic to facilitate a smooth extubation with the patient awake.

III. EAR, NOSE, AND THROAT CONSIDERATIONS

A. PAPILLOMATOSIS

Laryngeal papillomatosis, a benign recurrent tumor of childhood, often presents as subtle hoarseness of unknown cause.[40] The extent of the lesions and airway obstruction vary from minimal to severe with stridor at rest. The papillomats are friable, bleed easily, and may become edematous.[41]

Treatment includes repeated surgical excision and laser coagulation. Tracheostomy is avoided whenever possible to prevent seeding of papillomas into the distal trachea.

Usually a slow, careful halothane induction by mask, maintaining spontaneous respiration, is adequate. The airway patency may worsen as the child loses consciousness. Instrumentation should be (1) gentle and (2) delayed until airway reflexes have been suppressed. Spontaneous breathing adds to the safety and also provides a dynamic larynx with motion, air bubbles, and breath sounds to help identify the correct placement for the small endotracheal tube.

When a small child has stridor rest, wake intubation may be indicated. Intubation with a rigid ventilating bronchoscope with the patient awake or asleep may also be useful. Muscle relaxants should be avoided unless airway management can be guaranteed. Since many of these cases are treated with carbon dioxide lasers, the usual precautions must be observed to avoid airway fires during laser surgery.[42, 43] This includes the use of a low FiO_2 (0.3 to 0.4) in nitrogen or helium, avoiding nitrous oxide (supports combustion),[44] using properly wrapped metal or special endotracheal tubes, and having the surgeon use the laser within safe power limits.[45]

These patients with pathologic conditions of the upper airway should be extubated when awake with airway reflexes intact. They should be given oxygen and close monitoring with a pulse oximeter and nurse observation in the postanesthesia care unit.

B. CYSTIC HYGROMA

Cystic hygroma is a benign, multilocular tumor of lymphatic origin occurring in young children. It usually involves the deep fascia of the neck, oral cavity, and tongue. As the tumor grows, it may cause symptoms from pressure on the trachea, pharynx, blood vessels, tongue, and nerves.[46] As the tumor fills the pharyngeal, retropharyngeal, and submandibular areas it severely compromises the airway.

Airway security is of the utmost importance. Often, a protruding, enlarged tongue makes oral intubation impossible. A marginally adequate airway while the patient is awake may become fully obstructed during a mask induction as muscles relax and the soft tissue tumor fills the airway. The safest approach in these children is nasal intubation,[47] either blind or with fiberoptic assistance, with the patient awake. Tracheostomy with the patient awake may be necessary, but it is difficult in a struggling child whose tumor involves the submandibular region.

C. WEGENER'S GRANULOMATOSIS

Wegener's granulomatosis is a disease of uncertain cause (hypersensitive, autoimmune) in which midline necrotizing granulomas and vasculitis lead to muscosal ulcerations of nose, palate, larynx, and orbit.[48] Symptoms include rhinorrhea, nasal pain, airway obstruction, and pulmonary congestion. Its three main features are necrotizing giant cell granulomata of the upper airway, generalized vasculitis, and glomerulonephritis.[49] In addition to upper airway, pulmonary, and renal problems, ocular complications are fairly common and include uveitis, vitreous hemorrhage, central retinal artery occlusion, and papilledema.[50]

Patients with Wegener's granulomatosis may present to surgery for nasal, laryngeal, or ocular problems early in the course of the disease. The anesthesiologist must be sensitive to the presence of underlying pulmonary or renal problems. Furthermore, unsuspected midline necrotizing granulomas of the airway may cause obstruction or bleeding at intubation. Therefore, careful preoperative attention to airway management and evaluation is necessary. Direct laryngoscopy and x-ray studies are useful. Some tracheal stenosis and bleeding should be expected. Pulmonary function may be limited; thus, end-tidal carbon dioxide, oxygen saturation, and lung compliance must be followed closely.

D. ACROMEGALY

Acromegaly is a rare chronic disease of midlife caused by oversecretion of adenohypophyseal growth hormone, causing enlargement of bone especially the hands, feet, face, mandible, and head—connective tissue, and viscera. An increase in subcutaneous connective tissue thickens the lips, skin folds, and tongue and often causes glossoptosis.

Associated problems include mild diabetes, hypertension, degenerative vascular disease, and heart disease.[52]

The status of the associated problems must be appreciated. The main concern for the anesthesiologist is difficult visualization of the glottic area resulting from a large tongue,

abundant soft tissue folds, and enlarged facial structures. A nasal fiberoptic approach may be indicated either with the patient awake or after mask induction.[53] During mask induction it may become more difficult to maintain an airway, as muscle and soft tissue relaxation cause further obstruction.

E. LUDWIG'S ANGINA

Any infection of the oral cavity can spread rapidly to cause significant cellulitis and edema of submandibular and sublingual areas, the floor of the mouth, and the anterior neck region.[54] The tongue may be pressed posteriorly against the pharyngeal wall and can cause stridulous airway obstruction, trismus, and dysphagia.[55, 56]

Tracheostomy with the patient awake and under local anesthesia is safe, but it may be difficult because of the location of infection. Visualization of the glottis via the oral route may be impossible because of trismus and sublingual swelling.[57] A nasal approach to intubation is more likely to succeed but must be done carefully to avoid bleeding and perforation of any abscess. Visual support (fiberoptics) is useful because of the distortion of normal airway anatomy. Patients should be allowed to find the best position (sitting up?) for easy breathing and handling secretions. For safety, a cricothyrotomy puncture or emergency tracheostomy set should be at hand during airway manipulation in these patients.

F. EPISTAXIS

Epistaxis is a symptom often associated with hypertension, nasal tumors, or bleeding dyscrasias. Patients with intractable, recurrent epistaxis may eventually present for surgical ligation of the internal maxillary artery and the anterior ethmoid artery.[58]

Patients with epistaxis who come to surgery must be considered to be hypovolemic and to have a full stomach (blood). Posterior nasal packing can cause edema, partial airway obstruction, and hypoventilation. These patients are frequently nervous, excitable, and hypertensive with increased catecholamine levels. They must be evaluated for bleeding dyscrasia. A well-functioning, large-gauge intravenous line is needed for good preinduction hydration and in the event of sudden blood loss when the packing is removed. Preoperative sedation should be given cautiously under observation, in consideration of fatigue and hypoventilation.

Precautions that would be taken for a patient with a full stomach are necessary at induction. A posterior pharyngeal pack should be placed. Before extubation, a nasogastric tube should be passed and removed to help empty the stomach. Extubation should occur when the patient is awake with protective airway reflexes intact.

G. COMPROMISED AIRWAYS

Airway management is the special expertise that anesthesiologists bring to the medical community; however, 14 per cent of deaths and brain damage associated with anesthesia involve failure to maintain oxygenation. This risk of airway obstruction and hypoxia is greater when a patient's condition has already compromised the airway to some degree.

Compromised airways can be associated with a wide variety of clinical situations, including congenital abnormalities, infection, tumor, benign masses, and trauma involving the head or neck area.[59, 60]

Congenital problems with craniofacial pathologic features, such as choanal atresia, tracheomalacia, cleft palate, and the Pierre Robin syndrome, the Treacher Collins syndrome, and the Hallermann-Streiff syndrome present special challenges for airway visualization and induction.[61]

Any infectious process of the head and neck area can compromise the airway because of edema, abscess, dysphagia, trismus, and pain.[62] The mucosal tissues and fascial spaces of these areas readily expand in response to infections of the tonsils, the epiglottis, the floor of the mouth, and the salivary glands. Abscesses that have formed in the floor of mouth (Ludwig's angina), retropharyngeal space,[55] or tonsils may need to be aspirated before laryngoscopy to lessen the risk of abscess rupture and pus spilling into an unprotected airway.

Airway tumors may be benign or malignant. Benign tumors such as supraglottic papillomas are friable and may become edematous. Subglottic lesions include the firm cricoid chondroma and intratracheal fibromas and angiomas. Supraglottic malignant tumors of the epiglottis or the pyriform fossa area may be friable and floppy and may narrow the airway to less than 4 mm and obliterate visualization of the glottic opening. Affected patients must be approached with careful evaluation and planning. Usually, a direct laryngoscopy with the patient awake will dictate the safest route to intubation (awake, asleep, nasal, fiberoptic, tracheostomy, spontaneous breathing, and so on). Irradiation for head and neck tumors can cause fibrotic trismus and considerable glottic edema.

Large neck tumors can cause extrinsic compression and a shift of the trachea. An enlarged goiter may in fact create a subglottic S curvature of the trachea that makes intubation difficult.

Direct trauma to the larynx can cause substantial damage and disarrangement of intralaryngeal structures without obvious external signs. Laryngeal injury should be suspected when an accident victim demonstrates unexplained vocal or airway dysfunction. Close examination of the neck may reveal hematoma, subcutaneous crepitus, a deviated trachea, or loss of cartilaginous prominences. If a laryngotracheal rupture is suspected, a direct tracheotomy under local anesthesia ensures patency of the airway, even though the vocal cords may not communicate with the lower trachea. Aspiration of foreign bodies into the trachea is a common cause of sudden unexplained wheezing, croup, and hoarseness in young children.[60, 63]

When dealing with known or suspected airway compromise, the best management decisions are based on thorough evaluation. A history of symptoms, a physical examination, direct laryngoscopy, and x-ray studies should help the anesthesiologist know what he or she is dealing with before a therapeutic commitment is made.

Most pathologic conditions of the upper airway can be classified according to size, location, and rigidity. Supraglottic lesions will present problems of actually visualizing the glottic airway, whereas with subglottic lesions, glottic visualization should not be a problem. A mobile soft tissue lesion is likely to cause increased obstruction as the patient is sedated or loses consciousness, whereas a rigid lesion (tracheal web, cricoid chondroma) will not.

Compromised airway situations in which glottic visualization will be a problem (trismus, abscess, supraglottic tumor, and so on) are a major concern, especially if airway patency may be lost during induction. Affected patients require examination and intubation or tracheostomy while awake.

Regardless of the cause of a compromised airway, basic safety guidelines apply.[64] Safe management options include intubation with the patient awake, either nasally or orally as indicated and with or without visual assistance (laryngoscope or fiberoptics) as is possible. This requires a careful topical laryngeal block and a cooperative patient. Narcotic sedation is preferred, since it can be reversed if necessary and calms the patient but does not put him or her to sleep or relax the muscles as benzodiazepines do. When indicated (e.g., a lesion that is not large, a fixed pathologic condition, visualization that is not too difficult, better patient cooperation needed, as with a child) a spontaneously breathing induction with a volatile anesthetic is useful. These inductions require patience (slower gas uptake with compromised breathing), attention to possible loss of airway patency during induction, and no laryngoscope insertion until the patient has no airway reflexes.

Instead of an endotracheal tube, a rigid ventilating bronchoscope may be passed with the patient awake or asleep.

No patient with a compromised airway should be allowed to become hypoxic during intubation. At the least, emergency cricothyrotomy can maintain oxygenation temporarily using flush oxygen flow from the anesthesia machine.[65]

H. SPECIAL SITUATIONS

Teflon Injection. It is sometimes necessary to inject Teflon into a paralyzed vocal cord to build up the cord and move it toward midline to increase the strength and quality of the voice and to prevent aspiration.[66] These procedures must be done under local anesthesia so that the patient can cooperate and the surgeon can determine the proper dose by listening to the patient vocalize. Thus, a solid topical laryngeal block is required to eliminate the gag reflex and allow placement of the endoscope. Careful sedation is achieved by titrating droperidol and fentanyl, 50:1 (Innovar) to 1 to 4 ml intravenously, or small amounts of fentanyl, 50 to 150 µg, and midazolam, 1 to 3 mg, until the patient is calm but aware and cooperative.

T-Tube Placement. Some patients with tracheolaryngeal stenosis have semipermanent T tubes placed to provide an optional airway through a tracheal stoma or via the oral cavity.[67] These polymeric silicone (Silastic) tubes are easily removed if necessary (simple pull), but they may be replaced by an endotracheal tube or standard tracheostomy tube through the stoma. If the T tube is to be left in place during anesthesia, the proximal limb may be sealed (to decrease oral leakage) by using a Fogarty catheter precisely placed and inflated. The extending limb of the T tube may be connected to an endotracheal tube connector and then to an anesthesia machine.

REFERENCES

General

1. Morris DA: Cataracts and systemic disease, Chap. 41. *In* Duane T (ed): Clinical Ophthalmology, Vol. 5. Philadelphia, Harper & Row, 1987.
2. Gellis SS, Feingold M: Oculocerebrorenal syndrome (Lowe's). Am J Dis Child 124:891, 1972.
3. LaPiana FG: Renal disease and ophthalmology, Chap. 31. *In* Duane T (ed): Clinical Ophthalmology, Vol 5. Philadelphia, Harper & Row, 1987, pp 3–4.
4. Ackerman AL: Retinal problems in systemic disease. *In* Duane T (ed): Clinical Ophthalmology, Vol. 5. Philadelphia, Harper & Row, 1987.
5. Ginsberg SP: Corneal problems in systemic disease, Chap. 43. *In* Duane T (ed): Clinical Ophthalmology, Vol 5. Philadelphia, Harper & Row, 1987.
6. McGoldrick KE: Congenital and metabolic diseases and ophthalmology. *In* McGoldrick KE, Bruce RA, Oppenheimer P (eds): Anesthesia for Ophthalmology. Birmingham, Aesculapius Press, 1982, pp 150–151.
7. Morrison JD, Mirakhur RK, Graig HJL: Anaesthesia for Eye, Ear, Nose, and Throat Surgery, 2nd ed. New York, Churchill Livingstone, 1985.

Marfan's Syndrome

8. Pyerity RE, McKusich VA: Marfan's syndrome: Diagnosis and management. N Engl J Med 300:772, 1979.

Graves' Disease

9. Schimek R: Surgical management of ocular complications of Graves' disease. Arch Ophthalmol 87:665, 1972.
10. Stehling LC: Anesthetic management of the patient with hyperthyroidism. Anesthesiology 41:585, 1972.
11. Kadis LB, Bennet EJ, Dalal FV, et al: Anesthetic management of thyrotoxicosis. Anesth Analg 45:145, 1966.

Incontinentia Pigmenti

12. Charney R: Incontinentia pigmenti: A world statistical analysis. Arch Dermatol 112:535, 1976.
13. Zelickson A: Incontinentia pigmenti. *In* Dennis D (ed): Clinical Dermatology, Vol 2. Hagerstown, Harper & Row, 1979.
14. Whitmore PV: Skin and mucous membrane disorders, Chap. 27. *In* Duane T (ed): Clinical Ophthalmology, Vol. 5. Philadelphia, Harper & Row, 1987.

Homocystinuria

15. Stanbury JB, Wyngaarden JB, Friedrickson DS: Metabolic Basis of Inherited Disorders, 4th ed. New York, McGraw-Hill, 1978, pp 458–503.
16. Brown BR, Walson PD, Taussig LM: Congenital metabolic disorders in pediatric patients: Anesthetic implications. Anesthesiology 43:197, 1975.
17. Crooke JW, Towers JF, Taylor WH: Management of patients with homocystinuria requiring general anesthesia. Br J Anaesth 43:96, 1971.
18. McGoldrick KE: Anesthetic management of homocystinuria. Anesth Rev 8(3):42, 1981.
19. France NK: Anesthesia for pediatric ENT. In Gregory GA (ed): Pediatric Anesthesia. New York, Churchill Livingstone, 1973, p 794.
20. Holmgren G, Falkner S, Hambreus L: Plasma insulin and glucose tolerance in homocystinuria. Ups J Med Sci 78:215, 1975.

Hemoglobin Diseases

21. Dean J, Schechter A: Sickle cell anemia: Molecular and cellular basis of therapeutic approaches. N Engl J Med 299:752, 1978.
22. Condon P, Sergent G: Ocular findings in homozygous sickle cell anemia in Jamaica. Am J Ophthalmol 73:533, 1972.
23. Janik J, Seeler RA: Perioperative management of children with sickle cell anemia. J Pediatr Surg 15:117, 1980.

Retinopathy of Prematurity

24. Patz A: Retrolental fibroplasia (review). Surv Ophthalmol 14:1, 1969.
25. Merritt JC, Sprague DH, Merritt WE: Retrolental fibroplasia: A multifactorial disease. Anesth Analg 60:109, 1981.
26. Lucey JF, Dangman B: A reexamination of the role of oxygen in retrolental fibroplasia. Pediatrics 73:82, 1984.
27. Brann AW, Cefalo RC: Guidelines for Perinatal Care. Evanston, IL, American Academy of Pediatrics and American College of Obstetrics and Gynecology, 1983, pp 202, 212–216.
28. McGoldrick KE: Complications associated with prematurity. Chap. 13. In McGoldrick KE, Bruce RA, Oppenheimer P (eds): Anesthesia for Ophthalmology. Birmingham, Aesculapius Press, 1982.
29. Liu LMP, Cote C, Goudsouzian NG: Life threatening apnea in infants following anesthesia. Anesthesiology 59:506, 1983.

Retinitis Pigmentosa

30. Savovets D: Ketamine: An effective general anesthetic for use in electroretinography. Ann Ophthalmol 10:1510, 1978.
31. Chi OZ, Field C: Effects of isoflurane on visual evoked potentials in humans. Anesthesiology 65:328, 1986.
32. Sebel PS, Ingram DA, Flynn PJ, et al: Evoked potentials during isoflurane anesthesia. Br J Anaesth 58:580, 1985.

Eye Trauma

33. Cunningham AJ, Barry P: IOP-physiology and implications for anesthetic management. Can Anaesth Soc J 33:195, 1986.

34. Donlon JV: Anesthesia for ophthalmology surgery, Chap. 7. In Barash PG (ed): ASA Refresher Course, Vol. 16. Philadelphia, JB Lippincott, 1988.
35. Libonati MM, Leahy JJ, Ellison N: The use of succinylcholine in open eye surgery. Anesthesiology 62:635, 1985.
36. Mahajan RP, Grover VK, Sharma SL, et al: Lidocaine pretreatment in modifying IOP increases. Can J Anaesth 34:41, 1987.
37. Ghignone M, Noe S, Calvillo O, et al: Effects of clonidine on IOP and perioperative hemodynamics. Anesthesiology 68:707, 1988.
38. Badrinath SK, Braverman B, Ivankovich AD: Alfentanil and sufentanil prevent the increase in IOP from succinylcholine (Abstract). Anaesth Analg 67:S5, 1988.
39. Abbott MA: High dose vecuronium to control IOP during the induction of anesthesia. Anesthesia 42:1008, 1987.

Papillomatosis

40. Szpunar J: Juvenile laryngeal papillomatosis. Otol Clin North Am 10:67, 1977.
41. Hawkins DB, Udall JN: Juvenile laryngeal papillomas with cardiomegaly and polycythemia. Pediatrics 63:156, 1979.
42. Hermens JM, Bennett MJ, Hirshman CA: Anesthesia for laser surgery. A review. Anesth Analg 62:218, 1983.
43. van der Spek A: The physics of lasers and their use during airway surgery. Br J Anaesth 60:720, 1988.
44. Pashayan AG, Gravenstein N: Use of nitrous oxide and laser surgery of upper airway (letter). Anesth Analg 67:488, 1988.
45. Weisberger EC, Miner JD: Apneic anesthesia for endoscopic removal of laryngeal papillomata. Laryngoscope 98:693, 1988.

Cystic Hygroma

46. MacDonal DJ: Cystic hygroma. Anesthesia 21:66, 1966.
47. Weller RM: Anesthesia for cystic hygroma in a neonate. Anesthesia 29:588, 1974.

Wegener's Granulomatosis

48. Fauci AS, Haynes BF, Katz P, et al: Wegener's granulomatosis: Clinical and therapeutic experience. Ann Intern Med 98:76, 1983.
49. Olf S, Fauci AS, Horn R, et al: Wegener's granulomatosis. Ann Intern Med 81:513, 1974.
50. Straatsma BR: Ocular manifestations of Wegener's granulomatosis. Am J Ophthalmol 44:789, 1957.

Acromegaly

51. Melmed S, Braunstein GD, Horvath E, et al: Pathophysiology of acromegaly. Endocrinol Rev 4:271, 1983.
52. Jadresic A: Recent developments in acromegaly. A review. J R Soc Med 76:947, 1983.
53. Ovassapian A, Doka JC, Romsa DE: Acromegaly—uses of fiberoptic laryngoscopy to avoid tracheostomy. Anesthesiology 54:529, 1981.

Ludwig's Angina

54. Hirschmann JV: Localized infections and abscesses, In Braunwald E, et al. (eds): Principles of Internal

Medicine, 11th ed. New York, McGraw-Hill, 1987, p 481.

55. Koopmann CF, Coulthard SW: Retropharyngeal abscess. Laryngoscope 94:455, 1984.

56. Khilanani V, Khatib R: Acute epiglottis in adults. Am J Med Sci 287:65, 1984.

57. Baxter A, Dunne J: Acute adult epiglottis. Can J Anaesth 35:428, 1988.

Epistaxis

58. Rosnagle RS: Epistaxis. A review, Chap. 25. *In* English GM (ed): Otolaryngology, Vol. 2. Philadelphia, JB Lippincott, 1988.

Compromised Airways

59. Donlon JV: Anesthesia for eye and ENT surgery. *In* Miller R (ed): Anesthesia, 2nd ed, Vol. 3. New York, Churchill Livingstone, 1983.

60. Lopez NR: Mechanical problems of the airway. Clin Anaesth 3:8, 1968.

61. Cotton R, Reilly JS: Congenital malformations of the larynx. *In* Bluestone CD, Stool SE (eds): Pediatric Otolaryngology, Vol. 2. Philadelphia, WB Saunders, 1983.

62. Maze A, Block E: Stridor in pediatric patients. Anesthesiology 50:132, 1979.

63. Wilson RD, Putnam L, Phillips MT, et al: Anesthetic problems in surgery for respiratory obstruction in children. Anesth Analg 53:878, 1974.

64. Donlon JV: Anesthetic management of patients with compromised airways. Anesth Rev 7:22, 1980.

65. Thomas TC, Zornow MH, Scheller MS, et al: Efficacy of percutaneous trans-tracheal ventilation (Abstract). Can J Anaesth 35:S61, 1988.

Special Situations

66. Levine H: Surgical management of voice disorders. Teflon injection of vocal cords. In English GM (ed): Otolaryngology, Vol. 3. Philadelphia, JB Lippincott, 1988, pp 12–14.

67. Montgomery WM: Silicone tracheal cannula. Ann Otol Rhinol Laryngol 89:521, 1980.

CHAPTER 3

Respiratory Diseases

John P. McCarren

I. INTRODUCTION

This chapter discusses a number of uncommon respiratory diseases that could be encountered by every practicing anesthesiologist during the course of a career in anesthesia. Each section describes the salient features of the respiratory disease and concludes with a brief discussion of the anesthetic considerations.

Preoperative evaluation of patients with respiratory diseases serves to identify those at greater risk for intraoperative and postoperative complications and to help the anesthesiologist manage the patient's perioperative care and avoid complications. In the role of consultant, the anesthesiologist may even recommend deferring surgery until the patient is better evaluated or prepared for surgery. This chapter discusses a number of interventions outside the traditional scope of an anesthesiologist's practice that could be recommended to better prepare the patient for surgery: nutritional support, corticosteroid therapy, and a course of antibiotics are but a few of the medical interventions recommended.

Most patients with significant respiratory dysfunction can benefit from preoperative pulmonary evaluation. At minimum, testing should include simple spirometry, arterial blood gases, and chest radiography. The findings from these tests enable the anesthesiologist optimally to manage the perioperative care of these patients. Specific interventions may include chest physiotherapy, instruction in the use of an incentive spirometer, hydration, bronchodilator treatment, smoking cessation, and intensive perioperative monitoring of respiratory status.

The anesthesiologist can assist the intensivist with the postoperative care of patients by making simple physiologic respiratory measurements and calculations intraoperatively: Estimates of the degree of shunting or ventilation-perfusion mismatch [$P_{(A-a)}O_2$ gradients, P_aO_2/P_AO_2 ratios], wasted ventilation or alveolar dead space

$$\frac{VD}{VT} = \frac{P_aCO_2 - P_eCO_2}{P_aCO_2},$$

and lung compliance (leak inspiratory pressures at specified tidal volumes) are easily measured and calculated. If right heart catheterization is performed, the relevant findings should be clearly communicated to the physician who cares for the patient postoperatively.

II. DISEASES THAT AFFECT THE PULMONARY CIRCULATION

A. PULMONARY ARTERIOVENOUS FISTULAS

Pulmonary arteriovenous fistulas are abnormal communications between the pulmonary arteries and the pulmonary veins that bypass the pulmonary capillaries and, as a consequence, do not participate in gas exchange. This creates an intrapulmonary shunt that decreases P_aO_2. Raising the F_iO_2 may not significantly improve arterial oxygenation; furthermore, any increase in the overall pulmonary vascular resistance may increase flow through the low-resistance arteriovenous fistula and result in a higher shunt fraction and lower P_aO_2. Secondary polycythemia often results from the chronic hypoxemia caused by the shunt. Congenital arteriovenous fistulas may be associated with hereditary hemorrhagic telangiectasia (Rendu-Osler-Weber) and acquired fistulas with trauma, hepatic cirrhosis, or schistosomiasis.

Grossly, the fistulas appear as thin-walled sacs. The congenital fistulas typically are located adjacent to the visceral pleura of the lower lobes of the lung. Rupture of these thin-walled fistulas into the bronchi or the pleura causes hemoptysis or hemothorax, respectively. Thrombotic material may develop within these sacs and embolize to the central nervous system (CNS) and cause seizures or strokes. Septic emboli can lead to brain abscesses.

1. Anesthetic Considerations

Issues related to gas exchange and systemic emboli are the principal concerns of the anesthesiologist. Maneuvers that reduce the flow through the fistula tend to improve oxygenation. These maneuvers are analogous to those employed during one-lung ventilation. Positioning the patient with the fistula in a nondependent position reduces blood flow through the fistula. Similarly, nongravitational factors that tend to increase pulmonary vascular resistance, such as hypoxia, hypercarbia, acidosis, hypothermia, and lung hyperinflation, should be avoided. Positive end-expiratory pressure (PEEP) may redistribute some blood flow from the normal areas of the lung to the fistula and thus increase the shunt fraction.

Arteriovenous fistulas are right-to-left shunts that lack the filtering capacity of the normal pulmonary vasculature. Consequently, any particulate matter or air introduced into the venous circulation can "paradoxically" embolize into the systemic circulation and possibly cause stroke or myocardial infarction. The anesthesiologist should scrupulously eliminate all air in intravenous infusion lines, side ports, and stopcocks.

Resection of the pulmonary fistulas may result in much blood loss; therefore, adequate intravenous access for rapid blood infusions should be secured. Blood-salvaging techniques should also be considered. A double-lumen endotracheal tube (ETT) should also be considered, which can improve surgical exposure and protect the dependent lumen from possible endobronchial bleeding.

B. WEGENER'S GRANULOMATOSIS

Wegener's granulomatosis (WG) is a systemic necrotizing granulomatous vasculitis that predominantly affects the upper and lower respiratory tract and the kidneys and less commonly the eyes, skin, and musculoskeletal, nervous, cardiac, gastrointestinal, and genitourinary systems. One study revealed the following prevalences of abnormal bronchoscopic findings in patients with WG: endobronchial lesions, 59 per cent; subglottic stenosis, 17 per cent; ulcerating tracheobronchitis, 60 per cent; tracheal or bronchial stenosis, 13 per cent; and hemorrhage, 4 per cent.[1] Glomerulonephritis is the sine qua non of generalized WG. Renal involvement may result in nephrotic syndrome or systemic hypertension. Common clinical manifestations include rhinorrhea with nasal ulceration, sinusitis, and otitis media. Fever, malaise, and anorexia are common constitutional symptoms. Cardiac manifestations occur in about 20 per cent of patients with WG and include pericarditis, cardiomyopathy, pancarditis, and coronary arteritis. Neurologic manifestations include cranial neuropathies, cerebral hemorrhage, cerebritis, seizures, and peripheral neuropathies. Nonspecific disease markers for WG include antineutrophil cytoplasmic antibody (c-ANCA) and antibodies against a serine protease found in neutrophils (PR-3).[2] Chest films often show infiltrates, nodules, cavities, interstitial changes, and pleural effusions.[3]

Treatment with corticosteroids and cyclophosphamide has changed WG from an invariably fatal disease (1-year survival rate only 20 per cent) to one with 90 per cent partial remissions and 75 per cent complete remissions and an overall mortality rate of 13 per cent.[4]

1. Anesthetic Considerations

In general, nasotracheal intubation should be avoided in patients with sinusitis, nasal ulceration, a perforated septum, or saddle nose deformities. If subglottic stenosis is suspected, the diagnosis can be confirmed by bronchoscopy or by radiographic studies, and the functional limitation assessed by pulmonary function studies (flow-volume loops). In cases of severe subglottic stenosis, a smaller-caliber ETT may be required. Ophthalmologic consultation should be sought for any eye involvement (e.g., corneal ulceration, conjunctivitis, scleritis, uveitis, retinal vasculitis, and obstruction of the nasolacrimal ducts).

Stress doses of corticosteroids are recommended for patients treated with steroids within the preceding year. The selection and dosages of other medications may need to be adjusted if renal insufficiency is present.

C. LYMPHOMATOID GRANULOMATOSIS

Lymphomatoid granulomatosis (LG) is a necrotizing granulomatous angiitis that affects predominantly the lungs. The blood vessels are infiltrated with atypical lymphoid and plasmacytoid cells that form a granuloma. The vessels in lung, skin, kidneys, and central nervous system are most commonly affected. LG presents during the fourth or fifth decade of life with complaints of fever, cough, weight loss, dyspnea, and chest pains. Patients occasionally present with hepatosplenomegaly and lymphadenopathy. Cavitary lung lesions, nodular densities, and alveolar infiltrates may be seen on chest radiographs. A focal vasculitis occasionally occurs in the skin and kidneys, but, unlike in WG, glomerulonephritis is not a feature of this disease. CNS involvement occurs rarely and is associated with multiple cranial nerve palsies. Diabetes insipidus also has been reported in LG. Endocrine disorders associated with LG include hypoadrenalism, hypercalcemia, hypothyroidism, and hypogonadism.[5]

Benign variants of LG have an excellent long-term prognosis, but the disease in some patients undergoes malignant transformation into an atypical disseminated histiocytic lymphoma or an angiocentric immunoproliferative disorder; both have a poor prognosis. Although chemotherapeutic protocols vary, drug regimens often include cyclophosphamide, vincristine, and prednisone.

1. Anesthetic Considerations

Preoperative pulmonary function studies and arterial blood gases help to assess the severity of the lung disease. Ventilator management must be individualized.

The potential neurologic disorders and endocrine dysfunction are varied. The anesthesiologist should carefully review the patient's laboratory studies and perform a neurologic examination. Specific intravenous precautions are dictated by any neurologic deficit or endocrine dysfunction. The patient should be evaluated for potential complications of chemotherapy: myelosuppression from cyclophosphamide, peripheral neuropathy from vincristine, and adrenal suppression from corticosteroid therapy.

D. CHURG-STRAUSS SYNDROME

Churg-Strauss syndrome is an allergic granulomatosis and angiitis that is almost invariably associated with allergic rhinitis and asthma. Respiratory system involvement may also include nasal polyps, transient pulmonary infiltrates, and pleural effusions. Although the upper and lower airways are the predominant sites of involvement, practically any organ system can be involved. Cardiovascular involvement sometimes presents with pericarditis, endocarditis, coronary vasculitis and myocardial infarctions, myocarditis, and congestive heart failure. In fact, before steroid therapy, the leading cause of death from Churg-Strauss syndrome was heart disease. Renal manifestations occasionally include renal arteritis and glomerulonephritis, which, in turn, may lead to systemic hypertension. One study reported neurologic system involvement in 62 per cent of patients with Churg-Strauss syndrome.[7] Lesions included

peripheral neuropathies, cerebral infarcts, radiculopathies, bilateral trigeminal neuropathy, and ischemic optic neuropathy.

1. Anesthetic Considerations

The medical management of asthma should be optimized before elective surgery. Preoperative cardiac, renal, and neurologic evaluations should be individualized and guided by the patient's history and physical examination findings. Large nasal polyps and nasal mucosal edema can obstruct the nasal passages and make nasal intubations impossible.

Patchy pneumonitis reduces lung compliance in some lung segments and creates areas of low ventilation-perfusion ratios. Positive-pressure ventilation in patients with patchy pneumonitis tends to increase alveolar distention in the more compliant alveoli and to magnify the gas exchange problems caused by asthma. Consequently, when appropriate, intubation of the trachea and positive-pressure ventilation should be avoided in favor of regional or mask anesthesia. If positive-pressure ventilation is needed, then it should be adjusted to avoid alveolar overdistention. Longer expiratory times or a pressure-control mode of ventilation may help to limit alveolar overdistention. Corticosteroid coverage should be considered for patients at risk of adrenal suppression from steroid therapy.

III. OBSTRUCTIVE DISEASE

A. CYSTIC FIBROSIS

Cystic fibrosis (CF) is a lethal genetic disease that is transmitted in an autosomal-recessive pattern. It occurs with a frequency of about 1 in 2000 in Whites; in other races it is uncommon. The genetic defect is a mutation on chromosome 7 that codes for a protein involved in chloride transport at epithelial cell surfaces.[8, 9] Altered chloride transport reduces the normal transluminal potential differences and osmotic gradients.[10] This lowers the water content of secretions. As a consequence, the mucus is more viscous and the mucociliary apparatus is impaired. The majority of patients affected by CF survive into adulthood.[11]

CF is a multisystem disease, but the major clinical features that affect anesthesia involve the respiratory and gastrointestinal systems.

Chronic sinusitis and nasal polyps occur in the majority of adults with CF, and patients frequently need to undergo otolaryngologic procedures such as nasal polypectomy and antrostomy. The lungs of CF patients are normal at birth, but early in life viscid secretions begin to obstruct the small airways. Mucus plugging causes micro- and macroatelectasis, impedes ciliary clearance, and predisposes to bacterial colonization and infection. This, in turn, often leads to bronchiectasis and airway hyperreactivity. Ventilation-perfusion abnormalities ensue, gas exchange deteriorates, and chronic hypoxemia occurs. Right ventricular failure complicates chronic hypoxemia in some patients. The onset of arterial carbon dioxide retention signals ventilatory failure. Airway hyperreactivity is common and contributes to lung hyperinflation and abnormal gas exchange. Alveolar overdistention may result in alveolar rupture and pneumothorax or pneumomediastinum. Bronchiectasis and chronic infection inflame the airways and cause many minor episodes of hemoptysis and, rarely, major ones.

Pancreatic exocrine dysfunction causes malabsorption, steatorrhea, and, if untreated, malnutrition. Severe malnutrition compromises wound healing and impairs coagulation. Pancreatic endocrine dysfunction affects insulin secretion and often leads to glucose intolerance, but, unlike type I diabetes, not to ketosis. Oral hypoglycemic drugs are ineffective, and insulin is required to control hyperglycemia. CF patients are at increased risk of gastroesophageal reflux and constipation. Gastroesophageal reflux occurs in as many as 26 per cent of children[12] and in 12 per cent of adults. Intermittent small bowel obstruction occurs in 20 per cent of patients and causes constipation. Opioids can exacerbate this problem and thus create a serious complication.[13]

1. Anesthetic Considerations

Retained secretions and recurrent respiratory infections cause the respiratory status of patients with CF to change dramatically over relatively short periods of time, even over the course of a day. Adult patients are very knowledgeable about their disease, and they often know at what time of day their respiratory function is optimal. Surgery should be scheduled at that time, whenever possible. At times, it may be prudent to delay surgery until the respiratory therapist has an opportunity to mobilize the patient's retained secretions with chest physical therapy and mucolytic agents. Improved pulmonary toilet lowers airway resistance and the risk of postoperative pneumonia.

Sedative-hypnotic and opioid premedications should be used sparingly in patients with respiratory insufficiency. Treated patients should receive supplemental oxygen, and they should not be left unattended. Premedication with a H_2-histamine receptor antagonist and a nonparticulate antacid is recommended because of the high incidence of gastroesophageal reflux. A recent chest film could reveal asymptomatic pneumothorax, atelectasis, pulmonary bullas or blebs, or signs of occult pneumonia, findings that would affect anesthesia management, and should be reviewed by the anesthesiologist preoperatively.

Local and regional anesthesias minimize the risks of aspiration, bronchospasm, and barotrauma and are preferred whenever they are acceptable to the patient and suitable for the operation. Local and regional anesthetics may reduce the need for opioid analgesia and the associated risk of postoperative constipation.

General anesthesia occasionally presents a number of challenges for the anesthesiologist. Difficulty with intravenous access may require inhalation induction, but if the patient has a small tidal volume and an increased functional residual capacity (FRC) induction will be slowed. Gas trapping, bullas, and the risk of pneumothorax make the use of nitrous oxide imprudent in patients with severe CF. The potential risk of aspiration in patients with gastroesophageal reflux needs to be balanced against the risk of bronchospasm that may occur whenever the airway is instrumented before an adequate depth of anesthesia is achieved. Neither spontaneous ventilation nor controlled ventilation is ideal. Prolonged spontaneous ventilation may fatigue the respiratory muscles of patients with severe disease, whereas controlled ventilation may cause excessive alveolar distention and increase the danger of pneumothorax. In general, controlled ventilation is the technique of choice. Careful management of airway pressure, adequate expiratory time, humidification of inspired gases, and good pulmonary toilet help to reduce the risks of controlled ventilation.

IV. INFILTRATIVE AND INTERSTITIAL DISEASES

A. IDIOPATHIC PULMONARY HEMOSIDEROSIS

Idiopathic pulmonary hemosiderosis (IPH) is an interstitial lung disease of unknown cause and pathogenesis that affects children primarily and, less commonly, young adults. Repeated episodes of pulmonary hemorrhage can lead to interstitial fibrosis and cause iron deficiency anemia. Immune mechanisms do not seem to be involved in the pathogenesis of this disorder. Similarly, there is no apparent association between IPH and a bleeding disorder or a vasculitis. Specifically, there is no evidence to suggest a coagulopathy or platelet disorder. Histologic findings are nonspecific. Patients typically present with acute dyspnea, fever, and episodic bouts of hemoptysis. Intrapulmonary bleeding may remain clinically silent and slowly lead to iron deficiency anemia. Occasionally, massive pulmonary hemorrhage results in asphyxia and death. Pulmonary function studies show a restrictive pattern. The carbon monoxide diffusion capacity (D_LCO) is elevated following active pulmonary bleeding because the test gas is avidly taken up by the intraalveolar hemoglobin. Chest films are normal early in the course of this disease. During episodes of acute pulmonary hemorrhage, serial chest films may show transient perihilar and basilar infiltrates with a mottled appearance. A fine reticular or netlike pattern can be seen in the bases of the lungs when interstitial fibrosis is present.

1. Anesthetic Considerations

Patients should be evaluated for iron deficiency anemia. Because of the insidious onset of anemia, many patients are well-compensated and do not require blood transfusion preoperatively. However, these patients have reduced oxygen-carrying capacity and also may have abnormal gas exchange in their lungs and be unable to tolerate significant hemodynamic trespass. Platelets and clotting factors do not play a pathogenic role in pulmonary hemorrhage, and, consequently, prophylactic transfusion of platelets or clotting factors is never indicated.

Massive pulmonary hemorrhage is a life-threatening event that may require tracheal intubation and ventilator support. Because of the diffuse nature of the hemorrhage, attempts to isolate the bleeding segment of the lung with double-lumen ETTs and bronchial blockers are usually ineffective. A larger-sized single-lumen ETT enables the anesthesiologist to provide optimal pulmonary toilet (suctioning, lavage, and bronchoscopy).

B. PRIMARY PULMONARY HISTIOCYTOSIS X

Primary pulmonary histiocytosis X (HX) is one of a group of benign diseases with overlapping clinical presentations that are characterized by *Langerhans' cell histiocyte* proliferation. Other presentations include eosinophilic granuloma, Letterer-Siwe, and Hand-Schüller-Christian disease. HX, as the X suggests, is a disease of unknown cause that predominantly affects young adults. Cigarette smoking is the major risk factor. The most common presenting symptoms are nonproductive cough, dyspnea, and chest pain. Approximately 10 to 20 per cent of patients with HX develop diabetes insipidus, pneumothorax, or eosinophilic granuloma of bone. Pulmonary function studies may be normal but often show a restrictive, obstructive, or mixed pattern. Chest films may initially show a nodular or reticulonodular pattern but can progress to a cystic or honeycombed appearance.

1. Anesthetic Considerations

Most patients with HX present no special anesthetic considerations. Those with severe cystic and bullous changes in the lungs are at risk of developing pneumothorax from air trapping during positive-pressure ventilation. Consequently, for high-risk patients, preoperative planning should include appropriate preparations for treating pneumothorax and airway pressures should be carefully monitored intraoperatively. Longer expiratory times help to prevent hyperinflation of the lungs and the higher airway pressures that result from decreased lung compliance.

Diabetes insipidus, a deficiency of antidiuretic hormone (ADH), causes dilute polyuria that may result in urine output of up to 15 L a day. If urine losses are not adequately replaced preoperatively, the patient becomes hypovolemic and develops hypernatremia and hyperosmolality. Preoperative fluid restriction should be avoided in these patients, and access to intravenous fluids should be provided if NPO status is rigorously enforced. Fluid balance can be maintained intraoperatively with intravenous fluids alone, but intravenous desmopressin is commercially available. Desmopressin therapy is usually continued until the day of surgery and then resumed postoperatively.

C. CHRONIC EOSINOPHILIC PNEUMONIA

Chronic eosinophilic pneumonia (CEP), as the name suggests, is a chronic inflammatory pneumonia consisting largely of an eosinophilic infiltration of the pulmonary interstitium. Unlike other eosinophilic pneumonias in which a parasitic infestation or drug reaction is the cause, the cause of CEP remains unknown. Patients with CEP typically present with high fevers, sweats, and severe dyspnea. The classic chest radiograph of CEP shows dense peripheral infiltrates with relatively clear hila and midlung fields. This radiographic picture has been called the "photographic negative" of cardiogenic pulmonary edema. Common laboratory findings include a high erythrocyte sedimentation rate and an elevated IgE level. Corticosteroid therapy results in a dramatic clinical and radiographic improvement within a few days.

1. Anesthetic Considerations

Elective surgery should be postponed until the patient is well. Unlike patients with bacterial or viral pneumonia, who require several weeks of therapy before they recover, patients with CEP are often dramatically better within only a few days of corticosteroid therapy. Patients undergoing emergent surgery manifest the same physiologic disturbances as patients with other pneumonia: areas of ventilation-perfusion mismatch, abnormal gas exchange, decreased lung compliance, and higher metabolic rates secondary to fevers. When patients must undergo surgery before resolution of their pneumonia, the anesthesiologist should ensure adequate preoxygenation before induction of anesthesia, avoid positioning the areas of high ventilation-perfusion mismatch dependent, and optimize airway pressures.

Because of the inhomogeneity of pulmonary infiltrates, the use of PEEP to improve oxygenation may adversely affect lung perfusion and cause unintended deleterious effects.

D. LYMPHANGIO-LEIOMYOMATOSIS

Lymphangioleiomyomatosis (LAM) is a disease of unknown cause that occurs almost exclusively in women of childbearing age and is exacerbated by pregnancy.[1] It is characterized by a hamartomatous proliferation of smooth muscle within the alveolar walls, pleura, and lymph nodes. LAM is also associated with pleural thickening, tumors of the thoracic duct and lymph nodes, and large, thick-walled cystic cavities in the lung.[2] Three major clinical manifestations seen in LAM are due to obstruction of lymph channels: chylothorax, recurrent pneumothorax, and hemoptysis.[14] Chyle is bacteriostatic and nonirritating to the pleural surfaces. Consequently, fever, superinfections, formation of pleural peels, and pleuritic chest pain are uncommon with LAM. Pulmonary function studies show a combined obstructive and restrictive pattern. Lung volumes are characteristically increased because of the cystic changes and large blebs, but a large chylothorax can compress the lungs and acutely reduce lung volumes. Expiratory flow rates are reduced. Hypoxemia is common and is worsened by exertion. Chest films may show a fine, reticulonodular pattern, large cysts or blebs, and a honeycombed appearance, but, in contrast to other interstitial diseases, the lungs are hyperinflated. Progestational medication or surgical hormonal manipulations may induce a remission.

1. Anesthetic Considerations

Malnutrition and immunocompromise are major threats to the young women who must undergo repeated thoracocentesis for drainage of chylothoraces. Substantial amounts of protein, fats, electrolytes, and lymphocytes are contained in chyle and are lost from the body following chest drainage. Malnutrition adversely affects wound healing and virtually all components of the immune system. Malnutrition adversely affects energy stores, visceral proteins synthesis, myocardial function, and muscle strength and endurance. Preoperative hyperalimentation can improve the patient's nutritional status and should be considered prior to any major surgical intervention.

Large chylothoraces compress the lungs and cause atelectasis and ventilation-perfusion mismatches, and result in abnormal gas exchange. Preoperative thoracocentesis can improve ventilation-perfusion matching; however, immediately following thoracocentesis—and for several hours thereafter—the perfusion of the atelectatic segments increases more than the ventilation improves and the ventilation-perfusion mismatch is greater. In addition, an iatrogenic pneumothorax may not be radiographically apparent for several hours after thoracocentesis. For both of these reasons, the author recommends that preoperative thoracocentesis be performed at least several hours before the scheduled surgery time and that a chest film be obtained and reviewed just before surgery. Drugs that reduce hypoxic pulmonary vasoconstriction, such as nitroprusside, nitroglycerin, B$_2$-agonist, nitric oxide, and nimodipine, may worsen gas exchange and lower arterial oxygenation.[15]

LAM is a mixed obstructive and restrictive lung disorder, and the goals of ventilator management must be individualized. In general, the obstructive component dictates ventilator management (e.g., longer expiratory times and lower peak airway pressures) to minimize gas trapping and risk of pneumothorax. These recommendations need to be modified for patients with significant restrictive physiology.

E. PULMONARY ALVEOLAR PROTEINOSIS

Pulmonary alveolar proteinosis (PAP), a disorder of unknown cause, is characterized by the abnormal accumulation in the alveoli of an amorphous lipoproteinaceous material with a chemical composition similar to that of surfactant. It is hypothesized that the accumulation of this surfactant-like material may be caused either by an imbalance of surfactant homeostasis or by excessive proliferation and desquamation of the surfactant, producing type II pneumocyte into the alveoli. Inert dusts, toxins, immune factors, infectious agents, and genetic factors have been implicated in the pathogenesis of this disease. PAP has a peak incidence in middle-aged adults but occurs in all age groups; the male-female ratio is 3:1.

PAP typically has an insidious onset and presents with a mild cough and slowly progressive dyspnea. Occasionally, some patients develop chest pain, weight loss, and fever. The physical findings are essentially normal, and laboratory findings are nonspecific. Pulmonary function studies reveal a restrictive pattern with decreases in lung volumes, static lung compliance, and diffusing capacity. Chest films may show an alveolar filling pattern that mimics cardiogenic pulmonary edema.

PAP predisposes patients to superinfections with a variety of organisms; those most commonly associated with PAP are *Nocardia asteroides, Mycobacterium tuberculosis,* and *Mycobacterium avium–intracellulare.*

PAP resolves spontaneously in approximately 30 per cent of the patients. Expectant management is appropriate for the asymptomatic patient, but the symptomatic patient often requires pulmonary lavage.

1. Anesthetic Considerations[16]

Pulmonary lavage for PAP entails serially irrigating each lung with normal saline until the effluent is clear. The most severely affected lung, as assessed radiographically or by lung scan, is lavaged first. A rest period of 3 to 7 days between each lavage is customary and provides an opportunity for the lavaged lung to stabilize. The single-lung lavage is performed under general anesthesia with neuromuscular blockade using a left-sided double-lumen ETT. An arterial line is used to monitor the patient and for blood gas sampling. The patient is usually placed in the supine position. At least 20 L of normal saline should be warmed to body temperature before the procedure.

The risk of hypoxemia during induction of anesthesia is increased in these patients because of their decreased FRC, increased intrapulmonary shunt, and because extra time is often required to place a double-lumen ETT. Clearly, preoxygenation is very important and helps to minimize this risk. A left-sided double-lumen ETT is recommended for lavage of either the left or the right lung. The left-sided ETT is chosen for lavage of both lungs for two reasons. First, the left-sided ETT has a larger bronchial cuff than a right-sided ETT and therefore provides a better seal. Second, there is less chance of dislodging a left-sided ETT because the bronchus is longer on the left. Placement of the ETT should be confirmed by bronchoscopic examination of the ETT position, and the bronchial seal should be tested for leaks. This is done by submerging in water a catheter inserted into one side of the ETT while pressurizing the contralateral side to 50 cm H_2O. (Irrigation of the lung is performed using an instillation pressure of 30 cm H_2O; therefore, a 50-cm seal provides a margin of safety.)

An arterial line is placed, and a baseline arterial blood gas measurement is obtained on 100 per cent oxygen with single-lung ventilation. Warmed normal saline is infused by gravity from a surface height of 30 cm above the lung until the lung is filled (about 500 to 1000 mL) and then is drained through a Y connector to a collection bottle positioned 20 cm below the lung. Bubbles in the effluent, rales in the ventilated lung, or a significant disparity between the volumes of fluid infused and drained suggests a leak and demands rechecking the position and integrity of the bronchial cuff. Immediately following each drainage of lavage fluid, only partial reexpansion of the obstructed alveoli and the greatly improved perfusion of the poorly ventilated lavaged lung acutely exacerbate ventilation-perfusion mismatch and cause the arterial saturation to fall. Arterial saturation improves during each lung lavage fluid instillation phase because perfusion to the fluid-filled lung once again decreases. The desaturation is magnified if the patient is positioned with the lavaged lung dependent, because perfusion in the dependent lung is increased. Eventually, after the final lavage fluid drainage, alveolar stability returns and gas exchange improves. (Cardiopulmonary bypass or extracorporeal membrane oxygenation [ECMO] may be required for severely hypoxemic patients.)

Large volumes of irrigation fluid can cause hypothermia; consequently, body temperature should be closely monitored. Temperature measured in the esophagus may more accurately reflect the temperature of the irrigation solution than of the patient. The patient's temperature is best measured in the nasopharynx, tympanic membrane, or blood.

Following the procedure, the lungs are suctioned and ventilator support is continued until lung function recovers. The return of lung function is signaled by a return of lung compliance toward or above baseline and acceptable arterial saturation. Incentive spirometry is used to encourage deep inspiration, to reexpand the lungs, and to prevent atelectasis.

F. GOODPASTURE'S SYNDROME

Goodpasture's syndrome is an autoimmune disease of unknown pathogenesis. Recent experimental work indicates that the principal antigen is on the alpha-3 chain of type IV basement membrane collagen.[17, 18] It occurs predominantly in young adults and commonly presents with diffuse pulmonary hemorrhage and rapidly progressive glomerulonephritis. Untreated, the disease can lead rapidly to renal failure and to fatal hemoptysis. Antibodies directed against alveolar basement membranes (anti-ABM) and against glomerular basement membranes (anti-GBM) are found in the serum of these patients, but levels do not correlate with the severity of the disease. Epidemiologic studies suggest that lung injury from cigarette smoking, infection, and chemicals may expose antigens in the lung and initiate antibody production in susceptible individuals.[19] There is also the suggestion that subsequent lung damage may potentiate the disease. Pulmonary function studies show a restrictive pattern; the diffusing capacity increases during active bleeding owing to uptake of carbon monoxide by alveolar hemoglobin.[20] Blood loss from hemoptysis or hematuria may lead to a hypochromic, microcytic iron deficiency anemia.

Treatments are directed at reducing the circulating titer of anti-GBM antibodies and at suppressing antibody production. Plasmapheresis, large doses of corticosteroids, and cyclophosphamide are accepted therapies.

1. Anesthetic Considerations

Elective surgery should not be performed until the disease is quiescent. The preoperative evaluation should be tailored to the severity of the patient's disease. Pulmonary status can be assessed with chest radiographs, pulmonary function studies including carbon monoxide diffusing capacity, and arterial blood gases; renal status is evaluated by renal function studies, urinalysis, and blood chemistries. When hemoptysis is present and tracheal intubation is required, a larger than usual sized endotracheal tube may help provide better pulmonary toilet. Because of the theoretical possibility that any lung damage may subsequently exacerbate antibody-mediated lung injury, the anesthesiologist should avoid all unnecessary stresses to the lungs such as high airway pressure or the formation of pulmonary edema.

Although glomerulonephritis may be the sole cause of renal insufficiency, the anesthesiologist should nevertheless routinely assess every patient with renal insufficiency for potential prerenal factors such as hypovolemia or decreased cardiac output that could contribute to renal dysfunction and lead to renal failure. Potentially nephrotoxic drugs should be avoided whenever feasible. Drug selections and dosing guidelines often need to be modified when renal failure exists, and recommendations can be found in any standard textbook of anesthesiology. For patients with severe renal failure who require routine dialysis, preoperative dialysis should be performed close to the time of surgery to correct volume overload, hyperkalemia, and acidosis.

Knowing the patient's baseline weight helps to estimate the amount of fluid a patient can safely tolerate, but invasive monitoring with a pulmonary artery catheter is recommended whenever significant intraoperative volume shifts are anticipated. An arterial line is recommended for patients with pulmonary dysfunction, hypertension, or renal failure.

G. SARCOIDOSIS

Sarcoidosis is a noncontagious, multisystem granulomatous disease of unknown cause. The majority of cases occur between ages 20 and 50 years. Blacks are affected nearly 10 times more often than are Whites, and the prevalence of sarcoidosis in Black females is nearly twice that in Black males. Noncaseating granulomas are the histologic hallmark of sarcoidosis, but they are not specific for this disease. Clinical features that support the notion that immune factors play an important role in the pathogenesis of this disease are increased ratio of helper to suppressor T cells, the presence of activated lymphocytes and macrophages at sites of tissue involvement, hyperglobulinemia, and depressed cutaneous delayed hypersensitivity (anergy).

Clinical presentations vary according to the distribution of granulomas and the severity of disease. Many patients remain asymptomatic even after chest films become markedly abnormal and following widespread granulomatous involvement of many organs. Constitutional symptoms such as fever, weight loss, and fatigue do occur, but they are uncommon. Pulmonary function studies typically show a restrictive pattern characterized by reductions in lung volumes, lung compliance, and diffusing capacity. However, when only the small airways are involved, the routine spirometry studies may be normal, and more sensitive tests of the small airways may be needed to detect an abnormality (e.g., frequency dependence of compliance, helium-oxygen flow-volume loops, and maximum flow rates at low lung volume after correction for static lung elastic recoil pressure). Hypoxemia may be present at rest. Chest films are used to "stage" this disease. A characteristic early radiographic finding is bilateral hilar and paratracheal adenopathy. Other findings may include reticulonodular markings, fibrocystic and bullous changes, and extensive scarring.

1. Anesthetic Considerations

In general, an asymptomatic patient with sarcoidosis requires only routine monitoring and anesthesia care. Special anesthetic concerns derive from the nature and location of the granulomatous disease.

Virtually all the cranial nerves can be affected. Olfactory problems (I), visual disturbances (II), opthalmoplegia (III, IV, VI), facial nerve paralysis or Bell's palsy (VII),[21] deafness and vertigo (VIII),[22] depressed gag reflex and dysphagia (IX, X), and hoarseness and vocal paralysis (X) have been attributed to sarcoidosis.[23–26] In one study, abnormal visual and auditory evoked responses were noted in approximately 25 per cent of patients who lacked visual or brain stem symptoms.[27] Neurosarcoidosis can present as a mass lesion in the brain or spinal cord, and it has been reported to cause encephalopathy, seizures, sensory and motor peripheral neuropathies, meningitis, headaches, papilledema, personality changes, and neuroendocrine dysfunction (diabetes insipidus).[23] Any neurologic dysfunction should be documented in the medical record, and special care should be exercised in positioning the patient. The use of ophthalmic ointment is a reasonable precaution for patients with facial nerve paralysis. Furthermore, extubation in a reverse Trendelenburg position is recommended for patients with a depressed gag reflex or dysphagia.

More than 25 per cent of patients with sarcoidosis have cardiac involvement, but symptomatic cardiac involvement is rare.[28] Granulomatous infiltration and fibrotic reactions in the conduction system can lead to heart block, dysrhythmias, and sudden death. Other cardiac manifestations include pericardial effusions and cardiomyopathy. Medial therapies may include steroid and immunosuppressive drugs, a cardiac pacemaker, or an automatic implantable cardiac defibrillator. Preoperative evaluation should include electrocardiography (ECG), regardless of the patient's age or the absence of symptoms. All medical devices should be functioning properly, and the rationale for their use should be understood by the anesthesiologist. Preoperative stress doses of corticosteroids may be indicated.

Laryngeal sarcoid presents as dysphonia, dyspnea, or dysphagia, and laryngoscopic examination typically reveals diffuse supraglottic edema that is similar in appearance to "epiglottitis," but, unlike the patient with infectious "epiglottitis," the patient with laryngeal sarcoid is not toxic and the tissue is pink rather than beefy red.[29, 30] Neither direct laryngoscopy nor fiberoptic bronchoscopy is likely to cause complete airway obstruction, but any trauma to the supraglottic tissue could compromise the airway. Preoperative steroids are recommended, and a smaller-sized ETT should be considered. Sarcoid causes vocal cord granuloma and diffuse tracheal stenosis. Ventilator management needs to be individualized.

Hypercalcemia results from unregulated formation of 1,25 $(OH)_2D$ by the granuloma-associated macrophages and a potential complication of hypercalcemia is nephrocalcinosis and severe renal insufficiency. Sarcoid can cause renal failure that requires dialysis. Anesthetic concerns include issues related to fluid balance and cardiac status, electrolyte changes, and drug metabolism.

H. SYSTEMIC LUPUS ERYTHEMATOSUS

Systemic lupus erythematosus (SLE) is an autoimmune connective tissue disease of unknown cause that predominantly affects females between the ages of 20 and 50 years but is reported in all age groups. SLE is a multisystem disease with many diffuse protean manifestations (Table 3–1).

Therapeutic interventions for SLE include corticosteroids, cyclophosphamide, azathioprine, hydroxychloroquine, and nonsteroidal anti-inflammatory drugs (NSAIDs). In addition, major organ dysfunction may require specific therapy such as danazol, intravenous immune globulin, plasma exchange, and plasmapheresis for thrombocytopenia and thrombocytopenic purpura; anticonvulsants for seizures; anticoagulants for thromboses; and a variety of drugs and dialysis for renal insufficiency.

TABLE 3–1

Manifestations of Systemic Lupus Erythematosus by Organ System

Organ System	Specific Manifestations
Cutaneous	Malar ("butterfly facial rash"), discoid rash, alopecia, photosensitivity dermatitis, oral ulcers
Connective tissue	Arthritis, serositis, and myopathy
Renal	Glomerulonephritis
Hepatic	Hepatitis and jaundice
Cardiac	Libman-Sacks verrucous endocarditis with clinically silent valvular lesions, myocarditis with systolic and diastolic ventricular dysfunction, but congestive heart failure is uncommon, arrhythmia and conduction abnormalities, pericarditis (with and without) effusions that may rarely lead to constriction or tamponade
Pulmonary	SLE may affect all elements of the ventilator apparatus: muscles in the chest wall and diaphragm (myopathy), pneumonitis, alveolitis, pleuritis, pleural effusion, spontaneous pneumothorax, bonchiolitis obliterans with organizing pneumonia, interstitial fibrosis, alveolar hemorrhage, thromboembolic problems, and pulmonary hypertension. The pulmonary involvement usually results in a restrictive defect.
Neurologic	Cerebritis, seizures, transverse myelitis, psychosis
Hematopoietic	Anemia, leukopenia, lymphopenia, thrombocytopenia
Immune	ANA, anti-DNA, anti-Sm, positive VDRL, and lupus anticoagulant (associated with systemic arterial and venous thromboses)

1. Anesthetic Considerations

Anesthetic management depends on the type of surgery, the affected organs, the side effects of therapy, and the severity of the disease. The asymptomatic patient with mild disease typically requires only standard monitoring and anesthetic care. The symptomatic patient may benefit from a more thorough preoperative medical evaluation by a primary or specialty physician. The anesthesiologist should carefully review the available laboratory studies of renal function, pulmonary function tests, roentgenographic studies, and ECG.

Patients with restrictive lung disease and myopathy affecting diaphragm or chest wall muscles present a special management concern.[31, 32] Hypoxemia is often present in these patients, and they may be especially sensitive to nondepolarizing muscle relaxants. Peripheral nerve stimulation should be monitored closely, and the patient should be warned of the potential necessity for postoperative mechanical ventilation.

Adrenal insufficiency may be present in any patients who received corticosteroids within the preceding year, and perioperative steroid coverage should be considered. Other potential complications of medical therapy for SLE include interstitial infiltrates secondary to cyclophosphamide and hypersensitivity lung reaction from azathioprine.

Patients with a circulating lupus anticoagulant are at increased risk of developing systemic thrombosis, and prophylactic precautions against deep venous thrombosis are indicated.[33]

V. ARTHRITIC DISEASES CREATING UPPER AIRWAY PROBLEMS

A. RHEUMATOID ARTHRITIS

Rheumatoid arthritis (RA) is a chronic systemic inflammatory disease characterized by erosive symmetric polyarthritis. The pathologic hallmark of RA is proliferation of synovial membranes, erosion of articular cartilage, and resorption of subchondral bone. RA predominantly affects the proximal interphalangeal joints of the hands, metacarpophalangeal joints of the wrists, cervical spine, elbows, shoulders, and knees. Extraarticular manifes-

tations are reported in as many as 20 per cent of patients and affect the heart, lungs, nervous system, eyes, and skin. The overall prevalence of RA is approximately 2 per cent.

The onset of symptoms and the clinical course of RA are highly variable. Early symptoms often include morning stiffness, fatigue, and joint swelling and tenderness.

Medical treatments of RA include NSAIDs, gold salts, penicillamine, hydroxychloroquine, sulfasalazine, corticosteroids, and immunosuppressives (methotrexate, cyclophosphamide, chlorambucil, and azathioprine). Bone marrow suppression, renal injury, and hepatotoxicity are but a few of the potential side effects of some of these drugs. Reconstructive surgery is often required.

1. Anesthetic Considerations

a. Airway Considerations

Rheumatoid involvement of the cervical spine, laryngeal structures, and temporomandibular joints is of special concern to the anesthesiologist. The most common site of radiographic involvement is the atlantoaxial joint. Subaxial lesions occur less commonly, but these too can cause spinal cord compression and lead to cervical myelopathy. Symptoms correlate poorly with radiographic findings, and neurologic impairments correlate poorly with cervical instability. Studies have reported a prevalence of cervical spine involvement in 15 to 86 per cent of rheumatoid patients.[34] One community-based study using plain radiography detected anterior atlantoaxial subluxation in 33 per cent of patients with RA.[35] The study also detected 27 per cent vertical dislocations, 14 per cent lateral, 2 per cent posterior, and 21 per cent subaxial subluxations. Other studies have reported that up to 73 per cent of patients develop atlantoaxial subluxation within 10 years, and nearly 20 per cent significant subaxial disease.[36] Symptoms related to subluxation can vary over time, but it is surprising how rarely any symptoms are recognized. Overall, some 10 per cent of patients with unrecognized atlantoaxial subluxation may die from spinal cord or brain stem compression.[37] Common symptoms of cervical spine involvement include nonspecific neck pain and stiffness. Impingement of the second cervical nerve root causes occipital headache. Cervical myelopathy usually presents with paresthesias in a stocking-glove distribution and may be confused with peripheral neuropathy. Spastic paraparesis and abnormal bowel or bladder function are late findings.

The larynx is involved in 26 to 87 per cent of patients with RA.[38, 39] Rheumatoid nodules may occur on the vocal cords or arytenoids and cause significant airway obstruction. Cricoarytenoid synovitis may present as hoarseness, a sore throat and pain during speech, a sensation of a foreign body in the throat, and dysphagia. It may cause median fixation of the vocal cords. Case reports of acute, life-threatening upper airway obstruction due to rheumatoid involvement of the cricoarytenoid joints attest to the potential severity of this problem.[40] Temporomandibular joint involvement can severely limit jaw mobility and mouth opening.

The appropriate preoperative evaluation of the cervical spine for patients with RA should include a careful history and physical examination. Patients with evidence of myelopathy should be referred for neurologic evaluation and those with any symptoms suggestive of airway obstruction should be evaluated by an otolaryngologist. The practice of routine radiographic evaluation of the cervical spine in all patients with RA is controversial.[41, 42] Because cervical involvement is common even without signs or symptoms, the anesthesiologist could reasonably assume that the majority of patients with RA are at increased risk for neurologic injury from cervical manipulation, plan the anesthetic accordingly, and take the appropriate precautions; however, if cervical radiographs could affect management decisions, they should be obtained.

b. Systemic Considerations

The cardiovascular system is often affected by RA but is clinically silent. Cardiovascular features include pericarditis, myocarditis, disruption of the conducting system by rheumatoid nodules, valvular lesions, and, rarely, coronary arteritis.

The pulmonary system is affected in a number of ways by RA. Features of rheumatoid lung involvement include (1) diffuse interstitial pneumonitis and fibrosis, (2) pleurisy, (3) pleural effusions, (4) necrobiotic nodules, (5) bronchiolitis obliterans, (6) pulmonary arteritis, and (7) apical fibrocavitary lesions. Patients may develop pulmonary hypertension and pneumothorax as a consequence of some of these features. Lung involvement is common in RA. Pleural fibrosis or effusions occur in 50 per cent of patients, small airways disease in approximately 30 per cent of nonsmokers and 60 per cent of smokers with RA, and interstitial pneumonitis in fewer than 2 per cent of patients with RA.[43–45] Pulmonary function studies may demonstrate a restrictive, obstructive, or combined disorder. The diffusing capacity is often reduced, even when the chest films appear normal. Gold, methotrexate, or ibuprofen treatment can cause hypersensitivity pneumonitis.

The hematopoietic system is also affected by RA. Mild anemia is common. Felty's syndrome is the triad of chronic RA, splenomegaly, and neutropenia. Felty's syndrome may be accompanied by thrombocytopenia, fever, and hepatomegaly.

B. ANKYLOSING SPONDYLITIS

Ankylosing spondylitis (AS) is an inflammatory arthritic condition of the axial skeleton that affects predominantly young men between the ages of 20 and 40 years. Women tend to have milder disease than men and to be affected much less frequently, but they do have a higher incidence of isolated cervical spine disease. Pathologic changes in AS occur at the sites of ligamentous insertion into bone. In the lumbar spine, involvement of the ligamentous fibers of the annulus fibrosus causes squaring of the cephalad and caudad surfaces of the vertebral bodies. Squaring of the vertebral bodies, the loss of normal lordosis, and the bridging syndesmophytes combine to create the classic radiographic appearance of the "bamboo spine." Sacroiliitis occurs early in the course of the disease, but cervical spine involvement is a relatively late finding. Spontaneous odontoid process fractures have been reported in AS patients.[46] Atlantoaxial subluxation, a potential cause of cervical cord compression, was recently reported in 23 per cent of 103 patients with AS presenting to two outpatient clinics in Mexico.[47] The pulmonary system dysfunction is a consequence of both skeletal disease and of pleuropulmonary involvement. Fusion of the costovertebral joints decreases rib cage movement ("bucket-handle motion"), fixes the chest wall in a relatively inspiratory position, and increases the FRC of the lungs.[48] Increased diaphragmatic excursions compensate for the decreased movement of the thoracic cage, but ventilatory failure may ensue when diaphragmatic function is compromised.[49] In fewer than 2 per cent of patients, AS causes upper lobe fibrocavitary lung changes that may be radiographically indistinguishable from those seen with tuberculosis.[49] Peripheral joint manifestations occur in approximately 20 per cent of patients and involve the shoulders, hips, cricoarytenoids, and costochondral joints; extraarticular problems include plantar fasciitis, Achilles tendinitis, uveitis, and, rarely, cauda equina syndrome, aortitis, cardiac conduction abnormalities, pleural effusions, and interstitial fibrosis.[51]

1. Anesthetic Considerations

Rigidity of the spine and osteoporosis makes positioning and padding of pressure points especially important for patients with AS. Extra pillows under the head may be required for patient comfort and for adequate cervical support.

Cervical spine rigidity may prevent the anesthesiologist from placing the patient's head in a good sniffing position and thereby increase the difficulty of adequately exposing the larynx for tracheal intubation by direct laryngoscopy. Conversely, manipulation of a more mobile cervical spine may increase the risk of neurologic injury in patients with atlantoaxial subluxation. Temporomandibular joint and cricoarytenoid joint involvement may further hinder the ability of the anesthesiologist to intubate the trachea. The clinical spectrum of AS is broad, and many patients with AS can safely be intubated using direct laryngoscopy; however, the subset of patients with restricted cervical spine motion or with cervical spine subluxation or fractures should undergo awake flexible fiberoptic bronchoscopic intubation and positioning.

Diaphragmatic function is critically important to patients with limited thoracic cage movements. Especially vulnerable to diaphragmatic dysfunction are patients undergoing upper abdominal or thoracic surgery, and prolonged mechanical ventilatory support should be anticipated. The anesthesiologist should strive to optimize diaphragmatic function. The anesthesiologist should avoid placing the diaphragm at a mechanical disadvantage (lung hyperinflation), increasing its workload (small endotracheal tube, bronchospasm, retained endobronchial secretion, or abdominal binding), or decreasing its oxygen supply and metabolic substrate (low cardiac output, anemia, hypoxemia, or starvation).

Ossification of the interspinous ligaments and bony bridges between vertebrae (syndesmophytes) may limit flexion of the lumbar spine and make spinal or epidural anesthesia extremely difficult or impossible. Case reports of a lateral approach to spinal anesthesia for lower limb surgery and a caudal approach for hip surgery attest to the feasibility of these techniques.[51, 52]

VI. DRUG-INDUCED LUNG DISEASE

A number of pathophysiologic syndromes induced by drugs affect the lungs and concern anesthesiologists: aspiration pneumonitis, bronchiolitis obliterans with organizing pneumonia, bronchospasm, cough, hemorrhage, adenopathy, hypersensitivity reactions, pulmonary hypertension, hypoventilation, interstitial pneumonitis and fibrosis, lupuslike syndrome, pleural effusion, pleural thickening, pleuritis, pulmonary edema, pulmonary infiltrates with eosinophilia, and vasculitis.[53] Most of the drug-induced lung diseases, however, occur over a relatively long period of time and are more within the scope of practice of the pulmonologist than of the anesthesiologist.

Aspiration of gastric contents is a daily concern for every anesthesiologist. The more liberal acceptance of patients ingesting their usual medications preoperatively increases the risk of particulate aspiration. Aspiration of mineral oil laxatives typically causes no acute problem but can cause a chronic pulmonary infiltrate and should be proscribed preoperatively.

A number of medications may induce bronchospasm: NSAIDs such as ketorolac, beta-blockers, ophthalmic preparations, sulfating drugs (preservatives), and histamine releasers (morphine, tubocurare, atracurium).[54, 55] Even B_1-selective drugs in larger doses may provoke bronchospasm in susceptible individuals. Inhalation or instillation of lidocaine into the trachea can induce bronchoconstriction acutely.[56]

The angiotensin-converting enzyme (ACE)–inhibiting drugs (captopril, enalapril, and lisinopril) can cause tracheal irritation and an intractable chronic cough.[57] Concomitant use of a nonsteroidal medication appears to minimize the cough. Angioedema of the face and oropharyngeal structures is an important complication of ACE inhibitors and a special concern to the anesthesiologist. If the patient is known to have had this reaction to one ACE inhibitor drug, the anesthesiologist should not attempt to treat with another ACE inhibitor drug.

The anesthesiologist should consider the potential complications of thrombolytics and anticoagulant drugs before developing an anesthetic plan. Long-term use of some cephalosporins may induce hypoprothrombinemia. Cephalosporins with the *N*-methylthiotrazole and methylthiotrazole side chains (moxalactam, cefmenoxine, cefoperazone, cefotetan, cefamandole, and cefazolin) appear to inhibit the vitamin K–dependent hepatic enzyme epoxide reductase and thus interfere with prothrombin synthesis.[58]

Phenytoin, hydantoin, and methotrexate can each induce hilar adenopathy, but this problem is usually of little immediate concern to the anesthesiologist.

Hypersensitivity reactions are characterized by fever of acute onset, nonproductive cough, dyspnea, arthralgias, and peripheral eosinophilia. Pleuritic chest pains, pleural effusion, and pulmonary infiltrates are also features of hypersensitivity drug reactions. The list of drugs implicated in hypersensitivity reactions is long and grows longer as new drugs are introduced into the market. They include antibiotics such as ampicillin, isoniazid, nitrofurantoin, penicillin, sulfonamides, and tetracycline and a large variety of other drugs. Initially, it may be difficult to distinguish a hypersensitivity reaction from an infection. If a hypersensitivity reaction is recognized, the offending drug should be discontinued and the surgery deferred until the patient has improved.

Pulmonary hypertension may develop from intravenous and nasal cocaine abuse, intravenous injection of talc or starch by drug addicts, or protamine administered intravenously. The protamine reaction is seen most often during heparin reversal following cardiopulmonary bypass surgery. Protamine causes acute onset of pulmonary vasoconstriction with high pulmonary artery pressures and low left atrial pressures.[59]

Hypoventilation may be caused by narcotics, sedatives, and by inadequate reversal of neuromuscular blockade. It is well-recognized that aminoglycosides may prolong neuromuscular blockade, but clindamycin has also been reported to enhance nondepolarizing neuromuscular blockade.[60]

A number of chemotherapeutic drugs may cause interstitial pneumonitis: bleomycin, busulfan, BCNU, semustine, and lomustine. Of special interest to the anesthesiologist is bleomycin, which reliably causes fibrotic lung disease in experimental animals, and it is estimated that approximately 5 per cent of patients treated with this drug develop clinically recognized fibrotic lung disease. The major risk factors for pulmonary fibrosis with bleomycin are a cumulative dose greater than 500 mg, chest radiotherapy, and inhalation of increased oxygen concentrations. It is not clear how long after chemotherapy with bleomycin the increased risk from oxygen therapy persists, but there is concern that it may persist longer than a year. It is recommended that the fractional inspired oxygen concentration be kept as low as is safely feasible during surgery.[61–63]

VII. SLEEP APNEA SYNDROMES

Sleep apnea is defined as cessation of airflow during sleep. The sleep apnea syndrome is characterized by epochs of apnea that last 10 seconds or more and occur at least five times per hour. Three types of apnea have been described: obstructive, central, and mixed. Obstructive sleep apnea (OSA) is characterized by upper airway obstruction and cessation of airflow despite continued respiratory efforts. Central sleep apnea is characterized by absence of all respiratory effort during the apnea episodes. Mixed apneas have features of both the obstructive and central apneas. The major risk factor for obstructive sleep apnea is obesity, and especially upper body obesity. Other factors associated with a higher prevalence of sleep apnea include male gender, hypertension, cigarette smoking, alcohol consumption, and poor physical status.[64]

Patients with OSA often have a history of excessive daytime sleepiness, headaches, impotence, and enuresis. They may report falling asleep at work or while driving an automobile. Their bed partners commonly report that the patient snores loudly and appears to have a very disrupted sleep pattern. Chronic sleep deprivation can lead to excessive fatigue, neuropsychiatric symptoms, cognitive impairment, poor work habits, and sexual problems. Physical examination may disclose a deviated nasal septum, nasal polyps, an enlarged or elongated uvula, macroglossia, tonsillar hypertrophy, a floppy soft palate, retrognathia, or micrognathia. Repetitive episodes of nocturnal hypoxemia can cause polycythemia, pulmonary hypertension, cor pulmonale, and dysrhythmias.[65]

1. Anesthetic Considerations

During the preoperative evaluation, the anesthesiologist should seek information on the nature and severity of the patient's sleep disorder. If the site of airway obstruction is within the nasopharynx, oral intubation of the trachea may be preferred. The airway should be examined for tonsillar enlargement, macroglossia, redundant soft tissues, mouth opening, dentition, and oropharyngeal view. The patient should be evaluated for signs of pulmonary hypertension (tricuspid and pulmonic regurgitation), right ventricular failure (jugular venous distention, hepatomegaly, ascites, pitting edema of the legs), cardiomegaly, dysrhythmias, abnormal gas exchange, secondary polycythemia, and for neuropsychiatric symptoms that may affect perioperative care. ECG findings of pulmonary hypertension include right atrial enlargement, right axis deviation, and right ventricular hypertrophy. The precordial QRS complexes may be diminished in obese patients with a thickened chest wall. Chest films may also reveal evidence of pulmonary hypertension: enlarged right atrium, right ventricle, and pulmonary arteries. Conditions that elevate pulmonary vascular resistance, such as hypoxia, hypercarbia, acidosis, hypothermia, and high airway pressures, should be avoided in these patients.

A number of medications routinely used in anesthesia (benzodiazepams, narcotics, and volatile anesthetics) have been shown to decrease neural input to upper airway muscles and to the genioglossus muscle.[66, 67] The depressant effect of these drugs on pharyngeal muscle tone increases the tendency of patients with OSA to develop upper airway obstruction.[68, 69] There are anecdotal case reports of patients with OSA given benzodiazepines as a premedication who developed severe upper airway obstruction even while awake.[67, 70] It is recommended that all preoperative sedative-hypnotic and narcotic medications be used sparingly, if at all, and that the treated patient not be left unattended.

The method chosen to intubate the trachea must be individualized. If any difficulty is anticipated in ventilating the patient by mask or with direct laryngoscopy, awake fiberoptic bronchoscopic intubation should be seriously considered. Awake tracheostomy may be required for some patients, and it may be the most appropriate method of securing the airway in select patients undergoing uvulopalatopharyngoplasty. Similarly, preoperative precautions for aspiration should be tailored to the anticipated risks. When indicated, metoclopramide, nonparticulate antacids, and histamine H_2 antagonists are prescribed preoperatively. Preoxygenation before induction of anesthesia is especially important for obese patients with OSA. Their lower FRC, higher oxygen demand, increased central blood volume, and increased cardiac output tend to reduce the interval between apnea and the onset of hypoxemia and thus reduce the safety interval for intubation attempts. Furthermore, decreased chest wall compliance makes mask ventilation more difficult in obese patients. Routine monitors suffice for the "uncomplicated patient" with sleep apnea. Morbidly obese patients and those with pulmonary hypertension and heart failure are best monitored with arterial catheters and pulmonary artery catheters.

Restriction of postoperative analgesic medications reduces the risk of respiratory depression and of airway compromise, but it also may expose the patient to the risk of inadequate pain relief and needless anxiety. Continued mechanical support of the airway with an endotracheal tube or close monitoring in an intensive care unit safely permits more liberal use of sedative-hypnotic and analgesic drugs postoperatively. It also affords an opportunity to monitor the patient for cardiac dysrhythmias and gives more time for airway swelling to subside before extubation. Many patients can be safely extubated immediately following surgery and tolerate routine postoperative medications without complications. The application of nasal continuous positive airway pressure (nasal CPAP) to patients before surgery and then immediately after extubation appears to allow most patients with obstructive sleep apneas to "freely use sedative, analgesic, and anesthetic drugs without major complications."[71]

VIII. INFECTIOUS DISEASES

A. ECHINOCOCCAL DISEASES OF THE LUNG

Echinococcosis or hydatid disease is caused by the tapeworm *Echinococcus granulosus.*

These parasites divide their life cycle between two hosts. Dogs and other canines are the definitive host and harbor the mature tapeworm in the intestinal lumen. Eggs from the tapeworm are passed into the environment via the host's feces. Humans become infected by ingesting the eggs in contaminated water or foodstuffs. The eggs hatch in the human intestinal lumen, mature into oncospheres, and migrate into the liver, peritoneum, and mesentery, where they form cysts. The hydatid cysts that form contain an immature organism called a *protoscolex*, which reproduces by asexual budding. The liver is the most common visceral organ infected. Hematogenous spread to the lungs, mediastinum, brain, or bones is rare.

Symptoms may result from the mass effect of the cyst or from leakage of its contents. Enlargement of hepatic cysts may cause abdominal discomfort. Erosion of bone cortex by bony cysts causes pathologic fractures, and brain involvement with hydatid cyst can cause hydrocephalus and seizures. Within the lung, the unrupted cyst may remain asymptomatic; however, rupture of the intrathoracic cyst is a serious clinical concern. Rupture of the cyst may spread the infection throughout the thorax and may evoke an acute hypersensitivity reaction manifested by severe bronchospasm and anaphylaxis. Pulmonary cysts can grow large enough to fill an entire hemithorax.

Asymptomatic, calcified cysts may resolve spontaneously, and expectant management is often chosen. Symptomatic or enlarging cysts are best managed by complete surgical excision. During surgery but before resection, some surgeons aspirate the cyst and replace the fluid with a cidal agent such as 2 per cent formalin, hypertonic saline, or ethanol. Unresectable cysts are treated with antihelmintic drugs (mebendazole or albendazole).

1. Anesthetic Considerations[72]

The anesthetic goal is to optimize the conditions for surgical exposure and to be prepared to manage the potential complications. Anesthesia for surgical resection of small cysts located in the basilar segments of the lungs can often be managed using routine monitors and a single-lumen ETT. Large cysts and those located closer to the apexes of the lungs are best managed with a double-lumen ETT or with a bronchial blocker, both to facilitate surgical exposure and to safeguard the contralateral lung from contamination. Spillage of the contents of large cysts into the contralateral lung is potentially fatal. An arterial line should be inserted whenever the need for single-lung ventilation is anticipated. Patient movement or coughing during delivery of the cyst or after cyst rupture should be avoided. Although an adequate depth of anesthesia may suffice to achieve this goal, neuromuscular blockade is generally recommended.

REFERENCES

Wegener's Granulomatosis

1. Daum TE, Specks U, Colby TV, et al: Tracheobronchial involvement in Wegener's granulomatosis. Am J Respir Crit Care Med 151(2, Pt 1):522, 1995.
2. Allen NA: Wegener's granulomatosis. In Bennett JC, Plum F (eds): Cecil Textbook of Medicine, 20th ed. Philadelphia, WB Saunders, 1996, pp 1495–1498.
3. Landman S, Burgener F: Pulmonary manifestations of Wegener's granulomatosis. AJR 122:750, 1974.
4. Hoffman GS, Kerr GS, Leavitt RY, et al: Wegener's granulomatosis: An analysis of 158 patients. Ann Intern Med 116:488, 1992.

Lymphomatoid Granulomatosis

5. Collins S, Helme RD: Lymphomatoid granulomatosis presenting as a progressive cervical cord lesion. Aust NZ J Med 19(2):144, 1989.
6. Benumof JL: Special respiratory physiology of the lateral decubitus position, the open chest, and one-lung ventilation. Vasodilator drugs. In Benumof JL (ed): Anesthesia for Thoracic Surgery, 2nd ed. Philadelphia, WB Saunders, 1995, pp 137–140.

Churg-Strauss Syndrome

7. Sehgal M, Swanson JW, DeRemee RA, Colby TV: Neurologic manisfestations of Churg-Strauss syndrome. Mayo Clinic Proc 70(4):337, 1995.

Cystic Fibrosis

8. Koch C, Hoiby N: Pathogenesis of cystic fibrosis. Lancet 341:1065, 1993.
9. Davis P: Molecular and cell biology of cystic fibrosis. J Appl Physiol 70:2331, 1991.
10. Knowles M, Gatzy J, Boucher R: Increased bioelectric potential difference across respiratory epithelia in cystic fibrosis. N Engl J Med 305:1489, 1981.
11. Elborne JS, Shale DJ, Britton JR: Cystic fibrosis: Current survival and population estimates for the year 2000. Thorax 46:881, 1991.
12. Scott RB, O'Loughlin EV, Gall DG: Gastroesophageal reflux in patients with cystic fibrosis. J Pediatrics 106:223, 1985.
13. Stringer DA, Spragg A, Joudis E, et al: The association of cystic fibrosis, gastroesophageal reflux, and reduced pulmonary function. Can Assoc Radiol J 39:100, 1988.

Lymphangioeiomyomatosis

14. Corrin B, Liebow AA, Friedman PJ: Pulmonary lymphangiomyomatosis. Am J Pathol 79:348, 1975.
15. Carrington CB, Cugell DW, Gaensler EA, et al: Lymphangioleiomyomatosis. Physiologic-pathologic-radiologic correlations. Am Rev Respir Dis 116:977, 1977.

Pulmonary Alveolar Proteinosis

16. Alfrey DD, Benumof JL, Spragg RG: Anesthesia for bronchpulmonary lavage. *In* Kaplan J (ed): Thoracic Anesthesia. New York, Churchill Livingstone, 1982, pp 403–420.

Goodpasture's Syndrome

17. Turner N, Mason PJ, Brown R, et al: Molecular cloning of the human Goodpasture antigen demonstrates it to be the alpha-3 chain of type IV collagen. J Clin Invest 89(2):592, 1992.
18. Kalluri R, Sun MJ, Hudson BG, Neilson EG: The Goodpasture autoantigen. Structural delineation of two immunologically privileged epitopes on alpha3 (IV) chain of type IV collagen. J Biol Chem 271(15):9062, 1996.
19. Kelly PT, Haponik EF: Goodpasture syndrome: Molecular and clinical advances. Medicine 73(4):171, 1994.
20. Ewan PW, Jones HA, Rhodes CG, et al: Detection of intrapulmonary hemorrhage with carbon monoxide uptake: Application in Goodpasture's syndrome. N Engl J Med 295:1391, 1976.

Sarcoidosis

21. Keane JR: Bilateral seventh nerve palsy: Analysis of 43 cases and review of the literature. Neurology 44(7):1198, 1994.
22. O'Reilly BJ, Burrows EH: VIIIth cranial nerve involvement in sarcoidosis. J Laryngol Otol 109(11): 1089, 1995.
23. Jaffe R, Bogomolski-Vahalom V, Kramer MR: Vocal cord paralysis as the presenting symptom of sarcoidosis. Respir Med 88(8):633, 1994.
24. Stern BJ, Krumholz A, Johns C, et al: Sarcoidosis and its neurological manifestations. Arch Neurol 42(9):909, 1985.
25. Oksansen V: Neurosarcoidosis. Sarcoidosis 11(1):76, 1994.
26. Heck AW, Phillips LV 2d: Sarcoidosis and the nervous system. Neurol Clin 7(3):641, 1989.
27. Oksan V, Salmi T: Visual and auditory evoked potentials in the early diagnosis and follow-up of neurosarcoidosis. Acta Neurol Scand 74(1):38, 1986.
28. Shammas RL, Movahed A: Sarcoidosis of the heart. Clin Cardil 16(6):462, 1993.
29. Benjamin B, Dalton C, Croxson G: Laryngoscopic diagnosis of laryngeal sarcoid. Ann Otol Rhinol Laryngol 104(7):529, 1995.
30. Mariotta S, Valeri B, Guidi L, Bisetti A: Endoscopic findings in arytenoid sarcoidosis. Sarcoidosis 11(1): 40, 1994.

Systemic Lupus Erythematosus

31. Scano G, Goti P, Duranti R, et al: Control of breathing in a subset of patients with systemic lupus erythematosus. Chest 108(3):759, 1995.

32. Orens JB, Martinez FJ, Lynch JP 3rd: Pleuropulmonary manifestations of systemic lupus erythematosus. Rheum Dis Clin North Am 20(1):159, 1994.
33. Gluek HI, Kant KS, Weiss MA, et al: Thrombosis in systemic lupus erythematosus. Relation to the presence of circulating anticoagulants. Arch Intern Med 145(8):1389, 1985.

Rheumatoid Lung

34. Bland JH: Rheumatoid subluxation of the cervical spine. J Rheumatol 17:134, 1990.
35. Kauppi M, Hakala M: Prevalence of cervical spine subluxations and dislocations in a community-based rheumatoid arthritis population. Scand J Rheumatol 23:133, 1994.
36. Pellicci PM, Ranawar CS, Tsairis P, Bryan WJ: A prospective study of the progression of rheumatoid arthritis of the cervical spine. J Bone Joint Surg 63A:342, 1981.
37. Mikulowski P, Wolheim FA, Rotmil P, Olsen I: Sudden death in rheumatoid arthritis with atlanto-axial dislocation. Acta Med Scand 198:445, 1975.
38. Lofgren RH, Montgomery WW: Incidence of laryngeal involvement in rheumatoid arthritis. N Engl J Med 267:193, 1962.
39. Bienenstock H, Ehrlich GE, Freyberg RH: Rheumatoid arthritis of the cricoarytenoid joint: A clinicopathologic study. Arthritis Rheum 6:48, 1965.
40. Bamshad M, Rosa U, Padda G, Luce M: Acute upper airway obstruction in rheumatoid arthritis of the cricoarytenoid joints. South Med J 82:507, 1989.
41. Macarthur A, Kleiman S: Rheumatoid cervical joint disease—a challenge to the anesthetist. Can J Anaesth 40:154, 1993.
42. Campbell RSD, Wou P, Watt IA: Continuing role for pre-operative cervical spine radiography in rheumatoid arthritis? Clin Radiol 50:157, 1995.
43. Walker WC, Wright V: Pulmonary lesion and rheumatoid arthritis. Medicine 47:501, 1968.
44. Collins RL, Turner RA, Johnson AM, et al: Obstructive pulmonary disease in rheumatoid arthritis. Arthritis Rheum 19(3):623, 1976.
45. Helmers R, Galvin J, Hunninghake G: Pulmonary manifestations associated with rheumatoid arthritis. Chest 100:235, 1991.

Ankylosing Spondylitis

46. Kremer P, Despaux J, Benansour A, Wendling D: Spontaneous fracture of the odontoid process in a patient with ankylosing spondylitis. Nonunion responsible for compression of the upper cervical cord. Rev Rheum [English Edition] 62(6):455, 1995.
47. Ramos-Remus C, Gomez-Vargas A, Guzman-Guzman JL, et al: Frequency of atlantoaxial subluxation and neurologic involvement in patients with ankylosing spondylitis. J Rheumatol 22:(11):2120, 1995.
48. Grimby C, Fugl-Meyer AR, Blomstrand A: Partitioning of the contributions of rib cage and abdomen to ventilation in ankylosing spondylitis. Thorax 29:179, 1974.
49. Rosenow EC III, Strimlan CV, Muhm JR: Pleuropulmonary manifestations of ankylosing spondylitis. Mayo Clin Proc 52:641, 1977.
50. Luthra HS: Extraarticular manifestations of ankylosing spondylitis. Mayo Clin Proc 52:655, 1977.
51. Kumar CM, Mehta M: Ankylosing spondylitis: Lateral approach to spinal anaesthesia for lower limb surgery. Can J Anaesth 42(1):73, 1995.

52. DeBoard JW, Ghia JN, Guilford WB: Caudal anesthesia in a patient with ankylosing spondylitis for hip surgery. Anesthesiology 54:164, 1981.

Drug-Induced Lung Diseases

53. McCarren JP: Drug-induced lung disease. *In* Bordow RA, Moser KM (eds): Manual of Clinical Problems in Pulmonary Medicine, 4th ed. Boston, Little, Brown and Company, 1996, pp 394–409.
54. Hunt LW Jr, Rosenow EC 3rd: Drug-induced asthma. *In* Weiss EB, Stein M (eds): Bronchial Asthma: Mechanisms and Therapeutics. Boston, Little, Brown and Company, 1993.
55. Mecker DP, Wiedemann HP: Drug-induced bronchospasm. Clin Chest Med 11:163, 1990.
56. McAlpine LG, Thomson NC: Lidocaine-induced bronchoconstriction in asthmatic patients: Relation to histamine airway responsiveness and effect of preservative. Chest 96:1012, 1989.
57. Sebastian JL, McKinney WP, Kaufman J, Young MJ: Angiotensin-converting enzyme inhibitors and cough: Prevalence in an outpatient medical clinic population. Chest 99:36, 1991.
58. Shearer MJ, Bechtold H, Andrassy K, et al: Mechanism of cephalosporin-induced hypoprothrombinemia: Relation to cephalosporin side chain, vitamin K metabolism, and vitamin K status. J Clin Pharmacol 28:88, 1988.
59. Levy JH, Schwieger IA, Zaidan JR, et al: Evaluation of patients at risk for protamine reactions. J Thorac Cardiovasc Surg 98:200, 1989.
60. Becher LD, Miller RD: Clindamycin enhances a nondepolarizing neuromuscular blockade. Anesthesiology 45:84, 1976.
61. Goldiner PL, Carlon GC, Cvitkovic E, et al: Factors influencing postoperative morbidity and mortality in patients treated with bleomycin. Br Med J 1:1664, 1978.
62. Van Barneveld PWC, et al: Natural course of bleomycin-induced pneumonitis: A follow-up study. Am Rev Respir Dis 135:48, 1987.
63. Waid-Jones MI, Coursin DB: Perioperative consideration for patients treated with bleomycin. Chest 99:993, 1991.

Sleep Apnea

64. Patinen M, Telakivi T: Epidemiology of obstructive sleep apnea. Sleep 15(6 Suppl):S1, 1992.
65. Guilleminault C, Van Den Hoed J, Mitler MM: Clinical overview of sleep apnea syndrome. *In* Guilleminault C, Dement WC (eds): Sleep Apnea Syndromes. New York, Alan R Liss, 1978.
66. Krol RC, Knuth SL, Bartlett D: Selective reduction of genioglossal muscle activity by alcohol in normal human subjects. Am Rev Respir Dis 129:247, 1984.
67. Guilleminault C, Cummiskey J, Dement WC: Sleep apnea syndrome. Recent advances. Adv Intern Med 26:347, 1980.
68. Keamy MF III, Cadieux RJ, Kofke WA, Kales A: The occurrence of obstructive sleep apnea in a recovery room patient. Anesthesiology 66:232, 1987.
69. Rafferty TD, Ruskis A, Sasaki C, Gee JB: Perioperative considerations in the management of tracheotomy for the obstructive sleep apnea patient. Br J Anaesth 52:619, 1980.
70. Simmons FB, Hill MW: Hypersomnia caused by upper airway obstructions: A new syndrome in otolaryngology. Ann Otol 83:670, 1974.
71. Rennotte MT, Baele P, Aubert G, Rodenstein DO: Nasal continuous positive airway pressure in the perioperative management of patients with obstructive sleep apnea submitted to surgery. Chest 107:367, 1995.

Infectious Diseases

72. Benumof JL: Hydatid cyst of the lung. *In* Benumof JL (ed): Anesthesia for Thoracic Surgery, 2nd ed. Philadelphia, WB Saunders, 1995, pp 513–514.

Uncommon Cardiac Diseases

Tameshwar Ammar
David L. Reich
Joel A. Kaplan

I. INTRODUCTION

The anesthetic management of uncommon cardiovascular disease states differs in no fundamental way from the management of the more familiar problems, since it rests on the same principles of management. These include (1) understanding the disease process and its manifestations in the patient; (2) thorough understanding of anesthetic and adjuvant drugs, including their cardiovascular effects; (3) proper use of monitoring; and, (4) an understanding of the requirements of the surgical procedure.

Certainly, the most common major cardiovascular diseases encountered are atherosclerotic coronary artery disease, rheumatic valvular disease, and essential hypertension. Experience with these disease states has made the anesthesiologist familiar with both the pathophysiology and management of cardiac patients. While the disease states discussed in this chapter are not often encountered, they can be reduced to familiar patterns of physiology and pathophysiology.

The principle of understanding a disease state and its manifestations in a patient remains the same whether the disease is common or uncommon. An evaluation of the degree of cardiovascular involvement using available clinical and laboratory information is necessary to make a rational assessment of the disease state of each individual patient. A thorough understanding of the cardiovascular effects of the anesthetic and adjuvant drugs to be employed allows the patient to be managed using a rational anesthetic plan. Recent advances in cardiovascular pharmacology, anesthetic drugs, and new techniques of circulatory support have provided great flexibility in the management of the patient with impaired cardiovascular function.

The use of hemodynamic monitoring provides the best guide to intra- and postoperative treatment of patients with uncommon cardiovascular diseases. Monitoring is certainly no substitute for an understanding of physiology and pharmacology or for clinical judgment; rather, monitoring provides data that inform clinical decisions. Since the diseases to be discussed are rare, extensive knowledge of their pathophysiology, particularly in the anesthetic and surgical setting, is largely lacking, and monitoring helps bridge this gap. An understanding of the requirements of the surgical procedure and good communication with the surgeon are necessary in all operations to anticipate intraoperative problems, but especially with the diseases considered here.

This chapter does not provide an exhaustive list or consideration of all the uncommon diseases that affect the cardiovascular system, though it covers a wide range. No matter how bizarre a disease entity is, it can affect the cardiovascular system in only a limited number of ways. It can affect the myocardium, the coronary arteries, the conduction system, the pulmonary circulation, or valvular function or it can impair cardiac filling or emptying. Subsections in this chapter follow this basic pattern. Each section is accompanied by tables of uncommon diseases that may produce a cardiomyopathy, coronary artery disease, pulmonary hypertension, or another cardiac disorder, along with various comments and caveats for each disease. This method of presentation provides a reasonable approach to the anesthesia management of uncommon diseases.

II. CARDIOMYOPATHIES

A. GENERAL CLASSIFICATION

Diseases of the myocardium can be classified in a number of ways. On an etiologic basis, they are usually thought of as primary myocardial diseases, in which the basic disease locus is the myocardium itself, or secondary myocardial diseases, in which the myocardial pathology is associated with some systemic disorder. On a pathophysiologic basis, myocardial disease can be broken down into three categories: dilated (congestive), hypertrophic/obstructive, and restrictive/obliterative (Fig. 4–1). Unfortunately, there is often no sharp division among these three, and a particular patient may have features suggestive of any or all three categories. Dilated cardiomyopathies encompass both inflammatory and noninflammatory forms, and their most prominent clinical feature is myocardial failure manifested as ventricular dilatation, elevated filling pressures, and pulmonary edema. This, for example, is the usual response in cases of severe myocarditis. For the following discussion, the myocarditides are included with inflammatory dilated cardiomyopathies. The obstructive form of myocardial diseases consists of hypertrophy of the myocardial muscle that may result in impaired filling and obstruction to ventricular outflow. Restrictive cardiomyopathies usually result from infiltration of the myocardium by fibrous tissue or some other substance that decreases the compliance of the ventricle and

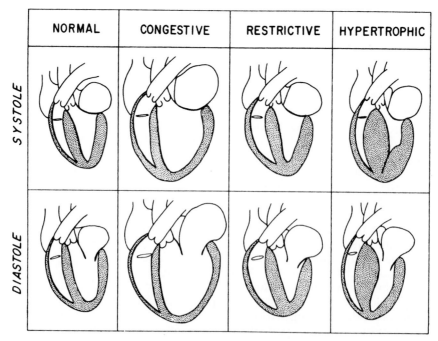

FIGURE 4–1. Illustration of the 50-degree left anterior oblique view of the heart in various cardiomyopathies at end-systole and end-diastole. (From Goldman MR, Boucher CA: Value of radionuclide imaging techniques in assessing cardiomyopathy. Am J Cardiol 46:1232, 1980. Reproduced with permission.)

impedes filling. They usually present a picture that mimics the physiology of constrictive pericarditis, often coupled with myocardial failure owing to loss of muscle mass.

B. DILATED CARDIOMYOPATHY

1. Inflammatory (Myocarditis)

Dilated (congestive) cardiomyopathies exist in both inflammatory and noninflammatory forms (Tables 4–1 and 4–2).[1, 2] The inflammatory variety, or myocarditis, is usually the result of infection. Myocarditis presents with the clinical picture of fatigue, dyspnea, and palpitations, usually in the first weeks of the infection, progressing to overt congestive heart failure with cardiac dilatation, tachycardia, pulsus alternans, and pulmonary edema.[3] Between 10 and 33 per cent of patients with infectious heart diseases have electrocardiographic (ECG) evidence of myocardial involvement. Mural thrombi often form in the ventricular cavity and may result in systemic or pulmonary emboli. Supraventricular and ventricular dysrhythmias are common. Fortunately, complete recovery from infectious myocarditis is usually the case, but there are exceptions, such as myocarditis associated with diphtheria or Chagas' disease. Occasionally, acute myocarditis may even progress to a recurrent or chronic form of myocarditis, resulting ultimately in a restrictive type of cardiomyopathy secondary to fibrous replacement of the myocardium.[4]

In the bacterial varieties of myocarditis, isolated ECG changes or pericarditis are common and usually benign, whereas congestive heart failure is unusual. Diphtheritic myocarditis is generally the worst form of bacterial myocardial involvement, since, in addition to inflammatory changes, its endotoxin is a competitive analogue of cytochrome B and can produce severe myocardial dysfunction. The conduction system is especially affected in diphtheria, producing either right or left bundle-branch block, which is associated with 50 per cent mortality. When complete heart block supravenes, the mortality rate approaches 80 to 100 per cent. Syphilis and leptospirosis represent two examples of myocardial infection by spirochetes. Tertiary syphilis is associated with multiple problems, including dysrhythmias, conduction disturbances, and congestive heart failure.

Viral infections manifest themselves primarily with ECG abnormalities, including PR prolongation, QT prolongation, ST and T-wave abnormalities, and dysrhythmias; however, each viral disease produces slightly different ECG changes, complete heart block being the most significant. Most of the viral diseases have the potential to progress to congestive heart failure if the viral infection is severe. Especially noteworthy in this regard is the coxsackie B virus, which most commonly produces severe viral heart disease. Presenting as fulminating cardiac failure with severe atrioventricular (AV) nodal involvement and respiratory distress, viral myocarditis is common in nursery epidemics of coxsackie B infection. Recovery from coxsackie B myocarditis is usual, but the condition may have constrictive pericarditis as a sequela. Primary atypical pneumonia has the unusual feature of producing Stokes-Adams attacks secondary to AV node involvement.

Mycotic myocarditis has protean manifestations that depend on the extent of mycotic infiltration of the myocardium and may present as congestive heart failure, pericarditis, ECG abnormalities, or valvular obstruction.

Of the protozoal forms of myocarditis, Chagas' disease, or trypanosomiasis, is the most significant one and the most common cause of chronic congestive heart failure in South America. ECG changes of right bundle-branch block and dysrhythmias occur in 80 per cent of patients. In addition to the typical inflammatory changes in the myocardium that produce chronic congestive failure, a direct neurotoxin from the infecting organism, *Trypanosoma cruzi,* produces degeneration of the conduction system, often causing severe ventricular dysrhythmias and heart block with syncope. The onset of atrial fibrillation in these patients is often an ominous prognostic sign.

Helminthic myocardial involvement may produce congestive heart failure, but more commonly symptoms are secondary to infestation and obstruction of the coronary or pulmonary arteries by egg, larval, or adult forms of the worm. Trichinosis, for example, produces myocarditis secondary to an inflammatory response to larvae in the myocardium, even though the larvae themselves disappear from the myocardium after the second week of infestation.

2. Noninflammatory

The noninflammatory variety of dilated cardiomyopathy also presents the picture of

Text continued on page 79

TABLE 4-1

Inflammatory Cardiomyopathies (Dilated)

Disease Process	Mechanism	Associated Circulatory Problems	Miscellaneous
1. Bacterial		Dysrhythmias, ST-T wave changes	
a. Diphtherial	Endotoxin competitive analogue of cytochrome B	1. Conduction system, especially BBB 2. Rare, valvular endocarditis	Temporary pacing often required
b. Typhoid	Inflammatory changes* with fiber degeneration	1. Dysrhythmias 2. Endarteritis, endocarditis, pericarditis, ventricular rupture	
c. Scarlet fever β-hemolytic strep	Inflammatory changes	Conduction disturbances and dysrhythmias	
d. Meningococcus	Inflammatory changes and endotoxin, generalized and coronary thrombosis	1. Disseminated intravascular coagulation 2. Peripheral circulatory collapse (Waterhouse-Friderichsen syndrome)	
e. Staphylococcus	Sepsis, acute endocarditis		
f. Brucellosis	Fiber degeneration and granuloma formation	Endocarditis, pericarditis	
g. Tetanus	Inflammatory changes, cardiotoxin	Severe dysrhythmias	Apnea
h. Melioidosis	Myocardial abscesses		
2. Spirochetal leptospirosis	Focal hemorrhage and inflammatory changes	1. Severe dysrhythmias 2. Endocarditis and pericarditis	Temporary pacing
3. Rickettsial		ECG changes, pericarditis	
a. Endemic typhus	Inflammatory changes	Dysrhythmias	
b. Epidemic typhus	Symptoms secondary to vasculitis and hypertension	Vasculitis	

Disease	Pathology	Cardiac manifestations
a. Coxsackie B	Inflammatory changes	1. Constrictive pericarditis 2. AV-nodal dysrhythmias
b. Echovirus Mumps Influenza Infectious mononucleosis Viral hepatitis Rubella Rubeola Rabies Varicella Lymphocytic Choriomeningitis Psittacosis Viral encephalitis Cytomegalovirus Variola Herpes zoster	Inflammatory changes 1. Primary atypical pneumonia—associated Stokes-Adams attacks 2. Herpes simplex—associated with intractable shock 3. Arbovirus—constrictive pericarditis is reported sequela	1. Dysrhythmia 2. Heart block 3. Pericarditis
5. Mycoses a. Cryptococcosis Blastomycosis Actinomycosis Coccidiodomycosis	Usually obstructive symptoms Reported congestive heart failure	Valvular obstruction Constrictive pericarditis
6. Protozoal a. Trypanosomiasis (Chagas' disease—see text)	1. Inflammatory changes 2. Neurotoxin of *T. cruzi*	1. Severe dysrhythmia secondary to conduction system degeneration 2. Mitral and tricuspid insufficiency secondary to cardiac enlargement Pacing often required
b. Sleeping sickness	Inflammatory changes	Cardiac tamponade
c. Toxoplasmosis	Inflammatory changes	Unusual manifestations of disease
d. Leishmaniasis Balantidiasis	Inflammatory changes Inflammatory changes	Dysrhythmias Unusual manifestations
7. Helminthic Trichinosis	Inflammatory changes Usually secondary to adult or ova infestation of myocardium or coronary insufficiency secondary to same	
Schistosomiasis Filariasis	Cor pulmonale—secondary pulmonary hypertension	

*Inflammatory type usually has myofibrillar degeneration, inflammatory cell infiltration, edema.

TABLE 4–2

Noninflammatory Cardiomyopathies (Dilated)

Disease Process	Mechanism	Associated Circulatory Problems	Miscellaneous
1. Nutritional disorders a. Beriberi	Thiamine deficiency Inflammatory changes	1. Peripheral AV shunting with low SVR 2. Usually high output failure with decreased SVR, but low output with normal SVR may occur	
b. Kwashiorkor	Protein deprivation	Degeneration of conduction system	
2. Metabolic disorders a. Amyloidosis	Amyloid infiltration of myocardium	1. Associated with restrictive and obstructive forms of cardiomyopathy 2. Valvular lesions 3. Conduction abnormalities	
b. Pompe's disease Glycogen storage disease Type II	Alpha glucuronidase deficiency Glycogen accumulation in cardiac muscle	Septal hypertrophy Decreased compliance	
c. Hurler's syndrome	Accumulation of glycoprotein in coronary tissue and parenchyma of heart	Mitral regurgitation	
d. Hunter's syndrome	Same	Similar to but milder than Hurler's	
e. Primary xanthomatosis	Xanthomatosis infiltration of myocardium	1. Aortic stenosis 2. Advanced coronary artery disease	
f. Uremia	Multiple metastatic coronary calcifications Hypertension Electrolyte imbalance	1. Anemia 2. Hypertension 3. Conduction defects 4. Pericarditis and cardiac tamponade	Most cardiac manifestations dramatically improve after dialysis
g. Fabry's disease	Abnormal glycolipid metabolism secondary to ceramide trihexosidase with glycolipid infiltration of myocardium	1. Hypertension 2. Coronary artery disease	
3. Hematological diseases a. Leukemia	Leukemic infiltration of myocardium	1. Dysrhythmias 2. Pericarditis	
b. Sickle cell	Intracoronary thrombosis with ischemic cardiopathy	1. Coronary artery disease 2. Cor pulmonale	Usually resolves with successful therapy
4. Neurological disease a. Duchenne's muscular dystrophy	Muscle fiber degeneration with fatty and fibrous replacement	Conduction defects possibly secondary to small vessel coronary artery disease	50% incidence of cardiac involvement
b. Friedreich's ataxia	Similar to Duchenne's with collagen replacement of degenerating myofibers	1. Conduction abnormalities 2. ? HOCM	
c. Roussy-Lévy hereditary polyneuropathy	Similar to Friedreich's		
d. Myotonia atrophica	Similar to above	Conduction abnormalities, possibly Stokes-Adams attacks	

76

	Pathology / Mechanism	Clinical features	Comments
5. Chemical and toxic			
a. Doxorubicin (see text)			
b. Zidovudine (see text)			
c. Ethyl alcohol (see text)	Myofibrillar degeneration secondary to direct toxic effect of ETOH and/or acetaldehyde		
d. Beer drinker's cardiomyopathy	Probably secondary to the addition of cobalt sulfate to beer with myofibrillar dystrophy and edema		Acute onset and rapid course
e. Cobalt intoxication	Similar to beer drinker's cardiomyopathy		CNS symptoms and aspiration pneumonitis are usually the predominant symptoms. Relatively unresponsive to adrenergic agents
f. Phosphorus	Myofibrillar degeneration secondary to direct toxic effect of phosphorus, which prevents amino acid incorporation into myocardial proteins	Cyanosis	
g. Fluoride	1. Direct myocardial toxin 2. Severe hypocalcemia secondary to (F)– binding of calcium ion		
h. Lead	1. Secondary to nephropathic hypertension 2. Direct toxin	Hypertension	
i. Scorpion venom	Sympathetic stimulation with secondary myocardial changes		Adrenergic blockade probably indicated
j. Tick paralysis	?		
6. Radiation	Hyalinization and fibrosis due to direct effect of x-radiation	Toxic myocarditis 1. Conduction abnormalities secondary to sclerosis of conduction system 2. Coronary artery disease 3. Constrictive myo- and pericarditis	
7. Miscellaneous systemic syndromes			
a. Rejection cardiomyopathy	Lymphocytic infiltration and general rejection phenomena	Dysrhythmias and conduction abnormalities	After heart transplantation
b. Senile cardiomyopathy	Unrelated to coronary artery disease		
c. Rheumatoid arthritis	1. Rheumatoid nodular invasion 2. Secondary to coronary arteritis	1. Mitral and aortic regurgitation 2. Coronary artery disease 3. Constrictive pericarditis	
d. Marie-Strumpell (ankylosing spondylitis)	Generalized degenerative changes	Aortic regurgitation	

Table continued on following page

TABLE 4-2 (Continued)

Noninflammatory Cardiomyopathies (Dilated)

Disease Process	Mechanism	Associated Circulatory Problems	Miscellaneous
e. Cogan's syndrome (nonsyphilitic interstitial keratitis)	Fibrinoid necrosis of myocardium	1. Aortic regurgitation 2. Coronary artery disease	
f. Noonan's syndrome (male Turner's)	? (No detectable chromosome abnormality)	1. Pulmonary stenosis 2. Obstructive and nonobstructive cardiomyopathy	
g. Pseudoxanthoma elasticum (Grönblad-Strandberg)	Connective tissue disorder with myocardial infiltration and fibrosis	1. Valve abnormality 2. Coronary artery disease	
h. Trisomy 17–18	Diffuse fibrosis		
i. Scleredema of Buschke	Myocardial infiltration with acid mucopolysaccharides		? Viral etiology Self-limited with good prognosis
j. Wegener's granulomatosis	Panarteritis and myocardial granuloma formation	1. Mitral stenosis (?) 2. Cardiac tamponade	
k. Periarteritis nodosa	1. Panarteritis 2. Changes secondary to hypertension	1. Conduction abnormalities 2. Coronary artery disease	
8. Postpartum cardiomyopathy			
9. Neoplastic diseases			
a. Primary mural cardiac tumor	Mechanical impairment of cardiac function	Obstructive symptoms	
b. Metastases—malignant (especially malignant melanoma)			
10. Sarcoidosis	1. Cor pulmonale secondary to pulmonary involvement 2. Sarcoid granuloma leading to ventricular aneurysms	1. Cor pulmonale 2. ECG abnormalities and conduction disturbances 3. Pericarditis 4. Valvular obstruction	

myocardial failure, but in this case secondary to idiopathic, toxic, degenerative, or infiltrative processes in the myocardium (see Table 4–2).[2, 5]

Alcoholic cardiomyopathy is a typical hypokinetic noninflammatory cardiomyopathy associated with tachycardia and premature ventricular contractions that progresses to left ventricular failure with incompetent mitral and tricuspid valves. This cardiomyopathy is probably due to a direct toxic effect of ethanol or its metabolite acetaldehyde, which releases and depletes cardiac norepinephrine.[6, 7] Alcohol may also affect excitation-contraction coupling at the subcellular level.[8] In chronic alcoholics, acute ingestion of ethanol produces decreases in contractility, elevations in ventricular end-diastolic pressure, increases in systemic vascular resistance and systemic hypertension.[9, 10]

Alcoholic cardiomyopathy is classified in three hemodynamic stages. In stage I, cardiac output, ventricular pressures, and left ventricular end-diastolic volume are normal, but the ejection fraction is decreased. In stage II, cardiac output is normal, though filling pressures and end-diastolic volume are increased and ejection fraction is decreased. In stage III, cardiac output is decreased, filling pressures and end-diastolic volume are increased, and ejection fraction is severely depressed. Generally speaking, all of the noninflammatory forms of dilated cardiomyopathy probably undergo a similar progression.[9]

Doxorubicin (Adriamycin) is an antibiotic with broad-spectrum antineoplastic activity; however, the clinical usefulness of this drug is limited by its cardiotoxicity. Doxorubicin produces dose-related dilated cardiomyopathy. It has been suggested that doxorubicin disrupts myocardial mitochondrial calcium homeostasis. Patients treated with this drug usually have serial evaluations of left ventricular systolic function.[11]

3. Pathophysiology

The key hemodynamic features of the dilated cardiomyopathies are elevated filling pressures, failure of myocardial contractile strength, and a marked inverse relationship between afterload and stroke volume.

Both the inflammatory and noninflammatory forms of dilated cardiomyopathies present a picture identical to that of congestive heart failure produced by severe coronary artery disease, even to the extent that, in some conditions the coronary arteries are also involved by the process that has produced the cardiomyopathy. The pathophysiologic considerations are familiar ones. As the ventricular muscle weakens, the ventricle dilates to take advantage of the increased force of contraction that results from increasing myocardial fiber length. As the ventricular radius increases, however, ventricular wall tension rises, increasing both the oxygen consumption of the myocardium and the total internal work of the muscle.

As the myocardium deteriorates further, cardiac output falls, and a compensatory increase in sympathetic activity occurs to maintain organ perfusion and cardiac output. One feature of the failing myocardium is the loss of its ability to maintain stroke volume in the face of increased afterload. Figure 4–2 shows that, in the failing ventricle, stroke volume falls almost linearly with increases in afterload. The increased sympathetic outflow that accompanies left ventricular failure initiates a vicious cycle of increased resistance to forward flow, decreased stroke volume and cardiac output, and further sympathetic stimulation in an effort to maintain circulatory homeostasis.

Mitral regurgitation is common in severe dilated cardiomyopathies, owing to stretching of the mitral annulus and distortion of the geometry of the chordae tendinae (see later

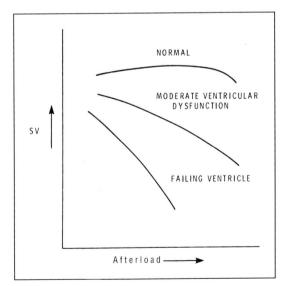

FIGURE 4–2. Stroke volume (SV) as a function of afterload for a normal left ventricle, for a left ventricle with moderate dysfunction, and for a failing left ventricle.

discussion). The forward stroke volume improves with afterload reduction, even though there is no increase in ejection fraction. This suggests that reduction of mitral regurgitation is the mechanism of the improvement. Afterload reduction also decreases left ventricular filling pressure, which relieves pulmonary congestion and should preserve coronary perfusion pressure.[12]

The clinical picture of the dilated cardiomyopathies falls into the two familiar categories of "forward" failure and "backward" failure. The features of "forward" failure, such as fatigue, hypotension, and oliguria, are due to decreases in cardiac output with reduced organ perfusion. Reduced perfusion of the kidneys results in activation of the renin-angiotensin-aldosterone system, which increases the effective circulating blood volume through sodium and water retention. "Backward" failure is related to the elevated filling pressures required by the failing ventricles. As the left ventricle dilates, "secondary" mitral regurgitation occurs. The manifestations of left-sided failure include orthopnea, paroxysmal nocturnal dyspnea, and pulmonary edema. The manifestations of right-sided failure include hepatomegaly, jugular venous distention, and peripheral edema.

4. Anesthetic Considerations

ECG monitoring is essential in the management of patients with dilated cardiomyopathies, particularly those with myocarditis. Ventricular dysrhythmias are common, and complete heart block, which can occur from these conditions, requires rapid diagnosis and treatment. The ECG is also useful in monitoring ischemic changes when coronary artery disease is associated with the cardiomyopathy, as in amyloidosis. Direct intra-arterial blood pressure monitoring during surgery provides continuous blood pressure information and a convenient route for obtaining arterial blood gases. Left-sided filling pressures are useful in the management of patients with congestive heart failure with severely compromised myocardial function. Monitoring right-sided filling pressures is of equal importance in patients whose cardiomyopathy is concomitant with pulmonary hypertension or cor pulmonale. In addition to measuring filling pressures, a thermodilution pulmonary artery catheter can be used to obtain cardiac outputs and calculate systemic and pulmo-

nary vascular resistances, which allow serial evaluation of the patient's hemodynamic status. Pacing pulmonary artery catheters and external pacemakers provide distinct advantages in managing the patient with myocarditis and associated heart block. Transesophageal echocardiography provides useful data on filling, ventricular function, severity of mitral regurgitation, and the response of the impaired ventricle to anesthetic and surgical manipulations.

The avoidance of myocardial depression still remains the goal of anesthesia management for patients with dilated cardiomyopathy (Table 4–3), although, paradoxically, carefully titrated beta-adrenergic blockade has been associated with improved hemodynamics—and possibly improved survival—in patients with dilated cardiomyopathy.[13, 14] All of the potent volatile anesthetic agents are myocardial depressants, and, for this reason, high concentrations of these agents are probably best avoided for this group of patients. An anesthetic based primarily on a combination of narcotics and sedative-hypnotics (with or without nitrous oxide) can be employed instead. For the patient with severely compromised myocardial function, the synthetic piperidine narcotics (fentanyl, sufentanil, and alfentanil) are useful, since myocardial contractility is not depressed. Chest wall rigidity associated with this technique is treated with muscle relaxants. Bradycardia associated with high-dose narcotic anesthesia may be prevented by the use of pancuronium for muscle relaxation, anticholinergic drugs, or pacing. For peripheral or lower abdominal surgical procedures, the use of a regional anesthetic technique is a reasonable alternative, provided filling pressures are carefully controlled and the hemodynamic effects of the anesthe-

TABLE 4–3

Treatment Principles of Dilated Cardiomyopathies

Clinical Problem	Treatment	Relatively Contraindicated
↓ Preload	Volume replacement	Nodal rhythm
	Positional change	High spinal
↓ Heart rate	Atropine	
	Pacemaker	Verapamil
↓ Contractility	Positive inotropes	Volatile
	Digoxin	anesthetics
↑ Afterload	Vasodilators	Phenylephrine
		Light anesthesia

tic are monitored. For shorter procedures, high-dose opioid anesthesia using remifentanil may prove to be advantageous because of the cardiovascular advantages of opioid anesthesia and the extremely short duration of action of the new drug.

In planning anesthetic management for the patient with dilated cardiomyopathy, associated cardiovascular conditions, such as coronary artery disease, valvular abnormalities, outflow tract obstruction, and constrictive pericarditis should also be considered. Patients with congestive heart failure often require circulatory support intra- and postoperatively. Inotropic drugs such as dopamine or dobutamine have been shown to be effective in low-output states and produce modest changes in systemic vascular resistance at lower doses. In severe failure, more potent drugs such as epinephrine or isoproterenol may be required. Amrinone and milrinone are phosphodiesterase III inhibitors with inotropic and vasodilating properties that may improve hemodynamic performance. As noted above, stroke volume is inversely related to afterload in the failing ventricle, and reduction of left ventricular afterload with vasodilating drugs such as nitroprusside is also effective in increasing cardiac output. In patients with myocarditis, especially of the viral variety, transvenous or external pacing may be required should heart block occur. Intra-aortic balloon counterpulsation and left ventricular assist devices are further options to be considered in the case of the severely compromised ventricle.

There is a definite increase in the incidence of supraventricular and ventricular dysrhythmias in myocarditis and the dilated cardiomyopathies.[15] These dysrhythmias often require extensive electrophysiologic workup and may be unresponsive to maximal medical therapy. Some patients present for automatic internal cardioverter-defibrillator implantation. Originally, cardioverting pads were sewn to the epicardial surface via a median sternotomy and the device was implanted in the abdominal wall. The procedure has become markedly less invasive. Presently, a transvenous coil electrode is placed in the superior vena cava, the device is implanted in the subcutaneous tissue near the deltopectoral groove, and a transvenous pacing/sensing electrode is placed in the right ventricle.[16] Intraoperative attempts to elicit dysrhythmias are necessary to test the device, and, for this reason, antidysrhythmic medications are often discontinued before surgery. Thus, proper ECG monitoring and access to a charged external cardioversion device are important details. The use of short-acting antidysrhythmia drugs, such as esmolol and intravenous lidocaine, are appropriate for treating problems encountered during the procedure.

C. HYPERTROPHIC CARDIOMYOPATHY

Hypertrophic cardiomyopathies (HCM) usually result from asymmetric hypertrophy of the basal ventricular septum and occur in either obstructive or nonobstructive forms (Table 4–4). A dynamic pressure gradient in

TABLE 4–4

Cardiomyopathies (Hypertrophic)

Disease Process	Mechanism	Associated Circulatory Problems
1. Idiopathic concentric hypertrophy	Symmetrical hypertrophy of left ventricle and outflow tract (usually nonobstructive)	
2. Hypertrophic obstructive cardiomyopathy (IHSS, ASH*)	(See text)	
3. Systemic syndromes		
a. Glycogen storage disease type II (Pompe's)	Glycogen infiltration of septal walls	1. Dilated cardiomyopathy
b. Noonan's syndrome	Left ventricular outflow obstruction	2. Coronary artery disease
c. Lentiginosis	Right and left AV-septal hypertrophy	Pulmonary stenosis

*IHSS = idiopathic hypertrophic subaortic stenosis; ASH = asymmetrical septal hypertrophy.

the left ventricular outflow tract (LVOT) is present in the obstructive forms.[17, 18] Other conditions can also produce the picture of obstructive cardiomyopathy, such as massive infiltration of the ventricular wall, as in Pompe's disease, where an accumulation of cardiac glycogen in the ventricular wall produces LVOT obstruction. The following discussion concentrates on the obstructive form.

Hypertrophic obstructive cardiomyopathy (HOCM), *asymmetric septal hypertrophy* (ASH), and *idiopathic hypertrophic subaortic stenosis* (IHSS) are all synonymous terms applied to a form of an idiopathic hypertrophic cardiomyopathy. However, it presents a picture that is typical of the problems encountered in virtually all forms of obstructive cardiomyopathy. The salient anatomic feature of HOCM is hypertrophy of ventricular muscle at the base of the septum in the LVOT. Histologically, this is a disorganized mass of hypertrophic myocardial cells extending from the left ventricular septal wall, often involving the papillary muscles. Intramural ("small-vessel") coronary artery disease has been identified in autopsy specimens, especially in areas of myocardial fibrosis. This may represent a congenital component of the disease and probably plays some role in the development of myocardial ischemia in these patients.[19]

Obstruction of the LVOT is caused by the hypertrophic muscle mass and systolic anterior motion of the anterior leaflet of the mitral valve. The systolic anterior motion may be caused by a Venturi effect. A subaortic pressure gradient is present in symptomatic patients. The outflow tract obstruction can result in hypertrophy of the remainder of the ventricular muscle secondary to increased pressures in the ventricular chamber. As the ventricle hypertrophies, ventricular compliance decreases, and passive filling of the ventricle during diastole is impaired. For this reason, the ventricle becomes increasingly dependent on atrial contraction to maintain adequate ventricular end-diastolic volume. Occasionally, HOCM is associated with a right ventricular outflow tract obstruction as well.

The determinants of the functional severity of the ventricular obstruction in HOCM are (1) the systolic volume of the ventricle, (2) the force of ventricular contraction, and (3) the transmural pressure distending the outflow tract. Large systolic volumes in the ventricle distend the outflow tract and reduce the obstruction, whereas small systolic volumes narrow the outflow tract and increase the obstruction. When ventricular contractility is high, the outflow tract is narrowed, increasing the obstruction. When aortic pressure is high, there is an increased transmural pressure that distends the LVOT. During periods of hypotension, however, the outflow tract is narrowed. This results in markedly impaired cardiac output and sometimes mitral regurgitation, as the mitral valve becomes the relief point for ventricular pressure.

The medical therapy of HOCM has been based on beta blockers; however, it is still not clear if life expectancy is prolonged by this treatment. In the past several years, verapamil has been used with increasing frequency. Its beneficial effects are likely due to depression of systolic function, and an improvement in diastolic filling and relaxation. Disopyramide, verapamil, and amiodarone are also administered to HOCM patients for control of supraventricular and ventricular dysrhythmias.[20]

Approximately 85 per cent of HOCM patients are treated with only medical therapy. The surgical therapy of HOCM is either myotomy/myomectomy, mitral valve replacement, or a combination of the two. While mitral valve replacement results in the greatest reduction in outflow tract pressure gradient, there remain all the potential complications associated with valve prostheses. The potential complications of myotomy or myomectomy include complete heart block and late formation of a ventricular septal defect due to septal infarction.[21]

In recent years, dual-chamber (atrioventricular sequential) pacing has been shown to result in delayed improvement in HOCM-associated LVOT obstruction.[22, 23] Dual-chamber pacing, therefore, should not be considered as a therapeutic option for the acute perioperative management of patients with HOCM.

1. Anesthetic Considerations

Patients with HOCM may be extremely sensitive to small changes in ventricular volume, blood pressure, heart rate, and rhythm. Accordingly, monitoring should be established that allows continuous assessment of these parameters, particularly in patients whose obstruction is severe. In patients with HOCM coming to surgery for mitral valve replacement and/or septal myomectomy, the ECG, an indwelling arterial catheter, and a pulmonary artery catheter are necessary monitors. Transesophageal echocardiography also provides useful data on ventricular function and filling and on the severity of LVOT obstruction.

In patients with HOCM coming for other procedures, the hemodynamic monitors should provide some indication of ventricular volume, force of ventricular contraction, and transmural pressure distending the outflow tract. An indwelling arterial catheter is almost always indicated for beat-to-beat observation of ventricular ejection during major regional or general anesthesia in patients with symptomatic HOCM. Intraoperative echocardiography is the most accurate monitor of ventricular loading conditions and performance in HOCM.

In the anesthetic management of patients with HOCM, special consideration should be given to those features of the surgical procedure and anesthetic drugs that can produce changes in intravascular volume, ventricular contractility, and transmural distending pressure of the outflow tract. Decreased preload, for example, can be produced by blood loss, sympathectomy secondary to spinal or epidural anesthesia, the use of nitroglycerin, or postural changes. Ventricular contractility can be increased by hemodynamic responses to tracheal intubation or surgical stimulation.

Transmural distending pressure can be decreased by hypotension secondary to anesthetic drugs, hypovolemia, or positive-pressure ventilation. In addition, increases in heart rate are poorly tolerated by patients with HOCM. Tachycardia decreases systolic ventricular volume and results in a narrowed outflow tract. As noted above, the atrial contraction is extremely important to the hypertrophic ventricle. Nodal rhythms should be treated aggressively, using atrial pacing if necessary.

Halothane has major hemodynamic advantages for the anesthetic management of patients with this condition. Halothane decreases heart rate and myocardial contractility, and tends to minimize the severity of the obstruction when volume replacement is adequate. Sevoflurane, isoflurane, and enflurane cause more peripheral vasodilation than halothane and are less desirable for this reason. Agents that release histamine, such as morphine and many benzylisoquinolinium neuromuscular blockers, are not recommended owing to the venodilatation and hypovolemia they produce. Agents with sympathomimetic side effects (i.e., ketamine and desflurane) are not recommended. High-dose

TABLE 4–5

Treatment Principles of HOCM

Clinical Problem	Treatment	Relatively Contraindicated
↓ Preload	Volume replacement Phenylephrine	Vasodilators Spinal, epidural
↑ Heart rate	Beta blockers Verapamil	Ketamine Beta-agonists
↑ Contractility	Halothane Enflurane	Positive inotropes Light anesthesia
↓ Afterload	Phenylephrine	Isoflurane Spinal, epidural

opioid anesthesia causes minimal cardiovascular side effects along with bradycardia, and thus may be a useful anesthetic technique in these patients. Preoperative beta-blocker and calcium channel–blocker therapy should be continued. Intravenous propranolol, esmolol, diltiazem, or verapamil may be administered intraoperatively to improve hemodynamic performance. Table 4–5 summarizes the anesthetic and circulatory management of HOCM.

Anesthesia for management for labor and delivery in the parturient with HOCM is quite complex. Beta-blocker therapy may have been discontinued during pregnancy because of the association with fetal bradycardia and intrauterine growth retardation. Spinal and epidural anesthesia are relatively contraindicated because of the associated vasodilation. If hypotension occurs during anesthesia, the use of beta-agonists such as ephedrine may result in worsening outflow tract obstruction, while alpha-agonists such as phenylephrine could potentially result in uterine vasoconstriction. Successful management of cesarean section with both general and epidural anesthetics has been reported; however, careful titration of anesthetic agents and adequate volume loading (guided by invasive monitoring) are essential to the safe conduct of anesthesia in this clinical setting.[24, 25]

D. RESTRICTIVE/OBLITERATIVE CARDIOMYOPATHY

Restrictive cardiomyopathies are usually the end stage of myocarditis or of an infiltrative process of the myocardium such as amyloidosis or hemochromatosis (Table 4–6). When a restrictive cardiomyopathy occurs, it mimics constrictive pericarditis coupled with

TABLE 4–6

Cardiomyopathies (Restrictive/Obliterative—Including Restrictive Endocarditis)

Disease Process	Mechanism	Associated Circulatory Problems	Miscellaneous
1. End stage of acute myocarditis	Fibrous replacement of myofibrils		

2. Metabolic
  a. Amyloidosis
  b. Hemochromatosis
	Amyloid infiltration of myocardium
	Iron deposition and secondary fibrous proliferation
		1. Valvular malfunction
		2. Coronary artery disease
		Conduction abnormalities	

3. Drugs—methysergide (Sansert)	Endocardial fibroelastosis	Valvular stenosis	Similar to changes in carcinoid syndrome
4. Restrictive endocarditis	Picture very similar to constrictive pericarditis		
a. Carcinoid	Serotonin-producing carcinoid tumors—but serotonin is apparently not causative agent for fibrosis	1. Pulmonary stenosis 2. Tricuspid insufficiency and/or stenosis 3. Right-sided heart failure	
b. Endomyocardial fibrosis	Fibrous obliteration of ventricular cavities	Mitral and tricuspid insufficiency	
b. Loeffler's disease	Fibrosis of endocardium with decreased myocardial contraction	Subendocardial and papillary muscle degeneration and fibrosis	
d. Becker's disease	Similar to Loeffler's	Similar to Loeffler's	

myocardial dysfunction. Pulsus alternans occurs in both restrictive cardiomyopathies and constrictive pericarditis. Restrictive cardiomyopathies are characterized by impaired ventricular filling and poor ventricular contractility. Cardiac output is maintained in the early stages by elevated filling pressures and increased heart rate; however, in contrast to constrictive pericarditis, an increase in myocardial contractility to maintain cardiac output is usually not possible. Diseases such as endocardial fibroelastosis appear similar to restrictive cardiomyopathy in that there is impairment of diastolic ventricular filling but differ in that contractility is not usually impaired.[2]

1. Anesthetic Considerations

Anesthetic and monitoring considerations in restrictive cardiomyopathies are virtually identical to those of constrictive pericarditis and cardiac tamponade with the additional feature of poor ventricular function. The combination of a restrictive and a dilated cardiomyopathy results in a more precarious situation than either condition alone. The reader is referred to the section on constrictive pericarditis for a more detailed discussion of the physiology and management of restrictive ventricular filling, and to the section on dilated cardiomyopathy for the management of impaired ventricular function. The anesthetic management must be tailored for whichever feature, restrictive physiology or heart failure, is predominant in a particular patient.

III. CARDIAC TUMORS

A. INTRODUCTION

Primary tumors of the heart are unusual; however, the likelihood of encountering a cardiac tumor increases when metastatic tumors of the heart and pericardium are considered. For example, breast and lung cancer metastasize frequently to the heart. Two-dimensional echocardiography and angiography are the major modalities for preoperative diagnosis of these lesions. Primary cardiac tumors may occur in any chamber or in the pericardium, and may arise from any cardiac tissue. Of the benign cardiac tumors, myxoma is the most common, followed by lipoma, papillary fibroelastoma, rhabdomyoma, fibroma, and hemangioma (Table 4–7).[26]

The generally favorable prognosis for patients with benign cardiac tumors is in sharp

TABLE 4–7

Primary Neoplasms of the Heart and Pericardium

Type	Cases	Percentage
Benign		
Myxoma	130	29.3
Lipoma	45	10.1
Papillary fibroelastoma	42	9.5
Rhabdomyoma	36	8.1
Fibroma	17	3.8
Hemangioma	15	3.4
Teratoma	14	3.2
Mesothelioma of AV node	12	2.7
Granular cell tumor	3	0.7
Neurofibroma	3	0.7
Lymphangioma	2	0.5
Subtotal	319	72.0
Malignant		
Angiosarcoma	39	8.8
Rhabdomyosarcoma	26	5.8
Mesothelioma	19	4.2
Fibrosarcoma	14	3.2
Malignant lymphoma	7	1.6
Extraskeletal osteosarcoma	5	1.1
Neurogenic sarcoma	4	0.9
Malignant teratoma	4	0.9
Thymoma	4	0.9
Leiomyosarcoma	1	0.2
Liposarcoma	1	0.2
Synovial sarcoma	1	0.2
Subtotal	125	28.0
Total	444	100.0

Adapted with permission from McAllister HA Jr, Fenoglio JJ Jr: Tumors of the cardiovascular system. *In* Atlas of Tumor Pathology (Fascicle 15). Washington, D.C., Armed Forces Institute of Pathology, 1978.

contrast to the prognosis for those with malignant ones. The diagnosis of a malignant primary cardiac tumor is seldom made before extensive local involvement and metastasis have occurred, making curative surgical resection unlikely. An aggressive approach, including surgery, radiotherapy, and chemotherapy, has not significantly altered the poor outlook for these patients.[27]

B. BENIGN CARDIAC TUMORS

Myxomas are most frequently benign. They typically originate from the region adjacent to the fossa ovalis and project into the left atrium. They are usually pedunculated masses that resemble organized clot on microscopy, and may be gelatinous or firm. A left atrial myxoma may prolapse into the mi-tral valve during diastole. This prolapsing action results in a ball-valve obstruction to left ventricular inflow that mimics mitral stenosis and may also cause valvular damage by a "wrecking-ball" effect. More friable tumors result in systemic or pulmonary embolization, depending on their location and on the presence of any intracardiac shunts. Cerebral arterial aneurysms are associated with cerebral embolization of myxoma tissue. Pulmonary hypertension may be present, owing to mitral valve obstruction by a left atrial myxoma or pulmonary embolization in the case of a right atrial myxoma. Atrial fibrillation may be present secondary to atrial volume overload. Two-dimensional echocardiography can delineate the location and consistency of these tumors with good precision. Angiography is also valuable but may be complicated by catheter-induced embolization of tumor fragments. Surgical therapy requires careful manipulation of the heart before institution of cardio-pulmonary bypass to avoid embolization, and resection of the base of the tumor (with repair by patching) to prevent recurrence.[28]

Other benign cardiac tumors occur less frequently. In general, intracavitary tumors result in valvular dysfunction or obstruction to flow, and tumors localized in the myocardium cause conduction abnormalities and dysrhythmias. Papilloma (papillary fibroelastoma) is usually a single villous connective tissue tumor that results in valvular incompetence or coronary ostial obstruction. Cardiac lipoma is an encapsulated collection of mature fat cells. Lipomatous hypertrophy of the interatrial septum is a related disorder of elderly women that results in right atrial obstruction. Rhabdomyoma is a tumor of cardiac muscle that occurs in childhood and is associated with tuberous sclerosis. Fibroma is another childhood cardiac tumor.[29]

C. MALIGNANT CARDIAC TUMORS

Approximately 25 per cent of primary cardiac tumors are malignant, and almost all of these are sarcomas. The curative therapy of sarcomas is based on wide local excision, which is not possible in the heart. In addition, the propensity toward early metastasis contributes to the dismal prognosis. Rhabdomyosarcoma may occur in neonates, but most cardiac sarcomas occur in adults. Sarcomas may originate from vascular tissue, cardiac or smooth muscle, and any other cardiac tissue. Palliative surgery may be indicated to relieve symptoms due to mass effects. These tumors respond poorly to radiotherapy and chemotherapy.[27]

D. METASTATIC CARDIAC TUMORS

Breast cancer, lung cancer, lymphomas, and leukemia may all result in cardiac metastases. About one fifth of patients who die of cancer have cardiac metastases. Thus, metastatic cardiac tumors are much more common than primary ones. Myocardial involvement results in congestive heart failure and may be classified as a restrictive cardiomyopathy. Pericardial involvement results in cardiac compression because of tumor mass or tamponade due to effusion. Melanoma is particularly prone to cardiac metastasis.

E. CARDIAC MANIFESTATIONS OF EXTRACARDIAC TUMORS

Carcinoid is a tumor of neural crest origin that secretes serotonin, bradykinin, and other vasoactive substances. Hepatic carcinoid metastases result in right-sided valvular lesions, presumably from a secretory product that is metabolized in the pulmonary circulation. Recently, serotonin itself has been implicated in the pathogenesis of tricuspid valve dysfunction.[30, 31] The end results are thickened valve leaflets that may be stenotic or incompetent, although regurgitation is more common. Even though the tricuspid valve is most commonly involved, this process may involve both right- and left-sided valves.

Pheochromocytoma is a catecholamine-secreting tumor also of neural crest origin. Chronic catecholamine excess has toxic effects on the myocardium that may result in dilated cardiomyopathy.

F. ANESTHETIC CONSIDERATIONS

The presence of a cardiac tumor requires a careful preoperative echocardiographic assessment of cardiac morphology and function. A right-sided tumor (especially myxoma) is a relative contraindication to pulmonary artery catheter insertion because of the risk of embolization, although it may be possible to advance the catheter through the right ventricle after the tumor is resected. Two-dimensional transesophageal echocardiography is well-suited for the intraoperative monitoring of these patients (Fig. 4–3). Left atrial myxomas are well-visualized by this technique; however, caution should be exercised in the manipulation of the transesophageal probe to prevent embolization of friable tumors attached to the posterior wall of the left atrium, because of the proximity of the probe. The management of a left atrial myxoma is similar to that of mitral stenosis (see later discussion). A slow heart rate and high preload should maximize ventricular filling in the presence of an obstructing tumor.

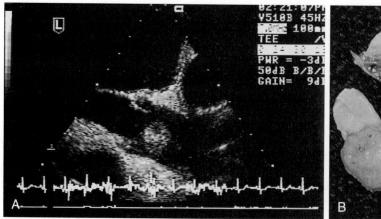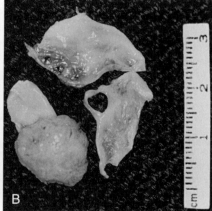

FIGURE 4–3. *A,* Transesophageal image of a mass on the right cusp of the aortic valve. *B,* Photograph of the resected aortic valve (from the same patient) with the tumor attached to the right cusp.

In the absence of a right-sided intracavitary tumor, pulmonary artery catheterization is useful for assessing cardiac function impaired by restrictive cardiomyopathy, pericardial tumor, pericardial effusion, or an obstructive lesion. Avoidance of myocardial depressants such as the potent volatile agents and the maintenance of an adequate heart rate are optimal in this scenario. Smaller induction doses of ketamine (0.25 to 1.0 mg/kg) or etomidate should minimize hypotension on induction with severely compromised ventricular function.

IV. ISCHEMIC HEART DISEASE

A. INTRODUCTION

The most important aspects of coronary artery disease remain the same no matter what the cause of the obstruction of the coronary arteries (Table 4–8). Like coronary artery disease produced by arteriosclerosis, the coronary artery disease produced by an uncommon disease retains the same key clinical features. Physiologic considerations remain

---

TABLE 4–8

Uncommon Causes of Coronary Artery Disease

I. Coronary artery disease associated with cardiomyopathy (poor left ventricular function)
  A. Pathologic basis—infiltration of coronary arteries with luminal narrowing
    1. Amyloidosis—valvular stenosis, restrictive cardiomyopathy
    2. Fabry's disease—hypertension
    3. Hurler's syndrome—often associated with valvular malfunction
    4. Hunter's syndrome—often associated with valvular malfunction
    5. Primary xanthomatosis—aortic stenosis
    6. Leukemia—anemia
    7. Pseudoxanthoma elasticum—valve abnormalities
  B. Inflammation of coronary arteries
    1. Rheumatic fever—in acute phase
    2. Rheumatoid arthritis—aortic and mitral regurgitation, constrictive pericarditis
    3. Periarteritis nodosa—hypertension
    4. Systemic lupus erythematosus—hypertension, renal failure, mitral valve malfunction
  C. Embolic or thrombotic occlusion of coronary arteries

    1. Schistosomiasis ⎫ cor pulmonale
    2. Sickle cell anemia ⎬ depending on length
                        ⎪ and extent of
                        ⎭ involvement

  D. Fibrous and hyaline degeneration of coronary arteries
    1. Posttransplantation
    2. Radiation
    3. Duchenne's muscular dystrophy
    4. Friedreich's ataxia—? associated with HOCM
    5. Roussy Lévy—hereditary polyneuropathy
  E. Anatomical abnormalities of coronary arteries
    1. Bland-White-Garland syndrome (left coronary artery arising from pulmonary artery)—endocardial fibroelastosis, mitral regurgitation
    2. Ostial stenosis secondary to ankylosing spondylitis—aortic regurgitation

II. Coronary artery disease usually associated with normal ventricular function
  A. Anatomic abnormalities of coronary arteries
    1. Right coronary arising from pulmonary artery
    2. Coronary AV fistula
    3. Coronary sinus aneurysm
    4. Dissecting aneurysm
    5. Ostial stenosis—bacterial overgrowth, syphilitic aortic
    6. Coronary artery trauma—penetrating or nonpenetrating
    7. Spontaneous coronary artery rupture
    8. Kawasaki's disease—coronary artery aneurysm
  B. Embolic or thrombotic occlusion
    1. Coronary emboli
    2. Malaria and/or malarial infested red blood cells
    3. Thrombotic thrombocytopenic purpura
    4. Polycythemia vera
  C. Infections
    1. Miliary tuberculosis—intimal involvement of coronary arteries
    2. Arteritis secondary to salmonella or endemic typhus (associated with active myocarditis)
  D. Infiltration of coronary arteries
    1. Gout—conduction abnormalities, possible valve problems
    2. Homocystinuria
  E. Coronary artery spasm
  F. Cocaine
  G. Miscellaneous
    1. Thromboangiitis obliterans (Buerger's disease)
    2. Takayasu's arteritis

essentially the same, as do treatment and anesthetic management.

In the preoperative assessment, the symptoms produced by the coronary artery disease should be determined. The obvious symptoms to look for in the history are angina, the patient's exercise limitations, and symptoms of myocardial failure, such as orthopnea or paroxysmal nocturnal dyspnea. The physical examination retains its importance, especially when quantitative data on cardiac involvement are not available. Physical findings such as S_3 and S_4 heart sounds are important, as are auscultatory signs of uncommon conditions such as cardiac bruits, which might occur in a coronary arteriovenous fistula. If catheterization data are available, the specifics of coronary artery anatomy and ventricular function, such as end-diastolic pressure, ejection fraction, and the presence of wall motion abnormalities are all useful. Information on ventricular perfusion and function can also be obtained by noninvasive means such as echocardiography and nuclear imaging.[32]

After the extent of coronary insufficiency is ascertained, the special aspects of the disease entity producing the coronary insufficiency should be considered. As an example, in ankylosing spondylitis, coronary insufficiency is produced by ostial stenosis, yet valvular problems often coexist and even overshadow the coronary artery disease. In rheumatoid arthritis, however, airway problems may be the most significant part of the anesthetic challenge. Hypertension, which frequently coexists with arteriosclerotic coronary artery disease, is also a feature of the coronary artery disease produced by Fabry's disease. Other features to consider are metabolic disturbances that coexist with the coronary artery disease, such as when systemic lupus erythematosus (SLE) produces both coronary artery disease and renal failure.[33]

B. PHYSIOLOGY OF CORONARY ARTERY DISEASE AND ITS MODIFICATION BY UNUSUAL DISEASES

The key to the physiology of coronary artery disease is the balance of myocardial oxygen supply and demand (Fig. 4–4). Myocardial oxygen supply depends on many factors, including the patency of the coronary arteries, hemoglobin concentration, P_aO_2, and the coro-

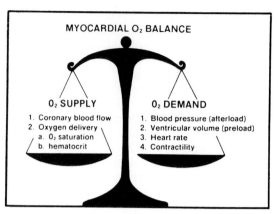

FIGURE 4–4. Myocardial oxygen supply and demand balance.

nary perfusion pressure. The same factors determine supply in uncommon diseases, but the specific manner in which an uncommon disease modifies these factors should be sought. A knowledge of the anatomy of the coronary circulation and how arterial patency can be affected by the disease process is a useful starting point. This information is usually gained from coronary angiography. In the assessment of the adequacy of coronary perfusion, the viscosity of the blood should be considered, since flow is a function both of the dimensions of the conduit and the nature of the fluid in the system. In disease processes such as thrombotic thrombocytopenic purpura, sickle cell disease, or polycythemia vera, the altered blood viscosity can assume critical importance.[34, 35]

Oxygen-carrying capacity must also be considered in certain uncommon disease states. Hemoglobin concentration usually is not a limiting factor in the supply of oxygen to the myocardium; however, in diseases such as leukemia, anemia may be a prominent feature, and the myocardial oxygen supply may be reduced accordingly. Another example is myocardial ischemia in carbon monoxide poisoning, when the hemoglobin, albeit quantitatively sufficient, cannot carry oxygen. Similarly, the P_aO_2 usually is not a limiting factor, but in conditions where coronary artery disease is intercurrent with cor pulmonale, as in schistosomiasis or sickle cell disease, the inability to maintain adequate oxygenation may limit the myocardial oxygen supply. In fact, in sickle cell disease, it may be the key feature, since failure to maintain an adequate P_aO_2, secondary to repeated pulmonary infarctions, further increases the tendency of cells containing hemoglobin S to sickle, compromising myocardial oxygen delivery through sludging in the coronary microcirculation.

The major determinants of myocardial oxygen demand include heart rate, ventricular wall tension, and myocardial contractility. Tachycardia and hypertension after tracheal intubation, skin incision, or other noxious stimuli are common causes of increased myocardial oxygen demand during surgery. In addition, complicating factors of an unusual disease may also produce increases in demand. Increases in rate may occur as a result of tachydysrhythmias secondary to sinoatrial (SA) or atrioventricular (AV) node involvement in amyloidosis or in Friedreich's ataxia. Increases in wall tension, for example, may occur in severe hypertension associated with SLE, polyarteritis nodosa, or Fabry's disease. Outflow tract obstruction with increased ventricular work can occur in primary xanthomatosis or in tertiary syphilis; and an increase in the diastolic ventricular radius with increased wall tension can occur in situations such as aortic regurgitation associated with ankylosing spondylitis.

Modern cardiac anesthesia practice should attempt to tailor the anesthetic management to the problems posed by the peculiarities of the coronary anatomy. For example, knowledge of the presence of a lesion in the left main coronary artery dictates great care during anesthesia to avoid even modest hypotension or tachycardia. Lesions of the right coronary artery are known to be associated with an increased incidence of atrial dysrhythmias and heart block, and steps must be taken either to treat these or to compensate for their cardiovascular effects.

In diseases such as primary xanthomatosis or Hurler's syndrome, the infiltrative process that produces coronary artery disease usually involves the coronary arteries diffusely, but some diseases may have features that can mimic either isolated left main coronary artery disease or right coronary artery disease. The Bland-White-Garland syndrome, which is anomalous origin of the left coronary artery from the pulmonary artery, or coronary ostial stenosis produced by an aortic valve prosthesis, may both behave as left main coronary artery disease. A similar syndrome could be produced by bacterial overgrowth of the coronary ostia, ankylosing spondylitis, a dissecting aneurysm of the aorta, or Takayasu's arteritis. Right coronary artery disease could

be mimicked by the syndrome of the anomalous origin of the right coronary artery from the pulmonary artery, or infiltration of the SA or AV nodes in amyloidosis or Friedreich's ataxia. In small-artery arteritis, which occurs in polyarteritis nodosa or SLE, the small arteries supplying the SA or AV node may be involved in the pathologic process, producing ischemia of the conduction system.

In Table 4–8, the uncommon diseases that produce coronary artery disease have been divided into those that produce coronary artery disease associated with good left ventricular function and those associated with poor left ventricular function. In any of these diseases, ventricular function can regress from good to poor. In some conditions, the coronary artery disease progression and ventricular function deterioration occur at the same rate, and left ventricular function is eventually severely depressed. In other situations, coronary insufficiency is primary, and left ventricular dysfunction eventually occurs after repeated episodes of ischemia or thrombosis. Ventricular function must be evaluated by clinical signs and symptoms, echocardiography, nuclear imaging, or cardiac catheterization. The converse is severe arterial disease coupled with relatively good left ventricular function. This is the picture of a cardiomyopathy associated with almost incidental coronary artery disease, as occurs in Hurler's syndrome, amyloidosis, or systemic lupus erythematosus. Most anatomic lesions, such as Kawasaki's disease, coronary AV fistula, and coronary insufficiency produced by trauma, are usually associated with good left ventricular function. There is a clinical gray zone in which coronary artery disease and poor left ventricular function coexist without either process clearly predominating, such as with tuberculosis and syphilis. These can be characterized only by investigating the extent of involvement of the coronary arteries and the myocardium in the disease process. What follows is a more detailed discussion of a few selected disease states that affect the coronary arteries.

C. SOME UNCOMMON CAUSES OF ISCHEMIC HEART DISEASE

1. Coronary Artery Spasm

The luminal narrowing of the coronary arteries secondary to spasm has been associated with angina and myocardial infarction.[36, 37] The mechanism of coronary artery spasm remains unclear. The smooth muscle cells of the coronary artery walls may contract in response to various stimuli. There may be abnormal response to various vasoactive substances,[38] and, in addition, there may be increased alpha-adrenergic tone.[39] Another theory is that vessels with eccentric atherosclerotic plaques have a segment of disease-free wall that may be a site for vasospasm, which can convert an insignificant obstruction into a critical lesion. Coronary artery vasospasm may respond to nitroglycerin and calcium channel blockers.

2. Cocaine Abuse

Cocaine can affect the heart in several ways, and the use of cocaine can result in myocardial ischemia, myocardial infarction, and sudden death.[40] Cocaine exerts its effects on the heart mainly by two mechanisms: its ability to block sodium channels, resulting in a local anesthetic or membrane-stabilizing property; and its ability to block reuptake of norepinephrine, resulting in increased sympathetic activity. It is not surprising, therefore, that cocaine when administered acutely has been shown to have a biphasic effect on left ventricular function with transient depression followed by a sustained increase in contractility.[41] Cocaine also induces coronary vasospasm and reduced coronary blood flow while at the same time increasing heart rate and blood pressure. These effects decrease myocardial oxygen supply and increase myocardial oxygen demand. In addition, cocaine and its metabolites can induce platelets to aggregate and release platelet-derived growth factor, which can promote fibrointimal proliferation and accelerated atherosclerosis.[42] Chronic users of cocaine also have an exaggerated response to sympathetic stimuli, which may contribute to the left ventricular hypertrophy frequently observed among long-time users.

3. Coronary Artery Dissection

When there is separation of the intimal layer from the medial layer of the coronary artery, there may be obstruction of the true coronary artery lumen with subsequent distal myocardial ischemia. Coronary artery dissection may be primary or secondary. Primary coronary artery dissection may occur during coronary artery catheterization or angioplasty and in trauma to the heart. Primary coronary artery dissection may also occur spontaneously. Spontaneous dissection is usually associated with coronary arterial wall eosinophils and is seen in the postpartum period. Secondary coronary artery dissection is more common and is usually caused by a dissection in the ascending aorta.

4. Inflammatory Causes

a. Infectious Causes

Infectious coronary artery arteritis may be secondary to hematogenous spread or to direct extension from infectious processes of adjacent tissue. The infectious process results in thrombosis of the involved artery with myocardial ischemia. Syphilis is one of the most common infectious agents to affect the coronary arteries. As many as 25 per cent of patients with tertiary syphilis have ostial stenosis of their coronary arteries.[43]

b. Noninfectious Causes

i. Polyarteritis Nodosa

This is a systemic necrotizing vasculitis involving medium-sized and small vessels. Epicardial coronary arteries are involved in the majority of cases of polyarteritis nodosa. Following the initial inflammatory response, the coronary artery may dilate to form small berrylike aneurysms that may rupture, producing fatal pericardial tamponade.

ii. Systemic Lupus Erythematosus

The pericardium and myocardium are usually affected in SLE. Patients with SLE, however, may suffer acute myocardial infarction in the absence of atherosclerotic coronary artery disease. The hypercoagulable state of SLE, together with a predisposition to premature coronary atherosclerosis, have been implicated. In addition, steroids used for the treatment of SLE may also predispose these patients to accelerated atherosclerosis.

iii. Kawasaki's Disease

Kawasaki's (or mucocutaneous lymph node syndrome) is a disease of childhood. A vasculitis of the coronary vasa vasorum leads to weakened walls of the vessels with subsequent coronary artery aneurysm formation. Thrombosis and myocardial ischemia can also occur. These patients are prone to sudden death from ventricular arrhythmias and occasionally from rupture of a coronary artery aneurysm. Thrombus in the aneurysm may also embolize, causing myocardial ischemia.

iv. Takayasu's Disease

Takayasu's disease leads to fibrosis and luminal narrowing of the aorta and its branches. The coronary ostia may be involved in this process.

5. Metabolic Disorders

a. Homocystinuria

There is an increased incidence of atherosclerotic disease in patients with high levels of homocysteine.[44] This process may involve intimal proliferation of small coronary vessels. Patients with high homocysteine levels are at increased risk of myocardial infarction.

6. Congenital Abnormalities of the Coronary Arterial Circulation

a. Left Coronary Artery Arising from the Pulmonary Artery

This lesion is also known as Bland-White-Garland syndrome. The right coronary artery arises from the aorta, but the left coronary arises from the pulmonary artery. Flow in the left coronary arterial system is retrograde with severe hypoperfusion of the left ventricle with myocardial ischemia and infarction. As such, most patients with this disease present in infancy with evidence of heart failure. Untreated patients usually die during infancy. Patients who survive childhood may present with mitral regurgitation from annular dilatation. The goals of medical therapy are to treat congenital heart failure and arrhythmias. The defect can be corrected surgically by primary anastomosis of the left coronary artery to the aorta. In older children, a vein graft or the left internal mammary artery may be used to establish antegrade flow in the left coronary arterial system. Improvement in left ventricular function can be expected of surgical survivors if this operation is performed early.[45]

b. Coronary Arteriovenous Fistula

There is an anatomic communication between a coronary artery and a right-sided structure such as the right atrium, right ventricle, or coronary sinus. The right coronary artery is more frequently affected and is usually connected to the coronary sinus. Most patients are asymptomatic; however, the left-to-right shunt created by the fistula may lead to pulmonary congestion and pulmonary hypertension. These patients are at risk for endocarditis, myocardial ischemia, and rupture of the fistulous connection. These fistulas should be corrected surgically.

D. ANESTHETIC CONSIDERATIONS

The functional impairment of the myocardium and coronary circulation dictates the extent and type of monitoring to be employed. The selection of ECG leads to monitor is dictated by knowledge of the coronary anatomy. Those diseases in which there is left coronary artery disease are best monitored using precordial leads, such as the V5 lead. In diseases with right coronary artery disease, ECG leads used to assess the inferior surface of the heart (leads II, III, or AVF) or the posterior surface (esophageal lead) are preferable.[46]

Knowledge of ventricular filling pressures is especially important in diseases associated with poor ventricular function. The use of a pulmonary artery catheter is preferable to central venous pressure monitoring in the assessment of left ventricular function. The cause of large V waves on the pulmonary capillary wedge pressure waveform that sometimes occur during myocardial ischemia is probably a decrease in diastolic ventricular compliance; however, large V waves did not correlate with other determinants of myocardial ischemia in a study of vascular surgical patients with coronary artery disease.[47]

Two-dimensional transesophageal echocardiography is an extremely important monitor of both ventricular function and myocardial ischemia. It can demonstrate regional changes in wall motion that are sensitive signs of myocardial ischemia.[48] Urine output is another important parameter, and is especially significant in diseases associated with nephropathy, such as long-standing sickle cell disease or SLE.

When severe cardiomyopathy associated with coronary artery disease exists, monitoring cardiac output and systemic vascular resistance is useful in evaluating both the effects of anesthetic drugs and therapeutic interventions. A pulmonary artery catheter is clearly indicated in patients requiring all but the most minor procedures. An indwelling arterial catheter for monitoring arterial blood gases is important, especially where pulmonary disease or cor pulmonale complicates the picture, as in schistosomiasis or sickle cell disease.

One caveat should be noted in the use of intra-arterial monitoring. When peripheral arterial monitoring is used in cases of generalized arteritis, the adequacy of collateral blood flow should be carefully evaluated before cannulation of the peripheral artery. In occlusive diseases, such as Raynaud's disease, Takayasu's arteritis, or Buerger's disease, or in cases of sludging in the microcirculation, as in sickle cell disease, the area distal to the cannulated artery should be checked frequently for signs of arterial insufficiency.

The anesthetic employed in these conditions should be tailored to the degree of myocardial dysfunction.[49] In cases of pure coronary insufficiency with good left ventricular function, anesthetic management is aimed at decreasing oxygen demand by decreasing myocardial contractility while preserving oxygen supply by maintaining blood pressure. Techniques commonly employed include the combination of a volatile anesthetic agent with nitrous oxide, or a nitrous-narcotic technique that employs intermittent use of vasodilators such as nitroprusside or nitroglycerin for control of hypertension.

When coronary vasospasm is considered, it is important to maintain a relatively high coronary perfusion pressure. Pharmacologic agents such as nitroglycerin and calcium channel blockers may also be used. Patients who are chronic users of cocaine should be considered at high risk for ischemic heart disease and arrhythmias. These patients may respond unpredictably to anesthetic agents and other drugs used in the perioperative period.

In patients with poor ventricular function, the anesthetic technique should maintain hemodynamic stability by avoiding drugs that produce significant degrees of myocardial depression. High-dose opioid techniques or opioid-benzodiazepine combinations have been found to be effective.[50, 51] In polyarteritis nodosa or Fabry's disease, hypertension is often associated with poor left ventricular function. In such situations, a vasodilator such as sodium nitroprusside or nitroglycerin can be used to control hypertension rather than a volatile anesthetic. The principles for the management of intraoperative dysrhythmias remain the same as for the treatment of dysrhythmias in the setting of atherosclerotic coronary artery disease. Regional anesthesia requires monitoring that will allow appropriate management of associated sympathetic blockade.

V. PULMONARY HYPERTENSION AND COR PULMONALE

A. PULMONARY HYPERTENSION

Pulmonary hypertension is defined as an elevation of the pulmonary artery pressure above the accepted limit of normal, regardless of the cause. The accepted upper limit of normal is about 35/15 mm Hg, or a mean pulmonary artery pressure of 20 mm Hg. Pulmonary hypertension has been further subdivided into mild, moderate, and severe forms by some authors.[52]

The normal pulmonary vasculature changes from a high-resistance circuit in utero to a lower-resistance circuit in newborns secondary to several concomitant changes: (1) the relief of hypoxic vasoconstriction that occurs with the first spontaneous breath; (2) the stenting effect of air-filled lungs on the pulmonary vessels, which increases their caliber and decreases their resistance; and (3) the functional closure of the ductus arteriosus, secondary to an increase in the P_aO_2. The muscular medial layer of the fetal pulmonary arterioles normally involutes in postnatal life. Assuming there is no severe active vasoconstriction, pulmonary artery pressure remains low owing to the numerous parallel vascular channels that accept increased blood flow as pulmonary blood volume is increased. For this reason, pressure is not normally increased in the pulmonary circuit, since increased pulmonary blood flow distends the pulmonary vessels, lowering their resistance.

Three general pathologic conditions can occur that will convert this normally low-resistance circuit into a high-resistance circuit: (1) increases in capillary or pulmonary venous pressures; (2) decreases in the cross-sectional area of the vasculature; or (3) increases in pulmonary arterial blood flow. Table 4–9, which lists causes of pulmonary hypertension, is arranged according to these three pathophysiologic mechanisms.

Increases in capillary or pulmonary venous pressure may be caused by conditions such as left ventricular failure, mitral regurgitation, and mitral stenosis. In addition to the passive increase in pulmonary blood volume, active vasoconstriction also occurs in the pulmonary vascular bed. Hypoxic vasoconstriction induced by ventilation-perfusion mismatch or reflex constriction occurring with the passive stretching of the muscular media of the pulmonary arterioles may be the basis of this phenomenon.

A decrease in pulmonary arterial cross-sectional area results in increased pulmonary vascular resistance, as dictated by Poiseuille's law, which states that resistance to flow is inversely proportional to the fourth power of the radius of the vessels. Very small decrements in pulmonary cross-sectional area can result in striking increases in resistance. There are a number of causes of decreased pulmonary arterial cross-sectional area. Filarial worms, the eggs of *Schistosoma mansoni*, or multiple small thrombotic emboli are typical of embolic causes of pulmonary hypertension. Primary deposition of fibrin in the pulmonary arterioles and capillaries is another cause of decreased cross-sectional area; and this, in fact, may be the mechanism of pri-

---

TABLE 4–9

Conditions Producing Pulmonary Artery Hypertension (PAH)

I. PAH produced by elevations of capillary and pulmonary venous pressure
  A. Mitral stenosis, mitral regurgitation, left atrial myxoma
  B. Hypertension, left ventricular failure
  C. Aortic stenosis or insufficiency
II. PAH produced by increases in pulmonary artery blood flow
  A. Congenital lesions: patent ductus arteriosus, atrial septal defect, ventricular septal defect, total anomalous venous return with right atrial or superior vena cava drainage, single ventricle, transposition of great vessels
  B. Acquired lesions: post-myocardial infarction ventricular septal defect
III. PAH produced by loss of arterial cross-sectional area
  A. Chronic hypoxia*
    1. Emphysema, chronic bronchitis, cystic fibrosis
    2. High altitude—mild PAH is a normal response—Monge's disease—chronic mountain sickness
    3. Chest and airway problems
      a. Pickwickian syndrome
      b. Kyophoscoliosis
      c. Chronic hypoxia secondary to enlarged adenoids
  B. Pulmonary fibrosis—produces fibrous occlusion and obliteration of small pulmonary arterioles with dilation of large pulmonary arteries
    1. Massive pulmonary fibrosis—silicosis and other pneumoconioses
    2. Interstitial fibrosis (fibrosing alveolitis)—abnormalities of alveoli and bronchi that extend to incorporate the pulmonary arterioles in the fibrotic process
      a. Collagen disease
        1) Scleroderma
        2) Dermatomyositis

      b. Metals
        1) Berylliosis
        2) Cadmium
        3) Asbestosis
      c. Primary pulmonary disease
        1) Hamman-Rich
        2) Sarcoidosis
      d. Iatrogenic
        1) Radiation
        2) Busulfan therapy
      c. Miscellaneous
        1) Letterer-Siwe
        2) Hand-Schüller-Christian
  C. Pulmonary emboli
    1. Recurrent
      a. Thromboemboli
      b. Parasitic
        1) Bilharzia
        2) Schistosomiasis
      c. Fat and tumor emboli
      d. Sickle cell
    2. Solitary emboli
      a. Massive thromboembolism
      b. Amniotic fluid
      c. Air
  D. ``Primary'' pulmonary hypertension—idiopathic
    1. Primary pulmonary arterial hypertension
    2. Primary pulmonary venous hypertension
  E. Dietary causes
    1. *Crotalaria labrunoides* seeds
    2. Aminorex fumarate—European appetite suppressant
    3. Oral contraceptives
  F. Hepatic cirrhosis—possibly secondary to development of plexiform and angiomatoid lesions in the lung
  G. Filariasis—adult worms in pulmonary circulation*
  H. Foreign body granulomas

*Conditions producing cor pulmonale.

mary, or idiopathic, pulmonary hypertension. Whatever the initiating cause of fibrin formation in this condition, there is increased thrombogenesis in the pulmonary arterioles and/or pulmonary capillaries, which can produce striking decreases in the total cross-sectional area. This also may be the cause of the pulmonary arterial hypertension that is rarely associated with the use of oral contraceptives, which are known to increase thrombogenesis.

Pulmonary arterial medial hypertrophy can occur if there is increased flow or pressure in the pulmonary circulation early in life. In this situation, the muscular media of the pulmonary arterioles undergo hypertrophy rather than the normal postnatal involution. As the muscle hypertrophies, there is increased reflex contraction in response to the elevations in pulmonary arterial pressure. This raises the pulmonary arterial pressure even higher by further reducing cross-sectional area. If this pulmonary arterial pressure elevation is of long standing, it results in intimal damage to the pulmonary arterioles, followed by fibrosis, thrombosis, and sclerosis, with an irreversible decrease in cross-sectional area of the arterial bed, as often occurs in long-standing mitral valve disease or emphysema. Pulmonary hypertension can also be caused by primary vasoconstrictors, such as the seeds of the crotalaria plant, or by hypoxia associated with high altitude or pulmonary parenchymal disease.

Pulmonary hypertension resulting from increases in pulmonary arterial flow is usually associated with various congenital cardiac lesions, such as atrial septal defect, ventricular septal defect, patent ductus arteriosus, or, in adult life, ventricular septal defect occurring after a septal myocardial infarction. Hypoxemia aggravates this situation. Evidence for this contention includes the observation that there is higher incidence of pulmonary hypertension in infants with congenital left-to-right shunting who are born at high altitudes than in similar infants born at sea level. Long-standing increases in flow with intimal damage may result in fibrosis and sclerosis, as noted above. An increase in pulmonary arterial pressure in these cases ultimately may result in Eisenmenger's syndrome, in which irreversibly increased pulmonary arterial pressure results in a conversion of left-to-right shunting to right-to-left shunting with the development of tardive cyanosis.

Like systemic arterial hypertension, pulmonary hypertension is characterized by a pro-longed asymptomatic period. As pulmonary vascular changes occur, an irreversible decrease in pulmonary cross-sectional area develops, and stroke volume becomes fixed as a result of the fixed resistance to flow. As such, cardiac output becomes heart rate dependent. This results in the symptoms of dyspnea, fatigue, syncope, and chest pain. The diagnostic dilemma presented by pulmonary hypertension is in differentiating primary pulmonary hypertension from secondary pulmonary hypertension. Usually, in secondary pulmonary hypertension, the symptoms of the primary condition are more prominent and the pulmonary hypertension is of secondary significance. When pulmonary hypertension exists alone, the key feature of its pathophysiology is fixed cardiac output. Right ventricular hypertrophy commonly occurs in response to pulmonary hypertension, which may progress to right ventricular dilatation and failure.[53]

B. COR PULMONALE

Cor pulmonale is usually defined as right ventricular hypertrophy, dilatation, and failure secondary to pulmonary arterial hypertension that is due to a decrease in the cross-sectional area of the pulmonary bed. This excludes, therefore, right ventricular failure, which occurs after increases in pulmonary arterial pressure secondary to increases in pulmonary blood flow, pulmonary capillary, or venous pressure. Both increases in pulmonary blood flow and passive increases in pulmonary venous and capillary pressure can produce right ventricular failure, but they do not, strictly speaking, produce cor pulmonale. The physiologic considerations in cor pulmonale and in right ventricular failure from other causes are similar. Given this restriction, though, there are still numerous causes of cor pulmonale, including pulmonary parenchymal disease, chronic hypoxia, and primary pulmonary arterial disease.

Cor pulmonale is divided into two types: acute and chronic. Acute cor pulmonale is usually secondary to a massive pulmonary embolus, resulting in a 60 to 70 per cent decrease in the pulmonary cross-sectional area associated with cyanosis and acute respiratory distress. With acute cor pulmonale, there is a rapid increase in right ventricular systolic pressure to 60 to 70 mm Hg, which slowly returns toward normal secondary to displacement of the embolus peripherally, lysis of the embolus, and increases in collateral blood flow. These changes often occur within 2 hours of onset of symptoms. Massive emboli may be associated with acute right ventricular dilatation and failure, elevated central venous pressure, and cardiogenic shock. Another feature of massive pulmonary embolization is the intense pulmonary vasoconstrictive response.[54]

Chronic cor pulmonale presents with a different picture. It is associated with right ventricular hypertrophy and a change in the normal crescent shape of the right ventricle to a more ellipsoid shape. This configuration is consistent with a change from volume work, which the right ventricle normally performs, to the pressure work required by a high afterload. Left ventricular dysfunction may occur in association with right ventricular hypertrophy. This dysfunction cannot be related to any obvious changes in the loading conditions of the left ventricle, but is probably due to displacement of the interventricular septum. Chronic cor pulmonale is usually superimposed on long-standing pulmonary arterial hypertension.[55]

Chronic bronchitis is probably the most common cause of cor pulmonale in adults, and its pathophysiology will be examined as a guide to understanding and managing cor pulmonale of all causes. Initially, the pulmonary vascular resistance in chronic bronchitis is normal or slightly increased because cardiac output increases. Later, there is a further increase in pulmonary vascular resistance or an inappropriately elevated pulmonary vascular resistance for the amount of pulmonary blood flow. Recall that, in the normal situation, there is a slight decrease in pulmonary resistance when pulmonary blood flow is increased that is probably secondary to an increase in pulmonary vascular diameter and in flow through collateral channels. In chronic bronchitis, the absolute resistance of the pulmonary circulation may not change, owing to the inability of the resistance vessels to dilate. A progressive loss of pulmonary parenchyma occurs and because of dilatation of the terminal bronchioles there is an increase in pulmonary dead space that causes progressively more severe mismatching of pulmonary ventilation and perfusion. In response to the ventilation-perfusion mismatch, the pulmonary circulation attempts to compensate by decreasing blood flow to the areas of the lung that have hypoxic alveoli. This occurs at the expense of a decrease in pulmonary arteriole cross-sectional area and an elevation in pulmonary arterial pressure.[56]

Long-standing chronic bronchitis results in elevations in pulmonary arterial pressure, with resulting right ventricular hypertrophy. In any form of respiratory embarrassment, whether it be infection or simply progression of the primary disease, further increases in pulmonary vascular resistance heighten pulmonary arterial pressure, and right ventricular failure supervenes. With the onset of respiratory problems in the patient with chronic bronchitis, a number of changes occur that can make pulmonary hypertension more severe and can precipitate right ventricular failure. A respiratory infection produces further abnormalities of blood gas values, with declines in P_aO_2 and elevations in P_aCO_2. Generally the pulmonary artery pressure is directly proportional to the P_aCO_2, although the pulmonary circulation also vasoconstricts in response to hypoxemia. With a fall in P_aO_2, there is usually an increase in cardiac output in an effort to maintain oxygen delivery to tissues. This increased blood flow through the lungs may result in further elevations in the pulmonary artery pressure, owing to the fixed decreased cross-sectional area of the pulmonary vascular bed. In addition, patients with chronic bronchitis and long-standing hypoxemia often have compensatory polycythemia. The polycythemic blood of chronic bronchitis increases resistance to flow through the pulmonary circuit because of its increased viscosity, and attempts to elevate cardiac output during respiratory compromise simply make the situation worse.

The patient with chronic bronchitis normally has an increase in airway resistance made worse during acute respiratory infection as a result of secretions and edema that further decrease the caliber of the small airways. These patients also have a loss of structural support from degenerative changes in the airways and from a loss of the stenting effect of the pulmonary parenchyma. For these reasons, the patient's small airways tend to collapse during exhalation, and there is a rise in airway pressure due to this "dynamic compression" phenomenon. In chronic bronchitis and emphysema the decrease in cross-sectional area of the pulmonary vessels results not from fibrotic obliteration of pulmonary capillaries or arterioles, but rather from hypertrophy of the muscular media of the pulmonary arterioles. The vessels become compressible but not distensible, so that with exhalation and an elevation in intrathoracic pressure, airway compression results in a further increase in pulmonary vascular resistance and an increase in pulmonary arterial pressure. The hypertrophic muscular media prevents the resulting greater pulmonary arterial pressure from distending the pulmonary vessels and maintaining normal pulmonary artery pressure. With the onset of respiratory embarrassment in the patient with chronic bronchitis there are increases in pulmonary artery pressure, afterload, and the work requirement of the right ventricle that may result in right ventricular failure.

A similar pattern may be observed in other forms of pulmonary disease, because the compensatory mechanisms are much the same as in chronic bronchitis. Chronic bronchitis, however, is somewhat more amenable to therapy, as the acute pulmonary changes are often reversible. Relief of hypoxemia, for example, may be expected to ameliorate the pulmonary hypertension. In pulmonary hypertension and cor pulmonale secondary to pulmonary fibrosis, relief of hypoxia probably has little to offer the pulmonary circulation, because the increase in pulmonary vascular resistance is due not to vasoconstriction of muscular pulmonary arterioles but rather to fibrous obliteration of the pulmonary vascular bed.

C. ANESTHETIC CONSIDERATIONS

Monitoring for patients with pulmonary hypertension and cor pulmonale should provide a continuous assessment of pulmonary arterial pressure, right ventricular filling pressure, right ventricular myocardial oxygen supply/demand balance, and some measure of pulmonary function. The ECG allows monitoring of dysrhythmias. In the setting of right ventricular hypertrophy when there is an increased possibility of coronary insufficiency, ECG monitoring allows observation of the development of ischemia or acute strain of the right ventricle, seen in the inferior, right precordial, or esophageal ECG leads.

Pulmonary artery pressure monitoring provides an indication of the workload imposed on the right ventricle in cor pulmonale. The pulmonary artery catheter affords the potential for monitoring the pulmonary artery pressure and also for monitoring the central venous pressure as an indication of the right ventricular filling pressure.

The pulmonary artery catheter can also aid in the distinction between left ventricular failure and respiratory failure. In left ventricular failure, an elevated pulmonary artery pressure occurs with an elevated pulmonary capillary wedge pressure, whereas in respiratory failure there is often an elevation of pulmonary artery pressure with a normal pulmonary capillary wedge pressure. The use of the pulmonary artery catheter allows for the determination of cardiac output and pulmonary vascular resistance. It is important to follow the pulmonary artery pressure in this setting, because an increase in pulmonary artery pressure is often the cause of acute cor pulmonale, and serial measurements of pulmonary artery pressure and the pulmonary vascular resistance allow the effects of therapeutic interventions to be evaluated.

Pulse oximetry and arterial blood gas sampling are simple ways of assessing pulmonary function. Capnography is not an accurate method of assessing P_aCO_2 when significant dead space ventilation is present. The use of an indwelling arterial catheter facilitates arterial blood sampling. Calculation of intrapulmonary venous admixture by using mixed venous blood samples obtained from the pulmonary artery, however, is a more sensitive indicator of pulmonary dysfunction than arterial P_aO_2 values alone. Currently, it is also possible to continuously monitor the arterial pH, P_aO_2, and P_aCO_2 using indwelling arterial catheters.

In the anesthetic management of patients with pulmonary hypertension and cor pulmonale, special consideration must be given to the degree of pulmonary hypertension, those factors that improve or worsen it, and the functional state of the right ventricle. For example, if pulmonary hypertension is coexistent with hypoxia in a patient with chronic bronchitis, administration of oxygen may afford significant relief of the pulmonary hypertension. If, however, the pulmonary hypertension is secondary to massive pulmonary fibrotic changes, little relief of pulmonary hypertension would be expected with the administration of oxygen. If the patient has an increase in blood viscosity, as in the polycythemia of chronic hypoxia, moderate hemodilution may be of some benefit in reducing the pulmonary vascular resistance if oxygen delivery can be maintained. When pulmonary hypertension is present without right ventricular failure, potent volatile anesthetics (that are pulmonary vasodilators in higher concentrations) may be the anesthetic drugs of choice. If, with high concentrations of potent volatile anesthetics, however, there is a decrease in hypoxic vasoconstriction, there is a theoretical risk of hypoxemia. Potent volatile agents or ketamine may also be indicated if pulmonary hypertension exists in patients who have pulmonary parenchymal disease with a significant bronchospastic component. In contrast to the volatile anesthetic agents, nitrous oxide might increase pulmonary artery pressure and should be used cautiously in this setting.[57]

When pulmonary hypertension coexists with cor pulmonale, the anesthetic technique should attempt to preserve right ventricular function. The anesthetic drugs that might have been useful in pure pulmonary hypertension are in these cases probably contraindicated because of their myocardial depressant effects. The primary concern is the maintenance of right ventricular function in the face of an elevated right ventricular afterload. In this setting, a technique that employs opioids, such as fentanyl, in combination with sedative-hypnotic drugs such as diazepam or midazolam probably provides the best cardiovascular stability.

Circulatory supportive measures in the setting of right ventricular failure do not differ in theory from measures employed in managing left ventricular failure (Table 4–10). Important concerns are ventricular preload, heart rate, the inotropic state of the ventricle, and ventricular afterload. Right ventricular preload can be assessed by measuring central venous pressure. Preload can be augmented by judicious fluid infusion or decreased with a vasodilator such as nitroglycerin that primarily affects venous capacitance in low doses. Ventricular preload can also be reduced by initiation of positive-pressure ventilation. The right ventricular contractile state and volumes can be estimated by the rapid-response thermistor calculations of right ventricular ejection fraction (RVEF) using specialized pulmonary artery catheters. This device can measure beat-to-beat RVEF but is affected by tricuspid regurgitation and cardiac dysrhythmias. RVEF catheters may be useful in the management of patients with cor pulmonale.

Inotropic support is often required in the setting of right ventricular failure with chronic cor pulmonale, and the patients usually come to surgery having been treated with a digitalis preparation. If further support is required, an inotropic agent should be selected only after consideration of its pulmonary effects, and the effects of the inotropic intervention should be monitored. For example, in the setting of right ventricular failure, norepinephrine may dramatically increase pulmonary artery pressure and pulmonary vascular resistance. On the other hand, isoproterenol, dobutamine, amrinone, or milrinone tends to reduce pulmonary artery pressure and pulmonary vascular resistance, and these would probably be the inotropic drugs of choice in right ventricular failure. Just as in left ventricular failure, when the reduction of left ventricular afterload can produce an increase in stroke volume and cardiac output, so in right ventricular failure, reduction in right ventricular afterload can produce similar effects. Vasodilators that have been found effective in reducing the afterload of the right ventricle include prostaglandin E_1, epoprostenol (formerly called *prostacyclin*), phentolamine, sodium nitroprusside, nitroglycerin, amrinone, milrinone, and enoximone.[58, 59] Inhaled nitric oxide selectively dilated the pulmonary vasculature and has been used to treat pulmonary hypertension in various clinical settings.[60, 61] Similarly, there has been some success with the use of inhaled epoprostenol.[62]

As noted previously, the use of positive-pressure ventilation and positive end-expiratory pressure (PEEP) may produce a decrease in right ventricular preload. Positive-pressure ventilation may produce an increase in pulmonary artery pressure by physically reducing the cross-sectional area of the pulmonary vasculature during the inspiratory phase of ventilation. Before PEEP is instituted, it must be remembered that the functional residual capacity is already increased in patients with chronic obstructive pulmonary disease, and the use of PEEP may have little to offer in terms of improving ventilation-perfusion matching.

VI. CONSTRICTIVE PERICARDITIS AND CARDIAC TAMPONADE

A. NORMAL PERICARDIAL FUNCTION

The pericardium is not essential to life, as is demonstrated from the benign effects of pericardiectomy; however, the pericardium normally provides resistance to overfilling of

TABLE 4–10

Abbreviated Pulmonary Vascular Pharmacopeia

Drug	PA Pressure	PCWP	Pulmonary Blood Flow	SAP	HR	PVR
α- and β-agonists						
1. Norepinephrine 0.10–0.20 μg/kg/min	↑	↑ to ↑↑	—*	↑↑	↓	NC† to ↑
2. Methoxamine 100–200 μg/kg	↑	↑	—	↑↑	↓↓	—
3. Phenylephrine 1–2 μg/kg	↑↑	—	↓	↑↑	↓↓	↑↑
4. Epinephrine 0.05–0.20 μg/kg/min	↑	NC or ↓	↑	↑↑	↑	↑
5. Dopamine 2–10 μg/kg/min	NC	NC or ↓	↑	NC or ↑	↑	NC
6. Dobutamine 5–15 μg/kg/min	—	↓	↑↑	NC or ↑	↑	↓
7. Isoproterenol 0.015–0.15 μg/kg/min	SL‡ ↓	↓	↑↑	↓	↑↑	↓
β-antagonist						
1. Propranolol 0.5–2 mg	—	NC to ↑	NC to ↓	NC to ↓	↓↓	NC to ↑
2. Esmolol 100–200 μg/kg/min	—	NC to ↑	NC to ↓	NC to ↓	↓↓	NC to ↑
α-antagonist						
1. Phentolamine 1–3 μg/kg/min	↓	↓	↑	↓	↑	↓
Smooth muscle dilators						
1. Sodium nitroprusside 0.5–3 μg/kg/min	↓	↓	↑↑	NC to ↓	↑	↓
2. Nitroglycerin 0.5–5 μg/kg/min	↓↓	↓↓	NC to ↑	↓	↑	↓
3. Prostaglandin E₁ 0.1 μg/kg/min	↓↓	↓	↑	NC to ↓	↑	↓
Phosphodiesterase III inhibitors						
1. Amrinone	—	↓	—	NC to ↓	↑	↓
2. Milrinone						
3. Enoximone						
Nitric oxide (1–40 ppm)	↓	—	↑	—	—	↓
Epoprostenol (Prostacyclin)	↓	—	↑	NC to ↓	↑	↓

*— = Data unavailable.
†NC = No change.
‡SL = Slight.

the ventricles in conditions such as tricuspid regurgitation, mitral regurgitation, or hypervolemic states. The intrapericardial pressure reflects intrapleural pressure and is a determinant of ventricular transmural filling pressure. The pericardium also serves to transmit negative pleural pressure, which maintains venous return to the heart during spontaneous ventilation.[63]

B. CONSTRICTIVE PERICARDITIS

Constrictive pericarditis results from fibrous adhesion of the pericardium to the epicardial surface of the heart (Table 4–11). Its key feature is resistance to normal ventricular filling. Constrictive pericarditis is a chronic condition that is usually well-tolerated by the patient until the disease is far advanced. Acute cardiac tamponade, in contrast, is a syndrome in which the onset of restrictive symptoms is rapid and dramatic.[64]

A number of characteristic hemodynamic features accompany constrictive pericarditis and pericardial tamponade. Rather than the slight respiratory variation in blood pressure seen in normal patients, dramatic respiratory variations in blood pressure (pulsus para-

TABLE 4–11

Conditions Producing Constrictive Pericarditis and Cardiac Tamponade

	Associated Cardiac Conditions
I. Constrictive pericarditis	
A. Idiopathic	
B. Infectious	
1. Can be sequela of most acute bacterial infections that produce pericarditis	Myocarditis
a. Tularemia	1. Cardiomyopathy
b. Tuberculosis	2. Valve malfunction
2. Viral—especially arbovirus, coxsackie B	
3. Mycotic	Valvular obstruction
a. Histoplasmosis	
b. Coccidioidomycosis	
C. Neoplastic	
1. Primary mesothelioma of pericardium	
2. Secondary to metastases—especially malignant melanoma	
D. Physical causes	1. Cardiomyopathy
1. Radiation	2. Coronary artery disease
2. Posttraumatic	
3. Postsurgical	
E. Systemic syndromes	1. Cardiomyopathy
1. Systemic lupus erythematosus	2. Coronary artery disease
2. Rheumatoid arthritis	1. Cardiomyopathy
	2. Coronary artery disease
	3. Aortic stenosis
3. Uremia	1. Cardiomyopathy
	2. Cardiac tamponade
II. Cardiac tamponade	
A. Infectious	
1. Viral—most	Myocarditis
2. Bacterial—especially tuberculosis	1. Cardiomyopathy
	2. Valve malfunction
3. Protozoal	
a. Amebiasis	
b. Toxoplasmosis	
4. Mycotic infection	Valvular obstruction
B. Collagen disease	
1. Systemic lupus erythematosus	1. Cardiomyopathy
	2. Coronary artery disease
	3. Constrictive pericarditis
2. Acute rheumatic fever	1. Cardiomyopathy
3. Rheumatoid arthritis	2. Coronary artery disease
	3. Aortic stenosis
C. Metabolic disorders	
1. Uremia	
2. Myxedema	Low cardiac output
D. Hemorrhagic diatheses	
1. Genetic coagulation defects	
2. Anticoagulants	
E. Drugs	
1. Hydralazine	
2. Procainamide (Pronestyl)	
3. Diphenylhydantoin (Dilantin)	
F. Physical causes	1. Cardiomyopathy
1. Radiation	2. Coronary artery disease
	3. Constrictive pericarditis
2. Trauma (perforation)	
a. Surgical manipulation	
b. Intracardiac catheters	
c. Pacing wires	
G. Neoplasia	
1. Primary—mesothelioma	
—juvenile xanthogranuloma	
2. Metastatic	
H. Miscellaneous	
1. Postmyocardial infarction—ventricular rupture	
2. Pancreatitis	
3. Reiter's syndrome	Aortic regurgitation
4. Behçet's syndrome	
5. Loeffler's syndrome—endocardial fibroelastosis with eosinophilia	Restrictive cardiomyopathy
6. Long-standing congestive heart failure	

doxus) are present. Kussmaul's sign (jugular venous distention during inspiration) is present. With adequate blood volume, the right atrial pressure in constrictive pericarditis is usually equal to or greater than 15 mm Hg and usually equals the left atrial pressure. The pulmonary artery systolic pressure is usually less than 40 mm Hg, which helps to distinguish constrictive pericarditis from cardiac failure. Both constrictive pericarditis and cardiac tamponade demonstrate a diastolic "pressure plateau" or "equalization of pressures." The right atrial pressure equals the right ventricular end-diastolic pressure, pulmonary artery diastolic pressure, and left atrial pressure. Early in the disease, cardiac output is normal, but with progression cardiac output falls. Most symptoms are related to this fall in cardiac output or to the elevated venous pressure that develops in response to the decreased cardiac output and restriction of right ventricular filling.

Constrictive pericarditis often resembles restrictive cardiomyopathy and occasionally presents a diagnostic dilemma; however, in contrast to constrictive pericarditis, cardiac output in restrictive cardiomyopathy is decreased primarily, left atrial pressure is increased, mean pulmonary artery pressure is increased, and there is no pulsus paradoxus.[65, 66]

Because constrictive pericarditis restricts ventricular diastolic filling, normal ventricular end-diastolic volumes are not obtained and stroke volume is decreased. Compensatory mechanisms include an increase in heart rate and contractility, which usually occur secondary to an increase in endogenous catecholamine release. This maintains cardiac output in the face of the restricted stroke volume until the decrease in ventricular diastolic volume is quite severe. As cardiac output falls, renal perfusion decreases. This results in increased liberation of aldosterone, providing for a compensatory increase in extracellular volume. The increase in extracellular volume increases right ventricular filling pressure, which eventually becomes essential for maintaining ventricular diastolic volume in the face of severe pericardial constriction.

C. CARDIAC TAMPONADE

Cardiac tamponade, like constrictive pericarditis, also restricts ventricular diastolic filling, but it is caused by extrinsic compression of the ventricular wall from fluid in the pericardium. Symptoms of cardiac tamponade are usually rapid in onset but depend on the rate and volume of pericardial fluid accumulation. With rapid fluid accumulation in the pericardium, a small volume can produce symptoms. With a more gradual accumulation of fluid, the pericardium stretches, and larger pericardial volumes are tolerated before symptoms occur. Once symptoms begin, however, they proceed rapidly because of the sigmoidal relationship between pressure and volume in the pericardial sac. As the limit of pericardial distensibility is reached, small increases in volume produce dramatic increases in intrapericardial pressure. As such, removal of small volumes of pericardial fluid in a situation of severe cardiac tamponade can produce very dramatic relief of symptoms as a result of a rapid fall in intrapericardial pressure.[67]

The clinical features of cardiac tamponade result from restriction of diastolic ventricular filling and increased pericardial pressure. The increased pericardial pressure is transmitted to the ventricular chamber. This decreases the atrioventricular pressure gradient during diastole and impedes ventricular filling. Thus, there is a decrease in the end-diastolic ventricular volume and in stroke volume. Increased diastolic ventricular pressure decreases coronary perfusion pressure and also results in early closure of the mitral and tricuspid valves, limiting diastolic flow and reducing ventricular volume. Figure 4–5 provides a diagrammatic summary of the pathophysiology of cardiac tamponade. The compensatory mechanisms in cardiac tamponade are similar to those of constrictive pericarditis. A fall in cardiac output results in an increase in endogenous catecholamines. The consequent elevations in heart rate and contractility help maintain cardiac output in the face of decreased stroke volume. Increased contractility heightens the ejection fraction, allowing more complete ventricular emptying. Echocardiography differentiates cardiac tamponade from constrictive pericarditis. Right ventricular and/or right atrial collapse is the echocardiographic hallmark of tamponade.

Cardiac tamponade can be seen in blunt chest trauma when there is rupture of a cardiac chamber; however, the most common cardiac involvement in blunt chest trauma is cardiac contusion. Cardiac contusion may mimic an evolving myocardial infarction, and specific markers for cardiac injury, such as

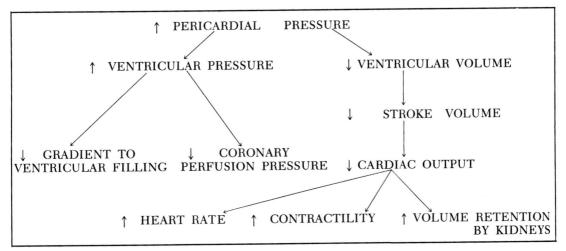

FIGURE 4–5. Schematic of physiology of tamponade.

troponin T and troponin I, are increased in both conditions. Blunt chest trauma may also result in tricuspid regurgitation from a ruptured papillary muscle, traumatic ventricular septal defect, and dissection or interruption of the aorta.[68]

D. ANESTHETIC CONSIDERATIONS

Monitoring should be aimed at the compensatory mechanisms in constrictive pericarditis and cardiac tamponade. The ECG should be observed for heart rate and ischemic changes, since the myocardial oxygen supply-demand ratio can be altered by the pathologic process and by therapeutic interventions.

Filling pressures should also be assessed. The decision to use a pulmonary artery catheter or a central venous pressure catheter is based on these variables: (1) the state of ventricular function, (2) the surgical procedure, and (3) the postoperative monitoring requirements. Central venous pressure monitoring is indicated in the following instances: (1) if cardiac tamponade is superimposed on an otherwise normal ventricle, as in trauma; (2) if the surgical procedure is only drainage of the tamponade fluid and an exploration of the pericardium in an effort to determine the cause of the tamponade (here central venous pressure adequately indicates the relief of cardiac tamponade); and, (3) if postoperative monitoring is aimed only at following the potential reaccumulation of pericardial fluid. The central venous pressure is probably more

sensitive than the pulmonary capillary wedge pressure in diagnosing reaccumulation of pericardial fluid.

The right ventricle has a very steep Starling curve with a relatively narrow range of filling pressures, which are lower than those of the left ventricle (Fig. 4–6). The filling pressures that would indicate reaccumulation of pericardial fluid are more widely divergent from the normal right ventricular filling pressures

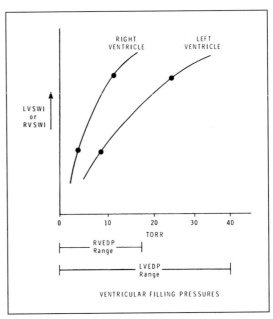

FIGURE 4–6. Right and left ventricular function curves where left or right ventricular stroke work index (LVSWI or RVSWI, respectively) is plotted as a function of right or left ventricular end-diastolic pressure (RVEDP or LVEDP, respectively).

than they are from the filling pressures of the left ventricle. Accordingly, monitoring right ventricular filling pressures is a more sensitive indicator of developing tamponade. On the other hand, with chronic cardiac tamponade coupled with cardiomyopathy, or in constrictive pericarditis of any cause, the pulmonary artery catheter probably provides more useful information. During pericardiectomy, the pulmonary artery catheter is useful for assessing myocardial depression secondary to cardiac manipulation and for assessing the volume status of the patient. Postoperative monitoring must address the problems of both reaccumulation of pericardial fluid and development of overt ventricular failure in patients with an underlying cardiomyopathy. Intra-arterial monitoring is nearly universally indicated in symptomatic constrictive pericarditis and pericardial tamponade.

Two-dimensional echocardiography is well-suited to monitoring patients with constrictive pericarditis or tamponade. Intraoperatively, this can be performed with a transesophageal probe. Qualitative estimation of the degree of tamponade and quantitative estimation of ejection fraction may be obtained with this technology.

The similar pathophysiology of cardiac tamponade and constrictive pericarditis creates similar approaches for circulatory support. Cardiovascular support may be required before definitive therapy can be undertaken for either condition, but especially for cardiac tamponade. Circulatory therapy should be directed toward the three main compensatory mechanisms in these conditions: (1) maintenance of adequate ventricular filling, (2) maintenance of heart rate, and (3) maintenance of myocardial contractility. Intravascular volume maintenance is crucial in these conditions, and a decline in filling pressures can result in dramatic decreases in cardiac output. Because an increased heart rate maintains cardiac output in the face of a decreased stroke volume, beta-agonists are the inotropic drugs of choice, as they increase heart rate and contractility. Drugs such as phenylephrine or methoxamine are contraindicated, because they elevate systemic vascular resistance and usually decrease heart rate because of baroreceptor reflexes. With inotropic drugs such as epinephrine and dopamine, myocardial contractility is also maintained, contributing to homeostasis by increasing ejection fraction.

The first step in the anesthetic management of cardiac tamponade is to assess its severity. The anesthesiologist must decide whether induction of anesthesia can be tolerated. In a patient who is tachycardic and hypotensive and has a high filling pressure, pericardiocentesis or a pericardial window performed under local anesthesia is probably needed before the induction of general anesthesia. After partial relief of severe cardiac tamponade, cardiac function should be reassessed. Usually, the hemodynamic situation is markedly improved. In the case of less severe symptoms, it is reasonable to induce general anesthesia using a smaller intravenous dose of ketamine (0.25 to 1.0 mg/kg) or etomidate. Thiopental is relatively contraindicated, as it can produce dramatic hypotension secondary to venodilatation. High-dose narcotic anesthesia does not depress myocardial contractility, but the associated bradycardia may not be tolerated. The tachycardia associated with the use of some muscle relaxants, such as pancuronium, may be advantageous in maintaining circulatory homeostasis.[69, 70]

In the presence of restricted ventricular diastolic filling, the initiation of positive-pressure ventilation may severely decrease venous return. When this occurs, intravascular volume must be increased in an effort to raise ventricular filling pressure. After the relief of tamponade, the physiologic situation tends to revert to normal, and further anesthetic requirements then depend on the degree of cardiac manipulation by the surgeon during exploration of the pericardium (for example, bleeding from a coronary graft may be the cause of the tamponade).

In constrictive pericarditis, the altered physiology remains throughout most of the surgical procedure, whereas in cardiac tamponade the altered physiology is often rapidly relieved by opening the pericardium. The features of anesthetic management are similar to those of unrelieved cardiac tamponade: maintaining the intravascular volume, heart rate, and myocardial contractility. In this setting, similar anesthetic techniques are also used, but a number of special problems may arise in the patient who comes to surgery for pericardiectomy. Dysrhythmias, often requiring medical therapy, are quite frequently associated with dissection of the adherent pericardial sac from the ventricular epicardial surface. Rapid changes in filling pressures occur with cardiac manipulation. Thus, it is important for the anesthesiologist to be in constant communication with the surgeon concerning the hemodynamic response to the various manipulations of the heart. During pericardiectomy, with frequent episodes of hypotension, it is often difficult to distinguish relative hypovolemia and transient myocardial depression, which occur with cardiac manipulation, from incipient myocardial failure. Here, the pulmonary artery catheter is particularly useful for distinguishing between hypovolemia and myocardial failure as the cause of hypotension.

Pericardiectomy is frequently associated with bleeding and coagulation problems. During the procedure, continuous oozing of blood from the raw pericardial and epicardial surfaces requires transfusion of packed red blood cells. If the patient cannot tolerate the vigorous cardiac manipulation, cardiopulmonary bypass with systemic heparinization is required for circulatory support during the procedure, particularly during dissection on the posterior cardiac surface. If cardiopulmonary bypass and heparinization are required, the coagulation problems become very complex. Platelet concentrates, fresh-frozen plasma, and cryoprecipitate may be required if the bleeding is massive. These bleeding problems often continue after heparin reversal by protamine. Prophylactic therapy with lysine analogue antifibrinolytics (aminocaproic acid or tranexamic acid) or aprotinin should be considered. Even without cardiopulmonary bypass, postoperative mechanical ventilation is probably the safest method of managing the postpericardiectomy patient with multiple intraoperative problems such as continued bleeding, dysrhythmias, and myocardial injury and depression.

VII. VALVULAR LESIONS

The normal function of the cardiac valves is to maintain one-way forward flow during the cardiac cycle. Valvular lesions interfere with this function, either by producing obstructions to forward flow or by allowing varying degrees of backward flow. In this section we consider the pathophysiology of uncommon causes of valvular lesions and how these diseases affect cardiac compensatory mechanisms.

Lesions that produce valvular stenosis are usually graded on the basis of valve area, according to Gorlin's formula, which states that flow across the stenotic valve is directly proportional to the square root of the differ-

ence in transvalvular pressures. This relationship states that the valve area is the key factor in determining flow across an obstruction. Flow is also influenced by such factors as blood viscosity and turbulence across the valve. Regurgitant lesions are usually evaluated on an echocardiographic or angiographic basis on a scale of 1 to 4+, depending on the rate of dye clearance.[71, 72]

Rheumatic valvular lesions often exist as isolated defects in a relatively normal cardiovascular system, and they can long be present without producing symptoms. In contrast, the uncommon diseases considered here produce valvular lesions that usually are not associated with an otherwise normal circulatory system, because these lesions frequently occur in the setting of cardiomyopathy, pulmonary hypertension, cor pulmonale, or coronary artery disease. The asymptomatic period for rheumatic lesions is related to the effectiveness of intrinsic cardiovascular compensatory mechanisms, and symptoms appear only when these compensatory mechanisms fail. With the diseases considered in this section, the normal methods of compensation are often severely compromised. Because anesthetic management of valvular lesions is directed at preserving the compensatory mechanisms, it is essential to understand how these diseases interfere with compensation and how anesthetic manipulations interact with them.

A. AORTIC STENOSIS
(Table 4–12A)

Aortic stenosis is due to narrowing of the aortic valve orifice, resulting in a pressure gradient across this narrow orifice. The obstruction to flow is proportional to the cross-sectional area of the obstructed outlet, for which the left ventricle compensates by increasing the transvalvular pressure to maintain flow. The ventricle undergoes concentric hypertrophy to force blood across the stenotic valve but suffers a decrease in compliance. As a result of hypertrophy, ventricular wall tension per unit area is decreased but total ventricular oxygen demand is increased because of an elevation in left ventricular mass. Another compensation for aortic stenosis is an increase in ventricular ejection time that decreases the turbulent flow across the valve, thus decreasing flow resistance and allowing more complete ventricular emptying.[67]

As ventricular compliance falls, passive

TABLE 4-12A

Uncommon Causes of Valvular Lesions

Disease	Features Affecting Compensatory Mechanisms		Associated Problems
	Atrial Transport and Rhythm	*Contractility and Hypertrophy*	
A. Aortic stenosis (AS)			
1. Congenital and degenerative diseases			
a. Congenital			
1) Valvular			
2) Discrete subvalvular			
3) Supravalvular			Coarctation of aorta, polycystic kidneys
b. Bicuspid valve			
c. Degenerative			
1) Senile calcification			
2) Mönckeberg's sclerosis			
2. Infectious diseases			
a. Syphilis		Dilated cardiomyopathy and outflow obstruction	
b. Actinomycosis		Dilated cardiomyopathy and outflow obstruction	
3. Infiltrative diseases			
a. Amyloidosis	SA and AV nodal infiltration	1. Dilated cardiomyopathy 2. Coronary artery disease	
b. Pompe's disease		1. Hypertrophic cardiomyopathy 2. Dilated cardiomyopathy Cardiomyopathy	
c. Fabry's disease		1. Dilated cardiomyopathy 2. Coronary artery disease	Hypertension
d. Primary xanthomatosis	Atrial dysrhythmias with rapid rate		
4. Miscellaneous			
a. Sarcoid	Dysrhythmias and inflammation of conduction system	1. LV dyssynergy with aneurysm 2. LV infiltration and cardiomyopathy	
b. Endocardial fibroelastosis		1. Restriction of ventricular filling 2. Interference with subendocardial blood flow with decreased oxygen delivery to myocardium	1. Mitral valve malfunction with stenosis producing poor ventricular filling 2. Regurgitation decreasing LV pressure development
c. Methysergide		Restriction of ventricular filling secondary to endocardial fibrosis	Similar to endocardial fibroelastosis
d. Paget's disease	1. Dysrhythmias with loss of atrial kick 2. Complete heart block		Possible mitral stenosis and poor ventricular filling

104

Classification	Findings	Associated conditions
B. Pulmonary stenosis (PS)		
1. Congenital		
a. Valvular		
b. Infundibular		
c. Supravalvular with peripheral coarctation		
2. Genetic—Noonan's syndrome		Aortic regurgitation
	Hypertrophic cardiomyopathy—obstructive and nonobstructive	
3. Infiltrative		
a. Pompe's	Dilated cardiomyopathy	Aortic stenosis and outflow tract obstruction
	Dysrhythmias secondary to conduction system infiltration	
b. Lentiginosis	Massive AV septal hypertrophy	Cor pulmonale
c. Sarcoid	Cardiomyopathy	
	Dysrhythmias secondary to conduction system involvement	
4. Infectious		
a. SBE	Heart block	Tricuspid insufficiency
b. Tuberculosis		Pulmonary insufficiency
c. Rheumatic fever	Usually associated with other valvular lesions	
5. Neoplastic		
a. Mediastinal tumors		
b. Primary tumors		
1) Sarcoma	Rhythm or cardiomyopathic complications will depend on extent of wall involvement in the neoplastic process	
2) Myxoma		
c. Malignant carcinoid syndrome	Endocardial fibrosis	1. Pulmonary hypertension 2. Pulmonary regurgitation 3. Tricuspid regurgitation and/or stenosis
6. Physical—extrinsic causes		
a. Aneurysm of ascending aorta or sinus of Valsalva		
b. Constrictive pericarditis	Picture of restrictive cardiomyopathy but usually with good ventricular function	
c. Postsurgical banding		Often associated with other congenital cardiac anomalies

filling of the ventricle during diastole is decreased and the ventricle becomes increasingly dependent on atrial augmentation of ventricular diastolic volume. In this setting, the atrial "kick" may contribute as much as 30 to 50 per cent to left ventricular end-diastolic volume. In aortic stenosis, ventricular filling pressures increase, in relation to both decreased ventricular compliance, where the same filling volume produces an elevation in filling pressure, and a real increase in intravascular volume. Left ventricular hypertrophy in aortic stenosis results in decreased wall tension overall, but the heightened intraventricular systolic pressure virtually eliminates systolic coronary flow. Diastolic subendocardial blood flow also drops as a result of a decrease in transmural pressures; and for this reason, perfusion pressures must remain elevated to provide adequate myocardial blood flow.

It is now appropriate to consider how a disease process might affect compensatory mechanisms. First, a disease could interfere with the compensatory mechanism of concentric hypertrophy and increased ventricular contractility. In Pompe's disease, left ventricular hypertrophy occurs but is secondary to massive myocardial glycogen accumulation, and for this reason ventricular strength is not increased to compensate for the outflow tract obstruction that commonly occurs in this disease. Another example would be amyloidosis, in which aortic stenosis is coupled with restrictive cardiomyopathy. Here, as in Pompe's disease, there is inability to increase either ventricular muscle mass or contractility. A disease process may also interfere with the crucial atrial augmentation of ventricular end-diastolic volume, as, for example, in sarcoidosis or Paget's disease. Diseases of this type infiltrate the cardiac conduction system, resulting in dysrhythmias or heart block, with loss of synchronous atrial contraction. The requirement for elevated ventricular diastolic filling pressure may be compromised in a situation such as methysergide toxicity, which can produce mitral stenosis coupled with aortic stenosis. This reduces both passive ventricular filling and ventricular filling resulting from atrial contraction.[2]

Diseases that affect the conduction system in addition to producing loss of atrial contraction can also produce tachydysrhythmias, which decrease ventricular ejection time and increase turbulent flow across the valves. Table 4–12A lists causes of aortic stenosis and key features of their pathophysiology that can adversely affect cardiac compensatory mechanisms.

B. PULMONIC STENOSIS
(Table 4–12A)

As in aortic stenosis, the valve area is the crucial determinant of transvalvular blood flow. Pulmonic stenosis produces symptoms that are similar to the classic clinical features of aortic stenosis: fatigue, dyspnea, syncope, and angina. The compensatory mechanisms in pulmonic stenosis are similar to those in aortic stenosis. Initially, under the stress of right ventricular outflow obstruction, the right ventricle dilates; however, it eventually undergoes concentric hypertrophy and changes from a crescent-shaped chamber best suited to handling volume loads to an ellipsoidal chamber best suited to handling pressure loads. Second, there is an increase in ejection time, which is maintained with a slow heart rate. Third, elevations in ventricular filling pressure occur as a result of increased intravascular volume and a change in the compliance of the right ventricle.

The presence of angina, which occurs occasionally in pulmonic stenosis, should especially be noted. Usually, the right ventricle is a thin-walled chamber with low intraventricular pressures. This normal situation results in a high transmural perfusion pressure and good subendocardial blood flow that limits development of ischemia of the right ventricle. Concentric hypertrophy raises both right ventricular mass and right ventricular pressures, increasing the potential for ischemia of the right ventricle, because right ventricular oxygen requirements are increased and coronary perfusion may be decreased. Cyanosis can occur with severe pulmonic stenosis accompanied by a low, fixed cardiac output. When right ventricular pressure rises, a patent foramen ovale may produce right-to-left interatrial shunting. Usually, isolated pulmonic stenosis is tolerated well for long periods, until compensatory mechanisms fail. When a second valvular lesion coexists with pulmonic stenosis, the potential effects of this lesion on compensatory mechanisms should be considered.[71]

Compensatory mechanisms can be altered in pulmonic stenosis in much the same way as in aortic stenosis. Decreases in right ventricular contractility occur in infiltrative diseases of the myocardium, such as Pompe's disease or sarcoidosis. The loss of the atrial "kick" and the development of tachydysrhythmias have the same implications for cardiac function in pulmonic stenosis as in aortic stenosis. In subacute bacterial endocarditis, tricuspid insufficiency may coexist with pulmonic stenosis, producing an impairment of pressure development in the right ventricle, especially when right ventricular failure supervenes. With the increase in right ventricular mass and the increased requirement for oxygen delivery to the right ventricle, the possibility should be considered that oxygen supply may be compromised, as in the coronary artery pathology of Pompe's disease.

Many of these patients are candidates for balloon valvuloplasty of the pulmonary valve. In this procedure, a balloon catheter is placed percutaneously, and the tip is guided across the pulmonic valve. The balloon is inflated, tearing the fused leaflets apart. A period of severe hypotension occurs during balloon inflation, and transient loss of consciousness, vomiting, and seizures may occur. Pulmonic regurgitation is invariably produced, but this is usually well tolerated hemodynamically. This procedure has reduced the number of patients needing operative valvuloplasty and valve replacement, although the long-term outcome for these patients has not been defined. In many institutions, anesthesiologists provided monitored care for these patients. Balloon valvuloplasty is also used for selected patients with aortic and mitral stenosis.[74]

C. AORTIC INSUFFICIENCY
(Table 4–12B)

The primary problem in aortic insufficiency is a decrease in net forward blood flow from the left ventricle that is due to diastolic regurgitation of blood back into the left ventricular chamber. The first question to ask in the setting of aortic insufficiency is whether the condition is acute or chronic, because this is often the main determinant of the degree of compensation. Aortic insufficiency represents an almost pure volume overload of the left ventricular chamber. The left ventricle responds initially with dilation to maximize the effects of increases in fiber length. Acutely, this may result in heart failure, as the increased ventricular diameter increases wall tension and end-diastolic pressure. An acute increase in ventricular volume may also compromise the anchoring of the mitral valve by changing the geometric relationship of the papillary muscles, resulting in mitral regurgitation and pulmonary edema.[73]

In chronic aortic insufficiency, however, a number of compensatory changes minimize the degree of diastolic regurgitation. The first compensatory mechanism is an increase in left ventricular chamber size with eccentric hypertrophy. The left ventricular compliance is elevated, which produces an increase in volume at the same filling pressure, thus reducing end-diastolic pressure and wall tension. The increase in ventricular volume allows full use of the Frank-Starling mechanism, whereby the strength of ventricular contraction is increased with greater fiber length. Ejection fraction is maintained, since both stroke volume and ventricular end-diastolic volume increase together. Despite these compensatory mechanisms, however, a number of studies have shown that ventricular contractility is depressed.[71]

In contrast to aortic stenosis, the augmentation of ventricular end-diastolic volume by the atrial contraction is not essential to ventricular compensation in aortic insufficiency. A rapid heart rate seems to be advantageous in aortic insufficiency, as the rapid heart rate in aortic insufficiency reduces the time for diastolic filling and helps prevent diastolic overdistention of the ventricle from regurgitant flow. In aortic insufficiency, the amount of regurgitant flow increases as systemic vascular resistance increases. Thus, the third major compensatory mechanism in aortic insufficiency is the maintenance of a low peripheral resistance, because forward flow in aortic insufficiency is inversely proportional to the systemic vascular resistance.

The increase in chamber size and eccentric hypertrophy, which help maintain cardiac function in aortic insufficiency, can be compromised in such conditions as ankylosing spondylitis, in which myocardial fibrosis limits the increase in chamber size to the degree that this disease produces a restrictive picture. Cogan's syndrome produces a generalized cardiomyopathy with coronary artery disease and can alter the compensatory mechanism by decreasing the ability of both the left ventricle to hypertrophy and of the coronary arteries to deliver oxygen to the ventricle. Increases in left ventricular compliance could be prevented in situations such as aortic insufficiency produced by methysergide,

TABLE 4–12B

Uncommon Causes of Valvular Lesions

Disease	Features Affecting Compensatory Mechanisms			Associated Cardiovascular Abnormalities
	LV Compliance and Contractility	Heart Rate and Rhythm	Vascular Resistance	
A. Aortic insufficiency				
1. Infiltrative disease				
a. Amyloidosis	Dilated and restrictive cardiomyopathy	Dysrhythmias with infiltration of conduction system		1. Coronary artery disease 2. Stenosis or insufficiency of other valves
b. Morquio's } c. Scheie's }	Usually isolated aortic insufficiency with mild mucopolysaccharidosis			
d. Pseudoxanthoma elasticum	Dilated cardiomyopathy			
2. Infectious disease				
a. Bacterial endocarditis		Complete heart block		Insufficiency of other valves
b. Syphilis	Dilated or restrictive cardiomyopathy	Infiltration of conduction system		1. Aortic stenosis 2. Aortic aneurysm
c. Rheumatic fever				
3. Congenital valve disease				
a. Bicuspid aortic valve	Usually intact compensatory mechanisms			
b. Aneurysm of sinus of Valsalva } c. Congenital fenestrated cusp }				
4. Degenerative				
a. Marfan's	Normal	Normal	Cystic medial necrosis of aorta with dissection	Pulmonic insufficiency
b. Osteogenesis imperfecta	Normal	Normal	Cystic medial necrosis	Mitral regurgitation
5. Inflammatory				
a. Relapsing polychondritis	Pericarditis and effusion			Mitral regurgitation
b. SLE			Hypertension secondary to renal disease	Mitral regurgitation
c. Reiter's syndrome				
d. Rheumatoid arthritis	Congestive cardiomyopathy	Complete heart block		1. Aortic stenosis 2. Mitral stenosis and/or insufficiency 3. Constrictive pericarditis 4. Cardiac tamponade

Lesion	Effect / pathophysiology	Conduction / vascular effect	Associated valvular lesion
6. Systemic syndromes			
a. Ankylosing spondylitis	1. Coronary artery disease 2. Dilated cardiomyopathy	Complete heart block	Aortic dissection
b. Cogan's syndrome		Generalized angiitis	
c. Noonan's syndrome	Cardiomyopathy		Pulmonic stenosis
d. Ehlers-Danlos			Spontaneous vascular dissection
7. Miscellaneous causes			
a. Aortic dissection	Interference with compensation depends on cause, e.g., syphilis, Marfan's, traumatic		
b. Methysergide	Endocardial fibrosis—restriction of LV filling		Mitral valve stenosis and/or insufficiency
c. Traumatic rupture	Acute dilatation and failure		
B. Pulmonic insufficiency			
1. Congenital			
a. Isolated	Usually tolerated as isolated lesion		
1) Hypoplastic			
2) Aplastic			
3) Bicuspid			
b. Associated with other congenital cardiac lesions	Toleration of PI depends on degree of myocardial dysfunction induced by other cardiac lesions		
2. Acquired	Dilated cardiomyopathy		
a. Syphilitic aneurysm of PA		Luminal narrowing	
b. Rheumatic	Tolerated well in isolation		
c. Bacterial endocarditis	Endocardial fibrosis		Endocarditis of other valves
d. Echinococcus cyst	Endocardial fibrosis		Tricuspid valve malfunction
3. Malignant carcinoid syndrome		Infiltration of conduction system / Complete heart block	Tricuspid valve malfunction
4. Physical			
a. Traumatic			
b. After valvotomy/valvuloplasty for pulmonic stenosis	Decreased ventricular compliance if RV hypertrophic from PS; Ventricular hypertrophy with decreased compliance		
5. Functional—secondary to pulmonary hypertension	Elevated pulmonary resistance due to pulmonary hypertension		1. Chronic obstructive pulmonary disease 2. Mitral stenosis 3. Primary pulmonary hypertension

which produces an endocardial fibrosis and thus decreased ventricular compliance. The usual ability of the left ventricle to maintain the ejection fraction in aortic insufficiency could be compromised by the cardiomyopathy of amyloidosis. The aortic insufficiency produced by acute bacterial endocarditis is occasionally associated with complete heart block, resulting in a slow heart rate with ventricular overdistention and a decrease in cardiac output. Aortic insufficiency due to conditions such as systemic lupus erythematosus associated with increased peripheral resistance can increase the regurgitant fraction in the face of the incompetent aortic valve.[2]

D. PULMONIC INSUFFICIENCY
(Table 4–12B)

Pulmonic insufficiency usually occurs in the setting of pulmonary hypertension or cor pulmonale but may exist as an isolated lesion, as in acute bacterial endocarditis in intravenous drug users. It may also be iatrogenic, as it frequently is a sequela of pulmonary valvuloplasty procedures. Pulmonic insufficiency is tolerated extremely well for long periods of time. Like aortic insufficiency, it represents a volume overload on the ventricular chamber, but the crescentic right ventricular geometry is such that volume loading is easily handled. Compensatory mechanisms for pulmonic insufficiency are the same as for aortic insufficiency: an increase in right ventricular compliance, rapid heart rate, and low pulmonary vascular resistance. The right ventricle is normally a highly compliant chamber, and with its steep filling pressure–stroke volume curve, it functions very well in the presence of volume increases.

The degree of pulmonic regurgitation is determined by the pulmonary arterial diastolic–right ventricular end-diastolic pressure gradient. For this reason, low pulmonary vascular resistance and low left-sided filling pressure are essential to maintaining forward flow. In general, there is less increase in ventricular end-diastolic volume than in aortic insufficiency. The ejection fraction, however, is not as well-maintained in pulmonic insufficiency as it is in aortic insufficiency. With severe pulmonic regurgitation, as in aortic insufficiency, eccentric hypertrophy of the ventricular chamber occurs.[74]

Disease states can interfere with the compensatory mechanisms of the right ventricle in several ways. Diseases that produce pulmonic insufficiency, such as the malignant carcinoid syndrome, also produce an endocardial fibrosis that decreases the ability of the right ventricular chamber to dilate in response to volume loading. Increases in right ventricular afterload increase the regurgitant fraction, especially when pulmonic insufficiency is secondary to pulmonary hypertension. Hypoxemia can increase pulmonary vascular resistance, as in the hypoxemia that results from pulmonary vascular dysfunction in carcinoid syndrome. It is unusual for a cardiomyopathy to coexist with isolated pulmonic insufficiency; thus, the potential for eccentric hypertrophy is usually left intact. However, syphilis could present a situation in which a cardiomyopathy exists along with pulmonic insufficiency, although this would depend on the extent of syphilitic involvement of the myocardium.

E. MITRAL STENOSIS
(Table 4–12C)

The primary defect in mitral stenosis is a restriction of normal left ventricular filling across the mitral valve. As in other stenotic lesions, the area of the valve orifice is the key to flow, and, as the orifice gets smaller, turbulent flow increases across the valve and total resistance to flow increases. The important features in compensation of mitral stenosis are (1) increasing the pressure gradient across the valve and (2) prolonging diastole. The compensatory mechanisms in mitral stenosis include (1) dilatation and hypertrophy of the left atrium, (2) increases in atrial filling pressures, and (3) a slow heart rate to allow sufficient time for diastolic flow with minimal turbulence.[75, 76]

Decompensation in rheumatic mitral stenosis usually occurs when atrial fibrillation occurs with a rapid ventricular rate. This causes a loss of the atrial contraction and decreased time for ventricular filling, which results in pulmonary vascular engorgement. Thus, altered left ventricular function usually is not the limiting factor in the ability of the heart to compensate for mitral stenosis. The observation has been made that cardiac index is decreased for 48 to 72 hours after mitral valve replacement, which may be secondary to either trauma to the left ventricle involved in excising the mitral valve or to chronic depression of left ventricular function, which occurs

TABLE 4–12C

Uncommon Causes of Valvular Lesions

Disease	Features Affecting Compensatory Mechanisms			
	Rhythm	Atrial Transport	LV Function	Associated Conditions
A. Mitral stenosis (MS)				
1. Inflammatory				
a. Rheumatic fever	Heart block	1. Pericardial constriction 2. Cardiac tamponade	Dilated cardiomyopathy	1. Aortic stenosis and insufficiency 2. Mitral insufficiency
b. Rheumatoid arthritis				
2. Infiltrative				
a. Amyloidosis	1. Heart block 2. Infiltration of conduction system	Atrial dilatation and hypertrophy	Dilated and restrictive cardiomyopathy	Malfunctioning of other valves
b. Sarcoidosis	Infiltration of conduction system		Dilated cardiomyopathy	1. Pulmonary hypertension 2. Cor pulmonale
c. Gout	Infiltration of conduction system			
3. Miscellaneous				
a. Left atrial myxoma	Normal compensatory mechanism			Mitral insufficiency
b. Parachute mitral valve				
c. Concentric ring of left atrium				
d. Methysergide	Dysrhythmias secondary to myocardial vasculitis	Myofibrillar degeneration	Endocardial fibrosis Dilated cardiomyopathy	
e. Wegener's granulomatosis				
B. Tricuspid stenosis				
1. Inflammatory				
a. Rheumatic fever	Usually associated with other valvular lesions		1. Coronary artery disease 2. Cardiomyopathy	
b. Systemic lupus erythematosus	Dysrhythmias secondary to pericarditis			
2. Fibrotic				
a. Carcinoid syndrome		Fibrosis evolving to hypertrophy and dilatation	1. Pulmonary hypertension with increased RV afterload 2. Endocardial fibrosis	Pulmonic stenosis
b. Endocardial fibroelastosis	Similar to carcinoid syndrome			
c. Methysergide	Similar to carcinoid syndrome			
3. Miscellaneous				
a. Hurler's	Infiltration of conduction system	Infiltration of atrial wall Usually normal compensatory mechanisms	Dilated cardiomyopathy	Mitral and aortic valvular abnormality
b. Myxoma of right atrium				Aortic stenosis

in mitral stenosis, even though the left ventricle is "protected."[77]

As in other valvular lesions produced by uncommon diseases, coexistent cardiovascular problems that interfere with compensatory mechanisms are very important. Diseases such as sarcoidosis or amyloidosis can infiltrate ventricular muscle, preventing left ventricular filling by decreasing compliance. Amyloidosis, gout, and sarcoidosis can also affect the conduction system of the heart, resulting in heart block, tachydysrhythmias, or atrial fibrillation.

F. TRICUSPID STENOSIS
(Table 4–12C)

Tricuspid stenosis is usually associated with mitral stenosis as a sequela of rheumatic fever. Usually the other valve lesions associated with tricuspid stenosis determine heart function and the tricuspid stenosis often exists as an almost incidental lesion. Isolated tricuspid stenosis is very rare. The problems in tricuspid stenosis are similar to those in mitral stenosis. There is a large right atrial–to–right ventricular diastolic gradient, and flow across the stenotic tricuspid valve is related to valve area.[78]

The compensatory mechanisms in tricuspid stenosis are also similar to those in mitral stenosis. An increase in right atrial pressure maintains flow across the stenotic valve, and this is associated with hepatomegaly, jugular venous distention, and peripheral edema. Also, the heart compensates with right atrial dilation and hypertrophy, increases in the strength of atrial contraction, improving the atrial transport of blood across the stenotic valve. The implications of slow heart rate in tricuspid stenosis are the same as in mitral stenosis. Ventricular contractility is usually well-maintained. The onset of atrial fibrillation in tricuspid stenosis is a less crucial event than in mitral stenosis. In tricuspid stenosis, it may produce symptoms such as an increase in peripheral edema, whereas in mitral stenosis it results in signs of left-sided failure.[79]

Diseases can interfere with cardiac compensation for tricuspid stenosis in much the same way as they can interfere with cardiac compensation for mitral stenosis. There may be further restriction of right ventricular filling in conditions such as malignant carcinoid syndrome that produce endocardial fibrosis that reduces right ventricular compliance. Tricuspid stenosis frequently coexists with pulmonic stenosis in the carcinoid syndrome, resulting in a severe restriction of cardiac output. Diseases that interfere with the conduction system of the heart can produce dysrhythmias.

G. MITRAL REGURGITATION
(Table 4–12D)

Mitral regurgitation, like aortic regurgitation, results from failure of the affected valve to maintain competence during the cardiac cycle. Mitral regurgitation occurs by one of three basic mechanisms: (1) damage to the valve apparatus itself, (2) inadequacy of the chordae tendineae–papillary muscle support of the valvular apparatus, or (3) left ventricular dilatation and stretching of the mitral valve annulus with a loss of the structural geometry required for valvular closure. Mitral regurgitation represents a volume overload of both the left atrium and the left ventricle, producing as much as a four- to fivefold increase in ventricular end-diastolic volume. In mitral regurgitation, ventricular ejection is usually well-preserved because of the parallel unloading circuit through the open mitral valve, which allows a rapid reduction of wall tension in the ventricle during systole. However, the volume overload results in an irreversible decrease in contractility. Ironically, mitral regurgitation serves as its own protective afterload reduction system.[75]

Compensatory mechanisms in mitral regurgitation include ventricular dilatation, elevations in ventricular filling pressure, and the maintenance of low peripheral resistance. As in aortic insufficiency, ventricular dilatation allows maximum advantage to be gained from the Frank-Starling mechanism. Low peripheral resistance maintains forward flow, whereas increases in peripheral resistance elevate the degree of regurgitant flow through the mitral valve. In mitral regurgitation, the heart benefits from a relatively rapid heart rate, because a slow rate is associated with increased ventricular diastolic diameter that may distort the mitral valve apparatus even further and result in increased regurgitation, in addition to heightening oxygen demand by increasing wall tension.[71]

A number of diseases can be cited that interfere with the compensatory mechanisms in mitral regurgitation. When mitral regurgitation is secondary to amyloid infiltration of

TABLE 4-12D

Uncommon Causes of Valvular Lesions

Disease	Features Affecting Compensatory Mechanisms			Associated Conditions
	Rate	LV Function and Compliance	Vascular Resistance	
A. Mitral regurgitation (MR)				
1. Conditions producing annular dilatation				
a. Aortic regurgitation			Elevated with low output	
b. Left ventricular failure		Usually in failure at this stage	Usually elevated	
2. Conditions affecting the chordae tendineae and papillary muscles				
a. Myocardial ischemia	Associated dysrhythmias, especially bradydysrhythmias	Often poor	Normal or elevated if cardiac output decreased	
b. Chordal rupture				
c. HOCM		Hyperkinetic with low ventricular compliance	Usually elevated	
3. Conditions affecting the valve leaflets				
a. Marfan's, Ehlers-Danlos, Osteogenesis imperfecta		Usually intact—these conditions also affect connective tissue of chordae tendineae		Other associated valve abnormalities
b. Rheumatic fever				Aortic regurgitation
c. Rheumatoid arthritis	Heart block	Dilated cardiomyopathy		Coronary artery disease
d. Ankylosing spondylitis				Coronary artery disease
e. Amyloidosis	AV dissociation; SA and AV nodal infiltration	Restrictive and dilated cardiomyopathy		
f. Gout	Urate deposits in conduction system	Usually normal		
B. Tricuspid regurgitation				
1. Annular dilatation				
a. RV failure		RV in failure or extremely dilated	Often secondary to pulmonary hypertension	
b. Pulmonic insufficiency			Often secondary to pulmonary hypertension	
2. Leaflets, chordae, and papillary muscles				
a. Ebstein's anomaly				
b. Acute bacterial endocarditis				
c. Rheumatic fever		Compensation intact		

the mitral valve, ventricular dilatation is compromised by coincident amyloid infiltration of the ventricular myocardium, which restricts ventricular diastolic filling. Amyloid infiltration of the conduction system can cause heart block and bradycardia, resulting in increased mitral regurgitation, for reasons already noted. In mitral regurgitation associated with left ventricular failure there is, in addition to poor left ventricular function, an elevation of endogenous catecholamine activity, which increases peripheral vascular resistance to forward flow, and regurgitant flow.

H. TRICUSPID INSUFFICIENCY
(Table 4–12D)

Tricuspid insufficiency is mechanically similar to mitral insufficiency. The most common cause of tricuspid insufficiency is right ventricular failure. Even in this setting, tricuspid insufficiency is usually tolerated well, just as it is when it exists in isolation. Tricuspid insufficiency represents volume overload of both the right ventricle and the right atrium, but because of the high compliance of the systemic venous system, pressure in the right atrium usually is not so elevated as it is in the left atrium in mitral insufficiency. This remains true until the right ventricle loses its compliance, as it might when faced with a high afterload, as in pulmonary hypertensive states.

The main compensatory mechanism in tricuspid insufficiency is adequate filling of the right ventricle. Because the right ventricle is constructed to efficiently handle a volume load, cardiac output is usually maintained. An increase in venous return, which occurs as a result of the negative intrapleural pressure resulting from spontaneous ventilation, helps maintain adequate right ventricular filling, even in the presence of tricuspid insufficiency. The main reason tricuspid insufficiency is tolerated well is that it is usually superimposed on a normal right ventricle. Tricuspid insufficiency usually becomes hemodynamically significant when there is coexisting right ventricular failure. In this situation, the loss of integrity of the right ventricular chamber owing to the incompetent tricuspid valve results in an increase in regurgitant flow at the expense of forward flow through the pulmonary circulation, decreasing the volume delivered to the left ventricle, with a resulting decrease in cardiac output.[71, 74]

I. MITRAL VALVE PROLAPSE

Mitral valve prolapse is not an uncommon condition per se, having a prevalence between 5 and 20 per cent in the general population; however, it does occur in association with uncommon diseases such as HOCM, left atrial myxoma, Wolff-Parkinson-White syndrome, long QT syndrome, Marfan's syndrome, and Ehlers-Danlos syndrome. In mitral valve prolapse, one or both mitral leaflet(s) are displaced into the left atrium during ventricular systole. Complications of mitral valve prolapse include bacterial endocarditis, mitral regurgitation, thromboembolism, dysrhythmias (both atrial and ventricular), syncope, and sudden death.

There is decreased prolapse of the valve leaflets when the left ventricle is dilated. Bradycardia, increased preload, increased afterload, and diminished contractility all tend to decrease the degree of prolapse. These patients are frequently treated with beta blockers for this reason. The patients also receive antibiotic prophylaxis against bacterial endocarditis for dental procedures, and surgery (or instrumentation) of the upper respiratory, genitourinary, or gastrointestinal tracts.[80]

J. ANESTHETIC CONSIDERATIONS

Perioperative problems arise from valvular lesions when compensatory mechanisms acutely fail. Monitoring should be selected to give continuing assessment of the status of these compensatory mechanisms. Certain aspects of monitoring should be considered common to all valvular lesions. The ECG is essential for monitoring cardiac rhythm and ischemic changes. Filling pressures should certainly be monitored, employing either the pulmonary artery catheter or a central venous pressure catheter, as appropriate to the specific lesion. Blood pressure can best be monitored with an indwelling arterial catheter. In addition, an arterial catheter provides for the monitoring of blood gases, which are important when pulmonary function is compromised. Pulse oximetry is valuable for determining that oxygenation is adequate. Transesophageal echocardiography is useful for assessing the changes in preload and contractility that result from anesthetic and surgical manipulations. Pulsed-wave Doppler and color-flow mapping are useful for determining the flow characteristics of valvular lesions and their response to pharmacologic or surgical manipulations.[71]

In lesions such as aortic or pulmonic stenosis in which high-pressure chambers have developed, monitoring of the appropriate ECG lead is mandatory for assessing ischemia.[81, 82] Monitoring of rate and rhythm is especially important. The reason for aggressive monitoring of filling pressures is clear if it is recalled that lesions such as mitral stenosis are exquisitely sensitive to preload.

In tricuspid and pulmonic stenosis, the pulmonary artery catheter may be difficult, if not impossible, to position. However, right-sided filling pressures indicate loading conditions in these lesions, and can be monitored with a central venous pressure catheter. If the chest is to be opened, then a pulmonary artery pressure catheter can be inserted under direct vision. A left-sided atrial pressure catheter may also be inserted to follow left-sided filling pressures.

In left-sided valvular lesions, a pulmonary artery catheter is indicated for monitoring both filling pressures and cardiac output. With the pulmonary artery catheter in place, vascular resistances for both the pulmonary and the systemic circulations can be calculated, allowing an assessment of therapeutic interventions, as has been mentioned before. Furthermore, changes in waveforms of the pulmonary capillary wedge pressure or central venous pressure tracings can often indicate increases in regurgitation or the development of regurgitation in situations of ventricular overdistention.

The anesthetic management of valvular lesions must avoid significant depression of contractility, as virtually all valvular lesions depend on good contractility as a major compensatory mechanism. This is especially true if the lesion coexists with cardiomyopathy, in which minor decreases in contractility can result in severe cardiac decompensation. For valvular lesions, a high-dose opioid technique probably represents the least trespass on physiologic reserves. Fentanyl, sufentanil, alfentanil, and remifentanil produce few cardiovascular changes, although bradycardia and chest wall rigidity may result.[83] Both of these problems are usually easily handled by the use of a muscle relaxant, such as pancuronium, which reduces chest wall rigidity and corrects the bradycardia; however, opioid-associated bradycardia may be advantageous in mitral and tricuspid stenotic lesions (see later discussion).

Nitrous oxide is a traditional supplement to narcotic analgesia, but it is a myocardial depressant and has the property of slightly increasing both pulmonary and systemic vascular resistance. This is usually not very significant, but it may be important in severe regurgitant lesions, when it may increase regurgitant flow.[84] Ketamine is probably not an unreasonable anesthetic for regurgitant lesions, owing to its slight sympathetic stimulating properties, but it is probably contraindicated for stenotic lesions because of the problems associated with tachycardia. Etomidate is an intravenous anesthetic that is tolerated well by patients with valvular lesions.[85] Thiopental and propofol must be administered slowly and titrated to effect if they are to be used safely in patients with valvular disease.

Muscle relaxants, when used with valvular lesions, should probably be selected according to their autonomic properties. For example, pancuronium may be useful in aortic insufficiency, owing to the increase in heart rate. In mitral stenosis, on the other hand, cisatracurium, rocuronium, vecuronium, atracurium, pipecuronium, and doxacurium do not produce detrimental increases in heart rate.[86]

Adjuvant drugs for sedation and amnesia can be selected on the basis of analogous considerations. Drugs such as the phenothiazines or the butyrophenones, which have mild alpha-adrenergic–blocking properties, may be usefully employed in lesions such as aortic or mitral insufficiency where decreases in systemic vascular resistance can increase forward flow. When sympathetic tone is increased and is important in maintaining cardiovascular homeostasis, or when elevated ventricular filling pressures are critical, these adjuvant drugs should be employed with care, because the loss of sympathetic outflow with anesthetic induction or the onset of alpha blockade may result in hypotension.

VIII. UNCOMMON CAUSES OF DYSRHYTHMIAS

A. IDIOPATHIC LONG QT SYNDROME

This rare syndrome is usually a familial disorder. The typical patient has a primary prolongation of the QT interval (QTc>440 msec) and syncopal episodes associated with physical or emotional stress. Congenital deafness is an associated condition.[87, 88] In untreated patients the mortality approaches 5 per cent per year, which is quite remarkable for a population with a median age in the twenties. The severity of the disease is judged by the frequency of syncopal attacks. These attacks may be due to ventricular dysrhythmias or sinus node dysfunction. The development of torsade de pointes is especially ominous and may be the terminal event for these patients. Torsades de pointes is a malignant variety of ventricular tachycardia with a rotating QRS axis that is resistant to cardioversion.[89]

The pathogenic mechanism for this syndrome is theorized as an imbalance of sympathetic innervation. Left stellate ganglion stimulation lowers the threshold for ventricular dysrhythmias, whereas right stellate ganglion stimulation is protective against ventricular dysrhythmias. Relief of syncope and diminished mortality have been demonstrated in patients receiving beta blockers and those who have had high left thoracic sympathectomies. It is not sufficient to ablate the left stellate ganglion, because the left sympathetic innervation to the heart also arises from the upper thoracic sympathetic ganglia.[90, 91]

1. Anesthetic Considerations

While the occasional patient presents for high left thoracic sympathectomy and left stellate ganglionectomy, these patients also may require surgery unrelated to their primary disorder. Because physical stress has been documented as a trigger for syncopal episodes, it is prudent to maintain beta blockade throughout the perioperative period.

The patient's usual oral dose of beta-adrenergic blocker should be given with a heavy premedicant to allay anxiety. The anesthetic technique should be tailored to minimize sympathetic stimulation. A large dose of opioid anesthetic is appropriate for this purpose and is effective at suppressing catecholamine elevations in response to noxious stimuli. Nitrous oxide causes mild sympathetic stimulation and should be avoided for this reason. In especially long procedures, supplemental intravenous doses of a beta blocker or a continuous infusion of esmolol should be used.

B. WOLFF-PARKINSON-WHITE AND LOWN-GANONG-LEVINE SYNDROMES

Wolff-Parkinson-White (WPW) and Lown-Ganong-Levine are pre-excitation syndromes that result in supraventricular tachycardias. The presence of accessory anatomic bypass tracts enables the atrial impulse to activate the His bundle in a shorter interval than it would through the normal AV nodal pathway. If there is an increase in the refractoriness of one of the pathways, reentrant tachycardia can be initiated. The ECG in WPW syndrome demonstrates a short PR interval (less than .12 sec), a delta wave (slurring of the R wave upstroke), and a widened QRS complex.[92]

Medications that produce more refractoriness in one pathway than in the other can create a window of functional unidirectional block. This initiates a circle of electrical impulse that results in a rapid ventricular rate. These patients are usually treated with drugs that prolong the refractory period of the AV node, such as beta blockers, verapamil and digoxin, or drugs that increase the refractory period of the accessory pathway, such as procainamide and amiodarone. However, the response of an individual patient varies, depending on the window of unidirectional block, and the different effects the same drug will have on both pathways. For example, verapamil and digoxin may perpetuate the dysrhythmia, especially when WPW is associated with atrial fibrillation.[93]

1. Anesthetic Considerations

The current treatment of choice for WPW is ablation of the accessory pathway, which is usually performed in electrophysiologic laboratories.[94] The anesthesiologist may be involved in an electrophysiologic diagnostic procedure (for young or uncooperative patients) or surgical ablative procedure.

The procedures often involve periods of programmed electrical stimulation in attempts to provoke the dysrhythmia before and after the ablation of the accessory pathway. Antidysrhythmic medications are usually discontinued before the procedure. Thus, the patient presents for an anesthetic in a relatively unprotected state. Heavy premedication is indicated to prevent anxiety, which could increase catecholamine levels and precipitate dysrhythmias. ECG monitoring should be optimal for the diagnosis of atrial dysrhythmias (leads II and V1). In patients undergoing general anesthesia, an esophageal ECG electrode provides the best "noninvasive" atrial complex.

If a dysrhythmia occurs, short-acting agents such as adenosine or esmolol should be used. The advantage of these drugs is that the effects can be terminated quickly and the procedure can continue in the absence of antidysrhythmia medications.

C. NEWER ANTIARRHYTHMIC AGENTS

1. Amiodarone

Amiodarone is structurally similar to thyroxine and procainamide. It is used to suppress a wide variety of ventricular and supraventricular arrhythmias by prolonging the refractoriness of the action potential duration in myocardial tissue. The drug has an active metabolite and a long half-life. Decreased cardiac contractility, heart rate, and systemic vascular resistance have been observed with intravenous administration of amiodarone. Many side effects are reported with the use of amiodarone. Interstitial pneumonitis, hypothyroidism, hyperthyroidism, and increased liver enzymes have all been reported with the use of amiodarone. Amiodarone and its metabolites can also inactivate cytochrome P450, resulting in the accumulation of drugs such as Coumadin.[95]

2. Sotalol (Betapace)

Sotalol is a beta-adrenergic antagonist used to treat ventricular and supraventricular arrhythmias. Unlike other beta blockers, sotalol prolongs the refractoriness of atrial and ventricular tissue. The drug has a long half-life and is proarrhythmic for the first few days after the initiation of therapy. The use of this drug has been associated with an increased incidence of torsades de pointes, especially in the presence of hypokalemia, bradycardia, and congestive heart failure.[95]

3. Propafenone (Rythmol)

Propafenone is similar in structure to propanolol but is only a weak beta-adrenergic antagonist. It is used to treat both supraventricular and ventricular arrhythmias. A decrease in left ventricular function and complete heart block have been associated with its use.[95]

4. Anesthetic Considerations

Patients receiving these newer antiarrhythmic agents will present for surgery. The decision to discontinue these long-acting medications preoperatively is controversial. Patients receiving amiodarone should have liver function and thyroid function studies. Amiodarone has been associated with intraoperative bradycardia and hypotension and postoperative pulmonary dysfunction.[96] The use of sotalol has been associated with torsades de pointes. The incidence of torsades de pointes is increased with hypokalemia and bradycardia. Propafenone depresses left ventricular function and may produce heart blocks.

IX. THE TRANSPLANTED HEART

For appropriate candidates with end-stage heart disease, heart transplantation has become a widely acceptable treatment modality, for improving both length and quality of life. The first human heart transplant was performed in the late 1960s, but this practice was discontinued shortly thereafter because of organ rejection and opportunistic infections. Since 1980, with the introduction of cyclosporine immunosuppression and improved survival, the procedure has emerged as a widely acceptable treatment modality for end-stage heart disease. By 1991, a total of 16,687 human heart transplants had been performed, and the 1-year postoperative survival rate had increased to about 90%.[97] These recipients of heart transplants may present for noncardiac surgery; therefore, the physiology of the denervated heart and the side effects of the immunosuppressive agents must be considered.

A. THE DENERVATED HEART

The recipient atrium (which usually remains after transplantation) maintains its innervation; however, this has no effect on the transplanted heart. Therefore, the transplanted heart is commonly referred to as being denervated. The efferent (to the heart) and afferent (away from the heart) limbs of both the parasympathetic and sympathetic nervous systems are disrupted during cardiac transplantation. This has significant impact on the physiology of the transplanted heart and the response to commonly used pharmacologic agents in the perioperative period.

B. IMMUNOSUPPRESSIVE THERAPY

The main agents used for chronic immunosuppression are cyclosporine, corticosteroids, and azathioprine. These drugs may interact with anesthetic agents, and they have side effects with anesthetic implications. Cyclosporine is nephrotoxic and hepatotoxic. Another important side effect associated with the use of cyclosporine is hypertension. Cyclosporine can also lower the seizure threshold. Chronic corticosteroid therapy is associated with glucose intolerance and osteoporosis, and azathioprine is toxic to the bone marrow.

C. ANESTHETIC CONSIDERATIONS

The physiology and response to pharmacologic agents are very different in the denervated heart. The vagus innervation of the heart is disrupted. This is seen by a lack of variation of heart rate with respiration[98] and vagal maneuvers. Cholinesterase inhibitors, such as neostigmine and edrophonium, do not produce bradycardia; however, the effects on other organ systems (e.g., salivary glands) remain intact, and these drugs must still be used in combination with anticholinergic agents. Similarly, because anticholinergic agents such as atropine do not increase the heart rate, bradycardia is treated with direct-acting agents such as isoproterenol or with pacing. Drugs with vagolytic side effects such as pancuronium do not produce tachycardia. The denervated sinus and AV nodes have been shown to be supersensitive to adenosine and theophylline.[99]

Sympathetic stimulation can originate from two sources: neuronal or humoral. In the denervated heart, the neuronal input is disrupted, but the increase in circulating catecholamines causes increased heart rate. The

Frank-Starling mechanism also aids in preserving the cardiac response to exercise or stress. Because of the denervation, indirect-acting cardiovascular agents have unpredictable effects. The response of the coronary circulation may also be affected: Bertrand and coworkers[100] reported cardiac autotransplantation to treat refractory coronary vasospasm in a 49-year-old man.

Sensory fibers in the heart play an important role in maintaining systemic vascular resistance (SVR). With rapid changes in SVR, the denervated heart may not respond appropriately, and these patients tolerate hypovolemia poorly. Sensory fibers in the heart are also important in the manifestations of myocardial ischemia. Thus, the patient with a denervated heart may not experience angina, although there are reports to the contrary.

Another factor that must be considered in the anesthetic management of these patients is that the transplanted heart is also predisposed to accelerated coronary artery disease. Fibrous proliferation of the intima of epicardial vessels may result from a chronic rejection process, and within 5 years of transplantation, many patients have developed significant occlusion of their coronary arteries. Therefore, these patients must be evaluated for coronary artery disease.

The immunosuppressive agents also should be considered in the anesthetic plan. Cyclosporine is nephrotoxic and hepatotoxic; therefore, these organ systems must be evaluated. Corticosteroids predispose patients to osteoporosis, and gentle positioning is required. Patients on azathioprine should have an appropriate hematologic workup in the preoperative period.

X. AIDS AND THE HEART

During the period from June 1981 to May 1991, 179,136 cases of acquired immunodeficiency syndrome (AIDS) were reported to the Centers for Disease Control. The current estimates indicate that more than 1 million persons in the United States and over 10 million worldwide may be infected with the human immunodeficiency virus (HIV).[101] All organ systems, including the cardiovascular system, are affected by HIV. The heart can be affected by (1) the HIV virus directly, (2) opportunistic infection secondary to the immunocompromised state, (3) malignancies common to the disease, and (4) drug therapy for the disease.

Left ventricular diastolic function is affected early in the course of HIV infection. Coudray and coworkers[102] performed an echocardiographic evaluation on 51 HIV-positive patients and compared the results with data obtained from age- and sex-matched controls and found that HIV-positive patients, regardless of the presence of symptomatic disease, had impaired left ventricular diastolic function. The mechanism of this dysfunction is unclear, but it may be secondary to viral myocarditis, and the clinical significance remains to be determined. In contrast to this diastolic dysfunction early in the course of the infection, systolic dysfunction has been reported late in the course of the disease. This systolic dysfunction may be caused by zidovudine (AZT).

AZT is an antiviral agent that inhibits HIV reverse transcriptase. Electron microscopic studies have demonstrated that AZT disrupts the mitochondrial apparatus of cardiac muscle.[103] Domanski and coworkers, in a randomized prospective study, found that children infected with HIV who were treated with AZT had a significant decrease in left ventricular ejection fraction as compared with children infected with HIV who had received no AZT.[104] They suggested that left ventricular function should be evaluated by serial examination. The effects of the newer antiviral agents on the heart have not yet been established.

Heart involvement was found in 45 per cent of patients with AIDS in an autopsy study.[105] Pericardial effusion, dilated cardiomyopathy, aortic root dilatation and regurgitation, and valvular vegetations were the more frequent findings. The pericardium is sometimes affected by opportunistic infections such as cytomegalovirus and by tumors such as Kaposi's sarcoma and non-Hodgkin's lymphoma. In addition, an autonomic neuropathy associated with HIV infection has been shown to cause QT prolongation, which may predispose these patients to ventricular arrhythmias.[106]

A. ANESTHETIC CONSIDERATIONS

Early in the course of HIV infection there is diastolic dysfunction that is usually clinically insignificant. As the disease progresses, and with prolonged treatment with AZT, there is reduction in left ventricular systolic function. Signs and symptoms of left ventricular failure may be masked by concurrent pulmonary disease. An echocardiographic evaluation may provide useful information in this setting. Patients with advanced disease may also have pericardial involvement with pericardial effusion and tamponade.

XI. CONCLUSIONS

Although the main focus of each of these sections has been on the cardiovascular pathology encountered in uncommon diseases, the clinician should remember that very few of these diseases have isolated cardiovascular pathology. Many of the diseases discussed are severe multisystem diseases, and an anesthetic plan must also consider the needs of monitoring dictated by other systemic pathology (e.g., measurements of blood sugar in diabetes secondary to hemochromatosis) and the potential untoward effects of drugs on unusual metabolic disturbances (e.g., the use of drugs with histamine-releasing properties such as atracurium or morphine in the malignant carcinoid syndrome).

Certainly, it cannot be stated categorically that one anesthetic technique is absolutely superior to all others in the management of any particular lesion, particularly those due to the unusual conditions discussed here. The key to the proper anesthetic management of any uncommon disease lies in an understanding of the disease process, particularly the compensatory mechanisms involved in maintaining cardiovascular homeostasis, the cardiovascular effects of anesthetic drugs, and appropriate monitoring of the effects of anesthetic and therapeutic interventions.

REFERENCES

Cardiomyopathies

1. Wenger NK, Abelmann WH, Roberts WC: Myocarditis. *In* Hurst JW (ed): The Heart. New York, McGraw-Hill, 1986, pp. 1158–1180.
2. Wenger NK, Goodwin JF, Roberts WC: Cardiomyopathy and myocardial involvement in systemic disease. *In* Hurst JW (ed): The Heart. New York, McGraw-Hill, 1986, pp. 1181–1248.
3. Wynne J, Braunwald E: The cardiomyopathies and myocarditides. *In* Braunwald E (ed): Heart Disease. Philadelphia, WB Saunders, 1988, pp. 1410–1469.
4. Billingham ME, Tazelaar HD: The morphological progression of viral myocarditis. Postgrad Med J 62:581, 1986.

5. Gravanis MB, Ansari AA: Idiopathic cardiomyopathies. Arch Pathol Lab Med 111:915, 1987.
6. Segel LD, Mason DT: Alcohol and the heart. *In* Advances in Heart Disease. Orlando, Grune & Stratton, 1977, pp. 481–489.
7. Rubin E: Alcoholic myopathy in heart and skeletal muscle. N Engl J Med 301:28, 1979.
8. Piano MR, Schertz DW: Alcoholic heart disease: A review. Heart Lung 23:3, 1994.
9. Bing RJ: Cardiac metabolism: Its contributions to alcoholic heart disease and myocardial disease. Circulation 58:965, 1978.
10. Regan TJ: The heart, alcoholism, and nutritional disease. *In* Hurst JW (ed): The Heart. New York, McGraw-Hill, 1986, pp. 1446–1451.
11. Solem LE, Henry TR, Wallace KB. Disruption of mitochondrial calcium homeostasis following chronic doxorubicin administration. Toxicol Appl Pharmacol 129:214, 1994.
12. Stevenson LW, Bellil D, Grover-McKay M, et al: Effects of afterload reduction on left ventricular volume and mitral regurgitation in severe congestive heart failure secondary to ischemic or idiopathic dilated cardiomyopathy. Am J Cardiol 60:654, 1987.
13. Fisher MI, Gottlieb SS, Plotnick GD, et al: Beneficial effects of metoprolol in heart failure associated with coronary artery disease. J Am Coll Cardiol 23:943, 1994.
14. Erlebacher JA, Bhardwaj M, Suresh A, et al: Beta-blocker treatment of idiopathic and ischemic dilated cardiomyopathy in patients with ejection fractions < or =20%. Am J Cardiol 71:1467, 1993.
15. Poll DS, Marchlinski FE, Buxton AE, et al: Sustained ventricular tachycardia in patients with idiopathic dilated cardiomyopathy: Electrophysiologic testing and lack of response to antiarrhythmic drug therapy. Circulation 70:451, 1984.
16. Shahian DM, Williamson WA, Svensson LG, et al. Transvenous versus transthoracic cardioverter-defibrillator implantation. J Thorac Cardiovasc Surg 109:1066, 1995.
17. Maron BJ, Bonow RO, Cannon RO, et al: Hypertrophic cardiomyopathy: interrelations of clinical manifestations, pathophysiology, and therapy (in two parts). N Engl J Med 316:780, 844, 1987.
18. Maron BJ, Epstein SE: Hypertrophic cardiomyopathy: A discussion of nomenclature. Am J Cardiol 43:1242, 1979.
19. Maron BJ, Wolfson JK, Epstein SE, et al: Intramural ("small vessel") coronary artery disease in hypertrophic cardiomyopathy. J Am Coll Cardiol 8:545, 1986.
20. Rosing DR, Epstein SE: Verapamil in the treatment of hypertrophic cardiomyopathy. Ann Intern Med 96:670, 1982.
21. Fighali S, Krajcer Z, Leachman RD: Septal myomectomy and mitral valve replacement for idiopathic hypertrophic subaortic stenosis: Short- and long-term follow-up. J Am Coll Cardiol 3:1127, 1984.
22. Fananapazir L, Epstein ND, Curiel RV, et al: Long-term results of dual-chamber pacing in obstructive cardiomyopathy. Evidence for progressive symptomatic and hemodynamic improvement and reduction of left ventricular hypertrophy. Circulation 90:2731, 1994.
23. Nishimura RA, Hayes DL, Ilstrup DM, et al: Effect of dual-chamber pacing on systolic and diastolic function in patients with hypertrophic cardiomyopathy. J Am Coll Cardiol 27:421, 1996.
24. Boccio RV, Chung JH, Harrison DM: Anesthetic

25. management of cesarian section in a patient with idiopathic hypertrophic subaortic stenosis. Anesthesiology 65:663, 1986.
25. Loubser P, Suh K, Cohen S: Adverse effects of spinal anesthesia in a patient with idiopathic hypertrophic subaortic stenosis. Anesthesiology 60:228, 1984.

Cardiac Tumors

26. Legler DC: Uncommon diseases and cardiac anesthesia. *In* Kaplan JA (ed): Cardiac Anesthesia. Orlando, Grune & Stratton, 1987, pp. 785–790.
27. Becker RC, Loeffler JS, Leopold KA, et al: Primary tumors of the heart: A review with emphasis on diagnosis and potential treatment modalities. Semin Surg Oncol 1:161, 1985.
28. Fine G: Neoplasms of the pericardium and heart. *In* Gould SE: Pathology of the Heart and Blood Vessels, 3rd ed. Springfield, IL, Charles C Thomas, 1968, pp. 851–883.
29. Kirklin JW, Barratt-Boyes BG: Cardiac Surgery: Morphology, Results, and Indications. New York, John Wiley & Sons, 1986, pp. 1393–1407.
30. Robiolio PA, Rigolin VA, Wilson JS, et al: Carcinoid heart disease. Correlation of high serotonin levels with valvular abnormalities. Circulation 92:790, 1995.
31. Jacobsen MB, Nitter-Hauge S, Bryde PE, Hanssen LE: Cardiac manifestations in mid-gut carcinoid disease. Eur Heart J 16:263, 1995.

Coronary Artery Disease

32. Mangano DT: Preoperative assessment. *In* Kaplan JA (ed): Cardiac Anesthesia. Orlando, Grune & Stratton, 1987, pp. 341-392.
33. Baim DS, Harrison DC: Nonatherosclerotic coronary heart disease. *In* Hurst JW (ed): The Heart. New York, McGraw-Hill, 1986.
34. Hoffman JI, Buckberg GD: The myocardial oxygen supply-demand ratio. Am J Cardiol 41:327, 1978.
35. Klocke FJ: Coronary blood flow in man. Prog Cardiovasc Dis 19:117, 1976.
36. Myerburg RJ, Kessler KM, Mallon SM, et al: Life-threatening ventricular arrhythmias in patients with silent myocardial ischemia due to coronary artery spasm. N Engl J Med 326:1451, 1992.
37. Kaski JC, Tousoulis D, McFadden E, et al: Variant angina pectoralis. Circulation 85:619, 1992.
38. Maseri A, Severi S, DeNes M, et al: "Variant" angina. One aspect of a continuous spectrum of vasospastic myocardial ischemia. Am J Cardiol 42:1019, 1978.
39. Hillis LD, Braunwald E: Coronary artery spasm. N Engl J Med 299:695, 1978.
40. Lange RA, Cigarroa RG, Yancy CW, et al: Cocaine induced coronary artery vasoconstriction. N Engl J Med 321:1557, 1989.
41. Stambler BS, Komamura K, Ihara T, Shannon RP: Acute intravenous cocaine causes transient depression followed by enhanced left ventricular function in conscious dogs. Circulation 87:1687, 1993.
42. Kugelmass AD, Shannon RP, Yeo EL, Ware JA: Intravenous cocaine induces platelet activation in the conscious dog. Circulation 91:1336, 1995.
43. Holt S: Syphilitic osteal occlusion. Br Heart J 39:469, 1977.
44. Selhub J, Jacques PF, Bostom AG, et al: Association between plasma homocysteine concentrations and

extracranial carotid artery stenosis. N Engl J Med 332:286, 1995.

45. Levitsky S, van der Horst RL, Hastreiter AR, Fisher EA: Anomalous left coronary artery from the pulmonary artery in the infant. J Thorac Cardiovasc Surg 79:598, 1980.
46. Griffin RM, Kaplan JA: Intraoperative myocardial ischemia. *In* Thys DM, Kaplan JA (eds): The ECG in Anesthesia and Critical Care. New York, Churchill Livingstone, 1987, pp. 139–154.
47. Haggmark S, Hohner P, Ostman M, et al: Comparison of hemodynamic, electrocardiographic, mechanical, and metabolic indicators of intraoperative myocardial ischemia in vascular surgical patients with coronary artery disease. Anesthesiology 70:19, 1989.
48. Smith JS, Cahalan MK, Benefiel DJ, et al: Intraoperative detection of myocardial ischemia in high-risk patients: Electrocardiography versus two-dimensional echocardiography. Circulation 72:1015, 1985.
49. O'Connor JP, Wynands JE: Anesthesia for myocardial revascularization. *In* Kaplan JA (ed): Cardiac Anesthesia. Orlando, Grune & Stratton, 1987.
50. Stanley TH, Webster LR: Anesthetic requirements and cardiovascular effects of fentanyl-oxygen and fentanyl-diazepam-oxygen anesthesia in man. Anesth Analg 57:411, 1978.
51. Wynands JE, Wong P, Townsend GE, et al: Narcotic requirements for intravenous anesthesia. Anesth Analg 63:101, 1984.

Pulmonary Hypertension and Cor Pulmonale

52. Kuida H: Pulmonary hypertension: Mechanism and recognition. *In* Hurst JW (ed): The Heart. New York, McGraw-Hill, 1986, pp. 1091–1099.
53. Kuida H: Primary pulmonary hypertension. *In* Hurst JW (ed): The Heart. New York, McGraw-Hill, 1986, pp. 1099–1104.
54. Dalen JE, Alpert JS: Pulmonary embolism. *In* Hurst JW (ed): The Heart. New York, McGraw-Hill, 1986, pp. 1105–1119.
55. Ross JC, Newman JH: Chronic cor pulmonale. *In* Hurst JW (ed): The Heart. New York, McGraw-Hill, 1986, pp. 1120–1129.
56. Harris P, Heath D: Pulmonary haemodynamics in chronic bronchitis and emphysema. *In* The Human Pulmonary Circulation. New York, Churchill Livingstone, 1977, pp. 522–546.
57. Tempe D, Mohan JC, Cooper A, et al. Myocardial depressant effect of nitrous oxide after valve surgery. Eur J Anaesthesiol 11:353, 1994.
58. Harris P, Heath D: Pharmacology of the pulmonary circulation. *In* The Human Pulmonary Circulation. New York, Churchill Livingstone, 1977, pp. 182–210.
59. D'Ambra MN, LaRaia PJ, Philbin DM, et al: Prostaglandin E1: A new therapy for refractory right heart failure and pulmonary hypertension after mitral valve replacement. J Thorac Cardiovasc Surg 89:567, 1985.
60. Goldman AP, Delius RE, Deanfield JE, Macrae DJ: Nitric oxide is superior to prostacyclin for pulmonary hypertension after cardiac transplantation. Ann Thorac Surg 60:300, 1995.
61. Chiche JD, Canivet JL, Damas P, et al: Inhaled nitric oxide for hemodynamic support after postpneumonectomy ARDS. Intensive Care Med 21:675, 1995.
62. Zobel G, Dacar D, Rodl S, Friehs I: Inhaled nitric oxide versus inhaled prostacyclin and intravenous versus inhaled prostacyclin in acute respiratory failure with pulmonary hypertension in piglets. Pediatr Res 38:198, 1995.

Constrictive Pericarditis and Cardiac Tamponade

63. Shabetai R: Diseases of the pericardium. *In* Hurst JW (ed): The Heart. New York, McGraw-Hill, 1986, pp. 1249–1275.
64. Hancock EW: Constrictive pericarditis. JAMA 232:176, 1975.
65. Field J, Shiroff RA, et al: Limitations in the use of the pulmonary capillary wedge pressure with cardiac tamponade. Chest 70:451, 1976.
66. Shabetai R, Fowler NO, et al: The hemodynamics of cardiac tamponade and constrictive pericarditis. Am J Cardiol 26:480, 1970.
67. Legler DC: Uncommon diseases and cardiac anesthesia. *In* Kaplan JA (ed): Cardiac Anesthesia. Orlando, Grune & Stratton, 1987, pp. 810–812.
68. Baum V: Anesthetic complications during emergency noncardiac surgery in patients with documented cardiac contusions. J Cardiothorac Vasc Anesth 5:57, 1991.
69. Kaplan JA, Bland JW, et al: The perioperative management of pericardial tamponade. South Med J 69:417, 1976.
70. Pories WJ, Gaudiani VA: Cardiac tamponade. Surg Clin North Am 55:573, 1975.

Valvular Lesions

71. Jackson JM, Thomas SJ: Valvular heart disease. *In* Kaplan JA (ed): Cardiac Anesthesia. Orlando, Grune & Stratton, 1987, pp. 589–634.
72. Braunwald E: Valvular heart disease. *In* Braunwald E (ed): Heart Disease. Philadelphia, WB Saunders, 1984.
73. Rackley CE, Edwards JE, Wallace RB, et al: Aortic valve disease. *In* Hurst JW (ed): The Heart. New York, McGraw-Hill, 1986, pp. 729–753.
74. Rackley CE, Edwards JE, Wallace RB, et al: Tricuspid and pulmonary valve disease. *In* Hurst JW (ed): The Heart. New York, McGraw-Hill, 1986, pp. 792–800.
75. Rackley CE, Edwards JE, Karp RB: Mitral valve disease. *In* Hurst JW (ed): The Heart. New York, McGraw-Hill, 1986, pp. 754–784.
76. Rackley CE, Edwards JE, Karp RB: Combined aortic and mitral valve disease. *In* Hurst JW (ed): The Heart. New York, McGraw-Hill, 1986, pp. 785–791.
77. Ross J Jr: Cardiac function and myocardial contractility: A perspective. J Am Coll Cardiol 1:52, 1983.
78. Keefe JF, Walls J, et al: Isolated tricuspid valvular stenosis. Am J Cardiol 25:252, 1970.
79. Morgan JR, Forker AD, et al: Isolated tricuspid stenosis. Circulation 44:729, 1971.
80. Keusch DJ, Hillel Z: Mitral valve prolapse: anesthetic considerations. Prog Anesthesiol 1(22):1, 1987.
81. Nadell R, DePace NL, Ren J-F, et al: Myocardial oxygen supply/demand ratio in aortic stenosis: Hemodynamic and echocardiographic evaluation of patients with and without angina pectoris. J Am Coll Cardiol 2:258, 1983.
82. Marcus ML: Effects of cardiac hypertrophy on the coronary circulation. *In* Marcus ML (ed): The Coronary Circulation in Health and Disease. New York, McGraw-Hill, 1983.
83. Bovill JG, Warren PJ, Schuller MH: Comparison of

fentanyl, sufentanil, and alfentanil anesthesia in patients undergoing valvular heart surgery. Anesth Analg 63:1081, 1984.

84. Schulte-Sasse U, Hess W, Tarnow J: Pulmonary vascular responses to nitrous oxide in patients with normal and high pulmonary vascular resistance. Anesthesiology 57:9, 1982.

85. Stoelting RK: Choice of muscle relaxants in patients with heart disease. Semin Anesth 4:1, 1985.

86. Lindeburg T, Spotoft H, Sorensen MB, et al: Cardiovascular effects of etomidate used for induction and in combination with fentanyl-pancuronium for maintenance of anaesthesia in patients with valvular heart disease. Acta Anaesthesiol Scand 26:205, 1982.

Unusual Causes of Dysrhythmias

87. Fraser GR, Froggatt P, James TN: Congenital deafness associated with electrocardiographic abnormalities. Q J Med 33:361, 1964.

88. Jervell A, Lange-Nielson F: Congenital deaf-mutism, functional heart disease with prolongation of the QT interval and sudden death. Am Heart J 54:59, 1957.

89. Moss AJ, Schwartz PJ, Crampton RS, et al: Hereditable malignant arrhythmias: A prospective study of the long QT syndrome. Circulation 71:17, 1985.

90. Schwartz PJ, Periti M, Malliani A: The long QT syndrome. Am Heart J 89:378, 1975.

91. Schwartz PJ: Idiopathic long QT syndrome: Progress and questions. Am Heart J 109:399, 1985.

92. Feinberg BJ: Anesthesia and electrophysiologic procedures. *In* Kaplan JA (ed): Cardiac Anesthesia. Orlando, Grune & Stratton, 1987, pp. 755–765.

93. Gulamhusein S, Do P, Carruthers SG, et al: Acceleration of ventricular response during atrial fibrillation in the Wolff-Parkinson-White syndrome after verapamil. Circulation 65:348, 1982.

94. Lowes D, Frank G, Klein J, Manz M: Surgical treatment of Wolff-Parkinson-White syndrome. Eur Heart J 14:99, 1993.

95. Woosley RL: Antiarrhythmic drugs. *In* Hurst JW (ed): The Heart. New York, McGraw-Hill, 1994, pp. 775–800.

96. Rooney RT, Marijic J, Stommel KA, et al: Additive cardiac depression by volatile anesthetics in isolated hearts after chronic amiodarone treatment. Anesth Analg 80:917, 1995.

Anesthetic Considerations for the Transplanted Heart

97. Kriett JM, Kaye MP: The registry of the International Society for Heart and Lung Transplantation: Eighth official report, 1991. Heart Lung Transpl 10:491, 1991.

98. Smith MI, Ellenbogen KA, Eckberg DI, et al: Subnormal parasympathetic activity after cardiac transplantation. Am J Cardiol 66:1243, 1990.

99. Ellenbogen KA, Thames MD, DiMarco JP, et al: Electrophysiological effects of adenosine on the transplanted human heart. Circulation 81:821, 1990.

100. Bertrand ME, Lablanche JM, Tilmant M, et al: Complete denervation of the heart to treat severe refractory coronary spasm. Am J Cardiol 47:1375, 1981.

AIDS and the Heart

101. Centers for Disease Control. The HIV/AIDS epidemic: The first 10 years. MMWR 40:357, 1991.

102. Choudry N, de Zuttere D, Force G, et al. Left ventricular diastolic function in asymptomatic and symptomatic HIV carriers: An echocardiological study. Eur Heart J 16:61, 1995.

103. Corcuera-Pindado A, Lopez-Bravo A, Martinez-Rodriguez R, et al: Histochemical and ultrastructural changes induced by zidovudine in mitochondria of rat cardiac muscle. Eur J Histochem 34:311, 1994.

104. Domanski MJ, Sloas MM, Follmann DA, et al: Effects of zidovudine and didanosine treatment on heart function in children affected with HIV. J Pediatr 127:137, 1995.

105. DeCastro S, Migliau G, Silvestri A, et al: Heart involvement in AIDS. Eur Heart J 13:1452, 1992.

106. Villa A, Foresti V, Confalonieri F: Autonomic neuropathy and prolongation of the QT interval in HIV infection. Clin Autom Res 5:48, 1995.

Renal Disease

Allen W. Burton
Richard I. Mazze
Donald S. Prough

I. INTRODUCTION

The purpose of this chapter is to provide the anesthesiologist with the background knowledge necessary to care for patients with uncommon renal diseases throughout the perioperative period. There are myriad uncommon renal diseases, so precise diagnosis of various syndromes is sometimes impossible. Despite the confusing array of conditions that affect the kidneys, the final common pathways of renal disease are loss of glomerular function and tubular dysfunction. Thus, we first present a brief overview of normal renal function, then review diagnostic methods used to assess renal function, and finally discuss specific pathologic states.

II. NORMAL RENAL PHYSIOLOGY: AN OVERVIEW

The kidneys perform two major functions: (1) regulation of the volume and composition of body fluids (including acid-base balance) and (2) regulation of certain systems (e.g., red blood cell formation and vitamin D metabolism).[1]

These processes are carried out by a combination of excretory and nonexcretory functions. The excretory functions consist of filtration and reabsorption, which ultimately form urine. Normal adult kidneys produce approximately 180 L per day of filtrate, generating approximately 1 to 2 L of urine. The tubules and collecting ducts reabsorb approximately 99 per cent of the filtered solute. The process can best be described by tracing the course of a single nephron (Fig. 5–1).[2]

A. THE NEPHRON: FORM AND FUNCTION

Afferent arterioles enter the glomeruli, where they branch to form the glomerular capillary network before exiting the glomeruli as efferent arterioles. The glomerular filtration rate (GFR) is a function of filtration pressure and the permeability characteristics of the membrane. Glomerular capillary pressure, the force driving the ultrafiltrate across the capillary membrane, is opposed by pressure within Bowman's capsule and the plasma oncotic pressure. The glomerular capillary wall is much more permeable than other systemic capillaries. Despite considerable interest, neither the precise mechanisms nor the sites of filtration (e.g., "pores") have been described. Two theories exist: the pore theory and the diffusion theory. The *diffusion theory* holds that the capillary membrane is gel-like and that substances diffuse through at different rates determined by transmembrane diffusion gradients. The diffusion theory is currently favored because pores have never been visualized, large proteins (presumably larger than the hypothetical pores) are found in trace amounts in the urine, and the membrane *is* gel-like. Large molecular size and electrical charge markedly restrict protein filtration.

Filtered fluid moves into the proximal convoluted tubule (PCT). In the PCT, glucose, potassium, uric acid, and amino acids are reabsorbed up to tubular threshold limits. Sixty-five per cent of filtered sodium is actively reabsorbed; water follows passively. Acid-base regulation begins in the PCT, with almost complete reabsorption of bicarbonate. The reduced volume of isoosmotic tubular fluid proceeds to the loop of Henle (LOH), which in some nephrons is short but in others is long and dips deeply into the medulla.

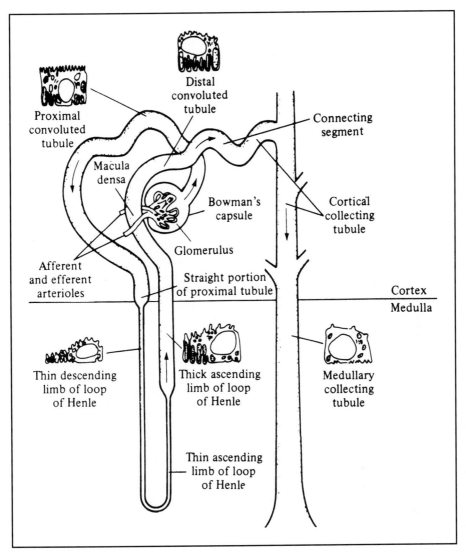

FIGURE 5–1. The nephron. (Reprinted with permission from Vander R: Renal Physiology, 2nd ed. New York, McGraw-Hill, 1980. Reproduced with permission of the McGraw-Hill Companies.)

Whereas cortical tissue contains the glomeruli, PCT, and distal convoluted tubules (DCT), the medulla consists of the LOH, collecting ducts (CD), vasa recta, and interstitium. The hypertonic medulla is crucial to the kidney's ability to conserve salt and water. Chloride is actively transported out of the tubular lumen in the medullary thick ascending LOH, resulting in hypotonic tubular fluid leaving the LOH and passing into the DCT.

In the DCT, sodium is variably reabsorbed in direct proportion to aldosterone levels. Antidiuretic hormone (ADH) acts on the DCT and the collecting duct to increase permeability to water, thus increasing water reabsorption and decreasing urine volume. In the absence of ADH, larger amounts of dilute urine are formed. Also in the DCT, the remaining bicarbonate continues to be reabsorbed as hydrogen ions are actively secreted. Finally, in the CD, the last concentration of urine occurs under the influence of ADH and the highly concentrated interstitium.

B. NEUROHUMORAL REGULATION OF RENAL FUNCTION

Several hormonal factors are involved in sodium and water balance: aldosterone,

ADH, atrial natriuretic peptide (ANP), and the renal prostaglandins.[3]

1. Aldosterone

This regulator hormone of sodium-potassium homeostasis is produced in the adrenal cortex as the result of a complex chain of endocrine events: First, renin is released from the juxtaglomerular apparatus in response to reduced arterial volume. Renin enters the circulation, where it catalyzes the conversion of circulating angiotensinogen to angiotensin I. Angiotensin I is transformed in the lungs by angiotensin-converting enzyme (ACE) into angiotensin II, which stimulates the adrenal cortex to release aldosterone. Acting on the DCT and CD, aldosterone influences the reabsorption of about 2 per cent of filtered sodium.[4–7] Overall, the renin-angiotensin system acts to preserve circulating blood volume by causing aldosterone-induced sodium retention during periods of intravascular volume depletion.

2. Antidiuretic Hormone

ADH secretion responds both to changes in serum osmolarity and to changes in intravascular volume. Release of ADH from the posterior pituitary gland occurs in response to increased blood osmolarity, mediated via osmoreceptors in the hypothalamus. ADH release is inhibited by increased activity of atrial baroreceptors in response to increased atrial stretch. ADH increases water reabsorption in the DCT and CD, resulting in the formation of small amounts of highly concentrated urine. Urine volume may vary 100-fold, depending on the ADH concentration.[3]

3. Atrial Natriuretic Peptide

ANP, secreted by the atria in response to increased atrial stretch (e.g., volume expansion), reduces blood pressure by relaxing vascular smooth muscle and increases sodium excretion by inhibiting renin and aldosterone secretion.[8, 9] ANP also exerts intrarenal effects; namely, constriction of efferent arterioles and dilatation of afferent arterioles, processes that lead to increased filtration and excretion of sodium.[8, 9]

4. Prostaglandins

Extensive renal synthesis of prostaglandins appears to mediate vascular tone and modulate other hormonal interactions in a complex manner, acting principally to maintain renal perfusion and GFR in the face of vasoconstricting influences.[10, 11]

C. NONEXCRETORY RENAL FUNCTIONS

The nonexcretory functions, which include regulation of red blood cell production,[12] vitamin D metabolism, and the kallikrein-bradykinin system, are controlled by a complex array of closely regulated secretory activity. Secretory products of the kidneys include renin, prostaglandins, erythropoietin, and 1,25-dihydroxycholecalciferol.

III. DIAGNOSIS OF RENAL IMPAIRMENT AND CLINICAL ASSESSMENT OF RENAL FUNCTION

The medical history is important in establishing the presence of renal disease. Physical findings may be minimal until renal disease has become advanced. In patients with renal failure, the physical examination should focus on determining volume status. Further assessment requires laboratory evaluation.

In the presence of renal disease it is important to estimate the degree of renal dysfunction. The GFR, the best clinical estimate of functioning renal mass, is normally 120 ± 25 mL/min in men and 95 ± 20 mL/min in women.[13–16] GFR normally declines with age, falling almost 1 mL/min per year after age 40. In infants, GFR is 15 to 30 per cent of normal adult values but reaches 50 per cent of adult normal values on the fifth to tenth days of life. By age one, an infant's GFR approximates normal adult values.[13]

A. BLOOD UREA NITROGEN AND SERUM CREATININE

Blood urea nitrogen (BUN) and plasma creatinine (Cr) concentrations are valuable indices of general kidney function. Plasma Cr, excreted primarily by glomerular filtration,

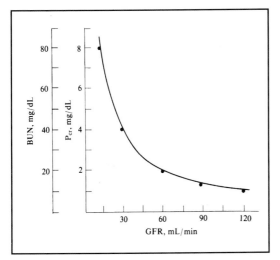

FIGURE 5–2. Steady-state relationship between the plasma creatinine concentration P$_{cr}$, blood urea nitrogen (BUN), and glomerular filtration rate (GFR). (From Rose BD: Clinical assessment of renal function. In Rose BD (ed): Pathophysiology of Renal Disease, 2nd ed. New York, McGraw-Hill, 1987. Reproduced with permission of the McGraw-Hill Companies.)

varies inversely with GFR (Fig. 5–2).[16] However, this relationship is valid only in the steady state. For example, in a patient who suddenly develops acute renal failure (ARF), plasma Cr lags behind the decrease in GFR, reaching a plateau only after 7 to 10 days. Because of the exponential shape of the curve relating GFR to plasma Cr, an apparently minor increase in plasma Cr from 1.0 to 2.0 mg/dL can represent a marked fall in GFR, from 120 to 60 mL per minute. In contrast, in a patient with advanced renal failure, a marked increase in the plasma Cr from 6.0 to 12.0 can reflect a reduction in GFR from 20 to 10 mL per minute. Thus, as chronic renal failure develops, the initial plasma Cr elevation represents the greater loss in GFR.

The relationship of GFR to plasma Cr depends on the rate of Cr production, which is largely a function of muscle mass. To account for the effects of body weight, age, and gender on muscle mass, the following equation estimates GFR from the plasma Cr in the steady state:

$$GFR^* = (140 - Age) \times Lean\ body\ weight \div Plasma\ Cr \times 72$$

Using this formula, a plasma Cr of 1.4 mg/dL represents a GFR of 100 mL/min in an 85-

kg, 20-year-old male, but that same plasma Cr of 1.4 mg/dL represents a GFR of only 20 mL/min in a 40-kg, 80-year-old female.

There is little potential for error in extrapolating the GFR from the plasma Cr. The following factors may cause an elevation in plasma Cr without impaired renal function: (1) Increased Cr production due to rhabdomyolysis or ingestion of large amounts of cooked meat or broth; (2) decreased Cr secretion induced by competition by cimetidine and trimethoprim for the same pump site as Cr; and (3) erroneous measurement of Cr by some assays of certain compounds, including acetoacetic acid (in ketoacidosis), cefoxitin, and flucytosine.

Changes in GFR are also reflected by alterations in BUN. Similar to Cr, urea is excreted primarily by glomerular filtration and varies inversely with GFR; however, BUN is less accurate than Cr because of variability in urea production and tubular reabsorption of urea. Urea production is increased by high protein intake, tissue breakdown, or gastrointestinal bleeding and is decreased by low protein intake or severe liver disease (which impairs urea synthesis). Urea reabsorption in the tubules is largely passive, accompanying sodium and water. Thus, in dehydrated states in which proximal sodium reabsorption is increased, enhanced urea reabsorption increases BUN. A normal value for BUN is 10 to 20 mg/dL, and the normal ratio of BUN to plasma Cr is 10:1 to 15:1. When the ratio exceeds 20:1, one of the conditions associated with enhanced urea production or enhanced tubular reabsorption should be suspected.

In summary, a reduction in GFR leads to an elevation in Cr and plasma BUN; however, due to variability of urea production and reabsorption, the plasma Cr is a more reliable reflection of the GFR. One exception to this occurs in patients with advanced renal failure (plasma Cr over 4.0 mg/dL, GFR under 30 mL/min) whose failing kidney begins to secrete Cr; thus, with advanced renal failure the GFR may be overestimated on the basis of the serum Cr value.

Additionally, it is important to note that patients with mild renal damage may maintain GFR with less functioning renal mass by compensatory glomerular hyperfiltration. As some nephrons are damaged, others compensate by increasing filtration. Thus, patients may have progressive renal damage with no change in GFR, BUN, or plasma Cr until approximately 33 per cent of the nephrons have

---

*Multiply value by 0.85 in women to adjust for higher body weight/muscle mass ratio.

been destroyed. For example, after donor nephrectomy, GFR stabilizes at about 70 to 80 per cent of baseline despite loss of 50 per cent of renal mass.[16]

B. URINALYSIS

Urinalysis is an important, inexpensive *diagnostic* tool that includes assessment of gross and microscopic appearance, pH, specific gravity, and protein and glucose content. In contrast to the GFR, the urinalysis provides little information about renal function or the severity of renal disease.

1. Appearance

Gross examination of the urine may suggest bleeding, infection, or systemic disease affecting the genitourinary tract. Microscopic examination of the urinary sediment may reveal cells, casts, crystals, and bacteria. Various findings in the sediment point to certain diseases (e.g., red-cell casts accompany glomerulonephritis).

2. pH

The urinary pH reflects acidification of the urine. The kidneys are responsible for excretion of approximately 60 mEq of nonvolatile acid generated each day by normal metabolism. Urinary pH can range between 4.5 and 8.0, but it is usually between 5.0 and 6.5, depending on systemic acid-base balance. The three main mechanisms of renal acid excretion are reabsorption of bicarbonate from the glomerular filtrate, acidification of buffers in the tubular urine, and production in the tubular cells of ammonia to be excreted as ammonium ion. Therefore, the ability to acidify urine is a gross measure of renal competence.

3. Specific Gravity and Osmolality

Specific gravity is a measure of urine-concentrating ability and thus is a test of tubular function. Specific gravity compares the weight of urine to that of distilled water, whereas osmolality is a measure of the number of particles per kilogram of urine. Although these two values often correlate well, large molecules, such as glucose, increase specific gravity much more than the osmolality; therefore, specific gravity unreliably estimates urine-concentrating ability.

Urinary osmolality is strongly influenced by neurohumoral factors. Tubular fluid is isosmotic in the proximal tubule but rapidly becomes hyperosmotic as it descends deep into the medulla in the LOH. As chloride is reabsorbed in the ascending LOH, tubular fluid becomes hyposmotic. In the DCT and CD, ADH controls osmolality. In the presence of ADH, sodium-free fluid passes into the interstitium of the renal medulla, resulting in the formation of small amounts of concentrated (i.e., high-osmolality) urine. When no ADH is present, sodium reabsorption continues in the DCT but water is not reabsorbed; so, large volumes of dilute urine are produced. Intact urine-concentrating ability indicates intact tubular function; however, owing to the variation in urine concentration produced by changes in systemic hydration, a random urinary osmolality or specific gravity test has little diagnostic value unless it correlates with clinical status.

In patients with acute oliguria, the two most common causes (hypovolemia and acute tubular necrosis) can be differentiated by examining the urinary osmolality or specific gravity. Because hypovolemia is a potent stimulus for ADH release, a hypovolemic patient usually has urinary osmolality greater than 500 mOsm/kg (or specific gravity above 1.020). In contrast, acute tubular necrosis impairs concentrating ability, resulting in urine osmolality usually around 300 mOsm/kg (or specific gravity about 1.010). Thus, high urine osmolality essentially excludes the diagnosis of acute tubular necrosis.

In contrast to urine-concentrating ability, the ability to dilute urine is better maintained as renal function declines, so urinary osmolality of 50 to 100 mOsm/kg may be found in the presence of advanced renal disease.

4. Proteinuria

Normally, less than 150 mg of protein is excreted in the urine per day. This amount may increase transiently after strenuous exercise or prolonged standing. Large molecules such as albumin normally are not filtered at the glomerulus. The glomerular capillary wall contains negatively charged proteoglycans that aid in electrostatic repulsion and limit filtration of macromolecules such as proteins. Glomerular damage generally leads to albuminuria. Tubular proteinuria occurs when low–molecular weight proteins, which normally are filtered, are incompletely reabsorbed (Fanconi's syndrome) or are filtered in large amounts that overwhelm tubular reabsorption capacity (multiple myeloma). Quantitation of proteinuria is usually done for a 24-hour period. A protein value of 3.5 g per day is virtually diagnostic of glomerular disease.

5. Glycosuria

Glucose is freely filtered by the glomerulus and is reabsorbed by the proximal tubule. Glycosuria usually indicates diabetes mellitus, but it may mean that the ability of the proximal tubule to reabsorb glucose has been temporarily exceeded by a heavy glucose load.

C. SERUM ELECTROLYTES

Potassium excretion is determined primarily by urinary output rather than GFR until GFR is lower than 10 mL per minute. Potassium concentration should be determined if impaired renal function is suspected. Hyperkalemia is common among patients with renal failure; chronic hyperkalemia is well-tolerated, but acute hyperkalemia is not; however, at potassium levels above 5.8 mEq/L hyperkalemia may lead to severe arrhythmias or cardiac arrest. Hemodialysis may be indicated, to reduce serum potassium to an acceptable range before elective surgery. Other measures used to treat hyperkalemia include co-administration of glucose and insulin, hyperventilation, intravenous sodium bicarbonate, and potassium-binding resins such as polystyrene sulfonate.

D. COMPLETE BLOOD COUNT

Hemoglobin should be measured preoperatively in patients with renal disease. These patients, anemic owing to reduced erythropoietin secretion, lose red cell mass gradually and generally adapt well. Recombinant erythropoietin is being used to treat anemia in some cases of renal failure.

E. ARTERIAL BLOOD GASES

Patients with severe renal disease develop metabolic acidosis as a result of their inability to excrete their daily acid load. An arterial blood sample and serum electrolytes enable quantification of the severity of the acidosis.

F. ELECTROCARDIOGRAPHY

The electrocardiogram (ECG) reflects the toxic electrophysiologic effects of hyperkalemia more accurately than a serum potassium value. Tall, peaked T waves, ST segment depression, QRS widening, and ventricular ectopy occur as hyperkalemia progresses. In addition, the ECG may be helpful in evaluating hypertensive and ischemic heart disease, which often accompany renal disease.

G. RADIOGRAPHIC STUDIES

A chest radiograph may indicate the presence of hypertensive cardiac disease, congestive heart failure, or pericardial effusion. Ultrasonography, computed tomography (CT), magnetic resonance imaging (MRI), and abdominal radiography are used to image the kidneys and urogenital tract for diagnostic purposes or to guide therapeutic procedures. Although radioisotope studies can be used to provide a real-time estimate of GFR, none are in routine clinical use.[17-19]

IV. EFFECTS OF ANESTHETIC AGENTS IN PATIENTS WITH NORMAL RENAL FUNCTION

All general anesthesia agents depress renal function—specifically, urine output, GFR, renal blood flow (RBF), and electrolyte excretion.[20-28] The depression in renal function caused by anesthetic agents is due to their direct effects on the kidney and their indirect effects on the circulatory, sympathetic nervous, and endocrine systems.[28] This consistent, generalized depression of renal function is influenced by many factors, including type and duration of surgical procedure; preoperative physical status (especially diseases of the cardiovascular and renal systems); preoperative and intraoperative blood volume and fluid and electrolyte balance; and choice of anesthetic agent.[28-44] Changes in renal function after spinal and epidural anesthesia tend to parallel the degree of hypotension associated with the anesthetic.[45] In most cases, changes in renal function associated with anesthesia and surgery are transient and resolve completely postoperatively.[28]

A. CIRCULATORY SYSTEM

During general anesthesia, RBF may be depressed as a consequence of renal vasoconstriction, systemic hypotension, or both.[46] Cyclopropane, diethyl ether, and ketamine evoke a sympathetic response, which increases renal vascular resistance, thus decreasing RBF and transiently depressing renal function.[47, 48] Isoflurane, enflurane, halothane, and thiopental are also associated with a moderate increase in renal vascular resistance, although the mechanism is unclear.[23-25, 49] Renal blood flow and GFR drop with these agents, but to a lesser extent than with drugs that cause catecholamine release. Desflurane affects RBF minimally.[41]

B. SYMPATHETIC NERVOUS SYSTEM

The renal vessels are sympathetically innervated with fibers that leave the spinal cord from T4 to L1 via the celiac and renal plexuses. There is no direct sympathetic or parasympathetic innervation of the renal parenchyma. Under a wide variety of physiologic conditions, RBF is regulated to maintain a stable GFR. Experimental evidence points to the role of the sympathetic nervous system in depressing RBF and renal function under general anesthesia. Berne[50] conducted experiments in dogs that had one normal kidney and a denervated one. Before induction of general anesthesia with Innovar, RBF and GFR of both kidneys were the same; however, after induction of anesthesia, RBF and GFR decreased in the normally innervated kidney, whereas no changes were seen in the denervated kidney. These changes were attributed to an anesthesia-induced increase in vasoconstrictor tone to the innervated kidney.[50]

Autoregulation of RBF and GFR occurs in unanesthetized animals, keeping RBF nearly constant between mean arterial pressures of 50 and 120 mm Hg. In animals, data about preservation of RBF autoregulation under general anesthesia are conflicting[51-53]; however, autoregulation appears to be impaired in humans undergoing inhalational general anesthesia.[22-24, 49]

C. ENDOCRINE SYSTEM

Endocrine effects on renal function during anesthesia are important and are closely tied to the circulatory effects. The most important anesthesia-related neuroendocrine response that regulates urinary volume is ADH.

The release of ADH is controlled by osmoreceptors in the carotid body and the pituitary gland, which are sensitive to osmolality changes of approximately 2 per cent.[54] An increase in the osmolality of blood causes reflex release of ADH. When the osmolality of plasma is lowered, ADH release is suppressed, resulting in formation of dilute urine. Decreased intravascular volume also causes ADH release, probably via reflex baroreceptor mechanisms.[55, 56] ADH release occurring during surgery, sometimes inappropriately, is most likely due to sympathetic stimulation and can be blunted by deep anesthesia.[57]

Epinephrine, norepinephrine, and the renin-angiotensin system are involved in control of RBF. Elaboration of these substances causes a marked increase in renal vascular resistance, with a decrease in RBF.[58] Renin secretion varies during anesthesia and surgery, but no patterns have been discerned.[56, 59, 60]

Aldosterone secretion is primarily controlled by renin release, and thus also varies during anesthesia and surgery, but with no discernible pattern.[56, 59, 60]

V. EFFECTS OF DRUGS ON REDUCED RENAL FUNCTION

In patients with renal impairment, the action of drugs may be changed owing to alterations in distribution and elimination[61] and by intercurrent anemia, hypoproteinemia, electrolyte abnormalities, and dialysis. Because patients with renal impairment often are debilitated, they may have impaired mechanisms of biotransformation, in addition to markedly decreased renal excretion of drugs (Table 5–1).

TABLE 5–1

Preferred Anesthetic Drugs for Patients with Compromised Renal Function			
Drug	**Safe**	**Use with Caution**	**Avoid**
Volatile agents	Isoflurane Desflurane Halothane	Sevoflurane Enflurane	Methoxyflurane
Intravenous anesthetic agents	Thiopental Propofol Etomidate	Midazolam	Diazepam Lorazepam
Neuromuscular blocking agents	Atracurium Cisatracurium	Succinylcholine Vecuronium	Pancuronium Gallamine Metocurine
Analgesic agents	Fentanyl Acetaminophen	Morphine Meperidine Ketorolac (All NSAIDs)	

A. INTRAVENOUS ANESTHETIC AGENTS

Almost all intravenous anesthetic agents, narcotics, and benzodiazepines are metabolized in the liver, usually but not invariably to inactive forms, and then are excreted in the urine. Therefore, most of these agents are suitable for use in patients with renal impairment, if one takes into account that often these patients have increased sensitivity to therapeutic and toxic effects. Uremia is often accompanied by central nervous system (CNS) depression, so drugs that cause CNS depression should be administered with caution.[62] A clinical rule of thumb is to reduce the initial dose by 25 to 50 per cent from normal using the response to the initial dose as a guide to maintenance dosing.

In uremic patients, thiopental produces more prolonged anesthesia, proportional to the severity of uremia.[63] This effect is most likely due to both the depressant effects of the uremia and to hypoalbuminemia, which leaves more unbound thiopental available to reach receptor sites. Although propofol has been used safely in renal failure patients, the dosage should probably be adjusted downward to limit hypotension after induction. Induction with etomidate, because of a reduced tendency to lower blood pressure,[64] may be beneficial in this hemodynamically labile patient population. Fentanyl is a suitable narcotic, owing to its lack of active metabolites. Both morphine and meperidine have active metabolites that may build up to dangerous levels in renal failure patients. Normeperidine can cause seizures, whereas morphine-6 glu-

curonide causes analgesia and sedation.[65] Benzodiazepines should be administered cautiously to patients with renal impairment. Midazolam is a good choice, as it has the shortest half-life and no active metabolites.[66, 67]

Both depolarizing and nondepolarizing muscle relaxants require careful use in patients with renal failure. Succinylcholine has been used without complications in many patients with moderately to severely impaired renal function. In most patients, succinylcholine transiently increases serum potassium by approximately 0.5 mEq/L.[68] The incremental rise is the same in renal failure; however, owing to the possibility of preexisting hyperkalemia, succinylcholine should be administered only after checking the serum potassium. The nondepolarizing agents of choice may be atracurium or cisatracurium because they do not undergo renal elimination. Pancuronium,[69] curare, gallamine, and metocurine should be avoided because of their dependence on renal elimination. Vecuronium, approximately 15 per cent eliminated renally, may be used if dosage is precisely managed and neuromuscular function monitored.[70] Excretion of cholinesterase inhibitors, used to reverse neuromuscular blockade, is also significantly impaired.[71–73]

Nonsteroidal antiinflammatory agents (NSAIDs), such as ketorolac, may induce a variety of acute and chronic renal pathologies.[74] Most renal syndromes associated with NSAID use can be attributed to prostaglandin inhibition.[75] Acute interstitial nephritis can occur with short-term NSAID use. Patients chronically taking NSAIDs can develop papillary necrosis, chronic interstitial nephritis, and end-stage renal disease (ESRD). Patients at risk for renal impairment from NSAID use are the elderly and those with preexisting renal insufficiency or heart disease.[74] Perioperative NSAID use should be avoided in these patient populations. Acetaminophen lacks significant peripheral prostaglandin inhibition and thus should be a first-line analgesic in patients at risk.[75]

B. INHALATIONAL AGENTS

Some volatile anesthetic agents are degraded to renally excreted metabolites.[76–78] However, because inhalational agents do not rely on renal excretion for reversal of anesthetic effects, they are generally more appropriate than "fixed" drugs for administration to patients with renal compromise. Isoflurane and desflurane are minimally metabolized and may be the best choices.[24] Halothane is not significantly defluorinated under normal clinical conditions and thus is not nephrotoxic.[79, 80] Enflurane is metabolized, releasing inorganic fluoride, although to a lesser extent than sevoflurane or methoxyflurane.[81] Some experimental models using enflurane have produced mild tubular defects with prolonged use, but no clinical impairment in renal function has been linked with enflurane. Sevoflurane and methoxyflurane are substantially metabolized, releasing inorganic fluoride ion for renal excretion.[82] Methoxyflurane caused a high-output renal failure syndrome resulting from high levels of inorganic fluoride ion produced during its biotransformation.[82–87] A newer inhaled agent, sevoflurane, is also metabolized to inorganic fluoride ion,[34, 88–90] but rapid elimination by the lungs reduces the duration of potentially toxic fluoride levels (Fig. 5–3). Sevoflurane also degrades in soda lime, releasing "compound A," which is nephrotoxic in rats.[90] Compound A levels are trivial if fresh gas flows greater than 2 L are used.[36] No evidence of clinically significant decreased renal function has been seen in human studies of sevoflurane.[35, 37, 39, 40, 43, 44] However, because there is some evidence of transient proximal tubular injury and transient impairment in concentrating ability after sevoflurane anesthesia,[43] this agent should be used with caution in patients with renal impairment.[38, 42, 91]

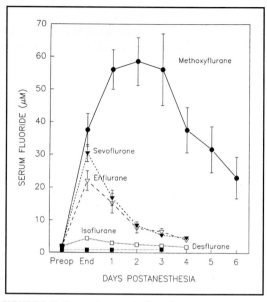

FIGURE 5–3. Serum inorganic fluoride concentrations before and after methoxyflurane, enflurane, sevoflurane, isoflurane, and desflurane anesthesia (3 hrs each). (From Kharasch ED: Biotransformation of sevoflurane. Anesth Analg 81:S27, 1995. Copyright by Williams & Wilkins.)

C. ANTIHYPERTENSIVE AGENTS AND VASOPRESSORS

In general, antihypertensive agents should be carefully titrated for clinical effect in these patients, owing to their labile blood pressure. Labetolol and esmolol are metabolized extrarenally and can safely be used in patients with renal impairment. Most of the clinically available calcium channel blockers are metabolized in the liver and are safe for use in renal patients. Nitroglycerin and nitroprusside may be used safely, with the caution that nitroprusside should be used only for short durations. Thiocyanate, a toxic metabolite of nitroprusside, accumulates after prolonged use in renal insufficiency.[92]

ACE inhibitors may precipitate renal failure in patients with bilateral renal artery stenosis. In these patients, glomerular filtration pressure is dependent on the actions of angiotensin II. Angiotensin II preserves glomerular filtration pressure distal to stenotic lesions by increasing systemic arterial pressure and by selective constriction of efferent arterioles. ACE inhibitors blunt these responses and precipitate acute renal failure (ARF), which is usually reversible, in approximately 30 per cent of these patients.[93] Calcium channel antagonists may decrease proteinuria and slow the progression of diabetic nephropathy. Calcium channel antagonists also have a poorly understood natriuretic effect.[94-96]

Because renal failure is associated with hypertension and dialysis-induced fluctuations of intravascular volumes, blood pressure in these patients is extremely labile. If vasopressors are required to treat acute hypotension, direct-acting agents such as phenylephrine are appropriate but may reduce renal perfusion.[97] Dopamine is metabolized in the liver and at lower doses (i.e., 0.5–5 µg/kg per minute) stimulates dopaminergic receptors that increase RBF; therefore, dopamine is a suitable choice as a vasopressor in patients with residual renal function.[98-101] When appropriate, it may be advantageous to substitute nonpharmacologic maneuvers such as fluid administration or reduction in the inspired concentration of volatile agents to improve blood pressure.

VI. RENAL DISEASES

Many primary and secondary renal diseases may influence anesthetic management. In this section, the pathophysiology and anesthetic implications of these disorders are discussed. There is a great deal of overlap in these syndromes.[102] Most of the conditions are progressive, and functional impairment is directly proportional to the severity of nephron damage. The eventual state of renal failure, GFR below 10 mL per minute, is known as ESRD, although this is not a specific pathologic diagnosis.[16] Chronic renal failure, ESRD, and ARF are important co-morbid conditions that anesthesiologists should consider in planning perioperative management.

A. PRIMARY RENAL DISEASES

1. Acute Glomerulonephritis

Acute glomerulonephritis (AGN) usually has an abrupt onset characterized by proteinuria, hematuria, and some degree of impaired renal function. Renal function tests accurately reflect the severity of AGN. The spectrum of cases ranges from mild, with slight elevation in BUN only, to oliguria with renal failure. Patients are treated with antihypertensive medications and corticosteroids.

Acute glomerulonephritis is most common in young males and is usually preceded by an upper respiratory tract infection. An immune mechanism has been implicated as the most common cause of AGN. Usually, immunoglobulin and complement are deposited within various sites in the mesangium, capillary walls, and basement membrane.

The two most serious complications of AGN are hypertensive encephalopathy and acute heart failure. Usually, the encephalopathy is reversible when blood pressure is lowered, suggesting that global cerebral vasoconstriction, not cerebral edema, is the cause. Heart failure associated with AGN, which occurs as a result of increased demand on the left ventricle secondary to hypervolemia and hypertension, is treatable by reducing blood pressure and inducing diuresis.

Ninety per cent of patients with AGN are asymptomatic within 4 to 7 days and recover completely in 3 to 4 weeks. About 2 per cent die in the acute phase, secondary to cerebral vascular accident, infection, or another complication of renal failure. Chronic glomerulonephritis develops in a small percentage of patients, with either rapid (2 to 10 years) or slow (10 to 40 years) progression to renal failure.

Membranoproliferative glomerulonephritis is an irreversible form of diffuse glomerulonephritis in which the glomerular lesion develops slowly throughout the course of the disease. Edema is the most prominent feature, with variably severe proteinuria. The nephrotic syndrome (proteinuria, hypoproteinemia, and edema) is often present, as is hypertension of varying severity.

There is no reported anesthetic experience with patients with glomerulonephritis. In general, patients suspected of having AGN should have elective surgery deferred until the condition resolves. If a patient with AGN needs emergency surgery, the main concerns are to control blood pressure and adjust drugs and dosages (as addressed earlier) consistent with the level of renal dysfunction.[103-107]

2. Nephrotic Syndrome

The nephrotic syndrome is not a specific disease entity; rather, the term describes a type of glomerular disorder characterized by profound proteinuria (greater than 3.0 gm per day), hypoproteinemia, and severe edema. Approximately 80 per cent of cases of nephrotic syndrome are secondary to AGN, with the remaining cases resulting from a variety of causes. Pathophysiologically, an in-crease in glomerular permeability allows al-bumin to be freely filtered into the urine. As hypoalbuminemia progresses, diminished intravascular colloid osmotic pressure results in sequestration of fluid into the interstitial space. For unclear reasons, about half of these patients are intravascularly hypovolemic, whereas half are hypervolemic. They have variable hypertension and renal dysfunction. Patients with long-standing nephrotic syn-drome often suffer from advanced atheroscle-rotic disease and are at risk for coronary ar-tery disease.

Recently, nephrotic syndrome has also been associated with infection with the human im-munodeficiency virus (HIV). HIV-associated nephropathy (HIV-AN) is present in approxi-mately 20 per cent of HIV-infected patients, if microalbuminuria is used as the criterion and in 2 to 15 per cent if substantial proteinuria is the criterion.[108] In 10 to 20 per cent of cases of HIV-AN, azotemia is a prominent feature; nephrotic-range proteinuria eventually occurs in approximately 90 per cent of patients.[108] This syndrome progresses inexorably to ESRD, although prednisone has recently been shown to reduce azotemia in most patients.[108] Meticulous sterile technique is necessary when performing procedures.

From the perspective of anesthetic manage-ment, it is crucial to assess intravascular vol-ume by clinical assessment or invasive moni-toring. Renal function and electrolytes should be evaluated preoperatively. Hypoproteine-mia necessitates careful dosing of highly pro-tein-bound drugs such as thiopental.[109-115]

3. Pyelonephritis

Acute pyelonephritis, characterized by bac-teriuria, chills, fever, leukocytosis, and flank pain, rarely necessitates surgery unless the infection is secondary to ureteral obstruction. Management of acute pyelonephritis should be directed at detecting and correcting dehy-dration and administering appropriate antibi-otics. Chronic pyelonephritis, the late stage of recurrent bacterial renal infection, occurs in patients with chronic ureteral reflux. Such pa-tients may require surgery for ureteral reim-plantation procedures. Because renal insuffi-ciency and loss of urine-concentrating ability occur with chronic pyelonephritis, these pa-tients should have renal function and electro-lytes checked preoperatively.[116-120]

4. Isolated Tubular Defects

There are several specific defects of tubular function. Nephrogenic diabetes insipidus re-sults from relative insensitivity of the collect-ing ducts to ADH. Proximal tubular defects lead to wasting of substances normally reab-sorbed in that segment of the nephron (i.e., sodium, bicarbonate, glucose, amino acids, and phosphate). Defects in the LOH result in sodium and potassium wasting. The most common distal tubular defect is renal tubular acidosis (RTA). There are at least four types of RTA, disorders in which renal excretion of acid (and reabsorption of bicarbonate) is reduced out of proportion to the reduction in GFR. They should always be considered when evaluating a non–anion gap acidosis. Type 1, or distal RTA, is inherited, whereas most other types are acquired (Table 5–2). Anesthetic management of the following two specific syndromes has been reported.

a. Fanconi's Syndrome

Fanconi's syndrome is a generalized proxi-mal tubular defect manifested as phosphate wasting, glycosuria, amino aciduria, and bi-carbonate wasting, resulting in proximal tu-bular acidosis. Excessive bicarbonate delivery to the DCT may lead to nephrogenic diabetes insipidus. Most patients progress to renal fail-ure and eventually require dialysis or renal transplantation.

A single case report of a patient with Fanconi's syndrome has been published.[121] In that patient, a 35-kg dwarf undergoing hip replacement, the only problem was main-taining adequate fluid balance. During the 4-hour operation, urine output was 1740 mL. The authors recommended that daily obliga-tory urinary water and electrolyte losses be established preoperatively and that appro-priate solutions be prepared for infusion dur-ing the perioperative period to avoid either hypovolemia or electrolyte imbalance. Cen-tral venous pressure measurement during surgery could facilitate fluid management.

b. Bartter's Syndrome

Bartter's syndrome consists of hypokalemic metabolic alkalosis[122, 123] accompanied by in-creased plasma renin and aldosterone, normal blood pressure, and, often, polyuria and poly-dipsia. Although the pathophysiology is un-known, there is an excess of prostaglandin

TABLE 5–2

Comparison of Three Types of Renal Tubular Acidosis

Finding	Type 1	Type 2	Type 3*
Non–anion gap acidosis	Yes	Yes	Yes
Minimum urine pH	>5.5	<5.5	<5.5
Filtered bicarbonate excreted (%)	<10	>15	<10
Serum potassium	Low	Low	High
Fanconi's syndrome	No	Yes	No
Stones/nephrocalcinosis	Yes	No	No
Daily acid excretion	Low	Normal	Low
Ammonium excretion	High for pH	Normal	Low for pH
Daily HCO_3 replacement needs	<4 mmol/kg	>4 mmol/kg	<4 mmol/kg

*Type 3 renal tubular acidosis is a rare form of a mixture of types 1 and 2.
From Coe FL, Kathpalia S: Hereditary tubular disorders. In Isselbacher KJ, Martin JB, Braunwald E, et al (eds): Harrison's Principles of Internal Medicine, 13th ed. New York, McGraw-Hill, 1994. Reproduced with permission of the McGraw-Hill Companies.

secretion; therefore, treatment with cyclooxygenase inhibitors (NSAIDs) has been advocated. Additionally, blockade of mineralocorticoid receptors with spironolactone and beta blockers has been attempted, with variable success.

Several case reports exist of surgical procedures in patients with Bartter's syndrome.[124, 125] These patients required careful observation of fluid and electrolyte balance owing to fluctuating serum potassium and copious diuresis.

5. Obstructive Nephropathy

Uncorrected urinary tract obstruction may result in marked structural and functional renal changes. Anesthetic management of these patients depends on the extent of renal insufficiency. The renal impairment seen in these patients is usually reversible with relief of the obstruction (e.g., bladder catheterization, transurethral resection of the prostate, or nephrostomy tube placement) unless renal damage is far advanced.[126]

B. SYSTEMIC DISEASES WITH RENAL INVOLVEMENT

Renal involvement is common in many systemic diseases. Assessment of renal function is critical in patients with all of the following systemic diseases.

1. Hypertension

The kidney plays an important, perhaps causative, role in essential hypertension. A current theory implicates the kidney in the pathogenesis of essential hypertension, smaller numbers of nephrons at birth being correlated with the risk of developing essential hypertension later in life. Smaller kidneys may alter sodium handling and vascular tone in some way that is still unelucidated.[127–129] Additional evidence of the kidney's crucial role in blood pressure control is seen with renal transplantation. Cross-transplantation of kidneys between genetically hypertensive and normal rats results in normalization of blood pressure in the hypertensive rats and hypertension in the normal rats.[130]

Renal artery stenosis accounts for 2 to 5 per cent of hypertension. This syndrome should be suspected when hypertension develops suddenly in a previously normotensive person over age 50 or under 30. Pathophysiologically, the affected kidney is underperfused distal to the stenosis and secretes renin in response. This in turn causes systemic hypertension. Angioplasty or surgery to correct the stenosis corrects the blood pressure.

The kidney is both damaged by hypertension and has a role in causing most types of hypertension (i.e., renovascular—and, probably, essential—hypertension). The role of hypertension in the loss of renal function is convincingly demonstrated only in a few experimental models, and in humans only in malignant hypertension and in diabetic nephropathy.[131] Thus, the kidney may be "victim or villain" in different subsets of patients with hypertension.[132] In patients with hypertension and renal impairment, controversy surrounds this core question: Are the observed changes in renal function a consequence of hypertension or the primary basis of the disease? Thus, the optimal blood pressure for individual patients with renal impairment is unclear.[133-138]

2. Diabetes Mellitus

Diabetes causes about 25 per cent of all renal failure in the United States. Diabetic nephropathy describes a spectrum of damage to the glomeruli, tubules, and arterioles. Most often, there is an accumulation of mesangial matrix components and a widening of the glomerular capillary wall resulting from thickening of the basement membrane. Diabetics are also prone to other renal conditions, such as acute pyelonephritis, acute papillary necrosis, and obstructive nephropathy.[139]

In type I diabetes, clinical signs of renal involvement usually do not appear until 10 or 15 years after diagnosis; however, during this period, the so-called first stage of diabetic nephropathy, there is a 20 to 40 per cent increase in the GFR (and RBF) as compared with readings in controls. Improvement in diabetic control returns the GFR to near normal in some patients. After the asymptomatic elevation in GFR, proteinuria heralds the second stage of diabetic nephropathy, during which the GFR falls into the normal range, then continues to fall. Proteinuria is initially intermittent, over a few years becoming constant and massive. This is accompanied by declining GFR and the development of hypertension and edema. The third stage is ESRD, in which the patient requires dialysis or transplant.[139] Preoperative assessment of renal function is mandatory in diabetes patients to determine whether renal insufficiency is present and, if present, to what degree.

C. COLLAGEN VASCULAR DISEASES

1. Systemic Lupus Erythematosus

Approximately 66 per cent of lupus (SLE) patients have clinical manifestations of glomerular disease, ranging from microscopic hematuria or proteinuria to AGN or the nephrotic syndrome. Patients with lupus-related nephropathy usually are hypertensive. Because the natural history of lupus is one of periods of active disease and remission, careful assessment and planning are necessary to ensure that elective surgery is done during a quiescent period. Corticosteroids are frequently used to treat this disorder. Other manifestations of SLE include fatigue, arthralgias, anemia, pleuritis, and cognitive dysfunction. Curiously, once end-stage lupus nephropathy develops, the other manifestations of lupus activity tend to decrease.[140]

2. Polyarteritis Nodosa

Polyarteritis nodosa is one of the syndromes, the other notable one being Goodpasture's syndrome, in which pulmonary hemorrhage is combined with renal failure. The pulmonary hemorrhage varies in severity from mild hemoptysis to life-threatening hemorrhage. Renal failure may progress rapidly. Patients usually become hypertensive as renal failure worsens. Treatment consists of cyclophosphamide and corticosteroids.

3. Rheumatoid Arthritis and Gout

Approximately 25 per cent of patients with rheumatoid arthritis suffer renal insufficiency from focal glomerulonephritis, amyloidosis, or interstitial nephritis secondary to analgesic use. Renal function studies should be obtained in patients with rheumatoid arthritis to determine whether renal involvement is present. Because renal involvement is also common in patients with gout, renal function should be evaluated preoperatively. Patients with gout and renal insufficiency may suffer an exacerbation perioperatively, as they are unable to excrete the increased uric acid resulting from surgically stimulated catabolism.

D. NEPHROTOXINS

The kidney is particularly susceptible to toxins, owing to its rich blood supply, the increased concentration of excreted compounds in various sites, and the progressive concentration of tubular fluid as it progresses through the nephron. Certain nephrotoxins are of particular interest.

1. Fluorinated Anesthetics

The classic anesthetic-induced nephropathy, methoxyflurane nephrotoxicity, was first reported in 1966 by Crandell and coworkers,[85] who observed a condition characterized by polyuria, hypernatremia, and the inability to concentrate urine. Mazze and Cousins[82-84, 86, 87, 141, 142] confirmed these findings and showed a dose-related effect caused by the metabolism of methoxyflurane to inorganic fluoride. (See section on Inhalational Agents above for details.)

2. Radiographic Contrast Media

ARF after the administration of radiographic contrast material is more likely to occur in the presence of dehydration or coexisting medical conditions. The incidence of renal failure after administration of contrast agents is around 1 per cent in all patients, whereas in nonazotemic diabetics it is around 16 per cent. Azotemic diabetics have an incidence of ARF of about 38 per cent.[143, 144] Because the mortality rate of contrast medium–induced ARF is approximately 34 per cent, elective surgery should be deferred.[143]

The pathogenesis of this condition has been elusive, but local renal vasoconstriction may be a key component. Vigorous hydration or mannitol- or furosemide-induced diuresis *may* prevent renal failure related to contrast media. Newer, nonionic contrast media also *may* lower the incidence of nephrotoxicity[145]; however, there is disagreement on these points.

E. OTHER TOXIC NEPHROPATHIES

Because of the kidney's role in concentrating and eliminating waste products from the body, it is often exposed to toxic concentrations of various substances, such as antibiotics and other medications, heavy metals, and organic solvents.

Medications known to be nephrotoxic include the aminoglycosides, vancomycin, amphotericin B, acyclovir, and several antineoplastic agents. Other medications specifically given to renal transplant patients are nephrotoxic, specifically cyclosporine and FK 506.[146] For other information on medications with nephrotoxic side effects see Effects of Drugs on Reduced Renal Function, above.

VII. ACUTE RENAL FAILURE

ARF, a highly lethal clinical syndrome seen perioperatively, is characterized by a rapid decline in glomerular filtration, perturbation of extracellular fluid volume, electrolyte and acid-base imbalance, and retention of nitrogenous wastes. Patients particularly at risk include those undergoing cardiopulmonary bypass, aortic surgery, extensive blood loss, and hypovolemic hypotension.[147] The mortality rate is as high as 42 to 88 per cent in a recent series.[147] This high mortality rate was thought to be due to co-morbid conditions, but a recent case-control study isolated ARF as a cause of increased mortality, regardless of co-existing diseases.[143] For purposes of diagnosis and management, ARF is subclassified as prerenal, intrarenal, and postrenal. Of all patients with ARF, about 70 per cent have a prerenal etiology, about 25 per cent intrarenal (often called *acute tubular necrosis),* and less than 5 per cent have a postrenal cause.[148] Frequently in the perioperative period, making a distinction between prerenal and intrarenal causes of ARF is difficult.

A. PATHOPHYSIOLOGY

The heterogeneous blood flow to the kidney explains its sensitivity to injury from hypoperfusion.[149] Although 20 per cent of the resting cardiac output is delivered to the kidneys, the bulk, about 90 per cent, of that flow is directed to the cortex, whereas metabolic demands are highest in the outer medulla.[150] If the ratio of oxygen uptake to delivery is calculated for various tissues, the lowest in the body, 18 per cent, would be in the overall kidney, while the highest, 79 per cent, would be in the outer medulla. Thus, severe local tissue hypoxia may develop in conditions of relatively adequate total blood flow.[151] There is convincing experimental evidence that the medullary thick ascending limb (mTAL) of LOH is selectively vulnerable to hypoxic injury (Fig. 5–4). Evidence suggests that oxygen deficiency is related not only to supply but also to demand. Thus, one can think of ARF as an oxygen supply versus demand disorder with the medulla exhibiting an "anginal" syndrome of ARF.[147] In prerenal ARF, there appears to be diversion of renal blood flow away from the medulla.[151]

Preglomerular vasoconstriction decreases glomerular and tubular perfusion. If vasocon-

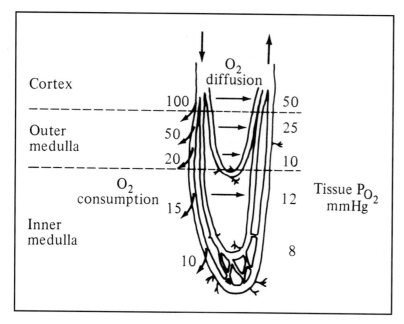

FIGURE 5–4. Development of medullary hypoxia due to the exchange of oxygen between the descending and ascending limbs of the vasa recta capillaries (straight arrows) and to oxygen consumption by the medullary cells (curved arrows). (From Brezis M, Rosen S, Silva P, et al: Renal ischemia: A new perspective. Kidney Int 26, 375, 1984. Reproduced with permission from Kidney International.)

striction is sustained, renal tubular cells slough, creating tubular obstruction.[152] This process compromises function and produces further ischemia and tubular endothelial necrosis.

B. CLINICAL FINDINGS

Generally, patients developing ARF demonstrate oliguria (urinary output below 20 mL/hour in a 70-kg adult), which persists for about 1 to 2 weeks. During this interval, likely complications include hypervolemia, hyperkalemia, hyponatremia, hyperphosphatemia, hypermagnesemia, hypocalcemia, and metabolic acidosis. Other common complications are malnutrition, infection, anemia, and platelet dysfunction. Uremia may lead to neuropsychiatric disturbances, pericardial effusion, anorexia, nausea, and vomiting. Renal replacement therapy must be started to treat volume overload, hyperkalemia, severe acidosis, pericardial effusion, or mental status changes related to uremia.[153] Fewer than 5 per cent of ARF patients will require long-term dialysis (i.e., most either succumb during ARF or survive by using dialysis until renal function improves spontaneously).[148] Most patients who survive begin to demonstrate recovery of renal function within 10 to 21 days and regain sufficient renal function to live without dialysis. During the recovery period the patient enters a diuretic phase, during which urinary volume may reach 5 L or more per day. Management requires close attention to avoid electrolyte abnormalities or hypovolemia. Meticulous sterile technique is necessary when performing procedures because of the risk of infection.

C. INTRAOPERATIVE RECOGNITION, TREATMENT, AND PREVENTION

When a patient develops intraoperative oliguria, the anesthesiologist should first consider whether ARF is a likely risk, then attempt to optimally hydrate the patient to rule out and treat prerenal azotemia.[154] Urinary specific gravity or osmolality may aid in the diagnosis of pre- versus intrarenal ARF but rarely can be used to guide therapy. Hypovolemia is a potent stimulus for ADH release; thus, a patient with prerenal ARF has urine osmolality greater than 500 mOsm/kg (or specific gravity greater than 1.020). In contrast, acute tubular necrosis impairs concentrating ability, usually resulting in urinary osmolality around 300 mOsm/kg (or specific gravity around 1.010). Thus, high urine osmolality essentially excludes the diagnosis of acute tubular necrosis.[148]

A patient with oliguria and questionable intravascular volume may benefit from invasive monitoring if that permits more aggressive fluid administration.[147] Oxygen-carrying capacity, (i.e., hemoglobin concentration) should be adequate. A small dose of dopamine (0.5 to 3.0 µg/kg per minute) may be added as a renal vasodilator.[100, 155] If cardiac filling pressures are normal or high, furosemide and mannitol may be given. Furosemide decreases cellular reabsorption of solute in the mTAL and distal tubule, thus decreasing oxygen demand.[147] Animal studies clearly show that furosemide increases RBF.[147] Mannitol may assist in flushing cellular debris out of the tubules[154, 156–159] and reducing endothelial swelling, which can further enhance renal perfusion. The oxygen free radical–scavenging effect of mannitol may also be of benefit.[147] Additionally, diuretics may convert oliguric into nonoliguric ARF, which eases management of volume status.[160]

Many different therapies and anesthetic techniques have been tried to modify or prevent the clinical course of established ARF; however, none have shown any advantage in lowering the incidence or modifying the natural history.[153, 161–165] In patients with established ARF, i.e., those in whom serum Cr has increased by least 1.0 mg/dL over the previous 24 to 48 hours, administration of small doses of dopamine (less than 3 µg/kg per minute) does not significantly attenuate the risk of death or dialysis, although there may be some minor effect.[166] Thus, treatment is supportive, centered around renal replacement therapy as needed to control intravascular volume and electrolyte concentrations and nutritional support.[148]

VIII. DIALYSIS AND RENAL TRANSPLANTATION

The artificial kidney was developed in 1944 by Kolff and Berk; by 1960, dialysis medicine was an established area of specialization.[167] Widespread hemodialysis was established in 1973, when Medicare extended coverage to all patients with ESRD. In 1995, patients enrolled in chronic hemodialysis programs in the United States numbered 205,000. Approximately 10,000 renal transplants are performed annually in the United States.[168]

A. DIALYSIS

Dialysis improves most of the medical complications of ESRD, including hypervolemia, metabolic acidosis, electrolyte imbalance,

muscle weakness, and hypertension. Patients with ESRD may also have peripheral neuropathies, altered mental status, and platelet dysfunction. A subset of patients with ESRD have persistent hypertension despite dialysis. These patients present numerous perioperative challenges. They require multiple surgical procedures, have a mean age of 63, and have co-morbid conditions such as diabetes, hypertension, and coronary artery disease. Because younger, more fit patients are more likely to undergo transplantation, the population remaining on chronic dialysis are generally older and have more coexisting conditions than the average ESRD patient.[168–171]

The dialysis principle involves equilibration of circulating blood constituents (e.g., catabolic products) with dialysate across a semipermeable membrane. Two dialysis techniques are used: peritoneal dialysis and hemodialysis. Peritoneal dialysis is usually performed daily at home via a peritoneal access catheter and uses the peritoneal lining as the semipermeable membrane. Thus, the need for vascular cannulas and their complications are avoided. The ion content and tonicity of the dialysate may be altered based on the patient's electrolyte and volume status. Peritoneal dialysis is less efficient than hemodialysis, so dialysis times are longer. Also, peritonitis is a known complication, and some patients experience abdominal pain during dialysis.

Hemodialysis is far more popular and widely used than peritoneal dialysis. Hemodialysis uses an extracorporeal circuit linked to the patient via an arteriovenous anastomosis. To prevent clotting of the dialysis circuit, heparin is given before dialysis and protamine for reversal after dialysis. The patient typically is dialyzed for 4 to 5 hours, three times per week. During a 5-hour treatment, the dialysate flow rates are about 500 mL/minute, so the blood is exposed to 150 L of dialysate.

The establishment and maintenance of acceptable vascular access frequently requires surgery. In 1994, vascular access placement and complications accounted for at least 25 per cent of all admissions for dialysis patients.[172] For acute hemodialysis, a double-lumen catheter may be placed into a central vein using standard venous access techniques. For chronic hemodialysis, subcutaneous arteriovenous fistulas have proved to be the best method of access. In patients with acceptably robust venous anatomy, a native arteriovenous fistula is created in the forearm. After this shunt is created, it must mature for 6 to 8 weeks before being used. In patients with inadequate venous anatomy, a synthetic arteriovenous fistula is created, usually using polytetrafluoroethylene (PTFE or Teflon) grafts, which require only 2 to 3 weeks to endothelialize before use. The native graft has a higher long-term patency rate, a lower rate of thrombosis, and a lower infection rate. Approximately 60 per cent of indwelling arteriovenous fistulas are patent after 1 year.[172]

ESRD patients who require surgery frequently have coexisting conditions, as noted above. In particular, the volume status and the need for preoperative dialysis should be assessed. In addition, serum potassium should be in an acceptable range, below approximately 5.8 mEq/dL. Because of the chronic nature of hyperkalemia in ESRD, patients tolerate relatively high serum potassium levels without symptoms.

Regional, general, and local anesthesia have been used successfully for creation of arteriovenous fistulas. If the surgeon is definitely operating on the forearm, a technique has been described to simply block the lateral and medial cutaneous branches of the musculocutaneous nerves at the elbow.[173] If the procedure is declotting a fistula, frequently this can be accomplished under local anesthesia. Although brachial plexus anesthesia increases brachial artery blood flow, the rate of early thrombosis appears to be independent of anesthetic technique.[174]

TABLE 5–3

Complications of Living Donor Nephrectomy in More Than 1500 Cases

Procedure/Complications	Prevalence (%)
Aortography	
Prolonged discomfort	0.5
Femoral thrombosis or aneurysm	0.4
Intraoperative	
Splenic laceration	0.3
Pancreatic injury, pseudocyst	0.2
Nephrectomy wound	3.2
Prolonged discomfort	2.1
Infection	2.0
Hernia	2.0
Hematoma	0.5
Pulmonary	
Atelectasis	13.5
Pneumothorax or pneumomediastinum	9.1
Pneumonitis or pleural effusion	4.3
Urinary tract	
Infection	8.6
Retention	1.6
Acute tubular necrosis	0.9
Late proteinuria	3.0
Others	
Prolonged ileus	2.6
Thrombophlebitis with or without pulmonary embolus	1.9
Peripheral nerve palsy	1.1
Hepatic dysfunction (late)	0.9
Acute depression	0.6
Hypertension (late)	15.0

From Cosimi AB: The donor and donor nephrectomy. In Morris PJ (eds): Kidney Transplantation: Principles and Practice, 4th ed. Philadelphia, WB Saunders, 1994.

B. RENAL TRANSPLANTATION

There are few contraindications, none absolute, to renal transplantation. In patients younger than 1 year or older than 65 years, the decision is based on the patient's fitness and ability to tolerate surgery and immunosuppression. Availability of a immunologically compatible kidney also may influence the decision. A living related donor is often the best match; this availability allows planning for the transplant.[135, 136, 175–182]

C. ANESTHETIC MANAGEMENT OF THE DONOR

Anesthesia for donor nephrectomy has been successfully managed using many different anesthetic techniques. The greatest risk is from surgical hemorrhage, so adequate intravenous access is essential, as is cross-matched blood. Relatively large amounts of crystalloid, furosemide, and mannitol are usually administered to ensure brisk diuresis from the donor kidney before removal. Drugs entirely dependent on renal elimination should be used with caution. Although the remaining kidney is usually sufficient for maintenance of excretory function, reserve is diminished. Perioperative mortality has been estimated at 0.06 per cent. See Table 5–3 for complications of donor nephrectomy.[183]

D. PREOPERATIVE TREATMENT OF THE RECIPIENT

Transplantation is usually accomplished before the complications of chronic renal failure, such as bone demineralization, muscle weakness, peripheral neuropathies, and anemia, have developed. Most recipients will be on dialysis and should be in stable condition when they present for transplant. Occasionally, recipients with progressive renal disease receive a transplant before they progress to ESRD, thus avoiding the need for dialysis. Acute abnormalities in fluid or electrolyte balance should be treated with dialysis before transplantation. The preservation time for cadaver kidneys has been extended to 48 hours by improved cadaver preservation solutions, so renal transplantation in a poorly prepared patient should be less common.[184, 185]

E. ANESTHETIC MANAGEMENT OF THE RECIPIENT

There are several detailed discussions of anesthesia for renal transplantation.[185] Preoperatively, serum potassium should be checked. It is probably safe to proceed with anesthesia if serum potassium is less than 5.8 mEq/L, unless there are hyperkalemic ECG changes (peaked T waves, widened QRS complex, or decreased P-wave amplitude). Owing to the anemia of renal failure, hemoglobin is often in the range of 6 to 8 g/dL, although severe anemia is now less prevalent, owing to the administration of synthetic erythropoietin.[12] Chronic anemia is generally tolerated well because of physiologic adaptations, including increased cardiac output and increased red cell 2,3-diphosphoglycerate. The incidence of preoperative hypertension is between 68 and 94 per cent of patients undergoing renal transplantation.[130, 133] Similarly, the incidence of ischemic heart disease is high, about 5 per cent in patients under 55 years old and higher in the elderly. Most patients will have been dialyzed on the day before surgery, so the patient should be presumed to be hypovolemic, a contributing factor in the labile blood pressures often seen during transplantation.

Premedication should be given in reduced doses or avoided. Strict asepsis is essential. A central venous catheter is useful to reflect intravascular volume in the absence of urine output, whereas an arterial catheter may be placed, depending on the severity and adequacy of preoperative control of blood pressure. Functional arteriovenous fistulas should be protected by careful positioning of the involved extremity and placement of the blood pressure cuff elsewhere. Venous catheters should be restricted, when possible, to the dorsum of the hand, thus preserving forearm and antecubital veins.

General or regional anesthesia may be successfully used.[186] For a general anesthetic, judicious doses of an intravenous induction agent are appropriate. The choice of muscle relaxants and narcotics should include compounds that are not excreted through the kidneys such as atracurium and fentanyl.

For a spinal or epidural anesthetic, several considerations are relevant. Because the kidney is implanted in the extraperitoneal space, a T10 level should be adequate for the surgery. Patients with ESRD have uremia-induced platelet dysfunction; prolonged postoperative sensory or motor changes should prompt the suspicion of an epidural hematoma.[187] It should also be recalled that recently dialyzed patients are hypovolemic and prone to hypotension as the sympathectomy develops.

During the surgical procedure, the donor kidney is placed in the iliac fossa, with the renal artery and vein anastomosed to the iliac artery and vein. The ureter is anastomosed to the bladder. Adequate hydration should occur by the time the anastomoses are opened. A regimen of antirejection drugs is given intraoperatively, based on the protocols of individual centers. These agents include prednisone, cyclosporine, azathioprine, and OKT3 in addition to diuretic agents. There is variable urine output postoperatively, as well as variable return of normal renal function.[185]

IX. SUMMARY

Although a variety of common and uncommon renal diseases may be present in patients who require surgery, the expression of those diseases is almost invariably reflected in abnormalities of glomerular or tubular function. Perioperatively, it is more important to evaluate the extent of renal dysfunction than it is to focus on specific diagnoses. The severity of renal dysfunction has important implications for management of fluids and electrolytes and choice of anesthetic and nonanesthetic drugs in the perioperative interval. Most important in the management of these patients is to avoid aggravation of renal dysfunction, particularly precipitation of renal failure, and to avoid prolonged effect of drugs that are excreted either in their original form or in active metabolites by the kidneys.

REFERENCES

Normal Renal Physiology: An Overview

1. Llach F: Structure and function of the kidney. *In* Llach F (ed): Papper's Clinical Nephrology, 3rd ed. Boston, Little, Brown, 1993.
2. Anderson S: Relevance of single nephron studies to human glomerular function. Kidney Int 45:384, 1994.
3. Franci CR: Aspects of neural and hormonal control of water and sodium balance. Braz J Med Biol Res 27:885, 1994.
4. Kamel KS, Quaggin S, Scheich A, et al: Disorders of potassium homeostasis: An approach based on pathophysiology. Am J Kidney Dis 24:597, 1994.
5. Vallotton MB, Rossier MF, Capponi AM: Potassium-angiotensin interplay in the regulation of aldosterone biosynthesis. Clin Endocrinol 42:111, 1995.
6. Laragh JH: Renin-angiotensin-aldosterone system for blood pressure and electrolyte homeostasis and its involvement in hypertension, in congestive heart failure and in associated cardiovascular damage (myocardial infarction and stroke). J Hum Hypertens 9:385, 1995.
7. Müller J: Aldosterone: the minority hormone of the adrenal cortex. Steroids 60:2, 1995.
8. Inagami T: Atrial natriuretic factor as a volume regulator. J Clin Pharmacol 34:424, 1994.
9. Ardaillou R, Dussaule JC: Role of atrial natriuretic peptide in the control of sodium balance in chronic renal failure. Nephron 66:249, 1994.
10. Schramek H, Coroneos E, Dunn MJ: Interactions of the vasoconstrictor peptides, angiotensin II and endothelin-1, with vasodilatory prostaglandins. Semin Nephrol 15:195, 1995.
11. Horton R, Zipser R, Fichman M: Prostaglandins, renal function, and vascular regulation. Med Clin North Am 65:891, 1981.
12. Kessler M: Erythropoietin and erythropoiesis in renal transplantation. Nephrol Dialysis Transplant 10:114, 1995.

Diagnosis of Renal Impairment and Clinical Assessment of Renal Function

13. Aviles DH, Fildes RD, Jose PA: Evaluation of renal function. Clin Perinatol 19:69, 1992.
14. Perrone RD, Madias NE, Levey AS: Serum creatinine as an index of renal function: New insights into old concepts. Clin Chem 38:1933, 1992.
15. Kellen M, Aronson S, Roizen MF, et al: Predictive and diagnostic tests of renal failure: A review. Anesth Analg 78:134, 1994.
16. Rose BD: Clinical assessment of renal function. *In* Rose BD (ed): Pathophysiology of Renal Disease, 2nd ed. New York, McGraw-Hill, 1996.
17. O'Malley JP, Ziessman HA: Quantitation of renal function using radioisotopic techniques. Clin Lab Med 13:53, 1993.
18. Rabito CA, Moore RH, Bougas C, et al: Noninvasive, realtime monitoring of renal function: The ambulatory renal monitor. J Nucl Med 34:199, 1993.
19. Ham HR, Peipsz A: Clinical measurement of renal

clearance. Curr Opin Nephrol Hypertens 1:252, 1992.

Effects of Anesthetic Agents in Patients with Normal Renal Function

20. Habif DV, Paper EM, Fitzpatrick HF, et al: The renal and hepatic blood flow, glomerular filtration rate, and urinary output of electrolytes during cyclopropane, ether, and thiopental anesthesia, operation, and the immediate postoperative period. Surgery 30:241, 1951.
21. Miles BE, de Wardener HE, Churchill-Davidson HC, et al: The effect on the renal circulation of pentamethonium bromide during anaesthesia. Clin Sci 11:73, 1952.
22. Mazze RI, Schwartz FD, Slocum HC, et al: Renal function during anesthesia and surgery. I. The effects of halothane anesthesia. Anesthesiology 24:279, 1963.
23. Cousins MJ, Greenstein LR, Hitt BA, et al: Metabolism and renal effects of enflurane in man. Anesthesiology 44:44, 1976.
24. Mazze RI, Cousins MJ, Barr GA: Renal effects and metabolism of isoflurane in man. Anesthesiology 40:536, 1974.
25. Deutsch S, Bastron RD, Pierce EC II, et al: The effects of anaesthesia with thiopentone, nitrous oxide, narcotics and neuromuscular blocking drugs on renal function in normal man. Br J Anaesth 41:807, 1969.
26. Auberger H, Heinrich J: Methoxyflurane und nierenfunktion. Anaesthetist 14:203, 1965.
27. Hayes MA, Goldenberg IS: Renal effects of anesthesia and operation mediated by endocrines. Anesthesiology 24:487, 1963.
28. Burchardi H, Kaczmarczyk G: The effect of anaesthesia on renal function. Eur J Anaesthesiol 11:163, 1994.
29. Barry KG, Mazze RI, Schwartz FD: Prevention of surgical oliguria and renal hemodynamic suppression by sustained hydration. N Engl J Med 270:1371, 1964.
30. Seitzman DM, Mazze RI, Schwartz FD, et al: Mannitol diuresis: A method of renal protection during surgery. J Urol 90:139, 1963.
31. Boba A, Landmesser CM: Renal complications after anesthesia and operation. Anesthesiology 22:781, 1961.
32. Hutchin P, McLaughlin JS, Hayes MA: Renal response to acidosis during anesthesia and operation. Ann Surg 154:161, 1961.
33. Mazze RI, Barry KG: Prevention of functional renal failure during anesthesia and surgery by sustained hydration and mannitol infusion. Anesth Analg 46:61, 1967.
34. Newman PJ, Quinn AC, Hall GM, et al: Circulating fluoride changes and hepatorenal function following sevoflurane anaesthesia. Anaesthesia 49:936, 1994.
35. Frink EJ Jr, Malan TP Jr, Isner RJ, et al: Renal concentrating function with prolonged sevoflurane or enflurane anesthesia in volunteers. Anesthesiology 80:1019, 1994.
36. Bito H, Ikeda K: Closed-circuit anesthesia with sevoflurane in humans: Effects on renal and hepatic function and concentrations of breakdown products with soda lime in the circuit. Anesthesiology 80:71, 1994.
37. Tsukamoto N, Hirabayashi Y, Shimuzu R, et al: The

effects of sevoflurane and isoflurane anesthesia on renal tubular function in patients with moderately impaired renal function. Anesth Analg 82:909, 1996.

38. Mazze RI, Jamison R: Renal effects of sevoflurane. Anesthesiology 83:443, 1995.

39. Conzen PF, Nuscheler M, Melotte A, et al: Renal function and serum fluoride concentrations in patients with stable renal insufficiency after anesthesia with sevoflurane or enflurane. Anesth Analg 81:569, 1995.

40. Malan TP Jr: Sevoflurane and renal function. Anesth Analg 81:S39, 1995.

41. Weiskopf RB, Eger EI II, Ionescu P, et al: Desflurane does not produce hepatic or renal injury in human volunteers. Anesth Analg 74:570, 1992.

42. Tinker JH, Baker MT: Sevoflurane, fluoride ion, and renal toxicity. Anesthesiology 83:232, 1995.

43. Higuchi H, Sumikura H, Sumita S, et al: Renal function in patients with high serum fluoride concentrations after prolonged sevoflurane anesthesia. Anesthesiology 83:449, 1995.

44. Higuchi H, Arimura S, Sumikura H, et al: Urine concentrating ability after prolonged sevoflurane anaesthesia. Br J Anaesth 73:239, 1994.

45. Papper EM, Ngai SH: Kidney function during anesthesia. Annu Rev Med 7:213, 1956.

46. Kenna JG, Jones RM: The organ toxicity of inhaled anesthetics. Anesth Analg 81:S51, 1995.

47. Deutsch S, Pierce EC II, Vandam LD: Cyclopropane effects on renal function in normal man. Anesthesiology 28:547, 1967.

48. Price HL, Linde HW, Jones RE, et al: Sympathoadrenal responses to general anesthesia in man and their relation to hemodynamics. Anesthesiology 20:563, 1959.

49. Deutsch S, Goldberg M, Stephen GW, et al: Effects of halothane anesthesia on renal function in normal man. Anesthesiology 27:793, 1966.

50. Berne RM: Hemodynamics and sodium excretion of denervated kidney in anesthetized and unanesthetized dog. Am J Physiol 171:148, 1952.

51. Shipley RE, Study RS: Changes in renal blood flow, extraction of insulin, glomerular filtration rate, tissue pressure and urine flow with acute alterations of renal artery blood pressures. Am J Physiol 167:676, 1951.

52. Bastron RD, Perkins FM, Pyne JL: Autoregulation of renal blood flow during halothane anesthesia. Anesthesiology 46:142, 1977.

53. Leighton KM, Koth B, Wenkstern BM: Autoregulation of renal blood flow: Alteration by methoxyflurane. Can Anaesth Soc J 20:173, 1973.

54. Robertson GL: Vasopressin in osmotic regulation in man. Annu Rev Med 25:315, 1974.

55. Moran WH Jr, Zimmerman B: Mechanisms of antidiuretic hormone (ADH) control of importance to the surgical patient. Surgery 62:639, 1967.

56. Hirose M, Hashimoto S, Tanaka Y: Effect of the head-down tilt position during lower abdominal surgery on endocrine and renal function response. Anesth Analg 76:40, 1993.

57. Philbin DM, Coggins CH: Plasma antidiuretic hormone levels in cardiac surgical patients during morphine and halothane anesthesia. Anesthesiology 49:95, 1978.

58. Jacobson WE, Hammarsten JF, Heller BI: The effects of adrenaline upon renal function and electrolyte excretion. J Clin Invest 30:1503, 1951.

59. Pettinger WA, Tanaka K, Keeton K, et al: Renin release, an artifact of anesthesia and its implications in rats. Proc Soc Exp Biol Med 148:625, 1975.

60. Miller ED Jr, Longnecker DE, Peach MJ: The regulatory function of the renin-angiotensin system during general anesthesia. Anesthesiology 48:399, 1978.

Effects of Drugs on Reduced Renal Function

61. Krishna DR, Klotz U: Extrahepatic metabolism of drugs in humans. Clin Pharmacokinetics 26:144, 1994.

62. Freeman RB, Sheff MF, Maher JF, et al: The blood–cerebrospinal fluid barrier in uremia. Ann Intern Med 56:233, 1962.

63. Dundee JW, Richards RK: Effect of azotemia upon the action of intravenous barbiturate anesthesia. Anesthesiology 15:333, 1954.

64. Fragen RJ, Caldwell N: Comparison of a new formulation of etomidate with thiopental—side effects and awakening times. Anesthesiology 50:242, 1979.

65. Bailey PL, Stanley TH: Intravenous opioid anesthetics. In Miller RD (eds): Anesthesia, 4th ed. New York, Churchill Livingstone, 1994.

66. Ziegler WH, Schalch E, Leishman B, et al: Comparison of the effects of intravenously administered midazolam, triazolam and their hydroxy metabolites. Br J Clin Pharmacol 16:63S, 1983.

67. Greenblatt DJ, Shader RI, Divoll M, et al: Benzodiazepines: A summary of pharmacokinetic properties. Br J Clin Pharmacol 11:11S, 1981.

68. Miller RD, Way WL, Hamilton WK, et al: Succinylcholine-induced hyperkalemia in patients with renal failure? Anesthesiology 36:138, 1972.

69. McLeod K, Watson MJ, Rawlines MD: Pharmacokinetics of pancuronium in patients with normal and impaired renal function. Br J Anaesth 48:341, 1976.

70. Orko R, Heino A, Bjorksten F, et al: Comparison of atracurium and vecuronium in anaesthesia for renal transplantation. Acta Anaesthesiol Scand 31:450, 1987.

71. Cronnelly R, Stanski DR, Miller RD, et al: Renal function and the pharmacokinetics of neostigmine in anesthetized man. Anesthesiology 51:222, 1979.

72. Cronnelly R, Stanski DR, Miller RD, et al: Pyridostigmine kinetics with and without renal function. Clin Pharmacol Ther 28:78, 1980.

73. Morris RB, Cronnelly R, Miller RD, et al: Pharmacokinetics of edrophonium in anephric and renal transplant patients. Br J Anaesth 53:1311, 1981.

74. Kleinknecht D: Interstitial nephritis, the nephrotic syndrome, and chronic renal failure secondary to nonsteroidal anti-inflammatory drugs. Semin Nephrol 15:228, 1995.

75. Whelton A: Renal effects of over-the-counter analgesics. J Clin Pharmacol 35:454, 1995.

76. Hitt BA, Mazze RI, Beppu WJ, et al: Enflurane metabolism in rats and man. J Pharmacol Exp Ther 203:193, 1977.

77. Mazze RI, Calverley RK, Smith NT: Inorganic fluoride nephrotoxicity: Prolonged enflurane and halothane anesthesia in volunteers. Anesthesiology 46:265, 1977.

78. Carter R, Heerdt M, Acchiardo S: Fluoride kinetics after enflurane anesthesia in healthy and anephric patients and in patients with poor renal function. Clin Pharmacol Ther 20:565, 1976.

79. McLain GE, Sipes IG, Brown BR Jr. An animal model of halothane hepatotoxicity: Roles of enzyme induction and hypoxia. Anesthesiology 51:321, 1979.

80. Jee RC, Sipes IG, Gandolfi AJ, et al: Factors influencing halothane hepatotoxicity in the rat hypoxic model. Toxicol Appl Pharmacol 52:267, 1980.

81. Sievenpiper TS, Rice SA, McClendon F, et al: Renal effects of enflurane anesthesia in Fischer 344 rats with pre-existing renal insufficiency. J Pharmacol Exp Ther 211:36, 1979.

82. Cousins MJ, Mazze RI: Methoxyflurane nephrotoxicity. A study of dose response in man. JAMA 225:1611, 1973.

83. Cousins MJ, Mazze RI, Kosek JC, et al: The etiology of methoxyflurane nephrotoxicity. J Pharmacol Exp Ther 190:530, 1974.

84. Mazze RI, Cousins MJ, Kosek JC: Dose-related methoxyflurane nephrotoxicity in rats. A biochemical and pathological correlation. Anesthesiology 36:571, 1972.

85. Crandell WB, Pappas SG, Macdonald A: Nephrotoxicity associated with methoxyflurane anesthesia. Anesthesiology 27:591, 1966.

86. Mazze RI, Shue GL, Jackson SH: Renal dysfunction associated with methoxyflurane anesthesia: A randomized prospective clinical evaluation. JAMA 216:278, 1971.

87. Mazze RI, Trudell JR, Cousins MJ: Methoxyflurane metabolism and renal dysfunction: Clinical correlation in man. Anesthesiology 35:247, 1971.

88. Kharasch ED, Hankins DC, Thummel KE: Human kidney methoxyflurane and sevoflurane metabolism: Intrarenal fluoride production as a possible mechanism of methoxyflurane nephrotoxicity. Anesthesiology 82:689, 1995.

89. Jin L, Baillie TA, Davis MR, et al: Nephrotoxicity of sevoflurane compound A [fluoromethyl-2,2-difluoro-1(trifluoromethyl)vinyl ether] in rats: Evidence for glutathione and cysteine conjugate formation and the role of renal cysteine conjugate β-lyase. Biochem Biophys Res Commun 210:498, 1995.

90. Kharasch ED: Biotransformation of sevoflurane. Anesth Analg 81:S27, 1995.

91. Brown BR Jr: Sevoflurane, fluoride ion, and renal toxicity. Anesthesiology 83:232, 1995.

92. Smith RP: Cyanate and thiocyanate: Acute toxicity. Proc Soc Exp Biol Med 142:1041, 1973.

93. Keane WF, Anderson S, Aurell M, et al: Angiotensin converting enzyme inhibitors and progressive renal insufficiency: Current experience and future directions. Ann Intern Med 111:503, 1989.

94. Zanchetti A, Leonetti G: Natriuretic effect of calcium antagonists. J Cardiovasc Pharmacol 7:S33, 1985.

95. Russell JD, Churchill DN: Calcium antagonists and acute renal failure. Am J Med 87:306, 1989.

96. Wagner K, Albrecht S, Neumayer HH: Prevention of posttransplant acute tubular necrosis by the calcium antagonist diltiazem: A prospective, randomized study. Am J Nephrol 7:287, 1987.

97. Churchill-Davidson HC, Wylie WD, Miles BE, et al: The effects of adrenaline, noradrenaline and methadrine on renal circulation during anaesthesia. Lancet 2:803, 1951.

98. Hollenberg NK, Adams DF, Mendell P, et al: Renal vascular responses to dopamine: Haemodynamic and angiographic observations in normal man. Clin Sci Molec Med 45:733, 1973.

99. Rosenblum R, Tai AR, Lawson D: Dopamine in man: Cardiorenal hemodynamics in normotensive patients with heart disease. J Pharmacol Exp Ther 183:256, 1972.

100. Parker S, Carlon GC, Isaacs M, et al: Dopamine administration in oliguria and oliguric renal failure. Crit Care Med 9:630, 1981.

101. Schwartz LB, Bissell MG, Murphy M, et al: Renal effects of dopamine in vascular surgical patients. J Vasc Surg 8:367, 1988.

Renal Diseases

102. Schlöndorff D, Dendorfer U, Brumberger V, et al: Limitations of therapeutic approaches to glomerular diseases. Kidney Int 48:S19, 1995.

103. Abbate M, Remuzzi G: Innovative strategies for pharmacological intervention in immune damage to the kidney. Nephrol Dial Transplant 10:1131, 1995.

104. Cattell V, Cook T: The nitric oxide pathway in glomerulonephritis. Curr Opin Nephrol Hypertens 4:359, 1995.

105. Abbate M, Remuzzi G: glomerulonephritis: From new knowledge on the mechanisms of tissue damage to novel therapies. Curr Opin Nephrol Hypertens 4:374, 1995.

106. Jardine AG: Angiotensin II and glomerulonephritis. J Hypertens 13:487, 1995.

107. Davison AM: Renal transplantation: Recurrence of original disease with particular reference to primary glomerulnephritis. Nephrol Dial Transplant 10:81, 1995.

108. Smith MC, Austen JL, Carey JT, et al: Prednisone improves renal function and proteinuria in human immunodeficiency virus-associated nephropathy. Am J Med 101:41, 1996.

109. Harris RC, Ismail N: Extrarenal complications of the nephrotic syndrome. Am J Kidney Dis 23:477, 1994.

110. Hopp L, Gilboa N, Kurland G, et al: Acute myocardial infarction in a young boy with nephrotic syndrome: A case report and review of the literature. Pediatr Nephrol 8:290, 1994.

111. Salcedo JR, Thabet MA, Latta K, et al: Nephrosis in childhood. Nephron 71:373, 1995.

112. Sagripanti A, Barsotti G: Hypercoagulability, intraglomerular coagulation, and thromboembolism in nephrotic syndrome. Nephron 70:271, 1995.

113. Kaysen GA: Nonrenal complications of the nephrotic syndrome. Annu Rev Med 45:201, 1994.

114. Tejani A, Ingulli E: Current concepts of pathogenesis of nephrotic syndrome. Contrib Nephrol 114:1, 1995.

115. Dorhout Mees EJ, Koomans HA: Understanding the nephrotic syndrome: What's new in a decade? Nephron 70:1, 1995.

116. Stein JP, Spitz A, Elmajian DA, et al: Bilateral emphysematous pyelonephritis: A case report and review of the literature. Urology 47:129, 1996.

117. O'Brien JD, Ettinger NA: Nephrobronchial fistula and lung abscess resulting from nephrolithiasis and pyelonephritis. Chest 108:1166, 1995.

118. Korman TM, Grayson ML: Treatment of urinary tract infections. Aust Fam Physician 24:2205, 1995.

119. Roberts JA: Mechanisms of renal damage in chronic pyelonephritis (reflux nephropathy). Curr Topics Pathol 88:265, 1995.

120. Bergeron MG: Treatment of pyelonephritis in adults. Med Clin North Am 79:619, 1995.

121. Joel M, Rosales JK: Fanconi syndrome and anesthesia. Anesthesiology 55:455, 1981.

122. Clive DM: Bartter's syndrome: The unsolved puzzle. Am J Kidney Dis 25:813, 1995.

123. Gitelman HJ: Unresolved issues in the pathogenesis of Bartter's syndrome and its variants. Curr Opin Nephrol Hypertens 3:471, 1994.

124. Abston PA, Priano LL: Bartter's syndrome: Anesthe-

tic implications based on pathophysiology and treatment. Anesth Analg 60:764, 1981.

125. Brimacombe JR, Breen DP: Anesthesia and Bartter's syndrome: A case report and review. J Am Assoc Nurse Anesth 61:193, 1993.

126. Klahr S, Purkerson ML: The pathophysiology of obstructive nephropathy: The role of vasoactive compounds in the hemodynamic and structural abnormalities of the obstructed kidney. Am J Kidney Dis 23:219, 1994.

127. Mackenzie HS, Brenner BM: Fewer nephrons at birth: A missing link in the etiology of essential hypertension? Am J Kidney Dis 26:91, 1995.

128. Brenner BM, Chertow GM: Congenital oligonephrophathy and the etiology of adult hypertension and progressive renal injury. Am J Kidney Dis 23:171, 1994.

129. Jelakovic B, Mayer G: A renocentric view of essential of hypertension: Lessons to be learnt from kidney transplantation. Nephrol Dial Transplant 10:1510, 1995.

130. Cowley AW Jr, Roman RJ: The role of the kidney in hypertension. JAMA 275:1581, 1996.

131. Fournier A, el Esper N, Makdassi R, et al: Hypertension and progression of renal insufficiency. Nephrol Dial Transplant Suppl 3:28, 1994.

132. Smith HT: Hypertension and the kidney. Am J Hypertens 6:119S, 1993.

133. Victor RG, Henrich WL: Autonomic neuropathy and hemodynamic stability in end-stage renal disease patients. *In* Henrich WL (eds): Principles and Practice of Dialysis. Baltimore, Williams & Wilkins, 1994.

134. Nisell H, Lintu H, Lunell NO, et al: Blood pressure and renal function seven years after pregnancy complicated by hypertension. Br J Obstet Gynaecol 102:876, 1995.

135. Sanders CE Jr, Curtis JJ: Role of hypertension in chronic renal allograft dysfunction. Kidney Int 48:S43, 1995.

136. Paul LC, Benediktsson H: Post-transplant hypertension and chronic renal allograft failure. Kidney Int 48:S34, 1995.

137. Hollenberg NK, Fisher NDL: Renal circulation and blockade of the renin-angiotensin system: Is angiotensin-converting enzyme inhibition the last word? Hypertension 26:602, 1995.

138. Frei U, Schindler R, Koch KM: Influence of antihypertensive therapy on renal function. Clin Invest 70:S120, 1992.

139. Osterby R: Renal pathology in diabetes mellitus. Curr Opin Nephrol Hypertens 2:475, 1993.

140. Mojcik CF, Klippel JH: End-stage renal disease and systemic lupus erythematosus. Am J Med 101:100, 1996.

141. Mazze RI, Cousins MJ: Combined nephrotoxicity of gentamicin and methoxyflurane anaesthesia in man. A case report. Br J Anaesth 45:394, 1973.

142. Barr GA, Mazze RI, Cousins MJ, et al: An animal model for combined methoxyflurane and gentamicin nephrotoxicity. Br J Anaesth 45:306, 1973.

143. Levy EM, Viscoli CM, Horwitz RI: The effect of acute renal failure on mortality: A cohort analysis. JAMA 275:1489, 1996.

144. Dunnick NR: Questions and answers. Am J Roentgenol 166:209, 1996.

145. Turney JH: Acute renal failure—a dangerous condition. JAMA 275:1516, 1996.

146. Ludwin D, Alexopoulou I: Cyclosporin A nephropathy in patients with rheumatoid arthritis. Br J Rheumatol 32:60, 1993.

Acute Renal Failure

147. Gelman S: Preserving renal function during surgery. Anesth Analg 74:88, 1992.

148. Brady HR, Singer GG: Acute renal failure. Lancet 346:1533, 1995.

149. Hollenberg NK, Epstein M, Rosen SM, et al: Acute oliguric renal failure in man: Evidence for preferential renal cortical ischemia. Medicine 47:455, 1968.

150. Regan MC, Young LS, Geraghty J, et al: Regional renal blood flow in normal and disease states. Urol Res 23:1, 1995.

151. Heyman SN, Fuchs S, Brezis M: The role of medullary ischemia in acute renal failure. New Horiz 3:597, 1995.

152. Racusen LC: The histopathology of acute renal failure. New Horiz 3:662, 1995.

153. Conger JD: Interventions in clinical acute renal failure: What are the data? Am J Kidney Dis 26:565, 1995.

154. Barry KG, Cohen A, Knochel JP, et al: Mannitol infusion. II. The prevention of acute functional renal failure during resection of an aneurysm of the abdominal aorta. N Engl J Med 264:967, 1961.

155. Reid PR, Thompson WL: The clinical use of dopamine in the treatment of shock. Johns Hopkins Med J 137:276, 1975.

156. Luke RG, Linton AL, Briggs JD, et al: Mannitol therapy in acute renal failure. Lancet 1:980, 1965.

157. Dawson JL: Postoperative renal function in obstructive jaundice: Effect of a mannitol diuresis. Br Med J 5427:82, 1965.

158. Behnia R, Koushanpour E, Brunner EA: Effects of hyperosmotic mannitol infusion on hemodynamics of dog kidney. Anesth Analg 82:902, 1996.

159. Gelman S: Does mannitol save the kidney? Anesth Analg 82:899, 1996.

160. Cantarovich F, Galli C, Benedetti L, et al: High-dose furosemide in established acute renal failure. Br Med J 2:449, 1973.

161. Colson P, Capdevila X, Cuchet D, et al: Does choice of the anesthetic influence renal function during infrarenal aortic surgery? Anesth Analg 74:481, 1992.

162. Mychaskiw G, II., Hines RL: Renal function during infrarenal aortic surgery. Anesth Analg 76:450, 1993.

163. Weinmann M: Natriuretic peptides and acute renal failure. New Horiz 3:624, 1995.

164. Bersten AD, Holt AW: Vasoactive drugs and importance of renal perfusion pressure. New Horiz 3:650, 1995.

165. Ito S, Carretero OA, Abe K: Nitric oxide in the regulation of renal blood flow. New Horiz 3:615, 1995.

166. Chertow GM, Sayegh MH, Allgren RL, et al: Is the administration of dopamine associated with adverse or favorable outcomes in acute renal failure? Am J Med 101:49, 1996.

Dialysis and Renal Transplantation

167. Schreiner GE: Acute renal failure. *In* Black DAK (eds): Renal disease, 2nd ed. Philadelphia, FA Davis, 1967.

168. Rettig RA: End-stage renal disease therapy: An American success story. JAMA 275:1118, 1996.

169. Moss AH: Dialysis decisions and the elderly. Clin Geriatr Med 10:463, 1994.

170. Chugh KS, Jha V: Differences in the care of ESRD

patients worldwide: Required resources and future outlook. Kidney Int 48:S7, 1995.

171. Port FK: End-stage renal disease: Magnitude of the problem, prognosis of future trends and possible solutions. Kidney Int 48:S3, 1995.

172. Fan P, Schwab SJ: Hemodialysis vascular access. *In* Henrich WL (eds): Principles and Practice of Dialysis. Baltimore, Williams & Wilkins, 1994.

173. Viscomi CM, Reese J, Rathmell JP: Medial and lateral antebrachial cutaneous nerve blocks. Reg Anesth 21:2, 1996.

174. Mouquet C, Bitker MO, Bailliart O, et al: Anesthesia for creation of a forearm fistula in patients with endstage renal failure. Anesthesiology 70:909, 1989.

175. Briggs JD: The recipient of a renal transplant. *In* Morris PJ (eds): Kidney Transplantation: Principles and Practice, 4th ed. Philadelphia, WB Saunders, 1996.

176. Hirschl MM: The patient with type II diabetes and uraemia—to transplant or not to transplant. Nephrol Dial Transplant 10:1515, 1995.

177. Carpenter CB: Long-term failure of renal transplants: Adding insult to injury. Kidney Int 48:S40, 1995.

178. Michielsen P: Recurrence of the original disease. Does this influence renal graft failure? Kidney Int 48:S79, 1995.

179. Garcia VD, Keitel E, Garcia CD, et al: Successful transplants using living donor kidneys with impaired function. Transplant Proc 24:2750, 1992.

180. Schweizer RT, Roper L, Hull D, et al: Measures to improve early results in kidney transplantation. Transplant Proc 24:2729, 1992.

181. Längle F, Sautner T, Grünberger T, et al: Impact of donor age on graft function in living-related kidney transplantation. Transplant Proc 24:2725, 1992.

182. Dantal J, Giral M, Hoormant M, et al: Glomerulonephritis recurrences after kidney transplantation. Curr Opin Nephrol Hypertens 4:146, 1995.

183. Cosimi AB: The donor and donor nephrectomy. *In* Morris PJ (eds): Kidney Transplantation: Principles and Practice, 4th ed. Philadelphia, WB Saunders, 1994.

184. Belzer FO, Kountz SL: Preservation and transplantation of human cadaver kidneys: A two-year experience. Ann Surg 172:394, 1970.

185. Sear JW: Kidney transplants: Induction and analgesic agents. Int Anesthesiol Clin 32:45, 1995.

186. Linke CL, Merin RG: A regional anesthetic approach for renal transplantation. Anesth Analg 55:69, 1976.

187. Cousins MJ: Hematoma following epidural block. Anesthesiology 37:263, 1972.

188. Brezis M, Rosen S, Silva P, et al: Renal ischemia: A new perspective. Kidney Int 26:375, 1984.

189. Coe FL, Kathpalia S: Hereditary tubular disorders. *In* Isselbacher KJ, Martin JB, Braunwald E, et al (eds): Harrison's Principles of Internal Medicine, 13th ed. New York, McGraw-Hill, 1994.

Hepatic Diseases

Leo Strunin
C. J. Eagle

The liver, the single largest parenchymal organ in the human body, is perfused by approximately 25 per cent of the cardiac output through a dual circulation from the portal vein and the hepatic artery. The liver has a central role in general metabolism and in carbohydrate, protein, and fat control essential to most body processes. Along with its role in normal metabolism, the liver biotransforms many exogenously administered compounds and has a major excretory role as a result of the production of bile. Chronic liver disease (cirrhosis), whatever the cause, leads to obstruction of blood flow through the liver and resultant portal hypertension. This, in turn, leads to the development of esophageal and gastric varices, and gastrointestinal hemorrhage may be a terminal event. Fulminant (acute) hepatic failure is defined by some authors as a condition that develops in a patient with a previously normal liver and no underlying liver disease. Onset typically occurs 3 to 8 weeks after an insult to the liver, with development of liver failure and encephalopathy. Recently, fulminant hepatic failure was more appropriately defined as a clinical syndrome evolving within 2 weeks, like that typically seen with hepatitis B virus (HBV) infection. Indeed, in the United States, some 75 per cent of cases of fulminant hepatic failure are viral in origin.

Interference with biliary secretion prevents bile salts from entering the gastrointestinal tract; since these salts are essential for the absorption of fat and fat-soluble vitamins (e.g., vitamin K) prothrombin production will be reduced. Disorders of bilirubin metabolism lead to retention of bilirubin in the blood and the clinical appearance of jaundice.

Despite these potentially serious complications of liver disease, liver damage must be considerable before any clinical signs appear. Indeed, many patients with well-compensated chronic liver disease will have few symptoms and only minimal changes in liver function tests; however, surgery and anesthesia may be sufficient to decompensate these patients and produce acute changes in the postoperative period.

Despite being at the center of most body processes, the liver has only a limited set of responses. Hepatic cells can be damaged chronically or acutely, blood and bile flow may be obstructed, and primary hepatoma of the liver can develop. The liver can become infected, most often with viruses, or can be the site of metastases from malignancies elsewhere in the body. Congenital abnormalities of the vascular and biliary systems may present at birth or in early childhood.

In this chapter, we focus on the relatively rare occasions when the anesthesiologist encounters patients with liver disease outside the operating room or when the disease process can affect the outcome after anesthesia and surgery. It should be remembered that these disease processes may be coincidental and unrelated to the operation or they may be the reason for the proposed surgery. It is not our intention to detail all possible causes of liver disease and their diagnosis and management; for these the reader is referred to the textbooks listed in the references.

I. GENERAL ASSESSMENT[1-7]

When hepatic disease is suspected, a careful history should be carried out with specific questions about drug and alcohol intake and exposure to viral and other infections, plus clinical examination of the patient and review of relevant liver function tests and imaging. Minor asymptomatic changes in liver function tests are not uncommon. Many of these patients are obese and consume much alcohol; diabetes mellitus is a common finding. Liver biopsy, the best method of determining the diagnosis, usually reveals a significant number of patients with either chronic active hepatitis or cirrhosis. In such patients, the most likely outcome after anesthesia and surgery is no major detrimental changes in hepatic function except for those related to the extent of the operation and other extraneous factors such as blood transfusion, unplanned hypoxia, and hypotension.

A. LIVER FUNCTION TESTS AND DIAGNOSTIC PROCEDURES

Table 6–1 lists some common liver function tests, and Table 6–2 shows their use in identifying various liver diseases. Albumin concentration is related to the synthetic capacity of the liver. With chronic liver disease, plasma albumin concentration is reduced and globulin concentration increased. Globulins are produced in the reticuloendothelial system, including the liver, and their levels rise in many forms of autoimmune liver disease. Reduced albumin concentration may enhance the action of drugs that are highly protein bound, allowing an increase in unbound fraction of the drug.

The international normalized ratio (INR) measures the rate at which prothrombin is converted to thrombin in the presence of thromboplastin, calcium, and blood clotting factors II, VII, IX, and X. The normal INR is 1. With liver disease, impaired synthesis of these factors causes an increase in the INR

TABLE 6–1

Liver Function Tests (Normal Ranges)

Protein	
Total	60–85 g/l
Albumin	35–50 g/l
Globulin	22–35 g/l
Enzymes	
Aspartate aminotransferase (AST)	0–4 U/l
Alanine aminotransferase (ALT)	2–22 U/l
Alkaline phosphatase (ALP)	30–115 U/l
Lactic dehydrogenase (LD)	60–200 U/l
Gamma-glutamyl transferase (GGT)	8–78 U/l
5'-Nucleotidase	1–11 U/l
Bilirubin	
Total	3–20 μmol/l
Conjugated	<8 μmol/l
Prothrombin time	
(always compared to a control; abnormal >3 seconds over control)	12–13 sec
Porphyrins (urine)	
Coproporphyrin	24–190 nmol/24 hr
Uroporphyrin	<36 nmol/24 hr
Ammonia (serum)	11–35 μmol/l
Ceruloplasmin	1.8–2.5 μmol/l
Immunoglobulins	
IgG	7.23–16.85 g/l
IgA	0.69–3.82 g/l
IgM	0.63–2.77 g/l
IgE (adult)	10,000–150,000 U/l

TABLE 6–2

Diagnostic Uses of Liver Function Tests

Enzyme	Clinical Considerations
Transaminases (AST; ALT)	Grossly raised in drug, viral, and ischemic hepatitis; nonspecific and not prognostic alone; may fall when liver failure occurs
Alkaline phosphatase (ALP)	Raised in cholestasis; measure 5'–nucleotidase and gamma-GT to distinguish hepatic ALP from nonhepatic origin (e.g., bone)
Glutathione S-transferase	May be sensitive marker for effects of volatile anesthetics
Gamma-glutamyl transferase (gamma-GT)	Used to assess alcohol, barbiturate, and phenytoin-induced liver damage
Lactate dehydrogenase (LDH)	LDH 5 is said to be liver specific, but like isocitrate dehydrogenase, (ICD), LDH is of limited use: both are elevated in hepatitis and hepatoma
Alpha-fetoprotein	Present in 70–90% of patients with hepatoma
Ceruloplasmin	A glycoprotein responsible for copper transport; is low in hepatolenticular degeneration (Wilson's disease)

to values greater than 1. This is a relatively nonspecific test because prolonged INR is also associated with nonhepatic disease. Nevertheless, it is a useful test in fulminant hepatic failure, as is a sensitive prognostic indicator. In biliary tract disease, supplementation by parenteral vitamin K should restore the prothrombin time to normal; however, this may require 12 to 24 hours of repeated intramuscular injections to be effective. In the presence of cellular disease, it may be impossible to return the INR to normal by administering vitamin K. In this circumstance fresh-frozen plasma should be considered, although the risk of viral and other infections or of sodium overload should be considered.

When bilirubin concentration exceeds 20 μmol/L, jaundice will be evident on clinical examination. Since many causes of jaundice are not amenable to surgical treatment, it is essential that a diagnosis be made before laparotomy is undertaken. Ultrasonography (Table 6–3) is the major imaging technique used to determine the pathway for further diagnostic tests or therapeutic maneuvers in the management of jaundiced patients. Nonoperative methods of relieving biliary obstruction include endoscopic retrograde cholangiopancreatography (ERCP), percutaneous biliary drainage, and papillotomy. In the presence of extrahepatic biliary obstruction, conventional intravenous cholangiography does not pro-

TABLE 6–3

Use of Ultrasound to Determine Further Diagnostic Procedures

Ultrasound indicates space-occupying lesion:
    Consider abscess, cyst, tumor
    Proceed to: hepatic scintigraphy, CT, MRI, liver biopsy
Ultrasound shows nondilated ducts:
    Consider intrahepatic disease
    Proceed to liver biopsy, ERCP
Ultrasound shows dilated ducts:
    Consider extrahepatic disease
    Proceed to: PTC, ERCP, hepatobiliary scintigraphy
Ultrasound shows portal hepatic vein obstruction:
    Proceed to arteriography/phlebography

duce adequate images. Percutaneous transhepatic cholangiography (PTC) and the use of computed tomography (CT) and magnetic resonance imaging (MRI) in combination with ultrasound should identify the site and cause of biliary obstruction. Unnecessary diagnostic laparotomy should be a thing of the past; the morbidity and mortality associated with such procedures, particularly in decompensated patients, are high.

Many enzymes present in the liver take part in the normal metabolic processes. In the presence of liver disease, these enzymes are released into the bloodstream in increased amounts and may help to determine the cause of hepatic damage. It should be noted that isolated measurements may have limited value; repeated measurements for trend analysis are more valuable. Table 12–2 shows the commonly measured enzymes and their diagnostic usefulness.

A number of other measurements may help determine the cause of liver dysfunction. For example, α-fetoprotein will be present in 70 per cent to 90 per cent of patients with primary carcinoma of the liver (hepatoma). Measurement of serum α-fetoprotein is also useful after operative resection of hepatomas to determine the success of the surgery. Blood ammonia is elevated with acute liver failure but is not helpful in determining the cause. Ninety per cent of patients with primary biliary cirrhosis have antimitochondrial antibodies present in their serum. In patients with Wilson's disease, an inherited disorder of copper metabolism, ceruloplasmin is low.

Finally, needle biopsy of the liver, percutaneous or laparoscopic, is a major diagnostic tool for determining various forms of cellular liver disease. Hemorrhage is the major risk of biopsy, so it should be undertaken only if the INR and platelet count are normal.

B. ESTIMATION OF HEPATIC RESERVE

The most valuable of the liver function tests is the INR. In addition, albumin concentration should be assessed as a measure of synthetic function and the various diagnostic procedures reviewed to determine a diagnosis. Elective surgery should be undertaken only in patients with well-compensated liver disease, since when deterioration of function is marked the outcome will almost certainly be poor, regardless of what anesthetic agents or techniques are used.

Tables 6–4 and 6–5 show two methods of assessing hepatic reserve using combinations of tests and observations. In general, only patients whose disease is in Child's classification A or at 5 to 6 points in that proposed by Pugh should be considered suitable candidates for surgical procedures. If there is any question that an elective surgery patient is incubating viral hepatitis, surgery must be delayed. Along with the conventional liver function tests reviewed above, hematologic profiles, tests for viral hepatitis, and assessment of renal, respiratory, and acid-base functions should be undertaken when there is evidence of liver disease.

C. DRUG METABOLISM IN LIVER DISEASE

One of the principal functions of the liver is to detoxify drugs by converting lipid-soluble compounds to more water-soluble ones, which can then be excreted in urine or bile. This metabolism is carried out by the microsomal enzymes in the endoplasmic reticulum of the hepatocyte. Most drugs undergo an initial step, such as oxidation or reduction, and are then conjugated with glucuronic or sulfuric acid. The microsomal enzyme system employs molecular oxygen and cytochromes; the entire system is often referred to as the *mixed function oxidase enzyme system.*

With chronic liver disease the number of liver cells is reduced, and therefore the amount of drug presented to each individual

TABLE 6–4

Clinical and Laboratory Classification of Patients with Cirrhosis in Terms of Hepatic Functional Reserve

	Group A	Group B	Group C
Bilirubin (μmol/l)	<40	40–50	>50
Albumin (g/l)	>35	30–35	<30
Ascites	None	Easily controlled	Poorly controlled
Neurologic disorder	None	Minimal	Coma
Nutrition	Excellent	Good	Poor (wasting)
Risk of operation	*Good*	*Moderate*	*Poor*

From Child CG: The liver and portal hypertension. *In* Child CG (ed): Major Problems in Clinical Sugery, Vol 1. Philadelphia, WB Saunders, 1964, pp 1–85.

cell for metabolism is increased. This overload actually increases the number of enzymes in the cell, a phenomenon called *substrate enzyme induction*. Therefore, only when hepatic damage is very severe is there an overall alteration in drug metabolism. There is no evidence that patients with liver disease are likely to develop side effects from potentially hepatotoxic drugs if the mechanism of toxicity is hypersensitivity; however, if the toxicity is dose related this principle does not hold; for example, cirrhosis patients are more likely to sustain liver damage from a drug such as pyrazinamide.

Centrally acting analgesic and sedative drugs may have prolonged action in patients with liver disease. This is not necessarily a reflection of altered hepatic metabolism but reflects the fact that brain metabolism is abnormal in such patients. This is particularly true in patients with acute liver failure, who should avoid all analgesics and sedative drugs.

The following additional factors should be borne in mind:

1. Coagulation factors are synthesized in the liver, so liver disease increases the risk of using anticoagulant drugs.

2. Fluid and sodium retention are common features of liver disease. Therefore, drugs that contain sodium or that have a sodium-retaining effect—for example, carbenoxolone and phenylbutazone—should be avoided if possible. During surgery, intravenous fluids containing sodium should be avoided, and 5 per cent dextrose should be the routine infusion fluid.

3. Protein abnormalities (low serum albumin and high globulin) may result in abnormal binding of drugs and may, for example, be responsible for the increased evidence of steroid side effects in patients with liver disease. Nondepolarizing relaxants are protein bound; it has been suggested that the increased amount of some of these drugs required during anesthesia reflects this binding.

TABLE 6–5

Grading of Severity of Liver Disease

Clinical and Biochemical Measurement	Points Scored for Increasing Abnormalities		
	1	*2*	*3*
Encephalopathy (grade)	None	1 and 2	3 and 4
Bilirubin (μmol/l)	<25	24–40	>40
Albumin (g/l)	35	28–35	<28
Prothrombin time (seconds prolonged)	1–4	4–6	>6

Using this system, patients who score 5 to 6 points are considered good operative risks (equivalent to Child grade A); patients with 7, 8, or 9 are moderate operative risks (equivalent to Child grade B); and patients with 10 to 15 points are poor operative risks (equivalent to Child C). Allowance should be made for the high bilirubin concentrations in patients with primary biliary cirrhosis relative to their other liver function tests.

From Pugh RNH, Murray-Lyon IM, Dawson JL, et al: Transection of the oesophagus for bleeding varices. Br J Surg 1973; 60:646–649.

4. When biliary obstruction is present, drugs that are usually excreted in the bile may either accumulate or cause toxicity. In addition, drugs that normally act on the biliary tree fail to reach their site of action.

5. The first pass effect is lost, probably as a result of spontaneous opening of portal-systemic shunts.

In summary, drugs that are known to be hepatotoxic should be avoided in patients with liver disease. Drugs that rarely cause hypersensitivity-type damage are acceptable if required. When possible, drugs that are normally excreted unchanged in the urine should be preferred. Drugs that have an effect on the central nervous system or blood coagulation should be used with caution; if necessary, the patient should first be given small doses and observed for ill effects.

II. CHRONIC LIVER DISEASE (CIRRHOSIS)[8–70]

Cirrhosis is a pathologic term denoting scarring of the liver. Table 6–6 shows some of the common and uncommon causes. Cirrhosis should be distinguished from hepatitis, which usually indicates infection of the liver and is more consistent with an acute disease episode. Pathologists also describe *chronic active* and *active chronic* hepatitis; these are histologic diagnoses related to autoimmune processes and viral infections. Biliary obstruction

alone, leading to jaundice, may not be associated with hepatocellular damage. *Cholestasis* is the pathologic term for biliary obstruction; however, jaundice may result from a combination of processes related to bilirubin metabolism, including transport, storage, liver cell damage, and excretion.

Chronic liver disease often produces little alteration in liver function and may be undetectable clinically and biochemically. Only when some additional insult, often iatrogenic, produces further deterioration in liver function does the underlying chronic liver disease become clinically obvious as jaundice, ascites, or encephalopathy. Therefore, the natural history of chronic liver disease is not necessarily progressive deterioration; with careful management, avoiding precipitation of complications, patients can be kept well for many years.

Cirrhosis is not a single entity; the characteristic pathologic changes of necrosis, fibrosis, and regeneration nodules can result from many causes. In addition, there may be histologic features specific to certain diseases. The size of the liver is very variable, ranging from shrunken to very large, and may change during the course of the disease; however, resistance to the flow of blood in the portal venous system is always increased, resulting eventually in congestive splenomegaly and collateral venous channels. This condition is usually described as portal hypertension. Another late complication of cirrhosis is the development of primary liver cell carcinoma (hepatoma).

Compensated cirrhosis is compatible with a feeling of complete well-being; when symptoms do occur they are usually vague, such as malaise, dyspepsia, weight loss, loss of libido, and menstrual disturbances. Physical signs are also often absent, and many of the skin changes described in cirrhosis, such as white spots, paper money skin, white nails, and palmar erythema, have little diagnostic value. Finger clubbing and cyanosis are occasionally seen but are nonspecific. Generalized pigmentation may indicate hemochromatosis or primary biliary cirrhosis. One of the most useful physical signs of cirrhosis is the presence of spider nevi on the skin of the face, arms, and upper torso; they may occur transiently with pregnancy or viral hepatitis but are particularly florid in alcoholic cirrhosis and chronic active hepatitis.

Chronic liver disease characteristically produces evidence of a high-output circulatory

---

TABLE 6–6

Causes of Cirrhosis

Common
   Cryptogenic (cause unknown): alcohol, HBV, and HBC may account for some
   Viral hepatitis—HBV and HCV; not HAV
   Alcohol
Rare
   Metabolic: hemochromatosis, Wilson's disease, alpha$_1$-antitrypsin deficiency, diabetes mellitus, galactosemia
   Prolonged cholestasis
   Hepatic (venous outflow obstruction): Budd-Chiari syndrome, venoocclusive disease, constrictive pericarditis
   Disturbed immunity: ``lupoid'' hepatitis
   Drug- and toxin-induced
   Primary biliary cirrhosis: progressive granulomatous destruction of intrahepatic bile ducts, probably immune-mediated: 90% of patients are female and antimitochondrial antibodies are present in 100%

state—flushed extremities, dilated veins, capillary pulsation, and a collapsing pulse. Although arteriovenous fistulas in the lungs have been demonstrated in liver disease (which may account for some of the changes, such as finger clubbing), the more likely explanation is that a vasodilator substance is either produced by or not inactivated by the damaged liver.

With cirrhosis, the proportion of blood supply derived from the portal vein diminishes gradually, and flow from the hepatic artery is relatively increased. Thus, the effects of portacaval anastomosis on the blood supply to the liver are less marked in cirrhosis patients, but the effects of systemic hypotension and hypoxemia are more marked. Since the regeneration nodules are supplied mainly by arterial blood, systemic hypoxemia may result in severe liver necrosis. Progressive distortion of the portal venous system by these regeneration nodules produces a rise in portal venous pressure, development of collateral channels bypassing the liver, splenomegaly, and hypersplenism.

A palpably enlarged liver is associated mainly with alcoholic cirrhosis or hemochromatosis, whereas a shrunken liver is more likely with cryptogenic cirrhosis. The cirrhotic liver is firm, and it may be possible to palpate irregularities on the surface in the macronodular type. Splenomegaly and venous collaterals on the abdominal wall are good indicators of portal hypertension. In the later stages of chronic liver disease, there may be progressive water retention, hyponatremia, azotemia, and oliguria due to reduced renal plasma flow, leading to hepatorenal failure. Signs that chronic liver disease has become decompensated include jaundice, edema, ascites, a flapping tremor, and other signs of impending hepatic coma. A change in size or shape of the liver may indicate a hepatoma.

It has been estimated that, for the 21 million anesthetics administered every year in the United States, approximately 11,000 patients present with alcoholic cirrhosis and 300,000 with gallbladder disease. Thus, cholecystectomy is one of the most common operations performed today. Cirrhosis patients are seen less often and, alcoholic cirrhosis aside, the other disease processes are rare.

A. PORTAL HYPERTENSION

It is assumed that patients with decompensated liver disease (those with 10 to 15 points in Pugh's system; see Table 12–5) will not be subjected to elective surgery; however, such patients may have to be anesthetized for management of some complication of their cirrhosis, most likely gastrointestinal bleeding associated with portal hypertension. In the past, portacaval anastomosis was carried out. Today, when surgery is indicated the distal spenorenal shunt (Warren's) is preferred. No data show unequivocally that any shunting procedure prolongs patients' life expectancy. Indeed, for many procedures the operative and immediate postoperative mortality rates are extremely high. Patients in Child's categories B and C are obviously also at great risk.

The initial treatment of esophageal variceal hemorrhage includes resuscitation, early endoscopy to determine the site of bleeding, and immediate injection sclerotherapy, if possible. Mechanical means of controlling hemorrhage—balloon tamponade (Linton-Nachlas tube, Sengstaken-Blakemore tube, or Minnesota tube) or administration of drugs (e.g., vasopressin, octreotide, somatostatin, propranolol) to lower portal venous pressure—are not as effective because they can be carried out only for a limited time. Vasopressin infusion may be associated with coronary artery vasoconstriction, but this may be offset by infusion of nitroglycerin. Interventional radiology may be used to embolize varices or to reduce portal pressure by placement of a transjugular intrahepatic shunt.

Gastrointestinal hemorrhage in association with esophageal varices, portal hypertension, and chronic liver disease is often dramatic. Clearly, if liver cell damage is extensive, it can be a terminal event. Nevertheless, if bleeding can be controlled and if the cause of the liver disease is reversible or its progress can be arrested, the outlook may not be hopeless. If patients with chronic alcoholic liver disease can be persuaded to abstain,[8] the 5-year survival rates are better than for those who persist in drinking. Rarer forms of hepatocellular damage, if progressive, may be amenable to liver transplantation.

B. ANESTHETIC CONSIDERATIONS

If the preoperative evaluation determines that vitamin K therapy or fresh-frozen plasma is indicated, it should be given preoperatively. Patients who are on steroid therapy for management of chronic liver disease may require additional steroids with their pre-medication. H_2 antagonists help reduce the risk of gastrointestinal hemorrhage. The presence of esophageal varices should be considered when passing nasogastric tubes. Clearly, if clotting ability is compromised, particular care should be taken with invasive monitoring and tracheal intubation. All patients with chronic liver disease should be considered potential carriers of HBV infection.

1. Neuromuscular Blocking Drugs

Patients with liver disease may require increased doses of nondepolarizing neuromuscular blocking drugs, and they exhibit apparent resistance. The most likely explanation for the resistance to these drugs is related to increased distribution volume in the presence of liver disease. Other possibilities include altered protein binding, sequestration in an enlarged liver or spleen, and reduced hepatic and urinary clearance.

Vecuronium has high biliary clearance in contrast to other nondepolarizing neuromuscular blocking drugs. In patients with cholestasis the elimination phase for vecuronium is prolonged. Since its hepatic uptake is rapid, however, action of the drug is not prolonged unless large doses are administered. Surgical manipulation of the liver and biliary tract may affect clearance of vecuronium and may prolong its action.

For patients who have both cholestasis and cirrhosis or hepatic failure, the muscle relaxant of choice is atracurium. This drug is relatively independent of hepatic metabolism, undergoes some nonenzymatic breakdown in plasma, and is excreted mainly in the urine. Since hepatic disease can be accompanied by renal dysfunction, however, any neuromuscular blocking drug may have a prolonged elimination phase. Monitoring of neuromuscular activity, avoidance of large dose increments, and institution of postoperative ventilation may be necessary when patients with liver disease are given nondepolarizing muscle relaxant drugs.

Pseudocholinesterase, a nonspecific esterase synthesized by the liver, has a half-life of about 15 days. When protein synthesis is decreased, as with hepatocellular damage, the plasma concentration falls. Since pseudocholinesterase is responsible for the metabolism of succinylcholine, it is often suggested that

the action of succinylcholine may be prolonged with liver disease. In practice, this does not seem to be a problem; genetically determined abnormalities of the enzyme are far more likely to be responsible. The action of mivacurium may also be prolonged in patients with a low pseudocholinesterase level. It should be remembered that fresh blood and plasma concentrates may contain pseudocholinesterase and thus interfere with plasma measurements. The enzyme has also been used to assess synthetic liver function before and after portacaval anastomosis and transplantation.

2. Opioids

Morphine elimination is increased in cirrhosis patients owing to a decreased hepatic extraction ratio or hepatic blood flow. Cholestasis does not interfere with morphine pharmacokinetics; however, renal impairment may prolong the action of the drug. Most textbooks devoted to liver disease indicate that morphine is unsuitable for cirrhosis patients. It is usually suggested that profound and prolonged effects are associated with conventional doses of morphine. Although some of these may be explained by altered pharmacokinetics, the presence of "coma factors" due to hepatic dysfunction can compound the normal effects of morphine and other opioids. In patients with well-compensated liver disease morphine is not contraindicated for postoperative pain. One complication, biliary tract spasm, is occasionally encountered in patients given morphine for pain relief in the postoperative anesthetic recovery area after cholecystectomy. The pain may be so severe as to mimic myocardial infarction; the diagnosis is confirmed by a normal electrocardiogram and immediate reversal of the pain after administration of a small dose of naloxone.

Fentanyl is probably the opioid of choice, since it seems least affected by changes in liver function; alfentanil and sufentanil may exhibit prolonged action with an extended elimination phase. In general, caution should be observed in administering opioids to patients with cirrhosis and in particular to those whose liver function is decompensated.

3. Intravenous Induction Agents

None of the currently available intravenous induction agents depends for its elimination on biliary excretion. In cirrhosis patients, however, the elimination phase of these drugs is prolonged as liver blood flow is reduced and hepatic clearance of the drugs is affected.[21] Patients with alcoholic cirrhosis frequently require larger doses of intravenous induction agents. This can be accounted for in part by alterations in protein binding, but many patients are obese, and when doses are calculated on the basis of weight the requirement may not be increased. If large doses are given, however, recovery may be prolonged, particularly if infusion techniques are used. Thiopental has been widely used and is subject to all the difficulties outlined above. Etomidate appears to have no advantages over thiopental, and propofol should be used with caution, as it can cause marked cardiovascular depression. The benzodiazepines may have extremely prolonged action; only small doses should be administered, preferably of oxazepam or lorazepam.

4. Hepatic Circulation and Volatile Anesthetics

Volatile anesthetics affect the liver principally through changes in the circulation. All currently available potent vapors decrease cardiac output and reduce liver blood flow in proportion to systemic arterial pressure. Although the liver is capable of some "autoregulation," this is limited. In general, systemic hypotension is associated with a drop in liver blood flow; however, compensation is usually good owing to increased hepatic oxygen extraction. Comparative studies of halothane, enflurane, and isoflurane suggest that the latter drug may be better for the liver because it has the least effect on hepatic circulation, which can be important for patients with liver disease. All volatile anesthetics undergo some metabolism in the liver, and nonvolatile metabolites may be demonstrated in the urine for many weeks after general anesthesia.

These potentially detrimental circulatory changes, as well as the presence of metabolites that could be hepatotoxic, have often been claimed as the basis of postanesthesia hepatitis. It should be recognized that postoperative jaundice (i.e., a rise in plasma bilirubin concentration without hepatitis) and any other changes in liver function tests indicative of cell damage have many possible causes (Table 6–7).

Rarely, hepatitis follows anesthesia and sur-

TABLE 6–7
Causes of Postoperative Jaundice

Excess bilirubin load
  Blood trransfusion
  Hemolysis
  Surgical trauma
Preexisting liver disease
  Chronic liver disease (cirrhosis)
  Hepatitis, alcoholic, viral, drug-induced
  Hereditary hyperbilirubinemias:
      Unconjugated: Gilbert's syndrome, Crigler-Najjar syndrome (type II), primary ``shunt'' hyperbilirubinemia
      Conjugated: Dubin-Johnson syndrome, rotor type
  Pulmonary/cardiac failure associated with hepatic congestion
Anesthesia
  Hypoxia
  Hypotension
Surgery
  Sepsis, biliary tree damage, retained gallstone, cholecystitis, cholangitis, pancreatitis, extensive liver surgery, liver trauma, benign postoperative cholestasis, hyperthermia
Drugs (Many of these are rare causes of jaundice but are listed to encourage the taking of an extensive drug history in all jaundiced patients, pre- or postoperative, before blaming the anesthetic postoperatively)
  Carbon tetrachloride, muscarine, acetaminophen, salicylates, mineral oil, yellow phosphorus, sodium valproate, tetracyclines, oxacillin, perhexiline maleate, amiodarone, isoniazid, rifampicin, alpha-methyldopa, ketoconazole, tienilic acid, disulfiram, verapamil, imipramine, diphenylhydantoin, dantrolene, azathioprine, vincristine and irradiation, estrogen, chlorpromazine, erythromycin, nitrofurantoin, cimetidine, ranitidine, halothane, ? other volatile anaesthetics

gery when all the causes listed in Table 6–7 have been ruled out. The incidence of this complication varies from 1 in 6000 to 1 in 30,000 anesthetics. The condition is rare in children and elders. It is usually seen in obese, middle-aged women after relatively minor surgery and uneventful anesthesia, most often with halothane and usually after repeated exposures to the drug at relatively short intervals. There have been individual case reports of similar postanesthetic hepatitis after exposure to enflurane, isoflurane, and sevoflurane; however, it is not clear at present specifically how these drugs cause hepatitis.

Most authorities agree that there is some risk of hepatitis associated with halothane under the circumstances described above. The mechanism has yet to be elucidated. Most likely, a combination of metabolism of the drug, an immune-mediated response to the metabolites, and perhaps some genetic factor is required before an acute halothane reaction occurs. This type of drug response is unpredictable, and there are no means for identifying susceptible persons ahead of time. In some patients, antibodies to halothane metabolites may be demonstrated during the acute phase of hepatitis, and sometimes later; however, cases of unexplained hepatitis following halothane (UHFH) have been described in which no antibodies were demonstrated. Clearly, for these patients the role of halothane is unclear. There is no evidence that patients with liver disease or cholestasis of known cause are susceptible in any way to UHFH, but in many parts of the world the medicolegal climate is such that most anesthesiologists hesitate to give halothane to any patient, with or without liver dysfunction. Indeed, there is no reason to do so, since alternatives such as enflurane, isoflurane, sevoflurane, and desflurane are available.

Isoflurane seems to be the drug of choice, since its effects on the circulation through the liver may be less pronounced than the other agents', the amount metabolized is small, and the case reports of unexplained hepatitis after isoflurane are limited. These observations notwithstanding, it seems sensible—particularly in patients with decompensated liver disease–to limit the concentration of isoflurane as much as possible. In addition, to minimize adverse cardiovascular effects, hypoventilation and hyperventilation should be avoided and arterial carbon dioxide pressure should be kept in the normal range. End-tidal carbon dioxide monitoring and vapor analysis of inspired and expired gases make these objectives easy to achieve.

5. Monitoring

When patients with cirrhosis undergo anesthesia and surgery, monitoring of vital signs should be carried out as shown in Table 6–8. Invasive vascular monitoring should be tempered with a knowledge of the patient's INR, and caution should be observed if it is prolonged.

III. BILIARY OBSTRUCTION (CHOLESTASIS)[71–74]

A. JAUNDICE

Although it is traditional to classify the causes of jaundice according to mechanism—

TABLE 6–8

Monitoring of Patients with Liver Disease During Anesthesia and Surgery

Noninvasive
  ECG
  Blood pressure
  Temperature
  Pulse oximeter
  End-tidal carbon dioxide (infrared)
  End-tidal volatile agents (infrared)
  Peripheral nerve stimulator
  Mass spectrometry end-tidal gas (air embolus
    detection, carbon dioxide, volatile agents)
Invasive*
  Arterial line (blood gas estimations)
  CVP catheter (volume status, transfusion)
  Pulmonary artery catheter (cardiac output,
    volume status)

*Invasive monitoring should be determined by the extent of the operative procedure and a review of the INR.

increased bile pigment production, defective uptake and transport within the hepatocyte, defective conjugation, defective excretion—in practice, in a given patient it may be difficult to attribute jaundice to any single mechanism. For example, hepatocellular damage may result in jaundice by all four mechanisms.

The capacity of the liver to handle bile pigment may increase considerably, so that even in chronic hemolytic states when production of bilirubin is greatly increased, the serum bilirubin concentration is rarely raised above 50 μmol/L. Higher levels usually indicate additional hepatocellular dysfunction.

The best example of defective bilirubin transport is Gilbert's disease, the commonest variety of familial, unconjugated, nonhemolytic hyperbilirubinemia, although the defect can also occur in patients with resolving virus hepatitis. Serum bilirubin is not raised above 50 μmol/L and is not affected by steroid therapy.

Defective conjugation by hepatic microsomes can result from two mechanisms: (1) enzyme deficiency such as that found in neonatal or "physiologic" jaundice and in the very rare (usually fatal) Crigler-Najjar hyperbilirubinemia, and (2) enzyme inhibition caused by a factor in maternal serum, probably a pregestational steroid that may inhibit glucuronyl transferase and cause neonatal jaundice. In both conditions bilirubin is unconjugated and does not appear in the urine.

Defective excretion can occur either within the bile canaliculi and small ducts of the liver (intrahepatic cholestasis) or in the main bile ducts between the liver and the duodenum (extrahepatic obstruction). Intrahepatic cholestasis may be the result of widespread hepatocellular damage, as in viral or alcoholic hepatitis or macronodular cirrhosis; in these instances, serum bilirubin concentration may be dramatically reduced by steroid therapy. The clinical picture of cholestasis may be seen in patients with the Dubin-Johnson syndrome (familial conjugated hyperbilirubinemia) and may be enhanced by ictogenic steroids (such as methyltestosterone or norethandrolone). Cellular reactions around the ductules and intralobular ducts may reflect drug sensitivity, for example to the phenothiazine group. Inflammatory reactions around the intralobular and septal bile ducts occur in primary biliary cirrhosis and biliary atresia; similar reactions around still larger ducts occur with ascending cholangitis. Extrahepatic obstruction in large bile ducts can result from gallstones, strictures, carcinoma of the bile duct, and carcinoma of the head of the pancreas. Hyperbilirubinemia—of either the intra- or extrahepatic obstructive type—is predominantly conjugated and is accompanied by bile in the urine. Unconjugated hyperbilirubinemia may occur later, because there is invariably a decrease in red cell survival with obstructive jaundice and because conjugation becomes defective.

B. RENAL FAILURE

Untreated biliary obstruction is eventually accompanied by renal failure. The cause is probably endotoxin that the damaged liver is unable to handle and that spills over into the systemic circulation. With long-standing biliary obstruction the bile is inevitably infected. Laparotomy in such patients used to be accompanied by a high incidence of postoperative renal failure. This can be prevented by adequate preoperative hydration, administration of antibiotics, and maintenance of diuresis before, during, and after operation. To achieve this diuresis, urine output of all jaundiced patients should be monitored. Those at particular risk have bilirubin concentrations in excess of 180 µmol/L preoperatively. Urine output should be at least 50 ml/hour. If adequate diuresis cannot be achieved by fluid loading alone or if this approach is not appropriate, then mannitol or furosemide should be used.

C. INTENSIVE CARE UNIT JAUNDICE

The prevalence of abnormal liver function tests in patients in the intensive care unit (ICU) who do not have liver disease may be as high as 50 per cent. In many of these patients jaundice may become clinically apparent 1 to 2 weeks after admission, and the precipitating event is often obscure. The diagnosis of ICU jaundice is one of exclusion. There is a progressive rise in bilirubin and a moderate rise in alkaline phosphatase, and transaminase values are significantly elevated only if there has been hepatic ischemia.

Many patients are in the ICU because of sepsis polytrauma, or major surgery. Many show a characteristic systemic inflammatory response syndrome (SIRS), and multiple organ failure or adult respiratory distress syndrome (ARDS) may develop. Three mechanisms for ICU jaundice have been postulated: hepatocellular ischemia, cytokine-induced inhibition of hepatocellular function, and oxidant injury. Treatment is supportive: infection should be controlled and early enteral feeding encouraged, and there may be a role for nitric oxide synthesis inhibitors.

IV. VIRAL HEPATITIS[75-101]

Table 6–9 lists the common and the less common viruses that can cause hepatitis. Although there are now serologic tests to identify carriers of many agents of viral hepatitis, the results of these tests may not be available at the time of surgery. It is now recommended that all body fluids be considered potentially infectious and that anesthesiologists take steps to apply "universal body fluid precautions." This will require fundamental changes in practice that are not yet widely applied.

A. HEPATITIS A VIRUS

Hepatitis A virus (HAV) infection most often affects children but is also responsible for some 20 per cent of adult viral hepatitis. The disease is commonly epidemic and has an incubation period of 15 to 45 days. Diagnosis of HAV[81] is made by a history of contact with the disease, which is usually spread by food or water. HAV is rarely transmitted by a

TABLE 6–9

Common and Uncommon Viruses That Cause Hepatitis

Virus	Serology
Hepatitis A (HAV)*	Anti-HAV IgM
	Anti-HAV IgG
Hepatitis B (HBV)*	HBsAg-HBcAg
	HBcAg-DNA
	polymerase
	Anti-HBs, Anti-HBc
Delta (hepatitis D (HDV))*	Anti-delta IgM
Hepatitis C (HCV)	Anti-HCV
Epstein-Barr (EBV*, infectious	EB IgM
mononucleosis)	
Cytomegalovirus (CMV)	Anti-CMV IgM
Herpes simplex I and II	Yes†
Coxsackie B	Yes†
ECHO	Yes†
Yellow fever*	Yes†
Adenovirus	Yes†
Varicella zoster virus	Yes†
Measles*	Yes†
Human immunodeficiency virus	Yes†
(HIV)	
Lassa fever/Marburg/Ebola virus	Yes†

*Vaccine available
†Serology or other tests available for diagnosis.

blood transfusion. In general, HAV infection is mild and infection does not result in a chronic carrier state. Only 4 per cent of fulminant hepatic failures are due to HAV. Approximately half the population show antibodies for HAV immunoglobulin M; these are found in the patient's plasma in rising titers shortly after infection.

In the event of possible transmission from an infected patient, the anesthesiologist who has not been vaccinated against HAV can be protected by a single dose of gammaglobulin, 0.02 ml/kg intramuscularly, within 2 weeks of exposure. This provides protection for approximately 3 months. Gammaglobulin is safe since it is heat and alcohol treated. The current HAV vaccine is very effective, and all anesthesiologists should consider its use.

B. HEPATITIS B VIRUS

Infection with hepatitis B virus may be identified by a number of serologic markers (see Table 6–9). The surface antigen (HBsAg) indicates the presence of infection; the appearance of anti-HBs indicates recovery and immunity to further infection. The hepatitis B cove antigen (HBcAg) is found only in the liver and is present in liver biopsy specimens from infected patients. The serologic markers found in the carrier state include HBsAg, (HBeAg), and (on occasion) DNA polymerase. If both HBsAg and HBeAg are present, the host is highly infectious.

HBV is transmitted principally by contact with body fluids, including transfused blood, and has a long incubation (up to 3 months). The commonest mode of transmission to anesthesiologists is accidental needle stick. HBV, unlike HAV, can cause chronic liver disease, cirrhosis, and hepatoma. The clinical course of the infection is that 90 per cent of infected persons recover fully without suffering untoward sequelae. Some of the remaining 10 per cent progress to a chronic carrier state, and approximately 1 per cent develop fulminant hepatic failure; some 60 per cent of these will die. The World Health Organization (WHO) has ascribed carrier status to any person who tests positive for HBsAg for more than 3 months; it is estimated that currently there are some 200 million carriers of HBV worldwide. Studies of anesthesiologists around the world have shown that many show evidence of exposure to HBV; antibodies to the surface antigen (anti-HBs) have been found in some 12 per cent to 23 per cent of anesthesiologists, and this indicates that there *is* an occupational risk. Although carriers are extremely rare, carrier status may constitute a legal bar in some jurisdictions to an anesthesiologist's performing invasive clinical procedures.

Although precautions for handling body fluids may protect from HBV infection, the most satisfactory protection is vaccination. Vaccines are now available, either of human origin or by DNA synthesis, that are extremely effective, have a low incidence of side effects, and carry no risk of other viral infections such as human immunodeficiency virus (HIV). Heptovax immunization consists of three intramuscular doses of 1 ml of vaccine, the second and third given 1 and 6 months after the initial one. Thereafter, some 90 per cent of vaccinated persons are protected by the development of adequate (anti-HBs) antibodies. The vaccine appears to be effective for approximately 5 years.

C. DELTA VIRUS

Delta virus is a defective RNA hepatotrophic virus. In the presence of HBV, delta virus can cause hepatitis; delta agent cannot act alone, so precautions against HBV also protect against delta. The clinical features of delta infection depend on whether the host is infected with HBV and delta together or whether a chronic hepatitis B carrier is superinfected with the delta agent. With coinfection the acute delta infection is self-limiting, since delta cannot outlive the HBs antigenemia; however, the attack can be fulminant. With superinfection, a stable HBsAg-positive patient may relapse or chronic hepatitis may be accelerated.

D. HEPATITIS C VIRUS

Three types of hepatitis C virus (HCV) have been described: blood-borne, coagulation factor–borne, and epidemic water-borne virus. HCV is responsible for approximately 90 per cent of posttransfusion hepatitis (PTH). The carrier state seems more common with HCV infection than HBV infection. Epidemic outbreaks of HCV (sometimes identified as *hepatitis E* by serology) have been reported. The incubation period varies from 2 to 26 weeks, and most cases follow transfusion of blood or blood products. Carriers of HCV are at high risk for progression to chronic liver disease and are more likely to develop hepatoma than HBV carriers. Fulminant hepatic failure is rare. As yet there is no vaccine for HCV infection, although the various types of virus can be identified serologically. Since carriers of HCV are becoming more common, infection of operating room personnel can occur during anesthesia and surgery.

E. OTHER VIRUSES

Table 6–9 lists some of the rarer causes of viral hepatitis, some of which may be encountered in the ICU. Exotic viruses are a particular problem, and patients with these infections should be cared for in a center familiar with stringent barrier nursing; otherwise, staff may be infected. Acquired immunodeficiency syndrome (AIDS) is caused by HIV. Although liver damage is not a primary symptom of AIDS, hepatic involvement can occur. In addition, homosexuals, one group at high risk for AIDS, are also at risk for HBV infection. AIDS is usually spread by sexual transmission, blood transfusion, or some other parenteral injection. Blood products that have not been screened or sterilized may transmit HBV, HCV, and HIV. Indeed, this has occurred in hemophiliacs. Drug addicts can also acquire all three infections by sharing unsterilized needles.

F. INFECTION CONTROL

Hepatitis is a recognized hazard for anesthesia personnel; however, simple measures are effective in preventing transmission from patients to staff. Awareness of the problem is important and implies that high-risk patients should be screened for serologic evidence of viral infection. In some jurisdictions this requires patient consent. Even if these facilities are not available, patients in high-risk categories should be regarded as potentially infectious until it is proved otherwise. These include persons who live in closed institutions, patients who have had multiple blood or blood product transfusions, infants of mothers with HBV, drug addicts, homosexuals, and persons with tattoos. Most cases of hepatitis among anesthesiologists follow accidental inoculation, and casual attitudes to spillage of blood and disposal of "sharps" should be tempered with restraint. Wearing gloves, a disposable gown, and a mask, use of disposable anesthesia equipment or in-line viral filters (when appropriate), and safe disposal of such equipment afterward are obvious precautions, as is hand washing between patient contacts. Hepatitis viruses are susceptible to heat, steam sterilization, ethylene oxide, aqueous formaldehyde, glutaraldehyde, and most proprietary bleach solutions, so sterilization of equipment should not be a problem.

Despite precautions, inadvertent inoculation of infectious material can occur. Hospitals should have an identified procedure for reporting and following all such contacts. In addition, in many parts of the world viral infections are "notifiable diseases." All anesthesiologists should consider vaccination their primary protection against HAV and HBV infection. HCV is a serious problem in many parts of the world; no vaccine is available; and it remains a risk for anesthesiologists.

G. ANESTHETIC CONSIDERATIONS

For patients with well-compensated chronic liver disease due to viral hepatitis or symptom-free carriers, anesthesia and surgery do not appear to carry any additional risk of postoperative deterioration in liver function. If viral hepatitis is in an acute stage, however, operation is extremely hazardous; deterioration in liver function is inevitable, regardless of what anesthetic technique is used. Therefore, elective surgery should be postponed until liver function returns to normal; this can take several months.

V. HYDATID DISEASE[102–104]

The adult worm of the parasite *Echinococcus granulosus* resides in the intestinal lumen of dogs and related carnivores. Sheep and cattle become infected by the fecal-oral route, and humans may become intermediate hosts by eating contaminated meat.

Ova from the parasite pass in the portal stream to the liver and form cysts for their larval colonies. These cysts are not toxic and do not injure the liver, but they can grow so large that they physically interfere with the host. Diagnosis is made by examining the abdomen and chest, abdominal radiography, bidirectional liver scintigraphy, ultrasonography, and CT and MRI. Casoni's skin test, which allegedly identifies allergy to hydatid fluid, is of limited usefulness. Calcified cysts do not usually require treatment since calcification indicates death of the parasite. Surgical resection of the liver is not necessary; simple drainage is sufficient. Depending on the location of the cyst, either laparotomy or thoracotomy is performed. Hydrocortisone should be given with the premedication to prevent an intraoperative anaphylactic reaction should hydatid fluid accidentally be spilled.

VI. LIVER DISEASES OF GENETIC CAUSE[105–120]

A. IDIOPATHIC HEMOCHROMATOSIS

Idiopathic hemochromatosis is an autosomal-recessive disorder that results in excessive intestinal absorption of iron commencing early in life. Secondary hemochromatosis can be produced by multiple transfusions and is associated with a variety of acquired and congenital hematopoietic disorders. The latter include thalassemia major, sickle cell disease, and sideroblastic anemia. Mild to moderate iron overload may also be associated with chronic alcoholic liver disease and porphyria cutanea tarda.

Most often the condition presents in males in the fifth or sixth decade of life. Clinical features include pigmentation, hepatomegaly, gonadal atrophy, and diabetes mellitus. About one third of patients also have cardiac symptoms, although only 15 per cent develop congestive heart failure. These latter patients tend to be younger, and they develop progressive right-sided heart failure, which can be associated with arrhythmias.

The clinical features arise from iron deposits in the tissues, which result in a fibrous reaction. The organs most commonly affected are the liver, pancreas, myocardium, and endocrine glands, including the adrenal cortex, anterior pituitary, and testes.

Laboratory investigations show little disturbance in liver function until late in the course of the disease. Plasma iron concentration and the proportion of saturated transferrin are both elevated. Needle liver biopsy is diagnostic. Marked iron overload can be detected by both CT and MRI, and these modalities may be useful for following therapy.

Repeated phlebotomy can slowly decrease tissue iron stores. Each 500 ml of blood collected removes only 250 mg of iron, but iron excess in the body can be as much as 20 to 60 grams. It is thus evident that a prolonged course of phlebotomy may be required. Patients with identified hormone deficiency are treated with specific replacement therapy—for example, testosterone and insulin. Cardiac complications may be reversible with phlebotomy.

There is little in the anesthesia literature that specifically addresses perioperative management of these patients. Attention should be directed to the extent of target organ damage. Liver function screening tests should be ordered preoperatively. Additionally, asymptomatic patients should be assessed for diabetes mellitus. Because of the frequency of cardiac abnormalities, a review of the patient's daily activity and exercise tolerance is important. Preoperative echocardiography may be particularly helpful in demonstrating limitations in left and right ventricular function.

B. WILSON'S DISEASE

Wilson's disease is a progressive, lethal, autosomal-recessive disorder that results from the absence of ceruloplasmin, an α_2-globulin responsible for transfer of copper in the plasma. Jews of eastern European origin and Orientals appear to be afflicted more frequently. The presentation of Wilson's disease varies with age of onset. Pediatric patients tend to present with symptoms and signs of progressive liver failure, older patients, with more marked neuropsychiatric changes. Deposition of copper in the brain results in dystonia, chorea, and psychosis.

Wilson's disease is characterized by development of cirrhosis, degeneration of the basal ganglia, and the presence of Kayser-Fleischer rings on the cornea (though these may not be observed in young children). Although the gene responsible for Wilson's disease has been located on chromosome 13, the precise mechanism of the disorder is not known. Abnormal deposition of copper in affected tissues results in liver disease, neuropsychiatric disturbance, and renal tubule dysfunction. Liver disease can be acute or chronic, acute fulminant hepatic failure presenting as a rare complication in children and young adults. In older patients, Wilson's disease may present as chronic active hepatitis. It can also present insidiously as cirrhosis. Laboratory findings include reduced plasma ceruloplasmin and copper concentrations. Elevated copper concentration is observed in liver biopsy specimens.

Penicillamine, an agent that chelates copper, is essential for reversing the progress of hemochromatosis, although improvement may require at least 6 treatments. Improvement in symptoms is possible, although patients with dystonia and cystic degeneration of the basal ganglia do poorly. Adverse reactions, including rashes and a lupuslike syndrome, occur with penicillamine but can be limited by restarting penicillamine therapy with steroid coverage. Fulminant hepatic failure is an indication for liver transplantation.

The extent of liver dysfunction should be evaluated preoperatively and the anesthetic management adjusted accordingly. Patients may be uncooperative owing to their neurodegenerative disease. Tremor and dystonia can make placement of peripheral intravenous lines difficult. As some patients can be extremely debilitated, care should be taken in positioning, hydration, and airway toilet.

C. GALACTOSEMIA

Galactosemia is a rare metabolic defect resulting from absence of the enzyme galactose-1-phosphate uridyltransferase, normally found in the liver and red cells. Deficiency of this enzyme results in accumulation of galactose-1-phosphate in the tissues, commonly leading to death in the first weeks of life. Clinically, these patients present with jaundice and rapid deterioration of liver function. Cataracts, mental retardation, and cirrhosis develop in survivors. Biochemical diagnosis is made by determining the concentration of galactose-1-phosphate uridyltransferase in red blood cells. Treatment consists of avoiding consuming milk products. Anesthetic management is determined by the degree of liver dysfunction.

D. HEREDITARY FRUCTOSE INTOLERANCE

Hereditary fructose intolerance is an autosomal-recessive defect of adolase B that results in accumulation of fructose-1-phosphate in the liver, renal cortex, and intestinal epithelium. After acute exposure to fructose, patients suffer abdominal pain and vomiting. Chronic exposure to fructose results in progressive liver dysfunction, cirrhosis, and renal tubular dysfunction. Diagnosis is made by enzyme assay after tissue biopsy. Treatment is avoidance of fructose and sucrose. There is no reported anesthesia experience with this disorder.

E. MUCOPOLYSACCHARIDOSES (HUNTER'S AND HURLER'S SYNDROMES)

The mucopolysaccharidoses are a group of disorders caused by deficiency of specific lysosomal enzymes required for degradation of polysaccharides. These disorders involve multiple organ systems with the abnormal deposition of polysaccharides. The disorders can be diagnosed by clinical presentation and the finding of increased urinary or leukocyte mucopolysaccharides. Most disorders are autosomal recessive, except for Hunter's syndrome, which is believed to be X linked. The liver is frequently large and firm. Liver biopsy shows vacuolated hepatocytes with lysozymes containing the mucopolysaccharides.

Hurler's syndrome is characterized by mental retardation, gargoyle facies, deafness, dwarfism, hepatosplenomegaly, mental retardation, limited joint movement, and severe myocardial, coronary, and valvular disease. Death usually occurs within the first decade of life. Hunter's syndrome is distinguished from Hurler's syndrome by the absence of corneal clouding and X-linked–recessive inheritance. Some patients with a mild form of Hunter's syndrome survive to adulthood.

Although disturbances in liver function are common in these patients, the life-threatening features of these disorders are related to cardiac and airway abnormalities. Although these are rare disorders, patients may present for a variety of surgical procedures—for example, corneal transplantation, hernia repair, or nerve entrapment release procedures. Liver function testing should be part of the preoperative assessment. Intraoperatively, management of the patient's airway may prove particularly challenging and positioning can be difficult.

F. HEPATIC PORPHYRIA

The porphyrias are a heterogeneous group of inherited enzyme deficiencies that affect either the bone marrow (erythropoietic) or liver (hepatic). The basic biochemical abnormality is overproduction of porphyrin or one of its precursors, depending on which enzyme is defective in the multistep sequence leading to the production of heme. Decreased production of heme results in lack of feedback inhibition of alpha-aminolaevulinic acid (ALA) synthetase, an early enzyme in the chain, and increased porphobilinogen. The erythropoietic porphyrias are characterized by hemolytic anemia and disfiguring cutaneous changes. Apart from the anemia, these conditions are not of major anesthetic concern.

The hepatic porphyrias include acute intermittent porphyria, coproporphyria, variegate porphyria, and porphyria cutanea tarda. The latter can be associated with hepatic disease but is not associated with exacerbation by barbiturates or neuropsychiatric disturbance. With the exception of porphyria cutanea tarda, clinical and anesthetic complications are similar for the hepatic porphyrias, although each is caused by a unique enzyme deficiency. All are autosomal-dominant conditions. Porphyria can also be an acquired disease and has been associated with heavy metal intoxication and exposure to certain chemicals, such as hexachlorobenzene.

Although acute attacks of hepatic porphyria have been characterized—manifested as vomiting, abdominal colic, constipation, peripheral neuropathy, neuropsychiatric disturbance—often only part of the symptom complex is present. Physical findings are commonly absent. A family history may reveal uncharacteristic neurologic or psychiatric symptoms. During an attack, large amounts of porphyrin precursors are excreted in the urine, and these are diagnostic.

Attacks can be prevented by avoiding enzyme-inducing drugs. Fasting, stress, and the hormonal changes of pregnancy have also been associated with precipitation of acute attacks. Treatment for an established attack consists of supportive care, hydration, analgesia, carbohydrate administration, and intravenous hematin or heme alginate to inhibit ALA synthetase.

The anesthesiologist presented with a patient with nonspecific abdominal pain and neurologic symptoms must consider the possibility of porphyria. Once the diagnosis is suspected, the most essential step is a careful family history. Thereafter the extent of hepatic involvement should be assessed.

Induction of anesthesia is commonly carried out in normal adults by intravenous injection of the barbiturate sodium thiopental. Since barbiturates can precipitate acute attacks of porphyria in susceptible persons thiopental and other barbiturates are contraindicated. Propofol and midazolam are probably safe induction agents. Nitrous oxide, succinylcholine, vecuronium, morphine, fentanyl, and atropine and neostigmine are safe for maintenance of anesthesia. For local anesthesia bupivacaine and procaine are considered safe. Extensive classifications of the perceived risks of anesthetic agents and other drugs were recently published. In this category, etomidate, halothane, and enflurane, along with barbiturates, are considered unsafe. With the exception of barbiturates, caution should be exercised in interpreting these lists too literally, as they are often based on anecdotal reports or single cases to which clear diagnostic criteria were not applied.

G. HEMOLYTIC ANEMIAS

Hemolytic anemias are diseases with multisystem involvement. In addition to the frequent associations with gallstones, these disorders may cause secondary liver disease.

Sickle cell disease is associated with intrahepatic vascular obstruction (secondary to sickling) that on rare occasions can cause acute hepatic failure. During an acute event, liver enzymes can be markedly elevated and plasma bilirubin concentration may also rise. After repeated crises, macronodular cirrhosis may develop. Liver abnormalities may also occur with thalassemia, and there may be hemosiderosis or intrahepatic fibrosis. It is important to expect patients with hemolytic anemias to have some degree of liver damage, which should be assessed preoperatively.

H. LIPID STORAGE DISEASES

Lipid storage diseases are a diverse family of specific enzyme defects that result in abnormal amounts of lipid products being stored in the cells of the reticuloendothelial system. The lipids include cholesterol (xanthomatosis), cholesterol esters, cerebroside (Gaucher's disease), and sphingomyelin (Niemann-Pick disease). These are most frequently autosomal-recessive disorders, although occasional families with Gaucher's disease have shown autosomal-dominant inheritance. The specific deficiency is confirmed by enzyme assay in peripheral white blood cells. Tissue biopsy may show cells of characteristic morphology in Gaucher's and Niemann-Pick disease. Both disorders are commonly associated with liver involvement.

Gaucher's disease is caused by an enzyme deficiency of β-glucocerebrosidase and affects predominantly Ashkenazi Jews. The enzyme deficiency causes accumulation of β-cerebroside throughout the reticuloendothelial system but especially in liver, bone marrow, and spleen. There are two forms of Gaucher's disease. The acute infantile form is associated with severe mental retardation and is usually fatal within the first 2 years of life. The chronic adult form is insidious, and patients usually present before age 30 years with unexplained hepatomegaly. Other clinical features include dermal pigmentation changes and orthopedic abnormalities. Gaucher's disease can cause gross abnormalities of liver function secondary to derangement of liver architecture. There may also be significant portal hypertension with ascites and esophageal varices.

Niemann-Pick disease results from deficiency of sphingomyelinase and is a rare familial disorder that also affects primarily the Ashkenazi. Type A disease is associated with mental retardation and death (usually in the first 2 years of life). Type B, the chronic nonneuropathic form, is associated with neonatal cholestasis, which is followed by insidious development of cirrhosis and portal hypertension.

I. GLYCOGEN STORAGE DISEASES

The glycogen storage diseases are a family of 10 disorders related to specific enzymes in the biochemical pathways of glycogen. Most are inherited, autosomal-recessive conditions. The final result is that the amount or molecular structure of glycogen in various tissues is abnormal. The organs most often affected are the liver, kidneys, heart, brain, and blood cells. The various disorders of this family differ markedly in clinical severity and organ involvement.

These disorders frequently present in infancy with complications of hypoglycemia. Hepatomegaly is a constant feature of all types of the disease. Some disorders, such as von Gierke's disease (type I), show marked mental retardation, whereas with others (Pompe's, type II; Covey's type III; and Her's, type VI) mental function is normal. Cirrhosis develops in only some of the disorders, particularly type IV or Anderson's disease. It is unusual for type I or type II to progress to cirrhosis, although hepatocellular adenomas can be a late development. Patients can be screened for these disorders by infusion of glycogen to stimulate blood glucose production. Specific diagnosis is usually made by enzyme assay after tissue biopsy.

J. ALPHA$_1$-ANTITRYPSIN DEFICIENCY

Alpha$_1$-antitrypsin is an acute-phase glycoprotein that is an inhibitor of proteases. Deficiency is a genetically determined disorder, and there are approximately 75 different alleles for the gene on chromosome 14, accounting for a wide variety of phenotypes, only a few of which are associated with significant liver disease. Alpha$_1$-antitrypsin deficiency is associated with a variety of extrahepatic manifestations, including pulmonary emphysema, membranous glomerulonephritis, and gastric ulcers. The mechanism of liver injury is unclear.

Some patients who develop liver problems present in the neonatal period with jaundice secondary to hepatitis and cholestasis. Such jaundice has an extremely poor prognosis; otherwise, the rate of progression of this disorder is very variable, and cirrhosis presents in some patients later in adult life. It is accepted that liver disease has a much greater effect on survival than does pulmonary disease. Alpha₁-antitrypsin deficiency should be considered in every patient with cirrhosis and a history of chest infections. Definitive diagnosis is made by measurement of serum alpha₁-antitrypsin concentration and phenotype determination by electrophoresis. Only supportive therapy is currently available, although the disease is obviously a candidate for gene therapy; some patients are suitable candidates for liver transplantation. Preoperative evaluation of patients with alpha₁-antitrypsin deficiency should include determination of liver and pulmonary damage.

K. CYSTIC FIBROSIS

Cystic fibrosis is a common (1 in 2000) autosomal-recessive disorder characterized by unusually viscid secretions from the skin, lungs, and pancreas. The gene for cystic fibrosis has been located on chromosome 7. Although major attention is directed to pulmonary and pancreatic functions in these patients, the frequency of liver abnormalities, including portal fibrosis and cirrhosis, should not be overlooked. Approximately 20 per cent of patients with cystic fibrosis develop these complications. In addition, intermittent biliary tract obstruction may cause biliary cirrhosis with general cirrhosis, esophageal varices, splenomegaly, and ascites in adolescence. Gene therapy for cystic fibrosis is just under way, but treatment is still mainly nonspecific and sometimes includes sclerosis of esophageal varices and liver transplantation.

L. TYROSINEMIA

Tyrosinemia is an autosomal-recessive disorder associated with a defect in the enzyme fumaryl acetoacetate hydrolase, which results in markedly elevated levels of tyrosine, phenylalanine, and methionine. Accumulation of these substances causes liver and renal tubule abnormalities. Diagnosis is made by measuring serum succinylacetoacetate concentration.

The acute form of tyrosinemia results in death in the first year of life from acute hepatic failure. The liver is initially infiltrated with fat, but this is followed rapidly by periportal fibrosis and cirrhosis. In the chronic form, dietary restriction of affected amino acids is employed, but the liver disease is frequently progressive. Liver transplantation is often indicated in the first decade of life, not only because of progressive loss of liver function but also because of the increased risk of hepatocellular carcinoma. When preparing patients with tyrosinemia for surgery, the extent of liver dysfunction should be assessed, as should any renal dysfunction that might have caused hypophosphatemia and rickets.

M. CHOLESTASIS SYNDROMES

The cholestasis syndromes are divided into two groups: *extrahepatic,* marked by obstruction in the main bile ducts, and *intrahepatic,* where the defect is in the microscopic bile ducts or the hepatocytes themselves. Extrahepatic obstruction can arise from a variety of congenital and acquired conditions. Patients may present with abdominal pain, fever, or hepatomegaly. The site of obstruction and the diagnosis may be determined by ultrasound examination of the liver and biliary tree, ERCP, CT, MRI, and liver biopsy.

While extrahepatic cholestasis can be associated with a number of common acquired conditions, including gallstones, cancer of the pancreas, and biliary strictures, extrahepatic cholestasis can also be due to rare congenital disorders. Congenital biliary atresia occurs in 1 in 10,000 births and affects more females than males. Affected babies present with unremitting progressive jaundice in the first week of life. Death usually occurs before age 3 years, often owing to intercurrent infection or liver failure or bleeding from esophageal varices. Ascites is a terminal event. Extrahepatic biliary atresia is surgically correctable with Kasai's procedure, in which the common hepatic duct is anastomosed to the intestine; however, even when the procedure is successful many of these patients subsequently require liver transplantation.

Intrahepatic cholestasis can arise from a variety of causes, including viral and alcoholic hepatitis, drugs, hormones, primary biliary cirrhosis, and sclerosing cholangitis. Rare congenital disorders include Watson-Alagille syndrome, Byler's disease, Zellweger's cerebrohepatorenal syndrome, and coprostanicoacidemia. Finally, prolonged parenteral hyperalimentation can also cause cholestasis in premature infants, although most recover when therapy is discontinued. Drugs that cause cholestasis include oral contraceptives, anabolic steroids, the chlorpromazine group and haloperidol, sulfonamides, various antibiotics, and some antithyroid medications.

The first stage of treatment involves removal of the precipitating cause of drug-related cholestasis, if possible, or correction of the underlying anomaly in congenital extrahepatic cholestasis. Supportive therapy includes adequate nutrition with fat-soluble vitamin supplementation, cholestyramine for pruritus, and management of any infection.

Neonates who present for the Kasai's procedure should be managed in a center that has much experience with anesthesia for neonates with liver dysfunction (and this implies adequate neonatal intensive care facilities). Intraoperative problems include fluid balance management, temperature control, and estimation of blood loss. Plasma potassium concentration can be elevated in these patients, so succinylcholine may be contraindicated. Atracurium has been recommended as the muscle relaxant of choice. If neomycin was used for preoperative bowel preparation and the drug was absorbed systemically, it could prolong neuromuscular blockade.

VII. LIVER DISEASE OF OTHER CAUSES

A. CARCINOID SYNDROME[121–134]

Approximately 25 per cent of patients with carcinoid tumors will develop carcinoid syndrome, which is associated with metastatic disease, usually involving the liver. The syndrome consists of a number of symptoms, including flushing attacks, diarrhea, bronchospasm, hypertension, and right-sided valvular heart lesions. Palliative treatment includes somatostatin analogs, ketanserin, and cyproheptadine. Removal of the primary tumor and debulking of liver metastases can also be beneficial. Recently, a long-acting somatostatin analog has proven useful for symptom control and management of hypertension.

In dealing with patients who present for hepatic resection of carcinoid tumors, the anesthesiologist should ensure that adequate means for rapid blood volume replacement are available and that the patient's symptoms are under optimal control. Dehydration should be specifically addressed preoperatively, if necessary. Right-sided heart lesions can be assessed clinically, but this assessment may be enhanced by echocardiography. Octreoide should be available in the operating room to treat hypertension during surgical manipulation of the tumor.

B. REYE'S SYNDROME[135–140]

Reye's syndrome, is an acute metabolic illness resulting from acquired mitochondrial dysfunction, and occurs predominantly in children aged 4 to 11 years. The syndrome consists of acute encephalitis and fatty infiltration of the viscera that occur during the recovery phase of an innocuous viral infection. In particular, treatment of influenza A or B or varicella with salicylates seems to be a precipitating cause; aflatoxin and insecticides have also been implicated. Liver biopsy shows vesicular fat, and there are increases in transaminase and blood ammonia values and a prolonged prothrombin time (INR). The differential diagnosis includes acute hepatic failure of other causes, infection (systemic sepsis, meningitis, encephalitis), inborn errors of metabolism, pancreatitis, drug overdose, and poisoning. The cause of death is cerebral edema; even with the best treatment the mortality rate is 10 per cent to 20 per cent.

Today, aspirin packages carry the warning that the drug should not be given to children younger than 12 years without medical advice. The Reye Syndrome Surveillance 1991 reported a decrease in incidence of the condition after insertion of the package warning. Interestingly, in Australia, where Reye first described the condition in 1963, no association with aspirin has been reported.

C. LIVER TUMORS

Primary or secondary tumors of the liver may be amenable to surgical removal, for example by partial hepatectomy or cryotherapy. The major anesthetic and surgical problem associated with such operations is hemorrhage. In addition, there may be a reduction in venous return from the inferior vena cava during certain parts of the surgical procedure.

There is also the risk of air embolus. Adequate intravenous lines and a rapid-transfusion device, availability of sufficient blood for transfusion, and careful monitoring of blood loss and patient temperature are clear requirements. All transfused blood should be warmed, and monitoring of central venous pressure and arterial blood pressure is essential. Tumors that are not amenable to surgical resection may be treated by hepatic artery ligation or infusion of cytotoxic agents. An infusion of glucose and insulin should be given before ligation of the hepatic artery to minimize subsequent liver damage. Severe deterioration in liver function can occur after hepatic artery ligation, particularly when cytotoxic agents have been infused.

D. CHRONIC AUTOIMMUNE HEPATITIS

Chronic autoimmune hepatitis occurs principally in women between ages 15 and 25 years or after menopause. It is a multisystem disease with associated arthralgia, hemolytic anemia, nephritis, and diabetes mellitus. The basic mechanism of the disease is a defect in suppressor T cells that results in production of autoantibodies against surface antigens of the hepatocytes. Patients also produce additional antibodies—antinuclear, smooth muscle, and mitochondrial.

Laboratory diagnosis is based on elevated plasma transaminase and gamma globulin values, elevated titers of antinuclear antibodies and antiactin antibodies, and active hepatitis on liver biopsy. Treatment with steroids produces symptomatic benefit and prolongs life. Sustained remission is possible, but eventually most patients develop cirrhosis.

As with other liver dysfunction, full preoperative investigation of liver function is essential. Renal function and hemoglobin concentration should be assessed. The patient's history of steroid use should be determined and steroid coverage provided, if warranted.

E. PRIMARY BILIARY CIRRHOSIS

Primary biliary cirrhosis, a disorder that mainly affects middle-aged women, is associated with profound changes in the immune system. Bile duct epithelium is destroyed by cytotoxic T cells in a manner suggestive of graft-versus-host disease.

Initial symptoms include pruritus and fatigue. Later, jaundice and malabsorption of fat-soluble vitamins occur. There is also an association with other autoimmune diseases, including mixed connective tissue disease, scleroderma, and thyroiditis. Skin xanthomas may develop, and plasma cholesterol can be markedly elevated. Bone disease is an important correlate and is exacerbated with advanced cholestasis.

Diagnosis is based on elevated gamma-glutamyl transpeptidase concentration, the presence of antimitochondrial antibodies, and a positive liver biopsy. Treatment consists of symptomatic and supportive therapy; for example, treatment for pruritus and vitamin deficiencies. Despite use of many therapies, including steroids and ursodeoxycholic acid, liver transplantation is often required.

F. VENOUS OUTFLOW OBSTRUCTION (BUDD-CHIARI SYNDROME)

Budd-Chiari syndrome is a disorder of multiple causes characterized by hepatomegaly, abdominal pain, ascites, and venous sinusoidal distension. Obstruction to venous drainage at any site, from the effluent vein of a hepatic lobule to the right atrium, can cause the disturbance. In the inferior vena cava and hepatic vein, tumor and thrombosis are possible causes. In the liver, obstruction may be caused by venoocclusive disease or alcoholic hepatitis. Oral contraceptives are a risk factor.

Laboratory investigations show prolonged INR and elevated plasma transaminase values. Liver biopsy shows characteristic congestion that is diagnostic. Treatment varies with the cause, but various portoasystemic shunts and balloon angioplasty have been used. Liver transplantation may benefit some patients.

VIII. THE LIVER IN PREGNANCY[141-145]

Liver function is not much altered in normal pregnancy. Although cardiac output increases by up to as much as 35 per cent, liver blood flow remains constant. Most liver enzymes stay within normal limits during pregnancy; however, there may be an increase in plasma alkaline phosphatase concentration, reflecting both placental and fetal production. Plasma albumin concentration may fall secondary to hemodilution. On biopsy, liver tissue looks normal.

Liver disease in pregnancy has been categorized into three groups. The first group includes diseases specific to pregnancy, for example hyperemesis gravidarum, intrahepatic cholestasis of pregnancy, and acute fatty liver of pregnancy. Preeclampsia patients may develop HELLP (*h*emolysis, *e*levated *l*iver enzymes, and *l*ow *p*latelets) syndrome. The second group is liver diseases exacerbated by pregnancy, usually viral infections. The third group is comprised of chronic liver disorders that may coexist with pregnancy; for example, chronic active hepatitis. This latter group of disorders are diverse, but advanced chronic liver disease, whatever the cause, is rarely compatible with pregnancy.

Although *hyperemesis gravidarum* has been associated with jaundice, elevation of the bilirubin concentration is usually modest. Raised transaminase levels are common, however. Strangely, hyperemesis is consistent with decreased fetal wastage and is more common in non-smokers and multiparas and with multiple gestations. Liver biopsy reveals normal histologic appearance in most cases, but some show fatty changes. It is important to rule out viral or drug-induced hepatitis.

Cholestasis of pregnancy is usually a mild, self-limited disease of unknown cause. Patients typically present with pruritus (frequently the most severe symptom) and mild jaundice in the last trimester of pregnancy. Diagnosis is made by laboratory findings of elevated conjugated bilirubin and alkaline phosphatase and normal or slightly increased plasma transaminase levels. Generally, these changes resolve rapidly within 2 to 3 weeks of delivery. The disorder can occur in subsequent pregnancies, and there is an association with increased fetal wastage. When liver biopsy has been performed, mild intrahepatic cholestasis has been found. Therapy consists of nutrition support, especially vitamin K supplements, and cholestyramine for pruritus. Cholestasis of pregnancy must be distinguished from viral hepatitis serologically. If the condition does not resolve after delivery, primary biliary cirrhosis should be considered.

Acute fatty liver of pregnancy is a rare but potentially fatal disease that most often occurs in the second half of gestation and that in the past had very high rates of maternal and fetal mortality (80 per cent to 90 per cent). Today, thanks to early recognition and treatment, mortality is only 20%. Patients may initially be asymptomatic, and symptoms are extremely variable but include jaundice, bleeding, and coma. Disseminated intravascular coagulation and renal failure can occur. On liver biopsy, fine, microvascular, fatty infiltration is observed. Treatment for both hepatic and renal dysfunction is supportive. Early delivery, vaginally or operatively, improves fetal and maternal survival. Any coagulopathy should be corrected preoperatively, particularly as epidural anesthesia has been recommended for this condition.

Liver involvement occurs infrequently with *preeclampsia* but is often associated with severe liver dysfunction. The mechanism of liver injury is hepatocellular necrosis following ischemia related to endothelial damage. Hepatic rupture can occur. Treatment for severe pre-eclampsia and HELLP syndrome is expedited delivery with supportive care. Anesthesiologists are often involved in the cardiovascular and neurologic management of these challenging patients. Fetal mortality is high (40 per cent to 70 per cent), but 90% of patients recover.

IX. LIVER DAMAGE CAUSED BY CHEMICALS

Drugs and chemicals can cause a variety of toxic effects in the liver. Since a quarter of cases of fulminant hepatic failure are caused by medications, a full drug history is essential when patients present with liver disease. The variety of drugs involved in liver reactions is shown in Table 6–10.

X. TRANSPLANTATION[146–148]

In the past few years liver transplantation has progressed from a rare, dramatic, often highly publicized event carried out in a limited number of centers to a relatively common procedure in both adults and children. Transplantation should be considered for any patient with fulminant hepatic failure; however the decision to transplant depends on certain prognostic factors. Age is relevant: mortality is highest in those older than 40 years. Bilirubin in excess of 300 μmol/L, an INR greater than 4, renal failure, sepsis, and bleeding are all bad prognostic signs. The interval between

TABLE 6–10

Compounds Toxic to the Liver

Anticonvulsants: Phenytoin, sodium valproate
Antiinflammatory Agents: Nonsteroidal antiinflammatory drugs, paracetamol, allopurinol, sulfasalazine
Antibiotics: Tetracyclines, isoniazid, rifampicin
Antihypertensive: Methyldopa
Miscellaneous: Amiodarone, vitamin A, azathioprine, chemotherapy cytotoxics, nitrofurantoin, quinidine, sex hormones, sulfonamides
Chemicals: Arsine gas, carbon tetrachloride, trichloroethylene, trichloromethane (chloroform), halothane, vinyl chloride
Pesticides: Gramoxone, paraquat
"Recreational" drugs: Toluene (glue sniffing), methylenedioxymethamphetamine (Ecstasy)

the appearance of jaundice and the onset of encephalopathy also appears to affect outcome: surprisingly, the prognosis is better when onset is rapid.

The cause of the fulminant hepatic failure is also an important determinant of survival. Transplantation may be the only treatment for fulminant Wilson's disease, halothane-induced hepatitis, and other idiosyncratic drug reactions; however, patients with HAV infection or pregnancy-induced hepatitis have a good chance of spontaneous recovery. Infection with HBV is more problematic, and HCV infection, although rare in fulminant hepatic failure, carries a high risk of mortality without transplantation. Patients who develop fulminant hepatic failure after acetaminophen (paracetamol) overdose tend to recover spontaneously; however transplantation is considered if metabolic acidosis persists, the INR at 48 hours is greater than 4, renal failure occurs, or there is persistent encephalopathy. No clear benefit has been shown for patients with primary hepatoma.

Anesthesia for liver transplantation has been well reviewed in the literature; the reader is referred to the specialty papers for detailed anesthesia management. Problems include the logistics of collection of donor organs, personnel and space requirements for intraoperative and postoperative management, severe hemorrhage, hypotension, obstruction of the inferior vena cava, hypothermia, and acid-base and electrolyte changes.

XI. ACUTE HEPATIC FAILURE[149–150]

Viral hepatitis is the commonest cause of fulminant hepatic failure. Many drugs can cause liver damage; rarely, acute liver failure follows general anesthesia and surgery. More rarely, known hepatotoxins such as that of the death's cap mushroom are ingested accidentally. The phrase *acute liver failure* is often used to describe both fulminant hepatic failure and severe encephalopathy secondary to chronic liver disease, although the management of the two entities is different.

Although fulminant hepatic failure is a rare event, for a condition that often affects young and previously healthy persons, worldwide mortality remains about 80 per cent. Treatment is therefore a serious challenge, and it is best provided in an intensive care area equipped to deal with these patients. The multiple clinical manifestations of liver failure include those directly related to hepatic damage and neurologic, acid-base, cardiac, renal, metabolic, and hematologic disturbances. Fetor hepaticus may be present, and the liver is often small to percussion. Clinical jaundice develops over a few days and in most acute cases is preceded by signs of encephalopathy.

A. COMPLICATIONS

1. Neurologic Disturbances

Deterioration in the level of consciousness is progressive and may go from a high of euphoria, through mild confusion to drowsiness and finally coma (grades 1 to 4). Decerebrate rigidity and convulsions are common. The causes of hepatic encephalopathy are probably multiple. Coma factors such as ammonia, mercaptans, free fatty acids, and biogenic amines have all been implicated, but as yet no clear picture has emerged of which (if any) of these compounds is responsible. Secondary factors that are particularly important because they may be prevented by correct management include hypoxia, hypoglycemia, hypovolemia, and hypotension. Administration of sedatives for control of restlessness during the early stages of encephalopathy may be responsible for deterioration in consciousness level. If liver function does return to normal and irreversible brain damage (e.g., secondary to hypoxia) has not occurred during the coma, the brain can also recover completely.

Cerebral edema can be a major problem; however, papilledema is seldom present and bradycardia and pyrexia are rarely seen, even

TABLE 6–11

Causes of Fulminant Hepatic Failure

Condition	Cause
Poisoning	Paracetamol
	Mushrooms (e.g., *Amanita phalloides*)
	Industrial solvents (e.g., carbon tetrachloride, chloroform, xylene (glue))
Viral hepatitis	Hepatitis A virus
	Hepatitis B virus
	Hepatitis C virus
	Other viruses (e.g., herpesvirus, cytomegalovirus, Epstein-Barr virus)
Drug reaction	Volatile anesthetic agents
	Antiepileptics (e.g., phenytoin, sodium valproate)
	Nonsteroidal antiinflammatory drugs
	Antidepressants
	Ketoconazole
	α-Methyldopa
	Recreational drugs (e.g., methylenedioxymethamphetamine (Ecstasy))
Miscellaneous	Wilson's disease
	Acute fatty liver of pregnancy
	Reye's syndrome
	Autoimmune chronic active hepatitis
	Malignant infiltration
	Acute hepatic ischaemia

though gross tentorial herniation may be found post mortem. If cerebral edema is present, sudden apnea, cardiac arrest, and hypothermia may occur.

2. Acid-Base Disturbances

Hyperventilation is a constant feature during the early stages of coma. Ammonia toxicity may be responsible for the respiratory stimulation. Alkalosis (respiratory or metabolic) is common. Hypokalemia, failure to alkalinize urine, and continuous gastric aspiration are contributing factors.

Respiratory alkalosis is associated with impaired oxygen dissociation, reduced cerebral and peripheral perfusion, and reduced cerebral oxygen consumption. In addition, respiratory alkalosis can result in neurologic or electroencephalographic changes that are similar in some respects to those of experimental ammonia toxicity and may be potentiated by intercurrent metabolic alkalosis. Correction of respiratory alkalosis, either by inhalation of carbon dioxide or by infusion of the carbonic anhydrase inhibitor acetazolamide, produces further clinical and biochemical deterioration, whereas intravenous administration of sodium bicarbonate produces improvement, correlating well with increased cerebral blood flow and oxygen consumption. This improvement is only temporary, however, and is limited by the adverse effects of a large sodium load.

Hypoxia, a frequent finding, may be due to pulmonary infection or edema, elevation of the diaphragm by ascites, or peritoneal dialysis. It is likely that pulmonary capillary permeability is abnormal with acute liver failure and results in interstitial and alveolar edema.

3. Cardiac Disturbances

Cardiac output is high and reflects low peripheral resistance and increased arteriovenous shunting. Cardiac irregularities are common and probably reflect changes in oxygenation, arterial carbon dioxide pressure, plasma potassium, or intracranial pressure. Hypotension, often associated with hemorrhage, is also seen frequently.

4. Renal Disturbances

Renal impairment is common in Grades 3 and 4 coma and often progresses to renal failure. This impairment may be classified into one of three groups: (1) prerenal uremia due to dehydration or absorption of nitrogenous compounds from the gut after gastrointestinal hemorrhage, (2) functional renal failure as a result of diversion of blood flow from the kidneys, or (3) that precipitated by an episode of hypotension. Renal failure is an extremely poor prognostic sign.

5. Metabolic Disturbances

Particularly important is hypoglycemia, which can develop rapidly and, unless treated by parenteral glucose administration, can lead to irreversible brain damage. Great care must be taken not to overlook hypoglycemia as the cause of a deteriorating level of consciousness. Oral feeding is not usually possible because of coma or gastrointestinal bleeding, and provision of adequate calories may be difficult. Amino acid solutions are contraindicated; fat emulsions and alcohols could further damage the liver, and the metabolic pathway for fructose can be so deranged that acute lactic acidosis occurs. In addition, solutions containing sodium should be avoided because of these patients' inability to excrete sodium. In practice, therefore, only glucose infusions are used. Solutions stronger than 10 per cent induce unacceptable osmotic diuresis and, even when combined with insulin, can produce lactic acidosis.

6. Hematologic Disturbances

As liver function deteriorates, synthesis of clotting factors declines and disorders of coagulation are inevitable. This is manifested as increased INR and depression of circulating levels of fibrinogen and factors II, VII, IX, and X. In addition, thrombocytopenia occurs. The usual sites of bleeding are the nasopharynx, esophagus, stomach, gastrointestinal tract, retroperitoneal space, and bronchial tree. Antacids or histamine antagonists may help reduce hemorrhage from the gastrointestinal tract.

B. MANAGEMENT

Acute liver failure requires general supportive measures aimed at the management of severely ill and unconscious patients. Ideally, transfer to a center experienced in dealing with acute hepatic failure should take place before the patient has lapsed into grade 3 encephalopathy, particularly if the patient is to be considered for transplantation. Early consultation with specialized units about patients with hepatic failure is recommended. Acetaminophen overdose should always be

considered, since antidote treatment with *n*-acetylcystine must be administered within 10 hours of ingestion of the drug. Avoidance of hypoxia, jugular vein compression, and hypercapnia reduces the risk of increased intracranial pressure (ICP).

Once the condition is diagnosed, monitoring of ICP with an indwelling extradural sensor is useful. This allows measurement of the cerebral perfusion pressure (mean arterial pressure minus ICP), which should remain above 50 mm Hg. When ICP reaches 30 mm Hg, active treatment should commence. This includes oncotic therapy using albumin and fresh-frozen plasma, moderate hyperventilation, osmotic diuresis using mannitol, and hemodialysis if renal failure is present. Steroid therapy is contraindicated as it can inhibit hepatic regeneration.

Cardiovascular disturbances are very common and require treatment by volume replacement, artificial ventilation, and limited use of vasoconstrictors, inotropes, and vasodilators. The latter drugs have not been shown to affect prognosis once tissue hypoxia and renal failure occur.

Complex deficiencies of the hemostatic system occur. Routine administration of histamine H_2 antagonists reduces the risk of hemorrhage from peptic ulcers but may be associated with increased incidence of nosocomial pneumonia or fungal colonization. Sucralfate may be more suitable for avoiding stress ulcers. Blood products, including fresh blood and fresh-frozen plasma, may be required. Infusion of these substances imposes further water and salt loads on the patient as well as a risk for other viral infections. Renal failure is a common feature of fulminant hepatic failure and occurs in up to 40 per cent of patients. Both dialysis and ultrafiltration techniques may be required for management of renal failure in these patients. Charcoal hemoperfusion, with prostacyclin infusion to reduce the risk of profound hypotension from platelet damage, has been helpful in the management of some patients. Perfusion through a column of cultivated hepatocytes is currently in clinical trials.

When hepatic decompensation is secondary to chronic liver disease, the clinical presentation may mimic an intra-abdominal surgical emergency, but exploratory laparotomy is a mistake, and liver function may deteriorate profoundly postoperatively. Most affected patients have alcoholic liver disease and are suffering from a superimposed bout of acute alcoholic hepatitis. Liver scintigraphy shows no isotope uptake, and careful questioning of relatives and friends may elicit a history of recent heavy alcohol consumption. When possible, anesthesia and surgery should be avoided in such patients.

REFERENCES

General Assessment

1. Hulcrantz R, Glauman H, Lindberg G, et al.: Liver investigation in 149 asymptomatic patients with moderately elevated activities of serum aminotransferases. Scand J Gastroenterol 1986; 21:109–113.
2. Schemel WH: Unexpected hepatic dysfunction found by multiple laboratory screening. Anesth Analg 1976; 55:810–814.
3. Aranha GV, Greenlee HB: Intra-abdominal surgery in patients with advanced cirrhosis. Arch Surg 1986; 121:774–778.
4. Powell-Jackson P, Greenway B, Williams R: Adverse effects of exploratory laparotomy in patients with suspected liver disease. Br J Surg 1982; 68:449–451.
5. Dobaneck RC, Sterling WA, Allison DC: Morbidity and mortality after operation in nonbleeding cirrhotic patients. Am J Surg 1983; 146:306–310.
6. Child CG: The Liver and Portal Hypertension. Philadelphia: WB Saunders, 1964, pp 1–85.
7. Pugh RNH, Murray-Lyon IM, Dawson JL, et al.: Transection of the oesophagus for bleeding varices. Br J Surg 1973; 60:646–649.

Chronic Liver Disease

8. Mezey E: Alcoholic liver disease. *In* Popper H, Schaffner F (eds): Progress in Liver Disease, Vol 7. New York: Grune & Stratton, 1982.
9. Lanza V, Demma I, Cali A, et al.: Correction of the unfavorable effects of vasopressin by nitroglycerin infusion. Can Anaesth Soc J 1982; 29:143–145.
10. Grossman RJ, Kranetz D, Bosch J, et al.: Nitroglycerine improves the hemodynamic response to vasopressin in portal hypertension. Hepatology 1982; 1:757–759.
11. Duvaldestin P, Lebrault C, Chauvin M: Pharmacokinetics of muscle relaxants in patients with liver disease. Clin Anesthesiol 1985; 3:293–306.
12. Bencini AF, Scaf AHJ, Sohn YJ, et al.: Hepatobiliary disposition of vecuronium bromide in man. Br J Anaesth 1986; 58:988–995.
13. Lebrault C, Duvaldestin P, Henzel D, et al.: Pharmacokinetics and pharmacodynamics of vecuronium in patients with cholestasis. Br J Anaesth 1986; 58:983–987.
14. Arden JR, Lynam DP, Castagnoli KP, et al.: Vecuronium in alcoholic liver disease: A pharmacokinetic and pharmacodynamic analysis. Anesthesiology 1988; 68:771–776.
15. Parker CJR, Hunter JM: Pharmacokinetics of atracurium and laudanosine in patients with hepatic cirrhosis. Br J Anaesth 1989; 62:177–183.
16. Shelly MP, Cory EP, Park GR: Pharmacokinetics of morphine in two children before and after liver transplantation. Br J Anaesth 1986; 58:1218–1223.
17. Mazoit J, Sandouk P, Zetlaovi P, et al: Pharmacokinetics of unchanged morphine in normal and cirrhotic subjects. Anesth Analg 1987; 66:293–298.
18. McQuay H, Moore A: Be aware of renal function when monitoring morphine. Lancet 1984; 2:284.
19. Haberer JP, Shoeffler E, Coyderc E, Duvaldestin P: Fentanyl pharmacokinetics in anaesthetised patients with cirrhosis. Br J Anaesth 1982; 54:1267–1270.
20. Ferrier C, Marty J, Bouffard J, et al.: Alfentanil pharmacokinetics in patients with cirrhosis. Anesthesiology 1985; 62:480–484.
21. Thompson IA, Fitch W, Hughes RL, et al.: Effects of certain IV anaesthetics on liver blood flow and hepatic oxygen consumption in the greyhound. Br J Anaesth 1986; 58:69–80.
22. Couderc E, Ferrier C, Haberer JP, et al.: Thiopentone pharmacokinetics in patients with chronic alcoholism. Br J Anaesth 1984; 56:1393–1397.
23. Van Been H, Manger FW, Van Boxtel C, et al.: Etomidate anaesthesia in patients with cirrhosis of the liver: Pharmacokinetic data. Anaesthesia 1983; 38:91S–92S.
24. Duvaldestin P, Chgauvin M, Lebraut C, et al: Effect of upper abdominal surgery and cirrhosis upon the pharmacokinetics of methohexital. Acta Anaesth Scand 1990; 35:159–163.
25. Servin F, Cockshott ID, Farinotti R, et al.: Pharmacokinetics of propofol infusions in patients with cirrhosis. Br J Anaesth 1990; 65:177–183.
26. Gelman S: Disturbances in hepatic blood flow during anesthesia and surgery. Arch Surg 1976; 111:881–883.
27. Hughes RL, Campbell D, Fitch W: Effects of enflurane and halothane on liver blood flow and oxygen consumption in the greyhound. Br J Anaesth 1980; 52:1079–1086.
28. Brown BR Jr, Gandolfi AJ: Adverse effects of volatile anaesthetics. Br J Anaesth 1987; 59:14–23.
29. Dale O, Brown BR Jr: Clinical pharmacokinetics of the inhalational anesthetics. Clin Pharmacokinet 1987; 12:145–167.
30. Allan LG, Hussey AJ, Howie J, et al.: Hepatic glutathione S-transferase release after halothane anaesthesia: Open randomised comparison with isoflurane. Lancet 1987; 1:771–774.
31. Hussey AJ, Aldridge LM, Paul D, et al.: Plasma glutathione S-transferase concentration as a measure of hepatocellular integrity following a single general anaesthetic with halothane, enflurane or isoflurane. Br J Anaesth 1988; 60:130–135.
32. Harper MH, Collins P, Johnson BH, et al.: Postanesthetic hepatic injury in rats: Influence of alterations in hepatic blood flow, surgery, and anesthesia time. Anesth Analg 1982; 651:79–82.
33. Christ DD, Saatoh H, Kenna JG, Pohl LR: Potential metabolic basis for enflurane hepatitis and the apparent cross-sensitization between enflurane and halothane. Drug Metab Dispos 1988; 16:135–140.
34. Hals J, Dodgson MS, Skulberg A, Kenna JG: Halothane-associated liver damage and renal failure in a young child. Acta Anaesth Scand 1986; 30:651–655.
35. Lewis RB, Blair M: Halothane hepatitis in a young child. Br J Anaesth 1982; 54:349–354.
36. Wark HJ: Postoperative jaundice in children. The influence of halothane. Anaesthesia 1983; 38:237–242.
37. Plummer JL, Van Der Walt JH, Cousins MJ: Reductive metabolism of halothane in children. Anaesth Intens Care 1984; 12:293–295.
38. Walton B, Simpson BR, Strunin L, et al.: Unex-

plained hepatitis following halothane. BMJ 1976; 1:1171–1176.

39. Elliott RH, Strunin L: Hepatotoxicity of volatile anesthetics. Implications for halothane, enflurane, isoflurane, sevoflurane and desflurane. Br J Anaesth 1993; 70:339–348.

40. Oikkonen M, Rosenberg PH: Liver damage after halothane anaesthesia: Analysis of cases in Finnish hospitals in 1972–1981. Ann Chir Gynaecol 1984; 73:28–33.

41. Paull JD, Fortune DW: Hepatotoxicity and death following two enflurane anaesthetics. Anaesthesia 1987; 42:1191–1196.

42. Foutch PG, Ferguson DR, Tuthill RJ: Enflurane-induced hepatitis with prominent cholestasis. Cleve Clin J Med 1987; 54:210–213.

43. Sigurdsson J, Hreidarsson AB, Thjodleifsson B: Enflurane hepatitis. A report of a case with a previous history of halothane hepatitis. Acta Anaesth Scand 1985; 29:494–496.

44. Zinn SE, Fairley HB, Glenn JD: Liver function in patients with mild alcoholic hepatitis, after enflurane, nitrous oxide-narcotic, and spinal anesthesia. Anesth Analg 1985; 64:487–490.

45. Dykes MH: Is enflurane hepatotoxic? Anesthesiology 1984; 61:235–237.

46. Lewis JH, Zimmerman HJ, Ishak KG, Mullick FG: Enflurane hepatotoxicity. A clinicopathologic study of 242 cases. Ann Intern Med 1983; 98:984–992.

47. Masone RJ, Goldfarb JP, Manzione NC, Biempica I: Enflurane hepatitis. J Clin Gastroenterol 1982; 4:541–545.

48. White LB, DeTarnowsky GO, Mir JA, Layden TJ: Hepatotoxicity following enflurane anesthesia. Dig Dis Sci 1981; 26:466–469.

49. Bennettes FE: Acute hepatitis following enflurane anaesthesia. Br J Anaesth 1981; 53:671–672.

50. Danielewitz MD, Braude BM, Bloch HM, et al.: Acute hepatitis following enflurane anaesthesia. Br J Anaesth 1980; 52:1151–1153.

51. Vacanti CJ, Lynch TC: Hepatitis following enflurane. Anesth Analg 1980; 59:890.

52. Ona FV, Patanella H, Ayub A: Hepatitis associated with enflurane anesthesia. Anesth Analg 1980; 59:146–149.

53. Douglas HJ, Eger EI, Biava CG, Renzi C: Hepatic necrosis associated with viral infection after enflurane anesthesia. N Engl J Med 1977; 296:553–555.

54. Eger EI, Smuckler EA, Ferrel LD, et al.: Is enflurane hepatotoxic? Anesth Analg 1986; 65:21–30.

55. McLaughlin DF, Eger EI: Repeated isoflurane anesthesia in a patient with hepatic dysfunction. Anesth Analg 1984; 63:775–778.

56. Carrigan TW, Straughen WJ: A report of hepatic necrosis and death following isoflurane anesthesia. Anesthesiology 1987; 67:581–583.

57. Stoelting RK: Isoflurane and postoperative hepatic dysfunction. Can J Anaesth 1987; 34:223–226.

58. Stoelting RK, Blitt CD, Cohen PJ, Merin RG: Hepatic dysfunction after isoflurane anesthesia. Anesth Analg 1987; 66:147–153.

59. Webster JA: Acute hepatitis after isoflurane anesthesia. Can Med Assoc J 1986; 135:1343–1344.

60. Gregoire S, Smiley RK: Acute hepatitis in a patient with mild factor IX deficiency after anesthesia with isoflurane. Can Med Assoc J 1986; 135:645–646.

61. Fisher NA, Iwata RT, Eger EI, Smuckler EA: Hepatic necrosis associated with herpes virus after isoflurane anesthesia. Anesth Analg 1985; 64:1131–1133.

62. McLaughlin DF, Eger EI: Repeated isoflurane anesthesia in a patient with hepatic dysfunction. Anesth Analg 1984; 63:775–778.

63. Plummer JL, Beckwith AL, Bastin FN, et al.: Free radical formation in vivo and hepatotoxicity due to anesthesia with halothane. Anesthesiology 1982; 57:160–166.

64. Varma RR, Whitesell RC, Iskandarani MM: Halothane hepatitis without halothane: Role of inapparent circuit contamination and its prevention. Hepatology 1985; 5:1159–1162.

65. Martin JL, Kenna JG, Pohl LR: Antibody assays for the detection of patients sensitised to halothane. Anesth Analg 1990; 2:154–159.

66. Hubbard AK, Roth TP, Gandolfi AJ, et al.: Halothane hepatitis patients generate an antibody response towards a covalently bound metabolite of halothane. Anesthesiology 1988; 68:791–796.

67. Kenna JG, Neuberger J, Williams R: Specific antibodies to halothane induced liver antigens in halothane associated hepatitis. Br J Anaesth 1987; 59:1286–1290.

68. Neuberger J: Halothane and hepatitis. Incidence, predisposing factors and exposure guidelines. Drug Safety 1990; 5:28–38.

69. Neuberger J, Williams R: Halothane hepatitis. Dig Dis 1988; 6:52–64.

70. Farrell G, Prendergast D, Murray M: Halothane hepatitis. Determination of a constitutional susceptibility factor. N Engl J Med 1985; 313:1310–1314.

Biliary Obstruction (Cholestasis)

71. Pain JA, Cahill CJ, Bailey ME: Perioperative complications in obstructive jaundice. Therapeutic considerations. Br J Surg 1985; 72:942–947.

72. Bailey ME: Endotoxin, bile salts, and renal failure in obstructive jaundice. Br J Surg 1976; 63:774–778.

73. Hunt DR, Allison ME, Prentice CR, et al.: Endotoxemia, disturbance of coagulation, and obstructive jaundice. Am J Surg 1982; 144:325–330.

74. Dawson JL: Postoperative renal function in obstructive jaundice: Effect of mannitol infusion. Br Med J 1965; 52:663–665.

Viral Hepatitis and Other Infectious Liver Diseases

75. Centers for Disease Control: Recommendations for prevention of HIV transmission in health care settings. MMWR 1987; 36:629–633.

76. Ping FC, Oulton JL, Smith JA, et al.: Bacterial filters—are they necessary on anaesthetic machines? Can Anaesth Soc J 1979; 26:415–419.

77. Craven DE: Contaminated condensate in mechanical ventilator circuits. Am Rev Respir Dis 1984; 129:625–628.

78. Cobo JC, Harley DP: The eyes as a portal of entry for hepatitis and other infectious diseases. Surg Gynecol Obstet 1985; 161:71.

79. Corey L, Spear P: Infections with herpes simplex viruses. N Engl J Med 1986; 314:686–757.

80. Browne RA, Chernesky MA: Infectious diseases and the anaesthetist. Can J Anaesth 1988; 35:655–665.

81. Browne RA, Chernesky MA: Viral hepatitis and the anaesthetist. Can Anaesth Soc J 1984; 31:279–286.

82. Decker RH, Kosakowski SM, Vanderbilt AS, et al.: Diagnosis of acute hepatitis A by NAVAB-M, a direct radioimmunoassay for IgM anti-HAV. Am J Clin Pathol 1981; 76:140–147.

83. Blumberg BS: Pleomorphisms of serum proteins and the development of isoprecipitins in transfused patients. Bull NY Acad Med 1964; 40:377–386.

84. Stephens CE, Aach RD, Hollinger FB, et al.: Hepatitis virus antibody in blood donors and the occurrence of non-A, non-B hepatitis in transfusion recipients: An analysis of the transfusion-transmitted viruses study. Ann Intern Med 1984; 101:733–738.

85. Carstens J, Macnab GM, Kew MC: Hepatitis B virus infection in anaesthetists. Br J Anaesth 1977; 49:887–889.

86. Cheresky MA, Browne RA, Rondi P: Hepatitis B antibody prevalence in anaesthetists. Can Anaesth Soc J 1984; 31:239–245.

87. Berry AJ, Isacson IJ, Hunt D, Kane MA: The prevalence of hepatitis B viral markers in anesthesia personnel. Anesthesiology 1984; 60:1–3.

88. Sinclair ME, Ashby MW, Kurtz JB: The prevalence of serological markers for hepatitis B virus infection amongst anaesthetists in the Oxford region. Anaesthesia 1987; 42:30–32.

89. Zuckerman AJ: Who should be immunised against hepatitis B? BMJ 1984; 289:1243–1244.

90. Oxman MN: Hepatitis vaccination of high-risk hospital personnel. Anesthesiology 1984; 60:1–3.

91. Blumberg BS, Millman I, London WT, et al.: Ted Slavin's blood and the development of HBV vaccine. N Engl J Med 1985; 312:189.

92. Zuckerman AJ: New hepatitis B vaccines. BMJ 1985; 290:492–496.

93. Stevens CE, Taylor PE, Rubinstein P, et al.: Safety of the hepatitis B vaccine. N Engl J Med 1985; 312:375–376.

94. Centers for Disease Control: Hepatitis B vaccine: Evidence confirming lack of AIDS transmission. MMWR 1985; 33:685–687.

95. Rizzetto M: The delta agent. Hepatology 1983; 3:729–732.

96. Wong DC, Purcell RM, Sreenivasan MA, et al.: Epidemic and endemic hepatitis in India; evidence for a non-A, non-B hepatitis virus etiology. Lancet 1980; 2:876–881.

97. Lee KG, Soni N: AIDS and anaesthesia. Anaesthesia 1985; 41:1011–1016.

98. Greene EF Jr: Acquired immunodeficiency syndrome: An overview for anesthesiologists. Anesth Analg 1986; 65:1054–1058.

99. McEvoy M, Porter K, Mortimer P, et al.: Prospective study of clinical, laboratory and ancillary staff with accidental exposure to blood or body fluids from patients infected with HIV. Br Med J 1987; 294:1595–1597.

100. Harville DD, Summerskill WHJ: Surgery in acute hepatitis. Causes and effects. JAMA 1963; 184:257–261.

101. Marx GF, Nagoyoshi M, Shoukas JA, et al.: Unexpected infectious hepatitis in surgical patients. JAMA 1968; 205:793–795.

Hydatid Disease

102. Kefi M, Sayed S, Henatati M, et al.: Anesthesia and resuscitation in the surgery of hydatid cysts. Tunis Med 1985; 63:559–562.

103. Baraka A, Slim M, Dajani A, Lakkis S: One-lung ventilation of children during surgical excision of hydatid cysts of the lung. Br J Anaesth 1982; 54:523–528.

104. Bacalbasa N, Nichiteanu C: Fatal anaphylactic shock (rupture of hydatid cyst) in the course of general anesthesia. Rev Chir 1980; 29:467–469.

Genetic Causes of Liver Disease

105. Rivers J, Garrahy P, Robinson W, et al.: Reversible cardiac dysfunction in hemochromatosis. Am Heart J 1987; 113:216–217.

106. Frydman M, Bonnie-Tamir B, Farrer LA, et al.: Assignment of the gene for Wilson disease to chromosome 13: Linkage to the esterose D locus. Proc Nat Assoc Sci 1985; 82:1819–1821.

107. Diaz JH, Belani KG: Perioperative management of children with mucopolysaccharidoses. Anesth Analg 1993; 77:1261–1270.

108. Belani KG, Krivit W, Carpenter BL, et al.: Children with mucopolysaccharidoses: Perioperative case, morbidity, mortality, and new findings. J Pediatr Surg 1993; 28:403–408.

109. Blekkenhorst GH, Harrison GG, Cook ES, Eales L: Screening of certain anaesthetic agents for ability to elicit acute porphyric phases in susceptible patients. Br J Anaesth 1980; 52:759–762.

110. Summer E: Porphyria in relation to surgery and anaesthesia. Ann R Coll Surg Engl 1975; 56:81–88.

111. Capouet V, Dernovoi B, Azagra JS: Induction of anaesthesia with ketamine during an acute crisis of hereditary coproporphyria. Can J Anaesth 1987; 34:388–390.

112. Harrison GG, Moore MR, Meissner PN: Porphyrinogenicity of etomidate and ketamine as continuous infusions. Screening in the DDC-primed rat model. Br J Anaesth 1985; 57:420–423.

113. Jensen NF, Fiddler DS, Striepe V: Anesthetic considerations in porphyrias. Anesth Analg 1995; 80:591–599.

114. Harrison GG, Meissner PN, Hift RJ: Anaesthesia for the porphyric patient. Anaesthesia 1993; 48:417–421.

115. McFarlane HJ, Soni N: Pompe's disease and anaesthesia. Anaesthesia 1986; 41:1219–1224.

116. Bevan JC: Anaesthesia in Von Gierke's disease. Current approach to management. Anaesthesia 1980; 35:699–702.

117. Alagille D: Alpha$_1$-antitrypsin deficiency. Hepatology 1984; 4:115–145.

118. Kasai M, Watanabe I, Ohi R: Follow-up studies of long-term survivors after hepatic portoenterostomy for "non-correctable" biliary atresia. J Pediatr Surg 1975; 10:173–180.

119. Simpson DA, Green DW: Use of atracurium during major abdominal surgery in infants with hepatic dysfunction from biliary atresia. Br J Anaesth 1986; 58:1214–1217.

120. Kasai M: Treatment of biliary atresia with special reference to hepatic portoenterostomy and its modifications. Prog Pediatr Surg 1974; 6:50–52.

Liver Disease of Other Causes

Carcinoid Syndrome

121. Padfield NL: Carcinoid syndrome: Comparison of pretreatment regimens in the same patient. Ann R Coll Surg Engl 1987; 69:16–17.

122. Galland RB, Blumgart LH: Carcinoid syndrome. Surgical management. Br J Hosp Med 1986; 35:168–170.

123. Houghton K, Carter JA: Perioperative management of carcinoid syndrome using ketanserin. Anaesthesia 1986; 41:595–599.

124. Simpson KH: Use of vecuronium in carcinoid syndrome. Br J Anaesth 1985; 57:934.

125. Jones RM, Knight D: Severe hypertension and flushing in a patient with a non-metastatic carcinoid tumour. Hypertension and flushing with a solitary carcinoid tumour. Anaesthesia 1982; 37:57–59.

126. Rawlinson WA, March RH, Goat VA: Anaesthesia for removal of carcinoid metastases. A case of serotonin-secreting secondary tumour in the lumbar spine. Anaesthesia 1980; 35:585–588.

127. Fleming FW: Carcinoid syndrome in a diabetic patient. Anaesthesia 1980; 35:589–592.

128. Miller R, Bopulukos PA, Warner RR: Failure of halothane and ketamine to alleviate carcinoid syndrome–induced bronchospasm during anesthesia. Anesth Analg 1980; 59:621–623.

129. Miller R, Patel AU, Warner RR, Parnes IH: Anaesthesia for the carcinoid syndrome: A report of nine cases. Can Anaesth Soc J 1978; 25:240–244.

130. Mason RA, Steane PA: Anaesthesia for a patient with carcinoid syndrome. Anaesthesia 1976; 31:243–246.

131. Mason RA, Steane PA: Carcinoid syndrome: Its relevance to the anaesthetist. Anaesthesia 1976; 31:228–242.

132. Neustein SM, Cohen E: Anaesthesia for aortic and mitral valve replacement in a patient with carcinoid heart disease. Anesthesiology 1995; 82:1067–1070.

133. Veall GR, Peacock JE, Bax ND, Reilly CS: Review of the anaesthetic management of 21 patients undergoing laparotomy for carcinoid syndrome. Br J Anaesth 1994; 72:335–341.

134. Gregor M: Therapeutic principles in the management of metastasizing carcinoid tumours: Drugs for symptomatic relief. Digestion 1994; 55:60–63.

Reye's Syndrome

135. Mowat AP: Reye's syndrome: 20 years on. Br Med J 1983; 286:1999–2003.

136. Reye RDK, Morgan G, Baral J: Encephalopathy and fatty degeneration of the viscera. A disease entity in childhood. Lancet 1963; 2:749–753.

137. Partin JC: Reye's syndrome (encephalopathy and fatty liver): Diagnosis and treatment. Gastroenterology 1975; 69:511–514.

138. Ede RJ, Williams R: Reye's syndrome in adults. BMJ 1988; 296:517–518.

139. Hurwitz ES, Mortimer EA: A catch in the Reye is awry. Cleve Clin J Med 1990; 57:318–320.

140. Reye Syndrome Surveillance—United States 1989. JAMA 1991; 265:960.

Liver in Pregnancy

141. Weinstein L: Syndrome of hemolysis, elevated liver enzymes, and low platelet count: A severe consequence of hypertension in pregnancy. Am J Obstet Gynecol 1982; 142:159–163.

142. Baska R, Waxman B: Ruptured liver associated with pregnancy: A review of the literature and report of two cases. Surg Gynecol Obstet 1976; 31:763–767.

143. Herbert WPN: Hepatic rupture in pregnancy. NY State J Med 1986; 86:286–291.

144. Gelman S: General anesthesia and hepatic circulation. Can J Physiol Pharmacol 1987; 65:1762–1779.

145. Riely CA: Hepatic disease in pregnancy. Am J Med 1994; 96:185–225.

Transplantation

146. Wall WJ: Liver transplantation: Current concepts. Can Med Assoc J 1988; 139:21–28.

147. Borland LM, Roule M, Cook DR: Anesthesia for pediatric orthotopic liver transplantation. Anesth Analg 1985; 64:117–124.

148. Borland LM, Martin DJ: Anesthesia considerations for orthotopic liver transplantation. Contemp Anesth Pract 1987; 10:157–182.

Acute Hepatic Failure

149. Ward ME, Trewby PN, Williams R, Strunin L: Acute liver failure. Anaesthesia 1977; 32:228–233.

150. Corall I, Williams R: Management of liver failure. Br J Anaesth 1986; 58:234–245.

FURTHER READING

Calne RY, Della Rovere GQ (eds): Liver Surgery. Philadelphia, WB Saunders, 1982.

Calne RY (ed): Liver Transplantation. London, Grune & Stratton, 1983.

Winter PM, Kang YG (eds): Hepatic Transplantation. New York, Praeger, 1986.

Brown BR Jr (ed): Anesthesia for Transplantation. Philadelphia, FA Davis, 1987.

Brown BR Jr: Anesthesia in Hepatic and Biliary Tract Disease. Philadelphia, FA Davis, 1988.

Gelman S (ed): Anesthesia and Organ Transplantation. Philadelphia, WB Saunders, 1987.

Millward-Sadler GH, Wright R, Arthur MJP: Wright's Liver and Biliary Diseases, ed 3. Philadelphia, WB Saunders, 1992.

Strunin L, Thomson S (eds): Clinical Anaesthesiology—The Liver and Anaesthesia. London, Baillière Tindall, 1992.

Hawker F: Critical Care Management—The Liver. Philadelphia, WB Saunders, 1993.

Peter K, Conzen P (eds): Clinical Anaesthesiology—Inhalational Anaesthesia. London, Baillière Tindall, 1993.

Sherlock S, Dooley J: Diseases of the Liver and Biliary System, ed 9. Boston, Blackwell Scientific, 1993.

Park G: Anesthesia and Intensive Care for Patients with Liver Disease. London, Butterworth-Heinemann, 1995.

CHAPTER 7

Gastrointestinal and Nutritional Disorders

Ahmed F. Ghouri
Mark Ezekiel

I. GENERAL CONSIDERATIONS

A. PREOPERATIVE CONSIDERATIONS

The principal function of the gastrointestinal (GI) tract is to supply the human organism with water, electrolytes, and energy. Therefore, essentially every organ system can be affected by GI disease. Although the anesthesiologist's primary focus during the preoperative assessment is most commonly related to a patient's cardiac and respiratory status, it must be appreciated that disorders of nutrition and the GI tract can have profound anesthetic implications.

Although thousands of unusual diseases have been described involving the GI tract, it is important for the consulting anesthesiologist to be aware that a seemingly straightforward procedure (e.g., resection of a bowel tumor of undetermined cause) can be fraught with challenges (e.g., if the tumor is endocrinologically active and liberates catecholamines). Thus, the assessment of patients with alimentary tract disease must take into consideration systemic effects of the disease and how these may affect intraoperative management and the postoperative course. Indeed, the anesthesiologist's role, once limited to intraoperative care, now includes preoperative optimization and postoperative management of patients.

Different portions of the GI tract serve different functions, and, consequently, the effects of disease in particular regions may vary significantly, depending on the area involved. However, before describing in detail the problems associated with specific disorders, it is worth reviewing the principal concerns in patients with GI disease, as it is the anesthesiologist's responsibility to optimize the patient's condition before surgery.

In a very general sense, the priorities for the body are (1) organ perfusion, (2) oxygenation, (3) electrolyte balance, and (4) acid-base homeostasis. Each of these can be significantly altered by GI pathology and must be addressed before all other concerns specific to the disease in question.

1. Hemodynamic Considerations

Alterations in volume status are common, and may be severe, in patients with GI disease. The most common problem, acute volume depletion, can result from GI bleeding, hypersecretion accompanied with inadequate fluid replacement, or third space losses. Anemia and/or hypotension due to bleeding can cause tissue hypoxia, myocardial (or other crucial end-organ) dysfunction, and death; however, too-rapid correction of volume can be deleterious in itself and can lead to cardiac decompensation or electrolyte disorders. Thus, if surgery can be delayed, it is recommended that optimization of volume status be progressive and cautious; however, oftentimes surgery cannot be deferred, in which case the anesthesiologist must consider invasive monitoring to help ensure cardiovascular stability.

The correction of volume depletion must take into consideration the nature of the deficit. For example, a villous adenoma of the colon can be associated with profound total body potassium deficit owing to its hypersecretory nature, and lethal hypokalemia may occur if a solution containing no potassium is administered rapidly in large volumes. Similarly, if a patient presents with an exsanguinating intra-abdominal mass with severe anemia, then whole blood is the replacement fluid of choice. In each circumstance it must be emphasized that, so long as oxygenation is accounted for, perfusion (i.e., preservation of arterial pressure) must take precedence over all other considerations during the time of initial resuscitation.

Hypotension can lead to central nervous system (CNS), myocardial, renal, or hepatic injury, and ultimately to death; therefore, the following causes must be considered when a patient with GI disease presents with hypotension: (1) hypovolemia due to bleeding; (2) hypovolemia due to third space losses or sepsis; (3) myocardial dysfunction due to electrolyte disturbances, anemia (leading to ischemia), or acid-base imbalance; and (4) effects of endogenous or exogenous substances related to the GI pathology (e.g., catecholamine-induced cardiomyopathy due to a hormonally active tumor, autonomic nervous system damage resulting from nutritional deficiency, or toxin ingestion).

Hypertension is less commonly life-threatening but may be associated with GI disease processes, as in a patient with a pheochromocytoma or even a benign tumor compressing a renal artery and leading to secondary renovascular hypertension. In summary, although rare GI diseases may present special concerns to the anesthesiologist, the fundamental priorities of the body must take precedence.

2. Pulmonary Considerations

GI and nutritional diseases can have dramatic implications with regard to the pulmonary system. Of foremost concern is the risk for aspiration, as patients with intra-abdominal lesions commonly have altered GI motility. With this in mind, the anesthesiologist must take into consideration aspiration prophylaxis (e.g., histamine H_2 antagonists, antacids, prokinetic agents), as well as the relative merits of (1) regional anesthesia, (2) general anesthesia following awake intubation, and (3) general anesthesia following rapid sequence induction and intubation. Also, it must be kept in mind that endotracheal intubation (even with a cuffed tube) does not guarantee against aspiration and that anesthetic mishaps can occur during any regional anesthetic requiring urgent intubation. Finally, it should be noted that *any* GI lesion proximal to the ligament of Treitz should alert the physician to the possibility of altered gastric emptying, even in the absence of clinical symptoms.

In addition to aspiration, a multitude of pulmonary problems must be anticipated in the patient with GI disease. These include alterations in oxygenation and ventilation resulting from (1) associated pleural effusions or empyema, (2) mediastinitis or mediastinal emphysema, (3) adult respiratory distress syndrome (e.g., pancreatitis or sepsis-related), (4) pneumothorax, (5) diaphragmatic compression due to abdominal masses with resultant atelectasis and decrease in functional residual capacity, (6) neuromuscular weakness due to electrolyte or nutritional imbalance, (7) pulmonary or mediastinal metastases related to malignancies, (8) drying and accumulation of viscous bronchial secretions in patients who may be hypovolemic, and (9) increased respiratory demands due to infection or any hypermetabolic state.

3. Electrolyte and Acid-Base Considerations

In addition to hypovolemia (discussed above), GI and metabolic diseases may lead to dramatic electrolyte and acid-base disturbances. The physiology of water and electrolyte movement varies according to location in the alimentary tract; consequently, GI disorders can lead to electrolyte disorders of considerable variety. In addition, electrolyte loss can be compounded by iatrogenic therapy (e.g., prolonged nasogastric suctioning, use of laxatives, and medication toxicity) or the presence of enterocutaneous fistulas. Moreover, electrolyte and fluid losses can be grossly underestimated because large amounts of fluid can be sequestered intraluminally and by intestinal wall edema. Furthermore, bowel distention may increase the rate of intestinal secretion, thus initiating a dangerous positive feedback mechanism.

GI fluid and electrolyte losses can lead to compensatory hormonal responses (e.g., antidiuretic hormone [ADH], aldosterone), which may themselves be deleterious, as in the case of aldosterone-induced paradoxical aciduria in dehydrated patients who already have a metabolic alkalosis. The entire spectrum of electrolyte and acid-base disturbances may be seen in patients with GI disorders, ranging from hypokalemic hypochloremic metabolic alkalosis in a patient with prolonged vomiting, to metabolic acidosis in patients with ulcerative colitis, pseudomembranous colitis, or Crohn's disease.

The invention of total parenteral nutrition (TPN) has allowed patients to survive the excision of large portions of bowel; however, pathologic states may result, such as hypomagnesemia and hypocalcemia after jejunoileal bypass. Hyperalimentation to treat malnutrition can induce disorders such as hypophosphatemia, which can cause respiratory failure due to weakness, and even cardiac arrest. Indeed, the astute clinician should appreciate that electrolyte disorders, although gastrointestinal in origin, may lead to dangerous alterations in drug effects, cardiac dysrhythmias, nervous system dysfunction, and mortality if appropriate corrective measures are not taken.

4. Immunologic and Nutritional Considerations

Patients with GI diseases are frequently treated with antibiotics, both prophylactically and therapeutically. Antibiotic therapy can affect drug pharmacokinetics and pharmacodynamics and lead to coagulation disorders and suprainfections. Sepsis is always a concern in immunocompromised patients, and often the first manifestation in a patient with an underlying malignancy may be a GI symptom (e.g., bowel obstruction in a patient with HIV-associated Kaposi's sarcoma of the intestine).

Malnutrition is a common feature of many GI disorders, since these patients typically have a lack of appetite, digestive impairment, or malabsorption coupled with increased metabolic demands due to illness. The relationship between surgical morbidity and malnutrition in patients has been described exhaustively during the past 50 years, and it is clear that nutritional support greatly improves patient outcome as well as mortality.[1]

The anesthetic implications of malnutrition are indeed immense. For example, malabsorption of vitamins or minerals may lead to anemia, psychosis, autonomic dysfunction, hepatic dysfunction, and coagulopathy, all of which affect perioperative management (uncommon hepatic diseases are discussed in Chapter 6). Chronic starvation, although rare in Western society, can lead to cardiomyopathy, hepatic failure, and renal failure. Finally, toxin ingestion (which may be the underlying cause of the patient's GI disease) can greatly potentiate drug effects and destroy virtually every organ system. Indeed, patients with GI lesions often present with major homeostatic derangements, and the implications of associated organ systems dysfunction must always be kept in mind.

Before describing specific alimentary or nutritional disorders, it is worth reviewing energy balance, metabolism, nutrition, and the function of the GI tract in general. Understanding the basic physiology of the GI system allows us to better appreciate the pathologic processes that can affect it. These are discussed in the following sections.

B. ENERGY BALANCE

1. General Considerations

Although nutritional assessment and support are rarely the primary responsibility of the anesthesiologist, it is important to appreciate the importance of nutritional optimization before surgery. As anesthesiologists become increasingly concerned with pre- and postoperative management, it is our responsibility to ensure that patients are medically "optimized" prior to surgery, no small part of which is nutritional assessment. Indeed, in all but the most dire emergencies, nutritional status must be taken into account before surgery, as malnutrition is clearly associated with increased perioperative morbidity and outcome.[2] This is particularly important for patients with coexisting GI disease, who are especially at risk for being inadequately nourished.

2. Energy Requirements

The catabolism of food liberates energy that becomes either (1) external work, (2) energy storage, or (3) heat. The peak efficiency of a mammalian organism is about 50%; that is, the maximum amount of useful work performed is nearly the same as the amount of heat produced in the process.[3] The standard measure of energy in living organisms—the *calorie*—is defined as the amount of heat that raises the temperature of 1 g of water (H_2O) 1°C. The unit commonly used in medicine is the kilocalorie or Calorie (upper case C) and equals 1000 calories. The caloric values of food components are measured with an apparatus known as the *bomb calorimeter*, in which food is combusted and the energy liberated is measured. Although high-temperature combustion by fire is different from oxidation in an organism at body temperature, the end-products (CO_2 and H_2O) are the same. Therefore, according to the first law of thermodynamics, the energy liberated must be the same regardless of the process.

The caloric content of food varies by substrate, and is 4.1 kcal/g of carbohydrate, 9.3 kcal/g of fat, and 5.3 kcal/g of protein.[4] Since the oxidation of protein in mammals in incomplete, however, the end-products of protein catabolism are urea and other nitrogen-containing substances (in addition to CO_2 and H_2O). Thus, the effective caloric content of protein is less, or about 4.1 kcal/g, and thus similar to that of carbohydrates.

The respiratory quotient (RQ) is the ratio of CO_2 production to oxygen consumption. The RQ for carbohydrates is 1.00 and for fat approximately 0.70.[5] Fat molecules contain relatively fewer oxygen atoms than carbohydrates; consequently extra O_2 is necessary for the production of CO_2 and water. In carbohydrates, O_2 and H_2 atoms are present in the same proportion as water, thus the RQ is equal to 1. The RQ of protein is about 0.82 and intermediate between fat and carbohydrate.[6] Factors other than metabolic rate may influence the RQ. For instance, in a patient with metabolic acidosis, the RQ may increase because expired CO_2 rises owing to pulmonary compensation. In severe acidosis, the RQ may exceed 1.0. Conversely, in metabolic alkalosis, RQ falls.

One can also infer much about the processes in an organ system based on the RQ. For example, in a nonstarved person, the RQ of the brain is 0.97, indicating that its principal source of energy is carbohydrate (i.e., glucose), not fat or protein. In the case of the stomach during active secretion, the RQ is negative, as it takes in more CO_2 from its arterial supply than it liberates into its veins.[7]

The metabolic rate is estimated by measuring the oxygen consumption of an organism, usually with a closed-loop spirometer and CO_2-absorbing system. Many factors affect the metabolic rate, muscle exertion like that during exercise being the most important. However, oxygen consumption is elevated not only during exercise but long afterward, as it is necessary to repay the oxygen "debt" that is incurred. Other factors that affect metabolic rate include environmental temperature, height, weight, surface area, recent ingestion of food, body temperature, sex, age, pregnancy, circulating thyroid hormones, circulating catecholamines, emotional state, and the disease states (e.g., sepsis or burns).[8]

The average 70-kg adult requires about 2000 kcal/day, with caloric requirements above that level depending on modifying factors, as already mentioned. For example, a sedentary person may require only an additional 500 kcal/day, but a world-class athlete may consume an additional 3000 kcal/day. However, since not all fuel sources are equivalent, one may have adequate caloric intake and still experience symptoms of malnutrition, as with deficiencies of essential amino acids, vitamins, minerals, and essential fatty acids. These are discussed in detail in subsequent sections.

The energy requirement for a healthy adult is estimated to be about 30 kcal/kg/day, which includes approximately 400 to 800 kcal/day above the basal metabolic rate (BMR) of a sedentary hospitalized patient. However, severity of coexisting illness must be taken into consideration. A gross estimate of energy consumption can be made as follows: (1) in mild illness, the additional calorie requirement is approximately 10 per cent above this value, (2) in moderate illness, approximately 25 per cent, and (3) in severe illness, 50 to 100 per cent higher.[9] Few patients, even the most severely stressed, manifest more than twice the normal energy utilization.

C. METABOLIC PROCESSES

1. Overview of Metabolism

The term *metabolism* means *change* and is broadly referred to when describing the chemical and energetic transformations that occur in the body. In animals, carbohydrates, proteins, and fats are oxidized, leading to the production of CO_2, H_2O, and high-energy phosphate compounds (e.g., adenosine triphosphate [ATP]) essential for life processes. However, since oxidation is a complex, multistep process, derangements are possible at many different locations.

The end-products of digestion are amino acids, fat derivatives, and hexoses (glucose, galactose, and fructose). The short-chain fragments produced by catabolism of these substances form a common metabolic pool of intermediates, which are either used to synthesize new carbohydrates, fats, or proteins, or else are broken down into hydrogen atoms, CO_2, and H_2O to provide energy for the organism via the citric acid cycle.

In a broad sense, the citric acid cycle is final common pathway for catabolism, and yields high-energy phosphates, the most important of which is ATP. Other high-energy phosphates include creatinine phosphate (found mostly in muscle), and pyrimidine and purine triphosphates (e.g., GTP, UTP, CTP, and ITP). Another group of high-energy substances are the thioesters, such as acetyl coenzyme A (aCoA), which are of profound importance in intermediate metabolic processes.[10] From the perspective of organism energetics, one molecule of aCoA is equivalent to one molecule of ATP.

Oxidation occurs when a substance combines with oxygen, loses electrons, or loses hydrogen. The reverse process is reduction. Oxidation is an enzyme-dependent process, in many cases requiring cofactors for a particular reaction. Cofactors are usually simple ions or nonprotein substances, and usually are carriers for products of a reaction. Coenzymes, as compared to enzymes, may catalyze a variety of reactions. Among the most important coenzymes are nicotinamide adenine dinucleotide (NAD) and related molecules and flavin adenine dinucleotide (FAD) and related molecules.

In mammalian mitochondria, the transfer of hydrogen atoms from NAD-related to FAD-related molecules results in the generation of ATP in a process known as *oxidative phosphorylation*. It should be noted that, in addition to being a source of energy, ATP is a precursor of cyclic adenosine 3'5' monophosphate (cAMP), an important cellular and hormonal second messenger.

2. Carbohydrate Metabolism

Dietary carbohydrates are most commonly polymers of hexoses, the principal ones being galactose, fructose, and glucose. The principal hexose circulating in the blood is glucose and is the primary energy source of the brain. The normal range of venous glucose concentration is 70 to 110 mg/dL in adults; arterial concentrations are approximately 15 to 30 per cent higher.

Upon entering cells, glucose is phosphorylated to glucose-6-phosphate by hexokinase. The glucose-6-phosphate is either polymerized into glycogen (the storage form of glucose) in a process called *glycogenesis* or undergoes catabolism via glycolysis. Glycolysis proceeds through the cleavage of hexoses into trioses (three-carbon sugars), and is also called the *Embden-Meyerhof pathway*.[11] Glycogen breakdown, called *glycogenolysis*, occurs primarily in the liver and is necessary prior to glycolysis.

The end-products of glycolysis are pyruvic acid, lactic acid, and ATP. Pyruvic acid is the "crossroads of metabolism" in that interconversions between fat, glucose, and protein may occur from this intermediate metabolite.[12] Pyruvate is broken down further into aCoA, which by way of the citric acid cycle leads to the most efficient generation of ATP for an organism in a process that requires oxygen. Glucose may also be converted into fats via aCoA, but the conversion of pyruvic acid to aCoA is irreversible.[13] Therefore, fat cannot be converted into glucose. Once glycogen stores are exhausted (e.g., as in a malnourished patient), protein must be catabolized to provide glucose to the brain, even if fat (and energy) stores remain enormous.

The *citric acid cycle* (also called the *Krebs cycle* or *tricarboxylic acid cycle*) is a series of reactions that convert aCoA to CO_2 and hydrogen atoms. This cycle, unlike glycolysis, requires O_2 and consequently does not function under anaerobic conditions. Unlike glycolysis, the citric acid cycle occurs only in the mitochondria of cells.[14]

When pyruvate is formed via glycolysis, there is a net production of only 2 moles of ATP per mole of glucose under anaerobic conditions; however, during aerobic conditions, the production of ATP is 19 times greater, as the citric acid cycle is utilized.[15] The inability to utilize pyruvate or lactate (end-products of glycolysis) as an energy source during anaerobic conditions leads to accumulation of these metabolites. Thus, lactic acidosis is a general indicator of oxygen deficiency at the cellular level.

Alterations in carbohydrate metabolism may lead to systemic consequences. For example, in galactosemia (deficiency of a galactose-cleaving enzyme), accumulation of galactose leads to growth and development disturbances.[16] In another disease known as *McArdle's syndrome,* a defect in the glycogenolytic enzyme myophosphorylase leads to accumulation of glycogen, resulting in profound fatigability of skeletal muscle.[17] Numerous enzyme defects related to carbohydrate metabolism have been described. Since glucose regulation is one of the principal functions of the liver and endocrine pancreas, these are described in detail in other chapters.

3. Protein Metabolism

Proteins are composed of amino acids linked by peptide bonds. Small groups of amino acids are called peptides or polypeptides, rather than proteins. Eight of approximately 20 amino acids are essential (phenylalanine, valine, tryptophan, threonine, lysine, leucine, isoleucine, and methionine) and cannot be synthesized de novo by humans.[18] Disease syndromes therefore occur when dietary intake is deficient in these substances. (Essential amino acid deficiency is discussed in subsequent sections.)

Small amounts of protein are absorbed from the intestine directly; however, most require digestion into amino acids before they can be absorbed. The average adult has an endogenous protein turnover of 100 g/day. In some diseases, such as Fanconi's syndrome, amino acids are spilled into the urine, dramatically depleting the amino acid pool and

leading to adverse consequences.[19] Such syndromes are discussed in detail in other chapters (see Chapter 14).

Apart from being the basis from which all proteins are synthesized, amino acids are often themselves associated with specific metabolic functions. For example, catecholamines, histamine, acetylcholine, creatinine, purines, pyrimidines, melatonin, neurotransmitters, and thyroid and other hormones are formed from specific amino acids.

Interconversion between amino acids can occur by the processes of deamination, amination, and transamination. In general, there is an equilibrium between the common metabolic pool, which contains intermediate metabolites (e.g., pyruvate, lactate) and a common amino acid pool, which contains amino acids. The amino acid pool obtains its constituents from one of three sources: (1) diet, (2) catabolism of body proteins, and (3) transamination or amination of common metabolic pool intermediates. Deamination of amino acids occurs in the liver, and leads to the generation of the waste products ammonia and urea, which are excreted in the urine. Protein degradation is a very complex, tightly regulated process, as is protein synthesis. The loss of protein in urine and stool is normally very low (less than 5 per cent of daily turnover).[20] The rate of degradation depends on a multitude of factors related to the function of the protein that is being degraded. For instance, denervated or unused skeletal muscle is destroyed rapidly.

The principal components of DNA (e.g., nucleotides) are synthesized from amino acids and are broken down to uric acid, which is excreted in the urine. Excess uric acid leads to deposition of urate crystals (gout) in a variety of anatomic sites.[21] Excess circulating uric acid may be due to (1) increased dietary intake, (2) excessive turnover of nucleic acid (e.g., tumor lysis or starvation), (3) inadequate elimination (renal dysfunction), or (4) specific enzyme dysfunction (e.g., congenital). Specific disorders of nucleotide metabolism are discussed in depth in other chapters.

The balance between protein degradation and synthesis is loosely termed *nitrogen balance,* because nitrogen is rarely (if ever) a significant constituent of fats or carbohydrates, the other fuel sources of the body. Because stool and urine losses of protein are normally very low, the amount of nitrogen in the urine is an approximate indicator of the amount of irreversible protein and amino acid catabolism. In malnourished states, nitrogen excretion (as measured in urine and stool) exceeds dietary intake, and the patient is therefore in negative nitrogen balance. During growth, recovery from illness, or following anabolic hormone therapy, nitrogen balance is positive. It should be noted that when any amino acid becomes unavailable for protein synthesis, other amino acids that would have gone into the molecule are deaminated into urea and excreted. Therefore, even if a single essential amino acid is absent from the diet, nitrogen balance will be negative, even if total calorie intake is adequate. This is exemplified by kwashiorkor, in which a diet adequate in calories but deficient in protein leads to a severe disease state characterized by edema, fatty infiltration of the liver, and anemia.[22]

Small amounts of glucose administered to a patient in negative nitrogen balance counteract protein catabolism dramatically. This is the so-called *protein-sparing effect* of glucose; this characteristic is a principal reason why postsurgical patients who are NPO are given intravenous solutions containing sugar. Indeed, 1 L of a solution containing 5 per cent dextrose (glucose) provides only about 200 calories but can have significant protein-sparing effect. The protein-sparing effect may be due to the release of insulin, which directly inhibits protein degradation.[23] Small amounts of intravenous amino acids and fats also exert a large protein-sparing effect.[24]

Most of the protein catabolized during starvation comes from skeletal muscles, liver, and visceral organs, to spare the brain and heart. Glycogen supply can only last about 1 day, and thereafter stored fat becomes the principal energy source; however, once fat supplies are exhausted, protein catabolism speeds up dramatically, and the organism soon dies. In studies of obese persons given only water, vitamins, and minerals, weight loss is approximately 1 kg/day for about 10 days, then 0.3 kg/day thereafter.[25] The average life expectancy of an adequately hydrated but starved person is approximately 60 days.[26]

4. Fat Metabolism

The term *lipid* is used to denote fats (triglycerides), phospholipids, and sterols. Triglycerides are composed of three fatty acids containing an even number of carbons bound to glycerol, a three-carbon backbone.[27] A saturated fat contains no carbon-carbon double bonds, whereas an unsaturated fat is composed of dehydrogenated fatty acids, which contain various numbers of double bonds.[28] Phospholipids are the major constituent of the cell membrane, and sterols comprise various hormones (e.g., cortisol, estrogen, testosterone) and cholesterol.

Fat is the principal source of energy storage in mammals, and fatty acids are broken down to aCoA, the principal substrate of the citric acid cycle, which occurs in the mitochondria. Carnitine is a lysine derivative that facilitates the crossing of fatty acids across the mitochondrial membrane, greatly enhancing fat oxidation. Therefore, carnitine deficiency greatly decreases the cellular availability of energy. The energy yield of fatty acid oxidation is very large—1 mole of a 6-carbon fatty acid yields 44 moles of ATP via the citric acid cycle under aerobic conditions.[29]

The synthesis of fatty acids is the reverse process, in which aCoA fragments combine, and requires large amounts of energy. Unlike oxidation, fatty acid synthesis can occur outside the mitochondria and takes place primarily in microsomes.[30] Humans do not generate fatty acids with more than 16 carbons in each chain.[31]

In several tissues, particularly the liver, aCoA units may combine to form the ketone bodies acetoacetic acid, beta-hydroxybutyrate, and acetone. In some conditions, ketone bodies become an important source of energy (except acetone, which is expired by the lungs). The normal level of ketone bodies in the circulation is low, as they are usually consumed as fast as they are formed; however, when the entry of aCoA into the citric acid cycle is decreased, ketone bodies accumulate, leading to ketoacidosis, which can be fatal. The cause of ketoacidosis is a deficiency of carbohydrate availability at the cellular level due to (1) starvation, (2) diabetes mellitus, or (3) a high-fat, low-carbohydrate diet. In diabetes, serum glucose may be very high, but its entry into cells is impaired. In starvation, an absolute deficiency of carbohydrate is present; however, exogenous glucose is antiketogenic in starvation although not in diabetes. Finally, a high-fat, low-carbohydrate diet leads to ketosis because there is no way for humans to synthesize glucose from fat. In such instances, hepatic dysfunction occurs owing to fatty infiltration of hepatocytes.[32]

The principal lipid moieties do not circulate

free in the blood. Free fatty acids are bound to serum albumin, whereas cholesterol, triglycerides, and phospholipids are bound together in complexes of lipoproteins called *apoproteins.*[33] Chylomicrons are formed in the intestinal mucosa following fat digestion and are very large micelles that enter the circulation via the lymphatic system. Lipoprotein regulation, the principal function of the liver, is very complex and subject to derangement in numerous disease states; however, for purposes of this chapter it is important to keep in mind that the GI tract is responsible for the exogenous portion of this system and is the ultimate source of chylomicrons.

Free fatty acids are transported to fat cells and other tissues by chylomicrons and apoproteins manufactured by the liver. Free fatty acids are also bound to serum albumin and serve as the primary energy source of the heart; however, the brain relies overwhelmingly on the passive diffusion of glucose, which is why serum glucose regulation is so critical. Three fatty acids (linoleic, linolenic, and arachidonic acid) are essential because they are the precursors of prostaglandins. Prostaglandins are 20-carbon unsaturated fatty acids that contain a cyclopentane ring, and have extremely diverse function, including mediation of inflammation, coagulation, red cell deformability, and regulation of multiple endocrine systems.[34] Cholesterol, the basis of all steroid hormones, bile acids, and cellular membranes, is absorbed and incorporated into chylomicrons in the intestinal mucosa. Cholesterol is also synthesized by various tissues and excreted into bile. The relationship of cholesterol excess to atherosclerosis is well-established and is related to genetic factors, diet, and GI pathology (e.g., biliary obstruction).

D. ABSORPTION AND DIGESTION OF NUTRIENTS

1. Carbohydrates, Proteins, and Fats

Products of digestion, rather than large molecules, are largely what are absorbed from the GI tract. The digestion of macromolecular foodstuffs is a complex process involving multiple enzymes. These enzymes are found not only in the intestinal lumen but also in the saliva, the stomach, and the exocrine pancreas. Furthermore, much of digestion is facilitated by acid produced by the stomach and bile produced by the liver. The glycocalyx is the brush border of the small intestine that lines the surface of the lumen, and is rich in digestive enzymes. The brush border serves to greatly increase the surface area available for digestion. Most digested food constituents in the lumen pass into mucosal cells by way of diffusion, facilitated diffusion, active transport, or pinocytosis (endocytosis). Substances may then enter the extracellular fluid, lymphatics, or the blood.

The principal dietary carbohydrates are poly-, di-, and monosaccharides. These are partially digested by ptyalin, the principal alpha-amylase in saliva and pancreatic amylase in the intestine.[35] Most dietary carbohydrates are glycogen, amylose, and amylopectins, which are converted by alpha-amylases to limit dextrans, maltotriose, maltose, lactose, and sucrose in the intestinal lumen.[36] Subsequently, they are broken down further in the intestinal villi by dextrinase, maltase, lactase, and sucrase to glucose, galactose, or fructose and subsequently absorbed into the portal venous blood.[37] Lactase is of special consideration, as lactase function may decline dramatically early in childhood and may lead to milk intolerance. Indeed, as many as 70% of Blacks may be lactose intolerant.[38]

Although hexoses and pentoses are readily absorbed across the intestinal lumen, the transport of some sugars is dependent on the amount of sodium present, higher sodium content facilitating absorption.[39] This is a consequence of the fact that the intestinal glucose transport molecule is the same as that for sodium, and requires energy (ATP). Fructose transport requires another transporter, which is independent of sodium. Although insulin is the principal regulator of blood glucose levels, it has no effect on the intestinal transport of sugars.[40]

The digestion of proteins begins in the stomach, not the mouth. The enzymes responsible are called *pepsins,* and are secreted in the forms of proenzymes (pepsinogens), which are subsequently activated by the presence of hydrochloric acid produced by the stomach. In the duodenum and jejunum, alkaline pancreatic secretions terminate the function of these enzymes; however, the pancreatic juice itself contains proteolytic enzymes, including trypsin, chymotrypsin, and elastase.[41] Some peptide digestion occurs in the cytoplasm of mucosal cells of the intestine, in addition to the intestinal lumen and the brush border of microvilli.

After digestion of proteins into amino acids, they are absorbed by four distinct transport mechanisms, D amino acids being passively absorbed and L amino acids actively absorbed.[42] There are also systems for allowing for the absorption of di- and tripeptides into mucosal cells of the intestine. Like glucose absorption, amino acids are coupled to sodium transport, and high sodium levels in the intestinal lumen favor absorption.[43] Absorption of proteins is highly efficient; less than 5 per cent of intestinal protein is found in the stool, and most is not of dietary origin but of microbial origin or mucosal cell debris. In humans, resection of portions of the intestine leads to hypertrophy of the brush border in other areas to compensate for the loss of surface area. Congenital defects of protein absorption include Hartnup's disease and cystinuria, which are discussed in subsequent sections.

The digestion of lipids begins in the duodenum owing to the presence of pancreatic lipase, leading to free fatty acids and 2-monoglycerides.[44] However, pancreatic lipase does not function without its colipase, which is also secreted by the pancreas.[45] Colipase is an emulsification agent that binds lipase to fat droplets. Most dietary cholesterol is esterified, and a pancreatic esterase digests (hydrolyzes) these substances.

Bile salts, lecithin, and monoglycerides are detergents that emulsify fats in the small intestine. These emulsifying substances are produced primarily in the liver and secreted into the duodenum via the common bile duct, and serve to form micelles, which solubilize lipids to allow for their transport into mucosal cells. Deficiency of pancreatic lipase or depression of micelle formation leads to steatorrhea (fat malabsorption), which is discussed in subsequent sections.

In persons who consume a typical Western diet, 95 per cent of fat is absorbed, mostly in the upper small intestine. However, the process of fat absorption is not functional in infancy (more than 15 per cent of ingested fat is found in the stool of newborns), and they are subject to fat malabsorption syndromes more readily than are adults when disease processes involve the GI tract.[46]

2. Water and Electrolytes

Water in the GI tract is 98 per cent conserved in the body. Of the 2000 mL which a typical adult ingests daily, another 7000 mL of intestinal secretions are added daily. Of the total 9000 mL that enters the GI tract, only 200 mL is found in stool.[47] Sodium- and glucose-rich diets greatly facilitate the absorption of water by the GI tract, which is the reason why oral rehydration therapies contain sodium chloride and glucose. Water moves into the mucosal cells until osmotic pressure in the lumen equals that of the blood. In general, absorption (sometimes active) of osmotically active particles in the GI tract produces a hypoosmolar luminal fluid which allows for the passive diffusion of water into the gut mucosa.

In the colon, sodium is actively pumped out and water moves passively along, following an osmotic gradient. Saline laxatives (e.g., magnesium) are salts that are relatively unabsorbed and retain water in the intestinal lumen, leading to diarrhea. There is a small amount of active secretion of potassium into the intestinal lumen, primarily in mucus, as well as passive diffusion. The movement of potassium is governed by the electrochemical potential difference between blood and the lumen of the intestine. This difference is largest in the colon and ileum; consequently, loss of colonic or ileal fluids may lead to hypokalemia. Chloride is actively absorbed in the ileum as a one-to-one exchange with bicarbonate (HCO_3^-).[48] This therefore tends to alkalinize the intestinal lumen.

3. Vitamins and Minerals

The absorption of water-soluble vitamins (B complex and C) is very rapid in the GI tract, but the fat-soluble ones (A, D, E, K) are not efficiently absorbed unless fat is absorbed.[49] For example, if pancreatic exocrine function is depressed, or if bile is deficient (e.g., common duct obstruction), then fat-soluble vitamin deficiency can occur. Although most vitamins are absorbed in the duodenum and jejunum, vitamin B_{12} is one exception, being absorbed in the terminal ileum. Vitamin B_{12} must bind to intrinsic factor, a protein secreted by gastric parietal cells, before being absorbed.[50] Deficiency of each vitamin presents with a characteristic syndrome; these are discussed in subsequent sections.

Approximately 50 per cent of ingested calcium is absorbed via active transport, indicative of the particular importance of this mineral. Transport of calcium is regulated by

1,25-dihydroxycholecalciferol, a vitamin D metabolite produced by the kidney via a negative feedback mechanism.[51] Calcium absorption is also increased by dietary lactose and protein (as is magnesium absorption) and reduced by phosphates and oxalates as they form insoluble complexes in the GI lumen.

Iron absorption is also very tightly regulated, since accumulation of excess iron is toxic to the body. Its daily absorption is only a small percentage of the ingested amount, as the amount of iron lost (e.g., in skin sloughing, menstruation, GI bleeding) is usually very minimal, averaging only 0.6 to 3.0 mg/day.[52] Iron absorption is facilitated by gastric secretions, and patients who have had gastrectomies (total or partial) may therefore manifest iron deficiency. As is the case with calcium, iron is absorbed in an active process, primarily in the upper small intestine. Mucosal transferrin binds iron and transports it into cells. Apoferritin and ferritin are also iron-binding proteins that are synthesized in mucosal cells of the intestine; their synthesis is a major regulatory mechanism for adjusting the amount of iron that is absorbed.[53] Hemosiderin is a complex composed of iron bound to ferritin in cellular lysosomes and is visible by light microscopy.[54] In iron overload states (e.g., hemochromatosis), hemosiderosis is a characteristic finding.

E. REGULATION OF GASTROINTESTINAL FUNCTION

1. Neural Components

Two major neural networks are intrinsic to the GI tract and are referred to as the *enteric nervous system.* The myenteric plexus (Auerbach's plexus) is located between the middle circular muscle layer and the longitudinal muscle layer, whereas the submucosal plexus (Meissner's plexus) is found between the middle circular muscle layer and the mucosa.[55] The two neural plexuses are heavily interconnected, however. The enteric nervous system contains many mucosal mechanoreceptors and chemoreceptors, which are linked via interneurons to hormone-secreting cells and smooth muscle cells, as well as integrated with sympathetic and parasympathetic neurons. It has been estimated that there may be more neurons in the GI tract than in the spinal cord itself, and peristalsis and coordinated motor activity occurs even if external innervation is removed.[56]

The automonic nervous system is the principal extrinsic innervation to the enteric nervous system, and parasympathetic activity augments peristaltic activity greatly. Sympathetic dominance leads to sphincter contraction and reduced gut activity. Autonomic fibers generally form synapses on cholinergic nerve cells associated with both the myenteric and submucosal plexuses. The parasympathetic input is primarily via the vagus tenth cranial nerve up to the splenic flexure of the colon; thereafter it is mediated by parasympathetic nerves that are sacral in origin.

2. Gastrointestinal Hormones

Venous return from the entire GI tract (with the exception of the mouth and lower anus) is a parallel system draining via the portal vein to the liver. As such, all liberated hormones that originate in the tract traverse the hepatic system. This has important implications in terms of GI diseases, which may liberate hormonally active substances.

There are two groups of GI hormones that are structurally very similar: gastrin-related (cholecytokinin [CCK] and gastrin) and secretin-related hormones (secretin, glucagon, glicentin, vasoactive intestinal peptide, and gastric inhibitory peptide).[57] In addition, other important hormones include motilin, substance P, gastrin-releasing peptide, enterogastrone, somatostatin, glicenin, and neurotensin. In large systemic doses, the effects of many of these hormones overlap, but in vivo they appear to have discretely defined functions. (The principal ones are discussed below.) Finally, many cells of the GI tract are members of the amine precursor uptake and decarboxylation (APUD) system, which are of neural crest origin and liberate biologically active amines related to epinephrine or serotonin.[58]

Gastrin is produced by the G cells of the stomach (probably elsewhere also), stimulates the secretion of gastric acid and pepsin, increases gastric motility, and increases lower esophageal sphincter tone. Gastrin also stimulates the secretion of insulin and glucagon. Luminal amino acids, distention, vagal activity (e.g., centrally mediated by the sight or smell of food), and calcium stimulate gastrin secretion, whereas luminal acidity, secretin, gastric inhibitory peptide (GIP), vasoactive intestinal peptide (VIP), glucagon, and somatostatin decrease it.[59] Gastrin is important in the pathophysiology of Zollinger-Ellison syndrome (discussed in subsequent sections).

CCK is secreted by the mucosa of the small intestine, and produces contraction of the gallbladder and increased secretion of alkaline pancreatic juices and enzymes.[60] It was previously thought that two separate hormones mediated each function, but now it is clear CCK does both. As a result, CCK is also called *cholecystokinin-pancreozymin* (CCK-PZ). Products of digestion and fatty acids in the duodenum stimulate CCK secretion. Finally, the cholekinetic effects of CCK are probably mediated by the second messenger, cyclic guanosine monophosphate (GMP).[61]

Secretin is the enzyme responsible for secretion of alkaline pancreatic juice, and its isolation in 1902 by Starling led him to coin the term *hormone*.[62] It also serves to inhibit gastric acid secretion. It is produced by cells of the upper small intestine, and its liberation is stimulated by the presence of acid and amino acids in the duodenum. Like those of CCK, its effects are indirectly mediated by cyclic adenosine monophosphate (cAMP).[63]

GIP is formed in the duodenum and jejunum and serves to inhibit gastric secretion and motility. It is produced in response to glucose and fat in the duodenum.[64] VIP is also found in the neurons of the GI tract and markedly increases the secretion of water and electrolytes and dilates peripheral blood vessels.[65] Tumors may actively secrete VIP-like substances, leading to severe diarrhea (discussed in subsequent sections). Somatostatin is secreted by the delta cells of the pancreatic islets and by the gastric mucosa. It is a very broad inhibitor of hormone secretion and greatly attenuates release of gastrin, VIP, GIP, and secretin. It also reduces pancreatic exocrine secretion, gastric motility, and gallbladder contraction.[66] Indeed, it is an important negative-feedback hormone, and pharmacologic analogues have been developed to stimulate these effects in cases of hormone overproduction.

The remaining hormones are discussed in the context of disease processes. In summary, the GI hormone system is a complex and very tightly regulated system. Moreover, several GI hormones (e.g., VIP, somatostatin, substance P) are also key regulators of the nervous system.[67] As such, imbalance of their regulatory function can have profound effects that extend beyond the GI tract.

3. Oral Cavity and Esophagus

Mastication breaks up food into smaller particles and is under voluntary control via the action of the mandibular branch of the trigeminal nerve (CN V_3). Digestion begins in the mouth with the action of saliva, which is produced in the submaxillary, sublingual, and parotid glands. An average adult produces about 1500 mL of saliva per day, of which 70 per cent is by the submaxillary glands and 25 per cent by the parotid glands.[68] The glossopharyngeal nerve stimulates parotid secretion, whereas the other salivary glands are stimulated by the facial nerve. Parasympathetic tone is primarily responsible for the amount of salivation that occurs; however, intentionally thinking of food can lead to salivation.

Saliva produced by the parotid is serous, whereas that produced by the sublingual glands is primarily mucous. Submaxillary gland secretion is of intermediate composition. Salivary alpha-amylase, also called ptyalin, digests starches.[69] Salivary mucin serves to lubricate food to allow its passage into the esophagus. The saliva also contains the antimicrobial lysozyme that prevents tooth decay and bacterial overgrowth in the oral cavity.[70] The neutral pH of saliva (7.0) prevents loss of calcium from the teeth and partially neutralizes gastric acid, preventing damage due to reflux.

Swallowing (deglutition) is a mixed voluntary-reflex mechanism mediated by a coordination of input from the trigeminal, glossopharyngeal, hypoglossal, and vagus nerves. The prevention of aspiration is markedly important in the regulation of swallowing. For example, swallowing is nearly impossible when one's mouth is open. Furthermore, during deglutition, respiration is inhibited and glottic closure commences. It should be emphasized that the principal function of the vocal cords is to prevent aspiration, not phonation.

4. Stomach

The stomach is an extremely vascular organ with an immense lymphatic supply. The sympathetic supply is via the celiac plexus, whereas the vagus mediates parasympathetic effects. Some 2.5 L of gastric juice is secreted daily in a typical adult, indicating the degree of activity of this organ.[71] Although gastric acidity is beneficial for digestive purposes, it also serves an antimicrobial function. The gastric mucosa is protected from acid damage by tight intracellular junctions between cells and the production of gastric mucus. Mucosal integrity depends on the presence of prostaglandin E_2, whose synthesis is inhibited by nonsteroidal antiinflammatory medications such as aspirin.[72] The principal stimuli for gastric acid secretion by parietal cells are vagal activity, gastrin, and histamine binding to gastric H_2 receptors.[73]

Provided that the peristaltic activity of the stomach and duodenum are intact, the pylorus has little effect on gastric emptying, despite the musculature that constitutes the pyloric sphincter. For example, patients who have had pyloromyotomy or resection of the pylorus usually have normal gastric emptying. The regulation of gastric secretion is broadly categorized into four components: (1) cephalic, (2) gastric, (3) intestinal, and (4) chemical, although there is overlap in terms of this classification.[74] Cephalic influences comprise vagally mediated responses which are dictated by the CNS (e.g., the smell of food). Gastric responses are local responses to the presence of food in the stomach. Intestinal influences result from the products of digestion entering the small intestine, via reflex arcs, and are hormonally mediated. Finally, chemical responses include the effects of alcohol, caffeine, and other substances that seem to have a direct effect on the gastric mucosa. Hyperactivity of any of these influences can lead to hypersecretion, gastric ulceration, and mucosal bleeding.

5. Exocrine Pancreas

Pancreatic juice is highly alkaline, and secretions of the exocrine pancreas are regulated primarily by secretin, CCK, and intestinal reflex mechanisms. By the time chyme reaches the jejunum, it has been neutralized by pancreatic, biliary, and intestinal secretions. The turnover of pancreatic fluid is enormous and can exceed several liters per day.[75] Normal pancreatic juice contains multiple cations, anions, digestive enzymes and proenzymes, albumin, and globulin.[76] Many protein-digesting enzymes liberated by the pancreas would destroy the pancreas itself, indicating the need for a very tightly regulated feedback system. For example, the pancreas contains trypsin inhibitors. In addition,

pancreatic juice contains phospholipase C, an enzyme that destroys lecithin, a principal component of cell membranes.[77] It is thought that the release of this substance leads to parenchymal destruction in patients with acute pancreatitis.

6. Hepatic and Biliary System

Diseases, function, and regulation of the hepatic and biliary system are reviewed in Chapter 6.

7. Small Intestine

The small intestine is the location of the majority of the products of digestion. About 9 L/day of fluid passes via the small intestine, of which 7 L is secretory in nature, but only 1 L is finally excreted in the stool.[78] The small intestine is therefore very long (approximately 25 feet in the typical adult), and its absorptive area is increased about 600 times (as compared with a cylindrical tube of equal length and diameter) by the presence of villi.[79]

Turnover in the small intestine is immense. About 20 billion cells are normally sloughed into the lumen each day, and each mucosal cell lives, on average, only 2 to 5 days.[80] Because mucosal cells proliferate so rapidly, they are among the most easily destroyed by antiproliferative agents, and GI distress is a common symptom in patients undergoing chemotherapy.

Two types of contractions are found in the small intestine: peristaltic and segmental. Peristaltic movements propel chyme toward the colon and occur in response to stretching of the lumen. Segmental contractions are circumferential and serve to increase the efficiency of digestion by exposing more chyme to mucosal surfaces. Both types of movement occur in the absence of external innervation. In mechanical bowel obstruction, peristaltic rushes occur, which are exaggerated contractions associated with hypersecretion and severe cramping pain. In adynamic ileus, these do not manifest; thus, abdominal pain is characteristically absent.

Vagal stimulation and GI hormones (e.g., VIP) dramatically increase secretion of the alkaline mucus that characterizes the small intestine. This mucus is produced largely by Brunner's glands, which help to protect the intestinal lining from gastric acidity.[81] In addition, large amounts of bicarbonate are produced by the intestinal mucosa, independent of Brunner's glands.

As many as half of the small intestine may be removed without consequence, as hyperplasia and hypertrophy of the remaining intestine occurs readily; however, certain areas are crucial for specific element absorption (e.g., the terminal ileum for vitamin B_{12}). Indeed, terminal small intestine resections are generally tolerated more poorly than proximal ones. If more than half of the intestine is removed, the malabsorption syndrome results, which may manifest as steatorrhea, deficiency of fat-soluble vitamins (A, D, E, K), hypocalcemia, hyperuricemia, and possibly cirrhosis due to fatty infiltration of the liver.[82]

8. Large Intestine

The principal function of the colon is the absorption of water, sodium, and minerals. It effectively removes at least 90 per cent of the fluid presented to it, leaving only about 250 mL of water in the stool per day.[83] Sodium is actively absorbed from the lumen of the colon, and water follows passively along its concentration gradient. There is also active secretion of potassium and bicarbonate ions into the lumen. Because the absorptive capacity of the colon is so high, the rectal medication route is practical for drug delivery. Finally, despite the importance of the colon in water resorption, humans can survive indefinitely following total colectomy, provided that fluid and electrolyte balance is carefully maintained.

The entry of chyme into the colon occurs through the ileocecal valve. Sympathetic stimulation increases the tone of the valve, whereas parasympathetic stimuli (vagally mediated) relax the valve, allowing for passage of chyme. As in the small intestine, both segmental and peristaltic contractions occur in the colon; however, mass action transport, a third form of motor activity, only occurs in the large bowel. In this type of motion, there is sustained and simultaneous contraction over large areas of the colon, which serves to make defecation rapid. Hormonal and neural activity only minimally affect the secretion of mucus by colonic epithelial cells. Moreover, no digestive enzymes are secreted into the lumen of the large intestine, as digestion is normally complete by this stage, except in pathologic conditions.

Although at birth the colon is sterile, in adults it contains a very large mass of bacteria, the principal species being *Escherichia coli, Enterobacter aerogenes, Streptococcus,* and *Bacteroides fragilis.*[84] Nearly all are pathogenic when they exceed the confines of the colon, as after perforation; however, some important vitamins are synthesized by colonic flora, such as B_{12} and vitamin K, and deficiency may occur if the colon is sterilized by the use of powerful broad-spectrum antibiotics. Ammonia, a product of protein metabolism, is produced in the colon by the action of bacteria. In patients with coexisting hepatic disease, hyperammonemia and encephalopathy can occur. However, resection of part of the colon improves symptoms only transiently, as the flora soon colonize the ileum. Nevertheless, oral neomycin is effective in hepatic encephalopathy, as it destroys many of the organisms in the gut and thus decreases the synthesis of ammonia. Oral lactulose leads to osmotic diarrhea and, so, decreases the time available for ammonia absorption.

F. ASSESSMENT OF NUTRITIONAL STATUS

1. Nutritional Assessment

In general, the goals of nutritional assessment are (1) to identify malnourished patients and those at risk and (2) to determine the efficacy of nutritional support. Nutritional status may be determined by history, physical examination, anthropometrics, and special tests. From the perspective of the anesthesiologist, the parameters selected to assess a patient's nutritional status should be realistically chosen and related to decisions that could alter management. History and physical exam are the most useful tools for the identification of a malnourished patient. A history of decreased food or water intake, emesis, and weight loss are the strongest indicators of nutritional compromise. Physical examination should pay special attention to decreased mobility, depletion of fat, muscle wasting, edema, cheilosis, and glossitis.

Anthropometric measures include weight, height, frame size, arm muscle circumference (AMC), and the triceps skinfold (TSF).[85] In addition, specific laboratory tests are employed that can also have prognostic value. These include measurement of visceral proteins (albumin, prealbumin, transferrin, retinol), creatinine-height index, total lymphocyte count, and delayed cutaneous hypersensitivity.[86] The relationship between these parameters and nutritional status is beyond the scope of this discussion, but it should be noted that they are useful in terms of overall nutritional assessment.

2. Consequences of Malnutrition

The implications of malnutrition extend to all organ systems. In general, and depending on the severity of the condition, there is significant deterioration of the functional status of the organism. Unlike fats and carbohydrates, there are no protein stores in the body; therefore, all existing protein serves some function and its loss has some consequence. In starvation, loss of muscle mass may lead to respiratory malfunction (due to loss of intercostal and diaphragmatic muscle strength), and even cardiac muscle atrophy leading to heart failure.[87] Indeed, bronchopneumonia is typically the preterminal event in severely malnourished patients.

The loss of skeletal muscle in starvation is about 30 times higher than the loss of visceral protein; ultimately, however, visceral sources are depleted also. Serum albumin is often regarded as a good measure of visceral protein status, and is easily measured. The consequences associated with hypoalbuminemia are diverse, and include decreased gastric emptying, intestinal ileus, decreased GI absorption of nutrients and medications, and altered resorption of electrolytes and water.[88] The distribution of body water is greatly affected in hypoalbuminemic states, which may manifest as edema and ascites and may impair ventilation and circulation. Finally, decreased albumin is strongly correlated with poor wound healing, decreased B- and T-cell–mediated immune function, and increased susceptibility to infections.[89] Ultimately, all these factors lead toward greatly increased morbidity and mortality in malnourished surgical patients.

II. SPECIFIC DISORDERS OF NUTRITION

A. PROTEIN-ENERGY MALNUTRITION

Protein-energy malnutrition (PEM) results when the requirements for protein, energy sources, or both are not met by the diet or owing to malabsorption. The spectrum of PEM includes three disease states that are subjectively characterized by their clinical presentation. These are kwashiorkor, marasmus, and marasmic kwashiorkor—described below.[90] All three disease states are characterized by markedly decreased physical strength and muscular endurance far exceeding that which would be expected from the degree of weight loss alone. Indeed, the most frequent terminal event in PEM is pneumonia, which results largely from inability to inspire deeply, cough, and clear secretions.[91] Thus, prolonged respiratory support may be necessary following general anesthesia until strength returns following adequate nutrition.

1. Kwashiorkor

Kwashiorkor was originally named by the Ga tribe in Ghana to describe a disease seen in older children suffering PEM. It is predominantly a protein deficiency that is disproportionate to calorie intake, which is also low. Edema is present and is accompanied by hypoalbuminemia, loss of lean body mass and often hepatomegaly, dyspigmentation of the skin and hair, and psychological disorders.[92] Anesthetic implications include hepatic and cardiac dysfunction (due to fatty infiltration and myocardial contractile protein catabolism, respectively), and the global consequences of edema resulting from hypoalbuminemia.

2. Marasmus

Marasmus is predominantly an energy deficiency. The clinical presentation may be impressive and includes a marked loss of weight and height. Seen most commonly in infants in geographic areas of malnutrition, the typical patient presents with a large-appearing head, staring eyes, and diminished trunk, limbs, and buttocks.[93] The significantly increased head size in proportion to the body may lead to difficulty in head positioning during laryngoscopy.

3. Combined Marasmus and Kwashiorkor

Marasmic kwashiorkor has clinical characteristics of marasmus and kwashiorkor.

Edema and lean body atrophy occur, accompanied by decreased growth rate, skin and hair pigmentary changes, psychological changes, and fatty infiltration of the liver with resultant hepatic synthetic dysfunction.[94]

B. NUTRIENT DEFICIENCIES

In general, deficiency of a nutrient may be due to (1) decreased intake, (2) decreased absorption, (3) decreased storage, (4) increased excretion, or (5) increased utilization of the nutrient. Important clinical consequences, such as anemia and bone disease, may result from deficiencies of vitamins, minerals, and other nutrients. Common deficiency syndromes (e.g., iron deficiency) have been excluded from the following discussion, for which numerous detailed references are available. Inadequate intake is the most common cause of nutrient deficiency, even in Western society. Adequate dietary intake is most important for those substances whose body stores are small, particularly folic acid, water-soluble vitamins (B complex and C), and protein. Nutrient deficiencies are most common in syndromes associated with a decreased mucosal surface leading to malabsorption, including short gut syndrome, celiac sprue, and Whipple's disease. Malabsorption of specific nutrients may also be due to the use of medications (e.g., cholestyramine, neomycin, sulfasalazine, antacids, colchicine) and should be anticipated and prevented, if possible.

Increased nutrient loss can occur without malabsorption. Common causes include diarrhea, enterocutaneous fistulas, emesis, and prolonged gastric suctioning. Chronic excessive bleeding (e.g., menses or GI) leads to iron deficiency. Excessive loss of nutrients in the urine is an important cause of nutrient deficiency (e.g., magnesium and zinc during severe illness). Sustained diaphoresis can lead to trace mineral loss, in addition to depleting sodium, potassium, chloride, and water. Increased utilization of nutrients occurs during illness, pregnancy, and lactation. In severely catabolic states, including sepsis, trauma, and burns, nutritional requirements may double owing to increased proliferation of phagocytes, leukocytes, fibroblasts, and other cells associated with stress, immune, and wound healing responses.

1. Trace Mineral Deficiencies

Approximately 15 trace minerals have been described as essential to the human diet.[95] With the exception of iron, these deficiencies are seldom diagnosed because they are exceedingly rare. Indeed, the majority of these syndromes are identified only in patients who have been on total parenteral nutrition (TPN) for prolonged periods. In current clinical practice, TPN is usually supplemented with trace minerals, including zinc, copper, chromium, manganese, molybdenum, iodine, and selenium, in hopes of preventing these rare deficiencies, which may be challenging to diagnose.

a. Chromium Deficiency

Chromium is known to affect lipoprotein metabolism and to potentiate the action of insulin at the cellular level.[96] In food it exists as a complex known historically as the *glucose tolerance factor.*[97] Following large intestine resections, in patients with prolonged TPN, chromium deficiency has been described.[98] The clinical presentation includes insensitivity to exogenous insulin with hyperglycemia, encephalopathy, peripheral neuropathy, and weight loss. Determination of deficiency is challenging because serum levels do not correlate with total body stores. Indeed, the best test may be improvement of glucose tolerance and peripheral neuropathy after dietary supplementation for 2 weeks.[99] It is not known if regional anesthesia exacerbates the neuropathy associated with chromium deficiency; thus it may be prudent to avoid it. The peripheral neuropathy is generally reversible with dietary supplementation.

b. Copper Deficiency

Cytochrome C, superoxide dismutase, ceruloplasmin, monoamine oxidase, and several other organometallic enzymes require copper to function. It is essential for normal skeletal and CNS development, leukocyte proliferation, erythropoiesis, iron absorption, and antioxidant formation.[100] In adults, copper deficiency generally occurs only in those receiving prolonged TPN without copper supplementation and in patients who chronically take metal chelators (e.g., D-penicillamine) or large doses of zinc or iron (which inhibit copper absorption).[101] In premature or malnourished infants, copper deficiency also can occur and may be due to Menkes's syndrome, resulting from a genetic defect in copper absorption.[102]

Laboratory diagnosis of copper deficiency is difficult because serum levels poorly reflect total body stores. Clinical manifestations of copper deficiency include hypochromic microcytic anemia, recurrent infections due to neutropenia and leukopenia, and skeletal anomalies similar to those seen in scurvy. The diagnosis is frequently made when anemia fails to correct with iron therapy but subsequently does with copper administration.[103] Anesthetic implications include those associated with anemia, skeletal anomalies, and increased susceptibility to infection.

c. Fluoride Deficiency

Fluoride is essential for normal development, reproduction, and the intestinal absorption of iron.[104] In Western societies, the major source is supplemented drinking water. A low intake is associated with an increased incidence of dental caries—and possibly increased risk of developing osteoporosis. Serious fluoride deficiency syndromes have not been described in humans, including those receiving prolonged TPN to which fluoride has not been added.

d. Iodine Deficiency

Iodine is an essential component of the thyroid hormones triiodothyroninine (T_3) and tetraiodothyronine (T_4). Although rare in Western societies, iodine deficiency continues to be a major problem worldwide, most commonly owing to inadequate dietary intake. It manifests as hypothyroidism, with thyroid hyperplasia and hypertrophy (goiter). Iodine status is best determined with thyroid function tests, including serum T_3, T_3 resin uptake (T_3RU), and thyrotropin (TSH) levels.[105] Iodine deficiency has not been reported in those on long-term TPN, even without iodine supplementation. Anesthetic implications are predominantly those related to hypothyroidism (e.g., lack of response to exogenous catecholamines, weight gain, autonomic instability) and goiter (e.g., difficult intubation).

e. Manganese Deficiency/Excess

Manganese (not to be confused with magnesium) is a cofactor in superoxide dismutase and pyruvate decarboxylase.[106] Manganese deficiency has been shown to exist in animals but its existence is controversial in humans. It is postulated that manganese deficiency may present as nausea, dermatitis, hypocholesterolemia, hair color changes, and symptoms typically associated with vitamin K deficiency (e.g., coagulopathy) based on a single case report.[107] Manganese excess may also be deleterious. A recent case report suggested possible manganese toxicity resulting in psychiatric symptoms and cholestatic jaundice in a patient on TPN with excessive manganese supplementation.[108]

f. Magnesium Deficiency

Magnesium is crucial for many enzymatic functions, maintenance of normal growth, phagocytosis and wound healing, neuromuscular transmission, cardiac contractility and conduction, and coagulation.[109] Deficiency of this nutrient is usually the result of decreased dietary absorption, especially in those with extensive small bowel resections. In addition, medications may promote renal losses, including diuretics, aminoglycosides, cyclosporin, amphotericin B, cisplatin, and digoxin.[110]

Deficiency of magnesium may manifest as muscle weakness, tremors of the extremities and tongue, ataxia, tetany, dysrhythmias (especially ventricular), hypotension, coma, and cardiac arrest.[111] Psychiatric disturbances may also result, including depression, delirium, and psychosis.[112] In summary, the major anesthetic implications of magnesium deficiency are serious cardiac disturbances, hemodynamic instability, coagulopathy, and neuromuscular weakness.[112] As magnesium may be administered intravenously and relatively rapidly, only in the most dire of circumstances should replacement therapy not be instituted prior to anesthesia.

g. Molybdenum Deficiency

Molybdenum is a key component of oxidases and is necessary for the metabolism of purines and sulfur-containing proteins. The use of serum molybdenum is an unreliable marker of total body deficiency, and some have argued for the measurement of xanthine oxidase and sulfite oxidase enzyme activity as surrogate markers. Molybdenum deficiency may result from prolonged parenteral nutrition without supplementation, manifesting as tachycardia, tachypnea, headache, night blindness, emesis, lethargy, and coma.[113] High serum levels of methionine and nearly indetectable levels of uric acid may also accompany molybdenum deficiency.

h. Selenium Deficiency

Selenium is an essential component of glutathione peroxidase, an enzyme that protects against peroxide tissue damage. Indeed, selenium is an antioxidant much like vitamin E. Selenium stores can be reliably estimated by serum, erythrocyte, or leukocyte level measurements.[114] In the United States, selenium deficiency is uncommon, but in China (where selenium content of the soil is low), it has been reported.[115] The principal manifestation of selenium deficiency is dilated cardiomyopathy, also known as Keshan disease. In patients receiving long-term TPN without selenium supplementation, myositis, muscular weakness, and cardiomyopathy have been described.[116]

i. Zinc Deficiency

Zinc is a cofactor for enzymes necessary for carbohydrate, fat, and protein metabolism. It is required for proper cell division, sexual maturation, reproduction, night vision, wound healing, and immune function.[117] Unlike other trace elements, zinc deficiency may be more common than is appreciated. In fact, even in the United States, inadequate dietary zinc may be responsible for childhood growth retardation.[118] Zinc deficiency may also be due to decreased intestinal absorption, even if dietary intake is adequate (e.g., in Crohn's disease, short gut syndrome, pancreatic insufficiency, or chronic diarrhea). Clinical manifestations of zinc deficiency are numerous and include growth retardation, scaly skin lesions, alopecia, diarrhea, night blindness, and poor wound healing. The skin rash in acute deficiency manifests principally around the mouth, nose, and groin.[119] Like many other trace elements, zinc serum levels correlate poorly with total body stores.

2. Fat-Soluble Vitamin Deficiencies

a. Vitamin A Deficiency

Vitamin A is a term used to denote retinol derivatives that are biologically active. Vitamin A is necessary for growth and differentiation of epithelial cells, stability of cell membranes, reproduction, and night vision.[120] Beta carotenes are precursors to vitamin A compounds and also function as antioxidants. Vitamin A deficiency is usually due to fat malabsorption, since it is fat soluble. It takes about 2 years for liver stores of vitamin A to be depleted, but in cirrhotics this can occur. Furthermore, worldwide it is estimated that 1 million people per year develop corneal disease due to vitamin A deficiency. The clinical symptoms of inadequate vitamin A stores are night blindness, dry eyes, follicular hyperkeratosis, altered taste and smell, increased cerebrospinal fluid pressure, and increased skin infections.[121] Therefore, one should probably avoid spinal neuraxial blockade if deficiency is suspected or is severe. Diagnosis may be confirmed by measurement of the serum beta carotene level.

b. Vitamin D Deficiency

Vitamin D is a broad term used to describe a class of sterols that prevent rickets, of which cholecalciferol (D_3) and ergocalciferol (D_2) are the most important.[122] Vitamin D, in conjunction with parathyroid hormone and calcitonin, regulates calcium homeostasis in humans. Vitamin D deficiency in children is almost nonexistent in the United States since milk is now fortified by most processors. Even if dairy products are minimally consumed, exposure to sunlight in adequate amounts can prevent vitamin D deficiency. Inadequate sun exposure may be seen in elderly patients, however, and may be responsible for a high incidence of bone fractures. Vitamin D deficiency may also been seen in patients with fat malabsorption, severe hepatic or renal disease, or following removal of large segments of the small intestine. Clinical manifestations of vitamin D deficiency are hypocalcemia, hypophosphatemia, and bone demineralization leading to rickets or osteomalacia.[123] Hypocalcemia may lead to cardiac rhythm disturbances, laryngospasm, and tetany, all of which may be life threatening. Abuse of vitamin D supplements is associated with hypercalcemia, hypercalciuria, and renal failure, which may be irreversible.

c. Vitamin E Deficiency

Vitamin E collectively refers to two fat-soluble substances: tocopherols and tocotrienes.

The principal function of vitamin E is as a free radical scavenger and antioxidant, and it is complementary to selenium in this regard.[124] Vitamin E deficiency is well-characterized in animals but not in humans. Premature infants are most at risk owing to poor GI absorption. Because vitamin E is fat soluble, deficiency may occur in those with cystic fibrosis, cirrhosis, biliary obstruction, steatorrhea, or secondary due to excessive mineral oil intake. Clinical manifestations of vitamin E deficiency include spinal cord and medulla degeneration associated with areflexia, gait disturbance, paresis of gaze, and loss of proprioception. In addition, erythrocyte hemolysis may occur, owing to increased red cell fragility.[125]

d. Vitamin K Deficiency

Total body stores of vitamin K are small, and turnover is rapid. Therefore, daily absorption of at least 1 μg/kg is necessary to prevent deficiency.[126] After intestinal absorption, vitamin K is taken up by the liver, where it is a required cofactor for the synthesis of coagulation cascade cofactors II, VII, IX, and X as well as other proteins involved in coagulation and fibrinolysis. Prolongation of the prothrombin time (and in severe deficiency, the partial thromboplastin time), which is correctable by vitamin K administration, is the primary clinical manifestation of deficiency. This is most commonly noted in critically ill patients who have been on broad-spectrum antibiotics that prevent vitamin K synthesis by colonic flora. In fact, healthy persons fed a vitamin K–deficient diet do not develop coagulopathy unless bowel-sterilizing antibiotics are administered concurrently.[127]

3. Water-Soluble Vitamin Deficiencies

a. Thiamine (B₁) Deficiency

Thiamine plays a key role in the function of numerous enzyme systems responsible for energy production. Thiamine deficiency is called *beriberi,* and while rare in the United States, occurs throughout the world where polished rice is a predominant source of food. In the United States, thiamine deficiency occurs primarily in alcoholics, in patients with severe malnutrition, those on chronic dialysis, or those with sepsis and prolonged pyrexia.[128]

The diagnosis of thiamine deficiency is made either by response to exogenous administration or by measurement of erythrocyte transketolase activity in vitro.[129]

The clinical manifestations of beriberi include easy fatigability, muscular weakness, paresthesias, and high-output congestive heart failure (owing to increased demands of the peripheral tissues).[129] Weakness and paresthesias are predominantly in the lower extremities. In severe thiamine deficiency, cerebellar degeneration, Wernicke's encephalopathy, and necrotizing encephalomyelopathy can occur. Wernicke's encephalopathy is characterized by delirium, weakness, photophobia, nystagmus, extraocular muscle paralysis, and ataxia.[129] Since congestive heart failure in beriberi is of the high-output type, therapy should be directed toward reducing total body oxygen consumption to decrease the work of the heart (e.g., antipyretics, sedation, paralysis). The presence of delirium may place patients at risk for aspiration, and weakness may contribute to respiratory failure.

b. Riboflavin (B₂) Deficiency

Flavin adenine dinucleotide (FAD) and flavin mononucleotide are essential coenzymes involved in host energetics, of which riboflavin is an essential component. Deficiency is typically seen in association with other B-complex deficiencies (e.g., as in alcoholics or with malabsorption syndromes). The clinical presentation includes a characteristic stomatitis with fissuring of the angle of the mouth, inflammation of the lips, glossitis, dermatitis with itching, and decreased vision.[130] Clinical diagnostic tests are rarely used, and therapy in suspected cases is usually started empirically; however, response to treatment may require several weeks.

c. Niacin (B₃) Deficiency

Niacin includes nicotinic acid and nicotinamide, also called niacinamide. Niacin is a key component of NAD and NADPH, two essential coenzymes involved in human energetics. Niacin deficiency does not occur unless there is a simultaneous deficiency of tryptophan, an essential amino acid.[131] Niacin deficiency is also termed *pellagra* and occurs mainly in alcoholics, those with severe malabsorption, and as a manifestation of carcinoid syndrome. In carcinoid syndrome, the tumor utilizes large amounts of tryptophan to synthesize serotonin. Finally, in Hartnup's disease, niacin deficiency may be due to a defect in tryptophan absorption.[132]

d. Pyridoxine (B$_6$) Deficiency

Pyridoxine comprises three compounds: pyridoxine, pyridoxal, and pyridoxamine, which are important components in transaminases and decarboxylases. Pyridoxine is also essential in the synthesis of porphyrin, arachidonic acid, bile acids, and the neurotransmitter acetylcholine. Deficiency is very rare in humans and occurs in alcoholics, with severe malabsorption, or as a consequence of therapy with isoniazid, hydralazine, and penicillamine.[133] The clinical presentation associated with deficiency includes peripheral neuropathy, periocular dermatitis, glossitis, angular stomatitis, sideroblastic anemia, and seizures. The diagnosis can be established by measurement of plasma pyridoxal phosphate, but therapy is usually empiric, as are most B-complex deficiencies. (Because of the water-soluble nature of B-complex and C vitamins, overdose is rarely a concern.) It should be kept in mind that pyridoxine deficiency usually occurs with other B-complex deficiencies.

e. Folate Deficiency

Deficiency of folate leads to megaloblastic anemia, which decreases oxygen-carrying capacity and alters the dynamics of microcirculatory blood flow. There is also an increased incidence of neural tube defects among children whose mothers are folate deficient during pregnancy.[134] Several drugs, including the chemotherapeutic agent methotrexate, the antimalarial pyrimethamine, trimethoprim, and triamterene inhibit the dihydrofolate reductase, the enzyme that converts dietary folate to the active tetrahydrofolate.[135] Sulfasalazine, phenytoin, and carbamazepine may also reduce folate levels by various mechanisms, leading to megaloblastic anemia in patients taking these medications. Finally, folate deficiency is common among malnourished alcoholics.

f. Cobalamin (B$_{12}$) Deficiency

Cobalamin is a generic term for all cobalamin species, including vitamin B$_{12}$ (cyanocobalamin).[136] Human dietary cobalamin requirements are met by the consumption of meats and eggs; however, cobalamin stores are approximately 3000 times the daily intake of cobalamin, so deficiency is generally seen only in strict vegetarians after years of inadequate intake.[137] B$_{12}$ deficiency leads to pernicious anemia (a megaloblastic anemia).

Intrinsic factor, secreted by the parietal cells of the stomach, is required for cyanocobalamin binding and absorption in the terminal ileum. The differential diagnosis of cobalamin deficiency is large and includes absence of intrinsic factor (e.g., after total gastrectomy or congenitally), inadequate release of food-bound cobalamin (due to histamine H$_2$ blockers), pancreatic exocrine insufficiency, Zollinger-Ellison syndrome, *Diphyllobothrium latum* (fish tapeworm) infection, ileal resection or bypass, abnormal ileal mucosa (HIV, celiac sprue, Crohn's disease), drugs (paraaminosalicylates, biguanide), and congenital defects in transileal transport (Imerslund-Graesbeck syndrome, congenital transcobalamin II deficiency).[138]

g. Vitamin C Deficiency (Scurvy)

Vitamin C (ascorbic acid) is an essential cofactor in hydroxylation reactions related to the synthesis of collagen, the principal component of connective tissue. Vitamin C deficiency (scurvy) develops after 2 to 3 months of dietary lack. Historically, scurvy was a common cause of death in sailors long at sea without perishable fruits and vegetables. In Western society, scurvy is seen only in alcoholism, Crohn's disease, severe malabsorption syndromes, and certain food faddisms. Initial symptoms of scurvy include weakness, irritability, myalgias, and weight loss. Subsequently, hyperkeratotic lesions and petechiae appear on the buttocks and lower extremities. With advanced disease, the gingivae become swollen, erythematous, and friable with hemorrhaging. Tooth loss is common. The muscles and skin may also hemorrhage. Although overt manifestations of scurvy are rare, in the critically ill, vitamin C deficiency is probably not uncommon.[139] It may be diagnosed by measurement of red cell or leukocyte ascorbic acid or response to empiric therapy (which is benign).

4. Deficiencies of Other Nutrients

a. Biotin Deficiency

Biotin is a cofactor in carboxylase enzymes in the body. Dietary deficiency is very rare, and seen only in those who consume excessive egg whites, which contain the biotin-binding protein avidin. Historically, biotin deficiency has also been reported in patients on prolonged TPN, but biotin is now a component of parenteral nutrition solutions.[140] The clinical symptoms associated with biotin deficiency include nausea, vomiting, anorexia, weight loss, alopecia, dermatitis, depression, and metabolic acidosis.[141] The diagnosis is usually made following empiric therapy.

b. Essential Fatty Acid Deficiency

By definition, essential fatty acids (EFA) cannot be synthesized by humans and must be provided by the diet. EFAs are precursors of the eicosanoids (e.g., prostaglandins, leukotrienes, prostacyclins) and key components of cell membranes. They are also important regulators of cholesterol transport.[142] The EFAs are linoleic acid and linolenic acid. EFA deficiency is seen only in patients receiving long-term fat-free TPN. It may develop with less than 10 days of continuous feeding, because those on TPN have elevated insulin levels, which is thought to inhibit the release of stores of EFAs in adipose tissue.[143] Clinical signs include scaly dermatitis of the lower extremities, axilla, and groin, alopecia, hepatomegaly, thrombocytopenia, diarrhea, infantile growth retardation, and diarrhea. EFA deficiency can be clinically indistinguishable from zinc deficiency.

c. Essential Amino Acid Deficiency

There are eight essential amino acids, from which all 20 may be subsequently synthesized: phenylalanine, valine, tryptophan, threonine, leucine, isoleucine, lysine, and methionine. If even a single essential amino acid is absent from the diet, protein cannot be synthesized de novo, negative nitrogen balance occurs, and the organism will die, regardless of total calorie intake. For this reason, essential amino acid deficiency syndromes are generally clinically synonymous with those associated with prolonged starvation.

5. Complications of Prolonged Total Parenteral Nutrition

Metabolic derangements are common in those on prolonged TPN. The most common problems are hyperglycemia, hypophosphatemia, and hypokalemia. In general, these are avoidable by frequent monitoring of patients on such therapy. However, dangerous levels of virtually all substances contained in TPN solutions have been reported to date. Less common complications of prolonged TPN include hypomagnesemia, hyponatremia, fluid overload, dehydration, hypoglycemia, hypercalcemia, fat intolerance, and liver dysfunction, steatosis, and calculous and acalculous cholecystitis.[144]

6. Gastrointestinal Bypass Operations

a. General Considerations

Most GI bypass procedures are performed in those with morbid obesity refractory to medical therapy, diet, and excercise. Morbid obesity generally is defined as three times ideal body weight according to population tables, with the weight remaining this elevated for several years. In general, surgery is restricted to those who have met the criteria for morbid obesity, have had all organic causes excluded, are free of psychiatric illness, are generally less than 50 years of age, and have tried dietary and exercise therapy without much success despite their motivation. The anesthetic implications associated with morbid obesity are profound (e.g., pulmonary hypertension, sleep apnea, chronic hypoxemia, congestive heart failure, and myocardial ischemia) and are described in detail in standard textbooks.[145]

b. Intestinal Bypass

Various strategies have been used in intestinal bypass procedures. The overall strategy tries to preserve the preferential absorptive capacity of the upper small bowel along with the fat and enterohepatic recirculation functions of the distal ileum, while bypassing enough of the absorptive area of the gut to allow for weight loss. Anchoring of structures is important to prevent postsurgical intussusception. In most surgical operations, panniculectomy and cholecystectomy are added to the procedure to eliminate the risk of postoperative cholecystitis, a potential problem. Because of the poor health of morbidly obese persons, complications are frequent postoperatively and include deep venous thrombosis, pulmonary embolism, coronary thrombosis, wound dehiscence, and peritonitis.

Patients are told they can expect to lose one third of preoperative weight, which steadily decreases for about 3 months after surgery until remaining bowel elongates and hypertrophies to compensate. Postoperative steatorrhea, diarrhea, and excessive weight loss are possible complications of surgery; however, they are usually manageable by medical therapy (e.g., diphenoxylate, paregoric, fat restriction, and medium-chain triglycerides). The most serious metabolic derangement following bypass procedures is hepatic fatty infiltration, which occurs in 60 to 90 per cent of patients.[146] Five per cent of patients may go into liver failure, necessitating reversal of the bypass procedure, if possible.[146] Liver failure in these cases is characterized by jaundice, coagulopathy, hypoprothrombinemia, edema, hypoalbuminemia, anorexia, and elevation of liver enzymes. There are also associated B_{12}, potassium, calcium, and magnesium deficiencies, as well as peptic ulceration, alopecia, calcium oxalate urolithiasis, and bypass enteritis secondary to bacterial overgrowth due to changes in pH.[146] Finally, altered GI anatomy predisposes to complications such as hernia, volvulus, and intussusception. Clearly, intestinal surgical bypass is a high-risk procedure.

c. Gastric Bypass

The high risks of intestinal bypass have led most surgeons to abandon the procedure, and gastric bypass, partition, or stapling is now the most commonly performed surgery for morbid obesity.[147] In a common technique, the proximal 10 per cent of the stomach is anastomosed to a Roux-en-Y limb of jejunum with a very small opening. Diarrhea is much less common with gastric operations, but nausea and vomiting are still frequent. Patients with gastric bypass do not seem to experience hepatic failure that is associated with intestinal bypass operations. Nevertheless, all the potential complications associated with morbid obesity, as already described, should still be anticipated.

d. Bypass for Hyperlipidemia

Nonobese patients with hyperlipidemia and atherosclerosis are candidates for ileal surgery in which the distal third of the small bowel is bypassed. This increases the loss of normally absorbed cholesterol and reduces the bile salt pool. Reductions in serum cholesterol up to 40 per cent have been described. Candidates are patients who do not respond to cholesterol-lowering medications, diet, or anion exchange resins. The success of the procedure is remarkable, in that regression of xanthelasma, and occasionally angina, claudication, and atherosclerosis has been reported.[148] The procedure is indicated in symptomatic patients with type III and IV hyperlipoproteinemias and a positive family history.[148] Despite the success of the procedure, operative morbidity remains high, as patients frequently have preexisting coronary and peripheral arteriosclerosis.

7. Systemic Diseases with Gastrointestinal Manifestations and Nutrient Deficiencies

a. Gastrointestinal Sarcoidosis

Although sarcoidosis of the GI tract is rare, the stomach is the most commonly affected organ. In addition, the esophagus, small bowel, and occasionally the colon, can be involved. Complications that have been reported include hemorrhage, obstruction, appendicitis, and protein-wasting enteropathy. Granulomas of the bowel may occur, and resemble Crohn's disease or Whipple's disease. GI sarcoidosis may also be associated with ascites and perforated appendicitis.[149, 150] It should be kept in mind that sarcoidosis may involve multiple organ systems, and these effects should be sought even if the primary presenting lesion or dysfunction is gastrointestinal. For example, sarcoidosis can lead to hepatic, myocardial, pulmonary, and marrow failure, all of which have immense anesthetic implications. These are discussed in greater detail in other chapters.

b. Progressive Systemic Sclerosis (Scleroderma)

Scleroderma (also called *progressive systemic sclerosis*) is a connective tissue disorder that manifests as systemic infiltration of all organ systems by fibrotic tissue. The cause is unknown, and there is no specific treatment; however, some patients with scleroderma are dependent on total parenteral nutrition owing to diffuse fibrosis of the alimentary tract. If such patients present for surgery, it should be kept in mind that the disease process is systemic and may involve multiple crucial organ systems, including the heart and lungs. Furthermore, patients may be at risk for complications of prolonged TPN (see previous sections). Scleroderma is discussed in detail in Chapter 11.

III. REGIONAL ANATOMIC DISORDERS

A. DISORDERS OF THE MOUTH

1. Temporomandibular Joint Syndrome

In general, temporomandibular joint (TMJ) syndrome is due to either "true" ankylosis of the joint or "false" ankylosis (e.g., from burns, trauma, radiation, or surgery). True ankylosis of the TMJ is most commonly seen in patients with rheumatoid arthritis, in which case immune complexes are deposited in the joint, leading to inflammation.[151] In patients following traumatic injury to the TMJ or who have an infection of the mouth or oral cavity, pain may be the limiting factor in mouth opening. The cause is crucial to ascertain because, once the patient is anesthetized or paralyzed, pain will not prevent mouth opening but joint dysfunction will, and intubation may be difficult. In some cases, forward pressure on the mandibular angle may allow for increased mouth opening and should be attempted if difficulty arises.

2. Xerostomia

Xerostomia is the symptom of decreased or absent saliva production in the oral cavity. It is commonly the result of anticholinergic medications, including antidepressants, antihypertensives, and antipsychotic medications. Other causes include nerve damage to salivary glands, diminished afferent input, salivary gland destruction (e.g., Sjögren's disease), or ductal stenosis (e.g., sialadenitis due to amyloidosis).[152] Head and neck radiation also damages salivary glands and can lead to xerostomia, which is irreversible. Xerostomia has many deleterious effects, including altered taste sensation, inadequate digestion of food, and increased dental caries. When the

condition is severe, malnutrition, depression, and weight loss can occur. Finally, there is an increased incidence of oral candidiasis and opportunistic infections of the GI tract, as saliva contains protective antimicrobial substances such as lysozyme. Also, saliva is a key component of mucosal tissue integrity, and its loss can lead to ulceration of membranes.

B. DISORDERS OF THE ESOPHAGUS

1. General Considerations

Of particular importance in patients with diseases of the esophagus is the presence of chronic malnutrition due to tumor obstruction of food passage or radiation changes. Esophageal perforations may occur if the esophageal wall is weakened, allowing contents to spill into the mediastinum and pleural space. Tumors, foreign bodies, severe vomiting, ulceration, and toxins all can cause this. Following perforation, mediastinitis or empyema may occur, both of which are associated with extremely poor prognosis. Mediastinitis in particular can lead to emphysema, pneumonitis, pericarditis, and tension mediastinum or tension pneumothorax. Cardiac and respiratory failure may ensue. Preparation for anesthesia must consider antibiotic therapy, drainage of pus and secretions, and cardiorespiratory optimization if possible.

Esophageal tumors may extend directly into the airways or bronchi, and this must be considered before induction of anesthesia. In such cases, fiberoptic bronchoscopy must be considered before intubation. If the mass is friable, manipulation may lead to profuse bleeding, which can be catastrophic if it occurs in the airway.

2. Esophageal Diverticula

In general, diverticula of the esophagus are classified by their site—pharyngoesophageal, thoracic, or supradiaphragmatic.

a. Zenker's or Pharyngoesophageal Diverticula (Pulsion). These outpouchings are due to protrusion of the pharyngeal mucosa posteriorly, between the inferior pharyngeal constrictor muscle and the cricopharyngeus muscle. The protrusion is thought to result from asynchronous coordination of the muscles of the pharyngoesophageal junction.[153] Zenker's diverticulum is rare in patients younger than 30 years of age. The clinical presentation is determined by the size and location of the diverticulum, but includes dysphagia, odynophagia, reflux of undigested food, a gurgling sensation in the throat when swallowing, or a swelling of the neck when eating.[153] Nighttime aspiration associated with regurgitation is possible, leading to pneumonia, weight loss, poor nutrition, and other pulmonary complications. Surgery is the only effective therapy; however, surgery should be delayed if foreign bodies, food, or barium are known to be present in the diverticulum, and the patient must be allowed a reasonable time to allow the material to be expelled.

b. Thoracic Diverticula (Traction). These diverticula are at or below the middle third of the esophagus, near the left mainstem bronchus. The cause is presumed to be traction on the esophagus due to lymph node enlargement and inflammation.[154] Symptoms are uncommon because food typically does not accumulate, owing to the broad base of the neck of the diverticulum. The indications for surgery are diverticulitis, perforation, hemorrhage, or the development of fistulas.

c. Supradiaphragmatic (Epiphrenic) Diverticula. These rare diverticula are also seen primarily in elderly patients and are characterized by dysphagia, odynophagia, and sometimes hemorrhage. They are located in the distal third of the esophagus and are associated with other esophageal motility disorders.[155] Surgery is uncommonly done unless symptoms are severe. Aspiration pneumonitis is possible but much less likely with Zenker's diverticulum.

3. Achalasia

Achalasia of the esophagus is also called *cardiospasm* (a misnomer). It is characterized by lack of peristaltic activity and esophageal relaxation after ingesting food. Although the cause is not known, the underlying problem is probably neural, involving Auerbach's (myenteric) plexus.[156] Alteration in the histology and physiology of the vagus nerve have been described in association with idiopathic achalasia.

Outside the United States, achalasia may not be idiopathic but may be due to Chagas' disease (infection by the parasite *Trypanosoma cruzi*).[157] This is an important distinction to make, since Chagas' disease may be associated with other physiologic problems, including cardiac conduction defects.[157] The peak incidence of idiopathic achalasia is 30 to 50 years of age, with no sex preference. Clinical symptoms are slow and progressive, the most important of which is dysphagia. Eventually, dysphagia becomes persistent, and pain is not common in later stages of the disease. Regurgitation with aspiration is possible, especially at night, and may lead to pulmonary complications. In severe disease, the esophagus becomes markedly dilated and adynamic, leading to stasis of food and a greatly enhanced risk of aspiration. With advanced disease, weight loss and malnutrition can occur.

Conservative medical management is possible and includes mechanical dilatation of narrowed segments of the esophagus. However, perforation is a potential complication, which may be lethal if it leads to mediastinitis or Boerhaave's syndrome. When the esophagus becomes completely dilated or immotile, surgery is the only effective therapeutic option. The most common surgical procedure is esophagomyotomy.

4. Diffuse Esophageal Spasm

The cause of this condition is not known, but it is probably neurogenic, since the only histologic abnormality is thickening of the smooth muscle.[158] It typically presents in middle age and has no sex predilection. Symptoms include dysphagia and odynophagia, which initially are intermittent. Chest pain resembling angina is possible, as the pain is substernal. Pain may be exacerbated by meals but can also occur at rest. Anxiety and nervousness are common associations with this disorder, and infrequently weight loss is a presenting symptom. Surgery is very rare, as it is indicated only for the most disabling symptoms.

5. Paraesophageal Hernia

In this disorder, portions of the stomach herniate along the esophagus into the thorax, but the esophagogastric junction remains below the hiatus.[159] Reflux is generally not a problem, however. Vascular congestion, ulceration of the mucosa, hemorrhage, and obstruction are possible and may require urgent operation. In addition, other important organs, including the spleen and the large or small intestine, may later become involved, and surgery is therefore commonly indicated for this condition.

6. Esophageal Perforation

The morbidity of esophageal perforation is very high, primarily owing to spillage of bacterial contents into crucial anatomic areas leading to overwhelming infection. It is usually due to ingestion of a foreign body, to retching and vomiting (Boerhaave's syndrome), external trauma, ulceration, or (traumatic or postsurgical) loss of the vascular supply to a portion of the esophagus.

The most common sites of perforation are the esophagopharyngeal junction and at the lower esophagus, just above the diaphragm.[160] The morbidity is much lower when perforation follows endoscopy, because the patient is usually NPO and the diagnosis is usually rapid.[161] Perforation of the cervical esophagus is associated with inflammation of the tissues of the neck; tears of the subdiaphragmatic esophagus may lead to peritonitis, and tears of the thoracic esophagus typically cause mediastinitis, pneumothorax, or pleural effusion. It should be noted that any of these entities is possible with perforation at any site, but they are more likely to be anatomically associated.

Mediastinitis is the most severe syndrome and may present as chest pain, fever, dyspnea, dysphagia, cyanosis, or cardiac and respiratory failure. In spontaneous rupture (Boerhaave's syndrome) pain is intense and may mimic pulmonary embolus or myocardial infarction, but a history of severe emesis usually helps in making a diagnosis. Surgical drainage, broad-spectrum antibiotics, hydration, electrolyte maintenance, and supportive care are the mainstays of therapy, but mortality may exceed 50 per cent even with aggressive treatment.[162] Complications include mediastinal or cervical abscesses, empyema, and mucocutaneous fistulas if the patient survives the initial insult.

7. Esophageal Moniliasis

Invasive infection of the esophagus by *Candida* species leads to destruction of the mucosa in this condition. Mycelial forms are characteristic of this disease, as yeast forms are thought to be noninvasive.[163] Major complications include erosion, ulceration, massive hemorrhage, perforation, and sepsis due to fungemia. Esophageal moniliasis is most common in immunosuppressed persons (e.g., with AIDS or after chemotherapy) but also occurs in otherwise healthy adults or after radiation to the neck. Presenting symptoms include odynophagia, dysphagia, pyrosis, and chest pain. Malnutrition is therefore a frequent finding. Surgery is indicated only for treatment of complications (e.g., bleeding), whereas antifungals remain the mainstay of therapy.

8. Corrosive Esophagitis

Corrosive esophageal disease is due to ingestion of toxic substances, particularly alkali (e.g., lye) or acid. Lye is the most common culprit, and is usually more caustic than acid in terms of tissue damage. Early complications of corrosive disease include aspiration, perforation, and mediastinitis; the major late complication is stricture. Chronic aspiration pneumonia with pulmonary parenchymal damage may also occur. Treatment includes irrigation with copious amounts of water, antibiotics, steroids, and possibly neutralization with an appropriate agent (although this may produce heat and further damage). Treatment of stricture involves serial esophageal dilatation, surgical resection, or GI bypass.[164]

9. Reflux Esophagitis

Reflux of acid gastric contents is the most common cause of esophagitis, and in 85 per cent of cases may accompany a hiatal hernia.[165] Esophagitis may also be due to ingestion of corrosive substances, such as lye and acid. Postsurgical esophagitis is also possible, owing to induced incompetency of the lower esophageal sphincter or motility mechanisms. Finally, operations that are intended to reduce gastric acidity (e.g., highly selective vagotomy) may also cause esophagitis since the esophageal mucosa is very sensitive to alkaline secretions.

The most common symptoms are nonspecific and include heartburn, dysphagia, odynophagia, and regurgitation. If stricture formation is evolving, dysphagia may be especially prominent. Although radiographic studies following the ingestion of contrast medium may demonstrate reflux, definitive diagnosis is possible only with esophagoscopy and tissue biopsy to demonstrate esophagitis. Other helpful diagnostic tools include manometry, acid perfusion measurements (Bernstein's test), pH monitoring, and acid elimination monitoring.

Conservative treatment prevents reflux or its effects and includes weight loss, dietary modification, antacids, elevation of the head at night, H_2 blockers, and mucosal protectives. It is important to identify refractory cases of esophagitis early and plan surgical therapy before fibrosis, stricture, or a malignant condition develops. Three common surgical treatments have been used: (1) Belsey Mark IV (horizontal gastric plication to the diaphragm), (2) Nissen fundoplication, and (3) Hill repair.[166] Some procedures are done transthoracically rather than intraabdominally. Most patients undergoing surgery for esophagitis are obese and also at increased risk for aspiration during anesthesia.

10. Esophageal Stricture

Stricture is most common following prolonged reflux with tissue damage and inflammation. The presence of an esophageal stricture greatly increases surgical morbidity and mortality. Therefore, before surgery, measures are undertaken to relieve the stricture, and include bougienage. Many persons who present for surgical correction of esophageal stricture are malnourished and probably should have TPN before surgery to achieve positive nitrogen balance, unless feeding is possible following bougienage.

Surgical procedures to treat stricture are quite extensive and associated with a high risk of morbidity. Consequently, preoperative nutritional optimization of patients cannot be overemphasized. Treatments include a Thal patch if the involved area of stricture is small, esophagogastrectomy, or esophagectomy with bowel interposition.[167] Almost all procedures include secondary pyloroplasty to enhance gastric emptying.

11. Barrett's Esophagus

The most distal portion of the esophagus is normally lined by columnar mucosal epithelial cells; however, in some persons columnar epithelium may line the entire lower esophagus and is thought to be a consequence of prolonged reflux of acid contents. This metaplasia, when associated with peptic ulcer or stricture, is also referred to as *Barrett's syndrome* and may be a premalignant condition.[168] Other complications of Barrett's esophagus include perforation, mediastinitis, and hemorrhage.

12. Benign Esophageal Neoplasms

Nonmalignant tumors of the esophagus are exceedingly rare. They usually present with dysphagia, and rarely pain. The majority are probably asymptomatic. The majority of tumors are leiomyomas, which can be intramural or extramucosal, pedunculated, or multiple. Other benign esophageal masses include cysts and papillomas.[169]

13. Esophageal Webs

A fibrous web may occur at any portion of the esophagus. Webs arising in the upper part are often associated with hypochromic, microcytic anemia, as occurs in Plummer-Vinson syndrome (also called Paterson-Kelly syndrome).[170] Plummer-Vinson syndrome manifests predominantly in middle-aged females with atrophic, dried oral mucosa. The clinical picture consists of dysphagia, glossitis, spooning of the fingernails, and iron-deficiency anemia. There is, however, some question about whether the concurrent pathology involving the oral cavity, esophagus, and gastric mucosa are coincidental or consitute the basis of the malnutrition and iron deficiency. Treatment is dilatation or surgical excision of the web and iron therapy to correct the anemia.

14. Lower Esophageal Rings

Also called *Schatzki's rings*, lower esophageal rings usually develop close to the squamocolumnar junction and are not associated with iron-deficiency anemia and may also occur in males.[171] About 15 per cent of persons with Schatzki's rings have an accompanying hiatal hernia. Dysphagia provoked by swallowing solid food is the principal complaint associated with lower esophageal rings. Pain is characteristically uncommon. Dysphagia is episodic, and there may be long, symptom-free intervals; however, discomfort may progress to the point at which soft or liquid food causes symptoms. Therapy includes dilatation of the esophagus and treatment of reflux.

15. Mallory-Weiss Tears

Tears of the mucosa of the gastroesophageal junction following vomiting or retching lead to the Mallory-Weiss syndrome.[172] The tear may lead to massive hemorrhage that presents as hematemesis. The syndrome is most common in chronic alcoholics following binge drinking episodes associated with prolonged vomiting. Lacerations of the gastroesophageal junction may also occur without a history of vomiting, so other mechanisms of injury apparently exist. Treatment include blood transfusion, vasoconstrictive medications, balloon tamponade, and surgical therapy for refractory cases.

C. DISORDERS OF THE STOMACH

1. General Considerations

Peptic ulceration is very common following any physiologic stress and may manifest as upper GI bleeding, aspiration, and perforation. Also, it should be kept in mind that gastric ulceration can be associated with other systemic illnesses, including hyperparathyroidism and steroid excess, which have immense anesthetic implications themselves.[173] Also, patients with gastric diseases often have macrocytic or iron-deficiency anemias due to B_{12} deficiency or bleeding, respectively.

2. Diseases Associated with Gastric or Duodenal Ulceration

a. Zollinger-Ellison Syndrome. This disease entity is characterized by severe ulceration of gastric or duodenal mucosa secondary to gastric hypersecretion or non–beta islet cell tumors of the pancreas.[174] It may also be associated with extremely copious diarrhea, also secretory in nature. Although it has been described in all age groups, the most typical presentation occurs during middle age. The major clinical features include (1) intractable ulcers, especially in atypical sites, (2) gastric hypersecretion (due to gastrin overproduction by the gastrinoma), (3) severe diarrhea, (4) fat malabsorption (steatorrhea), (5) hypokalemia (due to stool and urine losses of potassium secondary to dehydration), and (6) a tendency to recur even after surgical resection.[174] Not all findings are seen in all patients; for example, some may have hypersecretion with diarrhea but without ulceration. A histamine or betazole (Histalog) acid stimulation test is useful in establishing the diagnosis.[175] Following administration, acid secretion fails to significantly increase in patients with gastrinomas, as it is nearly maximal at all times.

The majority of patients with Zollinger-Ellison syndrome have malignant tumors, which may be found in the duodenum and pancreas, and have the potential to metastasize.[174] In addition, nearly one fourth have associated endocrine tumors that are commonly secretory and hormonally active.[174] These include tumors of the parathyroid gland, thyroid, and adrenal cortex, and may have significant anesthetic implications. Treatment includes long-term antacid therapy (e.g., H_2 blockers, omeprazole) to control symptoms, and total gastrectomy when the tumor cannot be found or is unresectable (e.g., owing to metastatic disease). In selected circumstances, metastatic gastrinomas have responded to antineoplastic therapy with 5-fluorouracil, streptozocin, and Adriamycin.[176]

b. Hyperparathyroidism. There is probably a relationship between hyperparathyroidism and peptic ulcer, but a definitive association has not been established. Hypercalcemia or large amounts of dietary calcium are known to stimulate gastrin secretion by antral cells in the stomach.[177] Furthermore, gastrin has been shown to be produced in ectopic cells located in the parathyroid glands. It has been estimated that 30 per cent of patients with ulcer-associated tumors of the duodenum are hyperparathyroid (Werner-Morrison syndrome or multiple endocrine neoplasia [MEN] syndrome type I).[178]

c. Steroid-Induced Ulceration. Cushing's syndrome, whether due to adrenal hyperfunctioning or excessive exogenous steroid use, is associated with an increased incidence of peptic ulceration.[179] The mechanism of steroid-induced ulcers is unclear, but an increase in acid secretion is not necessary for ulcer formation in such patients. Alteration in the quantity or chemical composition of protective mucus is probably the major factor. Patients with ulcerative colitis and rheumatoid arthritis who are taking exogenous steroids for control of the primary disease are particularly susceptible to peptic ulceration.[180] They may remain asymptomatic for long periods of time and present with a severe complication such as hemorrhage or perforation as the initial event. Surgical therapy is often suboptimal because of the primary disease and poor wound healing related to long-term steroid use.

d. Stress-Induced Ulcers. The term *stress* refers to situations associated with chronically elevated catecholamine levels, most typically seen after major surgery or trauma or during severe illness. These ulcers are most typical in the ICU in a patient who is already seriously ill. Consequently, the mortality in patients with stress-related gastric ulceration leading to hemorrhage is very high.

Curling's ulcers are an associated (but etiologically different) type of peptic ulceration and are seen in patients with large burns.[181] Stress ulcers are more common in the stomach than in the duodenum, are usually multiple, and may be superficial as well as deep and submucosal. Diagnosis is established by endoscopy, although the most common presenting symptom is hemorrhage. The best therapy is thought to be prophylaxis and correction of the underlying problem (e.g., sepsis). Intravenous vasopressin (Pitressin or DDAVP) is a temporary measure to control bleeding, and more definitive therapy (e.g., sclerosis or injection of epinephrine via endoscope, surgical resection of bleeding sites) is necessary in severe cases. Prophylaxis using H_2 blockers, omeprazole, antacids, sucralfate, or prostaglandins, in conjunction with gastric pH monitoring, has dramatically reduced the need for surgery in ICU patients.

e. Pulmonary-Associated Ulcers. Patients with chronic pulmonary disease of various causes (e.g., COPD, emphysema, bronchitis, cor pulmonale) are at increased risk of developing peptic ulcers. In this patient population, duodenal ulcers are far more frequent than gastric ulcers. Chronic hypoxemia is known to induce gastric acid hypersecretion, and this is the presumed mechanism in patients with chronic pulmonary disease who develop ulcers.[182]

f. Hepatic Disease. Patients with cirrhosis of any cause have an increased likelihood of developing peptic ulcer disease, as do those who have had portocaval shunting procedures. The mechanism is unknown, but it is postulated that the liver degrades a jejunal hormone that stimulates gastric output, and hepatic dysfunction therefore leads to elevated levels of the hormone.[183]

g. Pancreatic Exocrine Disease. Chronic pancreatitis, as seen in alcoholics, is known to be associated with increased risk of peptic ulcer disease.[184] Pancreatic endocrine dysfunction is not related, however. The mechanism is unclear.

h. Postsurgical Resection. It is known that the small bowel releases inhibitory factors that decrease gastric secretions, probably by inhibiting gastrin production. Generally, these inhibitory factors are produced in excess, but following massive resection of the small intestine they may be deficient. Indeed, in some patients, increased serum gastrin has been noted in patients following massive resection of the small bowel.

i. Drug-Induced Ulceration. In addition to exogenous steroids, many drugs are known to cause or exacerbate peptic ulcer disease. The mechanisms are diverse and specific to the class of drug involved. Common offenders include NSAIDs (e.g., aspirin, indomethacin), caffeine, ethanol, and nicotine. Unlike other NSAIDs, acetaminophen is not associated with peptic ulceration because it only acts centrally.

3. Phlegmonous (Necrotizing) Gastritis

Necrotizing gastritis is a rare infection of the wall of the stomach, usually caused by beta-hemolytic streptococci, fusiform, and spirochetal organisms normally found in the oral cavity.[185] Alcoholics with hypochlorhydria are most often afflicted with this disease, for reasons that are unclear. Symptoms are nonspecific and include abdominal pain, hematemesis, cellulitis of the abdomen, intraabdominal abscess, necrotizing gangrene of the gastric wall leading to perforation, and sepsis. As with necrotizing fasciitis, death can occur in a few hours after onset of disease. Therefore, treatment is aggressive, consisting of broad-spectrum antibiotics, surgery, and intensive supportive care.

4. Granulomatous Gastritis

The most common cause of granulomatous gastritis is *Myobacterium tuberculosis* infection, and is usually secondary to active pulmonary tuberculosis.[186] Gross findings include multiple gastric ulcers, with or without hypertrophic thickening of the wall of the stomach. Treatment is the same as for disseminated tuberculosis, and includes long-term therapy with multiple antituberculous agents, depending on sensitivities. Surgery may be necessary when GI obstruction or perforation occurs.

Tertiary syphilis may lead to gastric lesions similar to those of tuberculosis. Patients with this entity may present with symptoms of epigastric fullness, anorexia, weight loss, and iron-deficiency anemia due to chronic bleeding. The treatment is penicillin, but as before, obstruction or perforation may necessitate surgery. Eosinophilic infiltration of the stomach is another cause of focal or diffuse granuloma formation in the stomach wall, and its cause is unknown. It is managed in a similar manner as benign tumors, in that specific therapy is not necessary unless malnutrition, obstruction, hemorrhage, or perforation results.

5. Benign Gastric Neoplasms

Unlike the small intestine and colon, benign tumors of the stomach are very rare. Both mucosal and intramural benign lesions have been described involving the stomach. Gastric adenomas are described as either single or multiple, and polypoid or sessile. The most common location is the antrum of the stomach.[187] Risk factors include age over 60 years, achlorhydria, and the presence of atrophic gastritis. The majority of benign gastric neoplasms are asymptomatic and are found at autopsy. Rare symptoms include anemia (which may be microcytic if due to bleeding or macrocytic if pernicious), epigastric pain, nausea, vomiting, and intermittent partial obstruction. Complete gastric obstruction is unusual.

Intramural neoplasms of the stomach are also found in middle-aged or elderly patients. The following histologic types have been described: leiomyomas, fibromas, fibromyomas, schwannomas, neurofibromas, neuroblastomas, lipomas, hemangiomas, glomus tumors, and ectopic pancreatic tissue, which may be active.[188] The clinical presentation is nonspecific and includes hemorrhage, anemia, malnutrition, intermittent nausea and vomiting, epigastric distress, and obstruction if massive.

Treatment is directly related to severity of symptoms and may include total gastrectomy in the worst cases.

6. Malignant Gastric Neoplasms

a. Carcinoid Tumors (Argentaffinomas). These endocrine tumors are described in the section on the small intestine, where they are most commonly located, but rarely they occur primarily in the stomach.

b. Gastric Lymphoma. Gastric lymphoma may occur primarily in the stomach or can be a manifestation of systemic lymphoma that has metastasized. Lymphomas and related malignancies that have been noted to spread to the stomach include Hodgkin's disease, lymphosarcoma, and reticulum cell sarcoma. The treatment includes chemotherapy, if the tumor is known to be responsive, and/or total gastrectomy with radiation therapy. The overall 5-year survival for primary gastric lymphoma is about 40 per cent.[189]

c. Gastric Leiomyosarcoma. These malignancies are more common in children and may present with abdominal pain, weight loss, malnutrition, hemorrhage (acute or chronic), and perforation. Treatment is surgical resection if the tumor is confined to the stomach, and is associated with a 50 per cent 5-year survival; however, extragastric spread is associated with an ominous prognosis.[190]

d. Metastatic Tumors. Metastatic involvement of the stomach is very rare, and has been described for tumors of the breast, melanoma, generalized lymphomatosis, and leukemia. Unlike primary gastric lesions, they are multiple and usually affect the submucosa and muscularis primarily. Central ulceration is also typical.

7. Gastric Volvulus

Gastric volvulus may occur along two axial planes, either the long or transverse axis of the stomach.[191] Predisposing factors include loss or relaxation of supporting structures, as may occur in hiatal hernia, eventration of the diaphragm, ventral hernia, gastric neoplasms, gastric ulcers, or chronic dilatation of the stomach.[191]

The clinical presentation includes acute epigastric pain, nausea, and vomiting, which may be severe and associated with retching. The classical symptom triad includes (1) dry retching, (2) localized epigastric pain, and (3) inability to pass a nasogastric tube. The most severe complication associated with gastric volvulus is strangulation of the blood supply to the stomach, leading to ischemia and perforation. Sepsis and shock may subsequently result, and treatment may therefore be quite urgent. In the most urgent situations, gastrectomy and vagotomy may be performed, but in some cases detorsion with gastropexy may be sufficient. Some surgeons advocate a two-stage operation.

8. Gastric Vagotomy Procedures

Highly selective vagotomy is still a relatively common surgical procedure, despite dramatic advances in antacid therapy (e.g., omeprazole). Furthermore, many surgeons are now following vagotomy procedures to test for adequacy of acid control. These tests include electrostimulation of the vagus and monitoring changes in intragastric pressure. Other techniques include staining of the nerve and intraoperative use of vagal stimulants such as insulin and 2-deoxyglucose, which may be dangerous.[192] For this reason, they are rarely performed. The most common method used currently measures fundus mucosal pH using probes. If intraoperative postvagotomy testing is necessary, then major anesthetic considerations include the risk of aspiration and avoidance of medications that could interfere with testing, especially anticholinergics and antihistamines.

D. DISORDERS OF THE SMALL INTESTINE

1. General Considerations for Intestinal Disease

One of the most common surgical problems faced by the anesthesiologist is obstruction, which has multiple anesthetic implications. Hypovolemia, electrolyte abnormalities, anemia, and sepsis are possibilities, as mentioned earlier. In addition, increased intra-abdominal pressure may lead to respiratory embarrassment and increased work of breathing in a patient who is already malnourished and weak. A large bowel mass can also have profound circulatory effects, which are difficult to predict. Sudden decompression of a tense abdomen can lead to increased splanchnic venous flow, presenting as immediate hypoten-

sion and shock. On the other hand, intra-abdominal compression of the inferior vena cava can impede blood return to the heart, and decompression can dramatically increase preload. This may also lead to cardiac decompensation if it occurs too suddenly.

Although regional anesthesia is not absolutely contraindicated in bowel obstruction, the anesthesiologist must realize that its use is a high-risk proposition. Hypotension due to sympathetic blockade and the potential need to secure an airway rapidly in a patient with a full stomach are prime considerations. Combined regional-general anesthesia may offer many advantages over either technique alone; it is discussed in detail in standard textbooks of anesthesia. Finally, it should be restated that nitrous oxide should be avoided if the obstruction is active, as it dilates air-filled spaces considerably (e.g., may increase volume 100 per cent in 1 to 2 hours).

Diseases with systemic manifestations (e.g., Osler-Weber-Rendu disease, mucosal telangiectasias) may lead to unexpected complications, such as airway bleeding following endotracheal intubation or high-output cardiac failure due to massive arteriovenous fistulas.[193] The liver is commonly affected in intestinal disease, owing to its portal venous inflow from the bowel. For example, intestinal parasites commonly spread to and destroy the liver. Certain infectious organisms, such as amoebas, may also spread to the brain, liver, and lungs. Finally, tumors such as carcinoid may have considerable systemic effects, including valvular heart disease, paroxysmal hypotension, and bronchoconstriction. Therefore, systemic manifestations of what seems initially to be a localized instestinal process must be considered.

2. Celiac Sprue (Gluten-Sensitive Enteropathy)

Celiac sprue is also known as *celiac disease, adult celiac disease, nontropical sprue,* and *gluten-sensitive enteropathy.*[194] It is characterized by destruction of the mucosa of the small intestine and malabsorption of most nutrients. The disease waxes and wanes and is precipitated by dietary ingestion of wheat gluten, rye, barley, and oats. Symptoms may not appear until the third year of life, when such substances become a common component of the diet; however, the disease may also present spontaneously in adults during the third decade and is autoimmune. The clinical manifestations of celiac sprue are immensely variable and include diarrhea, steatorrhea, abdominal pain, and marked weight loss due to malabsorption. There is also a possible association of celiac disease with lymphoma of the GI tract. Adults may present with nonspecific symptoms, including lassitude, malaise, and lack of energy. Children typically have abdominal distention, failure to thrive, and foul-smelling stools.

Celiac disease may take a clinically unremarkable course for a long time and may finally manifest through an isolated abnormality, such as hemorrhage resulting from a vitamin K–deficient coagulopathy. Indeed, many of the symptoms of celiac disease may indicate abnormalities outside the GI tract, which result from nutrient deficiencies. These include anemia, osteogenic bone loss, neurologic symptoms, oligomenorrhea, mental status changes, and general failure to thrive.[196]

3. Neoplasms of the Small Intestine

Neoplasms of the small intestine are unusual, whether malignant or benign. Although the small bowel represents 75 per cent of the GI tract's length, and 90 per cent of its mucosal surface area, only about 5 per cent of GI tumors arise in this viscus.[197] Theories to explain the rarity of small bowel tumors include fluidity and alkalinity, short transport times (which causes limited contact with luminal carcinogens), lower bacterial population, protective enzymes, and high concentration of immunoglobulin A (IgA), which may destroy carcinogenic viruses.

Regardless of the cause, the most common clinical presentation involves symptoms attributable to bleeding, perforation, or liberation of endocrinologically active substances. Obstruction may occur by several mechanisms, including intussusception, volvulus, and luminal obstruction by the mass. In general, bleeding is usually slow, intermittent, and occult, leading to iron-deficiency anemia (i.e., hypochromic, microcytic). Occasionally, tumors may produce bloody stool (melena), but this requires brisk bleeding to manifest. Significant hemorrhage is typically noted for tumors that are either myomas or vascular in origin.

When perforation occurs, principal complications include peritonitis, fistula formation, and abscess formation. When these occur, symptoms are nonspecific and include nausea, vomiting, abdominal pain, mucous diarrhea, malnutrition, and weight loss.

a. Malignant Neoplasms. The most common cancerous lesions of the small bowel are adenocarcinomas; however, most malignant tumors involving the small intestine are metastases, not primaries. Among the areas of the small bowel, the duodenum is a more frequent site of metastasis than the ileum or jejunum. Duodenal tumors may bleed and lead to obstructive jaundice owing to their proximity to the common bile duct. Jejunal and ileal tumors present more commonly without jaundice but with symptoms of small bowel obstruction.

Chemotherapy and radiation therapy are unable to effect cure without surgery for malignancies of the small bowel. In hopes of cure, surgical therapy is also quite aggressive and includes wide resection along with a large segment of lymph nodes. Duodenal malignancies may require pancreaticoduodenectomy (e.g., Whipple's procedure) and are unresectable in about 60 per cent of cases. Even with negative margins following resection, the overall 5-year survival rate for small bowel malignancies is about 20 per cent.[198] While chemotherapy is evolving steadily, radiation to regions of the small bowel is probably of little benefit and is associated with high morbidity.

b. Carcinoid Tumors. Carcinoid tumors have provoked a great deal of interest because of their unpredictable behavior and clinical metabolic syndrome that produces profound systemic symptoms. They may be malignant or benign, and the malignant potential is related to both tumor location and size. Carcinoid neoplasms may also be found in teratomas. The most common sites are the appendix (46 per cent), the ileum (28 per cent), and the rectum (17 per cent).[199] Appendiceal tumors tend to have a low incidence of metastasis, whereas ileal tumors tend to be aggressive, especially if the primary lesion is large.

These submucosal tumors produce the carcinoid syndrome, caused by the liberation of serotonin and other vasoactive amines, including histamine, kallikrein, and adrenocorticotropin (ACTH). The tumor may be benign but is most commonly metastatic and may also arise at any portion of the GI tract, but the small bowel is the most typical location. Generally, the vasoactive hormones that are released are inactivated by the liver, but if the malignancy is metastatic to the liver, these substances are released into the systemic circulation. Manifestations include purplish skin flushing due to vasodilatation of smooth muscle, paroxysmal bronchospasm, arthralgia, pellagra-like skin changes, severe diarrhea, generalized edema, right-sided cardiac valvular and endocardial lesions, pulmonary stenosis, and vascular collapse.[200]

Tumor debulking of primary and metastatic lesions can be very helpful, and the anesthesiologist should anticipate dramatic intraoperative blood pressure lability and the possibility of coexisting heart failure. Right-sided heart lesions may result in difficult or dangerous pulmonary artery catheterization. Pharmacologic control of the tumor should be optimized before elective surgery. A multitude of regimens are employed, and the anesthesiologist should discuss with the endocrinologist the course of management before surgery. Strategies that have been employed, with varying degrees of success, include chemotherapeutic regimens, methysergide, α-methyldopa, phenothiazines, phenoxybenzamine, and octreotide.

c. Benign Neoplasms. The most common small bowel benign tumors are leiomyomas, lipomas, adenomas, polyps, hemangiomas, neurogenic tumors, and fibromas.[201] As with malignant tumors, the most common presenting signs are obstruction, hemorrhage (usually occult), and rarely perforation. Symptoms may include nausea, vomiting, abdominal pain, and melena. If perforation occurs, peritonitis, fistula formation, and abscess can develop. Despite their benign histology, they should be excised because some may have malignant potential or may grow to the point that obstruction occurs.

d. Peutz-Jeghers Syndrome. Peutz-Jeghers syndrome is characterized by polyposis of the GI tract, particularly the small intestine, and melanin pigmentation involving the oral and perianal mucosa, lips, hands, and soles of the feet.[202] The disease is familial and the inheritance is simple mendelian autosomal dominance. The polyps are tubular hamartomas and with malignant potential only in the rarest of cases. However, GI complications may occur, and include hemorrhage, obstruction, and intussusception. Surgical therapy is directed only toward areas of symptoms, as removing all polyps would leave the patient with severe short-gut syndrome.

4. Vascular Lesions

a. Osler-Weber-Rendu Syndrome (Hereditary Hemorrhagic Telangiectasia). This syndrome is characterized by telangiectasia of the mucous membranes of the nasal and oral cavities, viscera, and skin. It is an inborn progressive tendency to form dilated endothelial spaces and is transmitted as an autosomal dominant trait affecting both men and women. The principal problems are related to repeated hemorrhages. Telangiectasia, hemangiomas, fibrosis, and cirrhosis of the liver may develop.[203] Repeated GI hemorrhages may lead to iron-deficiency anemia requiring transfusion; however, surgery is indicated only for treatment of complications such as perforation, obstruction, or brisk bleeding. The anesthesiologist should be aware that associated arteriovenous shunting in the liver or lungs may lead to high-output cardiac failure in severe cases.

b. Hemangiomas. These vascular growths are described as being either capillary, cavernous, or mixed. The major complications are related to local tissue damage due to growth of the tumor, hemorrhage (which can be severe), GI obstruction, perforation, and sepsis. Despite the fact that these lesions can be very vascular, surgery is generally indicated only when complications occur.

5. Regional Enteritis (Crohn's Disease)

Crohn's disease is an inflammatory disease of unknown cause, possibly autoimmune or infectious, that involves the entire GI tract. Although Crohn's disease and ulcerative colitis are collectively categorized as *inflammatory bowel disease*, their pathophysiology is completely different (see subsequent section on ulcerative colitis).[204] Crohn's disease typically manifests in young adults, but its onset has been described in all ranges of age. The most common area of involvement in Crohn's disease is the terminal ileum. The disease is most often categorized by the segment of the bowel involved: ileocolitis (40 to 60 per cent), enteritis confined to the small bowel (30 per cent), and disease limited to the colon (10 per cent).[204] Diseased bowel demonstrates thickening of the bowel wall and granuloma formation in all layers, particularly the submucosa. Mesenteric fat tends to encroach around the bowel wall, and active enteritis is associated with hyperemia of the serosa, transmural wall thickening, and mesenteric edema.

The symptoms comprise a classic triad of nonbloody diarrhea, weight loss, and abdominal pain; however, other symptoms include fever, leukocytosis, lower GI bleeding, perianal involvement, and enterocutaneous fistula formation. Extraintestinal manifestations include arthritis and spondylitis, erythema nodosum, pyoderma gangrenosum, cholangitis, fatty degeneration of the liver, sclerosing cholangitis, iritis, episcleritis, and uveitis.[204] Medical management includes bowel rest, intravenous hyperalimentation, sulfonamide, azathioprine, steroids, and antibiotics for infectious complications. Nevertheless, most patients with Crohn's disease ultimately require surgery for complications such as fistula, abscess formation, obstruction, toxic megacolon, or perianal disease. Some patients present for surgery with frank malnutrition, weakness, steatorrhea, and the consequences of associated fat malabsorption (e.g., vitamin K deficiency–associated coagulopathy) or prolonged steroid therapy (e.g., Addison's disease, osteodystrophy, poor wound healing, infections). It should be remembered that the recurrence rate following surgery approaches 50 per cent, as Crohn's disease is generally a systemic illness.

Crohn's disease appears to predispose to the development of adenocarcinoma of the small intestine, the ileum being the most common site.[205] There is also a slight increase in the incidence of colon carcinoma, but it is far less than that associated with ulcerative colitis.

6. Cholera

Cholera is the classic form of enterotoxigenic diarrhea. It is caused by the bacterium *Vibrio cholerae* O-group 1, a member of the Vibrionaceae family, which also includes *Aeromonas* and other *Vibrio* species.[206] Although rare to nonexistent in the United States, it is endemic in Asia, Africa, and Latin America, where it remains a major cause of death, especially in children. Cholera is transmitted by stool contamination of drinking water; person-to-person transmission does not occur.

The cholera toxin is a protein that binds to adenylate cyclase molecules in the intestine, leading to excessive and unregulated production of cAMP, which manifests as profound and uncontrolled hypersecretion of chloride and bicarbonate from mucosal crypt cells.[206] Fluid loss occurs as water passively follows the electrolyte solutes into the lumen of the bowel.

Clinical symptoms include a wide spectrum of disease, comprising mild gastroenteritis to severe cholera leading to death from dehydration. Indeed, hypovolemic shock can occur within 1 hour of disease onset. The patient with advanced disease has metabolic acidosis, hyponatremia, hypokalemia, lethargy, mental status changes, and possibly seizures. The eyes may appear sunken into the orbits, the skin may be mottled, the extremities are usually cold, and mucous membranes are dry. In infants, fontanelles are depressed, the voice is weakened, and there may be hypotension. Fecal material resembles "rice water," which is characteristic of this disease, and can exceed 1 L per hour.

The treatment of cholera is usually only rehydration, which is remarkably effective if instituted early. Oral rehydration is acceptable in mild cases, and a specific solution is available from the World Health Organization. If intravenous hydration is necessary, then lactated Ringer's solution or balanced salt solution is the preferred electrolyte mixture. The rate of rehydration must exceed the rate of diarrhea production; many patients have a fluid deficit exceeding several liters, which must be replenished in addition to maintenance fluids. Antibiotic therapy may also be employed but is usually unnecessary. It may shorten the course of disease, however. Tetracycline 250 to 500 mg PO every 6 hours for 3 days is most commonly recommended. Chloramphenicol, ampicillin, and trimethoprim-sulfamethoxazole are also effective.

7. Typhoid Enteritis

Typhoid enteritis is caused by an acute systemic infection by *Salmonella typhi*. It is characterized by a rose-colored rash, prostration, headache, and fever in the early phase of infection. Approximately 3 weeks later, diarrhea and pyrexia may be marked. The illness can be serious and life threatening owing to bowel hemorrhage or perforation and associated cholecystitis/cholangitis. Moreover, pneumonia, hepatitis, bacteremia, and sepsis may occur in later stages.[207] *Salmonella* organisms can also cause osteomyelitis, endocarditis, meningitis, glomerulitis, and urinary tract infections.

Histologically, ulceration and erosion of blood vessels in Peyer's patches are noted. In fact, gross bleeding is noted in as many as 20 per cent of cases. Treatment includes surgery in severe cases, chloramphenicol, steroids, and supportive measures, including blood transfusion.

8. Tuberculous Enteritis

Tuberculosis of the intestine is commonly associated with systemic infection, and the anesthesiologist must therefore consider the implications of other involved organ systems. GI involvement of the ileocecal valve occurs in 85 per cent of tuberculous enteritis.[208] Tuberculous peritonitis may follow tuberculous enteritis, owing to spread of mycobacteria from adjacent lymph nodes. Clinically, it ranges from an insidious illness with local abdominal pain to a syndrome resembling frank bacterial peritonitis. The peritoneal exudate is characteristically mononuclear, which helps differentiate it from peritoneal carcinomatosis. Surgery is indicated only for management of complications (e.g., perforation, obstruction, abscess). The mainstay of therapy is medical and may include the administration of multiple antituberculous agents for up to 1 year.

9. Small Intestine Diverticulosis and Diverticulitis

Diverticula of the small bowel are false diverticula, as in the case of the large intestine. They are most commonly found in the jejunum, in patients older than 50 years, and there is no sex preponderance. Clinical manifestations include intermittent periumbilical or epigastric pain, profuse watery diarrhea, nausea, vomiting, and malnutrition in severe cases.

There may be hypertrophy and dilatation of the small intestine as well as hypermotility of the involved segment. Diverticula may also be associated with anemia, steatorrhea, and malabsorption in general. The anemia is usually megaloblastic, as vitamin B_{12} deficiency is the common cause. Medical management includes administration of exogenous B_{12}, folate, iron, and calciferol, but surgery may ultimately be needed. Diverticulitis is also a potential complication of diverticulosis. In this case, the risks are the same as those of colonic diverticulits, and include perforation, peritonitis, abscess formation, adhesion formation, and obstruction.

10. Radiation Enteritis

Radiation enteritis follows radiotherapy to the abdomen or exposure to high levels of ionizing radiation (e.g., in nuclear reactor accidents or thermonuclear blast) and is not associated with diagnostic radiographs. Radiation destroys the gut mucosa, which is comprised of a large proportion of rapidly dividing cells. Symptoms include anorexia, nausea, emesis, and diarrhea. Most symptoms respond to medical therapy and subside soon after radiation therapy ceases. In a small proportion of patients, symptoms may endure for months or may recur after quiescence. Occasionally, a mass may be palpable in the abdomen. There may also be malabsorption of fat, fat-soluble vitamins, vitamin B_{12}, and calcium, and loss of protein and blood. Anemia (iron-deficiency, megaloblastic, or both) and hypoalbuminemia may develop. In persons exposed to large doses of systemic radiation, associated marrow suppression should be anticipated (e.g., pancytopenia and infectious complications).

Some patients may respond to steroid therapy and supportive care alone, but operative treatment may be required if perforation, obstruction, abscess, bleeding, or fistulas result. Because patients are generally ill to begin with, operative mortality can be quite high (i.e., more than 15 per cent).

11. Pneumatosis Cystoides Intestinalis

Pneumatosis cystoides intestinalis is a rare condition characterized by gas-filled cysts in the wall and mesentery of the GI tract.[209] The vast majority (85 per cent) of cases are associated with other lesions of the GI tract, including peptic ulcer and diverticulitis. The cysts are submucosal or subserosal, and most common in the jejunum, ileocecal valve, and colon. Complications are uncommon but include hemorrhage, obstruction, volvulus, intussusception, external compression, perforation, malabsorption, and tension pneumoperitoneum. Cysts may disappear spontaneously, and treatment is administered only when complications occur. The disease should not be confused with pneumatosis intestinalis, a finding on plain radiographs associated with gut ischemia and death (as in necrotizing enterocolitis), which is a surgical emergency with extremely high mortality.

E. DISORDERS OF THE LARGE INTESTINE

1. Ischemic Colitis

Ischemia of the colon may result from thrombosis of the inferior mesenteric artery, embolization of inferior mesenteric artery (rare), inferior mesenteric vein thrombosis, accidental surgical ligation, abdominal aortic angiography, or low–cardiac output states (e.g., hypotension due to congestive heart failure or prolonged intraoperative hypotension). The syndrome can present as a transient episode with rapid healing or stricture formation, or as an acute, catastrophic disease with colonic necrosis and gangrene.

Patients generally have predisposing peripheral vascular disease and are commonly smokers or diabetics. The incidence of spontaneous ischemic colitis is highest in the sixth to eighth decades of life. Some patients may have intestinal angina (abdominal pain precipitated by eating), mild diarrhea, and cramping. However, in cases of acute arterial occlusion, severe pain, bloody diarrhea, fever, and left lower quadrant tenderness are common. Untreated disease progresses to perforation and peritonitis unless vascular supply is reestablished. In general, anticoagulation is not advised. Because patients with mesenteric artery thrombosis are usually elderly with extensive vascular disease and/or diabetes, surgical mortality in emergent operations is very high.

2. Ulcerative Colitis

Ulcerative colitis is an idiopathic inflammatory disease limited to the colon and rectum. There is strong evidence to suggest that the disease is autoimmune.[210] The disease is chronic and is characterized most commonly by bloody diarrhea. Like Crohn's disease, ulcerative colitis can affect patients of any age, but familial tendency is less significant. The age distribution is biphasic, with major peaks at 15 to 30 years and 50 to 70 years.[210] The disease usually begins near the rectosigmoid and extends proximally, eventually involving the entire colon. Ulcerative proctitis is a common but more benign form of the disease, being limited to the rectum in 90 per cent of cases. Pathologically, persons with ulcerative colitis exhibit degeneration of recticular fibers below the mucosal epithelium, capillary occlusion, and inflammatory cell infiltrates of the lamina propria.[210] Crypt abscesses, necrosis, and ulceration eventually develop.

Clinical symptoms include intermittent attacks of bloody and/or mucous diarrhea with variable intensity and duration. Fever, peritonitis, abdominal cramping, and profound toxemia are possible. In the most severe cases, patients may have more than 20 bowel movements per day, with severe tenesmus and distressing abdominal cramping, without relief during sleep. With extensive colitis, malaise, malnutrition, fever, anemia, leukocytosis, and increased erythrocyte sedimentation rate may be noted. Other potential systemic complications of particular importance to the anesthesiologist include B_{12} deficiency, folate deficiency, hyponatremia, iritis, arthritis, spondylitis, pericholangitis, hepatitis, cirrhosis, pancreatitis, thrombophlebitis, and acute psychosis.

Complications of ulcerative colitis include hemorrhage, toxic colitis, toxic megacolon, rectovaginal fistulas, and colon cancer. Toxic colitis is a severe local complication in which the ulceration extends transmurally and leads to localized ileus and peritonitis. In toxic megacolon (or toxic dilatation of the colon), loss of muscle tone leads the diameter of the transverse colon to exceed 6 cm, and can lead to perforation. Patients with toxic megacolon usually have high fevers, leukocytosis, severe abdominal pain, and involuntary guarding. When perforation and septicemia develop, the mortality rate may exceed 40 per cent. While rectovaginal fistulas are possible in patients with ulcerative colitis, they are small and unlike the large, abscess-related fistulas seen in Crohn's disease. The incidence of cancer in patients with ulcerative colitis is increased when the entire colon is involved and the disease is present longer than 10 years. After 10 years, the risk of colon carcinoma is estimated to be about 1 per cent per year.[211] Regular endoscopy with biopsy is warranted.

Treatment consists of steroids, sulfasalazine, azathioprine, antidiarrheals, dietary modification, vitamin and nutritional supplementation, and surgery. Almost all patients benefit from surgery, even those whose symptoms are intractable to medical therapy. Total proctocolectomy with ileostomy is the treatment of choice and is curative, but necessitates ileostomy or ileoanal pull-through. Rectal sparing has been advocated to preserve continence, but incidence of recurrence of disease in the rectal stump may be high. A continent ileal pouch (Kock's procedure) is probably the treatment of choice, but only in experienced hands, as complications are frequent.

The importance of excluding an infectious cause of acute colitis before commencing treatment for ulcerative colitis is crucial. Infectious causes that may mimic ulcerative colitis—especially in the first attack—include *Salmonella, Shigella,* and *Campylobacter* gastroenteritis.[212] *Entamoeba histolytica* and *Clostridium difficile* colitis may also produce symptoms similar to ulcerative colitis, including bloody diarrhea. Infectious proctitis due to gonorrhea, herpes simplex, or chlamydia should be excluded. Very rarely, oral contraceptive–induced colitis and ischemic colitis may mimic ulcerative colitis. Finally, colon cancer must be considered in the differential diagnosis of bloody diarrhea, but it rarely produces fever or purulent discharge.

3. Granulomatous Colitis

Granulomatous colitis is most commonly due to Crohn's disease involving the colon. Although Crohn's disease generally affects the terminal ileum, it may include any portion of the GI tract, including the colon. In fact, it may involve the colon alone as a variant of ulcerative colitis. As mentioned earlier, the cause is unknown, but autoimmune factors may play an important role. Clinical manifestations of the disease include diarrhea (usually not bloody, as in the case of ulcerative colitis), weight loss, malnutrition, abdominal pain, low-grade fever, anemia, and abdominal mass. Perianal (e.g., rectovesical and rectovaginal) lesions are common, unlike ulcerative colitis. Severe acute hemorrhage and toxic megacolon typically are not seen. The risk of colon cancer is increased, although not as much as in ulcerative colitis.[204] Recurrences are also more frequent. The anesthesiologist should be aware that many patients will have been taking large doses of steroids for a long time. Thus, steroid-associated complications

(poor wound healing, poor glycemic control, osteodystrophy, peptic ulceration, cataract formation, and increased risk of infection) should be kept in mind.

4. Pseudomembranous Colitis

Pseudomembranous colitis is a severe necrotizing inflammation of the colon and is associated with broad-spectrum antimicrobial therapy leading to suppression of the normal colonic flora. It encompasses a spectrum from transient, mild diarrhea to severe colitis characterized by exudative mucosal plaques (pseudomembranes). Bacterial invasion of the mucosa is not seen; however, severe ulceration of gut with diffuse friability may mimic ulcerative colitis.

Although broad-spectrum antibiotics may lead to overgrowth of many organisms, *C. difficile* is the one most frequently recognized in this disorder. Antimicrobials commonly implicated are clindamycin, lincomycin, ampicillin, broad-spectrum cephalosporins, penicillins, erythromycin, trimethoprim-sulfamethoxazole, tetracycline, and chloramphenicol.[213] Susceptibility increases with age, although even young children can be afflicted. Specific predisposing conditions increase the risk of pseudomembranous colitis, including recent bowel surgery, uremia, intestinal ischemia, and shock.

Clinical manifestations include severe, voluminous diarrhea, fever, tachycardia, hypotension, shock, volume depletion, oliguria, electrolyte imbalances, protein loss, distention and abdominal pain, weakness, malnutrition, and delirium.[213] The diarrhea is characteristically profuse, watery, and occasionally green or bloody. Stool volume can exceed 10 L per day. Diagnosis is established by clinical suspicion, presence of *C. difficile* toxin in the stool, or the presence of pseudomembranes on endoscopic examination. The treatment includes supportive care, with particular emphasis on restoring electrolyte and volume status, discontinuation of nonessential antibiotics, albumin, and blood as necessary. Oral (not intravenous) vancomycin or metronidazole is the preferred therapy for *C. difficile*; however, a few cases are refractory to medical therapy and require emergency colectomy. In these cases, mortality may range from 30 to 80 per cent.

5. Actinomycosis

This infection is caused by the fungus *Actinomyces israelii* and involves primarily the appendix and cecum.[214] The presentation may be one of appendicitis with perforation, and characterized by the usual findings, including right lower quadrant pain, spiking fever, chills, nausea, vomiting, and leukocytosis. Unlike in conventional appendicitis, weight loss and a palpable abdominal mass may be present, and the diagnosis is suggested by the presence of microscopic sulfur granules in the drainage fluid at surgery. Treatment includes surgical excision and drainage, and penicillin or tetracycline. Complications include abscess and fistula formation, and the development of sinus tracts.

6. Amebiasis

The protozoan *Entamoeba histolytica* may lead to infection of the cecum, ascending colon, and rectum characterized by the formation of mucosal ulcers.[215] Many patients may have asymptomatic infections, but others present with acute amebic dysentery. The disease usually presents as increasingly severe diarrhea over several days, associated with abdominal pain. The stools are semisolid with small tinges of blood-stained mucus, but occasionally may be frankly hemorrhagic.

Following an acute attack, the disease may become relapsing and recurring. The chronic form of amebic dysentery may include weight loss, malnutrition, intermittent bloody or mucoid diarrhea, abdominal cramping, and low-grade fever. The diagnosis may be established by endoscopic mucosal biopsy or amebic titers. Complications include perforation, hepatic abscess, or ameboma formation. Amebomas are large inflammatory masses that are most common in the cecum or sigmoid colon and can produce bleeding or obstruction.[215] Surgery without treatment of the underlying infection is dangerous and can lead to peritonitis, fistula formation, and abscess.

Pharmacologic treatment is complex but typically includes metronidazole, iodoquinol, diloxanide, emetine, dehydroemetine, and/or chloroquine.[216] The use of emetine and dehydroemetine may predispose the patient to tachydysrhythmias, hypotension, muscle weakness, and dermatoses and is contraindicated in pregnant patients or those with cardiac disease. Thus, patients receiving these two medications are generally restricted to continuous cardiac monitoring during the course of therapy.

7. Tuberculous Colitis

Tuberculosis of the colon is generally seen only in patients with pulmonary tuberculosis. The most frequent site of infection is the cecum and ascending colon. Patients may have no GI symptoms or may exhibit diarrhea, abdominal pain, and anemia. Complications are nonspecific and include perforation, bleeding, obstruction, and fistula formation. Surgery is generally limited to treatment of complications, and systemic antituberculosis therapy is the mainstay of therapy. Occasionally the patient with tuberculous colitis presents with GI complications necessitating emergency surgery. In this case, a preoperative chest film generally establishes a high index of suspicion for disseminated tuberculosis, and antimyobacterial therapy should be started immediately.

8. Schistosomiasis

Schistosomiasis is a parasitic disease caused by three major species of blood flukes: *Schistosoma mansoni, Schistosoma haematobium,* and *Schistosoma japonicum.*[217] Because freshwater snails indigenous to South America and Puerto Rico are the intermediate host for *S. mansoni,* infections by this species are most common there.[217] Clinical manifestations include pruritic dermatitis, fever, abdominal pain, cough, hemoptysis, urticarial rash, headache, tenesmus, hematuria, and hepatosplenomegaly.[218] With chronic infection, hematemesis, melena, ascites, weight loss, severe malnutrition, and alternating diarrhea and constipation can occur. Complications of infection include hepatic destruction, colonic polyps, and bowel strictures. Surgery is generally limited to treatment of complications, including perforation, hemorrhage, obstruction, or abscess formation. Treatment is usually with praziquantel or niclosamide.

9. Echinococcosis

This is an infection caused by *Echinococcus granulosa,* a worm found in the small intestines of dogs, wolves, and other canines. It produces cysts in the liver, where, after remaining asymptomatic for decades, it finally produces an abdominal mass or pain. Jaundice may occur if the bile duct is obstructed. Rupture may occur into the abdomen or lung, producing a serious anaphylactic reaction and death if untreated. Pulmonary cysts are usually discovered incidentally on routine chest films. Some may rupture, leading to cough, chest pain, hemoptysis, and anaphylaxis.[219] The treatment is surgical excision and mebendazole; however, the anesthesiologist must anticipate the possibility of anaphylaxis during cyst manipulation.

10. Ascariasis

Ascariasis is an infection caused by *Ascaris lumbricoides,* or giant intestinal roundworm. The geographic distribution of disease is cosmopolitan centers in almost all warm and moist climates of the Third World.[220] The source of the infection is fecal contamination of soil and vegetables. The most common symptoms of infection are colicky pains, but eosinophilia and bronchitis are common, as the parasite migrates to the lung parenchyma. The organism may also block the biliary duct, leading to cholangitis, or to the pancreatic duct, leading to acute pancreatitis.[220] Medical treatment is mebendazole or pyrantel.

11. Diphyllobothriasis

The fish tapeworm *Diphyllobothrium latum* is indigenous to Northern Minnesota, Michigan, and Canada. Infection may lead to pernicious anemia, as the parasite is a scavenger for ingested B_{12}.[221] Treatment is praziquantel or niclosamide; however, most patients have no symptoms.

12. Paragonimiasis

Paragonimus species, particularly *Paragonimus westermani* of Asia, are intestinal flukes that commonly invade the pulmonary system.[222] Infection may lead to GI disease, but patients may also present with peribronchiolar distress and hemoptysis. The geographic distribution of disease is broad, including Africa, Asia, Latin America, and rarely the United States and Canada.[222] The intermediate host is generally crabs or cray-fish, which are eaten by humans and thus spread the disease. Treatment is praziquantel.

13. Villous Adenomas

Villous adenomas occur in both the colon and rectum and in both sexes; incidence is highest in the sixth and seventh decades of life.[223] Clinical manifestations include rectal discharge of blood and mucus, constipation or diarrhea, and malnutrition with weight loss. In some patients, as much as 3 L per day of mucus may be produced by the tumor, leading to serious electrolyte depletion. Patients may present with hypokalemia, hypochloremia, hyponatremia, azotemia, dehydration, and shock.[223] Fluid and electrolyte replacement is crucial.

Invasive adenocarcinoma is present in as many as 30 per cent of lesions and is very likely in lesions larger than 6 cm.[224] Therefore, the entire tumor, including the base, must be completely excised. If malignancy is found, wide resection with node sampling is necessary, as with conventional colectomy for cancer. It should be noted that both benign and malignant tumors may recur.

14. Multiple Familial Polyposis (Familial Polyposis Coli)

Multiple familial polyposis, first described in the late 1800s, is a syndrome in which numerous tubular adenomas cover the entire large bowel and rectum.[225] The risk of malignant transformation is thought to be 100 per cent, and the average age at diagnosis of a malignancy is only 25 years.[225] The mode of inheritance is autosomal dominance with a high degree of penetrance. Polyps are not typically present at birth and appear around age 10 years. Symptoms include bloody diarrhea, abdominal pain, and malnutrition. The only effective treatment is total proctocolectomy at the time of diagnosis.[225] More recently, total colectomy with ileoanal pull-through has been employed if patients are motivated and willing to undergo frequent lower GI endoscopy for destruction of rectal polyps as they develop.

15. Gardner's Syndrome

Gardner's syndrome is a variant of multiple familial polyposis that includes sebaceous cysts, soft tissue tumors, and bony abnormalities.[226] Bone lesions are characteristic, and include osteomas of the mandible and skull and exostoses of the long bones. Soft tissue abnormalities are epidermoid cysts, fibromas, and thyroid carcinoma.

16. Cronkhite-Canada Syndrome

Cronkhite-Canada syndrome is characterized by GI polyposis, cutaneous hyperpigmentation, alopecia, and onychodystrophy.[227] The polyps involve the colon, stomach, and rarely the small intestine. The lesions are typically juvenile polyps that are cystically dilated with mucus. There is thought to be very little potential for malignancy, and polyps may regress before puberty.

17. Turcot's and Oldfield's Syndromes

Turcot's and Oldfield's syndromes are also thought to be variants of multiple familial polyposis and may be associated with CNS tumors as well as colonic polyps.[228, 229] Both are associated with a very high incidence of malignancy involving the large intestine. They are therefore treated aggressively with early total proctocolectomy or total colectomy with ileoanal pull-through.

18. Sigmoid and Cecal Volvulus

Rotation of a segment of bowel around its mesenteric axis (or other axis) can produce both obstruction and ischemia secondary to constriction of its blood supply. Volvulus occurs in areas of the colon that are freely mobile and elongated, whether congenitally or pathologically. About 80 per cent of cases of volvulus involve the sigmoid colon, 15 per cent the cecum, and 5 per cent the transverse colon.[230] Volvulus is not truly rare, as it is the third most common cause of intestinal obstruction in developed countries.

The majority of patients with volvulus (without frank ischemia of the bowel) report a history of chronic constipation associated with dilatation and elongation of the colon. Two groups of patients have been identified as being susceptible: (1) those with severe psychiatric or neurologic disease (e.g., Parkinson's, Alzheimer's) who are institutional-ized and often routinely take muscle relaxants and sedatives, and (2) inactive elderly patients with advanced cardiopulmonary disease.[231] Symptoms of volvulus include abdominal pain, increasing abdominal distention, lack of flatus or stool, and prostration. Nausea and emesis ensue after several hours, and distention may lead to respiratory failure in those with poor pulmonary reserve. Abdominal films following barium enema may demonstrate the classical bird's-beak appearance at the point of torsion.[232] In as many as 90 per cent of patients with sigmoid volvulus, detorsion is possible by proctoscopy and can be curative if instituted early, before bowel necrosis has occurred. Once strangulation of the blood supply of the bowel has occurred, perforation, bleeding, sepsis, and shock ensue; associated mortality is very high. It should be kept in mind that the group of patients who develop volvulus are generally elderly and frail. Therefore, despite aggressive and meticulous care, mortality remains high if surgical intervention is required.

In cecal volvulus, diagnosis by radiographic study is frequently inconclusive. In many cases, the disease presents as a small bowel obstruction. Detorsion is not possible owing to the location of the torsion, and strangulation is thus common and tends to occur early in the course of the disease. The treatment is generally right hemicolectomy or cecopexy.

19. Angiodysplasia

Vascular malformations are being recognized more often as the cause of gross hematochezia. This is particularly true among the elderly. Collectively, vascular ectasias include angiomas, angiodysplasias, and arteriovenous malformations. Generally, these are not associated with skin angiomas or systemic malformations, and most are located in the ascending colon and cecum. In addition, they tend to be small and multiple, and may be degenerative lesions associated with aging.[233] One theory proposes that many years of partial, intermittent obstruction of submucosal veins by years of muscle contraction leads to the dysplasia.[233]

Many patients with angiodysplasia have a history of diverticulosis, which in the past may have been confused with angiodysplasia as a source of GI bleeding. Bleeding from angiodysplastic lesions may be occult or massive and exsanguinating. At least one third of patients have had previous admissions related to lower GI bleeding. With the exception of massive bleeding, which is a surgical emergency, all patients should have upper and lower abdominal series radiographs, sigmoidoscopy, and coagulation studies. If time permits, selective angiography or red cell scans may identify the source of bleeding and may allow the interventional radiologist to stop the hemorrhage at its source by administering vasoconstrictive agents through a selectively placed catheter.

In many cases, bleeding stops spontaneously, which can be a great source of frustration for the physician, as the site of the lesion may never be identified. Rarely, empiric segmental, hemi-, or total colectomy without definite localization may be the only option.

F. DISORDERS OF THE PANCREAS

1. General Considerations

Patients with pancreatic disease may have complications due to both exocrine and endocrine insufficiency. For example, diabetes mellitus and all of its far-reaching sequelae may coexist. Conversely, insulinomas may lead to paroxysmal and severe hypoglycemia. Calcium and potassium homeostasis are also considerably altered in patients with pancreatic disease, the mechanisms of which are not well-established. Fluid derangements are quite frequent, which is not unexpected, given that the pancreas normally secretes as much as 3 L of pancreatic juice per day. Furthermore, exocrine pancreatic insufficiency may be associated with profound malnutrition and all of its consequences. Finally, it should be kept in mind that surgery of the pancreas is usually very protracted, technically difficult, and fraught with complications.

2. Acute Pancreatitis

Although the cause of pancreatitis has not been determined, several predisposing factors are known: cholelithiasis, alcoholism, operative trauma, external trauma, peptic ulcer disease, hyperparathyroidism, mumps, and hereditary forms of pancreatitis. Other factors that have been implicated but are not well-established causes include hyperlipidemia, hemochromatosis, toxins, autoimmune disease, and vascular disease.[234]

Clinical manifestations of acute pancreatitis encompass a wide spectrum. Pain is the most common presenting symptom and is usually epigastric, radiating to the back and relieved by assuming the sitting position while leaning forward.[235] Nausea and vomiting are also quite frequent; fever, tachycardia, jaundice, and cirrhosis may also be noted. In severe hemorrhagic pancreatitis, shock may be secondary to blood or fluid loss into the peritoneal cavity or retroperitoneum. Pleural effusions are also common. Hypocalcemia with spasm of the carpopedal muscles or even frank tetany is possible.

The treatment of acute pancreatitis is initially supportive and includes fluid and electrolyte resuscitation, blood component therapy if necessary, bowel rest with nasogastric suctioning, opioids for pain management, anticholinergics, antacids, antibiotics, insulin, and calcium (if necessary). If tetany is severe and life threatening, calcium, magnesium, and even parathyroid hormone may be administered. The use of H_2 antagonists is common, yet there are no data to demonstrate reduced mortality or morbidity in acute pancreatitis; however, TPN has been shown to be beneficial if the disease is prolonged.

The complications associated with pancreatitis include pseudocyst formation (discussed below), abscess, and necrosis of the stomach or duodenum.[236] If the pancreatitis is recurrent, diabetes mellitus and exocrine pancreatic insufficiency can develop in the most severe cases. If complications develop, then surgery is usually indicated, and in equivocal cases exploratory laparotomy may be necessary. Pancreatic abscess and retroperitoneal hemorrhage are extremely morbid complications associated with acute pancreatitis, carrying a mortality risk greater than 80 per cent.[236] The only treatment is peritoneal lavage during surgery with drainage of the retrogastric space, with or without total pancreatectomy.

Owing to liberation of multiple toxic factors (many of which are unidentified), pancreatitis may be associated with severe systemic complications. For example, renal failure, hepatic failure, CNS dysfunction, and respiratory or cardiac failure are possible, even without specific identifiable causes.[236] For example, the adult respiratory distress syndrome (ARDS) is especially frequent in patients with acute, severe pancreatitis, and carries a 50 percent mortality rate. The liberation of unknown toxic pancreatic factors that lead to noncardiogenic pulmonary edema and capillary leakage is postulated.

3. Chronic Pancreatitis

Chronic pancreatitis is slow, progressive inflammation of the pancreas due to recurrent episodes of acute pancreatitis. The causes are multiple, as with acute pancreatitis. Owing to its insidious nature, clinical manifestations include epigastric pain with radiation to the back, exacerbation of pain by eating, anorexia, weight loss, malnutrition, fat malabsorption, diabetes mellitus, and fat-soluble vitamin deficiencies (e.g., vitamin K–associated coagulopathy).[237] Frequently, affected patients are opioid-dependent because recurrent episodes of acute pancreatitis in the past necessitated narcotic therapy. Many patients are also alcoholics.

Therapy includes nutritional supplementation, pancreatic enzyme replacement if the patient is still able to tolerate enteral feeding, management of diabetes, and vitamin supplementation. Sedation and analgesia are also commonly required. Surgery may be necessary and is indicated for the treatment of intercurrent biliary tract disease, pseudocysts, abscess, or failed medical therapy. Most operations, including Puestow's procedure, pancreaticojejunostomy, sphincterotomy, and subtotal pancreatectomy, are unlikely to successfully control painful episodes without alcohol abstinence.

4. Pancreatic Cysts and Pseudocysts

a. Pancreatic Cysts. These are true cysts of the pancreas that are lined with epithelium and are congenital, parasitic, neoplastic, or "retention" cysts. Benign tumors of the pancreas, they present most commonly in women in the sixth and seventh decades of life.[238] The most common symptoms are related to abdominal mass, including discomfort, pain, difficulty breathing (if large), or, rarely, jaundice. The treatment is surgical excision.

b. Pseudocysts. These cysts have no epithelial lining, and are, therefore, false *(pseudo)* cysts. They are most commonly due to

trauma or recurrent episodes of pancreatitis. Tumors and parasitic infections are also rare causes. These represent the vast majority (more than 80 percent) of cystic formations involving the pancreas.[239] Clinical manifestations of pseudocysts include epigastric pain, fever, abdominal mass, nausea, emesis, anorexia, pleural effusion, and jaundice. Complications include obstructive jaundice, infection of the cyst with abscess or sepsis, and hemorrhage into the cyst, peritoneum, or viscus. The diagnosis is established by computed tomography (CT) or ultrasonography. The cysts may be followed over time and many disappear spontaneously. Large cysts that are symptomatic are uniformly operated on because of the high incidence of infections, hemorrhage, and development of a fibrous capsule within 6 weeks. The establishment of a fibrous capsule prevents subsequent self-resolution of the cyst, and thus requires an operation. Operative procedures must be individualized and include simple external drainage, extirpation, cystogastrostomy, cystoduodenostomy, Roux-en-Y cystojejunostomy, and transduodenal sphincterotomy.[239] Major complications following surgery include the formation of pancreatic cutaneous fistulas, which are difficult to heal owing to the content of the secretions.

5. Adult Cystic Fibrosis

Cystic fibrosis, an autosomal recessive disease involving the pancreas, is relatively common in children but exceptionally rare in adults. Fewer than 1 in 20 children with cystic fibrosis live to adulthood, owing to recurrent pulmonary infections and airway obstruction. Bronchiectasis, atelectasis, hemoptysis, pneumothorax, and cor pulmonale are common in these patients at an early age.[240] Pancreatic exocrine insufficiency is the other major manifestation of cystic fibrosis. On rare occasions, cirrhosis and diabetes may develop. Intestinal complications are very common and include obstruction, fecal impaction, and ileal and colonic intussusception.

REFERENCES

1. Studley HO: Percentage of weight loss: A basic indicator of surgical risk in patients with chronic peptic ulcer. JAMA 106:458, 1936.
2. Rombeau JL, Barot LR, Williamson CE, et al: Preop-

erative total parenteral nutrition and surgical outcome in patients with inflammatory bowel disease. Am J Surg 143:139, 1982.

3. Asimov I: Order! Order! *In* Asimov I (ed): Asimov on Physics. Garden City, NJ, Doubleday, 1976.

4. Kinney JM: Energy metabolism: Heat, fuel, and life. *In* Kinney JM, Jeejeebhoy KN, Hill GL, Owen OE (eds): Nutrition and Metabolism in Patient Care. Philadelphia, WB Saunders, 1988.

5. Elia M, Livsey G: Theory and validity of indirect calorimetry during net lipid synthesis. Am J Clin Nutr 47:591, 1988.

6. Weir JB: New methods for calculating metabolic rate with special reference to protein metabolism. J Physiol 109:1, 1949

7. Livesey G, Elia M: Estimation of energy expenditure, net carbohydrate utilization, and net fat oxidation and synthesis by indirect calorimetry: Evaluation of errors with special reference to the detailed composition of fuels. Am J Clin Nutr 47:608, 1988.

8. Owen OE: Regulation of energy and metabolism. *In* Kinney JM, Jeejeebhoy KN, Hill GL, Owen OE (eds): Nutrition and Metabolism in Patient Care. Philadelphia, WB Saunders, 1988.

9. Cunningham JJ: A reanalysis of the factors influencing basal metabolic rate in normal adults. Am J Clin Nutr 33:2372, 1980.

10. Stryer L: Biochemistry, 3rd ed. New York, WH Freeman, 1988, p 633.

11. Mayes PA: Regulation of carbohydrate metabolism. *In* Murray RK, Granner DK, Mayes PA, Rodwell VW (eds): Harper's Biochemistry. Norwalk, CT, Appleton and Lange, 1988.

12. McDonald I: Carbohydrates. *In* Shils ME, Young VR (eds): Modern Nutrition in Health and Disease, 7th ed. Philadelphia, Lea & Febiger, 1988.

13. Kinney JM: Clinical biochemistry: Implications for nutritional support. J Parenter Enteral Nutr 14:148, 1990.

14. Srere PA: The molecular physiology of citrate. Curr Topics Cell Regulation 33:261, 1992.

15. Olson MS: Bioenergetics and oxidative metabolism. *In* Devlin TM (ed): Textbook of Biochemistry with Clinical Correlations, 3rd ed. New York, Wiley-Liss, 1992.

16. Kint JA: Fabry's disease: Alpha-galactosidase deficiency. Science 167:1268, 1970.

17. Desnick RJ: Treatment of inherited metabolic diseases: An overview. *In* Kaback MM (ed): Genetic Issues in Pediatric and Obstetric Practice. Chicago, Year Book, 1981.

18. Laidlaw SA, Kopple JD: Newer concepts for the indispensable amino acids. Am J Clin Nutr 46:593, 1987.

19. Gale RP: Aplastic anemia: Biology and treatment. Ann Intern Med 95:477, 1981.

20. Rodwell VW: Catabolism of amino acid nitrogen. *In* Murray RK, Granner DK, Mayes PA, Rodwell VW (eds): Harper's Biochemistry. Norwalk, CT, Appleton & Lange, 1988.

21. Wyngaarden JB, Kelley WN: Gout. *In* Stanbury JB (ed): Metabolic Basis of Inherited Disease, 5th ed. New York, McGraw-Hill, 1982.

22. Alleyn GA, Hay RW, Picou DI, et al: Protein Energy Malnutrition. London, Edward Arnold, 1977.

23. Wolfe RR, Allsop JR, Burke JF: Glucose metabolism in man: Responses to intravenous glucose infusion. Metabolism 28:210, 1979.

24. Ganong WF: Review of Medical Physiology, 12th ed. Los Altos, CA, Lange, 1985, p 243.

25. Cahill GF: Starvation in man. N Engl J Med 282:668, 1970.

26. Young VR, Scrimshaw NS: The physiology of starvation. Sci Am 225:14, 1971.

27. Third JL, Bremner WF: Lipid and lipoprotein metabolism. *In* Fischer JE (ed): Surgical Nutrition. Boston, Little, Brown, 1988.

28. Hariharan JK: Essential fatty acids. Indian Pediatr 25:67, 1988.

29. Srere PA: The molecular physiology of citrate. Curr Topics Cell Regulation 33:260, 1992.

30. Devlin TM: Textbook of Biochemistry with Clinical Correlations, 3rd ed. New York, Wiley-Liss, 1992, p. 290.

31. Sardesai VM: The essential fatty acids. Nutr Clin Pract 7:179, 1992.

32. Alpers DH, Sabesin SM: Fatty liver: Biochemical and clinical aspects. *In* Schiff L, Schiff ER (eds): Diseases of the Liver. Philadelphia, JB Lippincott, 1987.

33. Tytgat GN, Rubin CE, Saunders DR: Synthesis and transport of lipoprotein particles by intestinal absorptive cells in man. J Clin Invest 50:2065, 1971.

34. Friedman Z: Essential fatty acids revisited. Am J Dis Child 134:406, 1980.

35. Keller PJ, Robinovitch M, Ivenson J, et al: The protein composition of parotid saliva and secretory granules. Biochim Biophys Acta 379:562, 1975.

36. Kelly JJ, Alpers DH: Properties of human intestinal glucoamylase. Biochim Biophys Acta 315:113, 1973.

37. Semenza G, Auricchio S: Small-intestinal disaccharidases. *In* Scriver CR, Beaudet AL, Sey WS, Valle D (eds): The Metabolic Basis of Inherited Disease, 4th ed. New York, McGraw Hill, 1989.

38. DiPalma JA, Narvaez RM: Prediction of lactose malabsorption in referral patients. Dig Dis Sci 33:303, 1988.

39. Wright EM: The intestinal Na^+/glucose cotransporter. Ann Rev Physiol 55:575, 1993.

40. Madara JL: Loosening tight junctions. J Clin Invest 83:1089, 1989.

41. Rinderknecht H: Activation of pancreatic zymogens. Dig Dis Sci 31:314, 1986.

42. Nicklin PL, Irwin WJ, Hassan IF, et al: The transport of acidic amino acids and their analogues across monolayers of human intestinal absorptive cells in vitro. Biochim Biophys Acta 1269:176, 1995.

43. Ferruzza S, Ranaldi G, Di Girolamo M, Sambuy Y: The transport of lysine across monolayers of human cultured intestinal cells depends on Na(+)-dependent and Na(+)-independent mechanisms on different plasma membrane domains. J Nutr 125:2577, 1995.

44. Blackberg L, Hernell O, Olivercrona T: Hydrolysis of human milk fat globules by pancreatic lipase: Role of colipase, phospholipase A2, and bile salts. J Clin Invest 67:1748, 1981.

45. Borgstrom B, Erlanson-Albertson C, Wielock T: Pancreatic colipase: Chemistry and physiology. J Lipid Res 20:805, 1979.

46. Smith LJ, Kamisky S, D'Souza SW: Neonatal fat digestion and lingual lipase. Acta Paediatr Scand 175:313, 1986.

47. Phillips SF: Diarrhea: A current view of the pathophysiology. Gastroenterology 63:495, 1972.

48. Fordtran JS: Speculations on the pathogenesis of diarrhea. Fed Proc 26:1405, 1967.

49. Carrey MC, Small DM, Bliss CM: Lipid digestion and absorption. Annu Rev Physiol 45:651, 1983.

50. Abels J, Schilling RF: Protection of intrinsic factor by vitamin B_{12}. J Lab Clin Med 64:375, 1964.

51. Auduran M: The physiology and pathophysiology of vitamin D. Mayo Clin Proc 60:851, 1985.

52. Conrad ME: Iron absorption. *In* Johnson LR (ed): Physiology of the Gastrointestinal Tract, 2nd ed. New York, Raven Press, 1987.

53. Finch CA, Huebers H: Perspectives in iron metabolism. N Engl J Med 306:1520, 1982.

54. Richter GW: The iron loaded cell—the cytopathology of iron storage. Am J Pathol 91:361, 1978.

55. Bennett A, Stockley HL: The intrinsic innervation of the human alimentary tract and its relation to function. Gut 16:443, 1975.

56. Furness JB, Costa M: The enteric nervous system: An overview. *In* Duchey WY (ed): Functional Disorders of the Digestive Tract. New York, Raven Press, 1983.

57. Conlon JM: Proteolytic inactivation of neurohormone peptides in the gastrointestinal tract. *In* Brown D (ed): Handbook of Experimental Pharmacology. Berlin, Springer-Verlag, 1993.

58. Mutt V, Jorpes E: Hormonal polypetides of the upper intestine. Biochem J 125:57, 1971.

59. Dockray GJ, Gregory RA. Gastrin. *In* Makhlouf GM (ed): Handbook of Physiology—The Gastrointestinal System. New York, Oxford University Press, American Physiology Society, 1989.

60. Mutt V, Jorpes JE: Structure of porcine cholecystokinin-pancreazymin. Eur J Biochem 6:156, 1968.

61. Birnbaumer L: G proteins in signal transduction. Annu Rev Pharmacol Toxicol 30:675, 1990.

62. Christ A, Werth B, Hildebrand P, et al: Human secretin. Biologic effects and plasma kinetics in humans. Gastroenterology 94:311, 1988.

63. Trimble ER, Bruzzone R, Biden TJ, et al: Secretin stimulates cyclic AMP and inositol triphosphate production in rat pancreatic acinar tissue by two fully independent mechanisms. Proc Natl Acad Sci USA 84:3146, 1987.

64. Brown JC, Dahl M, Kwauk S, et al: Properties and actions of GIP. *In* Bloom S, Polak J (eds): Gut Hormones. Edinburgh, Churchill Livingstone, 1981.

65. Mutt V, Said SI: Structure of the porcine vasoactive intestinal octacosanol peptide. Eur J Biochem 42:581, 1974.

66. Dharmsathaphorn K, Sherwin S, Cataland S, et al: Somatostatin inhibits diarrhea in the carcinoid syndrome. Ann Intern Med 92:68, 1980.

67. Emson PC, DeQuit ME: NPY—A new member of the pancreatic polypeptide family. Trends Neurosci Feb:31, 1984.

68. Jensen JL, Brodin P, Berg T, et al: Parotid secretion of fluid, amylase, and kallikrein during reflex stimulation under normal conditions and after acute administration of autonomic blocking agents in man. Acta Physiol Scand 143:321, 1991.

69. Parks HF: Morphological study of the extrusion of secretory materials by the parotid glands of mouse and rat. J Ultrastruct Res 6:449, 1962.

70. Vladez IH: Radiation-induced salivary dysfunction: Clinical course and significance. Special Care Dent 11:252, 1991.

71. Feldman M, Richardson CT: Total 24 hour gastric acid secretion in patients with duodenal ulcer. Comparison with normal subjects and effects of cimetidine and parietal cell vagotomy. Gastroenterology 90:540, 1986.

72. Olson GA, Leffler CW, Fletcher AM: Gastroduodenal ulceration in rabbits producing antibodies to prostaglandins. Prostaglandins 29:475, 1985.

73. Sachs G: The gastric proton pump: The H^+, K^+-ATPase. *In* Johnson LR (ed): Physiology of the Gastrointestinal Tract, 2nd ed. New York, Raven Press, 1987.

74. Soll HA: The actions of secretagogues on oxygen uptake by isolated mammalian parietal cells. J Clin Invest 61:370, 1978.

75. Case RM: Pancreatic secretion: Cellular aspects. *In* Duthe HL, Wormsley KG (eds): Scientific Basis of Gastroenterology. Edingburgh, Churchill Livingstone, 1979.

76. Gorelick FS, Jamieson JD: The pancreatic acinar cell—structure-function relationship of the pancreas. *In* Johnson LR (ed): Physiology of the Gastrointestinal Tract, 3rd ed. New York, Raven Press, 1994.

77. Smrcka AV, Hepler JR, Brown KO, Sternweiss PC: Regulation of polyphosphoinositide-specific phospholipase C activity by purified Gq. Science 251:804, 1991.

78. Devroede GJ, Phillips SF: Conservation of sodium, chloride, and water by the human colon. Gastroenterology 56:421, 1969.

79. Phillips SF, Giller J: The contribution of the colon to electrolyte and water conservation in man. J Lab Clin Med 81:733, 1973.

80. Moog F: The lining of the small intestine. Sci Am 245:154, 1981.

81. Misiewicz JJ, Bartram CI, Cotton PB, et al: Atlas of Clinical Gastroenterology. London, Gower, 1987.

82. Weser E: The management of patients after small bowel resection. Gastroenterology 71:146, 1976.

83. Binder HJ: Absorption and secretion of water and electrolytes by small and large intestine. *In* Sleisenger MH, Fordtran JS (eds): Gastrointestinal Disease: Pathophysiology, Diagnosis, Management, 4th ed. Philadelphia, WB Saunders, 1989.

84. Holdeman LV, Cato EP, Moore WEC: Human fecal flora: Variation in bacterial composition within individuals and a possible effect of emotional stress. Appl Environ Microbiol 32:359, 1976.

85. Huerta G, Viniegra L: Involuntary weight loss as a clinical problem. Rev Invest Clin 41:5, 1989.

86. Heizer WH: Weight loss. *In* Dornbrand L, Fletcher R, Hoole A, Pickard G (eds): Clinical Problems in Ambulatory Care Medicine. Boston, Little, Brown, 1992.

87. Levenson SM, Seifter E: Starvation: Metabolic and physiologic responses. *In* Fischer JE (ed): Surgical Nutrition. Boston, Little, Brown, 1983.

88. Davidson JD, Waldman TA, Goodman DS, Gordon RS Jr: Protein-losing enteropathy in congestive heart failure. Lancet 1:899, 1961.

89. Owen E: Starvation. *In* Degroot LJ, Besser GM, Cahill GF, et al (eds): Endocrinology. Philadelphia, WB Saunders, 1989.

Specific Disorders of Nutrition

90. Alleyn GA, Hay RW, Picou DI, et al: Protein-Energy Malnutrition. London, Edward Arnold, 1977, p 92.

91. Opper RH, Heizer WD: General nutritional principles. *In* Yamada T, Alpers DH, et al (eds): Textbook of Gastroenterology, 2nd ed. Philadelphia, JB Lippincott, 1995.

92. Alleyn GA, Hay RW, Picou DI, et al: Protein-Energy Malnutrition. London, Edward Arnold, 1977.

93. Torun B, Viteri FE: Protein-energy malnutrition. *In* Shils ME, Young VR (eds): Modern Nutrition in Health and Disease, 7th ed. Philadelphia, Lea & Febiger, 1988.
94. Viteri FE, Schneider RE: Gastrointestinal alterations in protein-calorie malnutrition. Med Clin North Am 58:1467, 1974.
95. Food and Nutrition Board Subcommittee on the Tenth Edition of the RDA's. *In* Recommended Dietary Allowances. Washington DC, National Academy Press, 1989.
96. Solomon NW: Trace elements. *In* Rombeau JL, Caldwell MD (eds): Parenteral Nutrition, 2nd ed. Philadelphia, WB Saunders, 1993.
97. Flodin NW: Pharmacology of micronutrients. *In* Albanese AA, Kritchevsky D (eds): Current Topics in Nutrition and Disease. New York, Alan R. Liss, 1988.
98. Kien CL, Veillan C, Pallerson KU, et al: Mild peripheral neuropathy but biochemical chromium insufficiency during 16 months of "chromium free" total parenteral nutrition. J Parenter Enteral Nutr 10:662, 1986.
99. Solomon NW: Trace elements. *In* Rombeau JL, Caldwell MD (eds): Parenteral Nutrition, 2nd ed. Philadelphia, WB Saunders, 1993.
100. Shike M: Copper in parenteral nutrition. Acad Med 60:132, 1984.
101. Prasad AS, Brewer GJ, Schoomaker EB, et al: Hypocupremia induced by zinc therapy in adults. JAMA 240:2166, 1978.
102. Groyens D, Brasseur D, Cadranez S: Copper deficiency in infants with celiac disease. J Pediatr Gastroenterol Nutr 4:677, 1985.
103. Shike M, Roulet M, Kurian R, et al: Copper metabolism and requirements in total parenteral nutrition. Gastroenterology 81:290, 1981.
104. Sweeney EA, Shaw JH: Nutrition in relation to dental medicine. *In* Shils ME, Young VR (eds): Modern Nutrition in Health and Disease, 7th ed. Philadelphia, Lea & Febiger, 1988.
105. Molitch ME, Dahms WT: Endocrinology. *In* Schneider HA, Anderson CE, Coursin DB (eds): Nutritional Support of Medical Practice, 2nd ed. Philadelphia, Harper & Row, 1983.
106. Solomon NW: Trace elements. *In* Rombeau JL, Caldwell MD (eds): Parenteral Nutrition, 2nd ed. Philadelphia, WB Saunders, 1993.
107. Doisy EA: Micronutrient controls on biosynthesis of clotting proteins and cholesterol. *In* Hemphill DD (ed): Trace Substances in Environmental Health. Columbia, University of Missouri Press, 1972.
108. Menta R, Reilly JJ: Manganese levels in a jaundiced long-term total parenteral nutrition patient: Potentiation of haloperidol toxicity? Case report and literature review. J Parenter Enter Nutr 14:428, 1990.
109. Graber TW, Yee AS, Baker FJ: Magnesium: Physiology, clinical disorders, and therapy. Ann Emerg Med 10:49, 1981.
110. Agurs Z, Wasseister A, Goldfarb S: Disorders of calcium and magnesium. Am J Med 78:473, 1982.
111. Graber TW, Yee AS, Baker FJ: Magnesium: Physiology, clinical disorders, and therapy. Ann Emerg Med 10:49, 1981.
112. Juan D: Clinical review: The clinical importance of hypomagnesemia. Surgery 91:510, 1982.
113. Abumrad NN: Molybdenum—is it an essential trace metal? Acad Med 60:163, 1984.
114. Solomon NW: Trace elements. *In* Rombeau JL, Cald-

well MD (eds): Parenteral Nutrition, 2nd ed. Philadelphia, WB Saunders, 1993.
115. Lane HW, Barosso AO, Englert D, et al: Selenium status of chronic intravenous hyperalimentation patients. J Parenter Enteral Nutr 6:246, 1982.
116. Brown MR, Cohen JH, Lyons JM, et al: Proximal muscle weakness and selenium deficiency associated with long term parenteral nutrition. Am J Clin Nutr 43:549, 1986.
117. Flodin NW: Pharmacology of micronutrients. *In* Albanese AA, Kritchevsky D (eds): Current Topics in Nutrition and Disease. New York, Alan R. Liss, 1988.
118. Hambridge KM, Hambridge C, Jacobs M, Baum JD: Low levels of zinc in hair, anorexia, poor growth, and hypergeusia in children. Pediatr Res 6:868, 1972.
119. Cousins RJ, Hempe JM: Zinc. *In* Brown MI (ed): Present Knowledge in Nutrition, 6th ed. Washington, International Life Sciences Institute, Nutrition Foundation, 1990.
120. Norum KR, Blomnoff R: Vitamin A absorption, transport, cellular uptake, and storage. Ann J Clin Nutr 56:735, 1992.
121. Sitren HS: Vitamin A. *In* Baumgartner TG (ed): Clinical Guide to Parenteral Micronutrition, 2nd ed. Melrose Park, IL, Lyphomed, 1991.
122. DeLuca HF: Vitamin D and its metabolites. *In* Shils ME, Young R (eds): Modern Nutrition in Health and Disease, 7th ed. Philadelphia, Lea & Febiger, 1988.
123. Goldsmith GA: Curative nutrition—vitamins. *In* Schneider HA, Anderson CE, Coursin DB (eds): Nutritional Support of Medical Practice, 2nd ed. Philadelphia, Harper & Row, 1983.
124. Sitren HS: Vitamin E. *In* Baumgartner TG (ed): Clinical Guide to Parenteral Micronutrition, 2nd ed. Melrose Park, IL, Lyphomed, 1991.
125. Farrell PM: Vitamin E. *In* Shils ME, Young VR (eds): Modern Nutrition in Health and Disease, 7th ed. Philadelphia, Lea & Febiger, 1988.
126. Olson RE: The function and metabolism of Vitamin K. Annu Rev Nutr 4:281, 1984.
127. Frick PG, Riedler G, Brogli H: Dose response and minimal daily requirement for Vitamin K in man. J Appl Physiol 23:387, 1967.
128. Food and Nutrition Board Subcommittee of the Tenth Edition of the RDA's. *In* Recommended Dietary Allowances. Washington, DC, National Academy Press, 1989.
129. McCormick DB: Thiamine. *In* Shils ME, Young VR (eds): Modern Nutrition in Health and Disease, 7th ed. Philadelphia, Lea & Febiger, 1988.
130. Vitamins. *In* Robbins SL, Cotran RS, Kumar V: Pathologic Basis of Disease, 3rd ed. Philadelphia, WB Saunders, 1984.
131. McCormick DB: Niacin. *In* Shils ME, Young VR (eds): Modern nutrition in health and disease, 7th ed. Philadelphia, Lea & Febiger, 1988, p. 370.
132. McCormick DB: Niacin. *In* Shils ME, Young VR (eds): Modern Nutrition in Health and Disease, 7th ed. Philadelphia, Lea & Febiger, 1988, pp. 371–372.
133. McCormick DB: Vitamin B6. *In* Shils ME, Young VR (eds): Modern Nutrition in Health and Disease, 7th ed. Philadelphia, Lea & Febiger, 1988.
134. Herbert V: Hematology and the anemias. *In* Schneider HA, Anderson CE, Coursen DB (eds): Nutritional Support of Medical Practice, 2nd ed. Philadelphia, Harper & Row, 1983.
135. Herbert VD, Colman N: Folic acid and vitamin B$_{12}$. *In* Shils ME, Young VR (eds): Modern Nutrition in

Health and Disease, 7th ed. Philadelphia, Lea & Febiger, 1988.

136. Linnell JC: The fate of cobalamin in vivo. *In* Babior BM (ed): Cobalamin: Biochemistry and Pathophysiology. New York, Wiley, 1975.

137. Baker SJ, Mathan VI: Evidence regarding the minimal daily requirement of dietary vitamin B_{12}. Am J Clin Nutr 34:2423, 1981.

138. Kapadia CR, Donaldson RM Jr: Disorders of cobalamin absorption and transport. Annu Rev Med 36:93, 1985.

139. Sauberlich HE: Ascorbic acid. *In* Brown ML (ed): Present Knowledge in Nutrition, 6th ed. Washington, DC, International Life Sciences Institute, Nutrition Foundation, 1990.

140. McCormick DB: Biotin. *In* Shils ME, Young VR (eds): Modern Nutrition in Health and Disease, 7th ed. Philadelphia, Lea & Febiger, 1988.

141. Heizer WD, Holcombe BJ: Approach to the patient requiring nutritional supplementation. *In* Yamada T, Alpers DH, et al (eds): Textbook of Gastroenterology, 2nd ed. Philadelphia, JB Lippincott, 1995.

142. Hariharan JK: Essential fatty acids. Indian Pediatr 25:67, 1988.

143. Gottschlich MM: Selection of optimal lipid sources in enteral and parenteral nutrition. Nutr Clin Pract 7:152, 1992.

144. Heizer WD, Holcombe BJ: General nutritional principles. *In* Yamada T, Alpers DH, et al (eds): Textbook of Gastroenterology, 2nd ed. Philadelphia, JB Lippincott, 1995.

145. Reisin E, Frohlich ED: Obesity: Cardiovascular and respiratory pathophysiological alterations. Arch Intern Med 141:431, 1981.

146. McLean LD, Rhode BM, Shizgal HM: Nutrition following gastric operations for morbid obesity. Ann Surg 198:347, 1983.

147. McLean LD, Rhode BM, Shizgal HM: Nutrition after vertical banded gastroplasty. Ann Surg 206:555, 1987.

148. Scott HW: Metabolic surgery for hyperlipidemia and atherosclerosis. Am J Surg 23:3, 1972.

149. Papowitz AJ, Li JKH: Abdominal sarcoidosis with ascites. Chest 59:692, 1971.

150. Munt PW: Sarcoidosis of the appendix presenting as appendiceal perforation and abscess. Chest 66:295, 1974.

Regional Anatomic Disorders

151. Redick LF: The temporomandibular joint and tracheal intubation. Anesth Analg 66:675, 1987.

152. Navazesh M, Christiansen C, Brightman V: Clinical criteria for the diagnosis of salivary gland hypofunction. J Dent Res 71:1363, 1992.

153. Ellis FH Jr: Pharyngoesophageal diverticula and cricopharyngeal incoordination. Mod Treat 7:1098, 1970.

154. Zboralske FF, Friedland GW: Medical progress: Diseases of the esophagus. Calif Med 112:33, 1970.

155. The Gastrointestinal Tract. *In* Robbins SL, Cotran RS, Kumar V (eds): Pathologic Basis of Disease, 3rd ed. Philadelphia, WB Saunders, 1984.

156. Cassella RR, Brown AL Jr, Sayre GP, et al: Achalasia of the esophagus: Pathologic and etiologic considerations. Ann Surg 160:474, 1964.

157. Bettarello A, Pinotti HW: Oesphageal involvement in Chagas' disease. Clin Gastroenterol 5:103, 1976.

158. Kramer P: Diffuse esophageal spasm. Mod Treat 7:1151, 1970.

159. Culver GJ, Pirson HS, Bean BC: Mechanism of obstruction in para-esophageal diaphragmatic hernias. JAMA 181:933, 1962.

160. Bruno MS, Grier WRN, Ober WB: Spontaneous laceration and rupture of the esophagus and stomach. Arch Intern Med 112:574, 1963.

161. Foster JH: Esophageal perforation. Mod Treat 7:1284, 1970.

162. Burford TH, Ferguson TB: Esophageal perforations and mediastinal sepsis. *In* Hardy JD (ed): Critical Surgical Illness. Philadelphia, WB Saunders, 1971.

163. Holt JM: *Candida* infection of the oesophagus. Gut 9:227, 1968.

164. Marchand P: Caustic strictures of the esophagus. Thorax 10:171, 1955.

165. Hiebert C: The recognition and management of gastroesophageal reflux without hiatal hernia. World J Surg 1:445, 1977.

166. Demeester T, Johnson L, Kent A: Evaluation of current operations for the prevention of gastroesophageal reflux. Ann Surg 180:511, 1974.

167. Mercer CD, Hill LD: Surgical management of peptic esophageal stricture: Twenty year experience. J Thorac Cardiovasc Surg 91:371, 1986.

168. Burgess JN, Payne WS, Andersen HA, et al: Barrett esophagus: The columnar epithelial–lined lower esophagus. Mayo Clin Proc 46:728, 1971.

169. Watson RR, O'Connor TM, Weisel W: Solid benign tumors of the esophagus. Ann Thorac Surg 4:81, 1967.

170. Klifto EJ, Allen SK, Metzman M, et al: Plummer Vinson syndrome: Report of a case and review of the literature. J Am Osteopath Assoc 83:56, 1983.

171. Schatzki R, Gary JE: The lower esophageal ring. Am J Roentgenol 75:246, 1956.

172. Michel L, Serrano A, Malt RA: Mallory-Weiss syndrome: Evolution of diagnostic and therapeutic patterns over two decades. Ann Surg 192:716, 1980.

173. Stehling LC: Anesthetic management of the patient with hyperparathyroidism. Anesthesiology 41:585, 1974.

174. Isenberg JI, Walsh JH, Grossman MI: Zollinger Ellison syndrome. Gastroenterology 65:140, 1973.

175. Romanus ME, Neal JA, Dilley WG: Comparison of four provocative tests for the diagnosis of gastrinoma. Ann Surg 197:608, 1983.

176. Moertel CG, Hanley JA, Johnson LA: Streptozocin alone compared with streptozocin plus fluorouracil in the treatment of advanced islet-cell carcinoma. N Engl J Med 303:1189, 1980.

177. Feldman M, Richardson CT, Taylor I, Walsh JH: Effect of atropine on vagal release of gastrin and pancreatic polypeptide. J Clin Invest 63:294, 1979.

178. Black BM: Primary hyperparathyroidism and peptic ulcer. Surg Clin North Am 51:955, 1971.

179. Messer J, Reitman D, Sacks HS, et al: Association of adrenocorticosteroid therapy and peptic ulcer disease. N Engl J Med 309:21, 1983.

180. Piper J, Ray W, Daugherty J, Griffin M: Corticosteroid use and peptic ulcer disease: Role of nonsteroidal anti-inflammatory drugs. Ann Intern Med 114:735, 1991.

181. Silen W: The clinical problem of stress ulcers. Clin Invest Med 10:270, 1987.

182. Skillman JJ, Silen W: Acute gastroduodenal "stress" ulceration: Barrier disruption of varied pathogenesis? Gastroenterology 59:478, 1970.

183. McCormack TT, Sims J, Eyre-Brook I, et al: Gastric lesions in portal hypertension: Inflammatory gastritis or congestive gastropathy? Gut 26:1226, 1985.

184. Worning H: Chronic pancreatitis: Pathogenesis, natural history, and conservative treatment. Clin Gastroenterol 13:871, 1984.

185. Gonzalez-Crussi F, Hackett RL: Phlegmonous gastritis. Arch Surg 93:90, 1966.

186. Chazan BI, Aichison JD: Gastric tuberculosis. Br Med J 2:1288, 1960.

187. Beard RJ, Gruebel Lee EC, Haysom AH, et al: Noncarcinomatous tumors of the stomach. Br J Surg 55:535, 1968.

188. Pack GT: Unusual tumors of the stomach. Ann NY Acad Sci 114:985, 1964.

189. Cogliatti SB, Schmid U, Schumacher U, et al: Primary B-cell gastric lymphoma: A clinicopathological study of 145 patients. Gastroenterology 101:1159, 1991.

190. Farrugia G, Kim CH, Grant CS, et al: Leiomyosarcoma of the stomach: Determinants of long-term survival. Mayo Clin Proc 67:533, 1992.

191. Gean AD, Deluca S: Acute gastric volvulus. Am Fam Physician 34:99, 1986.

192. Saik RP, Greenburg AG, Farris JM, et al: The practicality of the Congo red test or is your vagotomy complete? Am J Surg 132:144, 1976.

193. Weaver GA, Alpers DH, Davis JS, et al: Gastrointestinal angiodysplasia associated with aortic valve disease: Part of a spectrum of angiodysplasia of the gut. Gastroenterology 77:1, 1979.

194. Trier JS: Celiac sprue. N Engl J Med 325:1709, 1991.

195. Strober W: Gluten-sensitive enteropathy. *In* King RA, Rotter JI, Motulsky AG (eds): The Genetic Basis of Common Diseases. New York, Oxford University Press, 1992.

196. Ferguson A, Arranz E, O'Mahony S: Clinical and pathological spectrum of coeliac disease—active, silent, latent, potential. Gut 34:150, 1993.

197. Ostermiller W, Joergenson EJ, Weibel L: A clinical review of tumors of the small bowel. Am J Surg 111:403, 1966.

198. Nelson RL: Adenocarcinoma of the small intestine. *In* Nelson RL, Nyhus LM (eds): Surgery of the Small Intestine. Norwalk, CT, Appleton & Lange, 1987.

199. Wilson H, Cheek RC, Sherman R, Storer EH: Carcinoid tumors. Curr Probl Surg 7:1, 1970.

200. MacGillivray DC, Synder DA, Drucker W, ReMine SG: Carcinoid tumors: The relationship between clinical presentation and the extent of disease. Surgery 110:68, 1991.

201. Lowenfels AB: Why are small bowel tumors so rare? Lancet 1:24, 1973.

202. Jeghers H, McKusick VA, Katz KH: Generalized intestinal polyposis and melanin spots of the oral mucosa, lips, and digits. A syndrome of diagnostic significance. N Engl J Med 241:993, 1949.

203. Reilly PJ, Nostrant TT: Clinical manifestations of hereditary hemorrhagic telangiectasis. Am J Gastroenterol 79:363, 1984.

204. Farmer RG, Hawk WA, Turnbull RB: Clinical patterns in Crohn's disease: A statistical study of 615 cases. Gastroenterology 68:627, 1975.

205. Farmer RG: Clinical features and natural history of inflammatory bowel disease. Med Clin North Am 64:1103, 1980.

206. Rabbani GH: Cholera. Clin Gastroenterol 15:507, 1986.

207. Rubin RH, Weinstein L: Salmonellosis: Microbiologic, Pathologic, and Clinical Features. New York, Stratton, 1977.

208. Abrahams JS, Holden WD: Tuberculosis of the gastrointestinal tract. Arch Surg 89:282, 1964.

209. Kushlan SD: Pneumatosis cystoides intestinalis. JAMA 179:699, 1962.

210. Glotzer DJ, Gardener RC, Goldman H, et al: Comparative features and course of ulcerative and granulomatous colitis. N Engl J Med 282:588, 1970.

211. Thompson H, Waterhouse JAH, Allan RN: Cancer morbidity in ulcerative colitis. Gut 23:490, 1982.

212. Watts JM, de Dombal FT, Watkinson G, Goligher JC: Early course of ulcerative colitis. Gut 7:16, 1966.

213. Diagnosis and treatment of *Clostridium difficile* colitis. JAMA 269:71, 1993.

214. Axelrod FB, Fonda JN, Bradley EL III. Retroperitoneal actinomycosis: A rare manifestation of an uncommon disease. South Med J 75:1156, 1982.

215. Adams EB, MacLeod IN: Invasive amebiasis. I. Amebic dysentery and its complications. Medicine 56:315, 1977.

216. Ravdin JJ, Petri WA Jr: *Entamoeba histolytica. In* Mandell GL, Douglas RG Jr, Bennett JR (eds): Principles and Practice of Infectious Disease. New York, Churchill Livingstone, 1990.

217. Cheever AW, Kamel IA, Elwi AM, et al: *Schistosoma mansoni* and *S. haematobium* infections in Egypt. III. Extrahepatic pathology. Am J Trop Med Hyg 27:55, 1987.

218. Maddison SE: The present status of serodiagnosis and seroepidemiology of schistosomiasis. Diagn Microbiol Infect Dis 7:93, 1987.

219. Wilson JF, Rausch RL: Alveolar hydatid disease: A review of clinical features of 33 indigenous cases of *Echinococcus multilocularis* infection in Alaskan Eskimos. Am J Trop Med Hyg 29:1340, 1980.

220. Pawlowski ZS: Ascariasis: Host-pathogen biology. Rev Infect Dis 4:806, 1982.

221. Von Bonsdorff B: Diphyllobothriasis in Man. London, Academic Press, 1977.

222. Burt DRR: Platyhelminthes and parasitism: An introduction to parasitology. New York, American Elsevier, 1970.

223. Babior BM: Villous adenoma of the colon. Study of a patient with severe fluid and electrolyte disturbances. Am J Med 41:5, 1966.

224. Nicoloff DM, Ellis CM, Humphrey EW: Management of villous adenomas of the colon and rectum. Arch Surg 97:254, 1968.

225. Groden J, Thliveris A, Samowitz W, et al: Identification and characterization of the familial adenomatous polyposis coli gene. Cell 66:589, 1991.

226. Gardener EJ: Genetic and clinical study of intestinal polyposis, a predisposing factor for carcinoma of colon and rectum. Am J Hum Genet 3:167, 1951.

227. Daniel ES, Ludwig SL, Lewink J, et al: The Cronkhite-Canada syndrome: An analysis of clinical and pathological features and therapy. Medicine 61:293, 1982.

228. Turcot J, Despres JP, St. Pierre F: Malignant tumors of the central nervous system associated with familial polyposis of the colon. Dis Colon Rectum 2:465, 1959.

229. Jarvis L, Bathurst N, Mohan D, Beckly D: Turcot's syndrome. A review. Dis Colon Rectum 31:907, 1988.

230. Arnold G, Nance F: Volvulus of the sigmoid colon. Ann Surg 177:527, 1973.

231. Shoospow D, Berardi R: Volvulus of the sigmoid colon. Dis Colon Rectum 19:535, 1976.
232. Anderson A, Bergdohl L, Van Der Linden W: Volvulus of the cecum. Ann Surg 181:876, 1975.
233. Boley S, Sammartano R, Brandt L, et al: Vascular ectasias of the colon. Surg Gynecol Obstet 149:353, 1979.
234. Bradley EL: A clinically based classification system for acute pancreatitis. Arch Surg 128:586, 1993.
235. Anderson MC: Review of pancreatic disease. Surgery 66:434, 1969.
236. Marshall JB: Acute pancreatitis: A review with an emphasis on new developments. Arch Intern Med 153:1185, 1993.
237. Sarles H: Definition and classifications of pancreatitis. Pancreas 6:470, 1991.
238. Aranha GV, Prinz RA, Esguerra AC, et al: The nature and course of cystic pancreatic lesions diagnosed by ultrasound. Arch Surg 118:486, 1983.
239. Bradley EL, Clements JL, Gonzalez AC: The natural history of pancreatic pseudocysts: A unified concept of management. Am J Surg 137:135, 1979.
240. Marino CR, Gorelick FS: Scientific advancements in cystic fibrosis. Gastroenterology 103:681, 1992.

Diseases of the Endocrine System

Michael F. Roizen

A crucial factor in successful surgical treatment of endocrine diseases is a complete and accurate preoperative diagnosis. Sometimes the differential diagnosis is difficult, and often it requires the expertise of the endocrinologist, radiologist, and clinical pathologist. Armed with a complete and accurate diagnosis, the anesthesiologist and surgeon can offer the patient better relief of his or her symptoms and a more optimistic prognosis. Perioperative outcome in many of these conditions involves an understanding by the anesthesiologist of what the surgeon is trying to accomplish and, equally important, the end organ effect of the endocrine disorder. For example, diabetics often have renal and cardiac disease and peripheral and autonomic neuropathies. Understanding these consequences of diabetes and optimizing their treatment is crucial to the perioperative management of the diabetic, more so than is the finesse of managing insulin requirements by one of the many schemes available.

I. PARATHYROID GLANDS
A. PHYSIOLOGY

Total (bound and free) serum calcium concentration is maintained at the normal level of 9.5 to 10.5 mg/dl by the effects of both parathyroid hormone (PTH), calcitonin, and vitamin D.[1] When the ionized calcium concentration decreases or serum phosphate levels rise, release of PTH is stimulated. PTH is secreted by the four parathyroid glands, usually located behind the upper and lower poles of the thyroid gland.[2] PTH increases tubular reabsorption of calcium and decreases tubular reabsorption of phosphate to raise serum calcium concentration. A renal phosphate leak is the result of excessive PTH secretion. Calcitonin (produced in the C cells of the thyroid gland) antagonizes the effects of PTH and is released in response to high serum ionized calcium. Approximately 50 per cent of the serum calcium is bound to serum proteins (albumin). Forty per cent of the serum calcium is ionized, and the remaining 10 per cent is bound to such chelating agents as citrate. If the serum protein concentration decreases, the total serum calcium will also decrease. The rule of thumb is that for every 1-g decrement in albumin, a 0.8-mg/dl decrement in total serum calcium occurs. Likewise, if the serum proteins increase (as in myeloma), total serum calcium will increase. Acidosis tends to increase the ionized calcium, whereas alkalosis tends to decrease it. There may be a slight tendency for the serum calcium level to drop with age, with a concomitant elevation of the serum PTH, perhaps contributing to the osteoporosis associated with the aging process.[3]

The evaluation of disorders of calcium metabolism has been greatly helped by the measurement of PTH in blood. However, there have been problems with the radioimmunoassay of PTH, caused by the presence of various active and inactive fragments and forms of PTH in blood. Many laboratories now measure the biologically inactive C-carboxyl fragment accurately. Despite these problems, the PTH assay is extremely useful in evaluating patients with hypercalcemia.

Vitamin D plays an important role in calcium homeostasis. Cholecalciferol is synthesized in the skin by the effects of ultraviolet light. Cholecalciferol is hydroxylated in the liver to form 25-hydroxycholecalciferol. The 25-hydroxy derivative is further hydroxylated in the kidney to form 1,25-dihydroxycholecalciferol ($1,25(OH)_2D_3$). The 1,25-dihydroxy derivative is by far the most potent vitamin D compound yet discovered. $1,25(OH)_2D_3$ stimulates absorption of both calcium and phosphorus from the gastrointestinal (GI) tract.[4] Thus, vitamin D provides the substrates for the formation of mineralized bone. $1,25(OH)_2D_3$ may also directly enhance mineralization of newly formed osteoid matrix in bone. Vitamin D derivatives also seem to work synergistically with PTH in bringing about increased resorption of bone. Clinically, this is an important point because immobilization alone increases bone reabsorption, and if the patient is receiving a vitamin D derivative, bone reabsorption may be increased further. Evidence now indicates that the hydroxylation of 25-hydroxycholecalciferol is controlled in the kidney by PTH and the phosphorus level. Elevated PTH and hypophosphatemia tend to accentuate the synthesis of $1,25(OH)_2D_3$, whereas low levels of PTH and high levels of phosphate turn off the synthesis of $1,25(OH)_2D_3$ in the kidney. PTH maintains a normal calcium level in blood by increasing calcium reabsorption from bone and by promoting synthesis of $1,25(OH)_2D_3$, which in turn enhances calcium reabsorption from the gut. Finally, PTH directly increases calcium reabsorption from the renal tubule.

Thus, PTH accelerates the breakdown of bone by a complex mechanism that includes a fast component and a slow component (involving protein synthesis and cellular proliferation). In addition, PTH has an anabolic effect on bone formation, and in tissue culture it increases the number of active osteoblasts, the maturation of cartilage, and osteoid formation within the bone shaft.

B. HYPERCALCEMIA

Patients with hypercalcemia present with a variety of symptoms that are often nonspecific. The level of blood calcium is frequently related to the degree and severity of symptoms. With calcium levels above 14 mg/dl, signs and symptoms such as anorexia, nausea, vomiting, abdominal pain, constipation, polyuria, tachycardia, and dehydration may occur.[1] Psychosis and obtundation are usually the end results of severe and prolonged hypercalcemia. Band keratopathy is a most unusual physical finding. Patients with hyperparathyroidism occasionally present with a history of calcium-containing kidney stones or peptic ulcers. Bone disease in hyperparathyroidism, such as subperiosteal resorption, can also be seen in x-rays of the teeth and hands.[5, 6] Severe bone disease in hyperparathyroidism, such as osteitis fibrosa cystica, is only very rarely seen these days. It is usually seen only in older patients who have had long-standing disease (perhaps up to 20 years). The older patient with severe osteopenia, and perhaps vertebral compression fractures, should prompt suspicion of hyperparathyroidism. Many patients with hyperparathyroidism can tolerate blood calcium levels of 12 mg/dl without many symptoms.[5] This situation, often found by multiphasic screening, presents the dilemma of whether to operate on asymptomatic patients. The risk-benefit ratio is not clear at this point, and advocates of no treatment but watchful waiting appear to have the outcome data to at least present a reasonable argument.[5] Although surgical removal of a parathyroid adenoma is usually curative in asymptomatic patients, patients with mild, uncomplicated primary hyperparathyroidism may be followed medically if the serum calcium levels are less than 11.5 mg/dl and bone density and renal function are normal. Such patients should have quarterly check-ups of blood pressure, bone density, and renal function. Complications may be prevented by avoiding dehydration, thiazide diuretics, and immobilization. It was previously thought that a single parathyroid adenoma was the chief cause of the hypercalcemia of hyperparathyroidism.[7] However, it has been recognized that parathyroid hyperplasia, usually involving all four parathyroid glands, may be a major cause of the hyperparathyroid syndrome. Carcinoma of the parathyroid glands is extremely rare. Different institutions report varying incidences of parathyroid adenomas and of hyperplastic glands. It is conceivable that all adenomas begin as hyperplasia;[8] therefore, for any one patient, exactly where in the natural history of the disease an operation occurs may determine whether hyperplasia or an adenoma is found.

Patients with hyperparathyroidism have elevated calcium and low serum phosphate levels. Very mild hyperchloremic acidosis may be present. The PTH level is usually elevated but is certainly elevated for the level of calcium concentration.[5, 9] The only two situations in which hypercalcemia would be associated with a high PTH level are hyperparathyroidism and the ectopic PTH syndrome (usually secondary to a tumor of the lung or kidney that produces a biologically active fragment of PTH).[1] All other causes of hypercalcemia are associated with either normal or, more appropriately, low levels of PTH. When a patient presents with an extremely high blood calcium level (above 14 mg/dl), more likely than not, the patient has a distant cancer rather than hyperparathyroidism. Overall, about 50 per cent of all cases of hypercalcemia are due to cancer invading bone. In these cases, prognosis is poor: more than 50 per cent of patients die within 6 months. Treating hypercalcemia does not prolong survival but usually improves quality of life.[10, 11] The technetium diphosphonate bone scan is positive in a large percentage of cancers that have metastasized to bone. Myeloma is another important cancer that is associated with hypercalcemia. The isotope bone scan is sometimes normal in this disease.

A number of other anomalies have to do with excessive absorption of calcium from the GI tract. These abnormalities include (1) milk-alkali syndrome, which is usually due to excessive ingestion of calcium-containing antacids; (2) vitamin D intoxication; and (3) sarcoidosis, which is associated with hypersensitivity of the GI tract to vitamin D. Hyperthyroidism is occasionally associated with increased bone resorption, and hypercalcemia may be present. Many patients with hyperthyroidism also have hyperparathyroidism.

Some patients become hypercalcemic during treatment with thiazide diuretics. Thiazides increase renal tubular reabsorption of calcium and may even enhance the PTH effects on the renal tubule. Most patients who have significant hypercalcemia associated with thiazide diuretics have hyperparathyroidism. An important cause of increased bone reabsorption, and occasionally of mild hypercalcemia, is prolonged immobilization. Immobilization in any situation that is already associated with increased bone reabsorption, such as Paget's disease or ingestion of large quantities of vitamin D, can result in exaggerated hypercalcemia and excessive bone reabsorption. Table 8–1 lists the different causes of hypercalcemia and laboratory studies that differentiate them. In addition to the blood calcium and phosphate, the bony fraction of the alkaline phosphatase, creatinine, electrolytes, and urinary calcium level, as well as the appropriate skeletal x-ray studies and isotope bone scan, are often performed by endocrinologists to aid diagnosis.

Although the PTH level is elevated in both hyperparathyroidism and in patients with ectopic PTH syndrome, if the carboxyl terminal fragment is measured, PTH levels are higher for a given serum calcium in hyperparathyroidism than in cancers associated with PTH fragment production. There have been a few case reports of some lymphoproliferative malignancies associated with production of a prostaglandin that is in turn associated with increased bone reabsorption and hypercalcemia. Thus, cancer may produce hypercalcemia by at least three mechanisms: (1) metastasis to bone with increased bone reabsorption, (2) production by the cancer of a biologically active fragment of PTH, and (3) production of a prostaglandin that causes bone reabsorption.

Elevation of the bone fraction of alkaline phosphatase (heat labile) usually means excessive breakdown of osteoid tissue. It can be seen whenever either increased bone turnover or significant unmineralized osteoid is present. Very high alkaline phosphatase is seen in Paget's disease, where bone turnover is extremely high. Any state associated with excessive PTH can be associated with a high bone alkaline phosphatase value, such as hyperparathyroidism of renal disease. However, osteomalacia, in which bone turnover is extremely low but a large amount of unmineralized osteoid is present, is associated with a high rate of osteoid breakdown and therefore

TABLE 8–1

Differential Diagnosis of Hypercalcemia

	Serum Phosphorus	Serum Alkaline Phosphatase	Creatinine	Urinary Calcium	Blood Parathyroid Hormone	Comments
Cancer (metastatic)	N	↑	N	↑	N or ↑	Osteolytic lesion bone scan is +
Ectopic PTH production	↓	N or ↑	N	↑	↑ or N	Cancer of lung and kidney common
Myeloma	N	N or ↑	↑	↑	↓	Plasma protein ↑
Hyperparathyroidism	↓	N or ↑	N	N or ↑	↑	Subperiosteal resorption Kidney stones
Milk-alkali syndrome	N	N	↑	N	↓	Alkalosis; history of calcium intake
Vitamin D intoxication	↑	N or ↑	↑	↑	↓	Vitamin D levels ↑
Hyperthyroidism	N	N or ↑	N	↑	↓	T_4 or T_3 levels ↑
Sarcoid	N	N or ↑	N	↑	↓	Plasma proteins ↑
Thiazides	N or ↓	N or ↑	N	N or ↓	N or ↑	Coexistent hyperparathyroidism often
Adrenal insufficiency	N	N	N or ↑	N	↓	Hyponatremia Hyperkalemia
Immobilization	N	N	N	↑	N	If fracture, alkaline phosphatase ↑
Paget's disease	N	↑↑	N	↑	N	Bone scan is +

Key: ↑, elevated; ↑↑, markedly elevated; N, normal.

high alkaline phosphatase. Urinary hydroxyproline is also a specific measure of osteoid breakdown.

A number of patients have been described with renal stones, normal blood calcium, normal to mildly elevated PTH levels, and very high urinary cyclic AMP levels. It is now thought that these patients have normocalcemic hyperparathyroidism, and many have been found to have parathyroid disease at surgery. The high cyclic AMP levels in the urine are a reflection of PTH activity (perhaps a PTH fragment that affects only the kidneys and not bone).

Treatment. Severe hypercalcemia (especially above levels of 14–16 mg/dl) constitutes a medical emergency, and often treatment must be begun before the diagnosis is complete. There is no way to relate the signs and symptoms any one patient experiences to the level of blood calcium. In an extreme situation it is possible to have one patient who is almost asymptomatic, with a total blood calcium level of 14 mg/dl, while another who has an identical blood calcium level has severe polyuria, tachycardia, dehydration, and even psychosis. Age seems to be a factor; that is, for any given calcium level, the older patient is more likely to be symptomatic than a younger one. Tachydysrhythmias, including sinus tachycardia, are extremely common and usually out of pro-

portion to the degree of volume depletion. Occasionally heart block results. Extreme care must be exercised in the use of digitalis derivatives for patients with hypercalcemia. Digitalis intoxication occurs quite readily in the presence of hypercalcemia. Digitalis toxicity dysrhythmias are extremely common in this setting.

In general, any patient with a calcium level of 16 mg/dl should be considered a medical emergency and treated with saline hydration (with careful attention to the risk of precipitating congestive heart failure [CHF]) and furosemide. Salmon mithramycin (or human, if a patient is allergic), corticosteroids, intravenous phosphates, or indomethacin can also be used.[11] A few patients with calcium levels of 14 mg/dl (especially older patients) also qualify for emergency treatment.

1. Preoperative Considerations for Patients with Hyperparathyroidism

Patients with moderate hypercalcemia who have normal renal and cardiovascular function present no special preoperative problems. The electrocardiogram should be examined preoperatively and intraoperatively for shortened PR or QT interval.[12] Because severe hypercalcemia can result in hypovolemia, normal intravascular volume and electrolyte status should be restored before anesthesia and surgery are begun.

Management of hypercalcemia can include increasing urinary calcium excretion by means of hydration and diuresis.[11] Restoration of intravascular volume by augmentation of urinary sodium excretion and administration of diuretics (furosemide is commonly employed) usually increases urinary calcium excretion substantially. Complications of these interventions include hypomagnesemia and hypokalemia.

Phosphate should be given to correct hypophosphatemia, because hypophosphatemia decreases calcium uptake into bone, increases calcium absorption from the intestine, stimulates breakdown of bone, and can result in CHF or pump failure.[13] Hydration and diuresis, accompanied by phosphate repletion, suffice as management of most hypercalcemic patients. If additional intervention is needed, glucocorticoids, mithramycin, or calcitonin may be given. Corticosteroids inhibit further GI calcium absorption. Mithramycin lowers calcium levels by approximately 2 mg/dl after 36 to 48 hours through its effect on osteoclasts. Its toxic effects include thrombocytopenia, decreased levels of clotting factors, hepatotoxicity, azotemia, proteinuria, hypocalcemia, hypophosphatemia, and hypokalemia. Most of these can be reversed simply by discontinuation of the drug. Consultation with an endocrinologist or oncologist is advisable before mithramycin is given, because it has a narrow therapeutic-to-toxic ratio.

Calcitonin lowers serum calcium levels through direct inhibition of bone resorption. It can decrease serum calcium levels within minutes after intravenous administration. Calcitonin is less effective than phosphate or mithramycin, however, for patients with hypercalcemia caused by hyperparathyroidism. Side effects include urticaria and nausea.

It is especially important to know whether hypercalcemia has been chronic, as serious abnormalities in the cardiac, renal, or central nervous system may have resulted. Hypercalcemia associated with severe renal failure often can be treated successfully only by peritoneal dialysis or hemodialysis, with a low calcium concentration in the dialysis bath.

Finally, there are a few additional preanesthetic considerations. Aspiration precautions must be taken because the hypercalcemic patient with altered mental status may have a full stomach or be unable to protect the airway. The possibility of lytic or pathologic fractures warrants careful positioning. Radiographs of the cervical spine should be taken to rule out lytic lesions when hypercalcemia results from cancer.[14] Laryngoscopy in a patient with an unstable cervical spine may result in quadriplegia.

2. Intraoperative and Postoperative Considerations for Patients with Hyperparathyroidism

No controlled study has demonstrated clinical advantages of any one anesthetic drug over others. A review of cases at the University of California, San Francisco, and another at the University of Chicago from 1968 to 1982 revealed that virtually all anesthetic techniques and agents have been employed without adverse effects that could have been even remotely attributable to either the agent or the technique.

Maintenance of anesthesia usually presents little difficulty. No special intraoperative monitoring for patients with these conditions is required; a blood pressure cuff, lead II and/or MCL_5 ECG, temperature probe, and esophageal stethoscope typically are used. Because of the proximity of surgical retraction to the face, meticulous care is taken to protect the eyes. Response to neuromuscular blocking agents may be unpredictable when calcium levels are elevated;[15] reversal of the effects may be difficult.[14]

Failure to remove all the lesions at the first operation at times necessitates a second or third or even additional operation. Arteriography and venous localization with sampling of PTH levels in thyroidal venous beds at times provide useful information to the surgeon at reoperation. Unusual sites of parathyroid adenoma include areas behind the esophagus, in the mediastinum, and within the thyroid.

Of the many possible postoperative complications (nerve injuries, bleeding, and metabolic abnormalities), bilateral recurrent-nerve trauma and hypocalcemic tetany are feared most. Bilateral recurrent laryngeal–nerve injury (by trauma or edema) causes stridor and laryngeal obstruction as a result of unopposed adduction of the vocal cords and closure of the glottic aperture. Immediate endotracheal intubation is required in such cases, usually followed by tracheostomy to ensure an adequate airway. This rare complication occurred only once in more than 30,000 operations at the Lahey Clinic. Unilateral recurrent-nerve injury often goes unnoticed because of compensatory overadduction of the uninvolved cord. Since bilateral injury is rare and clinically obvious, laryngoscopy after thyroid or parathyroid surgery need not be performed routinely; however, one can easily test vocal cord function after surgery by asking the patient to say *"e"* or *"moon."* Unilateral nerve injury is characterized by hoarseness, and bilateral nerve injury by aphonia. Selective injury of adductor fibers of both recurrent laryngeal nerves leaves the abductor muscles relatively unopposed, and pulmonary aspiration is a risk. Selective injury of abductor fibers, on the other hand, leaves the adductor muscles relatively unopposed, and airway obstruction can occur.

Bullous glottic edema is edema of the glottis and pharynx, which occasionally follows parathyroid surgery. This is an additional cause of postoperative respiratory compromise; it has no specific origin, and there is no known preventive measure.

Unintended hypocalcemia during surgery for parathyroid disease occurs in rare cases, usually from the lingering effect of vigorous preoperative treatment. This effect is especially important for patients with advanced osteitis because of the calcium affinity of their bones. After parathyroidectomy, magnesium or calcium ions may be redistributed internally (into "hungry bones"), thus causing hypomagnesemia, hypocalcemia, or both.

Management following parathyroid surgery should include serial determinations of serum calcium, inorganic phosphate, magnesium, and PTH levels.[13, 16–18] Serum calcium levels should fall by several milligrams per deciliter in the first 24 hours. The lowest level usually is reached within 4 or 5 days. In some patients, hypocalcemia may be a postoperative problem. Causes include insufficient residual parathyroid tissue, operative trauma or ischemia, postoperative hypomagnesemia, and delayed recovery of function of normal parathyroid gland tissue. It is particularly important to correct hypomagnesemia in patients with hypocalcemia, because PTH secretion is diminished in the presence of hypomagnesemia.[17, 18] Potentially lethal complications of severe hypocalcemia include laryngeal spasm and hypocalcemic seizures.

In addition to monitoring total serum calcium or ionized calcium postoperatively, one can test for Chvostek's and Trousseau's signs. Because Chvostek's sign is present in 10 to 20 per cent of individuals who do not have hypocalcemia, an attempt should be made to elicit this sign preoperatively. Chvostek's sign is a contracture of the facial muscles produced by tapping the ipsilateral facial nerves at the angle of the jaw. Trousseau's sign is elicited by application of a blood pressure cuff at a level slightly above the systolic pressure for a few minutes. The resulting carpopedal spasm, with contractions of the fingers and inability to open the hand, stems from the increased muscle irritability in hypercalcemic states, which is aggravated by ischemia produced by the inflated blood pressure cuff. Because postoperative hematoma can compromise the airway, the neck and wound dressings should be examined for evidence of bleeding before a patient is discharged from the recovery room.

Hypophosphatemia may also occur postoperatively. It is particularly important to correct this deficiency in patients with congestive heart failure. In a group of patients with severe hypophosphatemia, correction of serum phosphate from 1.0 to 2.9 mg/dl led to significant improvement in left ventricular contractility at the same preload.[13] Other complications of hypophosphatemia include hemolysis, platelet dysfunction, leukocyte dysfunction (depression of chemotaxis, of phagocytosis, and of bactericidal activity), paresthesias, muscular weakness, and rhabdomyolysis.[19] In patients with both hypocalcemia and hypomagnesemia, correction of the hypomagnesemia may cause markedly increased PTH secretion, resulting in dramatic hypophosphatemia. Serum phosphate levels should be monitored closely in such patients.[17, 18]

Hypomagnesemia may occur postoperatively. Clinical sequelae of magnesium deficiency include cardiac dysrhythmias (principally ventricular tachydysrhythmias), hypocalcemic tetany, and neuromuscular irritability that is independent of hypocalcemia (tremors, twitching, asterixis, and seizures).[16] Both hypomagnesemia and hypokalemia augment the neuromuscular effects of hypocalcemia. Often, just restoring the magnesium deficit corrects the hypocalcemia. It is preferable to use oral calcium (1 or 2 g four times daily of calcium gluconate) when the patient is able to take oral fluids.

During the first week or 10 days after surgery, vitamin D derivatives are avoided to allow the suppressed parathyroid tissue (if present) to function. Vitamin D derivatives are always started if the patient has significant hypocalcemia 2 weeks following surgery. The older vitamin D derivatives include vitamin D_2 (ergocalciferol) and vitamin D_3 (cholecalciferol). Of these derivatives, 40,000 units is equal to approximately 1 mg. Therapy in the patient with permanent hypoparathyroidism is begun with 40,000 units daily of either vitamin D_2 or D_3. The dosage is increased by 20,000 units every 2 weeks until the desired calcium level is attained. Vitamin D is fat soluble, and the significant fat stores in adipose tissue, muscle, and liver must first be saturated before a therapeutic level is achieved.

Patients with surgical hypoparathyroidism sometimes require huge quantities of vitamin D derivatives (200,000 to 300,000 units or 5 to 7 mg daily) and thus appear to have an end-organ resistance to its effects.[20] In the hypoparathyroid patient it is best to aim for a calcium level of 8.5 to 9.0 mg/dl. While these patients have a urinary calcium leak because of the absence of PTH, in general it is best to keep the urinary calcium level below 300 mg per 24 hours. If the urinary calcium level is above 300 mg per 24 hours, the vitamin D dose should be dropped back by 25 per cent of the patient's initial dose. Another vitamin D derivative is dihydrotachysterol (Dygratyl). Doses of 250 to 2000 µg of dihydrotachysterol are required to control the hypocalcemia in hypoparathyroidism. The compound 25 hydroxycholecalciferol is 15 times more potent than the parent vitamin D_2 and $1,25(OH)_2D_3$ is about 1500 times more potent.

The management of hypoparathyroidism is not easy, and careful follow-up of patients is mandatory. Blood calcium and urinary calcium should be checked every 6 months after surgery. Vitamin D intoxication is an ever present danger.

C. HYPOCALCEMIA

Probably the most common cause of hypocalcemia is surgical removal of the parathyroids. However, the differential diagnosis of hypocalcemia should also include chronic renal insufficiency, malabsorption syndrome, pseudohypoparathyroidism, hypomagnesemia, osteoblastic metastasis to bone, pancreatitis, and the rare autoimmune abnormality of deficiency in multiple endocrine glands.

A very rare cause of hypocalcemia is thymic hypoplasia associated with hypoparathyroidism (Di George syndrome). Table 8–2 lists the differential diagnosis of hypocalcemia and some tests used to differentiate these cases. Measurement of PTH is not nearly as useful in differentiating the hypocalcemic states as it is in the hypercalcemic disorders. The vitamin D deficiency of the malabsorption syndrome, osteomalacia (in the adult) and rickets (in the child), is associated with a low serum phosphorus. In all other causes of hypocalcemia the serum phosphorus tends to be elevated. It is disproportionately elevated in chronic renal failure. Cataracts and basal ganglion calcification are seen in both hypoparathyroidism and pseudohypoparathyroidism. Subperiosteal resorption (the hallmark of excessive PTH secretion) is seen mainly in chronic renal failure associated with secondary hyperparathyroidism and in some forms of pseudohypoparathyroidism. The PTH level tends to be disproportionately elevated in chronic renal failure associated with secondary hyperparathyroidism, and there are a few patients with high PTH levels in blood who develop a high blood calcium level (so-called tertiary hyperparathyroidism). Most of these patients following renal transplantation develop normal calcium levels, and only a very few turn out to have an autonomous parathyroid adenoma.

Most of the clinical manifestations of hypoparathyroidism are attributable to hypocalcemia. Hypocalcemia occurs because of a fall in the equilibrium level of the blood-bone calcium relationship, in association with a reduction in renal tubular reabsorption and GI absorption of calcium. PTH inhibits renal tubular reabsorption of phosphate and bicarbonate; hence, serum phosphate and bicarbonate levels are elevated in patients with hypoparathyroidism.

Pseudohypoparathyroidism is an unusual entity associated with short stature, round facies, and short metacarpals, as well as parathyroid hyperplasia. It represents in part end-organ resistance to the action of PTH. $1,25(OH)_2D_3$ levels are low in pseudohypoparathyroidism, and replacement of this vitamin D derivative can partially reverse the end-organ resistance. Hypomagnesemia impairs PTH release and thus can cause profound hypocalcemia.[17, 18] Hypomagnesemia is common in patients with alcoholism, malnutrition, or chronic severe malabsorption states. The calcium level may be restored by

TABLE 8–2

Differential Diagnosis of Hypocalcemia

	Serum Phosphorus	Serum Alkaline Phosphatase	Creatinine	PTH	Comments
Hypoparathyroidism (usually surgical)	↑	N	N	↓ or 0	Cataracts; basal ganglia calcification; other endocrine gland hypofunction
Chronic renal disease (secondary hyperparathyroidism)	↑↑	↑	↑↑	↑↑	Impaired renal 1,25(OH)$_2$D$_3$ synthesis
Malabsorption syndrome vitamin D deficiency	↓↓	↑	N	N or ↓	Vitamin D malabsorption or deficiency (osteomalacia or rickets)
Pseudohypoparathyroid variants	↑	N	N	↑	Metastatic calcification, cataracts, short stature
Hypomagnesemia	↑	N	N	N or ↑	Malnutrition, alcoholism, and malabsorption
Osteoblastic metastasis	N	N or ↑	N	N or ↑	X-ray skeletal, seen in prostatic cancer
Acute pancreatitis	N	N or ↑	N	N or ↓	Mechanism unknown
Low plasma proteins	N	N	N or ↑	N	Ionized calcium may be normal; malnutrition nephrosis

Key: ↑, elevated; ↑↑, markedly elevated; N, normal.

replacing magnesium. Osteoblastic metastasis associated with increased acquisition of calcium can lower blood calcium. Relative parathyroid insufficiency may account for the persistent hypocalcemia observed in patients with acute pancreatitis.

The acute manifestations of acute hypoparathyroidism have already been discussed with postoperative management of hypercalcemia.

A nerve exposed to low calcium concentration has a reduced threshold of excitation, responds repetitively to a single stimulus, and has impaired accommodation and continuous activity. Tetany usually begins with paresthesias of the face and extremities, which increase in severity. Spasms of the muscles in the face and extremities follow. Pain in the contracting muscle may be severe. Patients often hyperventilate, and the resulting hypocapnia worsens the tetany. Spasm of laryngeal muscles can cause the vocal cords to be fixed at the midline, and this leads to stridor and cyanosis.

Chvostek's and Trousseau's signs (see above) are two classic signs of latent tetany. Manifestations of spasm distal to the inflated blood pressure cuff should occur within 2 minutes (see above).

Hypocalcemia delays ventricular repolarization, thus increasing the QT$_c$ interval (normal, 0.35 to 0.44). With electrical systole thus prolonged, the ventricles may fail to respond to the next electrical impulse from the SA

node, causing 2:1 heart block. Prolongation of the QT interval is a moderately reliable electrocardiographic sign of hypocalcemia, not for the population as a whole, but for individual patients.[21] Thus, following the QT interval as corrected for heart rate (Fig. 8–1) is a useful but not always accurate means of monitoring hypocalcemia. CHF may also occur with hypocalcemia, but this is rare. Since CHF in patients with coexisting heart disease is reduced in severity when calcium and magnesium ion levels are restored to normal, these levels should be normal before surgery. Sudden decreases in blood levels of ionized calcium (as with chelation therapy) can result in severe hypotension.[17]

Patients with hypocalcemia may have seizures. These may be focal, jacksonian, petit mal, or grand mal in appearance, indistinguishable from such seizures in the absence of hypocalcemia. Patients may also have a type of seizure called *cerebral tetany*, which consists of generalized tetany followed by tonic spasms. Therapy with standard anticonvulsants is ineffective and may even exacerbate these seizures (by an anti–vitamin D effect). In long-standing hypoparathyroidism, calcifications may appear above the sella, representing deposits of calcium in and around small blood vessels of the basal ganglia. These may be associated with a variety of extrapyramidal syndromes.

Other common clinical signs of hypocalcemia are clumsiness, depression, muscle

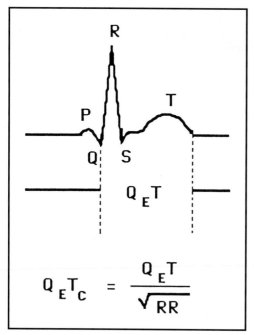

$$Q_ET_c = \frac{Q_ET}{\sqrt{RR}}$$

FIGURE 8–1. The QT_c interval (properly termed Q_ET_c, to indicate that it begins with the start of the Q wave, lasts for the entire QT interval, ends with the end of the T wave, and is corrected for heart rate) is measured as illustrated. (RR, RR interval in seconds.) (From Hensel P, Roizen MF: Patients with disorders of parathyroid function. Anesthesiol Clin North Am 5:294, 1987.)

stiffness, paresthesias, dry, scaly skin, brittle nails and coarse hair, and soft-tissue calcifications. Patients with long-standing hypoparathyroidism sometimes adapt to the condition well enough to be asymptomatic.

The symptoms related to tetany seem to correlate best with the level of the ionized calcium. If alkalosis is present, it is possible for the total calcium to be normal but the ionized calcium low, and symptoms of neuromuscular irritability may result (i.e., hyperventilation syndrome). With slowly developing chronic hypocalcemia, the symptoms may be very mild despite severe hypocalcemia, and this may in part be due to adaptive changes in the level of the ionized calcium. Even with calcium levels of 6 to 7 mg/dl, minor muscle cramps, fatigue, and mild depression may be the only symptoms. Many patients with a calcium level of 6 to 6.5 mg/dl are totally asymptomatic aside from some mild depression of intellectual function.

Vitamin D derivatives are used in the management of hypoparathyroidism (see preceding section), chronic renal insufficiency with secondary hyperparathyroidism, pseudohy-poparathyroidism, the malabsorption syndromes, and other vitamin D deficiency states. Malabsorption syndrome associated with fat malabsorption may require an intramuscular preparation of vitamin D (2000 to 4000 units daily IM) if adequate oral therapy fails. A high-calcium diet (2 g elemental calcium) is indicated whenever a vitamin D preparation is used. A low-phosphorus diet (including use of aluminum hydroxide) is useful in chronic renal failure, but a high-phosphate diet (calcium phosphate preparation may be used) is useful in patients with malabsorption syndrome and other vitamin D deficiency states (rickets and osteomalacia). In chronic renal disease the bone abnormalities due to excessive PTH levels (subperiosteal reabsorption) are essentially reversed by 1 or 2 µg of $1,25(OH)_2D_3$ (Rocaltrol); however, the osteomalacic changes in chronic renal disease may not be totally reversed by this potent vitamin D derivative. Pseudohypoparathyroidism and hypoparathyroidism are managed essentially in the same fashion (see preceding section). Phenothiazines should be used with caution in patients with hypocalcemia (especially hypoparathyroidism), since they may precipitate dystonic reactions or dysrhythmias. Furosemide may decrease calcium levels more in patients with hypoparathyroidism.

1. Perioperative Considerations for Patients with Hypoparathyroidism

Since treatment of hypoparathyroidism is not surgical, hypoparathyroid patients who come to the operating room are those who require surgery for an unrelated condition. Their calcium, phosphate, and magnesium levels should be measured both pre- and postoperatively. Patients with symptomatic hypocalcemia should be treated with intravenous calcium gluconate before surgery. Initially, 10 to 20 ml of 10 per cent calcium gluconate may be given at a rate of 10 ml per minute. The effect on serum calcium levels is of short duration, but a continuous infusion with 10 ml of 10 per cent calcium gluconate in 500 ml of solution over 6 hours may help to maintain adequate serum calcium levels.

The objective of therapy is to have symptoms under control prior to surgery and anesthesia. In patients with chronic hypoparathyroidism, the objective is to maintain the serum calcium level in at least the lower half of the normal range. A preoperative ECG can be obtained and the QT_c interval calculated. The QT_c value may be used as a guide to the serum calcium level if a rapid laboratory assessment is not possible. No special choice of anesthetic agents or techniques is indicated, with the exception of avoidance of respiratory alkalosis, since this tends to further decrease levels of ionized calcium.

D. SUMMARY

Physiologic derangements in patients with disorders of parathyroid function are caused principally by inappropriate serum calcium levels. Preoperative evaluation of these patients commonly includes determination of calcium, phosphate, and magnesium levels. An ECG with calculation of QT_c can be obtained preoperatively and can be followed intraoperatively. The patient's volume status may be affected, because both hypercalcemia and its treatment may lead to hypovolemia. If the patient has received steroids, steroid coverage might be provided perioperatively. If the patient has received mithramycin, it might be advisable to assess hepatic and renal function preoperatively and to obtain a platelet count and a coagulation profile.

There is no evidence supporting any particular anesthetic technique. In addition to the QT_c interval, the calcium level can be checked intraoperatively, if possible. Calcium, phosphate, and magnesium levels often vary postoperatively. The patient should be observed closely for evidence of nerve injury, hematoma, or hypocalcemic tetany.

II. THYROID GLAND

Perhaps no endocrine organ has contributed as much to the development of surgery as a specialty as has the thyroid gland. The Cleveland Clinic and the clinics of such prominent surgeons as Lahey, Crile, and the Mayo brothers had their beginnings as centers for the traditional "steal" of the hyperthyroid patient and for the safe removal of enlarged thyroid glands. These clinics were located in regions where the soil was deficient in iodine. As a result, both water and food contained less than optimal amounts of iodine, thus contributing to the development of endemic goiter.[22]

As with many other endocrinopathies, two themes emerge when anesthesia for patients with thyroid disease is discussed: (1) The organ system that most affects the anesthetic management of patients having any endocrinopathy is the cardiovascular system. (2) In almost all emergency situations, and certainly in all elective situations, any endocrine abnormality affecting the patient's preoperative state that can be stabilized may improve outcome. It is the task of the anesthesiologist to educate the primary care physician and surgeon about the hazards of not optimizing endocrine function preoperatively.[23, 24]

A. PHYSIOLOGY

Thyroid hormone biosynthesis involves five steps.[25, 26] They are as follows: (1) iodide trapping, (2) oxidation of iodide and iodination of tyrosine residues, (3) hormone storage in the colloid of the thyroid gland as part of the large thyroglobulin molecule, (4) proteolysis and release of hormones, and (5) conversion of less active thyroxine to more potent 3,5,3-triiodothyronine. The first four steps are regulated by pituitary thyrotropin-stimulating hormone (TSH). Proteolysis of stored hormone in the colloid is inhibited by iodide.

The major thyroid hormones are thyroxine (T_4, a product of the thyroid gland) and the more potent 3,5,3-triiodothyronine (T_3, a product of both the thyroid and the extrathyroidal enzymatic deiodination of thyroxine). Approximately 80 per cent of T_3 is produced outside the thyroid gland. Production of thyroid hormones is maintained by secretion of TSH by the pituitary gland, which in turn is regulated by secretion of thyrotropin-releasing hormone (TRH) in the hypothalamus. The production of thyroid hormone is initiated by absorption of iodine from the GI tract, where the iodine is reduced to an iodide and released into plasma. It is then concentrated up to 500-fold by the thyroid gland.

Once in the gland, the iodide is oxidized by a peroxidase to iodine (organification) and then bound to tyrosine, forming either mono- or diiodotyrosine. Both of these are then coupled enzymatically to form T_4 or T_3. T_3 and T_4 are bound to the protein thyroglobulin and stored as colloid in the gland. A proteolytic enzyme releases T_3 and T_4 from the thyroglobulin as these hormones pass from the cell to the plasma. T_3 and T_4 are transported through the bloodstream on thyroxine-binding globulin and thyroxine-binding prealbumin. The plasma normally contains 4 to 11 µg of T_4 and 0.1 to 0.2 µg of T_3 per 100 ml. Secretion of TSH and TRH appears to be regulated by T_4 and T_3 in a negative-feedback loop. Most of the effects of thyroid hormones are mediated by T_3; T_4 is both less potent and more protein bound, thus having lesser biologic effect.[26]

In peripheral tissues there exists a ubiquitous deiodinase that converts T_4 to T_3. Thus, T_4 appears to be a prohormone for T_3. Monodeiodinations can remove either the iodine at the 5' position to yield T_3 or the iodine at the 5 position to yield reverse T_3 (rT_3). Reverse T_3 is totally inactive biologically. In general, when T_3 levels are depressed, rT_3 levels are elevated. In a number of circumstances, rT_3 levels are increased, such as gestation, malnutrition, chronic disease, and surgical stress (Fig. 8–2).[27] A feedback circuit exists between the pituitary gland and the circulating thyroid hormones. High levels of thyroid hormones reduce release of pituitary TSH, while low levels result in more TSH release (Fig. 8–3).

Energy-dependent transport systems move T_3 across the target cell membrane into the cytoplasm. It then diffuses to receptors in the cell nucleus, where it alters the production of specific messenger-RNA sequences that result in physiologic effects. Thyroid hormone has anabolic effects, promotes growth, and advances normal brain and organ development. Thyroid hormone also increases the concentration of adrenergic receptors,[28] which may account for many of its cardiovascular effects.

Since T_3 has greater biologic effect than does T_4, one would expect the diagnosis of thyroid disorders to be based on levels of T_3. However, this is not usually the case.[26] The diagnosis of thyroid disease is confirmed by one of several biochemical measurements: levels of free T_4, total serum concentration of T_4, or by estimate of free T_4. The estimate is obtained by multiplying total T_4 (T_4-RIA) by the thyroid-binding ratio (formerly called the resin T_3 uptake).[26, 29]

B. THYROID FUNCTION TESTS

1. Total Thyroxine

Serum Thyroxine by Radioimmunoassay (T_4-RIA). The normal plasma range of the total T_4 is 4.5 to 10 µg/dl. The T_4 is high in hyperthyroidism and low in hypothyroidism. Most of the T_4 is bound to a plasma protein known as thyroid-binding globulin (TBG). Changes in TBG can affect the total T_4 level. Estrogens, infectious hepatitis, and genetic factors can elevate the level of the TBG and thus secondarily raise total T_4. Androgens,

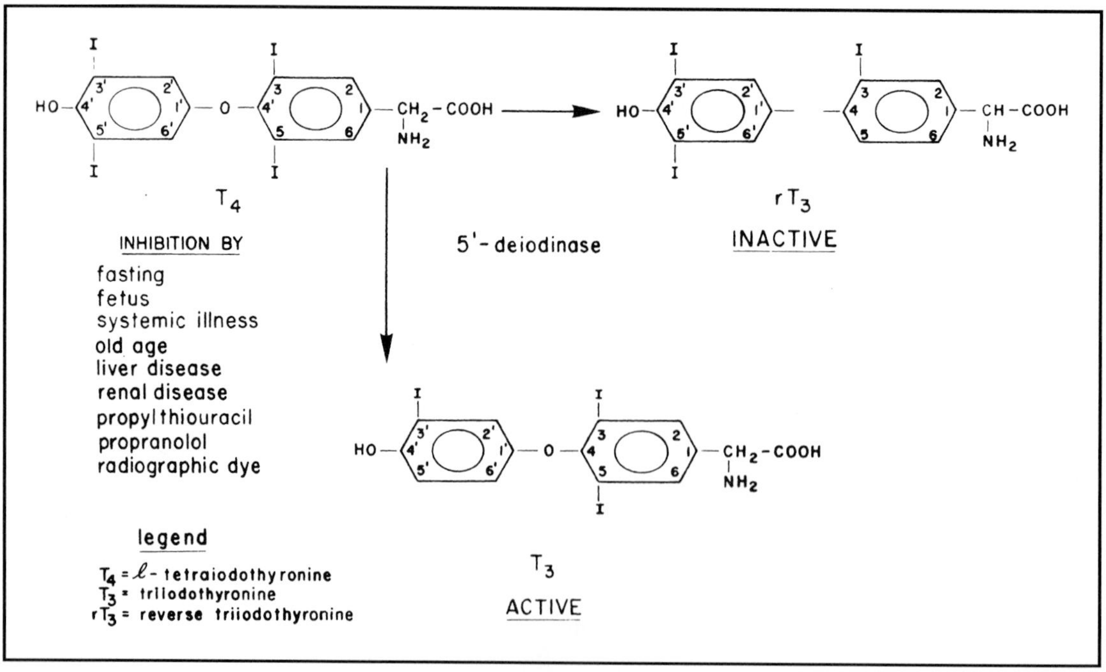

FIGURE 8–2. Peripheral deiodination of T_4.

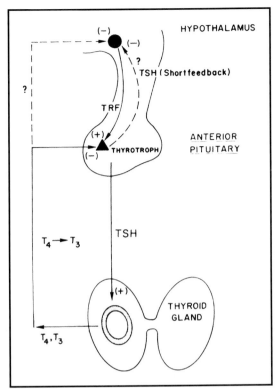

FIGURE 8-3. Hypothalamic pituitary thyroid axis. TRF, thyrotropin-releasing factor; TSH, thyroid-stimulating hormone; T_3, triiodothyronine; T_4, 1-tetraiodothyronine; +, stimulation; −, inhibition.

nephrosis, hypoproteinemia, and genetic factors can lower the TBG and thus secondarily lower the total T_4.

2. Thyroid-Binding Ratio

Resin Triiodothyronine Uptake (RT_3U). This important in vitro test depends upon the binding of a tracer amount of radioactive T_3 to an artificial resin. The amount of binding to resin is inversely proportional to the unoccupied binding sites of TBG. If the T_4 level is high because there is an excess of TBG (i.e., after estrogen administration), there will be an increase in the number of unoccupied binding sites and the thyroid-binding ratio will be low. The thyroid-binding ratio varies in different laboratories but the average is 20 to 25 per cent. If the ratio is multiplied by total T_4, an index is achieved. This index is usually called the "free T_4 estimate." The free T_4 estimate corrects the total T_4 level for any changes in TBG concentration or in unoccupied binding sites on the TBG molecule. It is very difficult to assay the free T_4 level directly, since it amounts to only about 0.5 per cent of

the total T_4 (approximately 1 to 2 ng/dl). The free T_4 estimate correlates directly with the metabolic status of the patient.

Serum Triiodothyronine by Radioimmunoassay (T_3-RIA). This extremely potent hormone normally is present in a concentration range of 75 to 200 ng/dl. It is important to note that the upper limit of normal tends to drop with each decade of life. Thus, a 20-year-old patient with a level of 190 ng/dl may be euthyroid while an 80-year-old patient with the same level may be hyperthyroid.

Serum Thyroid-Stimulating Hormone. In patients with primary hypothyroidism, the TSH level is high for the level of T_4 or T_3 in blood. Often serum concentrations of thyroid hormone are in the normal range, and only serum TSH levels are elevated.[29]

Radioactive Iodine Uptake. The radioactive iodine uptake (RAIU) is measured as the percentage of a tracer that is taken up by the thyroid in 24 hours. The normal range is 10 to 25 per cent. Patients with hyperthyroidism have values above 25 per cent. The major use of this test is to confirm the diagnosis of hyperthyroidism; however, patients with subacute thyroiditis can be hyperthyroid but have essentially no uptake. If a patient has used inorganic iodides or dyes (e.g., for gallbladder scans or intravenous pyelography) the RAIU may be low.

3. Ultrasound or Radioactive Thyroid Scan

Either of these scans is useful in diagnosis. Functioning thyroid nodules are rarely malignant, whereas "cold" or hypofunctioning nodules have a greater probability of malignancy.

4. Other Tests

The diagnosis of pituitary or hypothalamic disease can be quite complicated. The procedure is often aided by the use of TRH. This tripeptide is the hypothalamic factor that brings about release of TSH from the pituitary. It may also be used to confirm the diagnosis of hyperthyroidism. Thyroid antibodies (antithyroglobulin and antimicrosomal) are useful in arriving at the diagnosis of Hashimoto's thyroiditis. Serum thyroglobulin levels tend to be elevated in patients with thyrotoxicosis. Painless thyroiditis is associated with transient hyperthyroidism. This latter entity is a lymphocytic thyroiditis associated with low RAIU.

Measurement of the alpha subunit of TSH has been helpful in identifying the rare patients who have a pituitary neoplasm and who usually have increased alpha-subunit concentrations. Some patients are clinically euthyroid in the presence of elevated levels of total T_4 in serum. Certain drugs, notably gallbladder dyes, glucocorticoids, and amiodarone, block the conversion to T_3 of T_4, thus elevating T_4 levels. Severe illness also slows the conversion of T_4 to T_3. Levels of TSH are often high when the rate of this conversion is decreased. In hyperthyroidism, cardiac function and responses to stress are abnormal; return of normal cardiac function parallels the return of TSH levels to normal values.

C. PATHOPHYSIOLOGY OF THYROID DISEASE

1. Hyperthyroidism

Hyperthyroidism is usually caused by multinodular diffuse enlargement of the gland in Graves' disease that is also associated with disorders of the skin and eyes.[30] Hyperthyroidism can be associated with pregnancy,[31] thyroiditis (with or without neck pain), thyroid adenoma, choriocarcinoma, or TSH-secreting pituitary adenoma. Five per cent of women have been reported to suffer thyrotoxic effects 3 to 6 months post partum, and they tend to have recurrences with subsequent pregnancies.[31]

Major manifestations of hyperthyroidism are weight loss, diarrhea, warm moist skin, weakness of large muscle groups, menstrual abnormalities, nervousness, intolerance of heat, tachycardia, cardiac dysrhythmias, mitral-valve prolapse,[32] and heart failure. When the thyroid is functioning abnormally, the system threatened most is the cardiovascular system. Severe diarrhea can lead to dehydration, which can be corrected before a surgical procedure is undertaken. Mild anemia, thrombocytopenia, increased serum alkaline phosphatase, hypercalcemia, muscle wasting, and bone loss frequently occur in patients with hyperthyroidism. Muscle disease usually involves proximal muscle groups; it has not been reported to cause respiratory paralysis. In the apathetic form of hyperthyroidism (seen most commonly in persons over 60 years of age), cardiac effects dominate the clinical picture.[33, 34] The signs and symptoms include tachycardia, irregular heartbeat, atrial

fibrillation, heart failure, and occasionally papillary muscle dysfunction.[33–36] In fact, the presence of atrial fibrillation of unknown origin indicates the need to be concerned about apathetic hyperthyroidism. This concern is more than academic because "thyroid storm" can occur in such patients when they undergo operations for other diseases.

Although beta-adrenergic receptor blockade can control heart rate, its use is fraught with hazards in a patient who is already experiencing CHF. However, decreasing the heart rate may improve the cardiac pump function. Thus, hyperthyroid patients who have high ventricular rates, who have CHF, and who require emergency surgery are given propranolol in doses guided by changes in pulmonary artery wedge pressure and the overall clinical condition. If slowing the heart rate with a small dose of esmolol (50 μg/kg) does not aggravate heart failure, more esmolol (50 to 500 μg/kg) is administered. The aim is to avoid imposing surgery on any patient whose thyroid function is clinically abnormal. Therefore, only "life-or-death" emergency surgery should preclude making the patient pharmacologically euthyroid, a process that can take 2 to 6 weeks.

a. Preparation of the Hyperthyroid Patient for Surgery

In recent years surgery as treatment for the hyperthyroid patient has declined, especially in the patient with Graves' disease. This decline is probably due to the wider use and acceptance of radioactive iodine ^{131}I treatment. Nevertheless, 200,000 thyroid and parathyroid operations are performed annually in the United States. In general, the patients still considered appropriate for surgery are children, adolescents, women whose pregnancy is associated with Graves' disease, women of child-bearing age, and patients who have extremely large thyroid glands. A number of patients refuse radioactive iodine treatment, thereby becoming candidates for surgery. The traditional method for making the patient euthyroid involves giving one of the antithyroid drugs for 2 to 3 months before surgery to inhibit thyroid hormone synthesis. The drug that is still (after 30 years) most used is propylthiouracil, because it inhibits both thyroid hormone synthesis and the peripheral conversion of T_4 to T_3. The usual dosage is 300 mg daily in divided doses. Most patients will be euthyroid in 2 to 3 months on this dosage. If the patient is severely hyperthyroid or has an unusually large gland, larger doses may be used (up to 1 g daily). In general, the smaller the gland, the shorter the interval necessary to achieve euthyroidism. An alternative drug is methimazole (Tapazole). Doses of 30 to 60 mg daily are comparable to the above doses of propylthiouracil. About 10 days before surgery it is common to give the patient a potassium iodide solution (10 drops daily of a saturated solution) to decrease gland vascularity and block release of stored hormone. Lithium carbonate (300 mg four times daily) may be given in lieu of iodide, especially if there is a known allergy to iodine. Lithium carbonate, like iodide, blocks the proteolysis and release of stored thyroid hormone.

Published reports indicate a trend toward preoperative preparation with propranolol and iodides alone.[37-39] This approach is less time consuming (that is, 7 to 14 days versus 2 to 6 weeks); it causes the thyroid gland to shrink, as does the more traditional approach; and it treats symptoms, but abnormalities in left ventricular function may not be corrected.[34, 36, 38, 39] Regardless of the approach used, antithyroid drugs should be administered both chronically and on the morning of surgery. If emergency surgery is necessary before the euthyroid state is achieved or if the hyperthyroidism gets out of control during surgery, intravenous administration of 50 to 500 $\mu g/kg$ of esmolol can be titrated for restoration of a normal heart rate (assuming that CHF is absent; see previous discussion). Larger doses may be required, and in the absence of better data, the return of a normal heart rate and the absence of CHF serve as guides to therapy. In addition, intravascular fluid volume and electrolyte balance should be restored. It should be kept in mind that administering propranolol does not invariably prevent "thyroid storm."[38-41]

2. Management of Thyrotoxicosis During Pregnancy

The management of the thyrotoxicosis of Graves' disease during pregnancy presents some special problems. Radioactive iodine therapy is usually considered contraindicated since it crosses the placenta. The physician has a choice between antithyroid drugs and surgery. Antithyroid drugs also cross the pla-

cental barrier and can cause fetal hypothyroidism. This problem may theoretically be obviated by the simultaneous administration of L-thyroxine or T_3. However, most of the evidence indicates that neither T_4 nor T_3 crosses the placental barrier. The occurrence of fetal hypothyroidism when small doses of antithyroid drugs alone are used is quite unusual as long as the mother remains euthyroid. It is usually better to err on the side of undertreatment than overtreatment with antithyroid drugs. Small amounts of propylthiouracil (50 to 100 mg per day or even every other day) are often sufficient. Chronic use of iodide in the mother is usually considered contraindicated since fetal goiter and hypothyroidism may result. The use of propranolol during pregnancy is controversial. There have been case reports that babies whose mothers had received propranolol experienced intrauterine growth retardation and low Apgar ratings. Bradycardia and hypoglycemia also have been described in these infants. The thyrotoxicosis of pregnancy tends to be quite mild and often improves in the second and third trimester. Surgery is an acceptable alternative to treatment (this surgery is usually postponed until neural development and organogenesis of the first trimester are complete).[42]

Following pregnancy, it is impossible to predict the thyroid status of the mother. While some patients remain hyperthyroid, some become hypothyroid following delivery. Approximately 5 per cent of women suffer transient thyrotoxic effects 3 to 6 months post partum, and these mothers tend to have recurrences with subsequent pregnancies.[31]

The status of the neonate following delivery needs attention. Either hypothyroidism or hyperthyroidism may be present. Neonatal hypothyroidism is characterized by a low total T_4 (below 7 $\mu g/dl$) and an elevated TSH. At times the T_4 may be perfectly normal and only the TSH elevated. Amniotic fluid reverse T_3 levels tend to be low in the hypothyroid fetus in the third trimester, and likewise the blood reverse T_3 concentration is low after birth if hypothyroidism exists.

Management of neonatal hypothyroidism consists of the immediate replacement with L-thyroxine in the dose range of 9 μg per kg per day. This dose is relatively large, but it is often required to normalize the TSH level and T_4 concentration. Normally the total T_4 level (8–15 $\mu g/dl$) tends to be high in the first year of life and slowly but progressively drops until after puberty. Likewise, thyroid hormone replacement doses tend to be higher than in the average adult until puberty is complete.

Neonatal hyperthyroidism is most unusual and is always associated with high levels of thyroid-stimulating immunoglobulins. These immunoglobulins cross the placental barrier and are probably the cause of fetal hyperthyroidism. Consequently, it is common to measure these immunoglobulins in thyrotoxic women in the third trimester. Controlling maternal hyperthyroidism seems to prevent the development of hyperthyroidism in infants.

Thyroid storm refers to the clinical diagnosis of a life-threatening illness in a patient whose hyperthyroidism has been severely exacerbated by illness or operation. It is manifested by hyperpyrexia, tachycardia, and striking alterations in consciousness.[40, 41] No laboratory tests are diagnostic of thyroid storm, and the precipitating (nonthyroidal) cause is the major determinant of survival. Therapy usually includes blocking the synthesis of thyroid hormones by administration of antithyroid drugs, blocking release of preformed hormone with iodine, meticulous attention to hydration and supportive therapy, and correction of the precipitating cause. In fact, survival is directly related to the success of treatment of the underlying cause. Blocking of the sympathetic nervous system with alpha- and beta-receptor antagonists may be exceedingly hazardous and requires skillful management and constant monitoring of the critically ill patient.

3. Hypothyroidism

Hypothyroidism is a common disease, occurring in 5 per cent of a large adult population in Great Britain, in 3 to 6 per cent of a population of healthy elderly individuals in Massachusetts, and in 4.5 per cent of a medical clinic population in Switzerland.[43, 44] Many women with postpartum thyroiditis develop hypothyroidism, which is often mistaken for postpartum depression. Because this hypothyroidism is usually self-limited, it generally does not require treatment.

Hypofunction of the thyroid gland can be caused by surgical ablation, radioactive iodine administration, irradiation to the neck (e.g., for Hodgkin's disease), iodine deficiency or toxicity, genetic biosynthetic defects in thyroid hormone production, antithyroid drugs such as propylthiouracil, pituitary tumors, or

hypothalamic disease. Perhaps the most common cause of primary thyroid hypofunction is a form of thyroiditis, often chronic lymphocytic thyroiditis or Hashimoto's thyroiditis. The gland is usually enlarged, nontender, and extremely firm and indurated. A variety of antithyroid antibodies are found in the serum, including antithyroglobulin and antimicrosomal antibodies in high titer. Hypothyroidism seems to be the most common consequence of Hashimoto's thyroiditis and indeed is the most common cause of hypothyroidism in adults.[45] Patients with Hashimoto's thyroiditis are extremely susceptible to iodides and to antithyroid drugs, and overt severe hypothyroidism can be exacerbated by these maneuvers. Usually, symptoms of hypothyroidism are subclinical, serum concentrations of thyroid hormones are in the normal range, and only serum TSH levels are elevated.[25, 45, 46] In such patients, hypothyroidism may have little or no perioperative significance; however, a recent retrospective study of 59 mildly hypothyroid patients showed that more hypothyroid patients than control subjects required prolonged postoperative intubation (9 of 59 versus 4 of 59) and had significant electrolyte imbalances (3 of 59 versus 1 of 59) and bleeding complications (4 of 59 versus 0 of 59). Because only a small number of charts were examined, these differences were not statistically significant.[46]

In the less frequent cases of overt hypothyroidism, the deficiency of thyroid hormone results in slow mental functioning, slow movement, dry skin, intolerance to cold, depression of the ventilatory responses to hypoxia and hypercarbia,[47] impaired clearance of free water, slow gastric emptying, and bradycardia. In extreme cases, cardiomegaly, heart failure, and pericardial and pleural effusions are manifested as fatigue, dyspnea, and orthopnea.[48] Hypothyroidism is often associated with amyloidosis, which may cause enlargement of the tongue, abnormalities of the cardiac conduction system, and renal disease. The tongue may be enlarged in the hypothyroid patient even in the absence of amyloidosis, and this may hamper intubation.[49] Full-blown myxedema presents with a variety of symptoms including cold intolerance, apathy, hoarseness, constipation, retarded movement, anemia, hearing loss, and bradycardia.

a. Preparation of the Hypothyroid Patient for Surgery

Hypothyroidism decreases anesthetic requirements slightly.[50] Ideal preoperative management of hypothyroidism consists of restoring normal thyroid status: the normal dose of T_3 or T_4 should be administered routinely on the morning of surgery, even though these drugs have long half-lives (1.4 to 10 days). The usual daily replacement dose in adults is 0.1 to 0.2 mg of L-thyroxine (Synthroid). The T_4 level itself can be used as a guide to therapy. Both the T_4 and TSH serum level are usually in the normal range in adequately treated patients.

Myxedema coma is a rare complication that is associated with profound hypothyroidism. It is associated with extreme lethargy, severe hypothermia, bradycardia, and alveolar hypoventilation with hypoxia, and is occasionally accompanied by pericardial effusion and congestive heart failure. Hyponatremia associated with marked decrease in free water clearance by the kidney is also often part of the syndrome. This is the one single indication for intravenous T_4 therapy. For patients in myxedema coma who require emergency surgery, T_3 or T_4 can be given intravenously (with the risk of precipitating myocardial ischemia, however) while supportive therapy is undertaken to restore normal intravascular fluid volume, body temperature, cardiac function, respiratory function, and electrolyte balance. L-Thyroxine (Synthroid) is given in a single intravenous dose of 300 to 500 μg. Intravenous T_3 (Cytomel) may also be given in the dose range of 25 to 50 μg every 8 hours until the blood level of T_3 is normal. Intravenous T_3 probably is superior to intravenous T_4, since T_3 is the most physiologically active form of thyroid hormone therapy and since it bypasses the normal T_4 to T_3 peripheral conversion pathway, which tends to be markedly depressed in patients with serious systemic illnesses. The intravenous preparations should always be prepared fresh prior to use.

4. Hypothyroid Patients with Coronary Artery Disease

Treating hypothyroid patients who have symptomatic coronary artery disease poses special problems and may require compromises in the general practice of preoperatively restoring euthyroidism with drugs.[24, 51, 52] Although both T_4 and esmolol may be given, adequate amelioration of both ischemic heart disease and hypothyroidism may be difficult to achieve. The need for thyroid therapy must be balanced against the risk of aggravating anginal symptoms. One review suggests early consideration of coronary artery revascularization.[51] It advocates initiating thyroid replacement therapy in the ICU soon after the patient's arrival from the operating room after myocardial revascularization surgery. However, several deaths resulting from dysrhythmias and CHF as well as cardiogenic shock with infarction have occurred while patients who were not given thyroid therapy were awaiting surgery. Thus, there is a need to consider "truly" emergency coronary artery revascularization in patients who have both severe coronary artery disease and significant hypothyroidism. In fact, several large medical centers consider the presence of both diseases to be as important an indicator for immediate surgery as is left main coronary artery disease with unstable angina for immediate coronary revascularization.

In the presence of hypothyroidism, respiratory control mechanisms do not function normally.[48] However, the response to hypoxia and hypercarbia and the clearance of free water become normal with thyroid replacement therapy. Drug metabolism has been reported anecdotally to be slowed, and awakening times after administration of sedatives were found to be prolonged during hypothyroidism. However, no formal study of the pharmacokinetics and pharmacodynamics of sedatives or anesthetic agents in patients with hypothyroidism has been published. These concerns disappear when thyroid function is normalized preoperatively. Addison's disease (with its relative steroid deficiency) is more common in hypothyroid than in euthyroid individuals, and some endocrinologists routinely treat patients who have noniatrogenic hypothyroidism by giving stress doses of steroids perioperatively. The possibility that this steroid deficiency exists should be considered if the patient becomes hypotensive perioperatively.

5. Thyroid Nodules and Carcinoma

Identifying malignancy in a solitary thyroid nodule is a difficult and important procedure. Fine-needle aspiration biopsy has become a standard tool.[53] Males and patients with previous radiation to the head and neck have an increased likelihood of malignant disease in their nodules.[54] Twenty-seven per cent of all irradiated patients develop nodules. Often, needle biopsy and scanning are sufficient for the diagnosis, but occasionally an excisional biopsy is needed. If a cancer is found at surgery it is usually routine to do total thyroidectomy. Instead of starting these patients on exogenous thyroid immediately after surgery, this decision should be temporarily postponed until a decision is made as to whether massive amounts of radioactive ^{131}I therapy are indicated. A week after 50 to 100 millicuries of ^{131}I is given, exogenous replacement thyroid therapy can be instituted. Some internists prefer to start exogenous thyroid immediately after surgery, since it may have a cancer-suppressing effect.[55] However, before a radioactive iodine scan or definitive therapy with radioactive iodine can be accomplished, exogenous thyroid hormone must be stopped for at least 6 weeks. Papillary carcinoma accounts for more than 60 per cent of all carcinomas. Simple excision of lymph node metastases appears to be as efficacious for patient survival as are radical neck procedures.[56]

Medullary carcinoma is the most aggressive form of thyroid carcinoma. It is associated with familial incidence of pheochromocytoma, as are parathyroid adenomas. For this reason, a history should be obtained for patients who have a surgical scar in the thyroid and parathyroid region, so that the possibility of occult pheochromocytoma can be ruled out.

D. INTRAOPERATIVE ANESTHETIC CONSIDERATIONS AND POSTOPERATIVE PROBLEMS IN PATIENTS WITH THYROID DISEASE

The major considerations regarding anesthesia for patients with disorders of the thyroid are (1) attainment of a euthyroid state preoperatively, (2) preoperative preparation and attention to the characteristics of the diseases mentioned previously, and (3) normalization of cardiovascular function and temperature perioperatively.

No controlled study has demonstrated clinical advantages of any one anesthetic drug over another for surgical patients who are hyperthyroid. A review of cases at the University of California from 1968 to 1982 and at the University of Chicago from 1976 to 1984 revealed that virtually all techniques and anesthetic agents have been employed without adverse effects that could have been even remotely attributable to the agent or technique. In one animal study, liver enzyme induction by thyroid hormones was associated with hepatic centrilobular necrosis following halothane but not isoflurane anesthesia, despite the absence of arterial hypoxemia. Nevertheless, there are no data on human subjects to imply that the choice of anesthetic affects patient outcome in the presence of thyroid disease. Furthermore, although some authors have recommended that anticholinergic drugs (especially atropine) be avoided because they interfere with the sweating mechanism and cause tachycardia, atropine has been given as a test for adequacy of antithyroid treatment. Because patients are now subjected to operative procedures only when they are euthyroid, the traditional "steal" of the heavily premedicated hyperthyroid patient to the operating room has vanished.

A patient who has a large goiter and an obstructed airway can be treated like any other patient whose airway management is problematic. Preoperative medication need not include "deep" sedation, and an airway can be established, often with the patient awake. A firm armored endotracheal tube is preferable and should be passed beyond the point of extrinsic compression. It is most useful to examine computed tomographic (CT) scans of the neck preoperatively to determine the extent of compression. Maintenance of anesthesia usually presents little difficulty. Body heat mechanisms are inadequate in hypothyroid patients, and temperature can be monitored and maintained, especially in patients who require emergency surgery before the euthyroid state is attained.[44] Because there is an increased incidence of myasthenia gravis in hyperthyroid patients, it may be advisable to use a twitch monitor to guide muscle relaxant administration.

Postoperatively, extubation should be performed under optimal circumstances for reintubation, in case the tracheal rings have been weakened and the trachea collapses. Possible postoperative complications are those for hyperparathyroidism (see above).

E. SUMMARY

Preoperative normalization of thyroid function helps ensure that the patient with thyroid disease is at little additional risk of experiencing perioperative complications. The organ system most threatened by thyroid disease is the cardiovascular system. In apathetic hyperthyroidism, a rapid heart rate or idiopathic atrial fibrillation may be the only clue to such a diagnosis. Patients with hypothyroidism and myocardial ischemia also pose problems for perioperative management. No particular anesthetic techniques or agents have proved more beneficial or successful than others. Securing the airway and checking for nerve palsies, hematoma formation, hypothermia, and hypocalcemia must not be overlooked perioperatively. If a patient has a neck scar, the medical history should probably be reviewed because of the possibility of associated pheochromocytoma.

III. PITUITARY GLAND

A. PHYSIOLOGY

The pituitary gland is divided into an anterior and a posterior portion that have substantially different organizations. The anterior pituitary is connected to the hypothalamus via a complex portal vascular system. Hypothalamic releasing or inhibitory factors are synthesized in the hypothalamus, are secreted into the portal system, and reach the anterior pituitary gland in very high concentrations. Functional activity in the posterior pituitary has a different organization: specialized neurons in the hypothalamus synthesize vasopressin and oxytocin. These two hormones are then secreted through specialized axons down the stalk of the pituitary gland and are stored in the posterior pituitary gland.

Each pituitary hormone has a specific releasing factor associated with it—and in some cases a specific inhibitory factor. Except for the positive effect of TRH on both TSH and prolactin secretion and for disease states, generally there is no overlap in function of the hypothalamic hormones. For instance, in acromegaly, both somatotropin-releasing factor and thyrotropin-releasing factor can bring about release of growth hormone. In the normal state this would not occur. Specific hypothalamic-releasing hormones have been defined for TSH, adrenocorticotropin (ACTH), and the gonadotropins (both luteinizing hormone [LH] and follicle-stimulating hormone [FSH]). Both a releasing and an inhibitory hypothalamic factor have been discovered for

growth hormone (GH). Prolactin is primarily associated with an inhibitory hypothalamic factor (probably the neurotransmitter dopamine). An additional factor involving hypothalamic control of the pituitary is the pulsatile periodic operation of the hypothalamus. Probably the most important biological rhythm is the sleep or light-dark pattern. For instance, growth hormone and adrenocorticotropic hormones show specific nocturnal bursts in males. Prolactin also tends to increase in concentration in the blood immediately after sleep begins. LH shows a sleep pattern especially during puberty.

The three monoamine neurotransmitters, dopamine, norepinephrine, and serotinin, can profoundly affect hypothalamic function and are found in high concentration in major hypothalamic centers. There is essentially no blood–brain barrier in either the pituitary or the hypothalamus, and target organ products such as estrogen, testosterone, thyroid, and adrenal hormones can exert feedback at either the hypothalamic or pituitary level (Fig. 8–4).

B. DISEASES OF THE ANTERIOR PITUITARY GLAND

1. Hypofunction of the Pituitary Gland

All or several of the trophic hormones may be involved in hypopituitary states. The causes of hypopituitarism include chromophobe adenoma, Rathke's pouch cysts or craniopharyngioma in children, necrosis following circulatory collapse due to hemorrhage after delivery (Sheehan's syndrome), surgical hypophysectomy, irradiation to the skull or brain, granulomatous and other infectious diseases, and hemochromatosis.[57-59] Metastatic disease (especially from breast cancer) is only rarely seen. Destruction of the gland by tumor (i.e., chromophobe adenoma) is probably the most common cause of hypopituitarism. One third to half of all patients with chromophobe adenoma secrete excessive quantities of the hormone prolactin. Excessive secretion of prolactin may be associated with galactorrhea and amenorrhea (gonadotropin deficiency).[58] GH deficiency in a child results in severe growth failure. Loss of TSH or ACTH function usually occurs later in life, when variable features related to thyroid deficiency or cortisol lack inevitably manifest themselves. If a tumor exists, it may grow

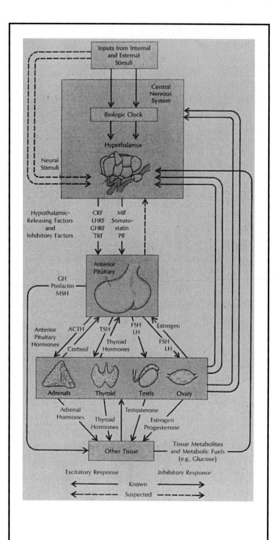

Pituitary Hormone	Hypothalamic Regulatory Hormones
Adrenocorticotropic hormone (ACTH)	Corticotropin releasing factor (CRF)
Thyroid stimulating hormone (TSH)	Thyrotropin releasing factor (TRF)
Follicle stimulating hormone (FSH) and luteinizing hormone (LH)	Gonadotropin releasing factor (GHRF)
Growth hormone (GH)	Growth hormone releasing factor (GHRF), somatostatin (inhibitory)
Prolactin	Prolactin inhibitory factor (PIF)

FIGURE 8–4. Basic feedback mechanisms in the neuroendocrine system. (Reprinted by permission of Hospital Practice *10*:60, 1975.)

above the sella (suprasellar extension), and headaches and visual field defects, notably bitemporal hemianopsia, will occur. Single isolated deficiencies of specific pituitary hormones have been described. The most common is gonadotropin deficiency. A well-known syndrome is gonadotropin deficiency associated with loss of the sense of smell (Kallmann's syndrome). This interesting hypothalamic entity is caused by failure of gonadotropin-releasing factor to function appropriately.

Diagnosis. It is possible to measure by radioimmunoassay virtually all of the hormones of the anterior pituitary gland. This includes measurements of GH, TSH, LH, FSH, prolactin, and ACTH. Low LH and FSH associated with estrogen deficiency in a female or low testosterone in a male points to a hypothalamic or pituitary deficiency.[60] Likewise low TSH with a low T_4 by radioimmunoassay also indicates either hypothalamic or pituitary deficiency. An elevated prolactin level is commonly associated with chromophobe adenomas.

An evaluation of the hypothalamic-pituitary-adrenal axis, however, can be quite difficult. The metapyrone test has long been a standard test for determination of the pituitary-adrenal axis. Metapyrone blocks the conversion of 11-deoxycortisol to cortisol. Normally 11-deoxycortisol is not measurable. The metapyrone test consists of giving a single oral dose of metapyrone (3 g) at midnight and measuring plasma cortisol and 11-deoxycortisol concentrations the following morning. If the 11-deoxycortisol level is greater than 10 µg/ml, ACTH stimulation must have occurred and the patient has a normal pituitary-adrenal axis. If both 11-deoxycortisol and cortisol are low, this means that ACTH was not stimulated and the patient has little or no ACTH pituitary reserve. The test can also be performed using the measurement of urinary 17-hydroxycorticoids while 750 mg of metapyrone is given every 4 hours for six doses.

Hypoglycemia induced by giving 0.1 unit of insulin per kilogram body weight intravenously can also be used to test not only ACTH reserve but also GH reserve. Hypoglycemia (blood sugar below 50 mg/dl) should result in significant rises in both plasma cortisol and GH if the pituitary gland is functioning normally. Failure of the plasma cortisol level to rise after intravenous insulin is an indication that ACTH reserve is low.

2. Hyperfunction of the Pituitary Gland

There are three major hyperfunctioning pituitary gland tumors: (1) prolactin-secreting chromophobe adenoma, (2) an ACTH-secreting tumor associated with Cushing's disease (see section on Adrenal Disease), and (3) acromegaly associated with excessive growth hormone secretion. Gonadotropin- and thyrotropin-secreting pituitary tumors are extraordinarily rare.

Acromegaly is a syndrome that presents with characteristic facies, weakness, enlargement of the hands (often to the point of rendering the usual oximeter probes difficult to use) and feet, thickening of the tongue (often to the point of making endotracheal intubation difficult), and enlargement of the nose and mandible with spreading of the teeth (often to the point of requiring larger than normal laryngoscope blades).[61–63] The patient may even appear myxedematous. Other findings include abnormal glucose tolerance and osteoporosis. The most specific test for acromegaly is measurement of GH before and after glucose. The typical acromegalic has very elevated fasting levels of GH (usually above 10 mg/ml), and the levels do not change appreciably after oral glucose. In the normal state, glucose markedly suppresses the GH level. A few patients with active acromegaly have normal levels of fasting GH but do not suppress with glucose. The drug L-dopa, which normally causes an elevation of GH in healthy subjects, in the acromegalic either has no effect or lowers GH levels. Therapy for acromegaly includes the options of pituitary irradiation (heavy particle or implants) and transsphenoidal hypophysectomy.[64] If suprasellar extension exists, conventional transfrontal hypophysectomy is often employed. The dopaminergic agonist bromocriptine can lower GH levels, but long-term follow-up with this drug is still lacking.[65]

Prolactin has been one of the most interesting markers for identifying patients with pituitary tumors.[58] Elevated prolactin levels are often (but not invariably) associated with galactorrhea. Females commonly have amenorrhea, and males impotence. Optimal therapy for prolactin-secreting tumors is still being evaluated: the dopamine agonist bromocriptine can be extremely effective in controlling the prolactin level and restoring gonadotropin function; however, in females who wish to get pregnant, the concern that pregnancy will cause rapid growth of these tumors may make a surgical procedure more desirable. Pituitary irradiation has not been uniformly successful.

3. Multiple Endocrine Adenomatosis Syndrome

Pituitary tumors are sometimes associated with multiple endocrine adenomatosis syndrome (MEA). Pituitary tumors are found more commonly in the MEA I syndrome where adenomas of the parathyroid glands and islets of the pancreas along with the Zollinger-Ellison syndrome may be associated.

4. Anesthetic Considerations for Patients with Abnormal Anterior Pituitary Function

The basic approach of rendering normal all abnormal endocrine functions before surgery holds for endocrine abnormalities originating in the pituitary as well as in the end organ. These considerations are dealt with in the individual sections in this chapter on thyroid and adrenal disorders and conditions with abnormal glucose metabolism or control. One special area—that of operations on the pituitary itself—deserves note here, however. The most common approach is now transsphenoidal hypophysectomy, performed on more than 30,000 patients in the United States each year.[63, 66]

For the patient undergoing craniotomy, the concerns common to any craniotomy, such as provision of patent airway, adequate pulmonary ventilation, control of circulating blood volume, inhibition of increase in brain size, and effective constant monitoring for adverse complications associated with posture, anesthesia, and operation are appropriate. Premedication, use of anesthetic agents and techniques, and monitoring indicated for operations on the pituitary gland are essentially measures that the individual anesthesiologist prefers for operations on other parts of the brain. The effects of anesthetic agents on secretion of pituitary hormones do not constitute an important factor in the selection of agents for use during operation on the pituitary gland. Disorders arising from this surgery include temperature deregulation and abnormalities of endocrine function, including the need for immediate treatment of steroid deficiency, hypoglycemia, and excessive or deficient secretion of vasopressin (also called antidiuretic hormone, ADH).

C. DISORDERS OF THE POSTERIOR PITUITARY GLAND

Deficiency of vasopressin synthesis results in the disease known as diabetes insipidus. Clinically, it is characterized by the excretion of a large volume of hypotonic urine, which in turn necessitates the intake of equally large amounts of fluid or prevention of hyperosmolarity of body fluids and dehydration.[67] Other causes of diabetes insipidus include compulsive water drinking and nephrogenic resistance to the action of vasopressin (Table 8–3).

The classic test to distinguish diabetes insipidus patients from compulsive water drinkers and patients with nephrogenic diabetes insipidus is the water deprivation test.[67, 68] Following dehydration, patients with diabetes insipidus can only minimally concentrate their urine. When the serum osmolarity rises to 295 mOsm/L (osmotic threshold), all normal patients release vasopressin into the blood and concentrate their urine to conserve water. Simultaneous measurements of urine and plasma osmolarity are made as water deprivation continues. Once the urine and plasma osmolarity have stabilized (usually with a 3 to 5 per cent loss in body weight), the patient is given an injection of vasopressin. If vasopressin is being maximally secreted by the posterior pituitary, then exogenous pitressin or vasopressin will have no effect. The patient with vasopressin deficiency never quite reaches stable plasma osmolarity, and the urine osmolarity rarely gets much above 500 mOsm/L. Moreover, even after severe dehydration, exogenous pitressin or vasopressin causes a significant increase in urine osmolarity only in patients with true diabetes insipidus. Thus, this sensitive test even distinguishes patients who have partial diabetes insipidus.

Compulsive water drinkers may at times present a diagnostic problem, since they often cannot concentrate their urine well, and the water deprivation test must be carried out until the osmotic threshold is reached. Tests employing hypertonic saline as a physiologic stimulus to antidiuretic hormone (ADH) are cumbersome and difficult to interpret. Adrenocortical insufficiency can mask the polyuria of partial diabetes insipidus, since it lowers the osmotic threshold for vasopressin release. Institution of steroid therapy in such patients unmasks the diabetes insipidus, and severe polyuria may result.

A number of drugs have been shown to alter the release and action of ADH.[67, 68] The sulfonylurea agents, notably chlorpropamide, have been shown to augment release of ADH and are used in the treatment of patients with partial nephrogenic diabetes insipidus. Likewise, clofibrate, carbamazepine (Tegretol), vincristine, and cyclophosphamide all either release ADH or potentiate its action on the renal tubule. Ethanol as well as phenytoin (Dilantin) and chlorpromazine inhibit the action of ADH and its release. Lithium, a drug widely used to treat manic-depressive disorders, can inhibit the formation of cyclic adenosine monophosphate (cAMP) in the renal tubule and probably even inhibit its synthesis of ADH directly and thus can result in a diabetes insipidus–like picture.

The treatment of diabetes insipidus usually consists of replacement of ADH. The preparation of ADH for intramuscular use is pitressin

---

TABLE 8–3

Causes of Diabetes Insipidus

Vasopressin deficiency (neurogenic diabetes insipidus)
  Acquired
  Idiopathic
  Trauma (accidental, surgical)
  Tumor (craniopharyngioma, metastasis, lymphoma)
  Granuloma (sarcoid, histiocytosis)
  Infectious (meningitis, encephalitis)
  Vascular (Sheehan's syndrome, aneurysm, aortocoronary bypass)
  Familial (autosomal dominant)
Excessive water intake (primary polydipsia)
  Acquired
    Idiopathic (resetting of the osmostat)
    Psychogenic
  Familial (?)
Vasopressin insensitivity (nephrogenic diabetes insipidus)
  Acquired
    Infectious (pyelonephritis)
    Postobstructive (prostatic, ureteral)
    Vascular (sickle cell disease, trait)
    Infiltrative (amyloid)
    Cystic (polycystic disease)
    Metabolic (hypokalemia, hypercalcemia)
    Granuloma (sarcoid)
    Toxic (lithium, demeclocycline, methoxyflurane)
    Solute overload (glucosuria, postobstructive)
  Familial (X-linked recessive)

tannate in oil, 5 units/ml, given intramuscularly every 48 hours. A synthetic lysine vasopressin, Diodid (50 units/ml in isotonic saline), is also used as a nasal spray. This agent is short acting and is given as an adjunct to pitressin tannate. A longer-acting nasal preparation, 1-deamino-8-D-arginine vasopressin (DDAVP), is most commonly used.

For patients with incomplete diabetes insipidus, a trial of thiazide diuretics or chlorpropamide can increase the renal adenyl cyclase response to low levels of ADH, and this can be used for control of urinary flow. Other agents used for incomplete diabetes insipidus are carbamazepine (Tegretol) and clofibrate.

Management of the patient with complete diabetes insipidus during surgery usually does not present difficult problems. A very small amount of aqueous vasopressin (10 to 20 units per ampule) can be given as a continuous intravenous infusion. Just before surgery, the patient is given an intravenous bolus of 100 milliunits aqueous vasopressin and then a constant intravenous infusion of 100 to 200 milliunits vasopressin per hour. In this situation isotonic fluids such as normal saline may be given safely, and there is little danger of water depletion or hypernatremia. The plasma osmolarity can be monitored during surgery and in the immediate postoperative period. The normal range for plasma osmolarity is 283 to 285 mOsm/L. Serum osmolarity can be calculated from the following formula:

$$\text{Osmolarity} = 2\,(\text{Na}^+\ \text{mEq/L}) + \frac{\text{Glucose (mg/dl)}}{20} + \frac{\text{Blood urea nitrogen (mg/dl)}}{3}$$

When blood glucose and blood urea nitrogen are normal, the plasma osmolarity may be calculated by multiplying the serum sodium concentration by 2. If the plasma osmolarity comes up much above 290 mOsm/L, then hypotonic fluids should be given and the amount of aqueous vasopressin given intravenously should be increased above 200 milliunits per hour. In patients who have only partial vasopressin or ADH insufficiency, nonosmotic stimuli such as volume depletion or the stress of surgery may stimulate large quantities of ADH, and it probably is not necessary to use aqueous vasopressin unless there is a demonstrated rise in plasma osmolarity above 290 mOsm/L during surgery or immediately postoperatively. Pitressin tan-

nate in oil (5 to 10 units daily) may be given intramuscularly or DDAVP intranasally in the immediate postoperative period until the intranasal preparations can be used.

1. Hypersecretion of Vasopressin

As first described by Bartter and Schwartz in 1967,[69] excessive secretion of ADH (syndrome of inappropriate secretion of ADH [SIADH]) is a disorder characterized by hyponatremia that results from water retention, which in turn is due to ADH release that is inappropriately high for the plasma osmolality or serum sodium concentration.[67, 70] Because patients with this syndrome are unable to excrete dilute urine, ingested fluids are retained and expansion of extracellular fluid volume without edema occurs. The hallmark of SIADH is hyponatremia in the presence of urinary osmolality that is higher than plasma osmolality.

The most common cause of SIADH is production of ADH by neoplasms. The ADH produced by neoplasms is identical to the arginine vasopressin secreted by the normal neurohypophysis. The most common of the neoplasms producing ADH are small cell and oat cell carcinomas of the lungs. SIADH is also associated with various nonmalignant and inflammatory conditions of the lungs and central nervous system (CNS). Any patient suspected of having SIADH should be screened for possible adrenal insufficiency or hypothyroidism.[70] The diagnosis is essentially one of exclusion. A wide variety of drugs can bring about hypersecretion or augmentation of ADH and result in the syndrome of inappropriate secretion. The most common drugs that cause inappropriate secretion of ADH are chlorpropamide, clofibrate, psychotropics, thiazides, and the antineoplastic agents vincristine, vinblastine, and cyclophosphamide.

Most of the clinical features associated with SIADH are related to hyponatremia and the resulting brain edema; these features include weight gain, weakness, lethargy, mental confusion, obtundation, and disordered reflexes and may progress, finally, to convulsions and coma. This form of edema rarely leads to hypertension.

SIADH should be suspected when any patient with hyponatremia excretes urine that is hypertonic relative to plasma. The following laboratory findings further support the diagnosis[67, 69]:

1. Urinary sodium >20 mEq/L.
2. Low BUN and serum levels of creatinine, uric acid, and albumin.
3. Serum sodium <130 mEq/L.
4. Plasma osmolality <270 mOsm/L.
5. Hypertonic urine relative to plasma.

The response to water loading is a useful means of evaluating the patient with hyponatremia. Patients with SIADH are unable to excrete dilute urine, even after water loading. Assay of ADH in blood can confirm the diagnosis.

Patients with mild to moderate symptoms of water intoxication can be treated with restriction of fluid intake to about 500 to 1000 ml per day. Patients with severe water intoxication and CNS symptoms may need vigorous treatment, with intravenous administration of 200 to 300 ml of 5 per cent saline solution over several hours, followed by fluid restriction.

Treatment should be directed at the underlying problem. If SIADH is drug induced, the drug should be withdrawn. Inflammation should be treated with appropriate measures, and neoplasms should be managed with surgical resection, irradiation, or chemotherapy, whichever is indicated.

At present, no drugs are available that can suppress release of ADH from the neurohypophysis or from a tumor. Dilantin and narcotic antagonists such as naloxone and butorphanol have some inhibiting effect on physiologic ADH release but are clinically ineffective in SIADH. Drugs that block the effect of ADH on renal tubules include lithium, which is rarely used because its toxicity often outweighs its benefits, and demethylchlortetracycline in doses of 900 to 1200 mg/day. The latter drug interferes with the ability of the renal tubules to concentrate urine, causing excretion of isotonic or hypotonic urine and thus lessening hyponatremia. Demethylchlortetracycline can be used for ambulatory patients with SIADH in whom it is difficult to accomplish fluid restriction.

D. ANESTHETIC CONSIDERATIONS FOR PATIENTS WITH ANTIDIURETIC HORMONE ABNORMALITIES

The abnormalities of ADH function that affect perioperative management are those of either a relative or an absolute lack of ADH or an excess of ADH. No matter what the cause of the ADH disorder, the perioperative management problems can be grouped into situations with *inadequate ADH* and situations with *excess ADH*.[70] This categorization or emphasis is not meant to minimize the importance of the diverse causes of perioperative management. Moreover, the cause of the ADH disorder should be sought and the potential perioperative problems evaluated; however, the focus in the remainder of this chapter is on "how to" and "why to" manage the ADH disorder perioperatively.

1. Inadequate Antidiuretic Hormone

Diabetes insipidus, and thus an inadequate ADH level, is the most significant complication following hypophysectomy. The severity and duration of diabetes insipidus depend on the degree of injury to the adjacent hypothalamus. The majority of patients who develop diabetes insipidus after hypophysectomy recover within a few days to 6 months. Patients with diabetes insipidus secondary to head trauma usually recover after a short period. Those who continue to have symptoms, and patients with a long history of diabetes insipidus who require surgery, present a challenge for the anesthesiologist with regard to perioperative management.

Perioperative management of patients with diabetes insipidus is based on the extent of the ADH deficiency. Management of a patient with complete diabetes insipidus and a total lack of ADH usually does not present any major problems as long as side effects of the drug are avoided and as long as that status is known before surgery. Just before surgery, such a patient is given the usual dose of DDAVP intranasally or an intravenous bolus of 100 milliunits of aqueous vasopressin, followed by constant infusion of 100 to 200 milliunits per hour. All of the intravenous fluids given intraoperatively should be isotonic, so that the risk of water depletion and hypernatremia is reduced. Plasma osmolality should be measured every hour, both intraoperatively and in the immediate postoperative period. If the plasma osmolality goes well above 290 mOsm/L, hypotonic fluids should be administered; the rate of the intraoperative vasopressin infusion should be increased to more than 200 milliunits per hour.

In patients who have a partial deficiency

of ADH, it is not necessary to use aqueous vasopressin perioperatively unless the plasma osmolality rises above 290 mOsm/L. Nonosmotic stimuli—for example, volume depletion, stress of surgery, and so on—usually cause release of large quantities of ADH in the perioperative period. Consequently, these patients require only frequent monitoring of plasma osmolality during this period.

Because of the side effects, the dose of vasopressin should be limited to that necessary for control of diuresis.[71–73] This limit is applicable especially to patients who are pregnant or who have coronary artery disease, because of the oxytocic and coronary artery–constricting properties of vasopressin.[73]

Another problem for anesthesiologists is the care for patients who come to the operating room with a pitressin drip for treatment of bleeding from esophageal varices. Although this situation is rare, the vasoconstrictive effect of vasopressin on the splanchnic vasculature is being used to decrease bleeding. Such patients are often volume depleted and may have concomitant coronary artery disease. Since vasopressin has been shown markedly to decrease oxygen availability, primarily because of a decreased stroke volume and heart rate, monitoring of tissue oxygen delivery may be useful. In 1982 Nikolic and Singh[74] reported on a patient with a history of angina pectoris who received a combination of cimetidine and vasopressin for esophageal varices and who developed bradyarrhythmias and atrioventricular block, requiring a pacemaker. Cessation of either of these drugs alleviated the symptoms on two occasions. This indicates that the combination of cimetidine and vasopressin could be deleterious to patients because of the combined negative inotropic and dysrhythmogenic effects of the two drugs.

2. Excessive Antidiuretic Hormone

Patients with SIADH resulting from malignancy have the usual problems present in malignancy, such as anemia and malnutrition, and often they have an imbalance of fluids and electrolytes.[70, 75] Perioperatively, they usually have low urine output, high urine osmolality, low serum osmolality, and delayed awakening from anesthesia or awakening with mental confusion.

When a patient with SIADH comes to the operating room for any surgical procedure, fluids are managed by measuring the central volume status by CVP or PA lines, by transesophageal echocardiography, and by frequent assays of urine osmolarity, plasma osmolarity, and serum sodium, often into the immediate postoperative period. Despite the common impression that SIADH is frequently seen in elderly patients in the postoperative period, studies have shown that the patient's age and the type of anesthetic have no bearing on the postoperative development of SIADH. It is not unusual to see many patients in the neurosurgical ICU suffering from this syndrome. The diagnosis is usually one of exclusion. Patients with SIADH usually require only fluid restriction; very rarely is hypertonic saline needed.

E. SUMMARY

There have been no controlled studies on the risks and benefits of various types of perioperative management for patients with either inadequate or excessive ADH.[75] Nevertheless, increasing knowledge of the pathophysiology of these endocrine aberrations and the use of pharmacologic treatment probably have led to improved clinical results. Inadequate levels of ADH secretion lead to a diabetes insipidus state, with production of large amounts of hypotonic urine, hypernatremia, and a resulting intravascular volume deficit (dehydration). Perioperative treatment consists of replacement of vasopressin by infusion or nasal spray. Since vasopressin causes vasoconstriction of arteriolar beds, monitoring of tissue oxygen delivery and of myocardial ischemia is commonly used. Excess levels of ADH lead to SIADH, which is manifested by low urine output, high urine osmolality, low serum osmolality, hyponatremia, and disordered nervous system functioning (ranging from confusion and delayed awakening from anesthesia to seizures). The perioperative procedures used for SIADH consist of fluid management with a central volume monitor (the author tends to restrict fluids and administer normal saline) and frequent assays for serum sodium level and osmolality and for urine volume and osmolality.

IV. ADRENAL CORTEX

A. PHYSIOLOGY

Cholesterol in the adrenal gland is converted to Δ^5-pregnenolone. This compound is changed either to progesterone or to 17-hydroxypregnenolone. Progesterone can be converted to aldosterone, the principal mineralocorticoid, only in the zona glomerulosa of the adrenal cortex. In the zona fasciculata and zona reticularis, progesterone is made into 11-deoxycortisol and finally to cortisol, the principal glucocorticoid. Sex hormones are also synthesized in the adrenal cortex. Testosterone is the most potent sex hormone synthesized; dehydroisoandrosterone and $^4\Delta$-androstenedione are weaker androgens but at times can contribute significantly to the androgen pool. Under certain circumstances, even estradiol, the female sex hormone, can be synthesized from its precursor hormone, testosterone. Thus, three major classes of hormones—glucocorticoids, mineralocorticoids, and androgens—are secreted by the adrenal cortex. An excess or a deficiency of each of these is associated with a characteristic clinical syndrome.[76–80] Medical use of steroids—now widespread—may render the adrenal cortex incapable of responding normally to the demands placed upon it by surgical trauma and subsequent healing.

More than 100 years ago, Brown-Séquard first demonstrated that bilateral adrenalectomy caused premature death. Over the last century, the central role of adrenal hormones in the maintenance of hemodynamic and metabolic homeostasis by regulation of volume and electrolytes has been defined.

1. Glucocorticoids

The principal glucocorticoid, cortisol, is an essential regulator of carbohydrate, protein, lipid, and nucleic acid metabolism.[78] Cortisol exerts its biologic effects by a sequence of steps initiated by its binding to stereospecific, intracellular cytoplasmic receptors. This bound complex stimulates nuclear transcription of specific messenger RNAs. These messenger RNAs are then translated to give rise to proteins that mediate the ultimate effects of these hormones.[78]

Most cortisol is bound to corticosterone-binding globulin (CBG, transcortin). It is the relatively small amounts of unbound cortisol that enter cells to induce actions or to be metabolized.[78] Conditions that induce changes in the amount of CBG include liver disease and nephrotic syndrome, both of which result in decreased circulating levels of CBG, and estrogen administration and preg-nancy, which result in increased CBG production. Total serum cortisol levels may become elevated or depressed under these conditions that alter the amount of bound cortisol and yet the unbound, active form of cortisol is present in normal amounts. The most accurate measure of cortisol activity is the level of urinary cortisol, that is, the amount of unbound, active cortisol filtered by the kidney.[79]

The serum half-life of cortisol is 80 to 110 minutes; however, since cortisol acts through intracellular receptors, pharmacokinetics based on serum levels is not a good indicator of cortisol activity. Following a single dose of glucocorticoid, serum glucose is elevated for 12 to 24 hours; improvements in pulmonary function in patients with bronchial asthma can still be measured 24 hours after glucocorticoid administration.[81, 82] Treatment schedules for glucocorticoid replacement are based, therefore, not on the measured serum half-life but on the well-documented, prolonged end-organ effect of these steroids. In the past, hospitalized patients who required chronic glucocorticoid replacement therapy were usually treated twice daily, with a slightly higher dose in the morning than in the evening to simulate the normal diurnal variations in cortisol levels.[83, 84] For patients who require parenteral "steroid coverage" during and following surgery (see later paragraphs), administration of glucocorticoid every 8 to 12 hours seems appropriate.[85–87] Relative potencies of glucocorticoids are listed in Table 8–4. Cortisol is inactivated primarily in the liver and is excreted as 17-hydroxycorticosteroid. Cortisol is also filtered and excreted unchanged into the urine.

The synthetic glucocorticoids vary in their binding specificity in a dose-related manner. When given in supraphysiologic doses (more than 30 mg per day), cortisol and cortisone bind to mineralocorticoid receptor sites and cause salt and water retention and loss of potassium and hydrogen ions.[88, 89] When these steroids are administered in maintenance doses of 30 mg per day or less, patients require a specific mineralocorticoid for electrolyte and volume homeostasis. Many other steroids do not bind to mineralocorticoid receptors, even in large doses, and have minimal mineralocorticoid effect (see Table 8–4).[89]

Control of Glucocorticoid Secretion. The hypothalamic-pituitary-adrenal axis is shown in Figure 8–4. Secretion of glucocorticoids is regulated exclusively by pituitary ACTH.[78, 90] ACTH is synthesized from a precursor mole-

TABLE 8–4

Relative Potencies and Biological Half-Lives of Cortisol and Its Synthetic Analogues

| Common Name | Other Name | Estimated Potency | | Biological Half-Life (hours) |
		Glucocorticoid	Mineralo-corticoid	
Cortisol	Compound F, hydrocortisone	1	1	8–12
Cortisone	Cortone	0.8	0.8	8–12
Prednisone	—	4	0.25	12–36
Methylprednisolone	Medrol	5	0.25	12–36
Triamcinolone	Aristocort Kenacort	5	0.25	12–36
Dexamethasone	Decadron	20–30	±	26–54
Fluorohydrocortisone	Florinef	5	200	—
Desoxycorticosterone	Percorten	0	15	—

cule (preopiomelanocortin) which breaks down to form an endorphin (β-lipoprotropin) and ACTH.[91] ACTH secretion has a diurnal rhythm; it is normally greatest during the early morning hours in men (afternoon in women) and is regulated at least in part by sleep-wake cycles.[80] Its secretion is stimulated by release of corticotropin-releasing factor (CRF) from the hypothalamus.[78] Cortisol and other glucocorticoids exert negative feedback at both pituitary and hypothalamic levels to inhibit secretion of ACTH and CRF.

Overproduction of glucocorticoids can be caused by adrenal tumors (primary Cushing's disease) or by overstimulation of normal adrenal glands by elevated levels of ACTH from pituitary microadenomas (secondary Cushing's disease). Inappropriately low levels of glucocorticoids may result from destruction or atrophy of the adrenal gland itself (primary adrenal insufficiency) or from diminished levels of ACTH in pituitary dysfunction (secondary adrenal insufficiency).[92]

2. Mineralocorticoids

Aldosterone, the major mineralocorticoid secreted in humans, comes from the zona glomerulosa of the adrenal cortex, causes reabsorption of sodium and secretion of potassium and hydrogen ions, and thus contributes to electrolyte and volume homeostasis. This action is most prominent in the distal renal tubules, but it also occurs in salivary and sweat glands. The main regulator of aldosterone secretion is the renin-angiotensin system.[93] Juxtaglomerular cells in the cuff of the renal arterioles are sensitive to decreased renal perfusion pressure or volume and consequently secrete renin. Renin splits the precursor angiotensinogen (from the liver) into angiotensin I, which is further converted by converting enzyme, primarily in the lung, to angiotensin II. Mineralocorticoid secretion is increased by increased levels of angiotensin.

3. Androgens

Androstenedione and dehydroepiandrosterone, which are weak androgens arising from the adrenal cortex, constitute major sources of androgens in women.[77] These androgens are converted outside the adrenal glands to testosterone, a potent virilizing hormone.[77, 94] Excess secretion of androgen in women causes masculinization, pseudopuberty, or female pseudohermaphroditism. Some tumors convert this androgen to an estrogenic substance, in which case feminization results.[98] Some congenital enzyme defects that cause abnormal levels of androgens in blood also result in glucocorticoid and mineralocorticoid abnormalities.[94] The altered sexual differentiation in the presence of such defects requires no specific modification of anesthetic technique. All syndromes related to abnormal androgen levels are associated with cortisol deficiency. In patients who have associated alterations in glucocorticoid or mineralocorticoid activity, anesthetic plans should be modified as outlined in the following sections.

B. EXCESSIVE ADRENOCORTICAL HORMONES: HYPERPLASIA, ADENOMA, CARCINOMA

1. Sex Hormone–Secreting Tumors of the Adrenal Glands

Hirsutism in females may be due to either adrenal or ovarian tumor. Adrenal virilizing tumors are almost always associated with markedly elevated 17-ketosteroid urinary excretion, whereas functioning ovarian tumors tend to produce very potent androgens such as testosterone or dihydrotestosterone, which are not measured as part of the 17-ketosteroids. Rarely, adrenal tumors produce only testosterone and are stimulated by human chorionic gonadotropin. Similarly, some androgen-producing ovarian tumors have been shown to respond to dexamethasone suppression. A common cause of hirsutism in females is polycystic ovarian disease, which is associated with bilaterally enlarged ovaries.[95] Extreme feminization in males can occasionally be due to an estrogen-producing tumor of the adrenal gland. Functioning sex hormone–producing tumors of the adrenal gland almost always tend to be unilateral. Pelvic B-mode ultrasonography, CT, and MRI are very useful modalities for localizing lesions. Most patients do not have to be managed with glucocorticoids during or after surgery. The only exception is the patient who has associated Cushing's syndrome with cortisol excess; management should be as outlined below for tumors of the adrenal gland.

Adrenal genital syndrome should be ruled out as a possible cause of hirsutism. These patients are not surgical candidates. Generally, in addition to high 17-ketosteroid levels in the urine, these patients have very high urinary pregnanetriol levels and elevated 17-OH progesterone blood levels. They are generally managed with mildly suppressive doses of corticosteroids.

2. Excessive Glucocorticoids

Glucocorticoid excess (Cushing's syndrome), resulting from either endogenous oversecretion or long-term treatment with large doses of glucocorticoids, produces a characteristic appearance and a predictable complex of disease states. The individual appears moon faced and plethoric, having a centripetal distribution of fat and thin extremities because of muscle wasting. The heart and diaphragm apparently are spared the effects of muscle wasting.[79] The skin is thin and easily bruised, and striae are often present. Hypertension (because of increases in renin substrate and vascular reactivity caused by glucocorticoids) and fluid retention are present in 85 per cent of patients.[79, 93] Nearly two of every three patients also have hyperglycemia resulting from inhibition of peripheral glucose use with concomitant stimulation of gluconeogenesis. These patients often have osteopenia as a result of decreased bone matrix formation and impaired calcium absorption. One third of the patients have pathologic fractures.

Special preoperative considerations for patients with Cushing's syndrome include regulating diabetes and hypertension and ensuring that intravascular fluid volume and electrolyte concentrations are normal.[96, 97] Ectopic ACTH production from sites other than the pituitary may cause marked hypokalemic alkalosis.[79] Treatment with the aldosterone antagonist spironolactone arrests the potassium loss and helps mobilize excess fluid. Because of the high incidence of severe osteopenia and the risk of fractures, meticulous attention to patient positioning is necessary.[76, 94] In addition, glucocorticoids are lympholytic and immunosuppressive, perhaps increasing the patient's susceptibility to infection.[98–100] The tensile strength of healing wounds decreases in the presence of glucocorticoids, an effect at least partially reversed by topical administration of vitamin A.[101, 102]

Specific considerations pertain to the surgical approach for each cause of Cushing's syndrome. For example, nearly three fourths of the cases of spontaneous Cushing's disease result from a pituitary adenoma that secretes ACTH.[79] Perioperative treatment for patients who have Cushing's disease and a pituitary microadenoma differs from that for patients who have a pituitary adenoma associated with amenorrhea and galactorrhea. The Cushing's patient tends to bleed more easily and (based on anecdotal evidence) tends to have a higher central venous pressure (CVP). Thus, during transsphenoidal tumor resection in such patients, we routinely monitor CVP or end-diastolic left ventricular volume on transesophageal echocardiography and maintain pressure and/or volume in the low end of the normal range. Such monitoring is needed only infrequently in other cases of transsphenoidal resection of microadenoma.[79]

Some 10 to 15 per cent of patients with Cushing's syndrome have adrenal overproduction of glucocorticoids (adrenal adenoma or carcinoma). If either unilateral or bilateral adrenal resection is planned, the author normally begins administering glucocorticoids at the start of the tumor resection, normally giving 100 mg of IV hydrocortisone phosphate every 24 hours.[97] This amount is reduced over the next 3 to 6 days until a maintenance dose of 20 to 30 mg per day in divided doses is reached. Beginning on about day 3, 9-alpha-fluorocortisone (a mineralocorticoid) is also given, 0.05 to 0.1 mg per day. Both steroids may require several adjustments in some patients. This therapy is continued for patients who have undergone bilateral adrenal resection. For patients who have had unilateral resection, therapy is individualized, based on the status of the remaining adrenal gland.

Patients with Cushing's syndrome who require bilateral adrenalectomy have a high incidence of postoperative complications. The incidence of pneumothorax approaches 20 per cent with adrenal carcinoma resection, and it is sought and treatment begun before the wound is closed. Ten per cent of patients with Cushing's syndrome who undergo adrenalectomy are found to have an undiagnosed pituitary tumor. After reduction of high levels of cortisol by adrenalectomy, the pituitary tumor enlarges (Nelson's syndrome).[103] These pituitary tumors are potentially invasive and may produce large amounts of ACTH and melanocyte-stimulating hormone, thus increasing pigmentation.

Adrenal adenomas are usually treated surgically, and often the contralateral gland will resume functioning after several months. Frequently, however, the effects of carcinomas are not cured by surgery. In such cases, administration of inhibitors of steroid synthesis such as metyrapone or o,p'-DDD[2,2-bis-(2-chlorophenyl-4-chlorophenyl)-1,1-dichloroethane] may ameliorate some symptoms but may not improve survival.[104] These drugs and the aldosterone antagonist spironolactone may alleviate symptoms in the case of ectopic ACTH secretion if the primary tumor proves unresectable. Patients given these adrenal suppressants are also given chronic glucocorticoid replacement therapy (with the goal of complete adrenal suppression). These patients should be considered to have suppressed adrenal function, and glucocorticoid replacement should be increased perioperatively as discussed earlier.

3. Excessive Mineralocorticoids

Excess mineralocorticoid activity leads to sodium retention, potassium depletion, hypertension, and hypokalemic alkalosis.[105–108] These symptoms constitute primary hyperaldosteronism, or Conn's syndrome (a cause of low-renin hypertension, as renin secretion is inhibited by the effects of the high aldosterone levels).

Primary hyperaldosteronism is present in 0.5 to 1 per cent of hypertensive patients who have no other known cause of hypertension. Primary hyperaldosteronism is most often the result of a unilateral adenoma, although 25 to 40 per cent of patients may have bilateral adrenal hyperplasia. Intravascular fluid volume, electrolyte concentrations, and renal function should be restored to within normal limits preoperatively by treatment with spironolactone. The effects of spironolactone are slow to appear and increase for 1 to 2 weeks. In addition, patients with Conn's syndrome have a high incidence of ischemic heart disease, and hemodynamic monitoring appropriate for their degree of cardiovascular impairment should be undertaken. A retrospective anecdotal study indicated that intraoperative stability, with preoperative control of blood pressure and electrolytes, was better with spironolactone than with other antihypertensive agents.[107] The efficacy for patient outcome of optimizing the preoperative status of patients with disorders of glucocorticoid or mineralocorticoid secretion, however, has not been clearly established.

C. ADRENOCORTICAL HORMONE DEFICIENCY

1. Glucocorticoid Deficiency

Withdrawal of steroids or suppression of their adrenal synthesis by steroid therapy is the leading cause of underproduction of corticosteroids.[78] The management of this type of glucocorticoid deficiency is discussed below (Patients Taking Steroids for Medical Conditions). Fewer cases of this potential problem are expected, in part because of a change from systemic steroids to inhaled ones for treatment of asthma.[81] Other causes of adrenocortical insufficiency include destruction of the adrenal gland by cancer, tuberculosis, hemorrhage, or an autoimmune mechanism; some forms of congenital adrenal hyperplasia (see previous discussion); and administration of cytotoxic drugs.

Primary adrenal insufficiency (Addison's disease) is caused by a local process within the adrenal gland that leads to destruction of all zones of the cortex and causes both glucocorticoid and mineralocorticoid deficiency if the insufficiency is bilateral. Autoimmune disease is the most common cause of primary (nonendogenous) bilateral ACTH deficiency.[78, 92] Autoimmune destruction of the adrenals may be associated with other autoimmune disorders, such as Hashimoto's thyroiditis. Enzymatic defects in cortisol synthesis also cause glucocorticoid insufficiency, compensatory elevations of ACTH, and congenital adrenal hyperplasia.[77]

Adrenal insufficiency usually develops slowly. Patients with Addison's disease can develop marked pigmentation (because excess ACTH is present to drive an unproductive adrenal gland) and cardiopenia (apparently secondary to chronic hypotension).

Secondary adrenal insufficiency occurs when ACTH secretion is deficient, often because of a pituitary or hypothalamic tumor. Treatment of pituitary tumors by surgery or radiation may result in hypopituitarism and consequent adrenal failure.

If glucocorticoid-deficient patients are not stressed, they usually have no perioperative problems.[97] However, acute adrenal (addisonian) crisis can occur when even a minor stress (for example, upper respiratory tract infection) is present.[109] In the preparation of such a patient for anesthesia and surgery, hypovolemia, hyperkalemia, and hyponatremia can be treated.[110, 111] Since these patients cannot respond to stressful situations, it was traditionally recommended that they be given a maximum stress dose of glucocorticoids (about 300 mg of hydrocortisone per 70 kg body weight per day) perioperatively. Symreng and colleagues[112] gave 25 mg of hydrocortisone phosphate IV to adults at the start of the operative procedure, followed by 100 mg IV over the next 24 hours. Since using the minimum drug dose that will cause an appropriate effect is desirable, this latter regimen seems attractive. Evidence is accumulating that less steroid supplementation does not cause problems, and the author now recommends giving 100 mg of hydrocortisone phos-

phate IV per 70 kg body weight over the next 24 hours.[109, 112]

Udelsman and colleagues[109] studied glucocorticoid replacement in primates. In that study, adrenalectomized primates and sham-operated controls were maintained on physiologic doses of steroids for 4 months. The animals were then randomized to receive subphysiologic (1/10 the normal cortisol production), physiologic, and supraphysiologic (10 times the normal cortisol production) doses of cortisol for 4 days before abdominal surgery (cholecystectomy). Hemodynamic variables were measured with arterial and pulmonary artery catheters. The animals were maintained on their randomized dosing schedules during and after surgery. The group receiving subphysiologic doses of steroid perioperatively had a significant increase in postoperative mortality. The death rates in the physiologic and supraphysiologic replacement groups were the same and did not differ from that for sham-operated controls. Death in the subphysiologic replacement group was related to severe hypotension associated with a significant decrease in systemic vascular resistance (SVR) and a reduced left ventricular stroke work index (LVSWI). The filling pressures of the heart were unchanged, as compared with those in control animals. There was, therefore, no evidence of hypovolemia or severe CHF. Despite the low SVR, the animals did not become tachycardic. All of these responses are compatible with the previously documented interaction of glucocorticoids and catecholamines, suggesting that glucocorticoids mediate catecholamine-induced increases in cardiac contractility and maintenance of vascular tone.

The investigators used a sensitive measure of wound healing by studying hydroxyproline accumulation. All treatment groups, including that which received supraphysiologic doses of glucocorticoids, had the same capacity for wound healing. Furthermore, there were no adverse metabolic consequences of supraphysiologic corticosteroid doses given perioperatively.[109]

This well-conducted study confirms several "old wives' tales" about patients who have inadequate adrenal function, either from underlying disease or secondary to exogenous steroids. Inadequate replacement of corticosteroids perioperatively can lead to addisonian crisis and death. Administration of supraphysiologic doses of steroids for a short time perioperatively caused no discernible complications. It is clear that inadequate corticosteroid coverage can cause death. What is not so clear is what dose of steroid for replacement therapy should be recommended.

2. Mineralocorticoid Deficiency

Hypoaldosteronism, a condition less common than glucocorticoid deficiency, can be congenital or can occur following unilateral adrenalectomy or prolonged administration of heparin.[108] It may also be a consequence of long-standing diabetes and renal failure. Nonsteroidal inhibitors of prostaglandin synthesis may also inhibit renin release and exacerbate this condition in patients with renal insufficiency.[113] Levels of plasma renin activity are below normal and fail to rise appropriately in response to sodium restriction or diuretics. Most of the patients have low blood pressure; rarely, however, a patient may be normotensive or even hypertensive. Most symptoms are due to hyperkalemic acidosis rather than hypovolemia. Patients with hypoaldosteronism can have severe hyperkalemia, hyponatremia, and myocardial conduction defects. These defects can be treated successfully with mineralocorticoids (9-alpha-fluorocortisone, 0.05 to 0.1 mg per day) preoperatively. Doses must be carefully titrated and monitored so that increasing hypertension can be avoided.

D. PATIENTS TAKING STEROIDS FOR MEDICAL CONDITIONS

1. Perioperative Stress and the Need for Corticoid Supplementation[76]

Many reports (mostly anecdotal) concerning normal adrenal responses during the perioperative period and responses of patients taking steroids for other diseases indicate that:

1. Perioperative stress is related to the degree of trauma and the depth of anesthesia. Deep general or regional anesthesia causes the usual intraoperative glucocorticoid surge to be postponed to the postoperative period.
2. Few patients who have suppressed adrenal function have perioperative cardiovascular problems if they do not receive supplemental steroids perioperatively.
3. Occasionally, a patient who habitually takes steroids will become hypotensive perioperatively, but this event has only rarely been documented sufficiently to implicate glucocorticoid or mineralocorticoid deficiency as the cause.
4. Although it occurs rarely, acute adrenal insufficiency can be life threatening.
5. There is little risk in giving these patients high-dose steroid coverage perioperatively.

What dose of steroids should one give and to whom? A definitive answer is not available; however, the recommendation of 100 mg per 70 kg body weight every 24 hours stands until a prospective, randomized, double-blind trial in patients receiving physiologic doses of steroids is performed. A smaller dose probably can be used. In any case, the author never supplements perioperatively with a dose lower than that the patient has already been receiving.

If in doubt, how can one determine a patient's need for perioperative supplementation with glucocorticoids? Since the risk is low, the author normally provides supplementation for every patient who has received steroids, including inhaled steroids, at any time during the previous year. It has been shown that topical application of steroids (even without the use of occlusive dressings) can suppress normal adrenal responses for as long as 9 months or a year.[114]

How can one determine whether the patient's adrenal responsiveness has returned to normal? The morning plasma cortisol level does not reveal whether the adrenal cortex has recovered sufficiently to ensure that cortisol secretion increases enough to meet the demands under stress. Insulin-induced hypoglycemia has been advocated as a sensitive test of pituitary-adrenal competence (see the section on Anterior Pituitary Disease), but its use is impractical and probably more dangerous than simply administering glucocorticoids. If plasma cortisol is measured during acute stress, a value greater than 25 μg/dl assuredly indicates and more than 15 μg/dl probably indicates normal pituitary-adrenal responsiveness.

The most sensitive test of adrenal reserve is the ACTH stimulation test. To test pituitary-adrenal sufficiency, one determines the baseline plasma cortisol level. Then 250 μg of synthetic ACTH (cosyntropin) is given, and the plasma cortisol is measured 30 to 60 minutes later. An increment in plasma cortisol of 7 to 20 µg/dl or more is normal. A normal response indicates a recovery of pituitary-adrenal axis function. A lesser response usually indicates pituitary-adrenal insufficiency, possibly requiring perioperative supplementation with steroids.

Usually, laboratory data defining pituitary-adrenal adequacy are not available before surgery. However, rather than delay surgery or test most patients, it is assumed that any patient who has taken steroids at any time in the preceding year has pituitary-adrenal suppression and will require perioperative supplementation.

Under perioperative conditions, the adrenal glands secrete 116 to 185 mg of cortisol daily. Under maximum stress, they may secrete 200 to 500 mg daily. A good correlation between the severity and duration of the operation and the response of the adrenal gland was shown during major surgery that included procedures such as colectomy and minor surgery procedures such as herniorrhaphy. In one study, the mean maximal plasma cortisol level during major surgery in 20 patients was 47 µg/dl (range 22 to 75 µg/dl). Values remained above 26 µg/dl for a maximum of 72 hours after operation. The mean maximal plasma cortisol level during minor surgery was 28 µg/dl (range, 10 to 44 µg/dl).[86]

Although the precise amount of glucocorticoid required has not been established, the author usually administers one third of the maximum amount that the body manufactures in response to maximal stress; that is, about 200 mg per 70 kg body weight per day of IV hydrocortisone phosphate. For minor procedures, the author usually gives hydrocortisone phosphate IV, 25 to 50 mg per 70 kg body weight per day. Unless infection or some other perioperative complication develops, this is decreased by approximately 25 per cent per day until oral intake can be resumed. At this point, the usual maintenance dose of glucocorticoids can be employed.

2. Risks of Supplementation

Rare potential risks of perioperative supplementation with steroids include aggravation of hypertension, hyperglycemia, fluid retention, the induction of stress ulcers, and psychiatric disturbances. Two risk factors associated with glucocorticoid administration to surgical patients have been described and reviewed:[98] abnormal wound healing and an increased rate of infection. However, the evidence is inconclusive since it relates to acute glucocorticoid administration and not to chronic administration of glucocorticoids with increased doses at times of stress. For example, in rats wounded before and after topical application of cortisone, delayed wound closure was found secondary to inhibition of granulation tissue and decreased proliferation of fibroblasts and of new blood vessels. Ehrlich and Hunt,[101] as well as Sandberg,[102] found that moderate to large doses of steroids exerted their morphologic effects maximally within 3 days after injury, and they postulated that the inhibition of the early inflammatory process by steroids after wounding was responsible for delayed healing. Vitamin A protected somewhat against delayed healing, presumably because of its effect in stabilizing lysosomes. In contrast to these studies that suggest a deleterious effect of perioperative glucocorticoid administration on wound healing in rats, a study on primates suggests that large doses of glucocorticoids, administered perioperatively, did not impair sensitive measures of wound healing.[109] An overall assessment of these results suggests that short-term perioperative steroid treatment has a small but definite deleterious effect on wound healing that is perhaps partially reversed by topical administration of vitamin A.

Information on the risk of infection as a result of perioperative supplement with glucocorticoids is also unclear. Winstone and Brook[100] reported four cases of septicemia among 18 surgical patients given perioperative supplementation with glucocorticoids, but no similar complications in 17 others who also took glucocorticoids but were not given perioperative supplementation. In a controlled study of 100 patients who received perioperative supplementation with glucocorticoids, there were 11 wound infections in the steroid-treated group and only one in the control group.[98] Test subjects and controls were not matched for underlying disease, however. In contrast, Jensen and Elb[115] found no change in the incidence of wound infections or other infections in an uncontrolled series of 419 patients subjected to surgery and perioperative supplementation with glucocorticoids. Oh and Patterson[116] found only one minor suture abscess among a group of 17 steroid-dependent asthmatic patients undergoing 21 surgical procedures. Thus, these data are inadequate to show that perioperative supplementation with steroids increases the risk of infection.

E. SUMMARY

Abnormalities in adrenal cortical function can be manifested as deficiencies or excesses of androgens, mineralocorticoids, or glucocorticoids. Deficiency of androgens is often accompanied by deficiency of the other hormones. Excess androgens result in no unusual perioperative problems for the anesthetist. Mineralocorticoid abnormalities can be associated with blood volume, electrolyte, and cardiac disturbances. The author routinely seeks and treats these abnormalities preoperatively as well as intra- and postoperatively.

Abnormal levels of glucocorticoids often cause mineralocorticoid disturbances, as well as suppressing healing and the capacity to combat infection. The author has presented data showing that it is probably better to give supplemental steroids to any patient who has received exogenous steroids in the previous year. The dose of steroids that provides the greatest benefit-risk ratio for supplementation appears to be declining (the author now uses 100 mg per 70 kg per day of hydrocortisone phosphate IV). Etomidate suppresses adrenal cortical steroid synthesis, and its use probably should be accompanied by steroid supplementation.[117] The author employs the previously discussed conclusions as derived from anecdotal studies; no controlled studies indicate that any one anesthetic practice or choice of drugs is better than any other for patients with adrenal disease. As with most other endocrinopathies, the focus of complications resides in the cardiovascular system.

V. ADRENAL MEDULLA: PHEOCHROMOCYTOMA

Cells of neural crest origin are capable of developing into catecholamine-secreting tumors. Indeed, pheochromocytomas, or catecholamine tumors, have been reported in neural-crest sites ranging from the neck to the inguinal ligament. Pheochromocytomas have been reported as part of the multiple endocrine adenomatosis syndrome and in association with neuroectodermal dysplasias, including neurofibromatosis, tuberous sclerosis, Sturge-Weber syndrome, and von Hippel–Lindau disease. Although pheochromocytomas cause fewer than 0.1 per cent of all cases of hypertension, they are important to the anesthesiologist. Some 25 to 50 per cent of hospital deaths of patients with pheochromocytoma occur during induction of anesthesia or during operative procedures for other disorders.[118]

Three issues are important in considering pheochromocytoma:[24, 119–122] (1) the organ system that most influences the anesthetic management of patients with pheochromocytoma is the cardiovascular system; (2) major reductions in morbidity associated with resection of pheochromocytoma occurred when the anesthetist was adequately informed about this disorder and when the patient had received adequate α-adrenergic blockade; and (3) no controlled studies have been done on almost any aspect of the diagnosis or treatment of pheochromocytoma; thus this summary is based on conclusions derived from the many published anecdotal studies.

A. PHYSIOLOGY AND DIAGNOSIS

The physiologic transmitters (catecholamines) are released from the terminals of the postganglionic sympathetic nervous system. Synthesis of catecholamines begins in the postganglionic nerve cell bodies when tyrosine is hydroxylated in the rate-limiting step to dopa; dopa is decarboxylated to dopamine; and, in most cells, dopamine is hydroxylated to norepinephrine. In the adrenal, in rare parts of the CNS, and at some ganglia, this norepinephrine can be converted by phenylethanolamine-N-transferase to epinephrine. The release of dopamine, norepinephrine, and epinephrine occurs both basally and in response to physiologic and pharmacologic stressors such as hypotension (through baroreceptors), low tissue perfusion, hypoxia, hypoglycemia, anger, determination, fear, and anxiety. Such release from the sympathetic nervous system can be generalized or localized. Most pheochromocytomas are independent of these physiologic stressors, however.

Some pheochromocytomas are under neurogenic control, with increased release of catecholamines stimulated by physiologic and pharmacologic stressors. However, much of the release of catecholamines from pheochromocytomas is not controlled by neurogenic influence. This lack of neurologic control is utilized in the clonidine suppression test for pheochromocytoma (see paragraphs that follow).[123]

Painful or stressful events such as intubation often cause an exaggerated catecholamine response in a less than perfectly anesthetized patient with pheochromocytoma. This response is caused by release of catecholamines from nerve endings that are "loaded" by the reuptake process. Stresses may cause catecholamine levels of 200 to 2000 pg/ml in normal patients. For the patient with pheochromocytoma, even simple stresses can lead to blood catecholamine levels of 2000 to 20,000 pg/ml. Squeezing the tumor, however gently, or infarction of the tumor with release of products onto peritoneal surfaces can result in blood levels of 200,000 to 1,000,000 pg/ml—a potentially disasterous situation that should be anticipated and avoided. The physician should ask for a temporary stay of surgery, if at all possible, during which the rate of nitroprusside infusion will be increased.

It has been found in several studies that the triad of paroxysmal sweating, hypertension, and headache is more sensitive and specific than any laboratory test for the diagnosis of pheochromocytoma. These are the symptoms that one experiences when given an infusion of epinephrine.[124] Physical examination of a patient with pheochromocytoma is usually unrewarding unless the patient is observed during an attack. Occasionally, palpation of the abdomen causes the bladder or rectum to rub against the tumor and stimulates release of catecholamines; however, the laboratory measurement of catecholamines or their metabolites has been the standard method of diagnosis.

Half of all patients with pheochromocytoma have continuous hypertension with occasional paroxysms, and another 40 per cent have paroxysmal hypertension. Labile hypertension or the triad of hypertension, headache, and sweating usually is an indication for urine testing.

In more than 85 per cent of cases, pheochromocytomas are sporadic tumors of unknown cause that are localized in the medulla of one adrenal gland; however, these vascular tumors can occur anywhere. They are found in the right atrium, the spleen, the broad ligament of the ovary, or the organs of Zuckerkandl at the bifurcation of the aorta. Malignant spread, which occurs in fewer than 15 per cent of cases of pheochromocytoma, usually proceeds via venous and lymphatic channels, with a predilection for the liver. Occasionally, this tumor is a familial autosomal-dominant trait. It may be a part of the pluriglandular-neoplastic syndrome known as multiple endocrine adenoma type IIa or type IIb. Type IIa consists of medullary carcinoma of the thyroid, parathyroid adenoma or hyperplasia, and pheochromocytoma. Type IIb consists of medullary carcinoma of the thyroid, a Marfanoid appearance, mucosal neuromas, and pheochromocytoma. Often, bilateral tumors are present in the familial form.

Urine tests have become a mainstay of diagnosis. The usual urine tests used measure 3-methoxy-4-hydroxymandelic acid, or metanephrines, or native catecholamines per milligram of creatine secreted. If the results of three 24-hour collections of urine are normal, the patient is considered not to have a pheochromocytoma.[122]

Although urine testing has been the standard for diagnosis, many more patients are found at autopsy to have had pheochromocytoma and to have died of its complications (often during operations for other problems) than have pheochromocytoma diagnosed while they are alive. If urine test results are normal, but the suspicion is strong enough, provocative tests with glucagon to promote catecholamine release by the tumor can be used, and the diagnosis is based on the blood pressure response and plasma catecholamine elevation. Catecholamine levels in urine and plasma are diagnostic when elevated to three times the normal median value. If plasma catecholamine levels are above normal, but below three times the normal median, a clonidine suppression test is recommended. Clonidine, by its α_2-adrenergic agonist activity in the brainstem, suppresses neurogenically controlled peripheral catecholamine release. Since most pheochromocytomas are not under neurogenic control, catecholamine release in patients with pheochromocytoma will not be suppressed, and their plasma level will remain elevated.[123]

Once the diagnosis of pheochromocytoma is made, the tumor must be localized and pretreated before surgical resection. The protocol for localizing these often small tumors has undergone radical revision. Plain radiographs or intravenous pyelograms that show lateral displacement of a kidney are a first approach. Recently, MRI has replaced CT, which itself replaced urography and venous sampling. When such techniques do not yield definitive results, scanning with ^{131}I-metaiodobenzylguanidine (a guanethidine analogue) can be tried.

B. ANESTHETIC CONSIDERATIONS FOR PATIENTS WITH PHEOCHROMOCYTOMA

There are many published reports on perioperative morbidity and mortality associated with pheochromocytoma, but little is known about the factors that affect the rates of morbidity and mortality.[125–129] Although no controlled, randomized, prospective clinical study has been done on the value of adrenergic blocking drugs, the preoperative use of these drugs for patients with pheochromocytoma is recommended because they are likely to reduce the incidence of the perioperative complications of hypertensive crisis, wide fluctuations in blood pressure during intraoperative manipulation of the tumor (especially until the venous drainage is obliterated), and perioperative myocardial dysfunction.[119, 124, 126–129, 137] Perioperative mortality associated with the excision of pheochromocytoma was reduced from 13 to 45 per cent to 0 to 3 per cent when α-adrenergic blockade was introduced as preoperative therapy and when it was recognized that these patients often had hypovolemia preoperatively[136, 137] (Table 8–5).[129, 130]

The presence of hyperglycemia preoperatively reflects the metabolic effects of catecholamines, resolves with tumor resection, and usually does not require insulin therapy pre- or perioperatively. Persistently elevated catecholamine levels may result in catecholamine myocarditis. This cardiomyopathy appears to pose an extra risk for patients, but it can be treated successfully by α-adrenergic blockade preoperatively (see paragraph that follows). Mortality for patients with pheochromocytoma is usually the result of myocardial failure, myocardial infarction, or hemorrhage (hypertensive) into the myocardium or brain. The incidence of all of these catastrophic situations appears to be reduced with α-adrenergic blockade.

Preoperative therapy consisting of α-adrenergic blockade with phenoxybenzamine, prazosin, or labetalol alleviates the patient's symptoms, favors a successful fetal outcome (that is, in patients whose pheochromocytoma is discovered during pregnancy),[131] and allows reexpansion of intravascular plasma volume by eradicating the vasoconstrictive effects of high levels of catecholamines. This reexpansion of fluid volume is often accompanied by a decreased hematocrit. Because some patients are sensitive to phenoxybenzamine, it should initially be administered in doses of 10 to 20 mg orally two or three times a day. Most patients require 60 to 250 mg per day. The efficacy of the therapy is judged by the reduction of symptoms (especially sweating) and by stabilization of blood pressure. For patients with catecholamine myocarditis as evidenced by often localized ST and T wave ECG changes, preoperative, long-term

TABLE 8–5

Perioperative Mortality for Pheochromocytoma Resection

Year	Investigator(s)	Mortality (%)	Number of Patients in Study
1951	Apgar (review)	45	91
1951	Apgar	33	12
1963	Stackpole et al.	13	100
Before 1960	Mayo Clinic	0–26?	101?
After 1960	Mayo Clinic	2.9?	44?
	Modlin et al.		
Before 1967	No alpha blockade	18	17
After 1967	Alpha blockade	2	41
1976	Scott et al.	3	33
1976–85	Roizen et al.	0	38

Data abstracted from Roizen MF: Anesthetic implications of concurrent diseases. In Miller RD (ed.): Anesthesia, Vol. 1, ed 4. New York, Churchill Livingstone, 1994, pp. 903–1014.

administration of α-adrenergic blockade (for 15 days to 6 months) has been shown to be effective in resolving the clinical and ECG alterations.[125]

Beta-adrenergic receptor blockade with concomitant administration of phenoxybenzamine is suggested for patients who have persistent dysrhythmias or tachycardia. It is recommended that β-adrenergic receptor blockade not be used without α-adrenergic blockade, however, lest the vasoconstrictive effects of the latter go unopposed and produce dangerous hypertension. The latter complication has been reported only rarely, however, and perhaps no firm rules are necessary.

To date, no one has investigated the optimal duration of preoperative phenoxybenzamine therapy. Most patients require treatment for 10 to 14 days, as determined by the time needed for stabilization of blood pressure and amelioration of symptoms. If the patient does not complain of nasal stuffiness, he or she is not ready for surgery, in the author's opinion. Because pheochromocytomas spread slowly, little is lost by waiting until the patient's preoperative condition has been optimized by means of medical therapy. The following criteria for an optimal preoperative condition are recommended:

1. No "in-hospital" blood pressure reading higher than 160/90 mm Hg should be evident for 24 hours before surgery. The author normally measures the blood pressure in each patient (as an outpatient) every minute for an hour in a recovery room setting during preoperative visits. This setting is most stressful to the medically naive, and thus a good test of inhibition of responses to sympathetic stimulation. If no blood pressure reading higher than 160/90 is recorded, the patient is scheduled for surgery, assuming the following three criteria are also met.

2. Orthostatic hypotension, with readings above 80/45 mm Hg, should be present.

3. The ECG should be free of ST-T abnormalities for at least a week; if abnormalities are persistent, two-dimensional echocardiography should reveal no evidence of global or regional dysfunction that cannot be attributed to a permanent deficit.

4. The patient should have no more than one premature ventricular contraction every 5 minutes.

Although specific anesthetic drugs have been recommended for patients with pheochromocytoma, optimal preoperative prepa-

ration, careful and gradual induction of anesthesia, and good communication between surgeon and anesthesiologist are most important. The author usually gives phenoxybenzamine in one half to two thirds of its normal dose immediately preceding surgery. Virtually all anesthetic agents, muscle relaxants, and techniques have been used successfully for patients with pheochromocytoma, and all are associated with a high rate of transient intraoperative dysrhythmias.[126] Although some agents may have advantages or disadvantages in theory, they have not been demonstrated clinically. For example, one might wish to avoid histamine release, since it can stimulate catecholamine release. Yet neither curare nor morphine has been associated with poor patient outcome. Case reports of hypertension after small doses of droperidol have appeared, but no study comparing variation in blood pressure after droperidol and after saline has been published. And it is very evident, on placement of an arterial line, that patients with pheochromocytoma have wide variations in blood pressure. In our randomized studies, use of Innovar (which contains droperidol) was not associated with greater blood pressure fluctuations than the other three agents tested.[126] (Patients with pheochromocytoma tend to be particularly sensitive to pain; we often have much more difficulty than in normal cases placing arterial and venous lines in such patients.)

Because both are easy to administer, phenylephrine or dopamine is used for treatment of hypotension, whereas nitroprusside is preferable when hypertension occurs.[24] Phentolamine, previously a mainstay of intraoperative therapy, has too long a period of onset and duration of action. After the venous supply has been secured, and if the intravascular volume is normal (as measured by pulmonary artery wedge pressure), the blood pressure usually becomes normal. The author usually does not treat abnormal blood pressure in α-adrenergically blocked patients unless it is below 75/40 mm Hg; however, some patients become hypotensive after tumor removal and occasionally require a relatively large infusion of catecholamines. On rare occasions, patients remain hypertensive intraoperatively. Postoperatively, about 50 per cent of patients have hypertension for 1 to 3 days and have markedly elevated but declining plasma catecholamine levels. After 3 to 10 days, all but 25 per cent become normotensive. Catecholamine levels do not return to normal for 10 days; therefore, early measurement of urine concentrations of catecholamines is usually not helpful in ensuring that all catecholamine has been removed from tissue.

Because pheochromocytomas may be hereditary, it is important to screen other family members and advise them that, should they require surgery in the future, they should inform the anesthesiologist about the potential for such disease.

C. SUMMARY

A lack of controlled studies precludes definitive statements about anesthetic management of patients with pheochromocytoma. It is known that the symptoms of paroxysmal hypertension, sweating, and headache are highly suggestive of the diagnosis. It appears that mortality can be reduced by preoperative α-adrenergic receptor blockade with progressively increasing doses of a blocking agent for 10 days to 2 months for treatment of symptoms, by treatment of myocarditis, and by restoration of intravascular volume. In fact, the largest decrease in mortality of patients following pheochromocytoma resection occurred with the introduction of preoperative α-adrenergic receptor blockade. The author believes that knowledge on the part of the anesthetist about the pathophysiology of pheochromocytoma, preoperative patient preparation, and communication between surgeon and anesthetist are more important to patient outcome than is the choice of the anesthetic or muscle-relaxing agent.

VI. PANCREAS

A. PHYSIOLOGY

Pancreatic islets are composed of at least three cell types: alpha cells that secrete glucagon, beta cells that secrete insulin, and delta cells that contain secretory granules. Insulin is first synthesized as proinsulin, converted to insulin by proteolytic cleavage, and then packaged into granules within the beta cells. A large quantity of insulin, normally about 200 units, is stored in the pancreas, and continued synthesis is stimulated by glucose. There is basal, steady-state release of insulin from the beta granules and additional release that is controlled by stimuli external to the beta cell. Basal insulin secretion continues in the fasted state and is of key importance in the inhibition of catabolism and ketoacidosis. Glucose and fructose are the primary and most important regulators of insulin release. Other stimulators of insulin release include amino acids, glucagon, GI hormones (gastrin, secretin, cholecystokinin-pancreozymin, and enteroglucagon), and acetylcholine. Epinephrine and norepinephrine inhibit insulin release by stimulating α-adrenergic receptors, and they stimulate its release at β-adrenergic receptors.

A normal plasma glucose level requires adequate endogenous substrate for glucose production, normal enzymatic mechanisms capable of converting glycogen and other substrates to glucose, and normal hormonal modulation of gluconeogenesis.[132, 133] The rise in glucose levels after a meal causes release of insulin from beta cells in the pancreas. The magnitude of the insulin response is governed in part by the action of other GI hormones that are secreted following food intake. The action of these other hormones accounts for the greater rise in insulin levels after oral than after parenteral administration of glucose. Release of insulin can also be triggered by β-adrenergic stimuli that are believed to act by increasing cAMP levels. Insulin release is inhibited by α-adrenergic stimuli. The action of insulin tends to return the levels of plasma glucose to normal within 1 to 2 hours after completion of a meal.

When endogenous nutrients are not available, plasma glucose levels are maintained by hepatic glycogenolysis and then gluconeogenesis.[133] In these situations, insulin levels are low and glucagon, growth hormone, cortisol, and catecholamines play important roles in gluconeogenesis. Insulin is normally secreted from the pancreas in response to elevated levels of blood glucose as a prohormone (proinsulin). This hormone is rapidly cleaved into C-peptide and insulin in the portal vein.[134] Patients with insulinoma tend to have high levels of proinsulin (more than 20 per cent of total insulin) in plasma and levels of C-peptide that parallel insulin levels.

B. HYPOGLYCEMIA AND HYPERINSULINISM (ISLET CELL TUMORS OF THE PANCREAS)

Almost all of the signs and symptoms in patients with insulinomas are directly related to prolonged hypoglycemic states. The word "hypoglycemia" means different things to different people. Hypoglycemia is a clinical syndrome that may have a variety of causes, and that results in plasma glucose levels sufficiently low to promote secretion of catecholamines and to impair the function of the central nervous system.[133] The diagnosis of hypoglycemia requires the presence of three findings: (1) symptomatic hypoglycemia (confusion, abnormal behavior, amnesia for the episode of hypoglycemia), (2) a plasma glucose level in the hypoglycemic range (less than 40 mg/dl for females and less than 45 mg/dl for males), and (3) amelioration of symptoms when plasma glucose is restored to normal levels.

The two major classifications of hypoglycemia can be distinguished by the relationship of symptoms to meals: (1) reactive, that is, if the hypoglycemia occurs within 2 to 4 hours after ingestion of food and is associated primarily with adrenergic symptoms, and (2) fasting, that is, if the hypoglycemia occurs more than 6 hours after a meal, is precipitated by exercise, and is often associated with central nervous system symptoms. Insulinomas usually cause fasting hypoglycemia.[132–138]

Reactive hypoglycemia can be caused by alimentation, impaired glucose tolerance, or functional causes. *Alimentary hypoglycemia* is associated with low levels of plasma glucose 2 to 3 hours after ingestion of food by patients who have rapid gastric emptying, for example, after subtotal gastrectomy, vagotomy, or pyloroplasty. It is postulated that rapid gastric emptying and rapid absorption of glucose may result in excessive release of insulin, falling glucose levels, and reactive hypoglycemia. *Impaired glucose tolerance* resulting in hypoglycemia, an early symptom of diabetes, usually occurs four to five hours after ingestion of food. *Functional hypoglycemia*, on the other hand, usually occurs three to four hours after ingestion of food and is associated with adrenergic symptoms.[137]

Because the brain is extremely sensitive to glucose utilization, CNS effects are often manifest. Of 1067 cases reviewed by Stefanini and coworkers,[136] 982 (92 per cent) showed CNS symptoms that included visual disturbances, dizziness, confusion, epilepsy, lethargy, transient loss of consciousness, and coma. Perhaps because of these many CNS manifestations of insulinomas, many patients with these tumors have been misdiagnosed as suffering from psychiatric illness.[137]

Less frequent but nevertheless important manifestations of insulinomas involve the cardiovascular system. Stefanini and coworkers[136] reported that more than 10 per cent of the insulinoma patients had palpitations, tachycardia, or hypertension, or all three. These symptoms are probably related to catecholamine release secondary to hypoglycemia. About 9 per cent of the patients reviewed by Stefanini and colleagues had either severe hunger or gastrointestinal upset, including cramping, nausea, and vomiting. Other investigators have noted obesity or weight gain as a symptom.[143]

The symptoms of hypoglycemia due to insulinoma may occur at a particular time of day that is associated with a low blood glucose level, especially 6 hours or more after eating, after fasting for a time, or in the early morning.

Fasting hypoglycemia results from inadequate hepatic glucose production or from overutilization of glucose in the peripheral tissues. The causes of inadequate production of glucose during the fasting state may be hormone deficiencies, enzyme defects, inadequate substrate delivery, acquired liver disease, or drugs. Overutilization of glucose may occur in the presence of either elevated or appropriate insulin levels.

In order to define the diagnosis of insulinomas, Whipple introduced a triad of diagnostic criteria, which have been modified to include (1) symptoms of hypoglycemia brought on by fasting and exercise, (2) blood glucose levels, while symptoms are present, of less than 40 mg/dl in females and less than 45 mg/dl in males, and (3) relief of these symptoms by administration of glucose, either orally or IV. If an insulinoma is suspected and Whipple's triad is confirmed, several tests may be done with which one can differentiate insulinoma from other causes of hypoglycemia.

In recent years, because it has been possible to determine insulin levels as well as glucose levels, the diagnosis has been made with even more certainty.[133, 137] During a prolonged fast, in patients with insulinoma, hypoglycemia develops because of a relative underproduction of glucose by the liver rather than because of increased glucose utilization.[135] High levels of C-peptide and proinsulin levels greater than 20 per cent of total insulin measured in blood are also helpful.

Selective celiac angiography or MRI of the pancreatic region is often used for localization of tumors prior to surgical exploration. However, the usefulness of angiography has been questioned for several reasons. A tumor must be larger than approximately 1 cm to be seen with this method, but insulinomas often are smaller. Islet cell adenomas of the pancreas are sometimes multiple and may have various sizes.

Medical management of insulin-secreting tumors is often difficult, but it is essential before surgery and in cases in which surgery fails to remove all of the tumor(s).

Glucose administration increases blood glucose for a short time in patients with symptomatic hypoglycemia. Long-term dietary therapy is aimed at maintaining blood glucose with frequent high-protein, low-glucose meals. Administration of diazoxide, which suppresses insulin release from beta cells, and corticosteroids, which increase the blood glucose concentration by causing increased gluconeogenesis, is also useful for both benign and malignant islet cell tumors. Streptozotocin, an antibiotic that inhibits the biosynthesis of insulin, is used principally for metastatic islet cell carcinoma. In large doses, streptozotocin is cytotoxic to beta cells. It may be given intravenously or, in patients with liver metastases, via the celiac and hepatic arteries.[136]

Surgical treatment of insulin-secreting islet cell tumors involves their removal, usually from the pancreas, where they are most often located. In 13 per cent of cases more than one adenoma has been present. Most insulinomas are benign; approximately one third of those that are malignant are found at laparotomy to have metastasized to the liver.

C. ANESTHETIC CONSIDERATIONS FOR PATIENTS WITH HYPOGLYCEMIA

Most patients who come to surgery with the diagnosis of reactive or fasting hypoglycemia do not require special intraoperative care other than frequent assays of blood glucose levels and adequate infusion of dextrose. The variations in plasma glucose levels are exaggerated in patients with functional islet cell adenoma, and the frequency of procedures to remove insulinomas has increased.[138–140]

Perioperative management of patients with insulinomas focuses on the control of blood glucose levels so that symptomatic pathologic

hypo- or hyperglycemia is prevented. Intravenous infusion of 5 per cent dextrose is useful in preventing hypoglycemia during the night before surgery. Several approaches to intraoperative glucose management have been advocated. In the first approach, an attempt is made to avoid the deleterious effects of hypoglycemia by administering glucose throughout the procedure, with frequent monitoring of blood glucose levels.

A rise in blood glucose, which is sometimes quite striking, is thought to be evidence of tumor removal.[138–140] Therefore, two other methods of intraoperative glucose management have been designed not to mask this hyperglycemic rebound. In the first of these, glucose infusion is stopped approximately 2 hours before surgery. Blood glucose is monitored frequently, but no glucose is administered unless the level drops below a certain value, usually below 40 to 50 mg/dl. A bolus of glucose is then given that is calculated to return the level in blood to more than 50 mg/dl, and constant glucose infusion is also started so that the blood glucose level is maintained at more than 50 mg/dl.

The second method makes use of the "artificial beta cell," or feedback-controlled dextrose infusion, during surgery. The artificial beta cell can be used either solely for monitoring of glucose or for monitoring and administering both glucose and insulin. A printout of the blood glucose level, amount of glucose infused, and amount of insulin infused can be obtained. This allows for frequent (every 60 seconds) determinations of the glucose level, so that any decrease in glucose requirement (the hyperglycemia response) can be observed.

Administration of insulin to hyperglycemic patients during and after surgery is aimed at short-term control of glucose levels. Intraoperatively, the author treats blood glucose levels above 300 to 400 mg/dl by administering regular insulin IV. Frequent monitoring of glucose is continued, and more insulin is given every 60 to 90 minutes if the hyperglycemia persists. Postoperatively, hyperglycemia, especially ketosis, is also treated with insulin. Blood glucose levels of 250 to 400 mg/dl may be treated by subcutaneous administration of insulin while blood glucose is monitored at fairly frequent intervals. Blood glucose levels higher than this are treated more aggressively, not with additional insulin (10 units per 70 kg maximum per hour), but with more frequent glucose monitoring, IV administration of insulin (either as a bolus or as a continuous infusion), and repletion of fluid, potassium, and phosphate.

Blood glucose also is monitored in the postoperative period because hyperglycemia and its complications can occur. Among 1012 patients reviewed by Stefanini and coworkers,[136] 101 (10 per cent) were described as having diabetes postoperatively.

Hyperglycemic rebound has been used as a diagnostic tool by several authors but may not be as effective as was once thought. Muir and coworkers[138] reviewed 39 patients who underwent surgery for insulinoma. After tumor removal, all patients but one had an increase in plasma glucose concentration. That patient subsequently proved to be cured, whereas a patient who had a hyperglycemic response was later shown not to be cured. Furthermore, in six patients whose blood glucose increased after tumor resection, the rise was less sharp than that prior to tumor removal.

Whether the perioperative control of glucose levels is aimed at euglycemia, with either glucose infusion or an artificial beta cell, or at slight hypoglycemia, one should try to keep the blood glucose level higher than the level at which the patient becomes symptomatic while awake. This aim is achieved more easily with euglycemic methods. Furthermore, although a hyperglycemic response is useful diagnostically when it occurs, it is not a substitute for careful exploration of the pancreas. Also, CPD (citrate-phosphate-dextrose preservative) or ACD blood contains dextrose, which may create a rise in blood glucose that could be confused with a hyperglycemic response.

1. Summary

The signs and symptoms of insulinomas are the signs and symptoms of hypoglycemia, which have predominantly CNS manifestations. The symptoms of hyperglycemia and hypoglycemia are masked by general anesthesia, but their deleterious systemic effects are not prevented. It is important to monitor blood glucose levels frequently in the perioperative period because either hyperglycemia or hypoglycemia may develop. Hypoglycemia is more dangerous, particularly because of its effects on the CNS. Hyperglycemia is deleterious because hyperosmolar coma and ketoacidosis may occur. A hyperglycemic response does not invariably occur after successful tumor resection, nor is it always diagnostic of cure. When hyperglycemia does occur postoperatively, it is treated with insulin until euglycemic levels are restored.

D. DIABETES MELLITUS

Although one thinks about diabetes in relation to glucose, recent data indicate that the end-organ disease that diabetes creates or with which it is associated should also be considered. This accent on problems other than hyperglycemia may seem strange at a time when lifelong tight control of blood glucose is being debated. The concern for the end-organ manifestations of diabetes originates in recent epidemiologic studies of surgical mortality.

Surgical mortality rates for the diabetic population are on average five times higher than those for the nondiabetic population.[141-143] However, in epidemiologic studies in which diabetes itself was segregated from the complications of diabetes (including cardiac and vascular disease) and old age, this finding was questioned.[142, 144, 146] Similarly, if diabetics undergoing major vascular surgery are compared with nondiabetics matched for type of surgery, age, sex, weight, and complicating diseases, there is no difference in the mortality rate or the number of postoperative complications.[144]

Diabetes mellitus is a heterogeneous group of disorders—present in more than 5 per cent of the population of developed countries—that have the common feature of a relative or absolute deficiency of insulin. Diabetes can be divided into two very different diseases, which share end-organ abnormalities.[147-154] Type I diabetes is associated with autoimmune diseases and has a concordance rate of 40 to 50 per cent (that is, if one of a pair of monozygotic twins has diabetes, the likelihood that the other twin also will have it is 40 to 50 per cent). In type I the patient is insulin deficient, has inadequate basal and stimulated insulin secretion, and is prone to ketoacidosis if exogenous insulin is withheld. Treatment with immunolytic agents once a viral infection has occurred appears to decrease the rate of development of type I diabetes.[155] For type II (non–insulin-dependent) diabetes, the concordance rate is 100 per cent (that is, the genetic material is both necessary and sufficient for the development of type II diabetes). Type II patients are not prone to develop ketoacidosis in the absence of insulin, and they have peripheral insulin resistance.

Type I and type II diabetes differ in other ways as well. Type I formerly was termed "juvenile-onset diabetes." The term may be a misnomer, because many older patients also fall into the same category. Most children and adolescents who are diabetic have type I diabetes; that is, they require insulin to prevent ketoacidosis. The maturity-onset diabetic is usually older and tends to be overweight; however, a younger person can develop type II and an older person type I diabetes.

Type II diabetics tend to be elderly, overweight, relatively resistant to ketoacidosis, and prone to the development of a hyperglycemic, hyperosmolar, nonketotic state. Plasma insulin levels are normal or elevated but are low relative to the level of blood glucose.[148]

Currently, therapy for type II diabetes usually begins with dietary management alone but may progress to oral hypoglycemic medications that act by stimulating release of insulin by pancreatic beta cells. The most common orally administered drugs are tolazamide (Tolinase) and tolbutamine (Orinase). The newer sulfonylureas include glyburide (Micronase) and glipizide (Glucotrol); these have a longer blood glucose–lowering effect, which persists for 24 hours or more. Oral hypoglycemic drugs may produce hypoglycemia for as long as 50 hours after intake (chlorpropamide [Diabinese] has the longest half-life). Occasionally, physicians advocating tight control of blood sugar levels will give insulin to type II diabetic patients twice a day or even more frequently.

Acute complications for the diabetic patient include hypoglycemia, diabetic ketoacidosis, and hyperglycemic, hyperosmolar, nonketotic coma. Diabetic patients also are subject to a series of long-term complications from cataracts, retinopathy, neuropathy, nephropathy, and angiopathy that lead to considerable morbidity and premature mortality. Many of these complications bring the diabetic patient to surgery. In fact, over 50 per cent of all diabetics come to surgery sometime in their disease.[156]

Hyperglcyemic, hyperosmolar, nonketotic diabetic coma[157] is characterized by elevated serum osmolality (over 330 mOsm/L) and an elevated blood glucose level (over 600 mg/dl) without acidosis. Blood glucose level, in milligrams per deciliter, divided by 18 yields the contribution of glucose to osmolality. Trauma or infection in type II diabetes patients usually leads to this state rather than to ketoacidosis.[157] Hyperglycemia induces marked osmotic diuresis and dehydration, enhancing the hyperosmolar state; this can result in failure to emerge from anesthesia and persistent coma. Serum electrolytes are often normal, although a widened anion gap (Na^+ [HCO_3] − [Cl^-] $\geq$ 16) may point to lactic acidosis or a uremic state.

The evidence that hyperglycemia itself accelerates complications or that tight control of blood sugar levels decreases the rate of progression of microangiopathic disease is now definitive. Glucose itself may be toxic because high levels can promote nonenzymatic glycosylation reactions, leading to formation of abnormal proteins that may decrease elastance—responsible for the stiff joint syndrome (and fixation of the atlantooccipital joint, making intubation difficult)—and wound-healing tensile strength. Glucose elevations may increase production of macroglobulins by the liver, increasing blood viscosity, and promote intracellular swelling by favoring production of nondiffusable, large molecules (like sorbitol). Newer drug therapies (such as aldose reductase inhibitors) aim to decrease intracellular swelling by inhibiting formation of such large molecules. Glucose can also inhibit the phagocytic function.

Glycemia disrupts autoregulation.[152–164] Glucose-induced vasodilatation prevents target organs from protecting against increases in systemic blood pressure. Glycosylated hemoglobin of 8.1 per cent is the threshold above which risk of microalbuminuria increases logarithmically. A person with type I diabetes with greater than 29 mg per day of microalbuminuria has an 80 per cent chance of developing renal insufficiency. The threshold for glycemic toxicity is different for different vascular beds. The threshold for retinopathy is a glycosylated hemoglobin value of 8.5 to 9.0 per cent (12.5 mmol/L or 225 mg/dl); for cardiovascular disease, an average blood glucose value of 5.4 mmol/L (96 mg/dl). Thus, different degrees of hyperglycemia may be required before different vascular beds are damaged, or certain degrees of glycemia are associated with other risk factors for vascular disease. Another view is that perhaps severe hyperglycemia and microalbuminuria are simply concomitant effects of a common underlying cause. Diabetics who develop microalbuminuria are more resistant to insulin;

insulin resistance is associated with microalbuminuria in first-degree relatives of patients with type II diabetes; and persons with normoglycemia who subsequently develop clinical diabetes have atherogenic risks before onset of disease.

Because of the known glucotoxicities, how tightly blood sugar levels should routinely be controlled was once controversial. It is now known that chronic tight control is a benefit. The controversy centers on whether attempts to attain normal blood sugar levels or levels that result in glycosylated hemoglobin values of less than 8.1 per cent in diabetic patients are of greater benefit than risk.

Perioperative management of the diabetic patient may affect surgical outcome. Physicians who advocate tight control of blood glucose levels point to the evidence of increased wound healing tensile strength and decreased wound infections in animal models of (type I) diabetes under tight control. Insulin is necessary in the early stages of the inflammatory response but seems to have no effect on collagen formation after the first 10 days. Healing epithelial wounds exhibit minimal leukocyte infiltration and, unlike deep wounds, are not dependent on collagen synthesis for the integrity of the tissue. Thus, simple epithelial repair is not inhibited in the diabetes patient, whereas the repair of deeper wounds is impaired with respect to collagen formation and defense against bacterial growth.

Infections account for two thirds of postoperative complications and about 20 per cent of perioperative deaths in diabetic patients. Experimental data suggest many factors that may make diabetics vulnerable to infection. Many alterations in leukocyte function have been demonstrated in hyperglycemic diabetics, including decreased chemotaxis and impaired phagocytic activity of granulocytes, as well as reduced intracellular killing of pneumococci and staphylococci. When diabetic patients are treated aggressively and blood glucose levels are maintained below 250 mg/dl (13.7 mmol/L), the phagocytic function of granulocytes is improved and intracellular killing of bacteria is restored to nearly normal levels. It has been thought that diabetic patients experience more infections in clean wounds than do nondiabetics. In a review of 23,649 surgical patients, the rate of wound infection in clean incisions was found to be 10.7 per cent for diabetics, as compared with 1.8 per cent for nondiabetics; however, when age is accounted for, the difference in the incidence of wound infection in diabetic and nondiabetic surgical patients is not statistically significant.

Recent information on the relationship between blood glucose and neurologic recovery after a global ischemic event may have important implications for perioperative diabetes management. In a study of 430 consecutive patients resuscitated after out-of-hospital cardiac arrest, mean blood glucose levels were found to be higher in patients who never awakened (341 ± 13 mg/dl) than in those who did (262 ± 7 mg/dl). Among patients who awakened, those with persistent neurologic deficits had higher mean glucose levels (286 ± 15 mg/dl) than did those without deficits (251 ± 7 mg/dl). These results are consistent with the finding that hyperglycemia during a stroke is associated with poorer short- and long-term neurologic outcomes. The possibility that blood glucose is a determinant of brain damage following global ischemia is supported by studies of global and focal CNS ischemia. Data are accumulating that suggest that a major effect of glycemia is to disrupt autoregulation, making arteries and arterioles (macro- and microvessels) vulnerable to the force disruption caused by increased blood pressure.[157–163] Glycemia appears to disrupt autoregulation by enhancing activation of protein kinase C.[152, 164] This activation may occur in anyone whose glucose level exceeds 96 mg/dl (5.7 mmol/L) and is a major factor in arterial degeneration (aging). Before long, we may all want to tightly control our glucose levels, not only perioperatively but throughout our lives. Until better data are available, most recommend that the diabetic patient about to undergo surgery in which hypotension or reduced cerebral flow may occur should have a blood glucose level below 225 mg/dl during the period of cerebral ischemia. Two other special situations can also affect how tightly one should manage the patient's glucose level: (1) surgery requiring cardiopulmonary bypass and (2) surgery in pregnant patients or in patients already suffering from diabetic ketoacidosis.

E. PERIOPERATIVE CONSIDERATIONS FOR PATIENTS WITH DIABETES

Before surgery, assessment and optimization of treatment of the potential end-organ effects of diabetes are at least as important as an assessment of the diabetic's current overall metabolic status. Special emphasis should be placed on history; autonomic, cardiovascular, renal, and drug therapy; and the status of skin care.[141-146, 165, 166] Basic laboratory examinations might include fasting blood sugar, blood urea nitrogen or creatinine, and ECG.

Patients with severe diabetic autonomic neuropathy are at increased risk for gastroparesis and consequent aspiration and for intraoperative and postoperative cardiorespiratory arrest. Recent data indicate that diabetics who exhibit signs of autonomic neuropathy, such as early satiety, lack of sweating, lack of pulse rate change with inspiration or orthostatic maneuvers, and impotence, have a very high incidence both of painless myocardial ischemia and gastroparesis.[143, 166-169]

Measuring the degree of sinus arrhythmia or beat-to-beat variability provides a simple, accurate test for significant autonomic neuropathy. The difference between maximum and minimum heart rate on deep inspiration, normally 15 beats per minute, was found to be five or less in all diabetic patients who previously sustained cardiorespiratory arrest.[166]

Other characteristics of patients with autonomic neuropathy include postural hypotension with a drop of more than 30 mm Hg, resting tachycardia, nocturnal diarrhea, and dense peripheral neuropathy. Diabetics with significant autonomic neuropathy may have impaired respiratory responses to hypoxia and are particularly susceptible to the action of drugs that have depressant effects. Such patients may warrant very close, continuous cardiac and respiratory monitoring for 12 to 24 hours postoperatively, although such logical treatment has not yet been tested in a rigorous, controlled trial.

1. Approach to Perioperative Management

There may be a relationship between blood glucose and neurologic recovery after a global ischemic nervous system event that has important implications for perioperative diabetic management.[169] In a study of 430 consecutive patients resuscitated after out-of-hospital cardiac arrest, mean blood glucose levels were found to be higher in patients who never awakened (341 ± 13 mg/dl) than in those who did (262 ± 7 mg/dl).[169] Among patients who awakened, those with persistent neurologic deficits had higher mean glucose levels (286 ± 15 mg/dl) than those without deficits (251 ± 7 mg/dl). These results are consistent with the finding in experimental models that hyperglycemia is associated with poorer short- and long-term neurologic outcomes.[161] If high glucose levels predispose to poor outcomes, the mechanism for the association of hyperglycemia with ischemic brain damage is not known. Until better data are available, there will be those who argue that the diabetic patient about to undergo surgery in which hypotension or reduced cerebral flow may occur should have a blood glucose level below 225 mg/dl during a period of cerebral ischemia; however, the risk of undetected hypoglycemia is much greater during surgery than while the patient is awake, since the normal physiologic responses are impaired and masked. Only frequent intraoperative monitoring of glucose levels can protect the patient. A popular approach, continuous insulin infusion for strict control of blood sugar during major surgery, has been highly recommended in some publications.[170, 171] This method does result in lower blood glucose levels but carries the risk of significant hypoglycemia in patients receiving 2 or more units of insulin per hour.

There are various methods of managing diabetes during surgery. The key to success includes individualized decision making for each patient, with the frequency of intraoperative monitoring appropriate to the tightness of control desired and with tailoring of insulin therapy to periodically measured blood glucose levels. The basic objectives of the perioperative management of diabetics include:

1. Achieving good control of blood glucose level with correction of any acid/base, fluid, or electrolyte abnormalities prior to surgery.

2. Providing an adequate amount of carbohydrate to inhibit catabolic proteolysis, lipolysis, and ketosis (this requires an average of 100 to 150 g of glucose per day for a 70-kg person during the operative period).

3. Providing insulin adequate to prevent hyperglycemia, glycosuria, and ketoacidosis while also avoiding hypoglycemia.

4. Keeping in mind problems associated with diabetes that require special perioperative attention or predispose to iatrogenic complications.

5. Remembering that the tighter the de-

sired control of blood glucose, the more frequently blood glucose must be measured.

Non–Insulin-Dependent Diabetes. Insulin is usually not required for minor surgery on patients whose diabetes is controlled by diet or small doses of oral agents. Short-acting oral hypoglycemic agents are omitted on the day of surgery, and long-acting agents are discontinued 2 days before surgery. Insulin may be required during and after surgery for major thoracic or abdominal operations or during prolonged parenteral alimentation. Given the potential of developing insulin allergy with intermittent insulin exposure, some physicians advocate the use of human insulin in this perioperative setting.

Insulin-Dependent Diabetes and Minor Surgery. There are many methods for managing insulin-dependent diabetics during surgery, but few comparisons of efficacy and safety have been published. Regular insulin given subcutaneously begins to act within 30 minutes, reaches peak effect in 2 to 4 hours, and has a duration of action of 6 to 8 hours. Intermediate-acting insulin (NPH or Lente) given subcutaneously begins to act within 100 to 120 minutes, reaches a peak effect in 6 to 12 hours, and has an 18- to 24-hour duration of action. The conventional preoperative therapy for the well-controlled, fasting diabetic consists of administration of half of the dose of insulin the patient usually takes. This insulin is given subcutaneously on the morning of surgery with a 5 per cent dextrose infusion at 100 to 150 ml per hour. Regular insulin is then given as a supplement to the intermediate-acting insulin when the need is indicated by blood glucose levels.[172]

Insulin-Dependent Diabetes and Major Surgery. Continuous intravenous insulin therapy similar to that used in the treatment of ketoacidosis is often administered to "brittle diabetics" during major surgery. Several methods of IV insulin therapy have been studied. Taitelman and coworkers compared constant IV insulin infusion with conventional subcutaneous administration of insulin in patients before orthopedic procedures.[171] They used 500 ml per hour of 5 per cent dextrose for the first hour, followed by 125 ml per hour plus 1 or 2 units per hour of regular insulin (0.16 or 0.32 unit of insulin per gram of infused glucose) in one group of patients. They compared the outcome with that for a group of patients who were given two thirds of their daily maintenance dose

of insulin subcutaneously immediately before surgery. The two methods resulted in equivalent diabetic control. At 2 units per hour, or 0.32 unit of insulin per gram of infused glucose, euglycemic levels were more readily achieved, but hypoglycemia requiring treatment occurred in several patients.

2. Guidelines for Continuous Intravenous Insulin Administration

The amounts of insulin and glucose that are administered need to be correlated. There is some argument about whether 5 or 10 per cent dextrose should be used. Infusion of 10 per cent dextrose provides more calories, thus favoring anabolism, but may lead to venous irritation and thrombosis. Concentrations of infused insulin vary from 0.2 to 0.4 units per gram of glucose (equal to 1 to 2 units/100 ml 5 per cent dextrose in water) under normal conditions. Higher levels of insulin may be required under certain circumstances, for example, in patients with liver disease, marked obesity, or severe infection, and in patients undergoing steroid therapy or coronary artery bypass surgery. Cessation of IV insulin may rapidly cause hyperglycemia, as insulin has a serum half-life of only 4 minutes and a biological half-life of 20 minutes. Since it may be necessary to adjust the amount of insulin or glucose independently, these solutions should be kept in separate bottles, with one line "piggy-backed" into the other. Separation of the IV line that contains the insulin and dextrose from all other IV fluids (these other IV fluids should contain no dextrose or lactate) reduces the risk of hypoglycemia or excessive hyperglycemia (Table 8–6).

Renal Transplant Surgery. The effectiveness of continuous IV administration of insulin has been compared to that of subcutaneous insulin in diabetics undergoing renal transplant surgery.[170] In this comparison, patients on IV insulin received 5 per cent dextrose in water, with the hourly dose of insulin controlled by an infusion pump according to the following equation:

Hourly insulin (U) = Plasma glucose value/100

(divided by 150 instead of 100 if the patient is thin or is not taking corticosteroids). Low-dose continuous insulin infusion maintained blood glucose levels at between 100 and 200

TABLE 8–6

Intravenous Insulin Regimen for "Brittle" Diabetics Undergoing Major Surgery

1. Obtain plasma glucose and potassium STAT on morning of surgery.
2. Begin IV infusion of 5% dextrose in water at 100–150 ml/hr and maintain dextrose infusion until the patient is taking oral nutrition.
3. "Piggy-back" to above an IV infusion of 50 units regular insulin in 500 ml 0.9% normal saline by using infusion pump; flush 60 ml to saturate insulin-binding sites of tubing.
4. Set infusion rate at Insulin (U/hr) =

$$\frac{\text{Last plasma glucose mg/dl}}{150}$$

   (Divide by 100 instead of 150 if patient is on steroids, is markedly obese, or has infection).
5. Determine glucose level every 2–3 hours; make appropriate insulin adjustments to obtain plasma glucose level of 80–150 mg/dl.

mg/dl and was more effective than endogenous control, on the average, in nondiabetics. Conventional subcutaneous insulin therapy was found to be grossly inadequate for maintenance of acceptable glucose levels in diabetic patients undergoing renal transplantation.

Cardiopulmonary Bypass Operations. For diabetics undergoing cardiopulmonary bypass surgery, the closed-loop "artificial pancreas" has been used in some studies for aggressive control of blood glucose level. Elliott and colleagues[167] compared the use of Biostator, a closed-loop glucose-controlled system for infusion of insulin during open-heart surgery, with simpler, open-loop, constant intravenous administration of insulin. A closed loop is characterized by automatic sensing and feedback control of insulin and glucose infusion. One intravenous line samples blood glucose levels by withdrawing blood at a rate of 1 ml per minute, while insulin or glucose is infused through the other intravenous line as dictated by this measurement. An open-loop requires physician-directed regulation of insulin and glucose infusion. With both methods, no glucose infusion was given during the procedure, and blood glucose was maintained at between 100 and 180 mg/ml throughout surgery. Insulin requirements increased during some phases of the operation, including cardiopulmonary bypass, transfusion of acid-citrate-dextrose stored blood, the rewarming phase, and

injection of inotropic agents. A peak infusion rate of 20 units per hour was required during rewarming.

Mechanical problems were encountered postoperatively with the use of the Biostator. These included difficulties caused by peripheral vasoconstriction, movement of the patient, and nursing procedures that resulted in interruptions in feedback and led to elevations in blood glucose. Open-loop systems currently remain superior to closed-loop techniques because of cost and mechanical problems.[174, 175]

3. Emergency Surgery and Ketoacidosis

Many diabetics who need emergency surgery for trauma or infection have significant metabolic decompensation, including ketoacidosis.[176] Often little time is available for stabilization of the patient, but even a few hours may be sufficient for correction of fluid and electrolyte disturbances that are potentially life threatening. It is futile to delay surgery in an attempt to eliminate ketoacidosis completely if the underlying surgical condition will lead to further metabolic deterioration. The likelihood of intraoperative cardiac dysrhythmias and hypotension resulting from ketoacidosis will be reduced if volume depletion and hypokalemia are at least partially treated.

Insulin therapy is initiated with a 10-unit intravenous bolus of regular insulin, which is followed by continuous insulin infusion. The actual amount of insulin administered is less important than regular monitoring of glucose, potassium, and pH. Because the number of insulin-binding sites is limited, the maximum rate of glucose decline is fairly constant, averaging 75 to 100 mg/dl per hour, regardless of the insulin dose.[150, 177] During the first 1 to 2 hours of fluid resuscitation, the glucose level may fall more precipitously. When the serum glucose reaches 250 mg/dl, the author usually adds 5 per cent dextrose to the intravenous fluid.

The volume of fluid required for therapy varies with overall deficits; it ranges from 3 to 5 L, but it can be as high as 10 L. Despite losses of water in excess of losses of solute, sodium levels are generally normal or reduced. Factitious hyponatremia caused by hyperglycemia or hypertriglyceridemia may result in this seeming contradiction. The plasma sodium concentration decreases by about 1.6 mEq/L for every 100 mg/dl increase in plasma glucose above normal. Initially, normal saline is infused at the rate of 250 to 1000 ml per hour, depending on the degree of volume depletion and on the cardiac status. Some measure of left ventricular volume should be monitored in diabetics who have a history of myocardial dysfunction. About one third of the estimated fluid deficit is corrected in the first 6 to 8 hours, and the remaining two thirds over the next 24 hours.

The degree of acidosis is determined by measurement of arterial blood gases and an increased anion gap [$Na^+ - (Cl^- + HCO_3^-)$]. Acidosis with an increased anion gap (at least 16 mEq/L) in an acutely ill diabetic may be caused by ketones in ketoacidosis, lactic acid in lactic acidosis, increased organic acids from renal insufficiency, or all three. In ketoacidosis, the plasma levels of acetoacetate, β-hydroxybutyrate, and acetone are increased. Plasma and urinary ketones are measured semiquantitatively with the Ketostix and Acetest tablets. The role of bicarbonate therapy in diabetic ketoacidosis is controversial. Myocardial function and respiration are known to be depressed at a blood pH below 7.0 to 7.10; yet rapid correction of acidosis with bicarbonate therapy may result in alterations in central nervous system function and structure. The alterations may be caused by (1) paradoxical development of CSF and CNS acidosis resulting from rapid conversion of bicarbonate to carbon dioxide and diffusion of the acid across the blood–brain barrier, (2) altered CNS oxygenation with decreased cerebral blood flow, and (3) development of unfavorable osmotic gradients. After treatment with fluids and insulin, β-hydroxybutyrate levels decrease rapidly, whereas acetoacetate levels may remain stable or even increase before declining. Plasma acetone levels remain elevated for 24 to 42 hours, long after blood glucose, β-hydroxybutyrate, and acetoacetate levels have returned to normal; the result is continuing ketonuria.[150] Persistent ketosis, with a serum bicarbonate level of less than 20 mEq/L in the presence of a normal glucose level, represents a continued need for intracellular glucose and insulin for reversal of lipolysis.

The most important electrolyte disturbance in diabetic ketoacidosis is depletion of total body potassium. The deficits range from 3 mEq/kg body weight up to 10 mEq/kg. Rapid declines in serum potassium level occur, reaching a nadir within 2 to 4 hours after the start of intravenous insulin administration. Aggressive replacement therapy may be required. The potassium administered moves into the intracellular space with insulin as the acidosis is corrected. Potassium is also excreted in the urine with the increased delivery of sodium to the distal renal tubules that accompanies volume expansion. Phosphorus deficiency in ketoacidosis caused by tissue catabolism, impaired cellular uptake, and increased urinary losses may result in significant muscular weakness and organ dysfunction. The average phosphorus deficit is approximately 1 mmol/kg body weight. Replacement may be needed if the plasma concentration falls below 1.0 mg/dl.[150]

4. Summary

Management of the diabetic surgical patient includes careful preoperative assessment, prevention of infection,[177, 178] frequent glucose and electrolyte monitoring, and above all, administration of adequate amounts of insulin and glucose based on that monitoring. The sine qua non of tight control is frequent determination of blood glucose levels. With good control of glucose levels, many of the metabolic problems associated with surgery in diabetics can be prevented or alleviated. However, such tight control may not be worth the risk incurred. Epidemiologic evidence indicates that the major risk factor for the diabetic is not the blood glucose level, but the end-organ effects of diabetes. Autonomic neuropathy often is associated with painless myocardial ischemia and gastroparesis. These problems, as well as myocardial and renal dysfunction, may need special perioperative treatment or monitoring. Whether or not tight control of blood glucose levels is warranted remains to be determined in future studies. As with most of the other endocrinopathies dealt with in this chapter, it is not the endocrinopathy per se that is associated with morbidity but its cardiovascular and/ or autonomic end-organ effects that appear crucial to patient outcome. Little is known about how the choice of anesthetic or anesthetic adjuvant drug(s) affects outcome;[179–197] consequently, attention might be directed to the cardiovascular and/or autonomic end-organ effects to optimize outcome.

Portions of this chapter have been revised from Pender, J.W., and Basso, L.V.: Diseases of the endocrine system. *In* Katz, J., Benumof, J., and Kadis, L.: Anesthesia and Uncommon Diseases, 2nd ed. Philadelphia, W.B. Saunders, 1981, pp. 155–220. Other portions have been adapted from Roizen, M.F. (ed.): Anesthesia for patients with endocrine disease. Anesthesiol. Clin. North Am. 5(2):245–548, 1987.

REFERENCES

1. Hensel P, Roizen MF: Patients with disorders of parathyroid function. Anesthesiol Clin North Am 5:287, 1987.
2. Aurbach GD, Marx SJ, Spiegel AM: Parathyroid hormone, calcitonin, and the calciferols. *In* Wilson JD, Foster DW (eds): Williams' Textbook of Endocrinology, ed 8. Philadelphia, WB Saunders, 1992, p. 8.
3. Thompson DL, Frame B: Involutional osteopenia: Current concepts. Ann Intern Med 85:789, 1976.
4. Parsons JA, Zanelli JM, Gray D, et al: Double isotope estimates of intestinal calcium absorption in rats; Enhancement by parathyroid hormone and 1,25 dihydroxycholecalciferol. Calcif Tissues Res 22(Suppl):127, 1977.
5. NIH conference. Diagnosis and management of asymptomatic primary hyperparathyroidism: Consensus development conference statement. Ann Intern Med 114:593, 1991.
6. Crocker EF, Jellins J, Freund J: Parathyroid lesions localized by radionuclide subtraction and ultrasound. Radiology 130:215, 1979.
7. Purnell DC, et al: Hyperparathyroidism due to single gland enlargement. Arch Surg 112:369, 1977.
8. Brennan MF, et al: Recurrent hyperparathyroidism from an autotransplanted parathyroid adenoma. N Engl J Med 299:1057, 1978.
9. Deftos LJ, Parthemore JG, Stabile BE: Management of primary hyperparathyroidism. Annu Rev Med 44:19, 1993.
10. Bilezikian JP: Clinical review 51: Management of hypercalcemia. J Clin Endocrinol Metab 77:1445, 1993.
11. Nussbaum SR: Pathophysiology and management of severe hypercalcemia. Endocrinol Metab Clin North Am 22:343, 1993.
12. Yu PNG: The electrocardiographic changes associated with hypercalcemia and hypocalcemia. Am J Med Sci 224:413, 1952.
13. O'Connor LR, Wheeler WS, Bethune JE: Effect of hypophosphatemia on myocardial performance in man. N Engl J Med 297:901, 1977.
14. Braunfeld M: Hypercalcemia. *In* Roizen MF, Fleisher LA (eds): Essence of Anesthesia Practice. Philadelphia, WB Saunders, 1997, p. 167.
15. Nahrwold ML, Mantha S: Hyperparathyroidism. *In* Roizen MF, Fleisher LA (eds): Essence of Anesthesia Practice. Philadelphia, WB Saunders, 1997, p. 174.
16. Anast CS, Mohs JM, Kaplan SL, et al: Evidence for parathyroid failure in magnesium deficiency. Science 177:606, 1972.
17. Zaloga GP, Chernow B: Hypocalcemia in critical illness. JAMA 256:1924, 1986.
18. Rude RK: Magnesium metabolism and deficiency. Endocrinol Metab Clin North Am 22:377, 1993.
19. Knochel JP: The pathophysiology and clinical characteristics of severe hypophosphatemia. Arch Intern Med 137:203, 1977.
20. Schneider AB, Sherwood LM: Calcium homeostasis and the pathogenesis and management of hypercalcemic disorders. Metabolism 23:975, 1974.
21. Rumancik WM, Denlinger JK, Nahrwold ML, et al: The QT interval and serum ionized calcium. JAMA 240:366, 1978.
22. Benson DW: Anesthesia for thyroid surgery. Semin Anesth 3:168, 1984.
23. Roizen MF, Hensel P, Lichtor JL, et al: Patients with disorders of thyroid function. Anesthesiol Clin North Am 5:277, 1987.
24. Roizen MF: Anesthetic implications of concurrent diseases. *In* Miller RD (ed): Anesthesia, Vol. 1. ed 4. New York, Churchill Livingstone, 1994, pp. 903–1014.
25. Murkin JM: Anesthesia and hypothyroidism: A review of thyroxine physiology, pharmacology, and anesthetic implications. Anesth Analg 61:371, 1982.
26. Larsen PR, Ingbar SH: The thyroid gland. *In* Wilson JD, Foster DW (eds): Williams' Textbook of Endocrinology, ed 8. Philadelphia, WB Saunders, 1992, pp. 414–445.
27. Chopra IJ: Reciprocal changes in serum concentrations of reverse T_3 and T_4 in systemic illness. J Clin Endocrinol Metab 41:1043, 1975.
28. Williams LT, Lefkowitz RJ, Watanabe AM, et al: Thyroid hormone regulation of β-adrenergic receptor number. J Biol Chem 252:2787, 1977.
29. Larsen PR, Alexander NM, Chopra IJ, et al: Revised nomenclature for tests of thyroid hormones and thyroid-related proteins in serum. J Clin Endocrinol Metab 64:1089, 1987.
30. Roizen MF: Hyperthyroidism. *In* Roizen MF, Fleisher LA (eds): Essence of Anesthesia Practice. Philadelphia, WB Saunders, 1997, p. 177.
31. Amino N, Morik H, Iwatani Y, et al: High prevalence of transient postpartum thyrotoxicosis and hypothyroidism. N Engl J Med 306:849, 1982.
32. Channick BJ, Adlin EV, Marks AD, et al: Hyperthyroidism and mitral-valve prolapse. N Engl J Med 305:497, 1981.
33. Davis PJ, Davis FB: Hyperthyroidism in patients over the age of 60 years. Clinical features in 85 patients. Medicine 53:161, 1974.
34. Forfar JC, Miller HC, Toft AD: Occult thyrotoxicosis: A correctable cause of "idiopathic" atrial fibrillation. Am J Cardiol 44:9, 1979.
35. Toft AD, Irvine WJ, Sinclair I, et al: Thyroid function after surgical treatment of thyrotoxicosis: A report of 100 cases treated with propranolol before operation. N Engl J Med 298:643, 1978.
36. Symons G: Thyroid heart disease. Br Heart J 41:257, 1979.
37. Forfar JC, Muir AL, Sawers SA, et al: Abnormal left ventricular function in hyperthyroidism. Evidence for a possible reversible cardiomyopathy. N Engl J Med 307:1165, 1982.
38. Eriksson M, Rubenfeld S, Garber AJ, et al: Propranolol does not prevent thyroid storm. N Engl J Med 296:263, 1977.
39. Trench AJ, et al: Propranolol in thyrotoxicosis. Cardiovascular changes during thyroidectomy in patients pretreated with propranolol. Anaesthesia 33:535, 1978.
40. Roizen MF, Becker CE: Thyroid storm: A review of cases at the University of California, San Francisco. Calif Med 115:5, 1971.

41. Burch HB, Wartofsky L: Life-threatening thyrotoxicosis. Thyroid storm. Endocrinol Metab Clin North Am 22:263, 1993.
42. Zuckerman R: Pregnant surgical patient. *In* Roizen MF, Fleisher LA (eds): Essence of Anesthesia Practice. Philadelphia, WB Saunders, 1997, p. 429.
43. Sawin CT, Castelli WP, Hershman JM, et al: The aging thyroid. Thyroid deficiency in the Framingham Study. Arch Intern Med 145:1386, 1985.
44. Butterworth J: Hyporthyroidism. *In* Roizen MF, Fleisher LA (eds): Essence of Anesthesia Practice. Philadelphia, WB Saunders, 1997, p. 185.
45. Singer PA: Thyroiditis. Acute, subacute, and chronic. Med Clin North Am 75:61, 1991.
46. Weinberg AD, Brennan MD, Gorman CA, et al: Outcome of anesthesia and surgery in hypothyroid patients. Arch Intern Med 143:893, 1983.
47. Bough EW, Crowley WF, Ridgway EC, et al: Myocardial function in hypothyroidism. Relation to disease severity and response to treatment. Arch Intern Med 138:1476, 1978.
48. Zwillich CW, Pierson DJ, Hofeldt FD, et al: Ventilatory control in myxedema and hypothyroidism. N Engl J Med 292:662, 1975.
49. Abbott TR: Anaesthesia in untreated myxedema. Br J Anaesth 35:510, 1967.
50. Babad AA, Eger EI II: The effects of hyperthyroidism and hypothyroidism on halothane and oxygen requirements in dogs. Anesthesiology 29:1087, 1968.
51. Levine HD: Compromise therapy in the patient with angina pectoris and hypothyroidism: A clinical assessment. Am J Med 69:411, 1980.
52. Paine TD, Rogers WJ, Baxley WA, et al: Coronary arterial surgery in patients with incapacitating angina pectoris and myxedema. Am J Cardiol 40:226, 1977.
53. Gharib H: Fine-needle aspiration biopsy of thyroid nodules: Advantages, limitations, and effect. Mayo Clin Proc 69:44, 1994.
54. National Cancer Institute: Information for physicians on irradiation-related thyroid cancer. Cancer 26:150, 1976.
55. Gharib H, James EM, Charboneau JW, et al: Suppressive therapy with levothyroxine for solitary thyroid nodules. A double-blind controlled clinical study. N Engl J Med 317:70, 1987.
56. Mazzaferri EL, et al: Papillary thyroid carcinoma. Impact of therapy in 675 patients. Medicine 56:171, 1977.
57. Jenkins JS, Gilbert CJ, Ang V: Hypothalamic pituitary function in patients with craniopharyngiomas. J Clin Endocrinol Metab 43:394, 1976.
58. Molitch ME: Pathologic hyperprolactinemia. Endocrinol Metab Clin North Am 21:877, 1992.
59. Jordan RM, Kendall JW: The primary empty sella syndrome. Am J Med 62:569, 1977.
60. Cohen KL: Metabolic, endocrine and drug-induced interference with pituitary function tests: A review. Metabolism 26:1165, 1977.
61. Kitahata LM: Airway difficulties associated with anaesthesia in acromegaly. Br J Anaesth 43:1187, 1971.
62. Southwick JP, Katz J: Unusual airway difficulty in the acromegalic patient: Indications for tracheostomy. Anesthesiology 51:72, 1979.
63. Wall RT III: Acromegaly. *In* Roizen MF, Fleisher LA (eds): Essence of Anesthesia Practice. Philadelphia, WB Saunders, 1997, p. 6.
64. Messick JM, et al: Anesthesia for transsphenoidal surgery of the hypophyseal region. Anesth Analg (Cleve) 57:206, 1978.

65. Spark RF, et al: Complete remission of acromegaly with medical treatment. JAMA 241:573, 1979.
66. Baker KZ: Transsphenoidal surgery. *In* Roizen MF, Fleisher LA (eds): Essence of Anesthesia Practice. Philadelphia, WB Saunders, 1997, p. 454.
67. Robertson GL: Thirst and vasopressin function in normal and disordered states of water balance. J Lab Clin Med 101:351, 1983.
68. Cannon JF: Diabetes insipidus: Clinical and experimental studies with consideration of genetic relationship. Arch Intern Med 96:215, 1955.
69. Bartter FC, Schwartz WB: The syndrome of inappropriate secretion of antidiuretic hormone. Am J Med 42:790, 1967.
70. Newfield P: Syndrome of inappropriate antidiuretic hormone secretion (SIADH). *In* Roizen MF, Fleisher LA (eds): Essence of Anesthesia Practice. Philadelphia, WB Saunders, 1997, p. 303.
71. Carlson DE, Gann DS: Effect of vasopressin antiserum on the response of adrenocorticotropin and cortisol to haemorrhage. Endocrinology 114:317, 1984.
72. Berardi RS: Vascular complication of superior mesentric artery infusion with pitressin in treatment of bleeding esophageal varices. Am J Surg 127:757, 1974.
73. Corliss RJ, McKenna DH, Sialers S, et al: Systemic and coronary hemodynamic effects of vasopressin. Am J Med Sci 256:293, 1968.
74. Nikolic G, Singh JB: Cimetidine, vasopressin, and chronotropic incompetence. Med J Aust 2:435, 1982.
75. Malhotra N, Roizen MF: Patients with abnormalities of vasopressin secretion and responsiveness. Anesthesiol Clin North Am 5:395, 1987.
76. Lampe GH, Roizen MF: Anesthesia for patients with abnormal function at the adrenal cortex. Anesthesiol Clin North Am 5:245, 1987.
77. Kaplan SA: Diseases of the adrenal cortex II. Congenital adrenal hyperplasia. Pediatr Clin North Am 26:77, 1979.
78. Orth DN, Kovacs WJ, Debold CR: The adrenal cortex. *In* Wilson JD, Foster DW (eds): Williams' Textbook of Endocrinology, ed 8. Philadelphia, WB Saunders, 1992, pp. 489–620.
79. Tyrell JB: Cushing's syndrome. *In* Wyngaarden JB, Smith LH, Bennett JC (eds): Cecil Textbook of Medicine, ed 19. Philadelphia, WB Saunders, 1992, pp. 1284–1288.
80. Migeon C, Keller A, Lawrence B, et al: DHA and androsterone levels in human plasma. Effect of age and sex: Day-to-day and diurnal variations. J Clin Endocrinol Metab 17:1051, 1957.
81. Cornbridge TC, Hall JB: The assessment and management of adults with status asthmaticus. Am J Respir Crit Care Med 151:1296, 1995.
82. Ellul-Micallef R, Borthwick RC, McHardy GJR: The time-course of response to prednisolone in chronic bronchial asthma. Clin Sci 47:105, 1974.
83. Moore-Ede MC, Czeisler CA, Richardson GS: Circadian time-keeping in health and disease. Part 1. Basic properties of circadian pacemakers. N Engl J Med 309:469, 1983.
84. Goldmann DR: The surgical patient on steroids. *In* Goldmann DR, Brown FH, Levy WK, et al (eds): Medical Care of the Surgical Patient. A Problem-Oriented Approach to Management. Philadelphia, J. B. Lippincott, 1982, pp. 113–125.
85. Hume DM, Bell CC, Bartter F: Direct measurement of adrenal secretion during operative trauma and convalescence. Surgery 52:174, 1962.

86. Plumpton FS, Besser GM, Cole PV: Corticosteroid treatment and surgery. An investigation of the indications for steroid cover. Anaesthesia 24:3, 1969.

87. Sampson PA, Brooke BN, Winstone NE: Biochemical confirmation of collapse due to adrenal failure. Lancet 1:1377, 1961.

88. Avioli LV: Effects of chronic corticosteroid therapy on mineral metabolism and calcium absorption. Adv Exp Biol Med 171:80, 1984.

89. Axelrod L: Glucocorticoid therapy. Medicine 55:39, 1976.

90. Taylor AL, Fishman LM: Corticotropin-releasing hormone. Med Progr 319:213, 1988.

91. Vale W, Spiess J, Rivier C, et al: Characterization of a 41-residue bovine hypothalamic peptide that stimulates secretion of corticotropin and beta-endorphin. Science 213:1394, 1981.

92. Werbel SS, Ober KP: Acute adrenal insufficiency. Endocrinol Metab Clin North Am 22:303, 1993.

93. Hollenberg NK, Williams GH: Hypertension, the adrenal and the kidney: Lessons from pharmacologic interruption of the renin-angiotensin system. Adv Intern Med 25:327, 1980.

94. Ross EJ: Symptomatology in adrenal diseases. *In* Keynes WM, Fowler PBS (eds): Clinical Endocrinology. London, William Heinemann Medical Books, 1984, pp. 148–194.

95. McKenna TJ: Screening for sinister causes of hirsutism. N Engl J Med 331:1015, 1994.

96. Lampe GH: Cushing's syndrome. *In* Roizen MF, Fleisher LA (eds): Essence of Anesthesia Practice. Philadelphia, WB Saunders, 1997, p. 97.

97. Symreng T: Steroids. *In* Roizen MF, Fleisher LA (eds): Essence of Anesthesia Practice. Philadelphia, WB Saunders, 1997, p. 545.

98. Engquist A, Backer OG, Jarnum S: Incidence of postoperative complications in patients subjected to surgery under steroid cover. Acta Chir Scand 140:343, 1974.

99. Dale DC, Fauci AS, Wolff SM: Alternate-day prednisone. Leukocyte kinetics and susceptibility to infections. N Engl J Med 291:1154, 1974.

100. Winstone NE, Brook BN: Effects of steroid treatment on patients undergoing operation. Lancet 1:973, 1961.

101. Ehrlich HP, Hunt TK: Effects of cortisone and vitamin A on wound healing. Ann Surg 167:324, 1968.

102. Sandburg N: Time relationship between administration of cortisone and wound healing in rats. Acta Chir Scand 127:446, 1964.

103. Moore TJ, Dluhy RG, Williams GH, et al: Nelson's syndrome: Frequency, prognosis, and effect of prior pituitary irradiation. Ann Intern Med 8:731, 1976.

104. Orth DN: Metapyrone is useful only as adjunctive therapy in Cushing's disease. (Editorial) Ann Intern Med 89:128, 1978.

105. Weinberger MH, Grim CE, Hollifield JW, et al: Primary aldosteronism: Diagnosis, localization, and treatment. Ann Intern Med 90:386, 1979.

106. Wagner RL: Hyperaldosteronism (secondary). *In* Roizen MF, Fleisher LA (eds): Essence of Anesthesia Practice. Philadelphia, WB Saunders, 1997, p. 166.

107. Hanowell ST, Hittner KC, Kim YD, et al: Anesthetic management of primary aldosteronism. Anesthesiol Rev 9:30, 1982.

108. Schambelan M, et al: Prevalence, pathogenesis and functional significance of aldosterone deficiency in hyperkalemic patients with chronic renal insufficiency. Kidney Int 17:89, 1980.

109. Udelsman R, Ramp J, Gallucci WT, et al: Adaptation during surgical stress: A re-evaluation of the role of glucocorticoids. J Clin Invest 77:1377, 1986.

110. Moore FD, Edelman IS, Olney JM, et al: Body sodium and potassium. Inter-related trends in alimentary, renal and cardiovascular disease; lack of correlation between body stores and plasma concentration. Metabolism 3:334, 1954.

111. Johnson JE, Hartsuck JM, Zollinger RM Jr, et al: Radiopotassium equilibration in total body potassium: Studies using ^{43}K and ^{42}K. Metabolism 18:663, 1969.

112. Symreng T, Karlberg BE, Kagedal B: Physiologic cortisol substitution of long-term steroid-treated patients undergoing major surgery. Br J Anesthesiol 53:949, 1981.

113. Zusman RM: Prostaglandins and water excretion. Ann Rev Med 32:359, 1981.

114. Rabinowitz IN, Watson W, Farber EM: Topical steroid depression of the hypothalamic-pituitary-adrenal axis in psoriasis vulgaris. Dermatologica 154:321, 1977.

115. Jensen JK, Elb S: Per-og postoperative komplikationer hos tigligere kortikosteroid behandlede patienter. Nord Med 76:975–978, 1966.

116. Oh SH, Patterson R: Surgery in corticosteroid asthmatics. J Allergy Clin Immunol 53:345, 1974.

117. Wagner RL, White PF, Kan PB, et al: Inhibition of adrenal steroidogenesis by the anesthetic etomidate. N Engl J Med 310:1415, 1984.

118. St. John Sutton MG, Sheps SG, Lie JT: Prevalence of clinically unsuspected pheochromocytoma. Review of a 50-year autopsy series. Mayo Clin Proc 56:354, 1981.

119. Roizen MF, Schreider BD, Hassan SK: Anesthesia for patients with pheochromocytoma. Anesthesiol Clin North Am 5:269, 1987.

120. Roizen MF: Pheochromocytoma. *In* Roizen MF, Fleisher LA (eds): Essence of Anesthesia Practice. Philadelphia, WB Saunders, 1997, p. 251.

121. Roizen MF: Adrenalectomy for pheochromocytoma. *In* Roizen MF, Fleisher LA (eds): Essence of Anesthesia Practice. Philadelphia, WB Saunders, 1997, p. 339.

122. Gifford RW Jr, Manger WM, Bravo EL: Pheochromocytoma. Endocrinol Metab Clin North Am 23:387, 1994.

123. Bravo EL, Tarazi RC, Fovad FM, et al: The clonidine suppression test: A useful aid in the diagnosis of pheochromocytoma. N Engl J Med 305:623, 1981.

124. Jensen JA, Jansson K, Goodson WH III, et al: Epinephrine lowers subcutaneous wound oxygen tension. Curr Surg 42:472, 1985.

125. Roizen MF, Hunt TK, Beaupre PN, et al: The effect of alpha-adrenergic blockade on cardiac performance and tissue oxygen delivery during excision of pheochromocytoma. Surgery 94:941, 1983.

126. Roizen MF, Horrigan RW, Koike M, et al: A prospective randomized trial of four anesthetic techniques for resection of pheochromocytoma. Anesthesiology 57:A43, 1982.

127. Cousins MJ, Rubin RB: The intraoperative management of pheochromocytoma with total epidural sympathetic blockade. Br J Anaesth 46:78, 1974.

128. Cooperman LH, Engelman K, Mann PEG: Anesthetic management of pheochromocytoma employing halothane and beta adrenergic blockade. Anesthesiology 28:575, 1967.

129. Desmonts JM, Le Houelleur J, Remond P, et al:

Anaesthetic management of patients with phaeochromocytoma. A review of 102 cases. Br J Anaesth 49:991, 1977.

130. Smith DS, Aukberg SJ, Levitt JD: Induction of anesthesia in a patient with undiagnosed pheochromocytoma. Anesthesiology 49:368, 1978.

131. Schaffer MS, Zuberbuhler P, Urlson G, et al: Catecholamine cardiomyopathy: An unusual presentation of pheochromocytoma in children. J Pediatr 99:276, 1981.

132. Service FJ: Hypoglycemia. Med Clin North Am 79:1, 1995.

133. Comi RJ: Approach to acute hypoglycemia. Endocrinol Metab Clin North Am 22:247, 1993.

134. Kitabchi AE: Proinsulin and C-peptide. A review. Metabolism 26:547, 1977.

135. Rizza RA, Haymond MW, Verdonk CA, et al: Pathogenesis of hypoglycemia in insulinoma patients, suppression of hepatic glucose production by insulin. Diabetes 30:377, 1981.

136. Stefanini P, Carboni M, Patrassi N, et al: Beta-islet cell tumors of the pancreas: Results of a study of 1,067 cases. Surgery 75:597, 1974.

137. Kavlie H, White TT: Pancreatic islet beta cell tumors and hyperplasia: Experience in 14 Seattle hospitals. Ann Surg 175:326, 1972.

138. Muir JJ, Enders SM, Offord K, et al: Glucose management in patients undergoing operation for insulinoma removal. Anesthesiology 59:371, 1983.

139. Schwartz SS, Horwitz DL, Zehfus B, et al: Continuous monitoring and control of plasma glucose during operation for insulinomas. Surgery 85:702, 1979.

140. Muir JJ: Insulinoma. In Roizen MF, Fleisher LA (eds): Essence of Anesthesia Practice. Philadelphia, WB Saunders, 1997, p. 191.

141. Walsh DB, Eckhauser FE, Ramsburgh SR, et al: Risk associated with diabetes mellitus in patients undergoing gallbladder surgery. Surgery 91:254, 1982.

142. Fowkes FGR, Lunn JN, Furow SC, et al: Epidemiology in anesthesia III. Mortality risk in patients with coexisting physical disease. Br J Anaesth 54:819, 1982.

143. Burgos LG, Ebert TJ, Asiddao C, et al: Increased intraoperative cardiovascular morbidity in diabetes with autonomic neuropathy. Anesthesiology 70:591, 1989.

144. Hjortrup A, Rasmussen BF, Kehlet H: Morbidity in diabetic and nondiabetic patients after major vascular surgery. Br Med J 287:1107, 1983.

145. Douglas JS, King SB, Craver JM, et al: Factors influencing risk and benefit of coronary bypass surgery in patients with diabetes mellitus. Chest 80:369, 1981.

146. Ransohoff DF, Miller GL, Forsythe SB, et al: Outcome of acute cholecystitis in patients with diabetes mellitus. Ann Intern Med 106:829, 1987.

147. Creutzfeldt W, Kabberling J, Neel JV: The Genetics of Diabetes Mellitus. New York, Springer-Verlag, 1976.

148. Archer JA, Gorden P, Roth J: Defect in insulin binding to receptors in obese man. J Clin Invest 55:166, 1975.

149. Kannel WB, McGee DL: Diabetes and cardiovascular disease. JAMA 241:2035, 1979.

150. Kreisberg RA: Diabetic ketoacidosis: New concepts and trends in pathogenesis and treatment. Ann Intern Med 88:681, 1978.

151. Diabetes Control and Complications Trial Research Group: The effect of intensive treatment of diabetes on the development and progression of long-term complications in insulin-dependent diabetes mellitus. N Engl J Med 329:977, 1993.

152. Porte D Jr, Schwartz MW: Diabetic complications: Why is glucose potentially toxic? Science 272:699, 1996.

153. Turner R, Cull C, Holman R: United Kingdom Prospective Diabetes Study 17: A 9-year update of a randomized, controlled trial on the effect of improved metabolic control on complications in non–insulin-dependent diabetes mellitus. Ann Intern Med 124:136, 1996.

154. Walters DP, Gatling W, Houston AC, et al: Mortality in diabetic subjects: An eleven-year follow-up of community-based population. Diabet Med 11:968, 1994.

155. Campbell PJ, Bolli GB, Cryer PE, et al: Pathogenesis of the dawn phenomenon in patients with insulin-dependent diabetes mellitus. N Engl J Med 312:1473, 1985.

156. Bagdade JD, Root RK, Bulger RJ: Impaired leukocyte function in patients with poorly controlled diabetes. Diabetes 23:9, 1974.

157. Clark CM Jr, Lee DA: Prevention and treatment of the complications of diabetes mellitus. N Engl J Med 332:1210, 1995.

158. Brenner BM: Hemodynamically mediated glomerular injury and the progressive nature of kidney disease. Kidney Int 23:647, 1983.

159. Forsblom CM, Eriksson JG, Ekstrand AV, et al: Insulin resistance and abnormal albumin excretion in non-diabetic first-degree relatives of patients with NIDDM. Diabetologia 38:363, 1995.

160. Krolewski AS, Laffel LMB, Krolewski M, et al: Glycosylated hemoglobin and the risk of microalbuminuria in patients with insulin-dependent diabetes mellitus. N Engl J Med 332:1251, 1995.

161. Lanier WL: Glucose management during cardiopulmonary bypass: Cardiovascular and neurologic implications. Anesth Analg 72:423, 1991.

162. Lanier WL, Stangland KJ, Scheithauer BW, et al: The effect of dextrose infusion and head position on neurologic outcome after complete ischemia in primates: Examination of a model. Anesthesiology 66:39, 1987.

163. Viberti G, Mogensen CE, Groop LC, et al: Effect of captopril on progression to clinical proteinuria in patients with insulin-dependent diabetes mellitus and microalbuminuria. JAMA 271:275, 1994.

164. Ishii H, Jirousek MR, Koya D, et al: Amelioration of vascular dysfunction in diabetic rats by an oral PKG beta inhibitor. Science 272:728, 1996.

165. Brenner WI, Lansky Z, Engelman RM, et al: Hyperosmolar coma in surgical patients: An iatrogenic disease of increasing incidence. Ann Surg 178:651, 1973.

166. Page MMcB, Watkins PJ: Cardiorespiratory arrest and diabetic autonomic neuropathy. Lancet 1:14, 1978.

167. Wright RA, Clemente R, Wathen R: Diabetic gastroparesis: An abnormality of gastric emptying of solids. Am J Med Sci 289:240, 1985.

168. Charlson ME, MacKenzie CR, Gold JP: Preoperative autonomic function abnormalities in patients with diabetes mellitus and patients with hypertension. J Am Coll Surg 179:1, 1994.

169. Longstreth WT, Inui TS: High blood glucose level on hospital admission and poor neurological recovery after cardiac arrest. Ann Neurol 15:59, 1984.

170. Meyer EJ, Lorenzi M, Bohannon NV, et al: Diabetic management by insulin infusion during major surgery. Am J Surg 137:323, 1979.

171. Taitelman U, Reece EA, Bessman AN: Insulin in the management of the diabetic surgical patient; continuous intravenous infusion vs subcutaneous administration. JAMA 237:658, 1977.

172. Campbell DR, Hoar CS, Wheelock FC: Carotid artery surgery in diabetic patients. Arch Surg 119: 1405, 1984.

173. Elliott MJ, Gill GV, Home PD, et al: A comparison of two regimens for the management of diabetes during open-heart surgery. Anesthesiology 60:364, 1984.

174. Johnson WD, Pedraza PM, Kayser KL: Coronary artery surgery in diabetics: 261 consecutive patients followed four to seven years. Am Heart J 104:823, 1982.

175. Alberti KG, Thomas DJ: The management of diabetes during surgery. Br J Anaesth 51:693, 1979.

176. Molitch ME, Reichlin S: The care of the diabetic patient during emergency surgery and postoperatively. Orthop Clin North Am 9:811, 1978.

177. Ammon JR: Diabetic ketoacids (DEA). *In* Roizen MF, Fleisher LA (eds): Essence of Anesthesia Practice. Philadelphia, WB Saunders, 1997, p. 110.

178. Nolan CM, Beaty HN, Bagdade JD: Further characterization of the impaired bactericidal function of granulocytes in patients with poorly controlled diabetes. Diabetes 27:889, 1978.

179. Kitabchi AT, Ayyagari V, Guerra SMO: The efficacy of low-dose versus conventional therapy of insulin for treatment of diabetic ketoacidosis. Ann Intern Med 84:633, 1976.

180. Clarke RSJ: Anaesthesia and carbohydrate metabolism. Br J Anaesth 45:237, 1973.

181. Greene NM: Lactate, pyruvate and excess lactate production in anesthetised man. Anesthesiology 22:404, 1961.

182. Greene NM: Insulin and anesthesia. Anesthesiology 41:75, 1974.

183. Paradise RR, Ko K: The effect of fructose on halothane depressed rat atria. Anesthesiology 32:124, 1970.

184. Mehta S: The influence of anesthesia with thiopentone and diazepam on the blood sugar level during surgery. Br J Anaesth 44:75, 1972.

185. Oyama T, Latto P, Holaday D: Effect of isoflurane anesthesia and surgery on carbohydrate metabolism and plasma cortisol levels in man. Can Anaesth Soc J 22:696, 1975.

186. Brandt M, Kehlet H, Binder C, et al: Effect of epidural analgesia on glucoregulatory endocrine response to surgery. Clin Endocrinol 5:107, 1976.

187. Cooper GM, Holdcroft A, Hall GM, et al: Epidural analgesia and the metabolic response to surgery. Can Anaesth Soc J 26:381, 1979.

188. Gurri JA, Burnham SJ: Effect of diabetes mellitus on distal lower extremity bypass. Am Surg 48:75, 1982.

189. Haff RC, Butcher RJ, Ballinger WF: Factors influencing morbidity in biliary tract operations. Surg Gynecol Obstet 132:195, 1971.

190. Halter FB, Pflug AE: Relationship of impaired insulin secretion during surgical stress to anesthesia and cataCholamine release. J Clin Endocrinol Metab 51:1093, 1980.

191. Fletcher J, Langman MJS, Kellock TD: Effect of surgery on blood-sugar levels in diabetes mellitus. Lancet 2:52, 1965.

192. Kalichman MW, Calcutt NA: Local anesthetic-induced conduction block and nerve fiber injury in streptozotocin-diabetic rats. Anesthesiology 77:941, 1992.

193. Metz S, Keats AS: Benefits of a glucose-containing priming solution for cardiopulmonary bypass. Anesth Analg 72:428, 1991.

194. Tsueda K, Huang KC, Dumont SW, et al: Cardiac sympathetic tone in anaesthetized diabetics. Can J Anaesth 38:20, 1991.

195. Dunnet JM, Holman RR, Turner RC, et al: Diabetes mellitus and anaesthesia. A survey of the perioperative management of the patient with diabetes mellitus. Anaesthesia 43:538, 1988.

196. Croughwell N, Lyth M, Quill TJ, et al: Diabetic patients have abnormal cerebral autoregulation during cardiopulmonary bypass. Circulation 82(suppl IV):IV407, 1990.

197. Eastwood DW: Anterior spinal artery syndrome after epidural anesthesia in a pregnant diabetic patient with sclerodema. Anesth Analg 73:90, 1991.

Hematologic Diseases

Jonathan L. Parmet
Jan Charles Horrow

I. INTRODUCTION

This chapter presents the anesthetic implications of significant hematologic disorders. Large published volumes already exist describing hematopathology, and separate works on hemostasis alone.[1, 2] For a large number of rare hematologic diseases, only a few patients or kindreds have been studied. An attempt even to summarize that wealth of information would overstep the scope of this text. Accordingly, this chapter presents in detail the pathophysiology and anesthetic considerations for the important hematologic diseases that may be encountered in anesthetic practice while merely touching on those rare entities that have perioperative implications. Very rare disorders with unknown anesthetic consequences or none remain unmentioned. The chapter separates the topics that meet these criteria into the anemias, the hemostatic disorders, and the diseases of white cells.

II. ANEMIAS

A. PHYSIOLOGY

Hemoglobin concentrations below 11.5 g/dL (hematocrit 36 per cent) for females and 12.5 g/dL (hematocrit 40 per cent) for males define anemia. Chronic anemias develop gradually permitting physiologic compensation. Indeed, patients with chronic anemia have "reasonably normal" lifestyles with hematocrits ranging from 18 to 20 per cent. Physiologic compensatory mechanisms that maintain oxygen transport, the product of cardiac output and arterial oxygen concentration, include increases in plasma volume to maintain euvolemia, in heart rate, and in stroke volume (Table 9–1). Decreased serum viscosity accompanied by an increase in heart rate yields increased cardiac output. Increased production of 2,3-diphosphoglycerate (2,3-DPG) shifts the oxygen-hemoglobin dissociation curve rightward, facilitating oxygen delivery (Fig. 9–1). When oxygen delivery to tissues is inadequate, the kidneys release erythropoietin to stimulate erythroid precursors. In physically active uncompensated anemic patients, fatigue and decreased exercise tolerance reflect an inability to increase cardiac output further to maintain tissue oxygenation.

Although some recommend a hemoglobin

TABLE 9–1

Compensatory Mechanisms in Chronic Anemia

Physiologic Variable	Effect of Chronic Anemia
Plasma volume	Increase
Cardiac output	Increase
Heart rate	Increase
Stroke volume	Increase
Afterload	Decrease
Blood viscosity	Decrease
Oxygen content	Decrease
Oxygen delivery	Maintained
2,3-DPG concentration	Increase
Erythropoietin secretion	Increase

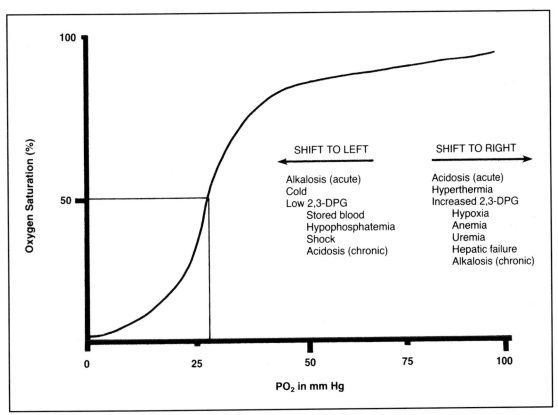

FIGURE 9–1. Oxyhemoglobin dissociation curve. Chronic anemia shifts the oxyhemoglobin dissociation curve rightward.

TABLE 9–2

Overview of Anemias

Hemolytic anemias
  Hereditary
    Sickle cell disease
    Thalassemias
    Spherocytosis
    G-6-PD deficiency
    Paroxysmal nocturnal hemoglobinuria
  Immune-mediated
    Drug-induced hemolytic anemia
    Autoimmune: paroxysmal cold
      hemoglobinuria
Nutritional anemias
  Iron deficiency
  Vitamin B_{12} deficiency
  Folate deficiency
Other causes
  Methemoglobinemia
  Felty's syndrome

concentration greater than 10 g/dL before elective surgery, no investigation has defined a minimal acceptable hemoglobin concentration for elective surgery,[3] nor has any study demonstrated an increase in postoperative morbidity in patients with mild to moderate chronic anemia. A hematocrit of 30 per cent does permit maximum oxygen transport (Fig. 9–2).[4] Oxygen transport varies by only 10 per cent between hematocrits of 20 and 50 per cent.[4]

Patients tolerate chronic anemia better than acute anemia. Animals can tolerate acute decreases in hemoglobin levels to between 3 and 5 g/dL.[5] Unpublished anecdotal reports claim survival of Jehovah's Witnesses with acute decreases in hematocrit to 10 per cent.[3] Maintenance of normovolemia remains crucial for patients to tolerate acute decreases in hematocrit. The authors support performing elective peripheral surgery in chronically anemic patients provided that they demonstrate no preoperative evidence of physiologic decompensation, such as dyspnea on moderate exertion as in climbing one flight of stairs. Elective surgical procedures associated with major blood loss should not proceed in patients whose anemia has a correctable cause (i.e., vitamin B_{12}, folate, or iron deficiency).

B. HEMOLYTIC ANEMIAS

Erythrocytes of patients with hemolytic anemia have an abbreviated life span (i.e., less than 120 days). The accelerated destruction of erythrocytes results in a compensatory increase in erythrocyte production, with attendant bone marrow hyperplasia. Hemolysis can occur either intravascularly or extravascularly. Extravascular hemolysis occurs in the reticuloendothelial system. Splenomegaly and jaundice appear on physical examination. Splenomegaly rarely occurs with intravascular hemolysis. Paradoxically, in some patients marrow suppression can occur even in the face of a maximally stimulated hematopoietic system. Two broad groups of hemolytic anemias become apparent hereditary defects that result in unstable erythrocyte cell membranes and immune-mediated hemolytic anemias (Table 9–2).

1. Sickle Cell Disease and Trait

Sickle cell disease, a disorder of abnormal hemoglobin synthesis, results from a single

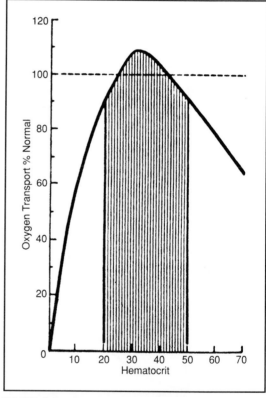

FIGURE 9–2. Oxygen transport versus hematocrit level. Hematocrits between 20 and 50 have a 10 per cent change in oxygen transport, which is the product of cardiac output and oxygen-carrying capacity. (From Cooper JF, Slogoff S: Hemodilution and priming solutions for cardiopulmonary bypass. In Gravlee GP, Davis RF, Utley JR (eds): Cardiopulmonary Bypass. Principles and Practice. Baltimore, Williams & Wilkins, 1993, with permission.)

nucleotide substitution in the β-globin gene on chromosome 11. Glutamate replaces valine in the sixth position, yielding a hemoglobin S β chain.[6] Persons homozygous for S β-globin chains have sickle cell disease. Those heterozygous have sickle cell trait.[7] Sickle cell anemia occurs in 0.5 to 1 per cent of the American black population. Sickle cell trait occurs in 8 to 10 per cent of American Blacks. Hemoglobin S (HbS) protects erythrocytes from malarial invasion, providing a survival advantage to the heterozygous carrier state, despite its genetic undesirability.

2. Sickle Cell Anemia

a. Pathophysiology

Four types of globin chains exist: α, β, δ, and γ. Hb A, composed of two α and two β chains (Fig. 9–3), accounts for 97 per cent of total adult hemoglobin in normal erythrocytes. Hb A_2 ($\alpha_2\delta_2$) accounts for the remaining 3 per cent and fetal hemoglobin ($\alpha_2\gamma_2$) for less than 1 per cent. Erythrocytes of patients with sickle cell anemia contain predominantly Hb S, no Hb A, and a small amount of Hb F. Hb S "sickles" when exposed to oxygen tensions below 40 mm Hg.[8] Desaturated Hb S, being 50 times less soluble than deoxygenated Hb A, aggregates into long stacks called *tactoids*. Tactoids alter the shape, function, and fluidity of the red blood cell. Initially reversible, multiple cycles of sickling and unsickling eventually damage the membrane components of the red cell, distorting erythrocytes. The reticuloendothelial system permanently elimi-

nates sickled erythrocytes. Hypoxia, hypothermia, low-flow states, and acidosis all contribute to erythrocyte sickling.

Sickling of erythrocytes produces hemolytic anemia as well as acute and chronic tissue damage from vasoocclusion.[9] Patients with sickle cell anemia have a baseline hematocrit of 18 to 25 per cent (hemoglobin concentration 6 to 8 g/dL).[10] The erythrocytes have a shortened life span of 10 to 20 days as compared with 120 days for normal red blood cells. On physical examination, patients may appear slightly jaundiced owing to an elevated total bilirubin value from intravascular hemolysis.

Systemic effects of sickling are numerous. First, vasoocclusion and thrombosis induced by sickling produce effects on the central nervous system. Cerebrovascular accidents occur in both adults and children, ranging from transient ischemic events to permanent neurologic deficits.[11] Young children suffer from thrombotic infarction, whereas adults more often have hemorrhagic infarcts. Preoperative physical examination should include a brief assessment of the nervous system.

Second, the heart and lungs are significantly affected. Patients with sickle cell disease develop left ventricular hypertrophy and cardiomegaly by age 20.[12] Like patients with chronic anemia, sickle cell patients have increased cardiac output and diastolic flow murmurs. Necropsy findings of sickle cell patients demonstrate moderate increases in wall thickness and dilatation of both ventricles.[12] Half of sickle cell patients demonstrate electrocardiographic evidence of left ventricular hypertrophy, and 10 to 15 per cent have evi-

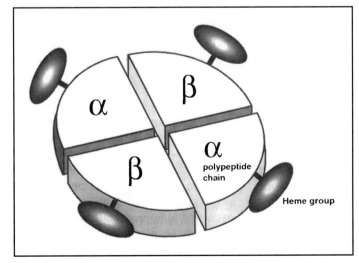

FIGURE 9–3. A schematic of normal human hemoglobin A, which is composed of two alpha (α) globin chains and two beta (β) globin chains (From Schloo BL: Normal development of the hematopoietic system. *In* Lake CL, Moore RA (eds): Blood: Hemostasis, Transfusion, and Alternatives in the Perioperative Period. New York, Raven Press, 1995, with permission.)

dence of right ventricular overload.[12] Surprisingly, sickle cell patients do not develop myocardial ischemia, despite the tendency for thrombosis and vasoocclusion.[12]

Patients with sickle cell anemia develop pulmonary infarctions and atelectasis. Necropsy findings have shown thrombotic obliteration of the pulmonary circulation.[13] Acute infarction of the lung may produce "acute chest syndrome," characterized by fever, chest pain, a rise in white blood cell count, and the appearance of a pulmonary infiltrate on chest films.[14] Arterial hypoxemia remains a characteristic finding, starting late in the second decade of life. Physiologic studies demonstrate ventilation-perfusion mismatch and venoarterial shunting. Over time, pulmonary vascular occlusions increase pulmonary vascular resistance and result in cor pulmonale.[15] Not surprisingly by the fourth decade of life many sickle cell patients develop right ventricular dysfunction.[12]

As with other anemias, the oxyhemoglobin dissociation curve shifts rightward to allow increased release of oxygen at the tissue level (see Fig. 9–1). Peripheral pulse oximetry may reveal lower oxygen saturation for a given arterial oxygen tension. Decreased affinity of oxygen to Hb S contributes to suboptimal oxygen loading at the pulmonary alveolus, resulting in the baseline hypoxemia observed in some patients. Measurement of arterial oxygen tension before surgery should help to determine the severity of pulmonary disease.

Third, the spleen's tortuous internal architecture and slow internal blood flow promote erythrocyte deoxygenation and stasis. Sickling and vasoocclusion result. During the first year of life most patients become hyposplenic.[16] Although autoinfarction of the spleen occurs at an early age, the spleen can enlarge and trap erythrocytes and platelets, producing a splenic sequestration crisis. Characterized by a hemoglobin concentration below 6 g/dL, such patients may require emergent splenectomy. Vinchinsky recommends splenectomy in patients that have had one major or two minor sequestration crises.[17]

Fourth, intrahepatic sickling with painful enlargement of the liver can occur. Hepatic transaminases are often elevated. Chronic hemolysis results in the formation of pigmented gallstones in this patient population. Several authors advocate cholecystectomy for asymptomatic patients with cholelithiasis, to avoid subsequent complications of cholecystitis and choledocholithiasis.[18, 19]

Fifth, anoxia, hyperosmolarity, and low pH which characterize the milieu of the renal medulla, all predispose to sickling and vasoocclusion, with resultant infarction of the renal medulla followed by papillary necrosis. Patients with sickle cell disease lose the ability to concentrate urine. Hematuria is frequent. Urinalysis may demonstrate isosthenuric specific gravity (1.010), reflecting the patient's inability to concentrate urine.[20]

Finally, chronic vasoocclusive sickling can cause infarction of the nutrient artery of the femur. Aseptic necrosis of the femoral head occurs in about 10 per cent of patients, of whom 17 per cent require total hip arthroplasty.[21] Necrosis of the marrow with subsequent marrow detachment can produce pulmonary emboli. Adults frequently develop ulceration of the malleoli, which requires surgical incision and drainage.

Hemoglobin SC disease is a double-recessive, mixed hemoglobinopathy disorder that behaves like a mild form of sickle cell anemia (i.e., SS disease) and thus is mentioned at this point. The following clinical considerations for sickle cell disease apply also to SC disease, but on a somewhat reduced scale. Decreased activity of serum cholinesterase occurs in some patients with Hb SC disease.[22] Chronic liver damage, rather than abnormal enzyme, may have produced this abnormality. Clinically, this should not affect administration of muscle relaxants to this patient population.

b. Preoperative Considerations

Patients with sickle cell anemia commonly present for the following surgical procedures: splenectomy, cholecystectomy, incision and drainage of peripheral ulcers, relief of priapism, and, occasionally, total hip arthroplasty. Patients in the third decade of life may have insidious underlying cardiovascular compromise. Preoperative electrocardiography and chest x-ray study should be obtained, along with arterial blood gas analysis before surgery. If physical examination and preoperative electrocardiography suggest evidence of cor pulmonale, echocardiographic or radionucleotide imaging should further assess ventricular function.

Sickle cell anemia patients have an increased frequency of perioperative complications, including painful vasoocclusive crises, acute chest syndrome, pneumonia, and pulmonary embolism.[23] Although no prospective randomized studies address the efficacy of preoperative transfusion therapy in reducing postoperative complications, investigators have reported a decrease in perioperative morbidity rates associated with preoperative blood transfusions. Lessins demonstrated that clinical vasoocclusion crises occur when Hb S comprises more than 50 per cent of total hemoglobin.[24]

Preoperative transfusion therapy attempts to increase the total hemoglobin concentration to 10 to 12 g/dL and to decrease the percentage of Hb S to less than 40 per cent.[10] Advocates of preoperative transfusion therapy recommend two transfusion methods: staged preoperative transfusion or partial exchange transfusion. Staged preoperative transfusions begin a month before surgery. Patients receive 15 mL/kg of packed erythrocytes to increase the total hemoglobin to 10 to 12 g/dL. After 2 weeks, patients receive a second transfusion to suppress erythropoiesis of Hb S and maintain Hb S levels below 40 per cent. Staged preoperative transfusions consume time and increase expense. Partial exchange transfusions, a more rapid (1 to 4 hours), less expensive method also decrease the percentage of Hb S and increase the concentration of Hb A. Some 10 to 15 mL/kg of whole blood is removed and then replaced by 15 to 20 mL/kg of packed erythrocytes. Bhattacharyya reported the successful use of partial exchange transfusions in pediatric patients undergoing elective and emergent cholecystectomy.[25] No vasoocclusive events related to sickle cell crises occurred in this group.

Recently, some have questioned the indiscriminate use of preoperative transfusion therapy in patients with sickle cell disease, citing the inherent risks of blood transfusions as well as the associated risk of transfusion reactions, including transmission of infectious agents and allosensitization against erythrocyte antigens. In Bischoff and colleagues' retrospective series, patients receiving transfusion therapy suffered an increased incidence of hypoxia and atelectasis.[26] The investigators also observed that patients with a total hematocrit below 30 per cent more frequently developed postoperative complications. Griffin and Buchanan reported on a large group of pediatric patients who did not receive preoperative transfusion therapy.[27] An increased incidence of complications occurred in patients undergoing thoracotomy, laparotomy, and tonsillectomy with adenoidectomy as compared with other minor surgical procedures such as herniorrhaphy, tympanotomy tube placement, and peripheral surgical procedures (Tables 9–3 and 9–4).[27, 147]

These data suggest that patients undergoing procedures involving invasion of the abdomen or thorax or resection of tonsils and adenoids should receive preoperative transfusion therapy.[28] Patients presenting for elective peripheral procedures other than adenotonsillectomy do not appear to require transfusion therapy.

C. Anesthetic Considerations

To the authors' knowledge, no randomized prospective studies address which is the best anesthetic technique for patients with sickle cell disease. Only retrospective series report successful administration of general anesthesia to sickle cell patients. The choice of anesthetic technique appears less important than the details of its performance. The goals of every anesthetic—avoidance of hypoxia, hypercarbia, acidosis, low-flow conditions, and

TABLE 9–3

Perioperative Complications in Patients with Sickle Cell Disease

Investigator	Cases (No.)	Prevalence of Complications		Comments
		Patients Transfused (%)	Patients not Transfused (%)	
Homi[147]	284	28	13	
Bischoff[26]	82	29	9	
Ware[28]	27	0	—	Cholecystectomy
Derkay[34]	10	0	—	Tonsilloadenoidectomy
Griffin[27]	66	—	27	(See Table 9–4)
Bhattacharyya[25]	22	18	—	

TABLE 9–4

Complications in Patients with Sickle Cell Disease Who Do Not Receive Preoperative Transfusion Therapy

	Major Procedures	Tonsilloadenoid-ectomy	Other Minor Procedures
Number of patients	20	9	37
Number without complications	10	4	35
Fever of no identified source	3	3	2
Atelectasis but no fever	2	0	0
Fever and atelectasis	2	1	0
Chest syndrome	3	1	0
Total with complications (rate)	10 (50%)	5 (56%)	2 (5%)

Adapted from Griffin TC, Buchanan G: Elective surgery in children with sickle cell disease without preoperative blood transfusion. J Pediatr Surg 28:681, 1993.

hypothermia—become more crucial when the patient has sickle cell anemia. Decreased sickling of erythrocytes during general anesthesia occurs with increased arterial oxygen tensions.[29]

A retrospective review of 45 patients undergoing general anesthesia showed no impact of the type of anesthetic on postoperative morbidity or mortality. All patients received perioperative hydration, vigorous intraoperative warming, and postoperative oxygen therapy.[30] Nevertheless, 46 per cent of patients receiving general anesthesia developed perioperative complications, including atelectasis, thrombophlebitis, and sickle cell crisis. The highest prevalence of complications, 85 per cent, occurred in patients receiving isoflurane, as compared with 59 per cent of patients receiving enflurane and 25 per cent of those receiving halothane; however, the isoflurane group had the highest incidence of upper abdominal surgery, atelectasis being the predominant postoperative complication. While those authors concluded that the operative procedure, not the anesthetic agent, appeared to be responsible for the perioperative complications, the confounding factors suggest that those data afford no conclusions.

Two case reports detail the successful use of epidural bupivacaine along with intrathecal opioids to control peripheral painful vasoocclusive crises.[31, 32] Peripheral vasodilation from epidural anesthesia, analgesia from the epidural opioids, or their combination could have terminated the painful crises. Central neural axis blockade when compared to general anesthesia, offers the advantages of maintained pulmonary function, decreased blood loss, and decreased incidence of thromboem-

bolic events. Central neural axis blockade, when feasible, appears to be the preferable anesthetic technique for patients with sickle cell anemia.

For orthopedic procedures, regional acidosis must be avoided along with hypothermia and the peripheral low-flow state produced by tourniquet inflation and positioning.[33] The successful use of an Esmarch tourniquet has been described; however, this practice appears questionable owing to the local cooling and intravascular stasis produced by a tourniquet.[33]

Most institutions employ a protocol to such patients. Some protocols include admission to the hospital 1 day before the surgery, to provide 1½ to 2 times calculated maintenance fluid requirements to prevent preoperative hypovolemia.[28, 34] All efforts to prevent intraoperative hypothermia should be exerted, including low fresh gas flows, heat and humidity exchangers, warming of the operative suite, warming of intravenous fluids, and convective warming of the patient. Postoperatively, the patient should receive supplemental oxygen therapy, and encouragement in active pulmonary toilet. Early ambulation is also recommended. While these form the basis for good anesthesia care for all patients, those with sickle cell disease have no tolerance for any compromise of these principles.

Some advocate prophylactic administration of bicarbonate to prevent acidemia. Such a maneuver would not restore sickled erythrocytes to their native state and could shift the hemoglobin-oxygen dissociation curve leftward, impairing delivery of oxygen to tissues. The authors reserve it for procedures in which acidemia is unavoidable and predictable.

3. Sickle Cell Trait

Sickle cell trait patients have 50 per cent Hb S in the erythrocytes and Hb A as the remainder of hemoglobin.[35] Unlike patients with sickle cell disease, sickle cell trait patients have an abundance of normal Hb A, which prevents the cell from sickling; however, the presence of some Hb S permits an oxygen tension of 15 mm Hg to produce sickling.[36] In vitro reducing agents induce sickling in sickle cell trait erythrocytes, providing the basis for the diagnosis of sickle cell trait.

Patients with sickle cell trait rarely "sickle." Inheritance of the sickle cell trait does not decrease the life span of either the patient or the erythrocyte; however sickling may occur in heterozygotes under severe hypoxic conditions. McCormick reported a 16 per cent prevalence of visceral infarcts on postmortem examination of patients with sickle cell trait.[37] All sickle cell trait patients by the fourth decade of life have autoinfarcted the renal medulla, leading to isosthenuria. Still, the morbidity and mortality associated with sickle cell trait are low and difficult to document. A study of 65,000 Black males documented a slightly higher incidence of hematuria and pulmonary embolism in those with sickle cell trait.[38] Anecdotal reports suggest that sickle cell trait contributes to cerebral thrombosis, sudden death, and anesthetic mishaps in patients with sickle cell trait.[39]

a. Anesthetic Considerations

With patients who have sickle cell disease, it is necessary to avoid hypoxemia, acidosis, stasis, and hypothermia with patients who have sickle cell trait. This includes physiologic perturbations such as hypoventilation, hemorrhage, low-flow states produced by tourniquet application, vascular cross-clamping, and cardiopulmonary bypass. The combination of stasis and extreme hypothermia attendant with bypass might predispose to sickling, even in these less sensitive heterozygotes. Despite accounts of open heart surgery being successfully performed in these patients,[40, 41] postanesthetic neurologic complications[36] as well as intraoperative death have occurred.

4. Thalassemias

These hereditary diseases arise from a defective rate of globin chain synthesis. Thalassemia minor, the heterozygous state, is a mild form of the disease. Two types of thalassemia major exist: β-thalassemia (decreased β-globin chain production) and α-thalassemia (decreased α-globin production). The consequences of impaired synthesis of α- or β-globin differ. In α-thalassemia, surplus β-globin chains can self-associate; in β-thalassemia, α chains cannot.[42] However in β-thalassemia other normally occurring globin chains (δ,γ) can combine with α chains. Thus the excess α chains combine with δ chains to form Hb A_2 or with γ chains to form fetal hemoglobin. Elevated levels of Hb A_2 characterize β-thalassemia minor. In α thalassemia minor no abnormal hemoglobins are present. These patients demonstrate mild hypochromic microcytic anemia. Occasionally these patients present for splenectomy to control hemolysis.

a. β-Thalassemia Major (Cooley's Anemia)

Clinical manifestations occur after the first 4 to 6 months of life, when the switch from γ-chain to β-chain synthesis occurs. Severe anemia then develops. Patients require multiple blood transfusions and can develop hemochromatosis with impaired cardiac, endocrine, and hepatic function. Erythrocytes become distorted and destroyed before leaving the marrow. Ineffective erythropoiesis results, with hemolysis and hyperplasia of the bone marrow. Accelerated hematopoiesis results in distortion of the craniofacial anatomy, as depicted by the "chipmunk" facies and "hair-on-end" skull radiographic patterns. These craniofacial anomalies can make laryngoscopy difficult.

b. α-Thalassemia Major

Failure to express three α loci results in α-thalassemia major. Hb H, a β-globin chain tetramer, predominates. Although severe anemia results, some normal hemoglobin is produced by the expression of the single remaining α gene. When none of the four α loci is expressed, hydrops fetalis or neonatal death results.

5. Hereditary Spherocytosis

Hereditary spherocytosis, an autosomal dominant disease, produces erythrocytes with abnormal cell membranes that permit sodium and water influx into the cell.[43] Consequently, erythrocytes swell and develop a spherical shape. Unlike the stable biconcave shape of normal erythrocytes, the spherical shape makes these erythrocytes so fragile that they rupture while passing through the spleen. Osmotic fragility testing documents the presence of these unstable erythrocytes (Fig. 9–4). Physical examination may reveal splenomegaly along with jaundice. Elective splenectomy in these patients increases erythrocyte life span. Children younger than 10 years do not undergo splenectomy owing to the risk of septicemia.[44] Tchernia and coworkers reported an increase in erythrocyte survival in children aged 2 to 13 after partial splenectomy.[45] Some investigators advocate elective cholecystectomy at the time of splenectomy because of a high incidence of cholelithiasis in these patients.

6. Hereditary Elliptocytosis and Hereditary Stomatocytosis

There are no clinical consequences of the red cell membrane defects hereditary elliptocytosis and hereditary stomatocytosis. Red cell survival time is nearly normal for each. Questions about cell survival under unusual conditions such as hypothermic cardiopulmonary bypass and suctioning with cell-saving devices remain incompletely answered.

7. Spur Cell Anemia

Redundant red cell membrane folds into spurlike projections in this disorder, which may occur in alcoholic liver disease. No anesthetic implications outside those potentially present with chronic alcoholism apply.

8. Glucose-6-Phosphate Dehydrogenase Deficiency

Glucose-6-phosphate dehydrogenase (G-6-PD) deficiency is a sex-linked disorder with incomplete penetrance.[46] In fact, 10 per cent of American Black males suffer from G-6-PD deficiency.

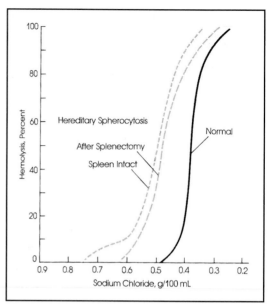

FIGURE 9–4. Osmotic fragility of normal red blood cells, hereditary spherocytes before splenectomy, after splenectomy. After splenectomy, a population of spherocytes exists that are less osmotically fragile than before splenectomy. (From Bunn HF: Disorders of hemoglobin. In Isselbacher K, Brunwald E, Wilson JD et al (eds): Harrison's Principles of Internal Medicine, 13th ed. New York, McGraw-Hill, 1994, with permission.)

G-6-PD reduces nicotinamide dinucleotide phosphate (NADP$^+$) to its reduced form (NADPH), which prevents hemoglobin oxidation. In this way, G-6-PD enables erythrocytes to combat oxidants. In G-6-PD deficiency, hemoglobin oxidizes, denatures, and precipitates into Heinz bodies in the erythrocyte. Heinz bodies represent denatured hemoglobin aggregates. Red blood cells with Heinz bodies cannot traverse the splenic pulp and are eliminated from the circulation. Deficiency of the G-6-PD enzyme renders erythrocytes vulnerable to the effects of oxidant drugs. Hemolytic anemia occurs in G-6-PD patients after administration of pharmacologic agents that form peroxides (Table 9–5).[148] Methemoglobinemia often accompanies the administration of these agents.[47] Therefore, some authors have implicated drugs that induce methemoglobin as a contributing factor to hemolysis in G-6-PD–deficient patients.

The presence of Heinz bodies in a peripheral blood smear indicates the possibility of G-6-PD deficiency. Assay of red cell G-6-PD diagnoses this disease. Treatment relies on discontinuing the offending agents. Splenectomy is generally ineffective.[48] Anesthetic considerations include avoiding agents listed

TABLE 9–5

Common Substances That Induce Hemolytic Anemia in G-6-PD–Deficient Patients

Acetanid	Niridazole
Doxorubicin	Nitrofurantoin
Furazolidine	Phenazopyridine
Methylene blue	Primaquine
Nalidixic acid	Sulfamethoxazole

Adapted from Beutler E: Glucose-6-phosphate dehydrogenase deficiency. N Engl J Med 324:169, 1991. Copyright 1991 Massachusetts Medical Society.

in Table 9–5 and others that have the potential to induce hemoglobin oxidation or methemoglobinemia. Because the anemia remains mild, most patients do not require red blood cell transfusions.

9. Paroxysmal Nocturnal Hemoglobinuria

Acute episodes of hemolysis superimposed on chronic hemolysis characterize paroxysmal nocturnal hemoglobinuria (PNH). In PNH, a cell membrane defect renders the cell susceptible to lysis by complement proteins. All cell lines can be affected, and an association with aplastic anemia exists. Patients may present with chronic hemolysis, iron deficiency, or recurrent thrombotic episodes. Young adults demonstrate hemoglobinuria upon first voiding after awakening, thus the name *PNH.*

Venous thrombosis accounts for 50 per cent of all deaths from the disease. Venous thrombosis can occur in hepatic, splenic, portal, and cerebral veins. The Budd-Chiari syndrome, hepatic vein thrombosis, can be fatal. Complement activation of platelets appears to be responsible for the predisposition to thrombosis.

Patients with PNH have successfully undergone regional, spinal, and general anesthesia. Specific clinical recommendations include avoiding hypoxemia, acidosis, and hypovolemia, initiating prophylactic red blood cell transfusion, administering corticosteroids to prevent and treat hemolysis, and avoiding drugs known to activate complement such as acetazolamide, magnesium compounds, drugs formulated in cremophor,[49, 50] and protamine.

10. Immune Hemolytic Anemia

The immune hemolytic anemias can be divided into drug-induced and autoimmune types. Regardless of the cause, antibodies directed against erythrocytes produce hemolysis. The direct and indirect Coombs' tests facilitate diagnosis. Agglutination of washed red cells from patients by animal antiglobulin serum (serum with antibodies to immunoglobulin G [IgG] and C3) defines a positive direct Coombs' test. Agglutination by the patient's serum of normal red cells defines an indirect Coombs' test. Antibodies that can react at body ("warm") temperature are usually IgG class, whereas those that react at colder temperatures are usually IgM class. Table 9–6 lists causes of warm-antibody hemolytic anemia and cold-antibody hemolytic anemia.

Drugs such as α-methyldopa, quinine, quinidine, paraaminobenzoate, sulfonamides, and phenacetin may induce antibody formation to the erythrocyte, or they may associate with the erythrocyte, inducing antibodies against the erythrocyte-drug complex (e.g., penicillin). An antihypertensive agent, α-methyldopa, produces hemolysis by warm IgG antibodies. Ten per cent of patients taking α-methyldopa demonstrate a positive direct

TABLE 9–6

Causes of Immune Hemolytic Anemias

Warm	Cold
Idiopathic	Cold agglutinin disease
Lymphomas	Acute infections
Chronic lymphocytic leukemia	*Mycoplasma* infection
Non-Hodgkin's lymphomas	Infectious mononucleosis
Hodgkin's disease	Chronic infections
Collagen vascular diseases	Idiopathic
Systemic lupus erythematosus	Lymphoma
Other collagen vascular diseases	Paroxysmal cold hemoglobinuria
Drugs	
α-Methyldopa	
Penicillin	
Quinidine	
Postviral infections	
Miscellaneous tumors	

Adapted from Bunn F: Disorders of hemoglobin. In Isselbacher K, Braunwald E, Wilson JD, et al. (eds): Harrison's Principles of Internal Medicine, 13th ed. New York, McGraw-Hill, 1994. Reproduced by permission of the McGraw-Hill Companies.

Coombs' test. Discontinuation of the pharmacologic agents permits resolution.

Patients with autoimmune hemolytic anemias may respond to glucocorticoid therapy. If this treatment fails, some authors recommend splenectomy. Most patients respond to the above treatment modalities. Patients whose disease is refractory to steroid therapy and splenectomy may receive immunosuppressive therapy with either azathioprine or cyclophosphamide.

11. Paroxysmal Cold Hemoglobinuria

Acute episodes of massive hemolysis following cold exposure characterize paroxysmal cold hemoglobinuria (PCH). Body cooling produces hemoglobinemia, hemoglobinuria, fever, joint pain, jaundice, and malaise. This disorder arises from the presence of cold-reactive autoantibodies. The cold-reactive antibody causes significant hemolysis. Tertiary syphilis, once the primary cause of PCH and now a rare disease, produces IgG antibody against the erythrocyte along with complement-mediated lysis. *Mycoplasma pneumoniae* and coxsackievirus produce IgM antibodies, which can mediate hemolysis. Other disease processes producing cold-reactive antibodies include cryoglobulinemia,

primary infectious mononucleosis, some lymphomas, and malignancies.

a. Anesthetic Considerations

Maintenance of body temperature above the critical temperature for antibody production or antibody agglutination is critical. No specific treatment exists for this disorder. Plasmapheresis can reduce the antibody titer, because the antibody remains intravascular.[51, 52] Since postinfectious forms of PCH terminate spontaneously within a few days to weeks after onset,[53] the authors recommend postponing elective surgical procedures until antibody titers have decreased. Splenectomy and glucocorticoid therapy have not successfully treated PCH.[54] Several authors have described the successful management of coronary artery revascularization in patients with cold agglutinin disease.[51, 52]

C. NUTRITIONAL ANEMIAS

1. Iron Deficiency Anemia

a. Pathophysiology

In iron deficiency anemia, one of the three most common causes of anemia (Fig. 9–5),[42] decreased total body content of iron, occurs.

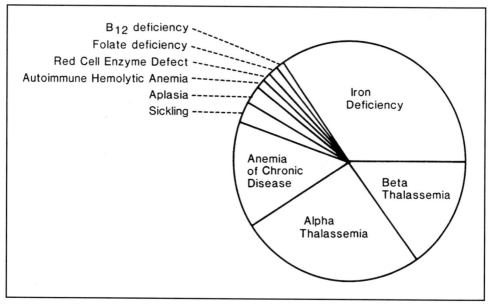

FIGURE 9–5. The estimated prevalence of different types of anemia in the United States. (From Stoelting RK, Dierdorf SF: Anemias. Anesthesia and Co-existing Disease, 3rd ed. New York, Churchill Livingstone, 1993, with permission.)

Iron deficiency results from inadequate iron intake, malabsorption of iron, chronic blood loss, pregnancy, or intravascular hemolysis. Gastrointestinal bleeding remains the most common cause of iron deficiency in the adult population and in postmenopausal women.

Decreased or absent iron stores in the bone marrow, low serum iron concentrations, low transferrin saturation, and low hemoglobin concentration and hematocrit values characterize iron deficiency anemia.[55] A decreased plasma ferritin concentration serves as a cost-effective way of diagnosing iron deficiency, because a linear relationship exists between plasma ferritin concentration and body total iron stores. Unsaturated iron-binding capacity increases in iron deficiency; its measurement permits the diagnosis of iron deficiency as the cause of anemia rather than anemia of chronic disease.[42] A microcytic, hypochromic peripheral red cell smear with anisocytosis and poikilocytosis also suggests the diagnosis of iron deficiency anemia.

b. Anesthetic Considerations

Oral ferrous sulfate therapy corrects the hemoglobin concentration halfway to normal in 3 to 5 weeks and fully in 2 months.[55] Thus, elective procedures associated with moderate to much blood loss in patients with moderate to severe iron deficiency can wait for endogenous erythrocyte replenishment to avoid the potential complications associated with red blood cell transfusions.

2. Megaloblastic Anemias

Folic acid and vitamin B_{12} deficiencies impair DNA synthesis and result in megaloblastic anemias. Pharmacologic agents that inhibit DNA synthesis can also produce megaloblastic changes in red blood cells. Megaloblastic red cells appear normochromic and macrocytic. Determining serum B_{12} and folate concentrations along with performing a Schilling test, which measures radiolabeled cobalamin absorption, distinguishes among the causes of megaloblastic anemia. One to two weeks' parenteral replacement of the deficient vitamin or vitamins yields hematologic improvement.

3. Vitamin B_{12} Deficiency

a. Pathophysiology

Vitamin B_{12} participates in two biochemical reactions: the conversion of L-methylmalonyl coenzyme A into succinylcoenzyme A, and the formation of methionine by methylating homocysteine (Fig. 9–6). The enzyme methionine synthetase, which has vitamin B_{12} as a cofactor, converts homocysteine to methionine and couples the conversion of N^5-methyltetrahydrofolate to tetrahydrofolate (FH_4). FH_4 eventually enables the formation of DNA precursors (Fig. 9–7). This combination of reactions, the "methylfolate trap," is the agreed mechanism of megaloblastic anemias.[56]

Vitamin B_{12} deficiency results primarily from malabsorption of vitamin B_{12} from the small intestine rather than from dietary deficiency. Surgical resections of the proximal small intestine can result in malabsorption of vitamin B_{12}. Intrinsic factor, a glycoprotein produced in the wall of the gastric mucosa, enables absorption of vitamin B_{12}. Atrophy of the gastric mucosa secondary to autoimmune disease decreases production and availability of intrinsic factor, thus impairing vitamin B_{12} absorption. *Pernicious anemia* is vitamin B_{12} deficiency that results from this autoimmune disease and is associated with hypothyroidism.

Vitamin B_{12} deficiency not only produces megaloblastic changes in red cells but also can produce bilateral peripheral neuropathies. Degeneration of the lateral and posterior columns of the spinal cord can occur. Patients may exhibit symmetric paresthesias, decreased proprioception, unsteady gait, and diminished deep tendon reflexes. Demye-

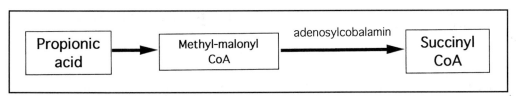

FIGURE 9–6. The cobalamin (vitamin B_{12})–dependent biochemical reaction in humans converting methylmalonyl CoA to succinyl CoA.

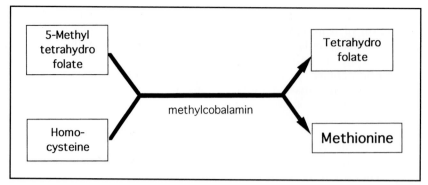

FIGURE 9–7. The transmethylation reaction utilizing cobalamin (vitamin B_{12}) as a cofactor for the enzyme methionine synthase. Nitrous oxide inhibits this reaction, preventing DNA production. This results in megaloblastic anemias.

lination occurs with the accumulation of odd-chain fatty acids secondary to impaired cobalamin-dependent degradation of methylmalonyl coenzyme A to succinyl CoA.[57] Progressive permanent neurologic deficits leading to paraplegia and bowel and bladder dysfunction can occur unless patients receive parenteral B_{12} therapy.

b. Anesthetic Considerations

Biologically active vitamin B_{12} contains cobalt in the reduced form (Co^+). Nitrous oxide administration irreversibly oxidizes Co^+ to Co^{++} and Co^{+++}, which inactivates vitamin B_{12} and methionine synthase (see Fig. 9–6). Patients with normal levels of vitamin B_{12} exposed to nitrous oxide rapidly replace inactivated vitamin B_{12} with active vitamin B_{12} stored in the body; however, patients with pre-existing vitamin B_{12} deficiencies exposed to nitrous oxide for less than 2 hours can develop megaloblastic anemia and severe neurologic deficits postoperatively.[58–60]

Nine documented cases have demonstrated postoperative exacerbations of unrecognized preoperative vitamin B_{12} deficiencies attributed to the intraoperative administration of nitrous oxide (Table 9–7).[58–63] All patients underwent brief exposure to nitrous oxide and developed neurologic deficits 2 1/2 to 6 weeks postoperatively. Before the surgical procedure, seven of eight patients had elevated mean corpuscular volume. Neurologic symptoms improved in all patients after they received parenteral vitamin B_{12} therapy. Since 5 to 10 per cent of patients have decreased serum cobalamin concentrations,[64, 65] Rabinowitz and colleagues recommend routine screening of vitamin B_{12} levels when contemplating nitrous oxide administration.[66]

However, the cost of routine vitamin B_{12} screening is prohibitive. The authors recommend substituting either desflurane or sevoflurane for nitrous oxide if red cell indices indicate increased mean corpuscular volume or if the history shows unexplained anemia or vitamin B_{12} deficiency.[60]

4. Folate Deficiency

Folate deficiency, unlike that of vitamin B_{12}, always develops from nutritional causes. Table 9–8 summarizes common causes of folate deficiency. Pharmacologic agents that contribute to folate deficiency include phenytoin, barbiturates, estrogen-containing oral contraceptives, and methotrexate, which inhibits folate reductase. Compared with the 2- to 12-year body reserve of vitamin B_{12}, stores of folate last only 4 to 5 months. Therefore, megaloblastic changes due to folate develop more rapidly. Clinical manifestations include a smooth tongue, hyperpigmentation, mental depression, and peripheral edema. Neurologic deficits do not occur with folate deficiency, in contradistinction to vitamin B_{12} deficiency. Treatment with oral folic acid affords hematologic improvement in 1 to 2 weeks.

D. OTHER CAUSES OF ANEMIA

1. Methemoglobin Anemia

Oxygen transport depends on maintaining intracellular hemoglobin in the reduced (Fe^{++}) state. Methemoglobin contains oxidized iron (Fe^{3+}), which cannot bind oxygen. Red cells contain less than 1 per cent methemoglobin. Methemoglobin reductase returns

TABLE 9–7

Vitamin B$_{12}$ Deficiency and Nitrous Oxide Administration*

Procedure	Hours of Exposure	Plasma B$_{12}$ Concentration	Outcome	Investigator	Symptoms
Hysterectomy	1.5	100 ng/L	Improved	Schilling[58]	Numbness, paresthesias, weakness
Laparotomy	1.5	180 ng/L	Improved	Schilling[58]	Paresthesias, weakness, loss of position and vibration senses
Anterior cervical fusion	2.25	<100 ng/L	Unknown	Berger[61]	Pain, numbness
Cervical decompression	2.3	<50 ng/L	Incomplete	Holloway[59]	Weakness, spasticity
L5-S1 disc	2.0	106 pg/mL	Resolved	Holloway[59]	Numbness in legs
Scalp, melanoma excision	3.5	<75 pm	Resolved	Flippo[61a]	Weakness, dizziness
Face, scalp	8	8 pg/mL	Resolved	Hadzic[60]	Paresthesias
Orthopedic	4	<40 pmol/L	Resolved	King[63]	Drowsiness, leg paresthesias
Uterine	2.25	<100 pg/mL	Improved	McMorrow[62]	Lower extremity paresthesias

*Each entry constitutes a single case of neurologic sequelae associated with nitrous oxide anesthesia in a patient with unrecognized vitamin B$_{12}$ deficiency.

methemoglobin to normal intracellular hemoglobin. If methemoglobin exceeds 15 g/L (1.5 g/dL) cyanosis will occur. A methemoglobin level greater than 35 per cent produces headache, weakness, and breathlessness. Oxidized hemoglobin affects the remaining hemoglobin by increasing its affinity for oxygen. This causes a shift of the oxyhemoglobin dissociation curve to the left, impairing unloading of oxygen bound to normal hemoglobin at tissues.

The presence of normal arterial oxygen tension with low measured arterial oxygen saturation along with a blood specimen having a chocolate-brown color regardless of exposure to air suggests the presence of methemoglobinemia. A significant amount of methemoglobin produces a pulse oximeter saturation reading of 85 per cent, regardless of P_aO_2.[67] Thus, the peripheral pulse oximetry reading may read spuriously low or high, depending on the arterial oxygen tension and the amount of methemoglobin (Fig. 9–8). Causes of methemoglobinemia include congenital absence of methemoglobin reductase, pharmacologic agents, and M hemoglobins. Administration of methylene blue, 1 to 2 mg/kg intravenously over 5 minutes, reduces ferric iron (Fe^{+++}) to the ferrous state (Fe^{++}) found in normal hemoglobin.

TABLE 9–8

Common Etiologies of Folate Deficiency

Increased requirement
   Infancy
   Pregnancy
   Hemolytic anemias
   Hyperthyroidism
Dietary
   Alcoholism
   Fad diets or other malnutrition
   Hyperalimentation (incomplete)
Malabsorption
   Alcoholism
   Small intestine disease
      Regional enteritis
      Sprue
      Small bowel resection (major)
      Lymphoma
      Congenital malabsorption of folate
Drug-induced
   Folate reductase inhibitors
   Antiepileptic agents
   Oral contraceptive and estrogens
   Sulfasalizine
Biochemical
   Congenital errors of folate metabolism

2. Sideroblastic Anemias

The sideroblastic anemias, inherited disorders of incorporation of iron into the hemoglobin molecule, have no anesthetic implications aside from the physiologic consequences of the anemia.

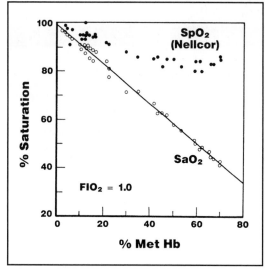

FIGURE 9–8. Measurement of per cent saturation of hemoglobin by a peripheral pulse oximeter and a co-oximeter at an inspired concentration of 100 per cent oxygen versus increasing concentration of methemoglobin. With increasing concentrations of methemoglobin, the peripheral pulse oximeter measures a saturation of 85 per cent. (From Barker SJ, Tremper KK, Hyatt BS, Zaccari J: Effects of methemoglobinemia on pulse oximetry and mixed venous oximetry. Anesthesiology 67:A171, 1987.)

3. Gaucher's Disease

An inherited disorder of glucocerebrosidase, Gaucher's affects phagocytic cells. Pancytopenia occurs, along with hepatosplenomegaly. The stomach may be encroached upon by the enlarged liver and spleen. Some patients may require platelet transfusion before surgery, but not of red cells, because the anemia is usually chronic and well-compensated.

III. HEMOSTASIS DISORDERS

A. OVERVIEW OF COAGULATION

1. The Coagulation Pathway

The coagulation factors participate in a series of activating reactions.[68] Most factors are glycoproteins synthesized in the liver that circulate as inactive molecules. Each factor serves as substrate in an enzymatic reaction catalyzed by the previous factor, which cleaves a polypeptide fragment, changing the inactive "zymogen" to an active enzyme

called a *serine protease* because its active site contains serine. The factors form four interrelated groups: contact activation, intrinsic, extrinsic, and common pathways (Fig. 9–9).

a. Contact Activation

Factor XII, high–molecular weight kininogen (HMWK), prekallikrein (PK), and factor XI form the contact, or "surface," activation group. Exposure of the negatively charged basement membrane of a vessel initiates coagulation protein surface activation when factor XII autoactivates upon binding to this negatively charged material. Factor XIIa then cleaves both factor XI (to form factor XIa) and prekallikrein (to form kallikrein) while HMWK assists in binding.

b. Intrinsic System

Factor XIa splits factor IX to form factor IXa, with calcium ion required. Then factor IXa activates factor X; calcium ion provides proximity of the reactants by binding them to

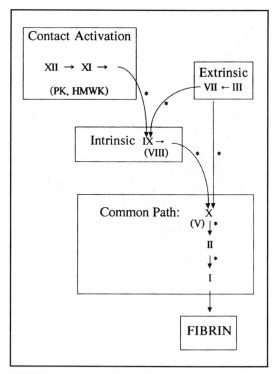

FIGURE 9–9. Procoagulant protein activation sequence divided into four groups. (Reproduced with permission from Horrow JC: Management of coagulation and bleeding disorders. In Kaplan JA (ed): Cardiac Anesthesia, 3rd ed. Philadelphia, WB Saunders, 1993.)

a phospholipid surface, while a glycoprotein cofactor, factor VIIIa, speeds the reaction.

c. Extrinsic System

This pathway begins with release into the vasculature of thromboplastin from tissues. It acts as a potent cofactor for initial activation of factor X by factor VIIa. Factor VIIa also activates factor IX, thus linking the extrinsic and intrinsic paths.

d. Common Pathway

With factor Va as cofactor, factor Xa splits prothrombin (factor II) to thrombin (factor IIa). Thrombin cleaves fibrinogen to form soluble fibrin monomer and small polypeptides, fibrinopeptides A and B. Fibrin monomers associate to form a soluble fibrin matrix, which factor XIII, activated by thrombin, cross-links into an insoluble clot. Factors II, VII, IX, and X depend on vitamin K to add γ-carboxyl groups to their glutamic acid residues, by which calcium tethers the factors to a phospholipid surface, thus facilitating molecular interactions. Some inhibitory coagulation proteins also depend on vitamin K.

2. Modulators of the Coagulation Pathway

a. Thrombin

Thrombin, the most important coagulation modulator, (1) activates factors V, VIII, and XIII; (2) cleaves fibrinogen to fibrin; (3) stimulates platelet recruitment; (4) releases tissue plasminogen activator (tPA) from endothelial cells; and, via thrombomodulin, (5) activates protein C, a substance that then inactivates factors Va and VIIIa.

b. Serpins

*Ser*ine *p*rotease *in*hibitors, or *serpins*, include α_1-antitrypsin, α_2-macroglobulin, and antithrombin (previously termed *antithrombin III*).[69] Antithrombin inhibits the activity of thrombin, of factors XIIa, XIa, IXa, and Xa, of kallikrein, and of the fibrinolytic molecule plasmin. Another serpin, protein C, degrades factors Va and VIIIa when it is activated by thrombin.

c. von Willebrand Factor

The von Willebrand factor (vWf) molecule is so massive that it is visible with the electron microscope. It protects circulating factor VIII from proteolytic enzymes in plasma and bridges normal platelets to damaged subendothelium by attaching to the glycoprotein Ib platelet receptor.

3. Platelet Function

Platelets provide phospholipid for coagulation factor reactions, contain their own coagulation factors, and secrete active substances that affect themselves, other platelets, the endothelium, and coagulation factors. Good hemostatic response depends on proper platelet adhesion, activation, and aggregation.

a. Adhesion

Exposure of the collagenous basement membrane beneath vessel endothelium allows vWf binding. Platelet membrane glycoprotein Ib attaches to vWf, anchoring the platelet to the vessel wall. Platelets so anchored then change shape, exposing glycoprotein receptor IIb/IIIa and releasing the contents of their dense granules (serotonin, adenosine diphosphate [ADP], and calcium), and α granules (platelet factor Va, β-thromboglobulin, platelet factor 4 [PF4], and adhesive proteins such as vWf, fibrinogen, vitronectin, and fibronectin).

b. Activation and Aggregation

Released ADP recruits additional platelets to the site of injury and stimulates formation of arachidonate, which platelet cyclooxygenase converts to thromboxane A_2. Serotonin and thromboxane A_2 are potent vasoconstrictors.[70] Sufficient agonist material results in platelet aggregation. Aggregation occurs when the adhesive proteins bridge the glycoprotein IIb/IIIa receptors of adjacent platelets.

4. Vascular Endothelium

What keeps clot from forming on the surface of the vascular endothelium? The answer is a combination of features: (1) negative charge; (2) heparan sulfate in the grid substance; (3) prostacyclin, adenosine, and protease inhibitors released by endothelial cells; (4) endothelial binding and clearance of activated coagulation factors; and (5) stimulation of fibrinolysis. Endothelium-derived *prostacyclin* opposes the vasoconstrictor effects of platelet-produced substances, inhibits platelet aggregation, and disaggregates clumped platelets.

The endothelial cell also helps clot formation. Like the platelet phospholipid surface, the endothelial cell surface facilitates factor activation. Thrombospondin, formed in endothelial cells and platelets, helps complete platelet aggregation and binds plasminogen, which decreases locally available plasmin, inhibiting fibrin breakdown.

5. Fibrinolysis

Normally, fibrin breaks down only in the vicinity of clot. This normal hemostatic process remodels formed clot, removing thrombus when endothelium heals. Like clot formation, clot breakdown occurs by intrinsic and extrinsic pathways, with the common end point of activating plasminogen, a serine protease circulating in zymogen form, to yield plasmin (Fig. 9–10). Plasmin splits fibrinogen or fibrin at specific sites. Plasma normally contains no circulating plasmin; thus, localized fibrinolysis, not systemic fibrinogenolysis, accompanies normal hemostasis.

Extrinsic Fibrinolysis. Endothelial cells release tPA. Both tPA and a related substance, urokinase plasminogen activator (uPA), are serine proteases that split plasminogen to form plasmin. tPA activity is negligible except in the vicinity of fibrin. Thus, plasmin formation remains localized to sites of clot formation.

Intrinsic Fibrinolysis. Factor XIIa can cleave plasminogen to plasmin. The physiologic importance of this pathway for fibrin breakdown has not been established and may be clinically irrelevant. *Streptokinase*, made by bacteria, and *urokinase*, found in human urine, both cleave plasminogen to plasmin, but with low fibrin affinity, allowing both systemic plasminemia and fibrinogenolysis in addition to fibrinolysis. Acetylated streptokinase plasminogen activator complex (ASPAC) possesses systemic lytic activity intermediate to that of tPA or streptokinase by requiring for its activity deacetylation in blood. Streptokinase, ASPAC, and tPA lyse thrombi associated with myocardial infarction, dissolving clots that form on atheromatous plaque. Clinically significant bleeding may result from administration of any of these exogenous activators.[71] Fibrinolysis also accompanies cardiopulmonary bypass. Clot lysis after operation contributes to postoperative hemorrhage and the need to administer allogeneic blood products. Fibrin degradation products intercalate between fibrin monomers, preventing cross-linking and exerting an antihemostatic effect.

B. PLATELET DISORDERS

1. von Willebrand Disease

Investigation of an autosomal dominant pattern of bleeding in a family of patients on an island off the coast of Finland resulted in the discovery of von Willebrand disease (vWd). This entity, caused by insufficient or abnormal von Willebrand factor (vWf) and now recognized as an entity distinct from hemophilia, requires a variety of different

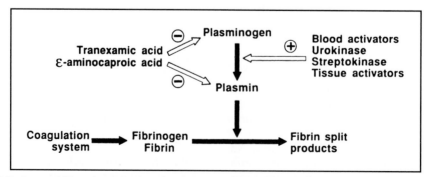

FIGURE 9–10. Pathway of fibrinolysis, showing the action of fibrinolytic activators and synthetic antifibrinolytic agents. (From Horrow JC: Management of coagulation and bleeding disorders. In Kaplan JA (ed): Cardiac Anesthesia, 3rd ed. Philadelphia, WB Saunders, 1993.)

therapeutic approaches. Most important, vWd is the most common inherited bleeding disorder.

a. Pathophysiology

Endothelial cells secrete vWf, an enormous protein composed of multimers of molecular weights ranging from 600 Kd to 20 million daltons. The vWf monomer weighs 250 Kd. Storage of vWf occurs in Weibel-Palade bodies in endothelial cells and in alpha granules in platelets. Thrombin releases vWf from platelets, and histamine releases it from endothelial cells.

vWf binds to the subendothelium. Intact endothelium prevents subendothelial vWf, bound to collagen, from contacting circulating platelets in the vasculature. Vessel injury destroys this barrier, thus exposing bound vWf to circulating platelets and their surface glycoprotein receptor GPIb. The resulting platelet adhesion initiates the platelet phase of coagulation, forming a platelet plug. Ristocetin, an antibiotic similar to vancomycin, facilitates GPIb–vWf interaction. It also thus provides an assay for vWf activity.

Von Willebrand factor has two actions on factor VIII. First, it associates with factor VIII via noncovalent interaction at the N terminals of both molecules. This association protects factor VIII from degradation and removal, prolonging its plasma half-life. Second, vWf facilitates secretion of factor VIII. vWf behaves as a transportation vehicle designed to bring factor VIII close to the phospholipid surface of platelets to facilitate factor VIII's hemostatic role.

There are several types of vWd. Classic vWd (type I) involves decreased amounts of vWf but the normal array of vWf multimers. In type II vWd an abnormal multimer pattern occurs, with selective depletion of those of the highest molecular weight. In type IIA both intermediate and large multimers are absent. In type IIB only the largest multimers are missing: they are synthesized and secreted but are abnormal. They bind spontaneously to normal platelets, accelerating clearance of both platelets and those large vWf multimers.

As compared with types I and II, in type III no vWf is synthesized. Lack of immune system exposure to vWf determinants places patients with type III vWd at risk for developing anti-vWf antibodies.

In *platelet-type vWd* the abnormality is of GPIb rather than vWf. This abnormality allows the larger vWf multimers to bind to GPIb, accelerating their clearance and inducing mild thrombocytopenia. Thus, clinically, platelet-type vWd resembles type IIB vWd. Table 9–9 summarizes the major types of vWd.

b. Clinical Features

Impaired platelet adhesion results in a bleeding diathesis. Patients present with mucocutaneous hemorrhages rather than hemarthroses or muscle hemorrhages as occurs in hemophilia. Ecchymoses, epistaxis, and excessive bleeding after trauma, at minor surgery, or with menses characterize vWd. Concentrations of vWf vary much with time, owing to its acute phase reactant nature: infection, pregnancy, birth control pills, surgery, and

TABLE 9–9

Major Types of von Willebrand Disease

| Classification | Prevalence (%) | Laboratory Findings | | Molecular Pathology |
		vWf:Ag	R:Co	
I (classic)	70–80	↓	↓	Normal multimers but all decreased in quantity
IIA	10–12	↓	↓↓	Intermediate and large multimers decreased
IIB	3–5	↓	Near nl	Abnormal large multimers that bind to platelets
III	1–3	None	None	No vWf present
Platelet-type	0–1	↓	↓	Normal vWf; platelet GPIb receptors bind large multimers*

*Treatment of platelet-type vWd is platelet transfusion rather than desmopressin (for type I) or with factor concentrate.

Modified from Montgomery RR, Coller BS: Von Willebrand disease. In Colman RW, Hirsh J, Marder VJ, Salzman EW (eds): Hemostasis and Thrombosis. Philadelphia, JB Lippincott, 1994.

Key: ↓, decreased; ↓↓, markedly decreased; vWf:Ag, vW antigen measurement; R:Co, ristocetin cofactor activity measurement; near nl, nearly normal.

other forms of stress increase vWf concentrations. This variable clinical expressivity may confound attempts at diagnosis.

c. Diagnosis

The hallmark of vWd is a prolonged bleeding time. Although vWf deficiency affects factor VIII concentrations, the activated partial thromboplastin time (aPTT) remains an insensitive test for vWd. A prolonged aPTT denotes moderately severe vWd. Confirmation of vWd obtains from measurement of its antigen by immunoassay (vWf:Ag) and by ristocetin cofactor activity (vWfR:Co). Because ristocetin induces binding of vWf to platelet membrane glycoprotein Ib, the amounts of vWf in plasma correlate with the degree of platelet aggregation caused by ristocetin (Fig. 9–11).[149] Various sophisticated tests can distinguish among the various types of vWd; immunoelectrophoresis permits identification of the various multimeric structures of vWf and thus constitutes the basis for such typing.

d. Incidence

Nearly all vWd demonstrates autosomal dominant inheritance. Estimates of the incidence of vWd vary widely, owing to biases of ascertainment in the populations studied; however, back-calculation of alleleic frequencies from the known prevalence of homozygous type III vWd produces an expected incidence of 1.4 to 5 cases per 1000 population. Most of these patients have type I vWd (70 to 80 per cent). Type IIA constitutes 10 to 12 per cent of vWd patients, whereas type IIB occurs in 3 to 5 per cent. The homozygous or compound heterozygous deficiency states (type III) constitute 1 to 3 per cent of patients, whereas platelet-type vWd is more rare.

Patients with group O blood exhibit slightly lower concentrations of vWf than others. For this reason, they may receive a misdiagnosis of vWd.[72]

e. Treatment and Anesthetic Considerations

Desmopressin, a synthetic variation of vasopressin, releases vWf and factor VIII from endothelium, usually tripling or quadrupling plasma vWf concentrations.[73] It is the therapy of choice for patients with mild or moderate type I vWd. A trial of desmopressin therapy, with confirmation of suitably increased ristocetin cofactor activity, should be pursued before it is used in patients presenting for surgery. The mechanism by which desmopressin releases vWf and factor VIII remains incompletely described; investigators postulate a secondary messenger, possibility from monocytes. Desmopressin may be administered either as an intravenous preparation, 0.3 µg/kg over 20 to 30 minutes, or as a concentrated intranasal preparation of desmopressin solution, 75 µg per nostril. Most patients respond to repeated desmopressin doses given every 12 to 24 hours without tachyphylaxis.

In patients with type IIA vWd, desmopressin releases only the lower–molecular weight monomers of vWf; thus, it is either transiently effective or ineffective. Likewise, release of the large abnormal multimers of vWf in patients with type IIB vWd results in accelerated thrombocytopenia. The extraordinarily rare patient with platelet-type vWd requires replacement therapy with normal platelets because the defect resides in the platelet and not with the vWf that is synthesized.

Patients with type III vWd have no vWf for desmopressin to release and thus require replacement vWf from plasma concentrates rather than desmopressin. Choices include cryoprecipitate and commercial concentrates.

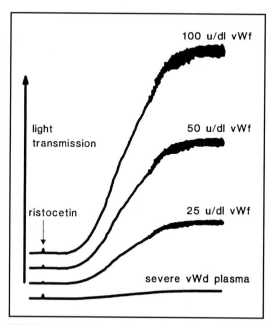

FIGURE 9–11. Platelet agglutination measurement using the ristocetin cofactor assay. Ristocetin agglutination of platelets depends on the presence of von Willebrand factor, thus forming the basis for an assay of vWf activity. (Reproduced with permission from Montgomery RR, Coller BS: Von Willebrand disease. In Colman RW, Hirsch J, Marder VJ, Salzman EW (eds): Hemostasis and Thrombosis. Philadelphia, JB Lippincott, 1994.)

Cryoprecipitate cannot be treated for viral attenuation, so there is risk for transmission of infectious disease. Patients with long-standing vWd may have designated donors who provide cryoprecipitate when needed via plasmapheresis to decrease infectious complications. Commercial factor VIII concentrates contain both vWf and factor VIII. They are treated via heat, solvents, and/or detergents to reduce infectious risk, and thus are preferred over cryoprecipitate.[74] However, the amount of vWf multimer present in these concentrates may vary widely. Currently, the concentrate product Humate P is most commonly used.

A patient undergoing major surgery requires a vWf concentration of 0.8 to 1.0 U/mL. The amount of vWf concentrate to administer is calculated by first determining the difference between the patient's plasma level of vWf and the target value. For every 0.02 U/mL of needed additional vWf plasma concentration, 1.0 U/kg body weight of vWf concentrate must be administered. Thus, assuming zero initial vWf, a dose of 40 U/kg would achieve the 0.8 U/mL target. Following surgery, vWf concentrations should remain at or above 0.4 U/mL. Likewise, factor VIII levels should remain above 0.4 U/mL for at least 5 days after operation. Consultation with a trusted hematologist is strongly advised when planning major surgery for a patient with vWd. Both vWf and factor VIII possess half-lives of approximately 12 hours.

Pregnant patients with vWd often require no therapy, owing to three- to fourfold increases in concentrations of vWf that occur by the third trimester. Hemostatic complications during labor and delivery are uncommon; however, treatment postpartum should be strongly considered, owing to rapidly decreasing plasma vWf concentrations, which can result in postpartum hemorrhage.

f. Acquired von Willebrand Disease

Von Willebrand disease can result from hypothyroidism; then, restoration of normal thyroid activity returns vWf concentrations to normal. Antibodies to vWf may occur in multiple myeloma, collagen vascular diseases, or lymphoproliferative disorders. Patients with ventricular septal defects may lack the larger molecular weight multimers of vWf; however, no bleeding disorder is associated with this loss. vWd may also accompany mitral valve prolapse or angiodysplasia.

g. Von Willebrand Disease As a Cause of Surgical Bleeding

Because patients with vWd may present first with abnormal bleeding at surgery, this most common hereditary bleeding disorder should form part of the differential diagnosis of excessive intraoperative surgical hemorrhage. Unfortunately, the hemostatic tests commonly performed in the operating room cannot yield a diagnosis of vWd. Fortunately, however, treatment with desmopressin improves hemostasis in most vWd patients and exacerbates it only in the 3 to 5 per cent of vWd patients who have type IIB. For this reason, patients who exhibit abnormal surgical bleeding and who respond to desmopressin deserve hematology consultation and an appropriate series of diagnostic tests once the stresses of surgery abate.

2. Heparin-Induced Thrombocytopenia and Thrombosis

Some patients develop decreased platelet counts with prolonged exposure to heparin. This heparin-induced thrombocytopenia (HIT) can be classified into two types: type I is a moderate, reversible decrease in platelet count without associated clinical complications. It is common. In contrast, the less frequent type II response consists of severe thrombocytopenia, immune responses, and significant morbidity and mortality. The latter disorder is addressed in this section.

a. Pathophysiology

Patients with type II HIT develop an IgG antibody to a complex composed of heparin and platelet factor 4 (PF4). This complex, localized to the platelet surface, binds that IgG antibody, which then activates the platelets via their FcγII receptors.[75] In addition, the IgG activates endothelium via the same heparin–PF4 complex.[76, 77]

In a subset of HIT patients platelet activation results in so-called white clot syndrome, in which clumps of platelets obstruct vascular channels, thrombosing those vessels. Thrombosis occurs rarely in the absence of an endothelial defect. Damaged endothelium, however, like that formed from a surgical or endovascular interventional procedure or endogenous pathologic event such as atheroma rupture, forms a locus for platelet adhesion, aggregation, and subsequent activation. Extrusion of PF4 from platelet granules upon activation then neutralizes heparin in its vicinity, thus no longer inhibiting coagulation events and amplifying antibody activity by providing additional antigen (i.e., heparin–PF4 complex; Fig. 9–12).

b. Prevalence

The prevalence of type II HIT remains controversial and is variously reported, owing to imperfect tests for the disorder; however, clinical trials utilizing respected diagnostic criteria yield a prevalence of 1 per cent after 7 days of unfractionated heparin therapy and 3 per cent after 14 days.[77] The prevalence of thrombosis accompanying HIT may be as high as 1 per cent of all patients receiving unfractionated heparin for more than 5 days.[77, 78] The high likelihood that HIT will progress to thrombosis dictates the need for prompt recognition and intervention upon its discovery.

The type of heparin affects the incidence of type II HIT: 5.5 per cent of patients who receive bovine heparin but only 1.0 per cent of those receiving porcine heparin develop the syndrome.[79] Although the incidence of HIT is dose related, the disorder can occur during

treatment of deep vein thrombosis, during prophylactic treatment with low doses, from heparin flush solution, from heparin-bonded intravascular catheters, and with administration of low–molecular weight heparins.[80–85]

c. Diagnosis

Type II HIT occurs within 2 weeks of commencing heparin therapy (median 10 days). The platelet count decreases steadily, usually to between $20 \cdot 10^9/L$ and $150 \cdot 10^9/L$. Daily platelet count determinations permit prompt recognition of the onset of HIT.

Three diagnostic methods exist to confirm clinical suspicion of HIT. First, the serotonin release assay, performed on the patient's plasma, incubated with heparin and washed donor platelets containing radiolabeled serotonin, detects the presence of antibody in the patient's plasma by release of serotonin from the donor platelets.[86] Second, donor platelets and the patient's plasma induce platelet degranulation in the presence of heparin in affected patients.[87] Third, an enzyme-linked immunosorbent assay (ELISA) can detect antibodies to the heparin–PF4 complex.[76] Although the serotonin release test is more sensitive and specific, platelet aggregation is more readily available but is less sensitive (81 per cent).[88] The type and formulation of heparin for testing in the serotonin release and platelet aggregation studies should duplicate those of the formulation given to the

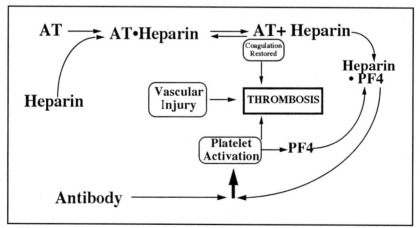

FIGURE 9–12. Depiction of the events leading to heparin-induced thrombosis. Heparin and antithrombin (AT) form a complex (AT • heparin). Platelet factor 4 (PF4) released on platelet activation inactivates heparin, driving the dissociation reaction of the AT • heparin complex to the right, thus restoring coagulation in the vicinity of platelets. In the presence of vascular injury, restored coagulation and activated platelets lead to thrombus formation. Prolonged exposure to heparin leads in some patients to formation of antibodies to the heparin • PF4 complex, activating platelets and releasing additional PF4, which can then fuel the reactions to produce more heparin • PF4 complex and increase thrombus formation.

patient. For example, in a patient diagnosed with type II HIT, a plan to administer low–molecular weight heparin instead of unfractionated heparin should begin with testing of the patient's plasma with low–molecular weight heparin before its administration.[84]

Clinicians should accept a diagnosis of HIT with great reluctance in the absence of an appropriate diagnostic test. Such behavior has served unnecessarily to increase artificially the presumed incidence of this disorder; nevertheless, prompt cessation of heparin exposure upon detection of a steadily decreasing platelet count remains an essential part of medical management.

Patients with baseline thrombocytosis may exhibit decreases in platelet count that reach a nadir within the normal range. Such decreases can herald the onset of HIT. For this reason, any substantial decrease in platelet count should raise concern about the development of HIT, even if the absolute platelet count is not below $150 \cdot 10^9/L$.

d. Treatment and Prevention

Because bleeding from the thrombocytopenia in HIT is uncommon, platelet transfusions are unnecessary and often are contraindicated, as they may induce or exacerbate thrombosis. The first action is to halt infusion of heparin. This includes removal of any heparin-bonded materials from the patient's vasculature[83] and removal of heparin flush solutions. Despite the formation of intravascular thrombus, these patients should not receive any form of heparin unless it has been proven safe by diagnostic testing in vitro.

In type II HIT venous thrombosis is much more common than arterial thrombosis; how-ever, the former often escapes detection, thus allowing arterial occlusive consequences to gain more clinical attention. The devastating sequelae of type II HIT with thrombosis cannot be understated: amputation of one or several limbs is often necessary, and death is not rare.

What should be done for the patients who require vascular surgery for thrombosis associated with HIT? Such surgery should either proceed without benefit of anticoagulant or employ an alternative to heparin (Table 9–10). These alternatives include ancrod, a snake venom, the heparinoid danaparoid (Orgoran), hirudin, plasmapheresis to deplete antibody levels, and antiplatelet drugs such as aspirin, dipyridamole, and Iloprost.[89–104] Patients may also receive oral anticoagulation with coumadin for suitable procedures.

Ancrod provides anticoagulation by cleaving fibrinogen abnormally. The resultant fragments clear via the reticuloendothelial system. This fibrinogen depletion requires a day for onset, and administration of banked products, fresh-frozen plasma, or cryoprecipitate to restore normal coagulation. Slow onset and prolonged bleeding render it a poor substitute for heparin.[105]

Danaproid consists of a mixture of low–molecular weight heparin fragments and dermatans. The latter are naturally occurring glycosaminoglycan polymers similar to heparins. They anticoagulate via activation of heparin cofactor II rather than antithrombin. Use of danaproid for hemodialysis[106] and for cardiopulmonary bypass[107, 108] has had varying success.

Plasmapheresis depletes antibodies by removing them from the circulation. The adverse response to heparin cannot occur with-

TABLE 9–10

Strategies for Anticoagulation in Heparin-Induced Thrombocytopenia

Modality	Cost	Labor	Advantages	Disadvantages
Ancrod	Moderate	Moderate	Effective	Slow onset, bleeding, need banked blood products
Danaproid	Unknown	Minimal	Effective	Reversibility unclear
Plasmapheresis	High	Intense	Effective	Time-consuming
Iloprost	Unknown	Low	Effective	Hypotension; drug not available
Aspirin + dipyridamole	Low	None	Simple	Not completely effective
Coumadin or warfarin	Low	Low	Simple	Difficult to reverse
Hirudin	Unknown	None	Effective	Not reversible
Delay of surgery	None	None	Simple	Urgent procedures cannot wait

out sufficient quantities of circulating antibody. Discontinuation of heparin also permits antibody concentrations to decrease with time. Thus, simply waiting several months following a type II HIT event may permit benign reexposure to heparin. In vitro testing of patient's plasma should precede such reexposure. In many instances, a single reexposure for vascular or cardiac surgery proves benign despite a diagnosis of type II HIT. Such instances may represent inappropriate diagnostic methods (i.e., false positives).

Antiplatelet drugs are useful as they block activation, thus preventing PF4 release. The most potent of these agents, Iloprost, also caused severe vasodilation. Iloprost is no longer available. Other agents such as aspirin, triclopidine, and dipyridamole may not provide sufficient protection in all cases.

Although low–molecular weight heparins may not cross-react, a growing list of case reports in which low–molecular weight heparins have induced type II HIT dictates in vitro diagnostic testing with the type and lot of drug proposed for administration to the patient.[109, 110]

3. Idiopathic Thrombocytopenic Purpura

An autoimmune disease, idiopathic thrombocytopenic purpura largely affects older children and young adults. An antiplatelet antibody, usually IgG, causes destruction of platelets in the spleen. Treatment consists of steroids and other immunosuppressive agents such as azathioprine and cyclophosphamide. In refractory cases, splenectomy is considered. Since platelet counts may be quite low (fewer than $20 \cdot 10^9/L$), mucosal bleeding constitutes a significant hazard requiring utmost care during airway instrumentation. Maternal antibodies may cross the placenta to cause neonatal thrombocytopenic purpura.

4. Thrombotic Thrombocytopenic Purpura

This uncommon, often catastrophic, abnormality features the triad of consumptive intravascular thrombocytopenia, microangiopathic hemolytic anemia, and various neurologic changes.[111] Fever and renal failure are less consistent additional features. A disease of middle age, it affects women twice as

often as men. In a similar disease that occurs mostly in children, the hemolytic-uremic syndrome (HUS), kidney involvement overshadows neurologic abnormalities.

a. Pathophysiology

Hyaline thrombi occlude the capillaries and precapillary arterioles of multiple organs, specifically heart, brain, kidneys, pancreas, and adrenals. The lungs and liver are usually spared. Neurologic symptoms include headache, paresis, dysphasia, aphasia, obtundation, seizures, paresthesias, and vision disturbances. When present, congestive heart failure usually is not severe. Unlike thrombotic lesions associated with consumptive coagulopathy, the thrombi of thrombotic thrombocytopenic purpura (TTP) contain large amounts of vWf and a predominance of platelets over fibrin.

The cause of TTP remains controversial. Theories involve defects in prostacyclin synthesis, inadequate suppression of platelet-activating factor, and inappropriate secretion of unusually large multimers of vWf. Those multimers can agglutinate platelets in the presence of small cationic molecules similar to the antibiotic ristocetin (see section on von Willebrand disease). Currently, most interest centers around vWf as a mediator, endothelial cell injury being the inciting cause. The HUS may result from injury to renal endothelium, which releases the abnormal vWf.

Treatment of HUS and TTP involves immediate infusion of fresh-frozen plasma, followed as soon as possible by exchange transfusion using fresh-frozen plasma. This presumably removes the substances that aggregate platelets. Glucocorticoids are administered because of the possibility of an autoimmune cause in some cases. Red cell transfusions should occur only if anemia is significant. Platelet transfusions may exacerbate the thrombosis. For this reason they are reserved only for hemorrhage or intracranial bleeding. Disorders refractory to these initial modalities may be treated with vincristine, azathioprine, and cryosupernatant, the product remaining once the vWf–rich cryoprecipitate is removed from plasma. Splenectomy is another option; however, TTP may not respond to splenectomy. Indeed, TTP has occurred in asplenic patients.

b. Anesthetic Considerations

Splenectomy or other surgery should not proceed until optimal control of the thrombotic process has been achieved with other modalities. Patients may require perioperative steroid infusion to compensate for adrenal suppression from long-term steroid administration. Desmopressin is contraindicated for treating intraoperative hemorrhage. Instead, fresh-frozen plasma or cryosupernatant should be administered and platelet transfusions withheld, if possible, when the platelet count is greater than $100 \cdot 10^9/L$.

5. Rare Inherited Platelet Disorders

Absence of the platelet membrane IIb/IIIa receptor *(Glanzmann's thrombasthenia)* prevents aggregation. Because ristocetin, an antibiotic, agglutinates platelets directly via Ib receptors and vWF, platelets of affected patients exhibit normal aggregation with ristocetin but none with adenosine diphosphate (ADP) or collagen. Absence of the Ib receptor *(Bernard-Soulier syndrome)* yields no agglutination with ristocetin, but aggregation to ADP is normal since the IIb/IIIa receptor is intact. vWd also exhibits impaired platelet adhesion but normal aggregation; decreased amounts of vWF antigen distinguish it from the Bernard-Soulier syndrome. In platelet *storage pool deficiency*, impairment of dense granule secretion yields no ADP upon adhesion. Addition of collagen in vitro does not aggregate platelets because ADP is not released, whereas added ADP initiates some aggregation (Table 9–11).

Patients known to have one of these diseases may present for surgery. The authors recommend transfusion of allogeneic platelets obtained from one or a few donors by plasmapheresis. The platelet count does not reliably reflect the contribution of circulating platelets to hemostasis and should not guide replacement therapy. The sophisticated tests mentioned above may not be readily available at most institutions. Consultation with a trusted hematologist and with a laboratory pathologist should facilitate surgical management of these patients.

6. Polycythemia Rubra Vera

Polycythemia rubra vera is addressed as a platelet disorder because its platelet component is the most clinically significant one. Increased production of all cellular blood elements results in hemoglobin concentrations exceeding 20 g/dL, platelet counts exceeding $800 \cdot 10^9/L$, and leukocyte counts greater than 25,000 per cubic millimeter. The platelets formed exhibit impaired aggregation, predisposing the patient to hemorrhagic events. Hyperviscosity from the excessive cellular elements leads to stasis and sludging in the vasculature, predisposing to thrombotic events. Appropriate preoperative interventions include phlebotomy to bring the hemoglobin concentration below 16 g/dL.

C. COAGULATION PROTEIN DISORDERS

1. The Hemophilias

Recognized since Talmudic times, the sex-linked bleeding disorders now known as the *hemophilias* are abnormalities of two different coagulation factors, factor VIII and factor IX. Next to vWd, they are the most common inherited disorders of hemostasis.

TABLE 9–11

Diagnosis of Some Inherited Platelet Disorders

Disorder Deficiency	Glanzmann's Thrombasthenia GP IIb/IIIa	Bernard-Soulier Syndrome GP Ib	Storage Pool Deficiency Dense Granule Secretion	von Willebrand Disease vWf
Platelet adhesion	Normal	Absent	Normal	Absent
Platelet aggregation	Absent	Normal	Impaired	Normal
Ristocetin agglutination	Occurs	Absent	Occurs	Absent or decreased
vWF:Ag level	Normal	Normal	Normal	Low

Key: GP, glycoprotein receptor: vWF, von Willebrand factor; vWF:Ag, von Willebrand factor antigen.
From Kaplan JA: Cardiac Anesthesia, 3rd ed. Philadelphia, WB Saunders, 1993.

a. Incidence

Both types of hemophilia occur worldwide in all cultures at similar rates. Approximately 2 males per 10,000 exhibit hemophilia (1 occurrence per 10,000 whole population). Approximately 85 per cent of these cases are hemophilia A, a defect in factor VIII; the remaining 15 per cent are hemophilia B, a defect in factor IX.

Despite the inherited nature of the hemophilias, about one third of hemophiliacs have no affected family members. This observation implies a high mutation rate for the disease. The rare female patient who acquires hemophilia is (1) the offspring of a male hemophiliac and female carrier, (2) a carrier female with extreme lyonization of the normal X chromosome, (3) a Turner's syndrome child (XO genotype) of a male hemophiliac or a female carrier, or (4) has a rare autosomal dominant form of hemophilia A.

b. Pathophysiology

In hemophilia A, the factor VIII molecule is synthesized but defective. Because the antigenic determinants are fully present, the carrier state yields normal factor VIII antigen levels but half as much factor VIII coagulant activity. Unlike hemophilia A patients, those with hemophilia B may or may not possess factor IX antigenic material. Factor IXa splits factor X, utilizing the phospholipid surface of the platelet as a meetingplace and factor VIII as a cofactor. Deficiency of either factor VIII or factor IX impairs activation of factor X, the first coagulation factor in the common pathways (Fig. 9–13).

c. Clinical Features and Anesthetic Considerations

Platelets maintain normal function in hemophiliacs. Thus, minor cuts and abrasions do not bleed excessively; however, hemarthroses affecting the knees, elbows, ankles, shoulders, hips, and wrists, in descending order of frequency, lead to disabling long-term sequelae. Some patients describe an aura of warmth, tingling, restlessness, or anxiety as much as 2 hours before joint hemorrhage symptoms appear. Intramuscular hematomas are also common. Hemophiliacs may present for surgery for presumed appendicitis, owing to lower quadrant abdominal pain secondary to a psoas muscle hematoma. Expertly performed ultrasonography may avoid such misdiagnosis. Bleeding into the tongue or muscles surrounding the airway can rapidly obstruct airflow, requiring prompt establishment of an artificial airway. Hematuria is common. If it is detected, antifibrinolytic medications that might prevent upper urinary tract clot lysis, thus inciting obstruction, must be avoided.

Epistaxis occurs only in moderate and severe hemophilia. About one quarter of hemophiliacs die from intracranial bleeding. Repeated hemarthroses cause joint instability, eventually resulting in chronic synovitis and then ankylosis of large joints. Protective measures taken by parents to prevent trauma injury often cause psychological sequelae and reactive risk-taking in adolescents. The excessive financial burden ($15,000 to $100,000 per year) creates tremendous social disruption.

Mild hemophilia is defined as more than 5 per cent normal factor coagulant activity. Such cases may not be diagnosed until adult life. Moderately severe hemophilia consists of between 1 and 5 per cent of normal activity and severe cases, less than 1 per cent of normal factor VIII or factor IX levels.

d. Treatment

Surgery requires factor VIII concentrations in plasma of 80 per cent to 100 per cent.

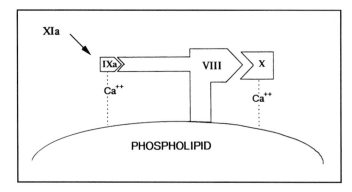

FIGURE 9–13. Cartoon of the "ten-ase" complex, composed of factors IXa, VIII, and X, calcium, and the phospholipid surface of platelets. (Reproduced with permission from Horrow JC: Desmopressin and antifibrinolytics. In Gravlee GP (ed): Blood Conservation. Int Anesth Clin 28:230, 1990.)

After surgery, levels above 30 per cent should persist 10 to 14 days. These concentrations are recommended for more extended periods (4 to 6 weeks) following extensive orthopedic procedures. For patients with hemophilia B, surgery requires plasma concentrations of 60 per cent of factor IX coagulant activity and at least 20 per cent for 10 to 14 days after surgery.

Hemophilia A patients may require only administration of desmopressin, which yields a two- to fourfold increase in factor VIII coagulant activity in patients with mild to moderate disease. Patients with severe disease do not respond to desmopressin. As with vWd, a trial of desmopressin therapy to confirm adequate factor VIII concentrations should be conducted before elective surgery.

When desmopressin is inadequate or inappropriate, factor VIII must be supplied from either concentrate or cryoprecipitate. Calculation of the replacement dose proceeds in a straightforward manner from the patient's deficiency: each infused unit per kilogram body weight of factor VIII yields a 2 per cent rise in plasma factor VIII coagulant activity. Fresh-frozen plasma alone cannot supply enough factor VIII because of the great volumes needed.

Replacement therapy in patients with hemophilia B requires allogeneic blood products. Desmopressin does not affect plasma concentrations of factor IX. The half-life of factor IX (about 24 hours) considerably exceeds that of factor VIII (8 to 12 hours), permitting less frequent factor IX replacement after the surgery; however, the bioavailability of factor IX is half that of factor VIII. Thus, each unit per kilogram body weight of factor IX administered yields only a 1 per cent increase in plasma IX activity. Following surgery, for which a level of 60 per cent is required, factor IX concentrations of 40 per cent activity should be sustained for several days, then at least 20 per cent activity for up to 14 days total. Longer periods of factor IX supplementation should accompany major orthopedic surgery. For examples of calculations of factor VIII or factor IX dosing, see Table 9–12.

Because the target levels of factor IX are substantially lower than those of factor VIII, fresh-frozen plasma may in some cases of mild hemophilia B provide appropriate replacement. Otherwise, prothrombin complex concentrates are used. These products contain factors II, VII, IX, and X and are obtained by absorption from plasma and subsequent elution followed by concentration. Some preparations add heparin to inhibit activation of the concentrated factors. Preparations recently marketed provide factor IX plus only minute amounts of factors II, VII, and X. These reduce the possibility of inducing consumptive coagulopathy in response to activated factors.

Deep venous thrombosis, with or without pulmonary embolism and other thrombotic consequences, may follow administration of prothrombin complex concentrate.[112–115] Some centers administer subcutaneous heparin every 8 hours along with the concentrate, even for major surgical procedures, to prevent thrombotic complications.

e. Other Anesthetic Considerations in Hemophilia

First, the expert consultation of an experienced hematologist should be obtained. Sec-

---

TABLE 9–12

Sample Calculations of Replacement Factors for Hemophilias

Hemophilia A

Initial plasma activity:	10%
Target plasma activity:	100% factor VIII
Patient's body weight:	80 kg
Calculation:	$(100 - 10) \times 80 \text{ kg} \times 1 \text{ U}/2\% = 3600 \text{ U}$

This can be provided by four vials of factor VIII concentrate, each vial containing 1000 U.

Hemophilia B

Initial plasma activity:	5%
Target plasma activity:	60% factor IX
Patient's body weight:	80 kg
Calculation:	$(60 - 5) \times 80 \text{ kg} \times 1 \text{ U}/1\% = 4400 \text{ U}$

This can be supplied by prothrombin complex concentrate.

ond, intramuscular medications are avoided and the patient must not take any aspirin compounds within 1 week of the planned surgery. Third, surgical colleagues and the scheduling office should schedule minor surgical procedures close in time to major ones, to obviate expensive repeat replacement therapy. Fourth, adjunctive use of antifibrinolytic medications such as aminocaproic acid or tranexamic acid is encouraged for oral surgery procedures.

Fifth, scheduled surgery should be early in the week to provide optimal laboratory services for factor assays. Likewise, availability of replacement concentrates must be ensured before commencing surgery, as well as at least 2 weeks' worth of replacement therapy to sustain coagulant levels after surgery. Finally, the anesthesiologist should be an active part of the patient's clinical team by maintaining frequent necessary communication with the primary physician, surgeon, and hematologist.

2. Factor XI Deficiency

Decreased plasma concentrations of factor XI occasionally cause bleeding after trauma or surgery, but not spontaneous bleeding. Because episodes rarely correlate with factor XI concentrations, prediction of hemorrhage for an individual patient is not possible. Inheritance follows an autosomal dominant pattern. This disease is most common in Jewish people of eastern European descent.[116]

Target plasma concentrations of factor XI for surgery are 20 per cent activity. Fresh-frozen plasma 10 mL/kg provides this level. Because the half-life of factor XI is 60 to 80 hours, daily or every other day infusions after surgery suffice. As with the hemophilias, administration of antifibrinolytic medications benefits oral surgery procedures.

3. Other Factor Deficiencies

A number of other known factor deficiencies are much more rare than those discussed previously. Each demonstrates autosomal-recessive inheritance.

Factor VII deficiency mimics hemophilia. Joint and muscle hemorrhages are the usual clinical presentation. Replacement is provided with either prothrombin complex concentrate or fresh-frozen plasma. Because

prothrombin concentrates are measured according to factor IX (not factor VII) activity, the exact amount patients with factor VII deficiency need must be estimated and an adequate factor VII concentration in blood subsequently verified.

Prothrombin deficiency yields prolongations of both prothrombin time and partial thromboplastin time. In contrast to hemophilia, hemarthroses are uncommon; easy bruising, gastrointestinal bleeding, and epistaxis do occur. Prothrombin complex concentrate or fresh-frozen plasma can replace the deficient factor.

Factor X deficiency presents similarly to prothrombin deficiency. Replacement with prothrombin complex concentrate or fresh-frozen plasma also applies. Factor X deficiency is extremely rare.

Factor V deficiency, another very rare coagulopathy, requires fresh-frozen plasma for treatment. The dose is 20 mL/kg every 12 hours.

Factor XIII deficiency presents with bleeding 12 to 36 hours after surgery or trauma. Routine coagulation test results are normal. Wound dehiscence or malformed scars may occur. Despite availability of factor XIII in cryoprecipitate, fresh-frozen plasma should replenish factor XIII deficiencies because the amount of factor XIII in cryoprecipitate is highly variable.

Abnormal fibrinogen or absence of fibrinogen requires replacement with cryoprecipitate. To increase the plasma fibrinogen concentration four bags of cryoprecipitate are administered for each 10 kg body weight. Because of the 3-day half-life of fibrinogen, replacement every other day suffices.

Abnormalities in the contact activation group (factor XII, high–molecular weight kininogen, and prekallikrein) have no clinical implications. This is consistent with the marginal importance of these substances to hemostasis.

4. Consumptive Coagulopathy

Every aspect of this disease is so controversial—even its name. The more common designation, *disseminated intravascular coagulation*, does a disservice because manifestations may be the reverse in all three of those spheres: *localized, extravascular,* and *hemorrhagic*! Although this syndrome arises from a host of inciting causes, which influence the manifestation of the disease as well as the approach to treatment, the common thread is the formation of thrombin. The degree to which plasmin elaboration responds to thrombin formation, and where that response occurs, determine where and whether thrombosis or bleeding predominates.[117]

a. Pathophysiology

The two fundamental lesions resulting in thrombin formation are endothelial injury and tissue injury. Table 9–13 categorizes some

of the causes of consumptive coagulopathy according to this overall scheme, along with generalizations about the descriptors associated with each manifestation of consumptive coagulopathy. These spheres of categorization include the time course of the disorder (i.e., acute or chronic), its extent (i.e., local or systemic, intravascular or extravascular), and the balance between thrombin effects (i.e., thrombosis) and plasmin effects (i.e., fibrinolytic bleeding).

The diagnosis depends on the clinical scenario and laboratory demonstration of de-

TABLE 9–13

Some Causes of Consumptive Coagulopathy

Entity	Tempo	Location	Thrombosis vs. Bleeding
Endothelial Cell Injury			
Infection	Acute	Disseminated, intravascular	Gram negative > gram positive; intravascular thrombosis; hemorrhage from consumption
Purpura fulminans	Acute	Skin	Vascular thrombosis; hemorrhagic infarction
Septic abortion	Acute	Systemic, fulminant	Endotoxin and hypovolemic shock
Renal allograft rejection	Variable	Donor kidney	Thrombosis of homograft kidney arterioles
Hypovolemic shock	Acute	Disseminated	Microvascular thrombosis, secondary fibrinolytic bleeding
Tissue Injury			
Abruptio placentae	Acute	Uterus and body	Localized intrauterine hemorrhage; systemic defibrination from thromboplastin
Amniotic fluid embolism	Acute	Systemic	Thrombosis via amniotic fluid debris; bleeding 1/2–3 hr later from consumption
Saline abortion	Acute	Systemic, mild	Placental thromboplastin enters circulation
Trauma	Acute	Systemic	Tissue thromboplastin enters circulation; thrombotic > hemorrhagic tendency
Heatstroke	Acute	Systemic	Tissue damage, especially liver
Adult respiratory distress syndrome	Acute	Lung/systemic	Platelet consumption
Pancreatitis	Acute	Systemic	Fibrinolytic action of pancreatic enzymes
Acute hemolysis	Acute	Systemic	Self-limited, requires impaired RES
Acute promyelocytic leukemia	Chronic	Systemic	Hemorrhagic > thrombotic tendency
Mucin-producing adenocarcinoma	Chronic	Systemic	Thrombotic > hemorrhagic tendency
Solid tumors	Chronic	Systemic	Microvascular fibrinolysis keeps pace with intravascular coagulation; larger vessel thrombi predominate
Retained dead fetus syndrome	Chronic	Systemic, mild	Compensated; hemorrhage after delivery if consumptive defects are not corrected
Other Sources of Thrombin/Other Causes			
Snakebite	Acute	Disseminated	Defibrination ± platelet consumption
Aortic aneurysm	Chronic	Localized	Aneurysmal clot incites platelet and fibrin deposition
Hemangiomas	Chronic	Localized	Convoluted vascular channels sequester platelets and consume fibrinogen
TTP/HUS	Chronic	Multiple organs or kidney	Only platelet agglutination
Fibrinogenolysis	Various	Systemic, but not microcirculation	Hemorrhage, not thrombosis, from circulating plasmin

pleted hemostatic elements. The prothrombin time and partial thromboplastin time are each prolonged, owing to inadequate concentrations of coagulation proteins, particularly factor V. The thrombin time is prolonged, owing to too little fibrinogen or the presence of fibrin degradation products, or both. Fibrinogen concentrations do not reliably afford the diagnosis, since the acute phase reactant nature of fibrinogen may result in spuriously normal concentrations despite significant consumption or spuriously decreased concentrations despite lack of consumption.

The platelet count, however, is decreased in nearly all patients with consumptive coagulopathy. Indeed, more than half the patients demonstrate a platelet count below 50 • 10^9/L. Fibrin degradation products are usually increased. Most hospital laboratories can now provide the D-dimer test, which measures breakdown products of cross-linked fibrin. More sophisticated laboratory tests can measure the concentrations of fibrinopeptides, which are released by the action of thrombin on fibrinogen, or release of plasmin as complexed with antiplasmin.

b. Treatment and Anesthetic Considerations

The treatment of consumptive coagulopathy is as varied as its causes; however, a few general rules can be stated. First, the cause of thrombin elaboration must be eliminated. The most common causes of intraoperative consumptive coagulopathy are hypovolemic shock and aortic aneurysm. The most common cause in the intensive care unit is sepsis.

Second, consumed factors must be replenished. Although some investigators maintain this merely "feeds the fire," hemorrhage and volume depletion are sure to continue unless platelets and fibrinogen are available to form fibrin clot. Appropriate management involves measurement of platelet counts and plasma fibrinogen on a regular basis. In the face of ongoing intraoperative blood loss, hourly determinations provide important feedback on the adequacy of hemostatic element replacements. When managing sepsis-related consumption, less frequent determinations usually suffice. On the other hand, if the patient is not bleeding and does not require an invasive procedure, replacement may be withheld. When replenishment cannot keep pace with consumption, heparin administration may slow consumption long enough to establish adequate concentrations of crucial hemostatic elements.

Third, normovolemia and normothermia must be maintained. Otherwise, a secondary cause for this disorder will take the place of the inciting one. Fourth, administration of heparin should be considered in special circumstances. Table 9–14 categorizes causes of consumptive coaguloapathy according to the usefulness of heparin in resolving the problem. In general, it is rare that improvement can clearly be ascribed to the administration of heparin.

Fifth, adjunctive treatments should be considered, including replacement of antithrombin, which should slow thrombin generation, administration of activated protein C (which has both anticoagulant effect and protection against endotoxic shock), and antifibrinolytic agents such as aminocaproic acid or tranexamic acid. The last should be used only when the physician is confident of the absence of ongoing microvascular coagulation, lest the antifibrinolytic halt the secondary fibrinolysis that is keeping vascular channels open. Two specific applications for antifibrinolytic therapy are selective local delivery to hemangiomas for deliberate embolization and for patients with amniotic fluid embolism who continue to bleed following resolution of the intravascular coagulation.

D. PROTHROMBOTIC DISORDERS

1. Antithrombin Deficiency

The serpin antithrombin serves as one of several restraining influences in a system otherwise designed to form large amounts of clot rapidly. Its deficiency thus results in an imbalance between coagulation and its inhibition, leading to inappropriate formation of clot (i.e., thrombosis).[118] Antithrombin deficiency has an autosomal dominant inheritance pattern and is of three types: absence of antithrombin molecules (type I); dysfunctional antithrombin (type II); and antithrombin with dysfunction limited to a reduced response to heparin (type III).

Clinical manifestations are rare before puberty; the incidence increases with age, beginning at age 15 years. Typically, patients present with venous thrombosis, often associated with another risk factor such as surgery, infection, prolonged bed rest, or pregnancy. The

TABLE 9–14

Role of Heparin in Treatment of Consumptive Coagulopathy

Condition	Rationale
Conditions That Warrant Heparin Therapy	
Retained dead fetus syndrome	Effective in restoring fibrinogen to normal before delivery
Giant hemangioma	Halts localized consumptive process
Aortic aneurysm	Halts localized consumptive process (withhold if leaking)
Solid tumor	Interrupts chronic, low-grade consumptive processes
Conditions for Which Benefit of Heparin Is Controversial	
Acute promyelocytic leukemia	
Septicemia, septic abortion	
Conditions for Which Heparin Is Not Helpful	
Most acute forms	Little chance to interrupt an ongoing consumptive process
Abruptio placentae	Exacerbates bleeding associated with delivery or hysterectomy
Amniotic fluid embolism	Accentuates bleeding aspects
Saline-induced abortion	Unnecessary since course usually mild
Liver disease	Fibrinolytic cause more likely than thrombotic one

normal range of concentrations of the coagulation inhibitors (0.8 to 1.2 U/mL) is more restrictive than that of the procoagulant proteins (0.5 to 1.5 U/mL, in general). Heterozygotes display antithrombin concentrations of 0.3 to 0.7 U/mL. Homozygotes probably die in utero.

The differential diagnosis of acquired antithrombin deficiency includes liver disease, in which production is decreased, consumptive coagulopathy, in which the protein cannot be replaced as quickly as it is consumed, nephrotic syndrome, in which renal clearance is increased, high-dose estrogen exposure, including high-dose birth control pills or diethylstilbestrol therapy,[119] and near term pregnancy. Heparin therapy also increases clearance of antithrombin, and this might explain the phenomenon of heparin resistance.

a. Heparin Resistance

Some patients develop tachyphylaxis in response to heparin infusions. They require more heparin to keep the aPTT in the therapeutic range or exhibit a much diminished activated coagulation time (ACT) response to heparin anticoagulation for cardiopulmonary bypass. Several observations suggest that alterations in antithrombin cause heparin resistance. First, a patient with congenital antithrombin deficiency displayed heparin resistance. Second, patients receiving heparin infusions display a 25 per cent shorter half-

life for antithrombin as compared with untreated patients. Third, plasma levels of antithrombin decrease by 17 to 33 per cent during heparin administration by the intravenous or subcutaneous route.

Accelerated elimination of antithrombin may arise from some modification of the protein during or after its interaction with heparin. Hemodilution accompanying extracorporeal circulation decreases antithrombin levels to about half of normal; however, supplemental antithrombin does not further prolong an ACT that already demonstrates a heparin effect.

Refractoriness of deep vein thrombosis and of pulmonary embolism to heparin therapy may be due to the release from thrombi of PF4, a known heparin antagonist. Thrombocytosis can decrease the ACT response to administered heparin.[120] The differential diagnosis also includes hypereosinophilia, oral contraceptive therapy, consumptive coagulopathy, thrombocytosis, nephrotic syndrome, and congenital antithrombin deficiency. Some presumed cases of heparin resistance may represent nothing more than normal individual anticoagulant response. Regardless of cause, measurement of each patient's anticoagulant response to heparin therapy for cardiopulmonary bypass appears warranted.[121] Measures of plasma heparin levels cannot substitute for clotting times because the goal of anticoagulation is not to achieve a heparin concentration in plasma but rather to inhibit the action of thrombin on fibrinogen.

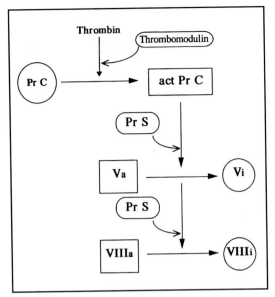

FIGURE 9–14. The protein C pathway. Thrombomodulin alters the activity of thrombin so that it activates circulating protein C (Pr C). The activated form of protein C (act Pr C) with the aid of its cofactor protein S (Pr S), then inactivates factors Va and VIIIa. Protein C and protein S depend on vitamin K for their activity. (From Horrow JC: Management of coagulation and bleeding disorders. In Kaplan JA (ed): Cardiac Anesthesia, 3rd ed. Philadelphia, WB Saunders, 1993.)

b. Anesthetic Considerations

Most often, additional heparin prolongs the ACT sufficiently for the conduct of surgery. Amounts up to 1000 U/kg may be needed to obtain an ACT of at least 480 seconds for cardiopulmonary bypass. While administration of fresh-frozen plasma, which contains antithrombin, should correct antithrombin depletion and prolong the ACT suitably, such exposure to transfusion-borne infectious diseases should be avoided whenever possible. This modality is reserved for the rare refractory case. Rather than administering fresh-frozen plasma, centers that normally accept only ACTs of at least 480 seconds for bypass might consider accepting a lower threshold, such as 400 or 350 seconds.

Commercial, pasteurized preparations of antithrombin can restore plasma antithrombin concentrations without exposing the patient to the infectious risks of banked blood products. They are used successfully to treat patients with ischemic heart disease receiving prolonged heparin infusions who become resistant to the anticoagulant effects of heparin.[122]

2. Protein C and Protein S Deficiencies

Protein C and protein S inactivate factors V and VIII and stimulate fibrinolytic processes. Figure 9–14 illustrates the pathway by which this occurs. Expression of thrombomodulin on the surface of intact endothelium alters the activity of thrombin itself, turning it from a procoagulant protein to one that activates circulating protein C. The activated form of protein C, with the aid of protein S as a cofactor, then inactivates factors V and VIII. Newborns exhibit decreased concentrations of protein C, which gradually increase to adult values by puberty.

Congenital deficiencies of these inhibitory proteins alter the balance between procoagulant and inhibitory processes, enabling thrombosis when circumstances permit. Homozygous protein C or protein S deficiencies appear at birth, often as neonatal purpura fulminans (microvascular cutaneous thrombosis). Heterozygous forms, in which protein C concentrations are 40 to 60 per cent of normal, usually manifest clinical effects beginning in adolescence.[123] Heterozygotes for protein S deficiency have concentrations of 30 to 60 per cent of normal for total protein S and 15 to 50 per cent for free protein S.[118]

Acquired protein C deficiency arises from liver disease, consumptive coagulopathy, adult respiratory distress syndrome, and vitamin K deficiency, including that secondary to oral anticoagulants. Acquired deficiencies of protein S occur in liver disease, consumptive coagulopathy, systemic lupus erythematosus, acute infections associated with purpura fulminans, and vitamin K deficiencies.

a. Anesthetic Considerations

Initiation of oral anticoagulant therapy in these patients is fraught with hazard, as synthesis of proteins C and S depends on vitamin K in a more sensitive manner than does synthesis of factors II, VII, IX, and X. As a result, initial depletion of the small amounts of the inhibitory protein worsens thrombotic tendencies, and may cause warfarin-induced skin necrosis unless heparin therapy antedates administration of oral anticoagulant by 24 to 48 hours. Warfarin administration then commences with a target internationalized ratio of 2.0 to 3.0, which may be decreased to 1.5 to 2.0 after several years without symptoms.

3. Antiphospholipid Syndrome

This disorder, misnamed *circulating lupus anticoagulant*, involves the appearance of an IgG or IgM antibody to the phospholipid portion of the prothrombinase complex, an association of phospholipid, calcium, factor Xa, and factor Va. It occurs in about 10 per cent of patients with SLE, in response to administration to procainamide, phenothiazines, hydralazine, and quinidine in some patients, after acute viral infection in some children, and in some patients infected with human immunodeficiency virus (HIV).[117] It usually comes to clinical attention because of a prolonged aPTT obtained for screening purposes.

More often, these patients suffer from thrombosis. Pregnant women risk fetal loss. Thrombocytopenia accompanies this disorder with increased incidence. The pathophysiology of thrombosis remains unclear, but platelet activation seems a likely factor in the process. In severe forms, corticosteroids afford improvement. Long-term oral anticoagulant therapy is needed to combat recurring thrombosis. Low-dose aspirin therapy may help reduce fetal wastage during pregnancy.

The anesthetic considerations involve steroid dependence, switching from oral anticoagulation to heparin perioperatively, and considerations associated with an underlying disorder, whether known or suspected.

4. Treatment and Anesthetic Considerations

Patients with coagulation inhibitor deficiencies who require surgery or invasive procedures need careful attention as to the timing of factor replacement. Many are receiving ongoing oral anticoagulant therapy. Switching to heparin entails significant risk, as antithrombin-deficient patients do not respond normally to heparin; more severe cases do not respond at all. For these patients, administration of antithrombin itself should precede dependence on heparin. Major invasive procedures may then require cessation of heparin therapy. Such a maneuver always risks thrombosis to achieve hemostasis. Thrombophilic patients require prophylactic perioperative administration of low-dose heparin or oral anticoagulants to prevent thrombosis. Consultation with a trusted hematologist should reveal an appropriate dosing scheme.

An alternative approach is to continue oral anticoagulant therapy without switching to heparin. In this case, prophylactic intraoperative administration of fresh-frozen plasma to counter the effects of oral anticoagulants may cause catastrophic thrombosis. The authors recommend proceeding with open surgical procedures without modifying oral anticoagulant therapy beforehand but ensuring availability of sufficient amounts of fresh-frozen plasma to restore procoagulant factors should abnormal surgical bleeding occur.

IV. DISEASES OF WHITE CELLS

A. THE LEUKEMIAS

The leukemias may be identified and classified as acute and chronic forms of myelogenous and lymphocytic diseases. Uncontrolled proliferation of hematopoietic stem cells gives rise to myeloblasts in myelogenous leukemia; lymphocytic stem cells produce lymphoblasts in lymphocytic leukemia. Myeloblasts reproduce in the bone marrow and spread to extramedullary organs in myelogenous leukemia; lymphoblasts originate from lymph nodes in lymphocytic leukemia. Both leukemias suppress normal hematopoietic cell differentiation and proliferation, eventually rendering the marrow aplastic. Normal erythrocyte, granulocyte, and platelet production decrease. Clinical manifestations of the leukemias include weakness, fatigue, and pallor as a result of anemia, infection as a result of granulocytopenia, and hemorrhage as a result of thrombocytopenia.

1. Acute Leukemias

The acute leukemias remain the 20th leading cause of death from cancer among all age groups and the most common malignant disease of children.[124] Acute myelogenous leukemia (AML) has a predilection for adults; acute lymphocytic leukemia (ALL) appears more often in children.[125] Mortality does not result from the proliferation of blast cells but rather from pancytopenia, infection, hemorrhage, and renal and hepatic insufficiency.

Morbidity relates to the blast cells' rapid production of nucleic acid metabolites and to release of intracellular electrolytes and biologically active enzymes upon cell death. Leukemia patients can develop uric acid nephropathy. In this case, production of uric acid, the result of human nucleic acid breakdown, exceeds renal clearance; it precipitates in the renal tubules, producing renal failure. Maintaining urine flow, inhibiting uric acid production by administering allopurinol, and solubilizing urate crystals with sodium bicarbonate helps prevent uric acid nephropathy.[124] Mannitol also helps promote diuresis.

Leukemic cells release phosphates, sulfates, and other organic anions. Hypocalcemia and hypomagnesemia result. Acute leukemic proliferation can produce infiltrates in anatomically confined spaces, resulting in mediastinal masses and superior vena caval obstruction.

2. Acute Myelocytic Leukemia

Eighty per cent of acute myelocytic leukemia (AML) cases occur in adults. Aggressive chemotherapy with anthracycline antibiotics (such as daunorubicin and doxorubicin) and cytosine arabinoside produce remission in 60 to 80 per cent of patients. Anthracycline antibiotics can impair ventricular function, resulting in ventricular tachydysrhythmias, heart block, and sudden death.[126] Whether or not a patient develops anthracycline-induced cardiomyopathy depends on the total dose administered. A dose of 500 to 700 mg/m^2 of doxorubicin produces a cardiomyopathy in 10 to 20 per cent of patients.[127] Patients with preexisting decreased cardiac function develop cardiomyopathy with smaller doses. Radionuclide angiography and echocardiography can monitor ventricular function in patients receiving these agents.[128] These anthracycline antibiotics also suppress the bone marrow, resulting in thrombocytopenia and infection.

Postremission therapy includes allogeneic and autologous bone marrow transplantation.[129, 130] Bone marrow transplantation produces sustained remission for longer than 2 years in 40 per cent of AML patients. In preparation for allogeneic bone marrow transplantation, the recipient receives total body radiation along with cyclophosphamide therapy, which can produce hepatotoxicity. Cyclophosphamide inhibition of cholinesterase can prolong the effect of succinylcholine.[131] Total body radiation can produce gastrointestinal symptoms such as nausea, vomiting, and diarrhea, oral mucositis, pulmonary fibrosis, and restrictive cardiomyopathy. The gastrointestinal perturbations often cause patients to present for surgery with decreased intravascular volume. Before induction of general or regional anesthesia the patient should receive adequate intravenous hydration.

3. Acute Lymphocytic Leukemia

Acute lymphocytic leukemia (ALL) has a more abrupt onset than AML. Largely a disease of children, ALL was the first disseminated malignancy to respond to chemotherapy.[132] Vincristine and prednisone therapy produce remission in 90 per cent of children, half of these patients enjoying long-term leukemia-free survival. This chemotherapeutic combination produces less morbidity from marrow suppression than does the therapy for AML. Studies to date in the pediatric population indicate a cure rate of 50 to 70 per cent of patients. Long-term survival rates for adults with ALL have not been as good.[133] ALL patients may relapse following remission. Allogeneic bone marrow transplantation has proved an option for both adult and pediatric patients, but it remains experimental.

4. Chronic Myelogenous Leukemia

Chronic myelogenous leukemia (CML), a disease of pluripotent stem cells, accounts for 20 to 30 per cent of all leukemias and generally affects middle-aged adults.[134] Initially it is asymptomatic; then, patients exhibit constitutional symptoms such as weakness, fatigue, and general malaise. Splenomegaly and hepatomegaly occur consistently.[135] Major complications include hemorrhage, thrombosis, and increased rate of infection. CML can undergo transformation, resembling AML or ALL. This accounts for two thirds of patients' deaths. Median life expectancy after diagnosis is 4 years, but survival is limited to 2 months in the uncontrolled blast crisis phase.

CML patients exhibit a 20 to 40 per cent increase in metabolic requirements, owing to excessive white cell production. Therapeutic modalities include busulfan, an alkylating agent, steroids, splenic irradiation, and radioactive phosphorus. Busulfan can produce bone marrow suppression, pulmonary fibrosis, and hypoadrenalism secondary to suppression of the pituitary adrenal axis. Allogeneic bone marrow transplantation is rarely performed for CML, owing either to the patient's advanced age or the lack of an adequately matched donor. Autologous bone marrow transplantation remains an option.

5. Chronic Lymphocytic Leukemia

Chronic lymphocytic leukemia (CLL), a monoclonal neoplasm, occurs usually in the sixth decade of life and accounts for 25 per cent of adult leukemias. Anemia, which is common, may be hemolytic. Lymphocytosis with lymphocytic infiltration of the marrow confirms the diagnosis. CLL may involve the liver, spleen, and lymph nodes. Classification is based on the number of lymph nodes involved and the presence of anemia or thrombocytopenia. Alkylating agents such as chlorambucil or cyclophosphamide are the treatment. Lymph node obstruction of the ureters may occur. Splenectomy may occasionally be necessary.

6. Anesthetic Considerations

Patients who present for surgery with acute leukemia should have their hemoglobin and hematocrit measured, along with serum electrolytes, blood urea nitrogen, and liver enzymes. Chest radiography helps detect a possible anterior mediastinal mass.[136] Physical examination may reveal evidence of superior venal caval obstruction, and patients so affected may develop upper airway edema, making endotracheal intubation difficult.

Common procedures performed on patients with leukemia include placement and removal of vascular access catheters and bone marrow transplantation. Frequently, patients with platelet counts less than $30 \cdot 10^9/L$ present for elective central venous access procedures. Should these patients receive platelet transfusion therapy? Such intervention in patients who subsequently receive allogeneic bone marrow transplantation may increase the risk for a graft-versus-host response. Therefore, patients who undergo central catheter placement not requiring extensive subcutaneous tunneling should not receive platelet transfusion therapy before surgery. Patients with a platelet count of less than $30 \cdot 10^9/L$ undergoing central catheter placement that requires the formation of a subcutaneous pocket may develop a hematoma in the pocket. These patients should receive platelet transfusion before the procedure to prevent hematoma formation.

B. BONE MARROW TRANSPLANTATION

1. Pathophysiology

Bone marrow transplantation provides treatment for patients with leukemia as well as other hematologic diseases and primary malignancies (Table 9–15). *Allogeneic bone marrow transplantation* is the process of harvesting bone marrow from a histocompatible donor and infusing that marrow into a recipient. Allogeneic marrow harvesting requires the aspiration of up to 1500 mL of marrow from the donor's posterior iliac spines and iliac crests. The recipient undergoes total body irradiation combined with cyclophosphamide treatment before receiving the donor's marrow. This preliminary treatment destroys the recipient's marrow and immune system, permitting engrafting of the new marrow.

In contrast to allogeneic marrow transplantation, autologous bone marrow transplantation requires the removal under general anesthesia of large volumes of the patient's own "postremission" marrow and reinfusion of this marrow following intensive chemotherapy. Autologous bone marrow transplantation, as compared with allogeneic marrow transplantation, has the advantage of

TABLE 9–15

Primary Malignant Neoplasms Treated with Bone Marrow Transplantation	
Neoplasm	Cases (No.)
Malignant melanoma	28
Neuroblastoma	13
Oat cell carcinoma	13
Pancreatic carcinoma	7
Ewing's sarcoma	7
Rhabdomyosarcoma	5
Ovarian carcinoma	4
Breast carcinoma	4
Wilms' tumor	4
Brain tumor	3
Osteosarcoma	3
Others	11

Adapted from Filshie J, Pollock AN, Hughes RG, Omar YA: The anesthetic management of bone marrow harvest for transplantation. Anaesthesia 39:480, 1984.

increasing the number of patients that can receive this therapy, avoiding the problems of histocompatibility, and eliminating graft-versus-host disease.

2. Safety

Multiple aspirations of large volumes of bone marrow during marrow harvesting produces pain. Therefore, marrow harvesting requires either general anesthesia or central neural axis blockade. Hypovolemia can result in hemodynamic instability. Filshie reported only minor complications in patients receiving general or spinal anesthesia for allogeneic and autologous marrow harvesting.[137] Fewer than 10 per cent of patients had postoperative nausea and vomiting. Some patients developed short-lived pyrexia of unknown cause. Ren Jin retrospectively reviewed 224 autologous bone marrow harvests. Of 171 procedures performed under general anesthesia, 48 procedures performed under spinal anesthesia, and 5 under caudal block, 23 patients developed postoperative fever of unknown origin. Other complications included one case of pneumonitis and one case of bradycardia in the postanesthesia care unit.[138] No study demonstrated any effect of anesthetic technique on outcome, however.

Cairo reported the safety of autologous bone marrow harvesting from children under general anesthesia. No child manifested postoperative pyrexia. One patient developed a pulmonary embolus in the postoperative period: tumor obstruction had produced venous stasis. Intraoperative packed red blood cell transfusions occurred in 20 per cent of patients.[139] Gild and Crilley reported sudden cardiac arrest during epidural anesthesia for bone marrow harvesting; however the authors cite hypercarbia as the cause of cardiac arrest.[140] Boortz-Marx, utilizing precordial Doppler monitoring, reported a 45 per cent rate of venous embolism during bone marrow harvest.[141] Because Doppler monitoring does not permit tissue characterization, the type of embolism detected (i.e., air or fat) and the significance of these emboli remain unknown. To the authors' knowledge, no case report documents the occurrence of fatal intraoperative venous embolism during bone marrow harvesting.

3. Anesthetic Considerations

Since rapid intravascular volume changes occur during bone marrow harvesting, the authors recommend insertion of a large-bore intravenous catheter, for rapid infusion of fluid, and placement of a Foley catheter to assess intravascular volume. Some marrow-harvesting protocols include the administration of 1500 U of subcutaneous heparin to facilitate aspiration of bone marrow.

Adult allogeneic marrow donors donate 1 to 2 U of autologous blood 1 to 2 weeks before the procedure. Most allogeneic donors receive 1 U of autologous blood intraoperatively.[137] Patients undergoing autologous bone marrow harvesting have 1 to 2 U cross-matched for the procedure. Transfused allogeneic blood for these patients undergoes irradiation with 15 Gy, to prevent activation of lymphocytes that might cause graft-versus-host disease. Filshie estimated average fluid requirements at 1838 mL of Ringer's lactated solution and 1 U of autologous blood for marrow-harvesting procedures.[137]

No study has shown definitively that central neural axis blockade improves outcome following bone marrow harvesting. Lavi retrospectively reviewed anesthesia records of 162 bone marrow harvests.[142] Patients who had regional anesthesia had greater intraoperative intravenous fluid requirements but fewer intraoperative autologous packed red blood cell transfusions as compared with those who had general anesthesia. The general anesthesia group required more postoperative analgesic medications than the regional anesthesia group. No difference in the duration of hospitalization was reported for the general anesthesia and the central neural axis groups. Other investigators have demonstrated a reduction in postoperative analgesic requirements in patients undergoing regional anesthesia for harvesting procedures.[142–144]

Should patients undergoing bone marrow harvesting receive nitrous oxide? Although nitrous oxide inactivates vitamin B_{12},[145] the clinical sequelae of cobalamin deficiency ensue with prolonged exposure (i.e., 7 to 12 hours).[146] Rabinowitz demonstrated mild DNA synthesis abnormalities in marrow harvested from patients who received nitrous oxide during harvesting procedures. Marrow from patients not exposed to nitrous oxide showed no such abnormalities.[66] Although that study suggests that nitrous oxide might have a deleterious effect on marrow engraftment, no recipient of marrow exposed to nitrous oxide had unsuccessful marrow engraftment, nor did any donor go on to develop symptoms of vitamin B_{12} deficiency. Nevertheless, because (1) 5 to 10 per cent of all surgical patients have low serum cobalamin levels preoperatively,[64, 65] (2) nitrous oxide potentially affects stem cell activity, and (3) patients undergoing bone marrow harvesting are susceptible to embolization of fat or air, the authors recommend avoiding nitrous oxide as an adjuvant to general anesthesia during bone marrow harvesting.

C. FELTY'S SYNDROME

Patients with chronic rheumatoid arthritis may develop hypersplenism and leukopenia. These elderly, debilitated persons experience frequent respiratory infections, which initially respond to steroid therapy. Once this syndrome ceases to respond to steroids, splenectomy may be scheduled, as it affords additional—but transient—improvement. Such patients may require steroid replacement perioperatively. The potential effects of rheumatoid arthritis on the airway require focused attention as well.

D. MULTIPLE MYELOMA

A disease of plasma cell proliferation, multiple myeloma results in urine spillover of the monoclonal substance, usually IgG, termed *Bence Jones protein*. The rheologic hyperviscosity effects of the massive amounts of protein poured into the blood each day result in sludging and organ failure. Cryoglobulinemia, hypercalcemia, and decreased platelet function occur with multiple myeloma. Death from renal failure usually follows. Treatment of the disease includes plasmapheresis to improve plasma viscosity.

Patients may present for surgery to stabilize the spinal column, which is invaded by lytic lesions. Anesthetic issues include the hypercalcemia, adequate intravenous hydration, airway issues if the cervical spine is unstable, and consideration of alternatives to central neuraxis anesthesia in the presence of lytic spinal lesions. Patients with cryoglobulinemia complicating their multiple myeloma require careful attention intraoperatively to preservation of body temperature.

E. AGRANULOCYTOSIS

Agranulocytosis can arise from toxins such as benzene, drugs such as phenothiazines, chloramphenicol, and antithyroid medications, radiation, infections, and immune-mediated phenomena. The anesthetic implications remain limited to ensuring strict aseptic techniques to minimize the opportunity for infection.

V. CONCLUSION

The uncommon hematologic diseases cover a wide array of disorders, ranging from those that threaten life on a nearly daily basis, such as heparin-induced thrombocytopenia and the severe forms of hemophilia, to those of little consequence in the absence of physician intervention, such as G-6-PD deficiency.

Even though many disorders are hereditary, they may escape detection until later in life, as when life-threatening intraoperative hemorrhage leads to the diagnosis of vWd. In other cases, the clinician expects dire consequences, only to observe a benign course of disease, as may occur with factor XI deficiency.

Only with a thorough understanding of the pathophysiology of these disorders and by learning the experience of others in treating them can a clinician serve his or her patients best. Consultation with a trusted hematologist and an oncologist facilitates this care and remains the hallmark of sound anesthesiology practice when caring for these patients.

REFERENCES

1. Williams W, Beutler E, Erslev A, Lichtman M: Hematology. New York, McGraw-Hill, 1990.
2. Colman R, Hirsh J, Marder V, Salzman E: Hemostasis and Thrombosis. Basic Principles and Clinical Practice. Philadelphia, JB Lippincott, 1994.

Anemias

3. National Institute of Health Consensus Conference: Perioperative red blood cell transfusion. JAMA 260:2700, 1988.
4. LeVeen HH, Ip M, Ahmed N: Lowering blood viscosity to overcome vascular resistance. Surg Gynecol Obstet 150:139, 1980.
5. Levine E, Rosen A, Sehgal L: Physiologic effects of acute anemia. Implications for a reduced transfusion trigger. Transfusion 30:11, 1990.
6. Ingram VM: Gene mutation in human haemoglobin:

The chemical difference between normal and sickle cell haemoglobin. Nature 180:326, 1957.

7. Neel JV: The inheritance of sickle cell anemia. Science 110:64, 1949.

8. Harris JW, Brewster HH, Ham TH: Studies on the destruction of red blood cells: The biophysics and biology of sickle cell disease. Arch Intern Med 97:145, 1956.

9. Kinney TR, Ware R: Sickle cell disease: Advances in sickle cell disease. Pediatric Consult 7:1, 1988.

10. Ware RE, Filston HC: Surgical management of children with hemoglobinopathies. Surg Clin North Am 72:1223, 1992.

11. Powars DR: Natural history of sickle cell disease: The first ten years. Semin Hematol 12:267, 1975.

12. Lindsay J, Meshel JC, Patterson RH: The cardiovascular manifestations of sickle cell disease. Arch Intern Med 133:643, 1974.

13. Oppenheimer EH, Esterly JR: Pulmonary changes in sickle cell disease. Am Rev Respir Dis 103:858, 1971.

14. Charache S, Scott JC, Charache P: Acute chest syndrome in adults with sickle cell anemia. Microbiology, treatment, and prevention. Arch Intern Med 139:67, 1979.

15. Powars D, Weidman, Odam-Maryon T: Sickle cell chronic lung disease: Morbidity and the risk of pulmonary failure. Medicine 67:66, 1988.

16. Pearson HA, McIntosh S, Ritchey AK: Developmental aspects of splenic function in sickle cell disease. Blood 53:358, 1979.

17. Vinchinsky E, Lubin BH: Suggested guidelines for treatment of children with sickle cell anemia. Hematol Oncol Clin North Am 1:483, 1987.

18. Stephens CG, Scott RB: Cholelithiasis in sickle cell anemia. Surgical and medical management. Arch Intern Med 140:648, 1980.

19. Rambo WM, Reines HD: Elective cholecystectomy for the patient with sickle cell disease and asymptomatic cholelithiasis. Am Surg 52:205, 1986.

20. Buckalew VM, Someren A: Renal manifestations of sickle cell disease. Arch Intern Med 133:660, 1974.

21. Milner PF, Krause AP, Sebes JI, et al: Sickle cell disease as a cause of osteonecrosis of the femoral head. N Engl J Med 325:1476, 1991.

22. Hilkowitz G, Jacobson A: Hepatic dysfunction and abnormalities of serum proteins and serum enzymes in sickle-cell anemia. J Lab Clin Med 57:856, 1961.

23. Flye MW, Silver D: Biliary tract disorders and sickle cell disease. Surgery 72:361, 1972.

24. Lessins LS, Kuranstin-Mills J, Klug PP: Determination of rheologically optimal mixtures of AA and SS erythrocytes. Blood 50:111, 1977.

25. Bhattacharyya BN: Perioperative management for cholecytectomy in sickle cell disease. J Pediatr Surg 28:72, 1993.

26. Bischoff RJ, Williamson A, Dalali MJ, et al: Assessment of the use of transfusion therapy perioperatively in patients with sickle cell hemoglobinopathies. Ann Surg 207:434, 1988.

27. Griffin TC, Buchanan G: Elective surgery in children with sickle cell disease without preoperative blood transfusion. J Pediatr Surg 28:681, 1993.

28. Ware R, Filston HC, Schultz W, Kinney TR: Elective cholecystectomy in children with sickle hemoglobinopathies. Successful outcome using a preoperative transfusion regimen. Ann Surg 208:17, 1988.

29. Guinee WS, Heaton JA, Barreras L: The effects of general anesthetics on sicklemic patients. Anesthesiology 29:193, 1968.

30. Gross ML, Schwedler M, Bischoff RJ, Kerstein M: Impact of anesthetic agents on patients with sickle cell disease. Am Surg 59:261, 1993.

31. Tobias JD: Indications and application of epidural anesthesia in a pediatric population outside the preoperative period. Clin Pediatr 32:81, 1993.

32. Finer P, Blair J, Rowe P: Epidural analgesia in the management of labor pain and sickle cell crisis—a case report. Anesthesiology 68:799, 1988.

33. Caputi R, Jacobs AM, Oloff LM: Sickle cell anemia in podiatric surgery. J Foot Surg 23:135, 1984.

34. Derkay CS, Bray G, Milmoe GJ, Grundfast KM: Adenotonsillectomy in children with sickle cell disease. S Med J 84:205, 1991.

35. Apthorp GH, Lehmann H: Sickle cell anemia. Proc R Soc Med 57:178, 1949.

36. Dalal FY, Schmidt GB, Bennett EJ: Sickle cell trait: A report of postoperative neurological complication. Br J Anaesth 46:387, 1974.

37. McCormick F: Abnormal hemoglobins II: The pathology of sickle cell trait. Am J Med Sci 92:329, 1961.

38. Heller P, Best WR, Nelson RB, Becktel J: Clinical implications of sickle cell trait and glucose 6 phosphate dehydrogenase deficiency in hospitalized black male patients. N Engl J Med 300:1001, 1979.

39. Sears DA: The morbidity of sickle cell trait. Am J Med 64:1021, 1978.

40. DeLaval MR, Taswell HF, Bowie EJW: Open heart surgery in patients with inherited hemoglobinopathies. Arch Surg 109:618, 1974.

41. Baxter MRN, Bevan JC, Esseltine DW, Bernstein M: The management of two pediatric patients with sickle cell trait and sickle cell disease during cardiopulmonary bypass. J Cardiothorac Vasc Anesth 3:477, 1989.

42. Beutler E: The common anemias. JAMA 256:2433, 1988.

43. Bertles JE: Sodium transport across the surface membrane of red blood cells in hereditary spherocytosis. J Clin Invest 36:816, 1957.

44. Singer D: Post-splenectomy sepsis. In Rosenberg HS, Bolande RP (eds): Perspectives in Pediatric Pathology. St. Louis, Mosby–Year Book, 1973.

45. Tchernia G, Gauthier F, Mielot F, et al: Initial assessment of the beneficial effects of partial splenectomy in hereditary spherocytosis. Blood 81:2014, 1993.

46. Beutler E: The hemolytic effects of primaquine and related compounds: A review. Blood 81:103, 1959.

47. Bunn E: Exchange of heme among hemoglobin molecules. Proc Natl Acad Sci USA 56:974, 1966.

48. Beutler E: Hemolytic Anemia in Disorders of Red Cell Metabolism. New York, Plenum, 1978.

49. Ogin GA: Cholecystectomy in a patient with paroxysmal nocturnal hemoglobinuria. Anesthetic complications and management in the perioperative period. Anesthesiology 72:761, 1990.

50. Taylor MB, Whitman JG, Worsley A: Paroxysmal nocturnal hemoglobinuria. Anaesthesia 42:639, 1987.

51. Shahian DM, Wallach SR, Bern MM: Open heart surgery in patients with cold-reactive proteins. Surg Clin North Am 65:315, 1985.

52. Diaz JH, Cooper S, Ochsner JL: Cardiac surgery in patients with cold autoimmune diseases. Anesth Analg 63:349, 1984.

53. Nordhagen R, Stensvold K, Winsnes A: The most frequent autoimmune hemolytic anemia in children. Acta Paediatr Scand 73:258, 1984.

54. Packman CH, Leddy JP: Cryopathic hemolytic syn-

dromes. *In* Williams W, Beutler E, Erslev A, Lichtman M (eds): Hematology. New York, McGraw Hill, 1990.

55. Fairbanks VF, Beutler E: Erythrocyte disorders: Anemia related to disturbances of hemoglobin synthesis. *In* Williams W, Beutler E, Erslev A, Lichtman M (eds): Hematology. New York, McGraw Hill, 1990.

56. Herbet V, Zalusky R: Interaction of vitamin B_{12} and folic acid metabolism: Folic acid and clearance studies. J Clin Invest 41:1263, 1962.

57. Metz J: Cobalamin deficiency and the pathogenesis of nervous system disease. Ann Rev Nutr 12:59, 1992.

58. Schilling RF: Is nitrous oxide a dangerous anesthetic for vitamin B_{12}–deficient subjects? JAMA 255:1605, 1986.

59. Holloway KL, Albercio AM: Postoperative myeloneuropathy: A preventable complication in patients with vitamin B_{12} deficiency. J Neurosurgery 72:732, 1990.

60. Hadzic A, Glab K, Sanborn KV, Thys DM: Severe neurologic deficit after nitrous oxide anesthesia. Anesthesiology 83:863, 1995.

61. Berger JJ, Modell JH: Megaloblastic anemia and brief exposure to nitrous oxide—a causal relationship? Anesth Analg 67:197, 1988.

61a. Flippo TS, Holder WD Jr: Neurologic degeneration associated with nitrous oxide anesthesia in patients with vitamin B_{12} deficiency. Arch Surg 128:1391, 1993.

62. McMorrow AM, Adamas RJ, Rubenstein MN: Combined system disease after nitrous oxide anesthesia: A case report. Neurology 45:1224, 1995.

63. King M, Coulter C, Boyle RS, Whitby RM: Neurotoxicity from overuse of nitrous oxide. Med J Austral 163:50, 1995.

64. Cooper BA, Fehedey V, Blanshay P: Recognition of deficiency of vitamin B_{12} using measurement of serum concentration. J Lab Clin Med 107:447, 1986.

65. Karnase DS, Carmell R: Low serum cobalamin levels in primary degenerative dementia: Do some patients harbor atypical cobalamin deficiency states? Arch Intern Med 147:429, 1987.

66. Rabinowitz CR, Mazunder A: Metabolic evidence of cobalamin deficiency in bone marrow cells harvested for transplantation. Eur J Haematol 50:228, 1993.

67. Barker SJ, Tremper KK, Hyatt BS, Zaccari BS: Effects of methemoglobinemia on pulse oximetry and mixed venous oximetry. Anesthesiology 67:A170, 1987.

Hemostasis Disorders

68. Colman R, Marder V, Salzman E, Hirsh J: Overview of hemostasis. *In* Colman R, Hirsh J, Marder V, Salzman E (eds): Hemostasis and Thrombosis. Philadelphia, JB Lippincott, 1994.

69. Salvesen G, Pizzo S: Proteinase inhibitors: Alphamacroglobulins, serpins, and kinins. *In* Colman R, Hirsh J, Marder V, Salzman E (eds): Hemostasis and Thrombosis. Philadelphia, JB Lippincott, 1994.

70. Kessler CM: The pharmacology of aspirin, heparin, coumarin, and thrombolytic agents. Implications for therapeutic use in cardiopulmonary disease. Chest 99:97S, 1991.

71. Goldberg M, Colonna-Romano P, Babins N: Emergency coronary artery bypass surgery following intracoronary streptokinase. Anesthesiology 61:601, 1984.

72. Gill JC, Endres-Brooks J, Bauer PJ, et al: The effect of ABO blood group on the diagnosis of von Willebrand disease. Blood 69:16915, 1987.

73. Mannucci PM: Desmopressin: A nontransfusional form of treatment for congenital and acquired bleeding disorders. Blood 72:1449, 1988.

74. Mannucci PM, Schimpf K, Brettler DB, et al: Low risk for hepatitis C in hemophiliacs given a high-purity, pasteurized factor VIII concentrate. Arch Intern Med 113:27, 1990.

75. Warkentin TE, Hayward CPM, Boshkov LK, et al: Sera from patients with heparin-induced thrombocytopenia generate platelet-derived microparticles with procoagulant activity: An explanation for the thrombotic complications of heparin-induced thrombocytopenia. Blood 84:3691, 1994.

76. Amiral J, Bridey F, Dreyfus M: Platelet factor 4 complexed to heparin is the target for antibodies generated in heparin-induced thrombocytopenia [letter]. Thromb Haemost 68:95, 1992.

77. Hirsh J, Raschke R, Warkentin TE, et al: Heparin: Mechanism of action, pharmacokinetics, dosing considerations, monitoring, efficacy, and safety. Chest 108:258S, 1995.

78. Bell WR, Royall RM: Heparin-associated thrombocytopenia: A comparison of three heparin preparations. N Engl J Med 303:902, 1980.

79. Warkentin TE, Kelton JG: Heparin and platelets. Hematol Oncol Clin North Am 4:243, 1990.

80. Godal HC: Report of the International Committee on Thrombosis and Haemostasis. Thrombocytopenia and heparin. Thromb Haemost 43:222, 1980.

81. Rizzoni WE, Miller K, Rick M, Lotze MT: Heparin-induced thrombocytopenia and thromboembolism in the postoperative period. Surgery 103:470, 1988.

82. Moberg PQ, Geary VM, Sheikh FM: Heparin-induced thrombocytopenia: A possible complication of heparin-coated pulmonary artery catheters. J Cardiothorac Anesth 4:226, 1990.

83. Laster J, Silver D: Heparin-coated catheters and heparin-induced thrombocytopenia. J Vasc Surg 7:667, 1988.

84. Ramakrishna R, Manoharan A, Kwan Y, Kyle P: Heparin-induced thrombocytopenia: Cross-reactivity between standard heparin, low–molecular weight heparin, dalteparin (Fragmin) and heparinoid danaparoid (Orgoran). Br J Haematol 91:736, 1995.

85. Vitoux J-F, Mathieu J-F, Roncato M, et al: Heparin-associated thrombocytopenia treatment with low–molecular weight heparin. Thromb Haemost 55:37, 1986.

86. Sheridan D, Carter C, Kelton JG: A diagnostic test for heparin-induced thrombocytopenia. Blood 67:27, 1986.

87. Kelton JG, Sheridan D, Brain M: Clinical usefulness of testing for a heparin-dependent platelet-aggregating factor in patients with suspected heparin-induced thrombocytopenia. J Lab Clin Med 103:6062, 1984.

88. Chong BH, Burgess J, Ismail F: The clinical usefulness of the platelet aggregation test for the diagnosis of heparin-induced thrombocytopenia. Thromb Haemost 69:344, 1993.

89. Zulys VJ, Teasdale SJ, Michel ER, et al: Ancrod (Arvin) as an alternative to heparin anticoagulation for cardiopulmonary bypass. Anesthesiology 71:870, 1989.

90. Demers C, Ginsberg JS, Brill-Edwards P, et al: Rapid

anticoagulation using ancrod for heparin-induced thrombocytopenia. Blood 78:21947, 1991.

91. Magnani HN: Heparin-induced thrombocytopenia (HIT): An overview of 230 patients treated with Orgoran (Org 10172). Thromb Haemost 70:554, 1993.

92. Vender JS, Matthew EB, Silverman IM, et al: Heparin-associated thrombocytopenia: Alternative managements. Anesth Analg 65:520, 1986.

93. Kappa JR, Fisher CA, Todd B, et al: Intraoperative management of patients with heparin-induced thrombocytopenia. Ann Thorac Surg 49:714, 1990.

94. Makhoul RG, McCann RL, Austin EH, et al: Management of patients with heparin-associated thrombocytopenia and thrombosis requiring cardiac surgery. Ann Thorac Surg 43:617, 1987.

95. Weiler JM, Freiman P, Sharath MD, et al: Serious adverse reactions to protamine sulfate: Are alternatives needed? J Allergy Clin Immunol 75:297, 1985.

96. Addonizio VP, Fisher CA, Kappa JR, Ellison N: Prevention of heparin-induced thrombocytopenia during open heart surgery with Iloprost (ZK36374). Surgery 102:796, 1987.

97. Kappa JR, Addonizio VP: Heparin-induced thrombocytopenia: Diagnosis and management. In Ellison N, Jobes DR (ed): Effective Hemostasis in Cardiac Surgery. Philadelphia, WB Saunders, 1988.

98. Kraezler EJ, Starr NJ: Heparin-associated thrombocytopenia: Management of patients for open heart surgery. Anesthesiology 63:336, 1988.

99. Ellison N, Kappa JR, Fisher CA, Addonizio VP: Extracorporeal circulation in a patient with heparin-induced thrombocytopenia. Anesthesiology 63:336, 1985.

100. Olinger GN, Hussey CV, Olive JA, Malik MI: Cardiopulmonary bypass for patients with previously documented heparin-induced platelet aggregation. J Thorac Cardiovasc Surg 87:673, 1984.

101. Riess FC, Lower C, Seelig C, et al: Recombinant hirudin as a new anticoagulant during cardiac operations instead of heparin: Successful for aortic valve replacement in man. J Thorac Cardiovasc Surg 110:265, 1995.

102. Matsuo T, Kario K, Chikahira Y, et al: Treatment of heparin-induced thrombocytopenia by use of argatroban, a synthetic thrombin inhibitor. Br J Haematol 82:627, 1992.

103. Kikta MJ, Keller MP, Humphrey PW, Silver D: Can low–molecular weight heparins and heparinoids be safely given to patients with heparin-induced thrombocytopenia syndrome. Surgery 114:705, 1993.

104. Nand S: Hirudin therapy for heparin-associated thrombocytopenia and deep venous thrombosis. Am J Hematol 43:310, 1993.

105. Lewis BE, Leya FS, Wallis DEG: Failure of ancrod in the treatment of heparin-induced arterial thrombosis. Can J Cardiol 10:559, 1994.

106. Greinacher A, Philippen KH, Kemkes-Matthes B, et al: Heparin-associated thrombocytopenia type II in a patient with end-stage renal disease: Successful anticoagulation with the low–molecular-weight heparinoid Org 10172 during haemodialysis. Nephrol Dial Transplant 8:1176, 1993.

107. Rowlings PA, Evans S, Mansberg R, et al: The use of low–molecular weight heparinoid (Org 10172) for extracorporeal procedures in patients with heparin dependent thrombocytopenia and thrombosis. Aust NZ J Med 21:52, 1991.

108. Tardy-Poncet B, Mahul P, Beraud A-M, et al: Failure of orgoran therapy in a patient with a previous heparin-induced thrombocytopenia syndrome. Br J Haematol 90:969, 1995.

109. Lecompte T, Luo S, Stieltjes N, et al: Thrombocytopenia associated with low–molecular-weight heparin. Lancet 338:1217, 1991.

110. Leroy J, Leclerc MH, Delahousse B, et al: Treatment of heparin-associated thrombocytopenia and thrombosis with low–molecular weight heparin (CY 216). Semin Thromb Hemostas 11:326, 1985.

111. Moake JL, Eisenstaedt RS: Thrombotic thrombocytopenic purpura and the hemolytic uremic syndrome. In Colman RW, Hirsh J, Marder VJ, Salzman EW (eds): Hemostasis and Thrombosis. Philadelphia, JB Lippincott, 1994.

112. Edson JR: Prothrombin-complex concentrates and thromboses. N Engl J Med 290:403, 1974.

113. Kingdon HS, Lundblad RL, Veltkamp JJ, Aronson DL: Potentially thrombogenic materials in factor IX concentrates. Thromb Diathes Heamorrh 33:6171, 1975.

114. Cederbaum AI, Blatt PM, Roberts HR: Intravascular coagulation with use of human prothrombin complex concentrates. Ann Intern Med 84:683, 1976.

115. Gruppo RA, Bove KE, Donaldson VH: Fatal myocardial necrosis associated with prothrombin-complex concentrate therapy in hemophilia A. N Engl J Med 309:242, 1983.

116. Asakai R, Chung DW, Davie EW, Seligsohn U: Factor XI deficiency in Ashkenazi Jews in Israel. N Engl J Med 325:153, 1991.

117. Marder V, Feinstein DI, Francis CW, Colman RW: Consumptive thrombohemorrhagic disorders. In Colman RW, Hirsh J, Marder VJ, Salzman EW (eds): Hemostasis and Thrombosis. Philadelphia, JB Lippincott, 1994.

118. Kitchens CS: Thrombophilia and thrombosis in unusual sites. In Colman RW, Hirsh J, Marder VJ, Salzman EW (eds): Hemostasis and Thrombosis. Philadelphia, JB Lippincott, 1994.

119. Litwack RS, Horrow JC: Lethal thrombosis during coronary artery bypass graft surgery. Anesthesiology 67:134, 1987.

120. Gravlee GP, Bauer SD, Roy RC, et al: Predicting the pharmacodynamics of heparin: A clinical evaluation of the Hepcon system 4. J Cardiothorac Anesth 1:379, 1987.

121. Jobes DR, Ellison N, Campbell FW: Limit(ation)s for ACT. Anesth Analg 69:142, 44, 1989.

122. Irani MS: Antithrombin concentrates in heparin-resistant cardiopulmonary bypass patients. Clin Appl Thromb Hemost 2:103, 1996.

123. Hirsh J, Prins MH, Samama M: Approach to the thrombophilic patient for hemostasis and thrombosis. In Colman RW, Hirsh J, Marder VJ, Salzman EW (eds): Hemostasis and Thrombosis. Philadelphia, JB Lippincott, 1994.

Diseases of White Cells

124. Henderson ES: Acute leukemia general considerations. In Williams W, Beutler E, Erslev A, Lichtman M (eds): Hematology. New York, McGraw Hill, 1990.

125. National Cancer Institute Monograph 70: Forty-five years of cancer incidence in Connecticut. Washington, DC: US Government Printing Office, 1986.

126. Couch RD, Loh KK, Sugino J: Sudden cardiac death following adriamycin therapy. Cancer 48:38, 1981.

127. Young RC, Ozolos RF, Myers CE: The anthracycline antineoplastic drugs. N Engl J Med 305:139, 1981.

128. Nitchi JL, Senger JW, Thorning D: Anthracycline cardiotoxicity: Clinical and pathological outcomes assessed by radionuclide ejection fractions. Cancer 46:1109, 1980.

129. Thomas E, Storb R, Clift RA: Bone marrow transplantation. N Engl J Med 291:832, 1975.

130. Thomas ED: Marrow transplantation for malignant disease. J Clin Oncol 1:517, 1983.

131. Dillman JB: Safe use of succinylcholine during repeated anesthetics in a patient treated with cyclophosphamide. Anesth Analg 66:351, 1987.

132. Mauer AM: Lymphocytic disorders: Malignant proliferative response leukemia. *In* Williams W, Beutler E, Erslev A, Lichtman M (eds): Hematology. New York, McGraw-Hill, 1990.

133. Marcu RE, DC, Johnson SA: Adult acute lymphoblastic leukemia: A study of prognostic features and response to treatment over a ten year period. Br J Cancer 53:175, 1986.

134. Gunz FW: The epidemiology and genetics of the chronic leukemia. Haematol 6:3, 1977.

135. Beattie JW, Seal RME, Crowther KV: Chronic monocytic leukemia. Q J Med 20:131, 1951.

136. Maile CW, Moore AV, Ulreich S, Putman CE: Chest radiographic-pathologic correlation in adult leukemia patients. Invest Radiol 18:495, 1983.

137. Filshie J, Pollock AN, Hughes RG, Omar YA: The anesthetic management of bone marrow harvest for transplantation. Anaesthesia 39:480, 1984.

138. Ren Jin N, Hill RS, Petersen FB, et al: Marrow harvesting for autologous marrow transplantation. Exp Hematol 13:879, 1985.

139. Cairo MS, Vande Ven C, Toy C, Sender L: Clinical and laboratory experience in marrow harvesting in children for autologous bone marrow transplantation. Bone Marrow Transplant 4:305, 1989.

140. Gild W, Crilley P: Sudden cardiac arrest during epidural anesthesia. Anesthesiology 73:1296, 1990.

141. Bootz-Marx RL, Palahniuk RJ, Lantz MS, Swaim SE: Venous air embolism is common during bone marrow harvest. Anesth Analg 82:S43, 1996.

142. Lavi A, Efrat R, Feigin E, Kadari A: Regional versus general anesthesia for bone marrow transplantation. J Clin Anesth 3:204, 1993.

143. Knudsen LM, Johnsen HE, Gaarsdal E, Jensen L: Spinal versus general anesthesia for bone marrow harvesting. Bone Marrow Transplant 3:486, 1995.

144. Tesno B, Jones MB, Yu L, Wall DA: Use of caudal block for pain control following bone marrow harvest in children. Am J Pediatr Hematol Oncol 16:305, 1994.

145. Blackburn R, Kyaw M, Swallow AJ: Reaction of cobalamin with nitrous oxide and cob(III)alamin. J Chem Soc 73:250, 1977.

146. Amess JAL, Burman JF, Rees GM, et al: Megaloblastic haemopoiesis in patients receiving nitrous oxide. Lancet 2:228, 1978.

Conclusion

147. Homi J, Reynolds J, Skinner A: General anesthesia in sickle cell diseases. Br Med J 1:1599, 1979.

148. Beutler E: Glucose-6-phosphate dehydrogenase deficiency. N Engl J Med 324:169, 1991.

149. Montgomery RR, Coller BS: Von Willebrand disease. *In* Colman RW, Hirsh J, Marder VJ, Salzman EW (eds): Hemostasis and Thrombosis. Philadelphia, JB Lippincott, 1994.

Muscle Diseases

Jordan D. Miller
Harvey Rosenbaum

I. CORI'S TYPE IX—DEFICIENT HEPATIC PHOSPHORYLASE-KINASE ACTIVITY WITH PREDOMINANT HEPATOMEGALY

J. CORI'S TYPE X—DEFICIENT CYCLIC 3',5'-ADENOSINE MONOPHOSPHATE–DEPENDENT KINASE

VII. **BLOCKS IN GLYCOLYSIS**

A. PHOSPHOHEXOISOMERASE DEFICIENCY

B. PHOSPHOGLYCERATE KINASE DEFICIENCY

C. PHOSPHOGLYCERATE MUTASE DEFICIENCY

D. LACTIC DEHYDROGENASE DEFICIENCY

VIII. **MYOADENYLATE DEAMINASE DEFICIENCY**

IX. **MYOSITIS OSSIFICANS PROGRESSIVA**

X. **MITOCHONDRIAL MYOPATHIES**

A. KEARNS-SAYRE SYNDROME, SPORADIC PROGRESSIVE EXTERNAL OPHTHALMOPLEGIA, "OPHTHALMOPLEGIA PLUS"

B. MYOCLONIC EPILEPSY WITH RAGGED RED FIBERS

C. MYOPATHY, ENCEPHALOPATHY, LACTIC ACIDOSIS, AND STROKE

D. LEIGH'S SYNDROME (SUBACUTE NECROTIZING ENCEPHALOMYELOPATHY)

XI. **DEFECTS OF OXIDATIVE PHOSPHORYLATION**

A. LUFT'S DISEASE

B. COMPLEX I—REDUCED NICOTINAMIDE ADENINE DINUCLEOTIDE–COENZYME Q REDUCTASE DEFECT

C. COMPLEX II—SUCCINATE–COENZYME Q REDUCTASE DEFECT

D. COENZYME Q DEFICIENCY

E. COMPLEX III—REDUCED COENZYME Q–CYTOCHROME C REDUCTASE DEFECT

F. COMPLEX IV—CYTOCHROME OXIDASE DEFICIENCY

G. COMPLEX V—MITOCHONDRIAL ADENOSINE TRIPHOSPHATASE DEFICIENCY

XII. **LIPID MYOPATHIES**

A. CARNITINE DEFICIENCY

B. SECONDARY CARNITINE DEFICIENCY

1. Long-Chain Acyl-Coenzyme A Dehydrogenase Deficiency

2. Medium-Chain Acyl-Coenzyme A Dehydrogenase Deficiency

3. Short-Chain Acyl-Coenzyme A Dehydrogenase Deficiency

4. Multiple Acyl-Coenzyme A Dehydrogenase Deficiency

C. CARNITINE PALMITOYLTRANSFERASE DEFICIENCY

XIII. **CONGENITAL MYOPATHIES**

A. CENTRAL CORE DISEASE

B. MULTICORE MYOPATHY

C. NEMALINE MYOPATHY

D. CENTRONUCLEAR (MYOTUBULAR) MYOPATHY

E. FINGERPRINT BODY MYOPATHY

XIV. **INFLAMMATORY MYOPATHIES AND "OVERLAP" SYNDROMES**

A. DERMATOMYOSITIS

B. ADULT DERMATOMYOSITIS AND POLYMYOSITIS

C. OVERLAP SYNDROMES

D. INCLUSION BODY MYOSITIS

E. VASCULITIDES

F. GRAFT-VERSUS-HOST DISEASE

XV. **INFECTIOUS DISEASES**

A. MYOPATHY OF HUMAN IMMUNODEFICIENCY VIRUS TYPE 1

B. INFLUENZA VIRUS AND OTHER VIRUSES

C. HELMINTHIC INFECTIONS: TRICHINOSIS AND ECHINOCOCCOSIS

D. BACTERIAL INFECTIONS

XVI. **MYOPATHY DUE TO DRUGS OR TOXINS**

A. NECROTIZING MYOPATHY AND ANTIHYPERLIPIDEMIA DRUGS

B. ε-AMINOCAPROIC ACID (AMICAR) MYOPATHY

C. ORGANOPHOSPHATE POISONING

D. ENVENOMATION: SNAKE, SPIDER, AND WASP VENOMS

E. HYPOKALEMIC MYOPATHY

F. LABETALOL MYOPATHY

I. INTRODUCTION

The muscle diseases are all intrinsic disorders of the skeletal muscle cell. Although the causes of these diverse diseases are frequently unknown, it has been possible in most cases to place the defect at or beyond the neuromuscular junction. Although most anesthesiologists have only limited experience with these diseases, the existing literature enables us to modify our anesthetic technique so as to decrease the risk to these patients.

Some general rules that apply to all patients with muscle diseases should be mentioned. Even patients who are capable of fairly normal activities may have decreased muscle reserves to compensate for the stress of anesthesia and operation. Thus, they are analogous to a partially "curarized" patient who seems normal but for whom any added stress may be catastrophic. Respiratory failure after upper abdominal surgery is more likely to occur in these patients, and the prognosis is more serious.

The anesthetic requirements are similar to those for any patient, but the margin of safety is reduced. One should use the smallest amounts of agents that provide satisfactory operating conditions. Fixed dosing schedules should be avoided, and continuous adjustments should be made according to the demands of the situation. Careful monitoring, of both objective and subjective parameters, must continue well into the postoperative period. It should be remembered that narcotics are as much a potential source of respiratory difficulty as are general anesthesia and muscle relaxants. The patient must demonstrate adequate respiratory reserve and an ability to handle secretions before leaving the recovery room. If either of these criteria is not met, mechanical ventilation via an endotracheal tube should be considered. If prolonged ventilatory assistance is required, tracheostomy may be necessary. Respiratory support using nasal continuous positive airway pressure (CPAP) may allow sicker patients to avoid tracheal intubation in the postoperative period; however, the use of nasal CPAP at home has allowed sicker patients to reach the operating room, and this could catch anesthesiologists off guard.

Preoperative use and teaching of chest physiotherapy may avoid many problems in the postoperative period. This is valuable even in patients whose surgical procedure is not usually associated with respiratory problems. Preventive measures can be life saving. Preoperative baseline measurements of respiratory reserve with at least simple tests of lung function (such as vital capacity and maximum inspiratory and expiratory force) and blood gas analysis will allow better postoperative assessment of these parameters. The use of the pulse oximeter while the patient is still breathing *room air* frequently reveals abnormal lung function before surgery. This readily available noninvasive tool is a much more sensitive way of identifying the patient with abnormal lungs than is the measurement when the patient's air is oxygen-enriched. We have frequently been surprised by the poor room air values and reserves of patients with muscle diseases.

Although the use of the nerve stimulator is always helpful, the results obtained must be interpreted cautiously in patients with muscle weakness and nonuniform muscle strength. Thus, the patient with proximal weakness and respiratory problems may have a totally normal response to muscle relaxants when tested in the distal arm; and, still, weakness potentiated by the relaxants may cause respiratory failure that would not be predicted by our normal criteria.

The measurement of serum enzymes derived from muscle is most abnormal in patients with ongoing muscle degeneration. When little muscle is left, the enzyme levels are reduced. Enzymes are frequently normal in severe muscle diseases that do not have continuous muscle destruction.

II. MUSCULAR DYSTROPHIES

Muscular dystrophies are a group of diseases of primary muscular atrophy of unknown cause. They are best characterized by the lack of any evidence of denervation,[1] and yet there is degeneration of the muscle fibers and increases in the content of fat and fibrous tissue in the muscle.

A. DYSTROPHINOPATHIES

Dystrophin is a membrane cytoskeletal protein that links the subsarcolemmal actin cytoskeleton to laminin, a component of the extracellular matrix. There are five dystrophin-associated glycoproteins (DAG), each defined by molecular weight (DAG 35, 43 doublet, 50 and 156 kd), and two proteins (25 and 59 kd). The absence of these components weakens the sarcolemma, which ruptures with mechanical stress. The ingress of extracellular components, particularly calcium, leads to necrosis.[2] The absence of one component may lead to reduced amounts of a second, thus confusing the picture. We are just learning to correlate the extent of the genetic defect with the severity of the disease process. Thus, complete absence of dystrophin, as in Duchenne's dystrophy (see below), produces the most severe form of the disease; whereas partial deletions cause Becker's dystrophy. The gene for dystrophin is on the X chromosome, so it is a sex-linked recessive entity. The associated proteins and glycoproteins are coded by genes on the autosomal chromosomes, so that inheritance is autosomal recessive.

B. DUCHENNE'S DYSTROPHY

The most common (1 in 3300 male births) and at the same time the most severe form of dystrophy is the childhood or Duchenne's type. This is characterized by onset of weakness between ages 2 and 6 years, usually in the pelvic girdle, followed rapidly by atrophy in the other proximal muscles.[1] The earlier the onset, the more rapid is the downhill course. Frequently, the atrophy is preceded by pseudohypertrophy, which occurs in the calf muscles. This is not true hypertrophy because the affected muscle is actually weaker than normal. On biopsy specimens, it can be seen that the enlargement is due to an increase in fat and fibrous tissue. This muscle, however, does not show the rapid loss of function seen in muscles that are only atrophic. Its level of function remains stable, although diminished, whereas other muscles become completely useless.

Because the inheritance is a sex-linked recessive trait[3] almost all of the reported patients are boys; however, there have been some well-documented cases in girls.[4] These "manifesting carriers" display a spectrum of severity, from full Duchenne's to mild weakness. Sex-linked recessive genes can produce disease in female offspring of normal fathers when (1) the paternal mutation occurs in the father's germ plasm but not elsewhere, (2) there is early inactivation of the normal X chromosome (Lyon hypothesis; see immediately below), (3) the paternally derived X chromosome mutates early in embryogenesis, or (4) the patient has Turner's syndrome with chromosomal anomalies (XO). The Lyon hypothesis states that, in any cell, only one X chromosome is active. The other X chromosome in females is inactivated early in embryonic growth and is a chance occurrence. Therefore, it would be expected that in the vast majority of the cells of some female heterozygotes the abnormal X chromosome would be the only active one. This would explain the existence of an occasional girl with the disease.[1] Female carriers typically show only elevated serum enzyme levels; those with the highest enzyme levels would be the ones with the largest proportion of abnormal cells. Thus, one can view manifesting carriers as being at one end of a spectrum of disease. Whether women heterozygous for the abnormal Duchenne's gene, such as mothers of Duchenne's patients, should be considered at risk for complications of anesthesia is not at present clear.

Elevated serum enzyme levels are derived from enzymes released by muscle injury. Aldolase and creatine kinase (CK; formerly called *creatine phosphokinase [CPK]*) are the ones most often measured. The MB fraction of CK, normally present only in heart muscle, is present in skeletal muscle in myopathies and thus cannot be used as a guide to cardiac injury.[5] The highest CK levels (50 to 100 times normal) occur up to age 3 years and then decrease by about 20 per cent per year as muscle atrophies.[6] This increase in serum enzymes is thought to result from increased permeability of the cell membrane. The finding that a specific cellular structural protein (dystrophin) is missing has increased our understanding of a number of related diseases, but this knowledge has yet to improve treatment. Dystrophin is a very large protein found on the inner surface of the sarcolemma. Its presence seems to protect cells from mechanical injury like that which occurs with usual exercise. Multiple deletions, duplications, and point mutations in the gene have been found, and DNA from leukocytes can be used to detect abnormalities, but the easiest test is to look for dystrophin in muscle biopsy specimens. It is almost completely absent from such specimens.[6] Approximately one third of all cases represent new mutations; the rest are from a maternal carrier.

The muscles turn pale early in the disease process, even before fat and fibrous tissue accumulate, since they lose their myoglobin through leaky membranes.[1] The fat that does increase during atrophy is quite resistant to mobilization, even in the presence of inani-

tion. The reason for this is not known. Cell degeneration is thought to be caused by leakage of calcium into the cell at a faster rate than the sarcoplasmic reticulum (SR) can handle, thus activating kinases, with a multitude of effects. The leakage of complement into cells would also cause injury.

Clinically, patients exhibit Gowers' sign—using their hands to "climb" up their legs to arise from the floor. This is necessary because of the early weakness of the pelvic girdle and the relative strength of the arms and shoulders. They cannot walk with the heels flat on the ground; they have a waddling gait and a lordotic stance—legs apart and shoulders back. They have difficulty lifting their heads from a pillow (flexing the neck), so this is not a good test of muscle relaxant reversal. The downhill course of the disease, although variable, is progressive, leading to a wheelchair existence after 3 to 10 years and to death after 5 to 20 years. A subgroup of about 15 per cent have a much slower disease course that seems to stabilize about the time of puberty. For these children, contractures are a major feature of their disability. If patients are bedridden for any length of time they may not recover their preoperative level of function. This is a major limitation to any surgery and emphasizes the need for physical therapy to prevent contractures.

Cardiac abnormalities occur in a large proportion of these patients—50 to 70 per cent[6, 7]—although they are clinically significant in only 10 per cent and in most of these only in the terminal phase of the disease. The severity of cardiac and skeletal disease does not correlate. Arrhythmias occur frequently, even after minor emotional trauma. Griggs reported atrial tachycardia in 65 per cent of his patients.[6] Complex ventricular premature beats have been noted and correlated with abnormal left ventricular function and increased incidence of sudden death.[8] One or more of the following electrocardiographic (ECG) abnormalities have been noted in more than 90 per cent of patients: (1) increased net RS voltage in lead V_1; (2) a deep, narrow Q wave in the left precordial leads; (3) RSR' in lead V_1; and (4) a polyphasic R wave in lead V_1. Mitral valve prolapse demonstrated by echocardiography is present in 10 to 25 per cent of the patients.[6, 7] Patients whose cardiac status was fully compensated have nevertheless died suddenly and unexpectedly. Although the usual picture at autopsy is that of cardiac dilatation, with or without hypertrophy, function of the ventricle as demonstrated by echocardiography shows posterobasilar hypokinesis in a thin-walled ventricle and a slow relaxation phase with normal contraction.[1,7] There is frequently a picture of increased connective tissue and fat, as in the skeletal muscle. Fibrosis of the myocardium typically is limited to the posterobasal and lateral free walls of the left ventricle in Duchenne's muscular dystrophy, unlike the fibrosis associated with other forms of muscular dystrophy. The ECG and echocardiographic findings can thus be used in the differential diagnosis—and even in carrier detection.[1]

Respiratory weakness and limitation are manifested by the end of the first decade of life, as seen by reductions in inspiration, expiration, vital capacity, and total lung capacity. Kyphoscoliosis secondary to the muscle weakness usually occurs after the patient needs a wheelchair, and this further limits lung function. The use of weight or arm span for predicting the correct vital capacity is important in these children with severe scoliosis. Respiratory problems usually result from respiratory tract infections. In one study of 48 patients who underwent Harrington rod insertion, all those whose vital capacity was greater than 35 per cent of the predicted value could be extubated immediately. Two of the three patients in this study whose vital capacity was less than 30 per cent had respiratory problems.[9] In a second study, one of nine patients had died from respiratory causes; again, 30 per cent vital capacity seemed to be the dividing line.[10] Late respiratory complications and cardiac arrest occurred in spite of apparently adequate ventilatory support. It was suspected that succinylcholine was the cause, but this was not proved.[11] In another study only 4 of 27 patients needed ventilatory support for as long as 2 days; all had forced vital capacity (FVC) less than 30 per cent of the value predicted.[7] Operative intervention for scoliosis does not cause any improvement: although it may slow the long-term deterioration of respiratory function, it is done principally for comfort.[6]

Although there is no effective treatment, there is some evidence that the disease is helped by verapamil. Concerns about this drug's myocardial effects and a report that the administration of verapamil was associated with respiratory arrest limit its use. A recent clinical trial using prednisone, 0.75 mg/kg daily, showed slowing of disease progression over a 3-year period; thus we may expect that many of the sicker patients will be taking steroids. The onset for therapeutic effect took at least 10 days, so short-term therapy in preparation for surgery has not been recommended.[6] Exercise is controversial because it may hasten muscle destruction; however, passive exercise to prevent contractures and resistive exercise of lungs to increase endurance may be helpful.[12] Recent randomized studies of the use of prophylactic nasal CPAP have produced conflicting results. In one study, there were more deaths among patients receiving "long-term" nasal CPAP; the explanation is not apparent.[13]

Several large series report the use of anesthetic agents. The two older studies listed drugs less commonly used today but are noteworthy in that they report no temperature rise or cardiac arrest. Cobham[14] described anesthetic use in 70 patients, and Richards[15] reported on 43 patients in whom 61 anesthetics were used. Virtually all anesthetic agents have been used. In Richards' study, halothane was used 37 times and succinylcholine 12 times, all without subsequent problems. The anesthetic difficulties seemed to parallel the severity of the illness, and patients with preexisting respiratory difficulties were most prone to postoperative problems; however, since that time, many case reports have described cardiac arrest in patients with Duchenne's muscular dystrophy, during or immediately after anesthesia.[16–23]

The most frightening aspect seems to be that, in many cases, the patients had minimal weakness at the time of operation. In several, the arrest first called attention to Duchenne's dystrophy. The reports do not give enough information to infer an explanation; however, elevated potassium (K^+), when measured, and CK levels and myoglobinuria (sometimes causing renal failure) occurred if the patients survived. These results should be interpreted with caution, since in this disease even walking can increase the CK level from 6000 to 25,000 U and the myoglobin level from 200 to 1000 ng/mL (Normal increases with vigorous exercise are 70 to 230 units for CK and 20 to 60 ng/mL for myoglobin, and both increases occur later in normal healthy persons than in patients with Duchenne's dystrophy.)[1] Acidosis was also common. Hyperpyrexia, hypermetabolism, and rigidity were less common in these patients. In at least one family, the inheritance was such that malignant hyperthermia (MH) and Duchenne's dystrophy were inherited independently.[24] It is speculated that the inherent membrane defect in Duchenne's muscular dystrophy, rather than an additional defect such as MH, renders the muscle more susceptible to injury induced by anesthesia. It must be remembered that there is no denominator to case reports and that several series reporting anesthetic experiences found no such events; however, at present, the risk of anesthesia with classic triggering agents such as the potent inhalational agents and succinylcholine tend to encourage use of anesthetic technique safe for patients with known MH. It is not known if the risks associated with using alternatives such as slower-onset, longer-acting relaxants or larger doses of narcotics, among others, might be the cause of an overall higher incidence of morbidity and mortality. Recent case reports[25] of the use of propofol in Duchenne's patients are encouraging, but, as with the earlier series of uneventful anesthetics with triggering agents, large series are required to document safety. Many patients tolerate agents that we later find cause an unacceptable number of serious complications.

The major predictable postoperative problem is respiratory depression in patients with minimal reserves; therefore, the lightest possible anesthetic levels should be aimed for. Minimal premedication should be used—with the understanding, however, that many affected children are hostile and withdrawn. Preoperative introduction to chest physiotherapy and nasal CPAP, and their use early in the postoperative period, should keep respiratory complications to a minimum. Regional anesthesia for muscle biopsy[26] and local anesthesia for dental work have been recommended.[27] Light general anesthesia combined with continuous spinal anesthesia, even though the patient had a Harrington rod in place, produced rapid return of preoperative pulmonary function.[28]

Several unusual postoperative complications have occurred in these patients. Gastric dilatation,[15] heralded by tachycardia and unobtainable blood pressure, occurred perioperatively in three patients. The combined effects of primary abnormalities in smooth muscle, inactivity, and anesthesia are all thought to lead to the dilatation. Prophylactic use of a nasogastric tube is recommended. Preoperative gastric dilatation and delayed gastric emptying may occur. Care, as for a patient with a full stomach, is warranted.[29] Another problem was difficulty in swallowing, which

led to aspiration, respiratory failure, and the death of two patients within 48 hours after minor operations.[30] If Pentothal is used, it should be given in small increments; with this regimen, no problems have been encountered.[31] Propofol has been recommended,[25] and the doses required may be even higher than normal:[32] however, some of these patients have significant cardiomyopathy, and the reduction in heart rate and decreased contractility may cause problems with tissue perfusion.

C. BECKER'S DYSTROPHY

A second "dystrophinopathy" is Becker's dystrophy. The gene is located at the same locus as that for Duchenne's; thus, it is an X-linked muscular dystrophy (incidence 1 in 18,000 to 33,000 male births)[33] that is distinguishable from Duchenne's by later onset (mean age 12 years) and a much more benign course. Instead of absence of the gene product, there are various exon deletions that allow translation of mRNA and lead to lesser amounts and abnormal forms of dystrophin. The clinical picture is much more varied and can be anything from that typical of Duchenne's to minimal disease. The average age at which patients become wheelchair bound is 30 years, and only 3 per cent require a wheelchair before age 11 years (versus more than 90 per cent with Duchenne's dystrophy). Death occurs at an average age of 42 years, pneumonia being the most common cause. Although cardiac involvement is much less common and less severe than in Duchenne's dystrophy, heart failure is still a common cause of death.[34] Pseudohypertrophy is common and helps distinguish the disease from limb girdle dystrophy. There have also been reports of cardiac arrest during and following anesthesia in Becker's dystrophy;[35, 36] it now seems likely that these patients, like those with Duchenne's dystrophy, are at risk of rhabdomyolysis. Unlike in malignant hyperthermia, neither hypercarbia nor elevated heart rate, blood pressure, or temperature is a premonitory sign of imminent arrest. The frequency of these events when using triggering agents is not known.

D. EMERY-DREIFUSS DYSTROPHY

Emery-Dreifuss muscular dystrophy is an X-linked genetic disorder with involvement of the biceps and triceps in the upper extremities and the distal muscles in the lower extremities. Contractures in elbow, ankles, and neck occur early and are the major cause of the disability, but the slow progression of the muscle disease distinguishes it from the Duchenne's and Becker's types. The patient's predominant risk is cardiac rather than skeletal muscle weakness. Atrial arrhythmias occur early in the disease and later progress to atrial arrest.[37] Sudden death is common between ages 30 and 60 years. The severity of the skeletal muscle disease does not correlate with the cardiac manifestations. Cardiomyopathy may be present; fibrosis of the entire ventricle has been reported.[6] Cardiomegaly is uncommon. The use of a prophylactic ventricular pacemaker early in the disease has been suggested.[38] Female carriers may also be at risk for sudden death.[39] Intubation may be a problem because of limitation of cervical motion, though flexion may be more limited than extension.

E. RIGID SPINE SYNDROME

A slowly progressive course much like that of Becker's dystrophy but with the addition of progressive, painless limitation of neck and trunk characterizes rigid spine syndrome. It occurs principally in boys; thus, it is thought to be a sex-linked recessive trait. Respiratory difficulty with severe restrictive disease and weakness of respiratory muscles occurs in many patients. Hypercapnic ventilatory failure may be a result.[40] Scoliosis accompanies the weakness, as does a cardiomyopathy in some patients. Although no anesthetic management has been described, the immobility of the neck might well create anesthetic problems, as would cardiac involvement. Many of these cases have been taken to be idiopathic scoliosis, so care must be exercised in their identification.

F. FACIOSCAPULOHUMERAL (LANDOUZY-DEJERINE) DYSTROPHY

Facioscapulohumeral (FSH) dystrophy is also known as the *benign dystrophy*. The incidence is 1 in 20,000, with autosomal dominant inheritance (boys and girls are equally affected). No clear-cut differentiation has been made between the heterozygous and homozygous forms of the disease, although it is assumed that the homozygous form is worse. Onset is usually in adolescence and progression is insidious if there is any progression at all. Patients have weak pectoral and facial muscles, especially the orbicularis, but the masseter and the extraocular muscles are spared. The pelvic muscles are much less affected than in Duchenne's dystrophy.[6] Occasional patients have signs of the disease at 6 years of age, but most have recognizable symptoms by age 12. More than 80 per cent seek medical help because of weakness of shoulder muscles, and winging of the scapula is seen on raising the arm away from the chest. Surgery may be performed to stabilize the scapula, to increase the lifting function of the arm. As many as 30 per cent of patients reach middle age without realizing that they have any abnormality. Life span is reduced minimally in most patients, but 20 per cent exhibit progression and need a wheelchair. Cardiac involvement is rare and probably the result of coincidence. The most abnormal respiratory finding is the vital capacity, owing to the involvement of the accessory muscles of respiration. In one study that followed patients for an average of 15 years after onset of disease (when two of eight patients were already in wheelchairs) the P_{CO_2} and the P_{O_2} values remained normal. The carbon dioxide response curve was also normal; however, many patients had recurrent bouts of upper respiratory tract infections.[41] If anesthesia and operation are required, one should focus on preventing respiratory complications. The report of a single patient with rapid return of function after atracurium does not allow us to generalize, because no explanation of the finding was made and the case may represent mere coincidence.[42]

G. LIMB GIRDLE DYSTROPHY

Limb girdle dystrophy is a "wastebasket" classification of predominantly autosomal recessive diseases that now includes five subtypes. Based on clinical presentation, two subdivisions are most common: *Erb's type*, of juvenile onset, in which the shoulder girdle is primarily involved, and the *Leyden-Möbius* late-onset type, with primarily pelvic girdle involvement. Onset occurs any time from the first to the third decade of life. The severity is midway between the Duchenne's and FSH types.[1] The involvement of the heart varies. Some estimates use 10 per cent for the prevalence of congestive heart failure.[6] The most common ECG abnormalities are sinus tachycardia and right bundle branch block. There may be early and severe weakening of the diaphragm, leading to hypoventilation. It is helpful to question the patient about symptoms related to nighttime hypercarbia, such as hypersomnolence and headache. These symptoms respond to mechanical ventilation. Becker's dystrophy and inclusion body myositis may be misdiagnosed as limb girdle dystrophy. In *severe childhood autosomal-recessive dystrophy*, the absence of the dystrophin-associated glycoprotein adhalin (50 kd) produces symptoms like those of Becker's dystrophy, with late onset, elevated CK, and weakness in the same distribution. There is greater variability in severity from sibling to sibling. The disease is most common in North Africa. The gene is located on 17q12–21. Cardiac disease may be much worse than the skeletal muscle component, and heart transplant has been used.[2, 6]

H. DISTAL MYOPATHIES

There are several less common varieties of muscular dystrophy. One unusual group are the four *distal* myopathies (since most myopathies present with proximal muscle weakness). In *Welander's (late adult–onset)*, myopathy, which occurs almost exclusively in Sweden, the hands are most frequently involved. Onset is after age 30 years, and the pattern of inheritance is autosomal dominant. It is only slowly progressive.[6] Similarly, *Markesberry's dystrophy* is slowly progressive. It starts in the fifth decade, but in the feet rather than the hands. It is seen in persons of French-English ancestry and is autosomal dominant. Some patients have cardiomyopathy secondary to interstitial fibrosis of the heart muscle.[6] *Early adult–onset myopathy* is another described but ill-understood disease whose subdivisions are based on involvement of anterior or posterior compartment of the legs.

I. OCULOPHARYNGEAL MUSCULAR DYSTROPHY

One of the most difficult problems in the classification of the muscular dystrophies is the exact position of *oculopharyngeal muscular dystrophy*. This type presents after the age of 30 years,[6] with weakness of pharyngeal muscles and ptosis and mild limb weakness. Extraocular muscle weakness is variable, but patients rarely have diplopia. Symptoms are similar to those of ocular myasthenia gravis.[43, 46] Confusion in classification occurs because biopsy specimens resemble those of muscular dystrophy, and progression is very slow, without episodes of severe weakness. Fatigue does not make the symptoms worse. Pharyngeal weakness is common and sometimes extension to the proximal limb muscles, but unlike in myasthenia gravis, there is no dysarthria or dyspnea. Dysphagia and aspiration are common, and dyscoordination of the posterior pharynx and involvement of the esophagus render these patients prone to aspiration and inanition.[6]

Despite these dissimilarities, many oculopharyngeal muscular dystrophy patients are exquisitely sensitive to muscles relaxants.[43–46] Patient weakness is not helped by anticholinesterase agents. In fact, several have been completely paralyzed by 5 to 10 per cent of the Effective Dose$_{95}$ (ED$_{95}$) and then could not have the paralysis reversed by edrophonium. In contrast, a recent case report found normal sensitivity to vecuronium in one patient;[47] nevertheless muscle relaxants must be used with extreme caution in these patients, and preparation must be made to ventilate them over many hours, particularly when muscles other than those around the eye are involved.

J. CONGENITAL MUSCULAR DYSTROPHY

Congenital muscular dystrophy is a wastebasket term used to denote onset of the disease at birth. It does not fit into one of the better-defined categories such as Duchenne's dystrophy. One group in this category exhibits slow progression or none and may or may not be associated with arthrogryposis (Batten-Turner congenital muscular dystrophy).[48] The degree of involvement is usually determined at birth, and the disease usually involves the proximal muscles more than the distal ones. The CK level is only slightly elevated. One case report[49] describes an episode of MH developing in an 18-month-old child that was responsive to dantrolene but required several days for resolution. A unique aspect of the episode was repeated hypoglycemia. The child eventually had a stroke, which was attributed to the episode.

The *Fukuyama form* of muscular dystrophy is seen frequently in Japan (incidence 1 in 18,000), but only rarely elsewhere. It involves proximal muscles, and its course is progressive, but unlike Duchenne's dystrophy it also involves the central nervous system (CNS): seizures occur in 50 per cent of patients, along with slow mental development. The latter is accounted for by abnormal migration and differentiation of the neurons during fetal development of the brain. The genetic trait is most likely autosomal recessive. The disease is progressive, and most patients die by age 10 years.[48]

III. MYOTONIAS

The myotonic phenomenon consists of persistent contraction after either voluntary use or mechanical stimulation of a muscle. This contraction, once started, does not require further stimulation by the motor nerve. In addition to the agonist muscles going into spasm, the antagonist muscles also contract as the patient tries to relax.[50] This has been referred to as *afterspasm.* Many clinically and genetically different muscle diseases display such a phenomenon. In some, the myotonia is the complaint, but often it is only a demonstrable sign. Using percussion of muscle, sustained contraction can be elicited in these patients. The muscles most often used to demonstrate myotonia are in the tongue, leading to a "napkin ring" appearance and the thenar eminence, leading to a depression in the muscle.

A. MYOTONIC MUSCULAR DYSTROPHY

The one type of muscular dystrophy that shows the greatest systemic involvement is *myotonic muscular dystrophy* (Steinert's disease or myotonia atrophica). This form of muscular dystrophy has myotonic symptoms that generally antedate the atrophy and weakness. This is one of the most common muscular dystrophies, with an incidence of 1 in 20,000 (though the regional incidence can be as high as 1 in 500, as in Quebec, Canada) and an autosomal-dominant mode of inheritance.[6] It is thought that the incidence of new mutations is low. The most common age of onset

is between the second and fourth decades of life, and the disease is slowly progressive. Death does not usually occur before the fifth or sixth decade. In spite of the myotonia, the major complaint is the atrophy, usually of the facial, sternocleidomastoid, and distal muscles. This leads to a classic appearance of hatchet face (secondary to temporalis and masseter atrophy), frontal baldness, and ptosis. There is pharyngeal weakness and nasal speech.

Measurements in vivo of membrane potential show values that are of smaller magnitude than is normal or than those typical of other forms of myotonia.[50] The resting levels of sodium are higher in the muscle cell, owing to larger Na^+ conductance. The defect in the Na^+ conductance is certainly not the only defect in this disease (as it is in some other myotonias). The gene, located on 19q13.2, has been isolated and is called *myotonin protein kinase,* since it resembles other protein kinases. Its function has not been worked out, but the phosphorylation of many proteins, including channels, can be responsible for the wide variety of defects seen in this disease.[51]

Historically, the properties of myotonic musculature have been elucidated by the use of various anesthetic techniques. Thus, it was shown that the abnormality was not neural in origin, because both spinal and regional blocks[52] failed to either prevent or terminate the contraction. Total neuromuscular block with curare also demonstrated the independence of the myotonia from the neuromuscular transmission. Instead, the local infiltration of procaine decreased the myotonia. This observation led to the use of quinine, procainamide (potentially dangerous in patients with cardiac conduction abnormalities),[53] and, more recently, phenytoin to decrease the myotonia.[50] These drugs are effective, both subjectively and objectively, in all forms of myotonia, with resultant improvement in electromyography (EMG) findings, a more stable resting potential, and less spontaneous muscle activity. The use of antiarrhythmics such as tocainide and mexiletine in this form of myotonia is not recommended because of the risk of worsening conduction abnormalities.[6] The anticholinesterases have been said to make the myotonia worse, but in one study there was no change in the EMG, except for some twitching in one patient.[53] The use of intra-arterial acetylcholine or choline in these patients gives a response to much smaller doses than in normal patients. The response looks like the response in denervated muscle.[54] The use of depolarizing muscle relaxants leads to sustained contraction. In nerve injury of short duration (less than 20 weeks), a similar response is seen in muscles beyond the point of injury. It is interesting that detailed studies of the motor end-plate in myotonic muscle show many end-plates with profuse subterminal ramifications of the nerves. The same picture is noted in bird and frog muscle, which also respond to succinylcholine with prolonged contraction.[54]

The truly systemic nature of myotonic dystrophy[6, 50] can be seen from the wide variety of systems involved. The most common of associated abnormalities is presenile cataract, which is characteristic of the disease. In many relatives of affected patients, this may be the only evidence of the disease. It was said that cataract occurred in the first generation, muscle abnormality in the second, and the full systemic manifestations in the third generation. This clinical observation was once thought to be an artifact of case selection. It is now known that the abnormality, an increasing number of CTG repeats at the noncoding 3' end of the gene, gets progressively worse generation to generation[55] and that this correlates with disease severity. Frontal baldness and testicular atrophy in males and intellectual and emotional changes are all common. The testicular changes are primary rather than secondary to pituitary abnormalities. Smooth muscle involvement is manifested in delayed gastric emptying and poor motility of the esophagus, colon, and uterus. The glucose tolerance test result is abnormal, with delayed utilization of glucose and slow return to normal serum glucose levels after the glucose load. Tolbutamide causes a greater than normal increase in insulin (by radioimmunoassay), but the decrease in glucose is only 65 per cent of normal. This would mean that these patients are resistant to insulin of endogenous origin and that the number of insulin receptors is reduced.[50] The control mechanisms for insulin release and inhibition are normal in these patients, and they do not suffer the problems associated with adult-onset diabetes.

The cardiorespiratory abnormalities are of particular concern to anesthesiologists. Cardiac arrhythmias were mentioned shortly after the original description of the disease. The most common ECG abnormalities are conduction defects (present in 57 per cent of patients in one series) and one third show an increased PR interval, which is unresponsive to both atropine and nitroglycerin. Greater degrees of heart block are common, but the criteria for insertion of a pacemaker have not been established.[6] The P wave has a decreased height, and ST elevations are common. Atrial flutter, which responds to quinidine, has been observed. Digitalis has also been used to control the heart rate associated with flutter. The blood pressure is usually low but rises when congestive heart failure intervenes. Of 37 patients in one series who died, 9 had cardiac failure as a primary cause. In one series, subclinical cardiac involvement occurred in 42 of 46 subjects, 70 per cent having left ventricular dysfunction.[56] One patient had documented cardiomyopathy with lesions similar to those in skeletal muscle.[57] Some patients had Stokes-Adams attacks, as would be expected from the frequent increase in the PR interval. After spinal anesthesia in one patient, the heart rate dropped to 40 beats per minute, but this responded to an anticholinergic agent and may not be representative of the disease.[58]

The use of a pacemaker is recommended if there are signs of a conduction abnormality, but sudden death may be related to tachyarrhythmias rather than to bradycardia.[56, 59] Transthoracic pacing as a backup measure in patients at risk for conduction abnormalities may obviate use of a temporary internal pacemaker, but one must remember that the loss of the atrial kick may cause a large reduction in cardiac output. Caution in the use of quinidine must be observed, as with any patient susceptible to Stokes-Adams attacks. The severity of the cardiac disease does not parallel that of the skeletal muscle disease.[56] An unusual form of cardiomyopathy is seen in many patients. Wall motion and ejection fraction are decreased, but they improve with exercise.[56] Using exercise stress testing, the maximum heart rate was less than 80 per cent of predicted value, and the maximum oxygen consumption only 40 per cent of predicted, indicating a major reduction in the patient's ability to tolerate stress.[60] Congestive heart failure is less frequent and is associated with cor pulmonale.[6] The value of Swan-Ganz catheters for intraoperative management of these patients is exemplified by the report of Meyers and coworkers.[61] One must not forget that many of these patients have risk factors for coronary disease, and thus some of the problems are caused by coronary insufficiency.

Respiratory problems can be classified into three categories: (1) abnormalities in pulmonary function test results; (2) central nervous system disease, leading to respiratory failure; and (3) problems of the oropharynx. Pulmonary function abnormalities include vital capacity, total lung capacity, and maximum voluntary ventilation that are frequently reduced; however, only 20 per cent are classified as moderate to severe impairment (less than 50 per cent FVC). Nevertheless, peak expiratory pressure is diminished on average to 27 ± 11 per cent of normal, whereas peak inspiratory pressure is 50 per cent of normal.[60] This is important since expiratory pressure is correlated with good cough. A history of pneumonia was found in 25 per cent, and there was some correlation with the severity of lung disease. The lungs themselves seem normal. Although this picture is similar to that in restrictive chest wall disease, the mechanism is different. Alternating dominance of the diaphragm and thoracic muscles, which is a normal pattern, was much more frequent, indicating muscle fatigue even with low ventilatory requirements. The most likely cause is the need for greater strength to overcome the myotonia of the respiratory muscles of the abdomen during inspiration.[62] The primary (diaphragm and intercostal) muscles as well as the accessory muscles of respiration have been shown to be abnormal in many of these patients. The diaphragm has been seen to move abnormally on fluoroscopy, and the intercostal muscles are myotonic.[63]

Many patients are somnolent, and the question arose whether this is a direct or a secondary CNS manifestation of the disease. Of the patients studied, several did have mild elevations of the P_{CO_2} and low oxygen saturation on room air. There was a shift in the carbon dioxide response curve to the right (lower sensitivity to carbon dioxide)[64] and an associated increase in the P_{CO_2} when patients breathed 100 per cent oxygen; however, with abnormal chest mechanics, one cannot be certain that these findings indicate abnormalities in central control of respiration. A more recent study of patients who were in the early course of their disease before the onset of carbon dioxide retention, using methods that were independent of muscle fatigue, failed to show any abnormality in central control of respiration.[62] The somnolence would not be expected just on the basis of these relatively mild changes in blood gases. In addition, one patient showed no change in somnolence

with improved respiratory function and restoration of P_{CO_2} to normal. Sleep caused an increase in P_{CO_2}, which produced pulmonary hypertension in the patient evaluated. The sleep apnea that occurs may be caused by upper airway obstruction, and this and hypersomnolence may be alleviated by tracheostomy;[65] however, only rarely can the somnolence be blamed on sleep apnea. One patient with somnolence described by Tsueda and coworkers could not be weaned from a respirator for 5 days postoperatively.[66] In short, somnolence, personality changes, and occasional CNS atrophy are thought to be primary CNS manifestations of the disease.

The frequency of pneumonia[60] has prompted investigation of the swallowing mechanism in some of these patients. Of four patients who died of pneumonia, two had pulmonary abscesses and one had evidence of aspiration.[67] Of 44 patients studied, all but one showed abnormal swallowing on cineradiography. Twelve patients had aspiration of radiopaque material without any cough.[68] Many patients without pulmonary symptoms had severe abnormalities demonstrated on cineradiography. Only males showed the aspiration, although there were many females in the study. Twenty-two patients had chronic cough, four had bronchiectasis, three tuberculosis, and three severe emphysema. The difficulty in swallowing was not improved by quinine, procainamide, or steroids. This is consistent with the observation that the swallowing abnormality parallels the atrophy rather than the myotonia. In addition to the esophagus, the stomach also shows poor motility. The smooth muscle involvement is thought to be responsible.[50] Poor gastric motility may decrease the absorption of oral medication and increase the danger of aspiration.

Therapy is limited, because the myotonia is not very symptomatic and there is no treatment for the atrophy.[6] Quinine was the first drug to be used, and although it is effective in many patients, toxic levels may be needed. Procainamide, in contrast, works without producing many of the toxic symptoms. It is given orally in a dose of 1 g four times a day. It is effective in blocking the myotonia after spontaneous effort but not percussion myotonia and thus may not enhance relaxation during surgery. It is also effective intravenously in doses up to 1000 mg given at a rate slower than 100 mg per minute. The use of this drug in patients with myotonic dystrophy is debatable, since they are prone to heart block.

Phenytoin has been advocated, as it does not increase the danger of heart block.[50]

As would be expected, this disease poses a very difficult problem to the anesthesiologist. Many serious problems are related to the systemic manifestations of the disease. Thus, one must be aware of the serious cardiac problems, and ECG monitoring is mandatory, not only intraoperatively but also postoperatively. The use of 24-hour monitoring to evaluate the frequency of rhythm disturbances is strongly recommended and may then indicate the use of antiarrhythmic agents or a pacemaker, or both.[56] The arguments for and against prophylactic "digitalization" are the same as in any other case of mild cardiac disease. Digitalization may increase the likelihood of heart block.[6] The respiratory problems require careful attention in the perioperative period, not only because of the anesthetic depression but also because of the inherent swallowing problems and weak cough associated with this disease.[60] The endocrine abnormalities should not pose any serious problem. If there is an episode of unexplained hypotension with poor response to vasopressors, steroids should be used. The psychological problems require a careful and thorough preoperative visit, to enlist the patient's cooperation. Because of the limited response to increased carbon dioxide, patients are more likely to require controlled ventilation during anesthesia and may well require postoperative ventilation, even after relatively minor surgery and relatively small amounts of short-acting narcotics.[69] Preoperative blood gas analysis should be obtained as a baseline value. Respiratory function tests should include a 1-second forced expiratory volume and maximum expiratory and inspiratory pressures, and, if possible, minute ventilation, maximum breathing capacity, and total lung volume.

It was reported as early as 1915[70] that myotonia patients did poorly after anesthesia. After an uneventful ether anesthesia procedure, a patient had cyanosis for the next 24 hours. Then, in the early 1950s, Dundee[71] reported that thiopentone produced severe apnea in these patients and was contraindicated. Careful studies have shown that this is not peculiar to thiopentone but that these patients are particularly sensitive to any respiratory depressant.[69, 72–80] The depression is not the result of a direct effect on muscle, as was once thought, but of a nonspecific effect of depressant medication in a patient with little

respiratory reserve, and probably CNS involvement, as mentioned earlier. The seriousness of the respiratory problem is well-documented by the deaths of four of five patients with respiratory depression in Kaufman's series.[81] In a comment on Kaufman's paper, Hunter described a patient who had Pentothal and curare anesthesia for a hysterectomy procedure and then required ventilation for 4 days and had difficulties handling secretions for four weeks.[82] Ravin and coworkers reported a patient with severe respiratory problems four hours postoperatively because of respiratory obstruction. This patient had appeared to do well in the immediate postoperative period.[83] This is obviously not just the result of a single anesthetic; rather, it demonstrates how easily these patients can undergo decompensation. Even doses of sedatives that usually produce little effect in normal persons may lead to prolonged and profound effects in these patients. Although newer drugs would seem to be safer, this has not reduced the number of reports of unexpected and adverse outcomes. If apnea occurs, the best therapy is ventilation rather than counteracting drugs such as neostigmine, naloxone, or doxapram.[84] The recent popularity of propofol in patients with muscle diseases has prompted case reports of increased sensitivity of myotonic dystrophy patients to this agent. What is clear is that there is a great range of sensitivity. Most are normal, but a few show extreme sensitivity.[85] One patient was reported to have the onset of myotonia with propofol, and relaxation occurred only after the use of isoflurane.[86] Other agents associated with myoclonus, including methohexital and etomidate, might be expected to produce similar responses. One must be prepared for both types of patients, and the sensitivity is not predictable at this time.[60, 79, 80] Although we pride ourselves on our ability to assess and treat respiratory failure, recent reports show that we continue to underrate the severity of the respiratory compromise in these patients.[71, 79, 80]

The production of muscle relaxation in a myotonic patient is one of the most difficult problems facing the anesthesiologist. Nerve blocks cannot guarantee relaxation, because the muscles are still subject to the equivalent of percussion myotonia, the stimulus of the surgeon, and electrocautery. Nerve blocks, however, are ideal if relaxation is not needed.[87–89] Nondepolarizing muscle relaxants have much the same problem: because they block only the motor nerve impulses, stimulation beyond the neuromuscular junction may still cause myotonia. The experience with muscle relaxants is best documented by Mitchell and coworkers.[90] It was shown that myotonic patients have normal sensitivity to curare.[90] Recently, shorter-acting nondepolarizing agents, such as atracurium, have been used with good effect and no unusual sensitivity.[63, 91–93]

Although neostigmine has been noted to increase myotonia, several reports indicate that its use to reverse nondepolarizing blocks has been uneventful.[83, 90] However, there have been some recent reports of delayed-onset weakness starting as long as 20 minutes after a dose of neostigmine,[94] as well as an increase in the myotonia as demonstrated by the capnogram,[95] as doses were increased incrementally within the usual dose range. This led to concerns about the use of reversal agents and might encourage the use of shorter-acting nondepolarizing agents and spontaneous recovery. Deep general anesthesia may also be used to produce relaxation;[96] however, if the general anesthesia is deep, cardiac function may be unacceptably depressed and residual effects on consciousness and respiration may be prolonged. The depolarizing muscle relaxants have the same limitations as the nondepolarizing type, but in addition there are many reports of widespread myotonia following their use. Involvement of the muscles of respiration as well as the larynx[97] has made it difficult or impossible to ventilate these patients. The myotonia seems to last as long as or longer than the effect of succinylcholine. Whether the use of procainamide, smaller doses, or pretreatment with a nondepolarizer would reduce the occurrence of this reaction is not known; however, with the presently available agents, succinylcholine would seem a poor choice. Its only indication might be rapid-sequence induction, but the possibility of myotonia rather than relaxation makes it unacceptable in this situation. Dantrolene has been tried for muscle relaxation during abdominal surgery. It was not effective and may even have increased muscle activity.[98] Intravenous lidocaine given distal to a tourniquet might be the ideal anesthetic for extremity surgery in which relaxation is necessary, because the direct effect of local anesthetics on the muscle might prevent myotonia. There are no reports in the literature of this being used. Althesin (not available in the United States) has been reported to prevent percus-

sion and surgical myotonia without affecting the EMG.[99] The postoperative shivering that is so frequently seen after a patient receives a potent inhalational anesthetic may also produce myotonia. Keeping the patient warm intraoperatively and using meperidine as the narcotic may lessen the incidence of shivering, even when inhalational agents are used. The relative risks of various techniques must be weighed.

Pregnancy may prove to be a hazard. Although there is some ovarian atrophy, many of the cases describing anesthesia for these patients relate to cesarean section.[58, 74, 87, 88, 100, 101] For patients who do become pregnant, regional anesthesia would seem ideal. Most of these patients have a normal first stage of labor, but it is preferable that they not strain in the second stage, to prevent skeletal muscle contracture and respiratory distress. Uterine atony has been reported to occur after delivery and may require oxytocic agents, massage, or massive blood transfusions, or all of these.[74, 87, 88] The injection of bupivacaine into the uterus during a period of uncoordinated contraction at cesarean section reduced blood loss and improved coordination of the contractions.[100]

Children born to mothers with myotonic dystrophy have a 25 per cent chance of having dystrophic symptoms at birth (for reasons that remain unknown) and this is called *congenital myotonic dystrophy.* They are at increased risk of perinatal death, usually because of poor respiratory function and feeding difficulties. The most common findings during pregnancy are reduced fetal movements and hydramnios; the neonate shows respiratory distress, an elevated hypoplastic diaphragm, mental retardation, and talipes (clubfoot). Myotonia is not present at birth, even on EMG. All neonates with the disease who are born prematurely need ventilation, in contrast to 50 per cent of term infants who need respiratory support.[102] The upper lip has a characteristic tent shape, and the jaw tends to hang open when the child is upright. Anesthesia may be needed, but it should be delayed, if possible, since the infant's strength improves over 4 to 6 weeks.[103] The use of caudal anesthesia in several of these children has been described.[102, 104] Even without sedatives, one infant had an increase in PCO_2.[102] As these children mature they have many of the symptoms of adult-onset disease but at an earlier age, although the rate of progression is slower. IQ test results are more than 2 SD below normal, and frequently it is the mental impairment that brings these subjects to medical attention.[60] The cause of the transient increased weakness is not known and is most like that produced by a circulating factor, but none has yet been found. The earlier onset seems to correlate with the increased number of CTG repeats in these patients.[6]

B. MYOTONIA CONGENITA

Myotonia congenita (which must be distinguished from congenital onset myotonia dystrophica) was first described by Thomsen in himself and several relatives.[105] It is a rather benign disease in that there are no occurrences of atrophy and no systemic symptoms other than those related to muscle. The myotonia is much more widespread than in myotonic dystrophy, and the muscles are frequently enlarged. Males are generally more severely affected than are females. This disease is much less common than is myotonic dystrophy. It is inherited as an autosomal dominant trait. The defect is now known to be in the skeletal muscle chloride channel, and one mutation (substituting one amino acid for another) accounts for 70 per cent of the cases. A recessive form of the disease called *Becker's myotonia* involves different changes in the gene.[106] Reduction in chloride conductance leads to repetitive propagated action potentials. Drug therapy and methods to produce relaxation in these patients are the same as for myotonic dystrophy patients. Therapy is used much more often in myotonia congenita, both because the patients complain about the myotonia more frequently and because the absence of cardiac disease makes the use of drugs safer. The use of oral lidocaine-like antiarrhythmic agents such as mexiletine is gaining popularity in the treatment of this disease.[50]

C. PARAMYOTONIA CONGENITA AND MYOTONIA FLUCTUANS

Myotonia followed by paresis, which is usually induced by exposure to cold, is characteristic of paramyotonia congenita. There is a resemblance both to hyperkalemic periodic paralysis and to myotonia congenita. In con-trast to myotonia congenita, the stiffness and weakness are worsened by activity; thus, the term *para* (doxical) *myotonia*. The exact place of this disease in the classification has been clarified by the understanding that paramyotonia congenita, hyperkalemic periodic paralysis, and sodium channel myotonia are all different defects in the alpha subunit of the skeletal muscle sodium channel. In paramyotonia, the resting membrane potential is normal at 37°C, but it rapidly drops to -40 mV as the muscle is cooled, and thus paralysis sets in. This seems to be caused by the increase in Na^+ conductance as the temperature is reduced.[107] It must be remembered that, as the membrane potential falls, propagated action potentials are easier to elicit, thus producing myotonia, but eventually the membrane potential falls so low that the membrane becomes inexcitable. Thus, small differences can produce myotonia or paralysis.[106] Use-dependent antiarrhythmic drugs such as lidocaine and its analogues prevent influx of Na^+, as the abnormally open channels will be blocked more than the normal channels, and in fact this allows function of muscle at reduced temperatures.[50, 107] An interesting case report discussed the use of potassium infusion, 11 mEq per hour, in a patient who required cardiopulmonary bypass at 28°C. This patient did very well and could be extubated in the early postoperative period.[108] (For a further discussion see section on Periodic Paralysis.)

Fortunately, this was classic paramyotonia congenita; a second type, called potassium-sensitive paramyotonia congenita, is very similar to the first, except that, in addition to cold inducing the weakness, increased serum potassium is a major trigger. Thus a diet rich in potassium provokes attacks, whereas in the classic variety increased potassium prevents episodes. This second type is very much like hyperkalemic periodic paralysis.[107]

Myotonia fluctuans is another sodium channel myotonia that shows prolongation of relaxation time 20 to 40 minutes after exercise. Potassium causes generalized myotonia. Cooling has no major effect on muscle function. Here, a correlation of masseter muscle rigidity and positive in-vitro halothane caffeine contracture test has been found.[109]

IV. FAMILIAL PERIODIC PARALYSIS

There are three distinct types of disorders in familial periodic paralysis—hypokalemic, hyperkalemic, and normokalemic.[105–107] The normal resting membrane potential is about -80 mV and is governed primarily by the intracellular-to-extracellular potassium concentrations. This is because the permeability of the membrane to potassium is much greater than its permeability to sodium. When the membrane is depolarized, sodium channels open and the membrane depolarizes further. If the membrane resting potential is less than -60 mV, the sodium channel cannot be activated. Although the hypo- and hyperkalemic forms of disease share many clinical similarities, there is a major difference in the underlying physiologic mechanisms, as shown by genetic analysis. Hyperkalemic periodic paralysis is caused by a decrease in the resting membrane potential as a result of high sodium permeability in the resting state. The defect in hypokalemic periodic paralysis is in the dihydropyridine receptor of the calcium channel of skeletal muscle.[106, 107]

A. HYPOKALEMIC PERIODIC PARALYSIS

The first case in the literature, reported by Schachnowitch in 1882, describes many of the symptoms of *hypokalemic periodic paralysis.* The attacks are precipitated by large carbohydrate-rich meals, characteristically a large evening meal, which lead to paralysis on awakening the next morning. The episodes usually last longer than 2 hours and frequently as long as 24 hours. Cold, mental stress, infections, exercise followed by rest, surgical or accidental trauma, and menstruation have all been implicated in the onset of these paralytic attacks. The paralysis is variable and usually asymmetric. Onset is proximal and progression distal, involving principally the lower and upper extremities and the trunk and neck, but only rarely the cranial nerve distribution or the diaphragm. The deep tendon reflexes are usually diminished. Most patients have symptoms before age 20 years, and the frequency increases with time until the fourth or fifth decade, when, after repeated episodes, permanent weakness may be found.[107] Transient bradycardia, cardiac dilatation, and the onset of an apical systolic murmur have been observed. Blood pressure rises, and arrhythmias can occur during attacks. Death has occurred from respiratory arrest or cardiac arrhythmias.[107] The ECG shows evidence of hypokalemia, with U waves in lead II and leads V_2 to V_4, a flattened T wave, and a depressed ST interval. Usually the ECG abnormalities are more severe than one would predict from the serum potassium levels. During the attack, the basal metabolic rate goes up. Whether this is solely because of the anxiety of the patient is not known. The EMG shows abnormal lengthening of the action potential as the patient goes into paralysis, until finally there is electrical silence and no direct or indirect stimulation of the muscle fiber is possible. Because of retention of water, sodium, potassium, and chloride, urine output falls during an attack. Improvement is preceded by diaphoresis and diuresis; total fluid loss is 1 to 3 kg. During recovery, the serum potassium level returns to normal before the EMG does. The actions of many drugs have been studied in these patients, in an attempt to understand the mechanism of the paralysis.

Potassium was found to be therapeutic before the mechanism was understood. If it is given and uptake is measured, there is first uptake into the muscles, then a paradoxical loss of potassium from the muscles, and recovery ensues. It is known that the potassium is not lost into the urine or the stool. In-vivo intracellular recording during the attacks has shown a reduction in the resting membrane potential,[107] which could be due to either increased sodium permeability or reduced potassium permeability. Although the defect in the dihydropyridine receptor is well-documented, how this change interferes with cellular potassium and sodium homeostasis is not yet known.

Insulin causes a decrease in the membrane potential in these patients (in normal healthy persons it causes hyperpolarization), thus potentiating the already low value present in these cells.[107] When the membrane potential is low enough, sodium channels do not open and the muscle becomes unresponsive to stimulation. Under these conditions, insulin administration leads to further hypokalemia, as does stimulation of beta receptors (in thyrotoxic patients) and rest. Increasing potassium externally restores excitability; however, an excessive increase in external potassium renders the muscle inexcitable. Large amounts of licorice, which causes hypokalemia by its mineralocorticoid-like activity, can induce attacks. Insulin and glucose are used to induce attacks for diagnosis. Further confirmation requires the weakness to respond to oral potassium. The only synthetic glucocorticoid that does not cause crisis is triamcinolone, which increases the sodium-to-potassium excretion ratio in the urine. Extreme limitation in sodium intake and the use of diuretics, plus potassium replacement, have prophylactic value.

More recently, the carbonic anhydrase inhibitor acetazolamide has been found to prevent attacks. The probable mechanism of action is its ability to produce metabolic acidosis. Other agents that produce metabolic acidosis are similarly protective.[107] The loss of potassium from diuresis may actually increase the risk of paralysis in 10 per cent of patients. Sodium bicarbonate induces attacks. The effects of respiratory acidosis and alkalosis have not been reported. It is thought that after repeated attacks atrophy ensues, but this is only a late occurrence and most patients are quite muscular.

While death is uncommon during episodes, when it occurs the most common cause is respiratory failure resulting from aspiration pneumonia or infection. Cardiac failure and shock have also been reported. Autopsies have shown no specific lesion, except for vacuoles in the SR of skeletal muscles, which increase during attacks. The contents of the vacuoles have not been identified. The disease, as the name implies, is familial. It is usually an autosomal dominant trait, and males display high penetrance and more severe attacks. There are also many sporadic cases, usually in males. These are more difficult to evaluate because affected persons may have only one attack in a lifetime, and the symptoms, particularly in females, may be minimal.

The thyrotoxic variety of periodic paralysis is clinically similar to that found in the hypokalemic type, except that the drop in serum potassium during an attack is usually greater. The incidence is much greater in males than in females and is found 10 times as frequently in Orientals as in others. Thyrotoxic symptoms may be mild and only demonstrable by blood tests. The cause may be related to sodium, potassium, adenosine triphosphatase (Na^+, K^+, ATPase), but this has not been fully worked out. The paralytic episodes are best treated by both blocking the effects of thyroid hormone (beta blockers acutely) and giving potassium. The episodes cease when the patient is made euthyroid.[107] Reports of postoperative appearance of paralysis in unsuspected thyrotoxic periodic paralysis have

stressed the difficulty of picking up the increased thyroid activity in these patients.[110]

There are several reports in the literature of anesthesia for patients with hypokalemic periodic paralysis.[111, 112] Two patients each had three anesthesia procedures, and one patient had two procedures. In addition, one paper reviewed the experience in a family of eight members who had 21 anesthesia procedures among them.[112] Single case reports have also appeared.[113, 114] All forms of anesthesia were used. Respiratory failure developed in one patient 6 hours after an appendectomy, and this patient required ventilatory assistance for 36 hours. This same patient had another episode of weakness after a second operation; this time, 18 hours postoperatively. In both cases, the patient's potassium level was less than 3.0 mmol/L and potassium chloride therapy was successful. Another patient who was given insulin, dextrose, and potassium as a cardioplegic agent, as well as sodium bicarbonate, had profound weakness of the extremities and a drop in potassium to 1.2 mmol/L. After administration of 180 mEq of potassium over 6 hours, strength returned and serum potassium levels normalized.[115] A third patient had weakness of the extremities on awakening from anesthesia, and only later was the history of hypokalemic periodic paralysis obtained.[113] A retrospective review of 21 anesthesia procedures in eight patients showed six episodes of weakness. In all episodes, the weakness was no greater than what was usually experienced by the patient. Four of six patients given cyclopropane anesthesia, one of two patients given halothane, and one of three patients given droperidol and fentanyl (Innovar) had episodes of weakness. The factors responsible for postoperative weakness cannot be determined from this report. Succinylcholine has been used, with no apparent problem. One patient given curare who had other unrelated problems seems to have had a mildly prolonged recovery. The majority of patients who experienced difficulties did so the first day postoperatively, although many did well immediately on awakening from anesthesia.

Guidelines for the anesthetic management of these patients should include warning the patient not to overeat the night before surgery, and an attempt should be made to decrease the patient's mental stress. If the patient is taking spironolactone, acetazolamide, or other diuretics, the serum electrolyte levels should be obtained. Abnormal results should not provoke hasty therapy; however, oral potassium therapy is indicated for patients on diuretics and those who have even the slightest degree of hypokalemia. Care must be used in giving potassium to patients taking spironolactone because this agent blocks the action of aldosterone and thus limits the ability of the kidney to excrete excess potassium. Use of dextrose should be limited, and supplementary potassium should be given to prevent hypokalemia because potassium accompanies the dextrose when it enters the cell. A large salt load can also precipitate paralysis, especially if the sodium is in the form of bicarbonate. Cold is a major cause of paralysis, so the patient must be protected. The best form of monitoring in the operating room is ECG, and changes in the T wave, signifying hypokalemia, should be watched for constantly. Central venous pressure or a Swan-Ganz catheter may be helpful, as cardiac failure is also a concomitant of paralysis in some patients.

The effects of muscle relaxants are not well documented, and unless absolutely necessary they should be avoided. Because during an attack the muscles are insensitive to even direct electrical stimulation, the nerve stimulator may not be helpful at that time; however, since respiratory muscles and face muscles are only rarely affected by the disease, the facial nerve can be used in the diagnosis of prolonged paralysis, and this was helpful in several cases.[112, 113, 115] The use of a nerve stimulator has been described in one patient.[112] Although the patient appeared normal at the time, the muscle response to electrical stimulation of the ulnar nerve was weak and showed marked posttetanic potentiation. No fade, however, was observed. Thus, a baseline measurement must be obtained before muscle relaxants are used. The possibility of respiratory failure encourages the use of respiratory assistance, chest physiotherapy, and intermittent positive-pressure breathing (IPPB). Since there is usually a decrease in the frequency and severity of the attacks in middle age, the patients who must be watched most carefully are those in the younger age groups. Care must also be used to recognize atrophy. Because this runs in certain families, a history of atrophy should be sought. Patients who suffer spontaneous attacks of paralysis rarely need ventilatory support or an endotracheal tube to prevent aspiration. The cough reflex is usually intact, and, in addition, gastric acid secretion is markedly diminished. The use of potassium chloride restores function within a few hours in most cases; however, the respiratory status should be checked and the adequacy of the cough evaluated.

It has been suggested that those with particularly severe symptoms undergo adrenalectomy. If steroids are necessary, triamcinolone would seem the best choice. If paralysis is found to have occurred, the use of 5 to 15 g of potassium chloride by mouth will abort the attack. A smaller dose is used intravenously (60 mEq potassium) over several hours. The use of mannitol as a carrier (rather than dextrose) has been suggested.[107] Frequent monitoring of serum potassium is mandatory, to prevent hyperkalemia. It may take 2 hours or more for the symptoms to disappear completely.

B. HYPERKALEMIC PERIODIC PARALYSIS

Hyperkalemic periodic paralysis (adynamia episodica hereditaria) was separated from the hypokalemic form in 1957. The pattern of inheritance is autosomal dominant, with high penetrance in both males and females. The age of onset is earlier, and symptoms are seen in infancy.[107] With age, the attacks become less frequent but more severe. They occur after exercise, but sooner than in the hypokalemic form. They are unrelated to high-carbohydrate meals and tend to occur when the person is hungry. The attacks are shorter, many lasting only an hour or less, instead of hours or days in the hypokalemic type. The attacks can be induced by administration of potassium, so the term *potassium-sensitive periodic paralysis* may be a better, more inclusive term. Cold also precipitates attacks; stress is less often a factor. The attacks start, as do those of the hypokalemic type, in the lower extremities, upper extremities, and trunk, but they then go on to include the facial muscles, including the tongue. Some patients have myotonic symptoms and others do not; this probably represents differences in the sodium channel defect. Although there are similarities between hyperkalemia periodic paralysis and paramyotonia congenita, there are enough clinical differences to separate these entities.

The defect is due to hypopolarization of the muscle membrane resulting from a defect in the sodium channel, and attacks occur because of further depolarization, which leads to inability to activate the sodium channel.

Lid lag was at one time thought to be the clinically distinguishing feature between this and hypokalemic periodic paralysis. Today this sign is known to be nonspecific. Respiratory muscles are spared. Pregnancy, especially during the last two trimesters, is associated with increased severity of the disease, which slowly remits post partum.[116] The potassium level rises during an attack—on average 20 per cent—but it may still be within normal limits.[107] In spite of this, the membrane potential is reduced during an attack. The hyperkalemia has been shown to result from an outpouring of potassium from muscles associated with increased permeability to sodium and increased intracellular chloride levels. The administration of potassium provokes the attack and is used to confirm the diagnosis.

Along with the paralytic episodes, many patients exhibit myotonia, which is most marked on percussion of the tongue and hypothenar muscles; in this respect, the disease is quite similar to paramyotonia congenita.

Neostigmine has been reported to increase the myotonia, so care should be taken when administering it to these patients. The EMG during an attack shows increased spontaneous activity, with marked myotonic discharges; however, with effort, the motor unit discharges are reduced in amplitude but remain of normal duration. As in hypokalemic paralysis, there is no propagation of the action potential along the muscle when it is fully paralyzed. The ECG shows peaking of the T waves before and during evidence of paresis. If one gives glucagon or epinephrine, or even inhalational salbutamol, paresis may be aborted, and the ECG shows signs of hypokalemia (U waves and small T waves), although the serum potassium level remains normal. At present, insulin and glucose therapy seem the best way to abort an attack. Use of calcium, epinephrine, thiazide, and glucagon has not been as successful. Prophylactic use of a high-sodium, low-potassium diet with frequent high-carbohydrate feedings decreases the severity of attacks. The low potassium level may increase the myotonia while reducing the attacks of paralysis. Acetazolamide decreases the number and severity of attacks; thiazide is likewise useful. Both are thought to work by kaluresis. The onset of atrophy depends more on the nature of the disease in a particular family than on any other factors now known.

Since the first report of anesthetic complications in patients with this disease appeared, when three anesthesia experiences were described,[116] several others have been presented that produced no untoward effects.[117] After Pentothal was given alone for dental extraction, a patient was paralyzed for several hours. A second patient who received general anesthesia for a vaginal delivery (the agent used was not reported) was paralyzed for several hours. The third case was uneventful spinal anesthesia for a vaginal delivery.[116] Fasting before the extraction may have provoked the episode in the first case; we cannot indict the Pentothal. The incidence of episodes of paralysis rises in the third trimester of pregnancy; thus the occurrence of paralysis after vaginal delivery in one patient does not indicate that the general anesthetic was responsible. In fact, recent cases using Pentothal and propofol have been successful.[117] In view of the limited experience, firm conclusions cannot be drawn and caution is indicated. The most important measure in preparing for anesthesia is to prevent carbohydrate depletion by loading carbohydrate the night before the operation and by using potassium-free and dextrose-rich fluids intraoperatively. Again, watching the ECG monitor for signs of increasing T-wave height intraoperatively would be of great assistance. Succinylcholine should be avoided if possible; because many of these patients may exhibit myotonia, nondepolarizing neuromuscular-blocking agents seem to elicit no unusual response.[117] When a neuromuscular stimulator is used, the absence of twitch may be either relaxant induced or secondary to hyperkalemic paralysis; it must be remembered that even facial muscles can be paralyzed by hyperkalemia. The ECG should give a clue to the diagnosis. One case of a patient with hyperkalemia periodic paralysis who responded abnormally to in-vitro contracture testing for malignant hyperpyrexia has been reported.[118] A history of masseter rigidity has been obtained in several other patients, and postoperatively these patients were weak for an extended time, although no other findings of malignant hyperthermia were noted.[117] The significance of this finding is not yet evident, and no cases of malignant hyperpyrexia have been reported.

C. NORMOKALEMIC PERIODIC PARALYSIS

The third and most difficult form of this disease to manage is *normokalemic periodic pa-*

ralysis. Onset is in early childhood, and the attacks are often severe and associated with loss of the cough reflex. An episode may last 2 to 21 days. Episodes are induced by rest after exercise, cold, or ingestion of alcohol or potassium. Like the attacks of hypokalemic periodic paralysis, these attacks occur in the morning, on awakening. In some but not all patients, cardiac arrhythmias occur during attacks, usually multifocal ectopic beats.[107] Potassium decreases arrhythmias but makes the weakness greater, and vice versa. Drugs have unusual effects in this condition. Digitalis preparations cause weakness, whereas quinidine reverses this effect, as does sodium loading. An increase in potassium provokes attacks. The use of 9α-fluorohydrocortisone and sodium loading is prophylactic against attacks. Owing to the nature of the spontaneous paralytic episodes, it would seem wise to protect the airway with an endotracheal tube. The same problems mentioned previously apply to anesthetic management, although the ECG monitor is now used to watch for arrhythmia rather than to diagnose paralysis. Arrhythmias that occur during anesthesia may result from the anesthetic or the primary disease. Use of large doses of sodium to correct or prevent both the paralysis and cardiac arrhythmias would seem indicated, although care must be taken not to overload these patients. The effects of quinidine make one wonder whether procainamide or intravenous lidocaine would be helpful in counteracting arrhythmias.

Cardiac arrhythmias have been seen in some families with hyperkalemic—and, less frequently, hypokalemic— periodic paralysis. Some have ended in sudden death. The arrhythmias are exacerbated by decreasing potassium levels and digitalis and are not helped by propranolol, phenytoin, or disopyramide. Imipramine has been useful in cases in which it has been tried.[107]

V. ENDOCRINE MYOPATHIES[119]

A. GLUCOCORTICOID EXCESS

Glucocorticoid-induced muscle atrophy is the most common endocrine myopathy. Patients with endogenous (Cushing's disease) or exogenous glucocorticoid excess may develop severe proximal muscle weakness and atrophy. The onset of weakness is usually insidious but may be accelerated by starvation or

immobilization. Muscles innervated by cranial nerves are usually spared. Patients taking large doses (1 to 1.5 mg/kg per day) of prednisone for extrapulmonary autoimmune disease may develop decreased inspiratory muscle strength within 4 weeks.[120] The fluorinated steroids (triamcinolone, dexamethasone, betamethasone) have a greater propensity to cause atrophy than equivalent doses of other steroids.[121] Corticosteroids produce selective type 2 fiber atrophy, especially 2b (fast glycolytic) fibers.[122] Glucocorticoids bind to cytoplasmic receptors, which are transported to the nucleus and affect DNA transcription. Corticosteroids decrease protein synthesis by decreasing translation and antagonizing the anabolic effect of insulin. Corticosteroids increase protein breakdown. This has been shown in patients taking more than 80 mg per day of prednisone;[123] increased protein degradation was measured by increased urinary excretion of 3-methylhistidine or creatine.

EMG findings in corticosteroid myopathy are variable. The EMG is usually normal; with severe atrophy, motor unit potentials typically have diminished amplitude and decreased duration (myopathic pattern).[124] Muscle biopsy shows type 2b fiber atrophy with increased glycogen in type 2b fibers. One must consider the underlying disease (e.g., inflammatory myopathy), for which steroids are prescribed when interpreting the EMG or muscle biopsy. In chronic corticosteroid myopathy CK levels are usually normal.

The primary treatment of steroid myopathy is reducing the steroid dose or converting to alternate-day dosing when possible. Recovery of strength may take weeks. Clinical improvement is preceded by decreased creatine excretion.[119] Patients with steroid myopathy may be at risk for complications associated with disuse atrophy, such as deep vein thrombosis and pulmonary embolism. Decreased inspiratory muscle strength may predispose patients to postoperative pulmonary complications. Succinylcholine-induced hyperkalemia has not been described in patients taking glucocorticoids for autoimmune disease outside an intensive care setting (see under Intensive Care Unit Myopathy, Neuromuscular Syndromes).

Investigators have described variable effects of steroid therapy on neuromuscular transmission. Durant and coworkers found that chronic hydrocortisone administration to cats had no effect on pancuronium-induced twitch depression; acute hydrocortisone administration had no independent effect on twitch depression but increased pancuronium-induced twitch depression.[125] Schwartz and coworkers found that acute steroid therapy did not alter nondepolarizing muscle relaxant (NDMR) effects in humans.[126] Preoperative therapy with hydrocortisone, prednisolone, or betamethasone has been associated with resistance to nondepolarizing muscle relaxants; a presynaptic effect with enhanced acetylcholine release may facilitate neuromuscular transmission.[127]

B. INTENSIVE CARE UNIT MYOPATHY, NEUROMUSCULAR SYNDROMES

Prolonged weakness has been observed in patients who require mechanical ventilation and who have received NDMR, often in combination with corticosteroids.[128] Prolonged weakness can be attributed to (1) prolonged neuromuscular blockade, (2) acceleration of steroid myopathy by NDMR functional denervation, (3) acute necrotizing myositis, sometimes seen in asthmatics receiving large doses of steroids, (4) motor neuropathy, and (5) critical illness polyneuropathy.

Prolonged neuromuscular blockade is characterized by persistent fade (decremental twitch tension) evoked by 2 Hz ulnar nerve stimulation. This has been most frequently observed after the aminosteroidal NDMRs vecuronium or pancuronium.[129–131] Vecuronium has an active metabolite, 3-desacetyl-vecuronium, which accumulates with renal failure or cholestatic jaundice;[132] little is removed by hemodialysis. Intensive care (ICU) patients with renal failure may have prolonged neuromuscular blockade because of accumulation of pancuronium, metocurine, vecuronium, or 3-desacetylvecuronium.

Myopathy with myosin loss has been observed following prolonged vecuronium infusion during steroid treatment.[133] Findings sometimes seen in steroid-associated ICU myopathy and not usually in chronic steroid myopathy include (1) atrophy of both type 1 and type 2 fibers, (2) abnormal EMG with fibrillation potentials and sharp positive spike activity, (3) significantly elevated CK levels (e.g. more than 1000 U/L), and (4) external ophthalmoplegia.[134, 135]

Axonal or preneuromuscular junction motor neuropathy is suggested by decreased motor-evoked response amplitude, preserved nerve conduction velocity, normal sensory examination, and muscle biopsy findings of denervation atrophy.[136] Critical illness polyneuropathy includes diminished sensory nerve action potentials; tendon reflexes are diminished or absent, and distal limb weakness is characteristic.[137]

Patients with these abnormalities of neuromuscular function may recover strength slowly (i.e., over several days to 1 or 2 months). Myopathy or motor neuropathy may result in difficult weaning from mechanical ventilation long after recovery from the acute pulmonary parenchymal disease. Succinylcholine-induced hyperkalemic cardiac arrest has been reported in a patient with muscle atrophy following 34 days of intensive care and a 10-day course of large doses of prednisolone,[138] and in another with severe intra-abdominal infection who had been ventilated for 17 days.[139] Prolonged weakness is observed less frequently after atracurium infusion than with vecuronium or pancuronium; it is not clear whether this is due to the lower frequency of atracurium use in the ICU or, possibly, to lower intrinsic toxicity.[140] It has been suggested that routine twitch monitoring reduces, but does not eliminate, prolonged weakness or myopathy in ICU patients receiving infusions of NDMRs.

C. HYPERTHYROIDISM

The majority of patients with untreated hyperthyroidism have clinical weakness. Thyrotoxic myopathy is characterized by proximal weakness and atrophy; 20 per cent of patients have distal weakness.[124] Some patients have bulbar myopathy, with dysphagia or aspiration resulting from oropharyngeal or esophageal dysfunction.[141] Myopathy may result from increased protein catabolism, reflected by increased urinary creatine excretion.[119] Other neuromuscular disorders associated with hyperthyroidism include myasthenia gravis (30-fold increased incidence) and periodic paralysis (predominantly in Oriental males). CK levels are usually normal in hyperthyroidism, although (rarely) rhabdomyolysis has been reported in thyroid storm.[142] Prominent fasciculations may occur, resulting in confusion with primary motor neuron disease. EMG may show motor unit potentials of decreased duration and amplitude with polyphasia (myopathic pattern). Muscle biopsy is usually normal. Successful therapy of hyperthyroidism usually improves strength, and that is followed by reversal of atrophy over several months. Unusual neuromuscular complications of therapy include aggravation of myasthenic weakness or myotonia by propranolol,[143] and myositis associated with propylthiouracil.[144] Thyroid storm or thyrotoxicosis factitia (overdose of thyroid supplement) may mimic malignant hyperthermia;[145, 146] rhabdomyolysis is very rarely observed in thyroid storm, and rigidity does not occur.

D. HYPOTHYROIDISM

More than 30 per cent of hypothyroid patients have symptoms of muscle cramps, pain, or stiffness. Both diminished rate of tension development and markedly slow relaxation ("hung-up" reflexes) are characteristic.[124] Slowed contraction correlates with reduced myosin adenosine triphosphatase (ATPase) activity; slowed relaxation is secondary to slower calcium uptake by the sarcoplasmic reticulum. Patients may have myoedema, which is an electrically silent, localized contracture produced by minor trauma. Hypothyroid patients usually have elevated serum CK; those with symptomatic myopathy often have 10-fold elevations. Protein catabolism is decreased.[119] Decremental response to repetitive nerve stimulation, responsive to edrophonium, has been described in hypothyroid patients without myasthenia gravis.[147] Miller and associates reported an acutely hypothyroid obese patient who had no response to peripheral nerve stimulation despite clinically adequate strength; 8 weeks of thyroxine therapy produced normal response to peripheral nerve stimulation.[148]

Two distinct syndromes include muscle hypertrophy: (1) Debré-Kocher-Sémélaigne syndrome in severely hypothyroid children and (2) Hoffman's syndrome in adults. Hypothyroidism rarely presents with rhabdomyolysis[149] or diaphragmatic dysfunction.[150] Patients who are clinically hypothyroid are at increased risk of postanesthetic hypoxemia or respiratory failure because of increased sensitivity to respiratory depressants, decreased ventilatory response to hypercarbia,[151] and predisposition to airway obstruction from macroglossia or obesity.

E. HYPERPARATHYROIDISM

Patients with hyperparathyroidism often have proximal weakness. Chronic hypercalcemia results in hyperreflexia (acute hypercalcemia results in hyporeflexia); fasciculations may occur. Patients with renal failure and osteomalacia may have secondary hyperparathyroidism associated with proximal myopathy. The degree of weakness may not correlate with serum levels of calcium or phosphorus. Muscle biopsy shows type 2 fiber atrophy. CK levels are normal or slightly elevated.[124] Decreased duration of relaxation with vecuronium has been reported in patients with primary and secondary hyperparathyroidism.[152, 153] Wooldridge and colleagues reported rhabdomyolysis 6 days after parathyroidectomy in a patient on chronic hemodialysis; this followed a grand mal seizure and was associated with hypophosphatemia (1.3 mg/dL).[154]

Parathyroid hormone (PTH) increases muscle cyclic adenosine monophosphate (cAMP) levels and protein degradation and could possibly elevate cytoplasmic calcium levels. In renal failure, $1,25(OH)_2D_3$ levels are decreased. Functional vitamin D deficiency results in diminished protein synthesis, depressed myofibrillar ATPase activity, and impaired SR function.[119] Patients with uremic myopathy and osteomalacia may benefit from treatment with $1,25(OH)_2D_3$ or $25(OH)D_3$.[155]

F. HYPOPARATHYROIDISM

Hypocalcemia results in hyperexcitability of peripheral nerve rather than true myopathy. Paresthesias, fasciculations, and sustained muscle spasm or tetanus may occur. Elevated CK levels may reflect sustained muscle contraction. Motor unit potentials are usually of normal amplitude and duration. Chronic hypocalcemia results in diminished tendon reflexes.[124] Hypoparathyroidism is sometimes noted in Kearns-Sayre syndrome (KSS).[156]

G. ADRENAL INSUFFICIENCY

Adrenal insufficiency usually results in mild weakness. Concomitant hyperkalemia can cause flaccid quadriparesis similar to that seen in hyperkalemic periodic paralysis.[124]

H. ACROMEGALY

Patients with acromegaly usually have slowly progressive mild proximal weakness without wasting. Myopathy is related to the duration of acromegaly, not to growth hormone level. Difficulties with mask ventilation, conventional laryngoscopy, and cardiovascular disease pose the chief anesthetic risks to patients with acromegaly.[157]

I. DIABETES MELLITUS

Proximal muscle weakness in diabetics is usually secondary to proximal neuropathy. Vascular disease may be associated with painful thigh muscle infarction; diagnosis may be confirmed with magnetic resonance imaging (MRI) or computed tomography (CT). Flier's syndrome—muscle pain, cramps, and fatigue—is associated with diabetes; patients have acanthosis nigricans (mossy, hyperpigmented plaques on the back of the neck or in the axillae or groins); CK levels may be elevated two- to five-fold; phenytoin often relieves myalgia.[124] Penn reported the development of myoglobinuria in two patients with extreme hyperosmolality (435 and 547 mOsm/L) associated with nonketotic hyperglycemic coma.[158] Singhal and coworkers found a direct correlation between serum osmolality (369 to 393 mOsm/L) and serum CK (4500 to 10,000 IU/L).[159] Myoglobinuria has been reported in two children with diabetic ketoacidosis,[160] and one adult during treatment of ketoacidosis.[161]

J. HYPOPHOSPHATEMIA

Severe hypophosphatemia (below 0.4 mM/L = 1.2 mg/dL) is often associated with rhabdomyolysis. This degree of hypophosphatemia is limited to the setting of acute illness (e.g., diabetic ketoacidosis, acute alcohol intoxication in a chronic alcoholic, or pursuant to major intra-abdominal surgery[162]). Continuous intravenous glucose infusion may decrease serum phosphate. Acute paralysis with hyporeflexia and paresthesias may be observed. Less severe hypophosphatemia may be associated with weakness; causes of hypophosphatemia may include phosphate-binding antacids, malnutrition (e.g., as in chronic alcoholism), or chronic diarrhea.[124] Hyperventilation may cause transient hypophosphatemia, which does not cause muscle injury. Rhabdomyolysis or persistent weakness associated with sustained serum phosphate less than 1.0 mM/L is treated with phosphate repletion.

VI. GLYCOGEN STORAGE DISEASES

Glycogen storage diseases are particularly interesting, from both clinical and biochemical points of view. Every enzyme deficiency that theoretically could lead to accumulation of glycogen has been found to occur. In addition, the theory that glycogen synthesis uses a different pathway from glycogen breakdown was based on a case of abnormal glycogen storage resulting from a lack of glycogenolytic enzyme. Glycogen is a very high–molecular weight polysaccharide that has many branches. It has two types of glucose-to-glucose bonds, which thus permit this branching (Fig. 10–1). The classification presented here of the glycogenoses is that of Cori.[163]

A. CORI'S TYPE I—VON GIERKE'S DISEASE, HEPATORENAL GLYCOGENOSIS

The enzyme defect is a lack of glucose-6-phosphatase. The mode of inheritance is autosomal recessive. This enzyme functions primarily in the liver to convert glucose-6-phosphate into glucose, which can then be mobilized and transported via the blood stream to the periphery. A variant, type Ib, is lacking the glucose-6-phosphate microsomal translocase, and cannot move the substrate to the inside of the microsome for further processing. In von Gierke's disease, enzymatic conversion is the rate-limiting step and glycogen is stored in excess in the liver. As the synthesis of glycogen continues, the liver increases in size, and a large, protuberant abdomen develops. Fasting produces profound hypoglycemia, as the liver cannot release glucose after stimulation with glucagon or epinephrine. The symptoms in the first year of life are secondary to the hypoglycemia.

Blood glucose levels between 16 and 36 mg/dL are not uncommon; thus, one may see convulsions, failure to thrive, and severe

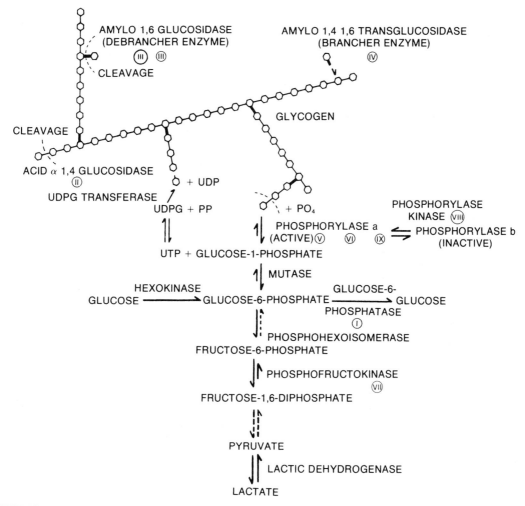

FIGURE 10–1. Schema of glycogen metabolism. The Roman numerals indicate where defects give rise to the individual types of glycogen storage disease. (Modified from Cornblath, M., and Schwartz, R: Disorders of Carbohydrate Metabolism, Philadelphia, W. B. Saunders, 1966.)

acidosis. There is massive hyperlipidemia, which must be taken into consideration when interpreting serum values such as sodium. Renal involvement presents as hyperuricemia and episodes of gout. The diagnosis is made by infusing glucagon and observing a smaller than expected rise in the blood glucose level. The rise that does occur is due to the debrancher enzyme, which frees glucose instead of glucose-6-phosphate. A more accurate test is to give fructose, which produces a rise in the blood glucose level in normal healthy persons, as fructose is rapidly transformed first into fructose-6-phosphate, then into glucose-6-phosphate, and finally into glucose. Since glucose-6-phosphatase is necessary for this conversion, there is no rise in glucose levels after the infusion of fructose in these patients.

The best therapy currently available is frequent, small carbohydrate feedings. Several investigators have used thyroxine and glucagon to limit the amount of glycogen synthesis, permitting the glucose to pass through the liver without being taken up and converted to glycogen. The glucose can then supply the brain and other organs. Similarly, portacaval bypass has recently been advocated to improve growth and decrease episodes of hypoglycemia. The mechanism is, again, based on allowing glucose to bypass the liver and thus reach the periphery.[164]

Cox[165] reported his experience with 11 surgical procedures performed over 10 years. One patient had cardiac arrest after a 1-hour tonsillectomy and could not be resuscitated. Although the remaining 10 patients survived, a single detailed case report emphasizes the serious anesthetic problems. The patient was a 17-year-old boy who weighed 32 kg and had had nothing by mouth for 7 hours before the operation. On arrival in the operating room his pH was 7.24 and he had lactic acidosis. The acidosis progressively worsened in spite of 5 per cent dextrose given intravenously. A total of 90 mEq of sodium bicarbonate was given to restore his pH from 7.08 to the preoperative value of 7.24. The pH slowly returned to normal by the next day. Cox believes that voluminous blood loss (18 per cent of predicted blood volume) associated with the surgery added to the acidosis. It would seem wise to continue feeding clear liquids using the short fasting guidelines recommended for pediatric patients, and to follow with a dextrose infusion as early as possible (0.25 to 0.5 g/kg per hour).[166] In a series of four patients, Casson[164] has used hyperalimentation preoperatively for at least a week both to improve the patient's general state and to decrease liver size before major surgery. Hyperalimentation is then continued postoperatively to allow optimal healing. Careful and frequent measurement of acid-base status is strongly recommended and is essential before and during any surgical procedure. Patients have been reported to develop severe acidosis without ketone bodies in the urine, so monitoring of ketones is not adequate. The type of anesthetic seems to make little difference. Cyclopropane, ether, halothane, propofol, and isoflurane have all been used successfully.[166]

B. CORI'S TYPE II—POMPE'S DISEASE, GENERALIZED GLYCOGENOSIS, (LYSOSOMAL) ACID MALTASE DEFICIENCY

Lysosomal acid maltase deficiency (α-1,4-glucosidase and α-1,6-glucosidase) is an autosomal recessive trait on chromosome 17.[167] The enzyme is produced initially as a high–molecular weight species modified in the endoplasmic reticulum; it then enters the Golgi apparatus and finally is incorporated into the lysosome. The function of the enzyme is not clear, since there is a neutral maltase in the cytoplasm that should perform much the same function. Any one of the steps outlined may be abnormal, but the clinical picture does not seem to correlate with the defect. Our incomplete understanding may be responsible for the seemingly striking clinical heterogeneity. Three forms of the disease are noted, based on age of onset and severity. The type is genetically transmitted.

The infantile form has a deficiency of this enzyme in all tissues. Storage of glycogen occurs in membrane-limited sacs (it may represent 8 to 15 per cent of the wet weight) and is seen in heart and skeletal muscle, including the tongue, and in the nervous system (the motor neurons in the brainstem and spinal cord are most severely affected).[167] The onset of symptoms—vomiting, anorexia, weakness, drooling, cyanosis, dyspnea—is at 2 to 6 months of age. The patient looks like a cretin. The primary symptoms are those of failure of the heart and neuromuscular system. The infants are hypotonic, but muscle bulk is good. The ECG shows (1) a short PR interval, (2) high QRS voltage, and (3) depressed ST segments and inverted or peaked T waves. The blood sugar levels and the glucose tolerance test results are normal. Death ensues—usually in the first year, but sometimes not until the third year of life—and is caused by congestive heart failure or aspiration pneumonia. The presence of increased ventriculoseptal wall thickness and outflow tract obstruction to both right and left sides has been reported and may contribute to congestive heart failure in these patients.[167, 168]

It is not clear how acid maltase deficiency causes muscle damage. One hypothesis is that the hypertrophy of the lysosomal apparatus occurs and rupture of these sacs by the accumulation of glycogen releases their contents and causes muscle destruction.[167] Kaplan recently reported the anesthetic experience in two patients with this disease. Both seemed to tolerate anesthesia with ether, ketamine, halothane and nitrous oxide, and succinylcholine on different occasions;[112, 168] however, only minimal monitoring was reported in these patients, and no information on changes in acid-base status, blood pressure, evidence of myocardial ischemia, or temperature changes was reported intraoperatively.

The late-onset forms of the disease do not occur in the same family as the infantile form, and so are thought to be unrelated genetic abnormalities.[163, 167] They can be divided into the childhood and adult forms. The childhood form has early onset, and death occurs by the third decade of life, with selective involvement of the respiratory muscles and proximal weakness but without cardiac or nervous system manifestations.

The adult form starts around age 20 years, and long-term survival is common. It looks much like limb girdle myopathy, and though there is EMG evidence of myotonia, no symptoms of myotonia are found. The patients have no cardiac or nervous system involvement. About a third have respiratory failure at presentation, and the diaphragm particularly is affected.[167] Diaphragmatic weakness reduces the supine vital capacity to about half of that when the patient is upright. The presence of small amounts (approximately 7 per cent) of normal enzyme activity in muscle may play a role in the later onset of the disease in these patients. The data on the levels of the enzyme in the heart or CNS and on whether the presence of enzyme in these tissues is, in fact, protective are very confusing.[167] The only anesthetic experience reported anesthesia for a noninvasive procedure. The patient had respiratory failure and required ventilatory support preoperatively. The patient did well and could return to baseline status 30 minutes after the anesthetic, which consisted of propofol, nitrous oxide, and atracurium for relaxation. The response to muscle relaxants was not specifically addressed.[169]

C. CORI'S TYPE III—FORBES' DISEASE, LIMIT DEXTRINOSIS, DEBRANCHER ENZYME DEFICIENCY

This autosomal-recessive disease looks like a milder form of Cori's type I, with hypoglycemia, failure to thrive, and hepatomegaly; however, cardiac and skeletal muscle are also involved. Signs and symptoms improve after puberty, for reasons unknown.[163] The fasting blood glucose level is depressed (35 to 50 mg/dL), although it is not as low as in Cori's type I. There is decreased response to epinephrine, and acetonuria is common. Glucose can be mobilized if it occurs after a branching point. As a result, the glycogen is much more branched than usual, and, once a branch occurs, that portion of the molecule can no longer be used. The debrancher enzyme has two functions: an α-1,4-transferase moves the oligosaccharide to expose a 1-6 linkage and thus allows hydrolysis. The enzyme also has an α-1-6-glucosidase activity. Both activities

are not always missing, and some investigators have subdivided the disease based on which activities are missing. No clinical utility has been found for this subdivision.

Unlike Cori's type I disease, infusion of fructose causes a rise in the blood glucose level, because the missing enzyme is not involved in the conversion of fructose to glucose. Because gluconeogenesis is possible, a high-protein diet is helpful.[170] The ECG is not a good indicator of the severity of cardiac involvement, nor can one see evidence of congestive heart failure even with a great deal of involvement. In a series of 99 patients, two thirds had deficient enzyme in both liver and skeletal muscle. Those who die young seem to be those with decreased activity in skeletal—and probably also cardiac—muscle.[170] The disorder is fairly common and accounts for approximately a quarter of the cases of glycogen storage disease.

Of the three patients in whom anesthetic use was reported, one patient had two general anesthesia procedures, both of which were uneventful except for an episode of laryngospasm. The first operation was open liver biopsy by open drop ether, and the second was open heart surgery with bypass to correct subvalvular aortic stenosis. In neither case were blood acid-base values reported. Severe acidosis was present in two patients, in spite of preoperative hyperalimentation and intraoperative use of a 15 per cent dextrose and bicarbonate solution. The acidosis, however, was not progressive. Pancuronium and halothane and nitrous oxide were tolerated well. The postoperative course in those patients undergoing portocaval shunts was benign.[164]

D. CORI'S TYPE IV— ANDERSEN'S DISEASE, BRANCHER DEFICIENCY, AMYLOPECTINOSIS

Cori's type IV is the rarest of these glycogenoses, although at least 31 cases are reported in the literature.[170] The mode of inheritance is autosomal recessive. In this disease, the glycogen is made abnormally, with few branches. All the enzymes needed for degradation are present; thus, the presence of excess glycogen is thought to be due to the precipitation of the unbranched polysaccharide, with tissue reaction and loss of glycogen availability to the tissues. The disease is characterized by hepatosplenomegaly, liver failure, and ascites. Some persons display cardiac failure and less commonly muscle weakness. Affected individuals die early, usually by age 4 years. There is no reported anesthetic experience with this disease. The severe liver involvement limits use of drugs that depend on this organ for metabolism. Bleeding may be a problem and can be treated with fresh-frozen plasma to restore clotting factors.

E. CORI'S TYPE V— McARDLE'S DISEASE, MYOPHOSPHORYLASE DEFICIENCY

There are multiple isoenzymes (distinct immunologic types) of phosphorylase.[171] The first is found in liver and leukocytes, a second in heart, and a third in skeletal muscle. If one is lacking, it is lacking in all tissues where it is normally found; however, the other types are still found in their usual sites. Tissues such as heart and brain have multiple isoenzymes, so even if one is missing these tissues function normally.

Characteristically, the onset of disease is before age 15 years, with diminished activity and cramping with exercise, followed by weakness. Weakness seems to increase with age and thus is thought to be a function of muscle damage.[171] Any muscle may be affected. If exercise continues, muscle contracture (contraction, but with EMG silence), and myoglobinuria occur. Although these symptoms would be expected to be attributable to decreased available energy sources, no documentation of this has been possible. Of 112 patients reported, 50 per cent had myoglobinuria, and a quarter subsequently had renal failure.[171] There is no muscle atrophy until the fifth decade of life. The CK level is variably elevated at rest, in contrast to the normal value in carnitine palmitoyltransferase deficiency, which also produces myoglobinuria.

The classic test for this disease is to determine venous lactate and pyruvate levels after ischemic exercise. A normal subject exhibits a two- to fivefold increase. In this disease there is a decrease, as the muscle cannot break down its glycogen and must use lactate and pyruvate for metabolism. Ischemic exercise tolerance is only 10 to 20 per cent of normal,

in spite of normal initial muscle strength. A "second-wind" phenomenon is observed when, after an initial period of activity followed by rest, a patient can sustain activity longer than the initial period of activity. The second-wind phenomenon may be related to the increase in blood glucose or free fatty acids or to increased blood flow. Blood glucose levels rise normally after glucagon or epinephrine, since glucose is released from the liver, which is not affected. Exercise tolerance can be increased by treatment with glucagon, dextrose, fructose, or lactate. For the long term, a high-protein diet is recommended.[172] In the one autopsy performed in this disease, the cardiac muscle was normal. It is not clear whether in another patient the uterine musculature was abnormal, but most likely smooth muscle is unaffected.[171] Although patients have a higher than expected incidence of seizures, they occur during strenuous exercise and may be related either to hyperventilation without the usual lactic acidosis or to the decrease in glucose caused by rapid muscle uptake.[173]

Variability in the expression of the disease is great; in newborns it can be lethal, whereas in adults it is of limited importance. Males are affected more than females, but whether this results from differences in the use of muscle is not known. Several patients were known to have done heavy work until middle age, at which time they experienced the classic symptoms and lack of myophosphorylase was proved on biopsy specimens. The evidence, however, strongly favors autosomal-recessive inheritance rather than acquired disease.

Because it is thought that repeated episodes of ischemia lead eventually to atrophy, it would seem unwise to use tourniquets for a prolonged period of time in these patients, either to reduce blood loss or to permit the use of intravenous local anesthesia. The use of an infusion of dextrose or glucagon to increase the blood glucose level would seem wise. Long-term feeding of a high-protein diet, with its supply of branched-chain amino acids, which can serve as an alternative fuel, might also be useful during anesthesia, especially at times of high muscle energy demand, as during shivering.[172] Myoglobinuria has been seen after prolonged ischemia and should be watched for (good hydration and mannitol administration may be necessary to prevent renal damage). Two uses of muscle relaxants[174] in this disease have been reported—one used atracurium and the other alcuronium. Both were uneventful. The use of a depolarizing agent would seem inadvisable, since severe fasciculations might lead to muscle injury, an exaggeration of the response normally seen after administration of succinylcholine and halothane.[175] The more serious stress would be postoperative shivering, and this should be avoided, if possible, by keeping the patient warm and giving meperidine to decrease the response to cooling. Muscle weakness is not very common and should not occur if perfusion is adequate and blood glucose levels are maintained.

F. CORI'S TYPE VI— HEPATOPHOSPHORYLASE DEFICIENCY, HERS' DISEASE

Mild to moderate degrees of hypoglycemia are caused by the deficiency of phosphorylase in the liver. There is usually a poor response to glucagon and epinephrine. The skeletal phosphorylase and cardiac muscle phosphorylase (being a different enzyme) levels are both normal, but leukocyte phosphorylase levels follow those of the liver. One patient had bleeding diathesis. Whether it was related to this disease is not known. Liver function usually is not impaired. Except for the prevention of hypoglycemia, there is no specific therapy.

G. CORI'S TYPE VII— TAURI'S DISEASE

Muscle phosphofructokinase deficiency is an autosomal-recessive trait, though it has marked male predominance.[176] Symptoms are similar to those in myophosphorylase deficiency. Again, ischemic exercise fails to elevate the lactate value. Muscle weakness on strenuous exercise and cramping of muscle and myoglobinuria can occur. To date 29 cases have been reported.[177] Phosphofructokinase, the enzyme that converts either fructose-6-phosphate or fructose-1-phosphate to fructose-1,6-diphosphate, is missing. Because this enzyme is necessary for the metabolism of glycogen, glucose, or fructose, none of these compounds should be expected to improve the picture.[168] The enzyme is also missing from erythrocytes, and this leads to hemolysis with increased reticulocytosis. The

reason that primarily muscle, and to a lesser extent red cells, is involved is that these two tissues are capable of synthesizing only one of the three isoforms. Other tissues have several types and can thus compensate for the absence of one. The muscle tissue in the fetus and in tissue culture has all the subunits, so the enzyme can be normal in muscle from these sources. The genetic defect is the production of an abnormal form of the M isoform from chromosome 1. Other subunits come from other chromosomes. Although red cell survival is reduced, anemia is not frequent because the reduction in 2,3-diphosphoglyceric acid (2,3-DPG) is a stimulus to red cell production. The shift in the oxyhemoglobin dissociation curve has not been found to account for other problems.[176, 177] Although the anesthetic experience is limited, no anesthetic problems have been reported. Recommendations are similar to those for myophosphorylase deficiency, but increased glucose would not be expected to improve muscle function.

H. CORI'S TYPE VIII— LOW HEPATIC PHOSPHORYLASE ACTIVITY

Patients with this condition show progressive CNS degeneration and die in childhood.

I. CORI'S TYPE IX—DEFICIENT HEPATIC PHOSPHORYLASE-KINASE ACTIVITY WITH PREDOMINANT HEPATOMEGALY

One patient underwent two anesthesia procedures.[178] The first, with halothane and succinylcholine, produced no reported problems. During the second anesthesia procedure, with enflurane after succinylcholine and ketamine for induction, the temperature increased 2°C in 2 hours and there was evidence of a hypermetabolic state with an increase in arterial P_{CO_2} and a base excess of -12 mEq/L. The acidosis was at least partially caused by ketosis, although adequate serum glucose was documented and extra glucose was given intravenously. No other findings of malignant hyperpyrexia were found in this patient, and only minimal changes in CK levels occurred. The child did well postoperatively.

A muscle form of the enzyme has been

found to be deficient in a small number of children and adults (22) and is related to a defect on chromosome 16. The symptoms are primarily exercise intolerance and myoglobinuria, with some distal weakness.[177]

J. CORI'S TYPE X—DEFICIENT CYCLIC 3',5'-ADENOSINE MONOPHOSPHATE–DEPENDENT KINASE

Excess glycogen is found in both skeletal muscle and liver. Hepatomegaly is a major sign.

VII. BLOCKS IN GLYCOLYSIS

The clinical picture resembles McArdle's syndrome in all patients with blocks in glycolysis who exhibit muscle abnormalities. Thus, there is normal initial strength, weakness with strenuous exercise, and pigmenturia if exercise is continued. Lactic acid production is reduced during ischemic exercise. All blocks are incomplete and are thus less effective than in phosphofructokinase deficiency.[179]

A. PHOSPHOHEXOISOMERASE DEFICIENCY

Phosphohexoisomerase is the enzyme needed to convert glucose-6-phosphate to fructose-6-phosphate. As expected, fructose relieves the symptoms and permits the production of lactate.[180]

In Cori's types V and VII, and in phosphohexoisomerase deficiency, high levels of glycolysis, without ischemia, would be expected to produce symptoms. Thus, anything that would produce a hypermetabolic state in muscle, such as shivering or hyperthermia, might lead to problems and even myoglobinuria. Careful avoidance of heat loss during the operation and continuous temperature monitoring are indicated. In the patient with proved phosphohexoisomerase deficiency intravenous fructose is warranted.

B. PHOSPHOGLYCERATE KINASE DEFICIENCY

Phosphoglycerate kinase deficiency is an X-linked recessive disease. A single gene is responsible for the enzyme. The enzyme converts 1,3-phosphoglycerate to adenosine triphosphate (ATP) and 3-phosphoglycerate. At present, 20 patients with various combinations of hemolytic anemia (65 per cent), CNS dysfunction (50 per cent), and myopathy (40 per cent) have been found; only one patient displayed all three. Exercise intolerance, cramps, and myoglobinuria have been reported, and continued exercise leads to muscle destruction and pigmenturia. Severe hemolytic anemia may occur and must be distinguished from myoglobinuria.[179] Why there are different expressions of this single enzyme disease is not known. Those with hemolytic anemia may undergo splenectomy and thus require anesthesia; however, no anesthesia experience is reported.[177]

C. PHOSPHOGLYCERATE MUTASE DEFICIENCY

Nine patients in seven families have been described with phosphoglycerate mutase deficiency since 1981.[181] In normal individuals, the enzyme catalyzes the conversion of 3-phosphoglycerate to 2-phosphoglycerate. The enzyme consists of two different monomers that combine to form dimers, the brain and muscle types being distinct. The muscle band is lacking in these patients, but the brain form is present, though there is not enough to return activity to near normal. All of these patients had primary muscle symptoms, with cramps and pigmenturia with exercise. Although the one patient who had cardiac symptoms had them for other reasons, the predominance of the muscle form of the enzyme in heart muscle makes it likely that some cardiac abnormality will be found.

D. LACTIC DEHYDROGENASE DEFICIENCY

The enzyme is a tetramer composed of two different monomers. Lactate dehydrogenase (LDH) M (muscle) deficiency has been reported in nine families. The activity in muscle is 5 per cent of normal if the muscle form is missing, whereas activity is more normal in other tissues, including the heart. The symptoms are exercise fatigue and intolerance, though exertional myoglobinuria requires severe exercise.[177] Renal failure thought secondary to myoglobinemia has occurred. The M isoform of LDH is predominant in muscle, uterus, and skin. Patients have a scaling, erythematous rash. Three patients had uterine stiffness during labor that required cesarean section. No anesthetic reports have appeared in the literature. When there is muscle destruction, serum CK rises without an increase in LDH.[182]

VIII. MYOADENYLATE DEAMINASE DEFICIENCY

Myoadenylate deaminase deficiency was first described in 1978, yet it may be the most common of the enzyme deficiency diseases of muscle. In the series of muscle biopsy specimens examined at the Armed Forces Institute of Pathology, 1.5 per cent were from patients with myoadenylate deaminase deficiency.[177] The enzyme is responsible for the conversion of AMP to inosine monophosphate and is most useful when phosphate reserves are less than half of normal and AMP is accumulating from the conversion of two molecules of adenosine diphosphate (ADP) to ATP and AMP. The symptoms are postexertional weakness associated with soreness and cramping. Weakness increases throughout the day. Limb and trunk weakness predominate, with sparing of facial and eye muscles. The symptoms usually are recognized after age 20 years. Autosomal inheritance is present, and roughly equal involvement of males and females is seen. There have been no reports of myoglobinuria. Affected children exhibit decreased muscle tone, but this is not seen in adults, who have tenderness to palpation and mild to moderate weakness with atrophy. The CK level is elevated mildly, and the EMG does not show a myasthenic pattern. The cardiac muscle type of deficiency is different from the skeletal form, though there is a report of two siblings with cardiomyopathy and AMP deaminase deficiency. There may also be a fetal form of the disease.

The diagnosis is made by looking at the ratio of lactate to ammonia after exercise (the LAER test): after drawing a blood sample and inflating a tourniquet midway between the systolic and diastolic pressures, the arm is exercised until fatigued. A blood sample is obtained from that arm before the tourniquet is released. For the test results to be valid, an increase of at least 4.5 mM of lactate should be obtained. An increase in the ammonia level

less than 0.7 per cent of the lactate increase is abnormal. Although muscle cramps occur, there is no evidence that permanent damage is done to the muscle by exercising, and no drug therapy is recommended, though dantrolene and verapamil produce symptomatic relief. There have been no anesthetic incidents, of either MH or other problems, in these patients, but considering the frequency of this defect it would not be unexpected to see associations of all kinds. Differentiating true relationships from those caused by chance is difficult. One family was reported with both the enzyme deficiency and MH, but the two diseases seemed to have been inherited independently.[24]

IX. MYOSITIS OSSIFICANS PROGRESSIVA

Another familial disease, myositis ossificans progressiva, usually starts in early childhood and is transmitted as an autosomaldominant trait. After minor trauma, a cystlike nodule is first felt under the skin. This is followed by the appearance of true bone in that area. The heart, diaphragm, sphincters, and larynx are spared in this otherwise widespread, progressive disease. The major problems are fixation of the muscles of mastication and the neck. In addition, three quarters of affected persons have other associated anomalies such as microdactyly, curved or ankylosed digits and other digital anomalies, missing teeth, and spina bifida, many of which lesions require surgical correction. Biopsies and other surgical intervention, however, can cause local formation of bone. Death is usually caused by limitation of motion over the trunk leading to secondary respiratory or cardiac failure. Although death usually occurs in the second to fourth decades of life, survival to the seventh decade has been reported.

Anesthetic problems are related primarily to the inability to open the mouth or bend the neck. This cannot be overcome by muscle relaxants once ossification has occurred. Blind nasal or fiberoptic intubation is preferred over tracheostomy, since ossification may occur at the tracheostomy site. Limitation of the chest wall can become a problem as the disease progresses. Steroids have been used for treatment, although their efficacy remains in question. Recently, use of ethane-1-hydroxy-1, 1-diphosphonic acid (EHDP) seemed to be effective in slowing the disease by preventing crystal growth.[183]

X. MITOCHONDRIAL MYOPATHIES[184-186]

Disorders of fatty acid utilization or mitochondrial function may affect skeletal muscle; more often, defective aerobic metabolism affects several organ systems. One frequently observes CNS involvement; thus the term *mitochondrial encephalomyopathy*. Other organ systems that may be involved include the peripheral nervous system, heart, liver, kidneys, endocrine glands, gastrointestinal tract, and bone marrow. Exercise intolerance and lactic acidosis are frequently observed. Mitochondrial myopathies can be classified according to histologic appearance, immunochemical and biochemical examination, or genetic analysis. The histologic hallmark of mitochondrial myopathies is the "ragged red fiber" (RRF): on Gomori-trichrome stain, muscle fibers with markedly increased numbers of structurally abnormal mitochondria have a "ragged, red" appearance. Skeletal muscle RRF may be observed in some mitochondrial diseases without clinical myopathy; conversely, RRF is not always demonstrated in mitochondrial myopathy. Immunochemical or biochemical examination may demonstrate deficiencies of pyruvate dehydrogenase (PDH), Krebs cycle enzymes, or respiratory chain proteins. Specific syndromes are associated with large deletions (e.g., Kearns-Sayre syndrome, nonfamilial progressive external ophthalmoplegia) or point mutations (e.g., MELAS or MERRF; see below) of mitochondrial DNA.

Most mitochondrial proteins are encoded by nuclear genes. Mitochondria are unique among organelles by virtue of their having a *maternally inherited* genome independent of the nuclear genome. The oocyte contributes exclusively to the mitochondrial DNA of the zygote. Each cell has numerous copies of mitochondrial DNA. The mitochondrial genome consists of double-stranded circular DNA with 16,569 base pairs. Mitochondrial DNA is transcribed into tRNA (for amino acid transfer), rRNA (ribosomal), and mRNA (messenger) for protein subunits of the respiratory chain. Protein subunits of respiratory chain complexes I, III, IV, and V are encoded by mitochondrial and nuclear genes; complex II (succinate dehydrogenase–ubiquinone oxido-reductase) is encoded by only nuclear DNA. In the mitochondrial myopathies, a detailed family history may demonstrate maternal inheritance, autosomal recessive or dominant inheritance, or sporadic occurrence. Spontaneous large-deletion mutations may alter mitochondrial (mt) DNA during embryogenesis, resulting in sporadic occurrence of KSS or progressive external ophthalmoplegia (PEO). The mother may contribute different numbers of normal and mutant mtDNA to different children. Mitotic distribution of variable proportions of mutant and normal ("wild-type") mtDNA during tissue differentiation and organogenesis may determine the disease phenotype. *Heteroplasmy* is the coexistence of mutant and normal mtDNA in a single tissue or cell. Marked variability in expression and age of onset, even in close relatives, is characteristic of heritable mitochondrial disorders.

Mitochondrial genotype may not correlate with only one specific disease.[187] The same point mutation may be associated with several different phenotypes. MELAS (*m*itochondrial *e*ncephalomyopathy, *l*actic *a*cidosis, and *s*trokes) is associated with a mutation of nucleotide pair (nt) 3243 of the tRNA[Leu] gene; the same point mutation has been noted in some families with maternally inherited diabetes mellitus and sensorineural deafness. A different point mutation of the same tRNA[Leu] gene is associated with maternally inherited adult-onset myopathy and cardiomyopathy. A large (4977 base pairs) deletion may be associated with sporadic PEO, KSS, or Pearson's disease (sideroblastic anemia with hepatic and pancreatic dysfunction). The size and site of mtDNA deletions do not correlate well with severity of disease. The following sections discuss mitochondrial diseases, which include skeletal myopathy.

A. KEARNS-SAYRE SYNDROME, SPORADIC PROGRESSIVE EXTERNAL OPHTHALMOPLEGIA, ''OPHTHALMOPLEGIA PLUS''

The KSS, PEO, and ophthalmoplegia plus syndromes are associated with large deletions of mtDNA; in any single patient, the size and site of the deletion are constant. Family history is negative in KSS or sporadic PEO, indicating that the deletion occurs during embryogenesis. Small duplications of mtDNA noted in KSS have been associated with in-creased incidence of diabetes.[188] Numbers of mitochondria are markedly increased in RRF; these mitochondria contain increased mutant mtDNA, decreased normal mtDNA, and are deficient in cytochrome C oxidase (COX, com-plex IV). It is postulated that deleted mtDNA has a replicative advantage over normal mtDNA, resulting in increased disease ex-pression over time.

KSS usually features PEO, pigmentary reti-nopathy, myopathy, and onset before age 20; it often includes cardiac conduction abnor-malities (e.g., heart block), elevated cerebro-spinal fluid (CSF) protein, ataxia, or diabetes. PEO is progressive and nonfluctuating; diplo-pia is uncommon, unlike in myasthenia gra-vis. Patients often present for surgical correc-tion of ptosis. Basal serum lactic acid levels are normal or elevated and increase to an abnormal degree with exertion. Depressed ventilatory response to hypercarbia or hy-poxia, independent of muscle weakness or sleep apnea, has been described in patients with various mitochondrial encephalomyopa-thies, including (1) KSS, (2) familial or spo-radic PEO with proximal myopathy, (3) my-oclonic epilepsy with RRF (MERRF), and (4) Leigh's syndrome (necrotizing encephalomy-elopathy of infancy or childhood).[189, 190] Marked sensitivity to intravenous induction agents, opiates, or sedative-hypnotics may be present.[191, 192] Difficulty in weaning from me-chanical ventilation has been described in pa-tients presenting with recurrent pneumonia and respiratory failure.[189] *Heart block may re-quire pacemaker insertion;* congestive cardiomy-opathy is rarely described. Deafness, demen-tia, and peripheral neuropathy can be other manifestations of nervous system degenera-tion. Abnormal mitochondria have been dem-onstrated in glial or Schwann cells. Autopsy studies show marked spongiform degenera-tion in deep white matter of the cerebral hemispheres, cerebellum, and brainstem. In addition to diabetes mellitus, other endocrine disturbances can include hypoparathy-roidism, hypothyroidism, and short stature. Administration of ubiquinone, or coenzyme Q (CoQ), is infrequently associated with im-provement in strength, lactic acidosis, or neu-rologic disease.[193] Progressive neurologic de-terioration usually causes death by age 40 years.

In addition to sporadic PEO, there are two forms of heritable PEO: (1) maternally inher-ited, without mtDNA deletion, and (2) an autosomal dominant type. Maternally inher-ited PEO lacks cardiac or CNS involvement. Autosomal-dominant PEO is characterized by the presence of multiple mtDNA deletions in a given patient; as in KSS, central and periph-eral nervous system involvement (e.g., ataxia, tremor, sensorimotor neuropathy, deafness) or myopathy may be prominent. PEO is also a feature of *MNGIE* (*m*yo *n*euro*g*astro*i*ntestintal disorder and *e*ncephalopathy) syndrome, which combines intestinal pseudoobstruction, demyelinating sensorimotor neuropathy, and mitochondrial myopathy. MNGIE has also been referred to as *POLIP* (*p*olyneuropathy, *o*phthalmoplegia, *l*eukoencephalopathy, *i*ntes-tinal *p*seudoobstruction). Multiple mtDNA deletions without PEO have been observed in two sets of brothers: one set had ptosis with-out other myopathy; the other set had recur-rent myoglobinuria.

B. MYOCLONIC EPILEPSY WITH RAGGED RED FIBERS

MERRF is a heritable mitochondrial en-cephalomyopathy characterized by myoclo-nus, seizures, ataxia, dementia, sensorineural deafness, optic atrophy, and myopathy. PEO, cardiomyopathy, retinopathy, and stroke are usually absent. Estimated incidence in Japan is 0.1 per 100,000.[194] Age of onset, expression of symptoms, and disease progression are highly variable. Serum lactate is usually in-creased. Most patients with MERRF have a point mutation of nucleotide (nt) pair 8344 (A to G) or nt-8356 (C to T) in tRNA^{Lys} of mtDNA.[187] The nt-8344 point mutation has also been found in PEO, Leigh's syndrome, and (in a small proportion of total mtDNA) in eye muscle of healthy elderly persons. Pa-tients are usually treated symptomatically with anticonvulsants, including clonazepam.

C. MYOPATHY, ENCEPHALOPATHY, LACTIC ACIDOSIS, AND STROKE

MELAS is characterized by strokelike epi-sodes resulting in hemiparesis, hemianopsia, or cortical blindness. Short stature, seizures, vascular headache, ataxia, hearing loss, PEO, and episodic vomiting may be observed. Early development may be normal. Serum lactate is usually increased. Arterioles that stain intensely for the mitochondrial enzyme SDH have been observed in brain and muscle of patients with MELAS. These abnormal arterioles, termed SDH-staining vessels (SSV), are postulated to play an important role in producing cerebral ischemia.[195] Most patients with MELAS have a point mutation of nt-3243 (A to G) or nt-3271 (A to G) in tRNA[Leu] of mtDNA. The nt-3243 mutation has also been found in familial PEO. Progressive neurologic deterioration usually causes death in adolescence or young adulthood.

D. LEIGH'S SYNDROME (SUBACUTE NECROTIZING ENCEPHALOMYELOPATHY)

Leigh's syndrome usually presents in infancy or early childhood with progressive psychomotor regression with hypotonia. Children often present with feeding difficulty, vomiting, respiratory abnormality (e.g., aspiration, stridor), ataxia, nystagmus, or seizures. Optic atrophy or hearing loss may be observed. Cerebrospinal fluid lactate and pyruvate are usually increased more dramatically than serum levels. Neuropathology typically shows gliosis and demyelination involving brain stem, basal ganglia, thalamus, and hypothalamus, cerebellum, optic chiasm, or spinal cord. RRF usually is *not* demonstrated with muscle biopsy. CT may demonstrate symmetric, hypodense lesions in the basal ganglia or thalamus. Enzyme abnormalities most often associated with Leigh's syndrome include (1) complex IV (COX) deficiency, (2) PDH deficiency, and rarely (3) complex V (H^+ ATPase subunit 6) deficiency. Inheritance may be autosomal recessive (e.g., COX deficiency), X-linked (e.g., PDH deficiency), mitochondrial (maternal; e.g., ATPase 6 mutation), or sporadic. Death usually occurs in early childhood from respiratory failure. Anesthesiologists may be asked to care for patients undergoing diagnostic muscle biopsy or CT. Grattan-Smith and colleagues reported three patients with a history of either stridor or aspiration who had postanesthetic respiratory failure; severe decompensation occurred 12 to 24 hours following general anesthesia.[196]

XI. DEFECTS OF OXIDATIVE PHOSPHORYLATION

A. LUFT'S DISEASE

Luft's disease was first described in 1959, and in 1962 a more detailed account of the metabolic abnormality was presented.[197] The patient was noted to have symptoms from at least age 7 years but was studied at age 35. At that time, she was noted to have many of the symptoms of hyperthyroidism, including hyperhidrosis, polydypsia, polyphagia, asthenia, and decreased weight; however, her growth and development were normal by history. She was first treated for hyperthyroidism medically, which initially produced a decrease in her basal metabolic rate. Later, after thyroidectomy, unmistakable signs of myxedema developed, despite a basal metabolic rate of +100 per cent. Although this was considerably less than her maximum of +270 per cent, she required thyroid replacement therapy. She had not only the expected increased minute ventilation but also increased functional residual capacity and increased residual volume–total lung capacity ratio. The pathologic picture was one of mitochondria of variable size with increased numbers of cristae; this is normal in mitochondria from liver, heart, and diaphragm but not in those from skeletal muscle. The nuclei were surrounded by a clear myofibril-free area. Her uterine and skin mitochondria were normal. A similar picture was seen in a second case reported and described in detail by both Haydar and Afifi and respective coworkers.[198, 199]

The clinical picture could be explained by biochemical studies that demonstrated loose coupling of oxidative phosphorylation, which is a situation in which the stepwise oxidation of hydrogen by the cytochrome system does not produce ATP from ADP in a stoichiometric relationship. ADP thus is not necessary for the production of water from hydrogen. Because ADP is produced from ATP during muscle contraction, its concentration is related to the work done by the cell; thus, the metabolic rate normally increases as available ADP increases. This patient's mitochondria, unlike normal ones, did not decrease the rate of oxidation when ADP was lacking from the medium. Thus, the fixed relationship no longer held. Her rate of oxidation of hydrogen is not dependent on the availability of ADP; however, her oxidative phosphorylation is not uncoupled, because ATP can be produced if ADP is present. This is mandatory for life, because energy, in the form of high-energy phosphate, must be stored if the body is to do useful work.

This patient had one anesthesia procedure, for thyroidectomy, which consisted of intravenous Narkotal (5,2-bromoallyl-*N*-methyl-5-isopropyl barbituric acid) and ether by endotracheal tube. There were no complications during or after the surgery.[200] Undoubtedly, this patient, having such a high metabolic rate, would benefit from the use of high concentrations of oxygen and a larger than usual minute ventilation. High-output respiratory failure might be expected, especially after major surgery, and postoperative ventilation might be required. Blood gas measurements would also be valuable, both before and during surgery, because normal amounts of shunt might produce arterial desaturation owing to the increased arteriovenous oxygen gradient. Short periods of apnea, or decreased perfusion, would be expected to be hazardous. Since this patient's blood volume was almost twice the predicted normal level, blood volume measurements would be of value in this disease. Hyperthermia, not seen in the single anesthetic experience, would be a concern, and means should be available to cool the patient rapidly.

In 1967, van Wijngaarden[201] reported on a patient whose onset of myopathy dated from at least age 4 years. At 11 years, she had slight deltoid weakness and a waddling gait (her basal metabolic rate was normal). At 15 years, the disease showed slow progression and the basal metabolic rate was now slightly elevated, at +24 per cent. The muscle mitochondria were seen to be elongated and annular, with tightly packed cristae. They also demonstrated loosely coupled oxidative phosphorylation but used a normal amount of glucose-6-phosphate for the oxygen consumed. How this disease is related to Luft's disease is not known, and the marked weakness relative to the metabolic abnormality certainly produced a quite different clinical picture. No anesthetic experience is reported.

The inner mitochondrial membrane contains the respiratory chain that is responsible for the oxidation of hydrogen to water with the production of ATP. For convenience, this chain has been broken down into five complexes, each made up of many polypeptides; thus, clinical heterogeneity is expected, since many different genetic defects would be expected to occur (Fig. 10–2). Mitochondrial genomic disorders consisting of large mtDNA deletions or point mutations in tRNA genes are often associated with defects in multiple respiratory chain complexes.

B. COMPLEX I—REDUCED NICOTINAMIDE ADENINE DINUCLEOTIDE–COENZYME Q REDUCTASE DEFECT

The enzyme requires a flavin mononucleotide for the transport of hydrogen from reduced nicotinamide adenine dinucleotide (NADH) to CoQ. It is fed from PDH and other sources of NADH (e.g., Krebs cycle or fatty acid oxidation). More than 100 patients have been described. Some patients die in infancy with systemic involvement, severe lactic acidosis, cardiomyopathy, and CNS

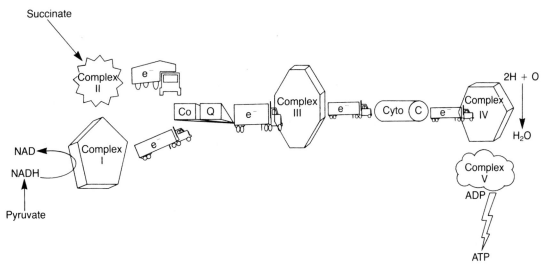

FIGURE 10–2. Mitochondrial oxidation of hydrogen to H_2O with production of ATP.

symptoms. Defects in complex I have also been described in patients with Leigh's syndrome, PEO syndromes and KSS, or progressive encephalomyopathy. The presentation of progressive encephalomyopathy is often similar to that of MELAS; in addition, cardiomyopathy has been observed in some patients. Other patients have a pure myopathy with exercise intolerance, variable lactic acidosis that worsens with exercise, and myalgia. One patient with a myopathy responded to riboflavin, 100 mg per day, whereas others have not.[202] Other suggestions, including some that have not been tried but should theoretically be useful, include administration of menadione, thiamine, prednisone, and as a last resort methylene blue, 2 mg/kg intravenously.[203]

C. COMPLEX II— SUCCINATE–COENZYME Q REDUCTASE DEFECT

A flavin dinucleotide is required for the transport of hydrogen from succinate to CoQ. The defect has not been as well-documented, but two patients had severe infantile myopathy with lactic acidosis, whereas several others also had encephalopathy. A 22-year-old man with episodic exertional myoglobinuria and a 14-year-old girl with generalized myopathy and exercise intolerance each had significantly reduced muscle SDH activity. The 22-year-old also had a defect of the Krebs cycle enzyme aconitase, which converts citrate to isocitrate.

D. COENZYME Q DEFICIENCY

Two sisters with severe muscle CoQ deficiency have been reported. They had myopathy with exercise intolerance and recurrent myoglobinuria. They also had encephalopathy; one sister had generalized seizures, the other had a progressive cerebellar syndrome. Lactic acidosis was present. Muscle biopsy demonstrated mitochondrial proliferation and lipid storage.

E. COMPLEX III—REDUCED COENZYME Q– CYTOCHROME C REDUCTASE DEFECT

This group transports electrons from coenzyme Q to cytochrome C. So far, 19 patients have been described with the defect, 11 with myopathy (6 cases were extraocular myopathy [PEO]). Since either vitamin C, 1 g by mouth four times per day, or vitamin K_3, 10 mg by mouth four times per day, can bypass this block, they have been given, and improvement has been seen. In the skeletal myopathy, the defect is not seen in cardiac muscle, but it can occur in cardiac muscle with normal skeletal values.[203] Of the six patients with PEO, four had large single deletions of mtDNA; one of the six had the point mutation at nt-3243 of mtDNA also found with MELAS. The sixth patient with PEO had multisystem (skin, IDDM, aminoaciduria, progressive encephalopathy) involvement and was found to have a maternally inherited partial duplication of mtDNA; she and her sister died before age 10.

F. COMPLEX IV— CYTOCHROME OXIDASE DEFICIENCY

Complex IV myopathy is a severe infantile type with lactic acidosis, respiratory insufficiency, and, usually, death before the first birthday. Renal tubule dysfunction (de Toni-Fanconi syndrome) with aminoaciduria and glycosuria may be observed. In the pure myopathy, the heart, liver, and brain are spared. Muscle biopsy usually shows RRF and lipid storage. Inheritance is usually autosomal recessive; recently, four patients have been described with severe depletion of mtDNA. A few patients with severe myopathy and acidosis improve with age so that the defect is gone by age 2 to 3 years. An encephalomyopathy called *Leigh's syndrome* (see above) may also be caused by a defect in this complex. Partial deficiency of muscle COX has also been noted in some cases of progressive encephalopathy (MELAS-like presentation), PEO (KSS or MNGIE), or MERRF. No specific recommendations for therapy can be made, but symptomatic treatment is warranted because of the few patients who improve spontaneously. The acidosis has been treated with bicarbonate, tris(hydroxymethyl)aminomethane (TRIS), or dialysis.

G. COMPLEX V— MITOCHONDRIAL ADENOSINE TRIPHOSPHATASE DEFICIENCY

Two patients have been described who had complex V deficiency. One, aged 37 years, had a very slowly progressive myopathy. The other had encephalomyopathy of slow onset.

In all of the complexes described, trials of agents that bypass the respiratory chain, such as vitamins C and K, have met with variable success. Methylene blue caused improvement in the blood lactate level in one patient, but the patient had cardiac arrest, which might have been caused by the drug. The use of drugs such as valproic acid, which uses carnitine; barbiturates, which inhibit the respiratory chain (though it is not clear whether primarily or secondarily); and antibiotics such as tetracyclines, which inhibit mitochondrial protein synthesis, might best be avoided. It must be remembered that these are theoretical considerations only, and no direct evidence is available to implicate them in patients' problems. Glucose is useful to prevent problems associated with fasting in many of these patients. It must be remembered that all forms of lactic acidosis are not helped by glucose loading, and in patients with pyruvate dehydrogenase deficiency the lactic acidosis may actually get worse if glucose is given.[203]

Preoperative evaluation of patients with mitochondrial myopathies should assess (1) acid-base status, (2) presence of feeding difficulties and history of vomiting or aspiration, (3) history of stridor or apnea, (4) history of recurrent pneumonia or respiratory failure, (5) cardiac function, including conduction system abnormalities,[204] (6) history of seizures and use of anti-convulsants, (7) endocrine disturbances, and (8) sensory or motor neuropathy. Prolonged preoperative fasting should be avoided; if oral intake is inadequate or prohibited, maintenance intravenous glucose should be promptly initiated.[205] Intra- and postoperative ventilation must be rigorously observed to avoid respiratory acidosis superimposed on any existing lactic acidosis.[206] Abnormal hemodynamics or tachypnea mandate measurement of blood gases. One should attempt to maintain body temperature to minimize postoperative shivering. Anesthetics (inhaled or intravenous), analgesics, and muscle relaxants should be titrated to effect whenever possible. While uneventful use of succinylcholine has been reported in some patients with mitochondrial myopathies,[207, 208] the additional metabolic stress imposed by succinylcholine could theoretically aggravate lactic acidosis. Patients with significant motor neuropathy should not receive succinylcholine. Ohtani and colleagues reported presumptive MH (generalized rigidity after halothane and succinylcholine, myoglobinuria, metabolic acidosis) in a 2-year-old with proximal myopathy; she was treated with dantrolene and bicarbonate and promptly recovered. Muscle biopsy showed marked subsarcolemmal accumulation of mitochondria; no specific respiratory chain complex deficiency was noted.[209] There was no description of other affected relatives. A strong association between malignant hyperthermia and mitochondrial myopathies has not been demonstrated; it is not reasonable to prohibit the use of halogenated anesthetics on the basis of one case report. Patients with a history of respiratory failure, stridor, apnea, aspiration, hypoglycemia, or cardiac involvement may require postoperative care in a closely monitored setting.

XII. LIPID MYOPATHIES

Another group of mitochondrial myopathies with abnormal metabolism of lipids has been found.[210] The normal metabolism of the muscle uses long-chain fatty acids. The fatty acids are esterified with coenzyme A (CoA) present in the outer mitochondrial membrane. Acyl-CoA is then attached to carnitine by acylcarnitine transferase (carnitine palmitoyltransferase [CPT] I), transported across the membrane by a translocase, and then reforms acyl-CoA by a second transferase (CPT II) located on the inner surface of the inner mitochondrial membrane. The repeated beta-oxidation produces shortening of the fatty-acid chain and free acetyl-CoA (Fig. 10–3). The inner membrane is impermeable to CoA and acyl-CoA and thus requires the translocase for movement of fatty acids in and out of the mitochondria. Most commonly, a slowly progressive myopathy is described.

A. CARNITINE DEFICIENCY

Carnitine (γ-amino-β-hydroxybutyric acid, trimethylbetaine) facilitates the transport of long-chain fatty acids into mitochondria. It is synthesized from lysine and methionine, principally in the liver, and is then transported to skeletal muscle, in which more than 90 per cent of the carnitine is found.[211] Approximately 75 per cent of carnitine requirements are derived from dietary sources. Its absence from muscle causes weakness; lipid granules are seen in the muscle. Fatty acids

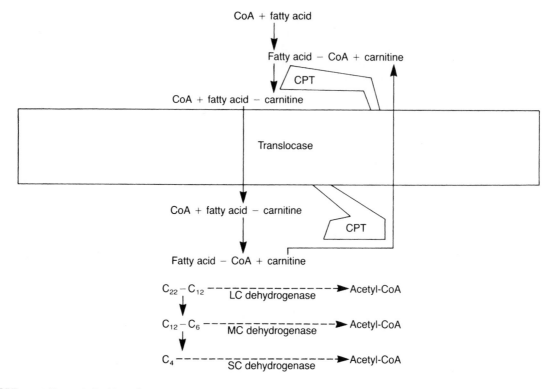

CoA + fatty acid

Fatty acid − CoA + carnitine

CPT

CoA + fatty acid − carnitine

Translocase

CoA + fatty acid − carnitine

CPT

Fatty acid − CoA + carnitine

$C_{22} - C_{12}$ ------------→ Acetyl-CoA
LC dehydrogenase

$C_{12} - C_6$ ------------→ Acetyl-CoA
MC dehydrogenase

C_4 ------------→ Acetyl-CoA
SC dehydrogenase

CPT = carnitine palmitoyl transferase
LC = long chain
MC = medium chain
SC = short chain

FIGURE 10–3. Transport of fatty acids into mitochondria in muscle.

account for approximately 70 per cent of the energy use of muscle at rest, and are the primary energy source during fasting or prolonged exercise. Carnitine-deficient muscle can be exercised, but not to the same extent as normal muscle. Medium-chain fatty acids (which do not require carnitine to get into mitochondria) and carnitine help most patients. In addition, steroids may be efficacious. It is thought that the steroids afford long-chain fatty acids access to the mitochondria without carnitine or that they afford carnitine access into the mitochondria.

Skeletal or cardiac muscle carnitine levels are normally 20- to 60-fold greater than the serum level; this reflects active uptake via high-affinity receptors. In primary systemic or myopathic carnitine deficiency, tissue uptake is impaired. There are systemic deficiencies of carnitine, with symptoms like those in Reye's syndrome, and myopathic forms with deficiency principally in muscle with weakness. Among 24 cases of the myopathic form reported between 1973 and 1981, the weak-

ness started between ages 1 and 38 years. More than 20 patients with dilated cardiomyopathy have been reported; the cardiomyopathy is reversible with oral L-carnitine therapy. Three patients had recurrent episodes of myoglobinuria. A few patients have been reported with respiratory insufficiency.

The anesthetic experience is limited to three case reports; one led to a fatal outcome,[212] and the others were uneventful,[213, 214] but the management is not described in enough detail to link management to outcome. Optimal preoperative preparation with carnitine and medium-chain fatty acids, maintenance of the glucose level with frequent checks, and possibly use of steroids might all contribute to a better outcome. The presence of a cardiomyopathy must be sought, and appropriate monitoring must then be instituted.

The number of causes of secondary carnitine deficiency has increased greatly in the past few years, and many of the cases originally reported as primary are now known to be secondary carnitine deficiency.

B. SECONDARY CARNITINE DEFICIENCY

Many organic acidurias cause a loss of carnitine, and thus deficiency. There are at least six acyl-CoA dehydrogenase deficiencies. These enzymes act on different length and branched and unbranched fatty acyl-CoAs. The defective fatty acyl-CoA dehydrogenase places a metabolic "roadblock," resulting in excessive accumulation of fatty acyl-CoA; the excess fatty acyl-CoA is converted to fatty acylcarnitine. The accumulation of acylcarnitine (fatty acid linked to carnitine) in the mitochondria leads to excessive loss from the cells and eventual excretion in the urine. Urinary excretion of the esterified carnitine causes the deficiency, but the low carnitine level frequently is not the only problem. The Reye's-like syndrome that is seen in the systemic form of the disease presents with vomiting, stupor, and coma. Increased liver enzyme levels, hepatomegaly, hypoglycemia, and hypoprothrombinemia are also seen, but, unlike in Reye's syndrome, the hypoglycemia occurs *without ketosis*. The product excreted in the urine is not acetyl carnitine, as in Reye's syndrome, but a longer-chain ester that is present because of the underlying enzyme defect.[215] Supplementation of carnitine works in some instances, and 100 mg/kg per day, to a maximum of 4 g per day, is frequently used. Fasting must be avoided, and the use of glucose loading in affected patients is important.

1. Long-Chain Acyl-Coenzyme A Dehydrogenase Deficiency

So far, nine patients have been reported with symptoms like those of systemic carnitine deficiency. It is thought to be an autosomal-recessive trait.[216] Onset is in the first months of life, and death comes early. Symptoms include encephalopathic metabolic crises (nonketotic hypoglycemia, hyperammonemia), hypertrophic cardiomyopathy, hypotonia, and hepatosplenomegaly. Fasting caused cardiorespiratory arrest in one patient. Carnitine is of some help, though most patients have died by age 1 year, in spite of treatment. Four infants who survived early metabolic crises developed myopathy with recurrent muscle pain, fatigue, and myoglobinuria.

2. Medium-Chain Acyl-Coenzyme A Dehydrogenase Deficiency

This is the most common defect of beta oxidation, with an estimated incidence of 1 in 10,000. More than 85 patients have been reported with this Reye's-type syndrome, having hypoketotic, hypoglycemic episodes brought on by any stress, followed by lethargy and coma. It is one of the more common causes of sudden infant death syndrome (SIDS). Muscle weakness is worse during an attack and improves only slowly. Onset is usually before 2 years of age.[215, 216] The use of frequent, high-carbohydrate meals or glucose loading during fasting is recommended. Carnitine helped the hepatomegaly and hypoglycemia without altering the deficiency in muscle. Children who survive early metabolic crises may develop mild myopathy with lipid storage. Susceptibility to metabolic crisis, muscle weakness, and association with SIDS suggest that postoperative care be given in a closely monitored setting.

The gene encoding medium-chain acyl-CoA dehydrogenase (MCAD) is located on the short arm of chromosome 1, band p31. Most patients with MCAD deficiency are homozygous for a point mutation at codon 985; this changes a lysine residue at position 329 to glutamate.

3. Short-Chain Acyl-Coenzyme A Dehydrogenase Deficiency

Only five patients with this condition have been described—two adults and three infants. In adults it seems that the enzyme deficiency is limited to muscle and is not improved by carnitine administration. Infants have evidence of hepatic involvement (e.g., nonketotic hypoglycemia).

4. Multiple Acyl-Coenzyme A Dehydrogenase Deficiency

These represent partial or complete defects in electron-transferring flavoproteins. The first step in fatty acid beta oxidation produces reduced flavin adenine dinucleotide (FAD); electrons are transferred from reduced FAD to CoQ via electron-transferring flavoprotein (ETF) and ETF-CoQ oxidoreductase (ETF-

QO). There are several variants of this disease, with congenital anomalies in one type and not in a second, but both types kill neonates in the first weeks of life. These patients show rapidly progressive myopathy that is lethal;[217] they may also have rapidly progressive cardiomyopathy. A third form presents with later onset, even into the second decade of life, with hypoglycemic episodes, vomiting, acidosis provoked by stress (e.g., pregnancy, fasting, infection), and proximal myopathy. It may be an autosomal-recessive trait, the homozygous form being lethal and the heterozygous form becoming manifest during severe stress. Storage of lipid is seen in muscle, liver, kidney, and myocardium. Although carnitine deficiency is present, a trial of carnitine was not successful in one case. An acute metabolic disorder was responsible for death in all these patients. Riboflavin, to 100 mg three times per day orally, is sometimes helpful in these patients, as is a high-carbohydrate, low-fat diet.[215]

Other mitochondrial enzyme CoA defects can also lead to the abnormally low carnitine levels and systemic disease.

C. CARNITINE PALMITOYLTRANSFERASE DEFICIENCY

Carnitine palmitoyltransferase (CPT) is the enzyme responsible for the addition and removal of carnitine from long-chain fatty acids at the inner mitochondrial membrane. Although there are two sites for the enzyme, one on the outside and one on the inside of the membrane, there is some evidence that the two enzymes are structurally identical. The mutant enzyme seems to show more substrate inhibition than the normal variant. This might explain the limited amount of lipid storage, as well as the fact that little damage is done with day-to-day activity. The enzyme activity is reduced in most tissues tested, even the liver, yet symptoms are related almost entirely to muscle.

Myoglobinuria and muscle cramps, frequently without pain, are associated with increased plasma triglyceride levels. Weakness usually is not present, and normal lactate production is encountered on ischemic exercise. On prolonged fasting, however, serum levels of muscle CK increase and myoglobinuria occurs. The onset of muscle cramps that occurs later than in glycogen storage disease and more frequent episodes of myoglobinuria are characteristic. Exercise enhances the fasting myoglobinuria, which may be severe enough to cause renal failure (seen in more than 20 per cent of patients).[218, 219] No second-wind phenomenon is seen, and myoglobinuria is more common after prolonged moderate exercise than after brief, vigorous exercise. Brief, strenuous exercise is dependent on glucose and glycogen stores, which are normal, whereas exercise for more than 40 minutes is associated with a switch to lipid substrate. In at least five patients, episodes of weakness were associated with respiratory weakness, and three patients required ventilatory assistance. Between attacks, the CK level is normal in most patients and no weakness is present. Although most patients remember having muscle pains since childhood, the age at diagnosis is usually 15 to 30 years.

Although at least 39 patients (male-female ratio 5:1) are known, the anesthetic experience is limited to three reported cases.[220] The first patient had general anesthesia for muscle biopsy, which was uncomplicated. The second patient, reported in the Japanese literature, presents the picture of MH after induction with halothane and succinylcholine. The patient became febrile and acidotic and had arrhythmias and muscle rigidity. The most recent report was of an asymptomatic 43-year-old patient who had halothane anesthesia for gastrectomy. Renal failure developed in the postoperative period secondary to myoglobinuria, though no apparent intraoperative problems occurred. Use of succinylcholine was followed by normal relaxation, and there was no increase in body temperature. No glucose was given in the fluids, and no mention was made of the degree of shivering experienced on awakening. Both of these factors would be expected to cause myoglobinuria in these patients. Glucose would seem to be mandatory to prevent glycogen depletion followed by muscle dependence on long-chain fatty acids. Excessive muscle activity, such as shivering, should be prevented if possible. Temperature must be tightly controlled. The ability to distinguish between muscle damage secondary to CPT deficiency and the afebrile form of MH is very difficult. The differentiation, however, may be of practical significance, since these two entities would be treated differently.

There are many cases of apparently abnormal lipid metabolism in which defects have yet to be determined.

XIII. CONGENITAL MYOPATHIES

There are many types of histologic abnormalities of skeletal muscle sarcoplasm. They are somewhat more common than the myopathies of mitochondrial origin but are still extremely rare. Although the histologic patterns are easily described and distinguished from one another, the abnormalities are not specific and may well have unrelated causes, such as infection or pressure necrosis.[221] These changes may even be found nonspecifically in other myopathies, for example, periodic paralysis. When no other cause is found, the patients are categorized by the description of the histologic lesion and the clinical and genetic picture.

A. CENTRAL CORE DISEASE

Central core disease was first described by Shy and colleagues in 1956. A second family was described in 1961, and many more in subsequent years. Some patients exhibit reduced fetal movement, breech presentation, or congenital hip dislocation, but most have a history of normal birth and present with hypotonia and symmetric proximal muscle weakness in the first year of life. There is a delay in physical development.[221] This weakness remains, without progression, throughout life. Lower extremity weakness is more pronounced than upper extremity weakness, and these patients have difficulty walking up stairs and rising from a sitting position. Lumbar lordosis is also increased. Wasting of muscles has not been prominent in most patients.

Histologically, nearly every muscle cell has a central area devoid of oxidative enzymes; this is most characteristic of type I cells. This core is a region without mitochondria and SR in an otherwise normal fiber. There is no increase in the connective tissue of the endomysium, nor is there evidence of regenerating fibers. Serum aspartate aminotransferase (AST) and CK levels have been normal or only slightly elevated in all of these diseases.[221] There is an autosomal dominant mode of inheritance, and three mutations in the ryanodine receptor on chromosome 19q have so far been identified. How the gene defect causes the disorder is not known.[221]

Denborough reported a patient from a family with malignant hyperpyrexia who was diagnosed as having central core disease. A muscle biopsy specimen responded abnormally to halothane in vitro.[222] In one series of ten patients who had abnormal results on in vitro testing, eight had central core disease.[223] In another series, only one patient of those who had positive results with associated diseases had central core disease;[224] however, almost all patients with central core disease test positive for MH in vitro, and several of these have had abnormal responses to general anesthetics.[225] Harriman reported two patients with central core disease who had no problems when they were given halothane anesthesia.[226] One of our patients with this disease had an uneventful open reduction of the hip at another hospital; however, considering the information presently available, avoiding agents known to trigger MH seems advisable.

B. MULTICORE MYOPATHY

The first report of multicore myopathy appeared in 1966—and many additional cases since then. As the name implies, there are many weak-staining foci throughout the fibers and a lack of striations and mitochondria in these areas. The disease presents as a slowly progressive or nonprogressive myopathy, weakness being greatest in the proximal muscles. A variety of other problems are associated, including cardiac defects, conduction abnormalities, and cardiomyopathy.[227] It is difficult to assess how often these are just random associations, because of the rarity of the disease. Multicore myopathy is also not specific, as it can occur in many other muscle diseases, including MH; however, a recent case of fever and death subsequent to an anesthesia procedure raises the possibility of susceptibility to MH.[227]

C. NEMALINE MYOPATHY

Since nemaline myopathy was first described in 1963 by Shy and associates, the diversity of features has increased, and there are now three distinct types.[221] The first type is congenital with a slow course; the second is congenital, but with rapidly fatal outcome; and the third has late onset with progression. The only common finding is the rods seen on muscle biopsy specimens.

The majority of reports describe a relatively nonprogressive symmetric muscle weakness without marked wasting that affects principally the proximal muscles. Hypotonia is severe in infancy, with resultant late acquisition of motor skills: only one in eight patients walked by 18 months of age. In one case the newborn was noted to be weak, and in two of four cases cyanosis was noted perinatally. Older patients with this disease exhibit facial dysmorphism—elongated face, open mouth, short jaw, and a narrow, high-arched palate. Other abnormalities seen are pes cavus, talipes, and severe kyphosis, which may lead to cord compression and further diminution in muscle power. One patient was reported to have a vital capacity of only 40 per cent of the predicted value, but with normal flow rates; her mother, who also had the disease, died of respiratory failure at 63 years of age after an upper respiratory track infection.[228] In numerous reported autopsies, with one exception, there was no involvement of cardiac or smooth muscle.[221] Cineradiography reveals an asymptomatic abnormality in swallowing.

There have been seven reports of the rapidly progressive type of disease. One such patient died of cardiac failure at 12 years of age,[221] but most died before age 12 months. Diaphragm, intercostal, and bulbar muscles are involved. Histologically, rods (0.3 to 3 μm in diameter by 1 to 7 μm long) are found between the normal myofibrils in 2 to 40 per cent of the muscle fibers. They originate from the Z band of the muscle cell. Because the smallest percentage of abnormal cells was found in the oldest patient, the number of affected cells probably does not increase with time. No biochemical abnormalities have been demonstrated to date, although fewer mitochondria were observed in the affected areas than in the normal persons. The rods themselves are not the abnormality responsible for the weakness, since weakness may be greater in proximal muscles although distal muscles show more rods. From the limited data available, this appears to be an autosomal-dominant disease with incomplete penetrance, although there is marked female predominance.[221]

Four reports describe anesthesia in these patients. One patient underwent four anesthesia procedures with halothane without problems. Her sister, who also had nemaline rod myopathy, had some difficulty with intubation but no other problems. Both patients had less than 50 per cent of predicted vital capacity on pulmonary function testing. Muscle relaxants were specifically avoided in these patients.[229] Another case report described the use of muscle relaxants. Succinyl-

choline showed delayed onset and some resistance to effects but no change in serum potassium levels and no problems. Pancuronium—and then neostigmine—produced the expected responses.[230] Three children had open heart surgery, and all had an increase in temperature though no triggering agents were used and no cause was found.[231] One patient had cesarean section with vecuronium used for intubation, and no problems were associated with the anesthesia or muscle relaxant reversal, though they needed a 4 MacIntosh blade for intubation because of an unexpectedly deep larynx.[232]

D. CENTRONUCLEAR (MYOTUBULAR) MYOPATHY

Centronuclear myopathy shows bilateral facial paralysis with an elongated, thin face and a high-arched palate and internal strabismus—the Mobius syndrome. In addition, cranial nerve function is lost. Neonatal respiratory distress is frequent. Scoliosis and talipes equinovarus become evident with time and may require surgical correction. Weakness persists, and most patients are wheelchair bound by early adult life. Seizures occur in almost 20 per cent. The muscle fibers are round, small, type I fibers, with a clear area devoid of myofibrils around the centrally placed nuclei.[221] The trait is inherited in an autosomal-recessive manner. Other forms are distinguishable on the basis of sex-linked recessive genetics and clinical history. The sex-linked variety is associated with high rates of neonatal deaths and cardiac involvement.[221] Two anesthetic reports have recently appeared. The first describes a hypermetabolic state during open heart surgery associated with difficulty cooling the heart on bypass. No triggering agents were used, and the patient responded to small doses of dantrolene.[233] The second used a propofol–nitrous oxide technique with no problems for bilateral orchidopexy in a child.[234] There are no published results of in vitro halothane caffeine contracture tests in these patients.

E. FINGERPRINT BODY MYOPATHY

Fingerprint body myopathy is a slowly progressive proximal myopathy with atrophy and hypotonia present from birth. Half the patients have subnormal intelligence, and two patients had febrile seizures. Cranial nerve musculature is generally spared. The histologic appearance of small, dark-staining bodies in the subsarcolemmal area looks like fingerprints on electron microscopy.[221]

In each of the aforementioned diseases, the weakness is relatively nonprogressive, and the expected life span is close to normal; however, as in the reported case of nemaline myopathy, upper respiratory tract infection,[228] musculoskeletal abnormalities, and weakness make these patients poor risks. Any operation associated with splinting of the diaphragm or chest or decreased motion secondary to pain may lead to respiratory failure. Preoperative evaluation of respiratory function would be helpful. Because these patients have been shown by cineradiography to have abnormalities of swallowing, they must be watched carefully to prevent aspiration, even after normal recovery from anesthesia. Muscle relaxants may be necessary for these patients, as their weakness may be only slight. If relaxants are required, a nerve stimulator should be placed before they are used, to obtain a baseline. Following oxygenation, a small initial dose should be used (and unless specifically indicated, succinylcholine should be avoided). Additional doses should be based on the response to the test dose and should be given sparingly; however, because of the nonuniform degrees of weakness, the degree of relaxation in the muscles of the hand may not give an accurate picture of the relaxation in the abdominal or respiratory muscles.

XIV. INFLAMMATORY MYOPATHIES AND "OVERLAP" SYNDROMES[235]

The majority of patients with inflammatory myopathy of unknown cause have polymyositis or dermatomyositis. Polymyositis and dermatomyositis are not identical; muscle injury is mediated by humoral mechanisms in dermatomyositis and by a cell-mediated immune response in polymyositis.

A. DERMATOMYOSITIS

Dermatomyositis can be divided into childhood-onset (age 5 to 14 years) and adult-onset (typically 40 to 60 years) types. Dermatomyositis has an overall incidence of less than 1 in 100,000. Dermatomyositis rarely affects siblings or twins. In childhood dermatomyositis, proximal weakness is accompanied by malar or periorbital rash and erythematous skin lesions over extensor surfaces. Patients often walk on tiptoes secondary to ankle contractures. Nail bed telangiectasia and digital ulcers may occur. Subcutaneous or intramuscular calcification (calcinosis cutis) is observed in up to 50 per cent of children. Gastrointestinal vasculitis may result in bleeding or perforation, particularly with childhood-onset disease. Pulmonary fibrosis may occur in adults or children. Abnormal oropharyngeal peristalsis or upper esophageal sphincter function may cause weight loss or recurrent pulmonary aspiration. Childhood dermatomyositis usually responds well to steroids; occasionally rapid deterioration leads to respiratory failure and death.

B. ADULT DERMATOMYOSITIS AND POLYMYOSITIS

In adults the inflammatory myopathies dermatomyositis and polymyositis usually have an insidious onset. In dermatomyositis, rash is often observed prior to onset of clinical myopathy. Skin involvement is similar in adult and childhood dermatomyositis. Symmetric proximal weakness is often accompanied by muscle pain and tenderness of the arms or legs. Other striated muscles may be adversely affected, including (1) those of the oropharynx and upper esophagus (see above), (2) neck flexors, and (3) respiratory muscles. Raynaud's phenomenon is sometimes present. Arthritis is observed in 25 to 50 per cent of patients with polymyositis.

Cardiac involvement has been described. Atrial arrhythmias or conduction abnormalities have been noted. In one series of 76 patients, 18 had congestive heart failure and 5, pericarditis.[236] Cardiac involvement was not necessarily limited to patients with advanced skeletal myopathy.[237]

Pulmonary function tests usually show a restrictive pattern. This can be due to respiratory myopathy, recurrent aspiration, or interstitial disease (overall frequency about 10 per cent, varying from 5 to 47 per cent in different series). Pulmonary involvement may have variable onset and progression; patients with acute pulmonary symptoms appear to respond better to steroids. Interstitial disease usually affects the lung bases. In 67 patients with interstitial lung disease, 40 per cent mortality was observed over follow-up of 31 ± 32 months.[238] In polymyositis, an antihistidyl tRNA synthetase (anti Jo-1) antibody is a marker for interstitial lung disease.

Malignancy is associated with adult dermatomyositis in 6 to 45 per cent of patients. The incidence of malignancy in dermatomyositis is increased five- to seven-fold over that in the general population. It has been suggested that this increased incidence is due to more intensive workup for malignancy in patients with dermatomyositis. In women with dermatomyositis, ovarian cancer is more likely to be diagnosed at an advanced stage. In China, nasopharyngeal cancer is the tumor usually associated with dermatomyositis.

CK levels are elevated in dermatomyositis and polymyositis; in active disease, CK levels may be increased 50-fold above normal.[239] Clinical myoglobinuria is rarely observed.[240] During steroid therapy, CK levels decline before strength returns. EMG demonstrates abnormal insertional activity and abnormal motor unit potentials, with decreased amplitude and duration with polyphasia (myopathic pattern).

In dermatomyositis, deposition of immunoglobulin and complement (membrane attack complex [MAC]) injures capillary endothelium. Decreased capillary density and thrombosis result in ischemic injury to muscle fibers at the periphery of the fascicle. Muscle fiber necrosis occurs before invasion by macrophages. B cells and helper T (CD4+) cells form a perivascular infiltrate. Muscle biopsy in dermatomyositis shows perifascicular atrophy, regenerating muscle fibers, and increased fibrous tissue. Electron microscopy may show large, distorted endothelial cells with microtubular inclusions. In polymyositis, injury is probably cell mediated. Cytotoxic (CD8+) T lymphocytes and macrophages invade nonnecrotic muscle.

The mainstay of therapy is corticosteroids. Some 58 to 73 per cent of adults improve with therapy. If the response is good, CK levels normalize within 4 to 8 weeks. Antimetabolites (Imuran, methotrexate, or Cytoxan) and, alternatively, cyclosporine A have been added to steroids in steroid-resistant patients. In pooled trials, intravenous immune globulin (IVIG) has produced improvement in most patients (20 of 23 with dermatomyositis, 11 of 14 with polymyositis).[241] Plasmapheresis has not proved beneficial for steroid-resistant disease. Passive range-of-motion therapy and mild exercise may help prevent disuse atrophy and joint contractures. Patients with dysphagia and mild impairment of pharyngeal peristalsis may benefit from cricopharyngeal myotomy; patients with recurrent aspiration may benefit from gastrostomy tube placement.[242]

Responses to NDMRs have not been systematically investigated in polymyositis or dermatomyositis.[243, 244] While of theoretical concern, severe hyperkalemia or gross myoglobinuria has not been documented following succinylcholine in these patients. This probably reflects the rarity of these diseases; one cannot conclude that it is safe to give succinylcholine to patients with significant muscle necrosis. Patients should undergo preoperative evaluation for swallowing disorders and possible pulmonary or cardiac involvement.

C. OVERLAP SYNDROMES[235]

A subgroup of patients with connective tissue disease have signs and symptoms that overlap with polymyositis. Some 77 per cent of these patients have antinuclear antibodies. Patients with scleroderma usually have little or no CK elevation and normal EMG findings. A subgroup with scleroderma-myositis have elevated CK, myopathic EMG findings, and severe proximal weakness; antipolymyositis-scleroderma (Anti-PM-Scl) antibody (antinucleolar) serves as a marker for this in North American patients. Endothelial hyperplasia and decreased capillary density in muscle may be more severe than in dermatomyositis. In Sjøgren's syndrome, muscle biopsy often shows myositis and vasculitis, even without clinical myopathy. Polymyositis and dermatomyositis are infrequently associated with systemic lupus erythematosus (SLE); dysphagia and Raynaud's phenomenon are much more common in the combined conditions than in SLE alone. In rheumatoid arthritis, neuropathy or myositis is caused by vasculitis; corticosteroids, joint pain, myelopathy, and radiculopathy may contribute to disuse atrophy.

D. INCLUSION BODY MYOSITIS[245]

Inclusion body myositis differs from poly- or dermatomyositis by the additional presence of *distal* weakness (e.g., wrist flexors) and poor response to steroid therapy. On light microscopy, basophilic rimmed vacuoles are observed. Muscle biopsy shows nonnecrotic muscle fibers invaded by mononuclear cells. Electron microscopy characteristically shows 15- to 17-nm microtubular filamentous inclusions. Dysphagia has been observed. Familial occurrence has been noted.

E. VASCULITIDES[245]

Vasculitis has been noted in skeletal muscle in (1) polyarteritis nodosa, (2) Churg-Strauss eosinophilic vasculitis (usually with a history of asthma), (3) Wegener's granulomatosis, (4) hypersensitivity vasculitis, and (5) temporal (giant cell) arteritis. Pain and weakness in vasculitides is usually due to peripheral neuropathy, not muscle necrosis.

F. GRAFT-VERSUS-HOST DISEASE[245]

Inflammatory myopathy with features of polymyositis has been observed in chronic graft-versus-host disease (GVHD), as has myasthenia gravis. Inflammatory myopathy of GVHD usually responds to corticosteroids.

XV. INFECTIOUS DISEASES

High fever from a variety of bacterial or viral infections is sometimes associated with myoglobinuria.[158] The following sections review viral, parasitic, and bacterial pathogens specifically associated with skeletal muscle involvement.

A. MYOPATHY OF HUMAN IMMUNODEFICIENCY VIRUS TYPE 1

An inflammatory myopathy, often associated with nemaline rods, occurs in patients with HIV-1 infection. Patients may develop painless proximal weakness. HIV-1 infection sometimes presents with myopathy. Certain neurologic disorders may coexist with or resemble myopathy, including (1) chronic inflammatory demyelinating polyneuropathy, (2) cytomegalovirus polyradiculopathy, and

(3) subacute combined degeneration (vitamin B_{12} deficiency). Other causes of myopathy in patients with HIV-1 include zidovudine (AZT) or rifampin toxicity and mycobacterial or disseminated fungal infection. Dysphagia and respiratory muscle weakness are unusual in HIV-1 myopathy. CK levels are elevated in most patients. Muscle biopsy shows muscle fiber necrosis and macrophage invasion; about 50 per cent of patients demonstrate nemaline rods and loss of myosin filaments on electron microscopy. Large doses of prednisone often produce clinical improvement of HIV-1 myopathy, but the physician must assess the risk of additional immunosuppression. Direct HIV-1 invasion of skeletal muscle has not been documented.[245] Exaggerated sensitivity to muscle relaxants or succinylcholine-induced hyperkalemia related to HIV-1 inflammatory myopathy has not been reported.

Zidovudine myotoxicity may occur with long-term therapy; myalgia usually accompanies weakness. Toxicity is dose related. RRF may be demonstrated by Gomori-trichrome stain of muscle biopsy specimens. RRF suggests mitochondrial myopathy. Zidovudine inhibits DNA γ-polymerase, which is essential for mitochondrial DNA replication. Decreasing or discontinuing zidovudine may result in improved strength; myalgia resolves rapidly after discontinuation.[246]

B. INFLUENZA VIRUS AND OTHER VIRUSES[247]

Most patients with acute influenza A or B infection describe myalgia. In the literature, 16 adults have been described with acute myositis during influenza infection; 13 of the 16 had myoglobinuria, and 10 developed renal failure. Four of the 16 died of cardiopulmonary complications. Other viruses implicated in adult acute myositis with myoglobinuria include Epstein-Barr virus, echovirus, parainfluenza virus, cytomegalovirus (CMV), HIV-1, and herpes simplex virus. *Benign acute childhood myositis* has been described in more than 100 children with influenza (most with influenza B). As prodromal symptoms recede, myositis presents with severe bilateral calf pain and tenderness (*myalgia cruris epidemica*). Other viruses have been associated with benign acute childhood myositis, including adenovirus, herpes simplex, parainfluenza, and respiratory syncytial virus. Only three children developed myoglobinuria; one of them had CPT deficiency. Myalgia usually resolves within a week. Antiviral agents have not been evaluated for treatment of acute myositis. Patients with X-linked recessive hypogammaglobulinemia may develop persistent echovirus infection with chronic meningoencephalitis and associated dermatomyositis-like syndrome ([DLS], 21 reported cases). Steroids are ineffective in treating DLS.

C. HELMINTHIC INFECTIONS: TRICHINOSIS AND ECHINOCOCCOSIS[245]

Trichinosis should be suspected whenever a patient presents with eosinophilia and inflammatory myopathy of 3 months' duration or less. Trichinosis is caused by the nematode *Trichinella spiralis*. Undercooked infected meat (usually pork) harbors larvae, which are released in the gut. Diarrhea and fever are common during the enteric phase of infection. Larvae enter the blood stream and migrate into blood vessels of skeletal muscle, provoking intense inflammation. Muscle pain, tenderness, and weakness begin during the first week after ingestion. Eosinophilia (5 to 90 per cent) is seen by the second week of illness. *Myocardial involvement may cause severe or fatal congestive heart failure.* Brain infestation may cause encephalitis. CK levels are elevated. Muscle biopsy usually demonstrates *Trichinella* larvae. Serologic tests (ELISA or bentonite flocculation) may be useful for diagnostic confirmation after several weeks. Prednisone improves myopathic symptoms even without specific anti-*Trichinella* treatment with albendazole. Brackmann and colleagues reported on a patient with florid trichinosis who had swelling of the tongue, floor of the mouth, and cheeks.[248]

In sheep-raising areas, larvae of the cestode *Echinococcus granulosus* may be ingested, and when they are they migrate to liver, lung, brain, or muscle. These larvae then produce cysts, which enlarge over months to years. In endemic areas, echinococcal cysts are the most common cause of mass lesions in muscle. *Anaphylaxis has been reported with cyst rupture during attempted excision.*[249]

D. BACTERIAL INFECTIONS[245, 250]

Exaggerated hyperkalemic response to succinylcholine has been reported in patients with severe intra-abdominal infections lasting more than 1 week.[251, 252] It is unclear whether the cause of hyperkalemia is exaggerated release from the liver and/or gut or skeletal muscle in this group of patients.[253] Khan and Khan reported that patients with severe osteomyelitis or gangrene had greater increases in serum potassium than controls (mean increase 1.5 mEq/L) following succinylcholine. Hyperkalemia correlated with duration of preoperative bed rest and duration (1 to 3 weeks) and severity of infection.[254] The following section discusses specific pathogens that often cause skeletal muscle injury or necrotizing fasciitis.

Clostridium perfringens and *Clostridium septicum* can cause gas gangrene after wound infection or colonic perforation. Most patients with gas gangrene have an underlying malignancy or peripheral vascular disease or are immunosuppressed; mortality is lower among previously healthy trauma patients. Involved muscle does not contract, and interfascical gas may be observed. Fulminant systemic toxicity with hemolysis or myoglobinuric renal failure may occur. Treatment usually consists of prompt surgical débridement. Infections often involve multiple enteric pathogens in addition to *Clostridium* species (e.g., *Bacteroides fragilis*, *Escherichia coli*, *Streptococcus faecalis*); broad-spectrum antibiotic coverage is recommended. Hyperbaric oxygen therapy may be beneficial.[255] *Clostridium tetani* may infect wounds and cause tetanus in unimmunized persons. Tetanus toxin is not inherently myotoxic, but violent muscle spasms invariably elevate CK levels. Succinylcholine-induced hyperkalemia was reported in three patients approximately 3 weeks after onset of severe tetanus.[256]

Vibrio vulnificus is a halophilic organism that can cause life-threatening sepsis and myonecrosis in two settings: (1) ingestion of raw oysters by persons with hepatic cirrhosis or immunosuppression (e.g., transplant recipients) or gastric achlorhydria, (2) wound infection with contaminated sea water. Persons in at-risk groups who eat raw oysters can become septicemic; disseminated intravascular coagulation (DIC), myonecrosis, and necrotizing fasciitis may ensue (expected mortality 50 per cent). Wounds infected by sea water may exhibit cellulitis, subsequent formation of bullae, and myonecrosis. Treatment requires surgical débridement and therapy with tetracycline and gentamicin.

Streptococcal myonecrosis is uncommon; it

presents with local muscle pain and swelling. Bullae, necrotizing fasciitis, and muscle necrosis may rapidly progress to fulminant septic shock with DIC. Prompt, aggressive surgical débridement is required. Fatalities have been noted even among previously healthy persons.[258] Anaerobic streptococci may infect muscle and overlying fascia; painless erythema and gas in muscle and fascia are observed. In contrast to *C. perfringens* infection, muscle remains contractile.

Staphylococcal toxic shock syndrome has been associated with elevated CK and myoglobinuria.[259] Toxic shock syndrome is rarely observed postoperatively; patients may present with fever and an erythematous truncal rash that often desquamates.[260] Staphylococcal pyomyositis presents as a firm, nonfluctuant mass in one or more muscles; patients complain of severe pain and tenderness. Surgical drainage may be required if antibiotic therapy is delayed.

Patients with leptospirosis often present with severe pain and tenderness of the thigh and paraspinous muscles. Aseptic meningitis is common. Hepatic and renal failure may develop in severe cases. CK levels are elevated in most patients, and rhabdomyolysis may occur.

Legionnaire's disease may cause proximal weakness, elevated CK levels (prevalence 78 per cent), or acute renal failure. Patients typically present with pneumonia. *Legionella* organisms may contaminate water used to humidify breathing systems.

In immunosuppressed patients with systemic fungal infection, skeletal muscle filters organisms from the blood stream. Asymptomatic granulomas or muscle tenderness may be observed. Muscle biopsy may be used to diagnose systemic candidiasis.

XVI. MYOPATHY DUE TO DRUGS OR TOXINS[261]

Recognition of drug- or toxin-associated muscle injury is important because muscle pain, weakness, or myoglobinuria often resolves when the drug is discontinued or the toxin removed. Toxins may produce muscle injury in several ways: by (1) direct toxicity; (2) electrolyte abnormality; (3) neural activation with excessive muscle activity; (4) ischemia; and (5) immune-mediated mechanisms. In most cases of toxic myopathy, the exact mechanism of injury is not known. Necrotiz-

ing myopathy is the most frequent syndrome, characterized by the development of muscle pain, tenderness, and weakness. CK levels are usually significantly increased. Drug- or alcohol-associated myoglobinuria accounts for more than 8 per cent of acute renal failure. Nonsteroidal antiinflammatory drugs should be avoided by patients with deteriorating renal function. Although specific sensitivity to muscle relaxants or succinylcholine-induced hyperkalemia has not been reported in most drug-induced myopathies, it may be prudent to avoid succinylcholine when motor neuropathy or significant rhabdomyolysis (e.g., CK value greater than 1000 IU/L) has been present for more than a week. Individual response to non-depolarizing muscle relaxants should be assessed carefully with the aid of peripheral nerve stimulation. For a discussion of toxic muscle effects of glucocorticoids see Section VB, on ICU Myopathy.

A. NECROTIZING MYOPATHY AND ANTIHYPERLIPIDEMIA DRUGS

Necrotizing myopathy has been associated with HMG-CoA reductase inhibitors (antihyperlipidemia drugs), fibric acid derivatives, and nicotinic acid. It is infrequent, but recognition is important since life-threatening rhabdomyolysis can be avoided by discontinuing the drug. The HMG-CoA reductase inhibitors include lovastatin (Mevacor), simvastatin (Zocor), and pravastatin (Pravachol); they inhibit cholesterol synthesis and reduce plasma low-density lipoprotein [LDL] cholesterol. Myalgia or moderate CK elevation often occurs transiently during initiation of therapy. Concurrent administration of lovastatin and certain other drugs has been associated with increased risk of severe myotoxicity. Four of 80 patients taking lovastatin with gemfibrozil (Lopid) developed severe toxic myopathy.[262] Administration of lovastatin with cyclosporine has been associated with rhabdomyolysis in heart transplant recipients.[263] Cyclosporine, HMG-CoA inhibitors, and the antifungal agents ketoconazole and itraconazole compete for metabolism by cytochrome P-450; concurrent administration may increase serum concentrations of cyclosporine and the HMG-CoA inhibitor.[264, 265] Recently, Kobashigawa and associates have shown that the combined use of small doses of pravastatin (maximum 20 mg per day) and cyclo-sporine reduced the incidence of acute severe rejection and coronary vasculopathy and improved 1-year survival in heart transplant recipients;[266] this combination has been associated with a low incidence of rhabdomyolysis.

Patients with chronic renal failure are at increased risk of toxic myopathy associated with fibric acid derivatives (clofibrate, gemfibrozil, bezafibrate, fenfibrate). Nicotinic acid (niacin) has been associated with myalgia and elevated CK levels in three patients; symptoms resolved rapidly after discontinuing nicotinic acid.[261]

B. ε-AMINOCAPROIC ACID (AMICAR) MYOPATHY[267]

The antifibrinolytic ε-aminocaproic acid (EACA) is rarely associated with myonecrosis and myoglobinura. *All cases have occurred after treatment for more than 4 weeks.* Symptoms include tenderness and weakness. Muscle biopsy usually does not show intravascular coagulation.

C. ORGANOPHOSPHATE POISONING

Organophosphate insecticide poisoning results in irreversible inhibition of acetylcholinesterase. Excess acetylcholine at the neuromuscular junction produces excessive muscle stimulation and muscle fiber necrosis. Tonic-clonic convulsions may contribute to muscle injury. An *intermediate syndrome* with proximal myopathy (especially neck flexors) and *weakness of respiratory muscles* or those innervated by cranial nerves may follow recovery from acute organophosphate poisoning.[268] Concomitant inhibition of pseudocholinesterase prolongs succinylcholine-induced neuromuscular block.[269]

D. ENVENOMATION: SNAKE, SPIDER, AND WASP VENOMS[158]

The venom of a number of crotaline (e.g., rattlesnake) and elapid (e.g., seasnake) snakes are potent myotoxins. Components of venom that are myotoxic include the single-chain peptides crotamine and myotoxin a and the A2 phospholipases. A2 phospholipases show high specificity for skeletal muscle. One may observe widespread muscle necrosis and myoglobinuria. Elapid venom is neurotoxic; death is caused by respiratory paralysis. Crotalid venom often produces hemolysis. Use of antivenin may be life saving.[270] The venoms of the Arkansas and Honduran tarantulas are intensely myotoxic and cardiotoxic. Brown spider bites have been associated with rhabdomyolysis. Black widow spider venom depletes presynaptic acetylcholine, resulting in permanent neuromuscular block.[271] There are reports of rhabdomyolysis and acute renal failure following multiple wasp or hornet stings.

E. HYPOKALEMIC MYOPATHY[261]

Severe hypokalemia (less than 2.5 mEq/L) may result in muscle weakness and severe muscle injury. Drugs or toxins associated with hypokalemia include: diuretics, laxatives, amphotericin B, aminophylline, excess mineralocorticoids, lithium, glycyrrhizic acid (in licorice), and toluene (produces renal tubular acidosis). Hypokalemia has been associated with acute alcoholic myopathy and with management of diabetic ketoacidosis. Hypokalemia is associated with three different myopathic syndromes: (1) flaccid proximal weakness, with preserved sensation and tendon reflexes and increased CK levels; (2) areflexic periodic paralysis; and (3) rarely, severe myonecrosis and myoglobinuria. Hypokalemia prevents the usual increase in skeletal muscle blood flow seen with exercise. Acute renal failure is rare in hypokalemic myopathy; it is postulated that associated metabolic alkalosis is protective. Muscle biopsy typically shows vacuoles derived from T tubules in scattered muscle fibers. Hypokalemic myopathy is easily treated with potassium repletion.

F. LABETALOL MYOPATHY

There are two case reports of patients with either weakness or myalgia and CK elevation associated with oral labetalol; symptoms resolved when labetalol was discontinued.

G. DRUG-INDUCED LYSOSOMAL STORAGE MYOPATHY

Amphiphilic drugs contain a hydrophobic region and an amine group that can interact with membrane acidic phospholipids. The drug-lipid complexes are resistant to lysosomal digestion and result in the formation of myeloid bodies, which appear as cytoplasmic vacuoles on light microscopy. Myeloid induction causes a generalized lysosomal storage disorder; peripheral neuropathy is often more prominent than myopathy. Amphiphilic drugs associated with myopathy include chloroquine and hydroxychloroquine, quinacrine, and amiodarone.

Chloroquine and hydroxychloroquine are well-known antimalarial agents. They have also been used to treat connective tissue diseases, sarcoidosis, and amebiasis. Side effects include corneal and macular degeneration, peripheral neuropathy, and myopathy. Muscle weakness is associated with daily dosing of 500 mg for 1 year or longer; current use of smaller doses has made chloroquine myopathy rare. One may observe cardiomyopathy; conduction abnormalities (fascicular to complete atrioventricular block) are observed more frequently than congestive failure or restrictive cardiomyopathy.[272] Skeletal muscle weakness resolves slowly after chloroquine is discontinued.

Amiodarone is associated with tremor, ataxia, and peripheral neuropathy. Peripheral neuropathy is a well-documented side effect; myopathy is rare. Amiodarone-induced hypothyroidism can be associated with proximal weakness (see Hypothyroidism).

H. EMETINE INTOXICATION

Emetine has been used as an amebicide and emetic agent (syrup of ipecac) for decades. Cardiotoxicity and muscle pain, stiffness, and weakness are well-known side effects of prolonged administration. Possible toxicity should be anticipated if the cumulative dose exceeds 500 to 600 mg over 10 days. Muscle biopsy shows atrophy and disruption of sarcomeres. Anorexics who abuse syrup of ipecac may develop emetine cardiotoxicity and myopathy; skin changes similar to those of dermatomyositis may confound diagnosis.

I. ANTIMICROTUBULAR MYOPATHY

Colchicine and vincristine disrupt microtubules, resulting in accumulation of autophagic vacuoles in muscle cells and clinical myopathy. Colchicine neuromyopathy most frequently develops in patients with gout and mild renal insufficiency. Renal impairment results in elevated colchicine levels. Proximal weakness coexists with distal sensory neuropathy. Myopathy usually resolves within 6 weeks of stopping colchicine. Vincristine-associated weakness is usually secondary to peripheral neuropathy; direct muscle toxicity is rare.

J. HYPERVITAMINOSIS E

Proximal myopathy with elevated CK levels has been observed with vitamin E toxicity. Muscle biopsies have shown necrotizing myopathy.

K. TOXIN-INDUCED INFLAMMATORY MYOPATHY

D-Penicillamine is used to treat rheumatoid arthritis, scleroderma, Wilson's disease, and cystinuria. Immune-mediated myositis has been observed in a small number of patients. Heart block has been reported in three patients with D-penicillamine–induced polymyositis.[273] Recovery occurs after withdrawal of D-penicillamine. Other adverse neuromuscular effects of D-penicillamine include reversible myasthenia gravis and one case report of fasciculations, which resolved when D-penicillamine was discontinued.[124]

Eosinophilia-myalgia syndrome (EMS) was associated with the ingestion of L-tryptophan manufactured by a single manufacturer before 1990. The L-tryptophan contained a contaminant synthesized from tryptophan and acetaldehyde. Patients with EMS presented with intense myalgias, skin changes, and marked blood eosinophilia. Patients frequently had cough, dyspnea, or dysphagia. Some patients presented with distal sensorimotor polyneuropathy. EMG was consistent with myopathy or denervation. Muscle biopsy usually showed eosinophilic inflammation, mainly in perimysium and fascia, with selective involvement of intramuscular nerves and muscle spindles. Prolonged latency from tryptophan ingestion to onset of symptoms and persistence of symptoms despite drug discontinuation were noted in some patients. Treatment consisted of large doses of glucocorticoids.[274] Patients with dysphagia may be at increased risk for aspiration. Succinylcholine should be avoided by patients with significant motor neuropathy. Other drugs occasionally associated with polymyositis include procainamide, phenytoin (Dilantin), cimetidine, propylthiouracil, and leuprolide (Lupron).[261]

L. SUBSTANCE ABUSE MYOPATHY

Intoxication with cocaine, amphetamines, phencyclidine ("PCP"), or heroin has been associated with rhabdomyolysis and myoglobinuric renal failure. Roth and coworkers reported on 39 patients with acute myoglobinuria after cocaine use; thirteen developed acute renal failure. The group who developed renal failure were characterized by greater incidence of hypotension and hyperthermia on admission and higher mean CK level (above 28,000). Seven of the 13 with renal failure had DIC; six of these patients died. Thirty-five of 39 were described as *combative* or *agitated;* four were comatose, but none had prolonged coma or status epilepticus.[275] The combination of hyperthermia, excessive muscle exertion (agitation, seizures, muscle rigidity), and toxic additives may contribute to rhabdomyolysis associated with cocaine, amphetamines, or phencyclidine. Muscle ischemia from vasoconstriction may be significant. Increased CK levels have been observed in unhospitalized crack cocaine abusers.[276]

Heroin abuse most often causes myoglobinuria in subjects who lose consciousness; sustained pressure causes ischemia of skeletal muscle. Rhabdomyolysis rarely occurs without loss of consciousness after self-injection of heroin-additive mixtures.

M. ALCOHOL-ASSOCIATED MYOPATHIES[261]

The most common cause of muscle weakness and wasting in an alcoholic is peripheral neuropathy. Other muscle syndromes associated with alcohol abuse include: (1) rhabdomyolysis associated with acute intoxication or withdrawal seizures, (2) acute hypokalemic myopathy, and (3) chronic myopathy. Acute rhabdomyolysis (necrotizing myopathy) usually occurs during acute intoxication in a chronic alcoholic; it sometimes occurs during withdrawal. Coma-associated "crush syndrome," fasting, or hypophosphatemia may contribute to alcohol myotoxicity. Severe muscle cramps, pain, and swelling are characteristic. Calf swelling and tenderness may mimic thrombophlebitis. Initial CK levels may be normal or significantly increased. It may take several days to reach peak CK levels, which decrease over approximately a week. Some cases are complicated by myoglobinuric renal failure. Recovery of muscle strength usually occurs within 2 weeks; weakness may occasionally persist for several months despite abstinence. Subjects with a history of acute alcoholic myopathy are prone to recurrent muscle injury on resumption of drinking. Elevated serum CK and serum and urine myoglobin values may be observed after acute intoxication not accompanied by myalgia or weakness. Anesthetic care of the alcoholic patient should include assessment of aspiration risk, metabolic derangement (e.g., measure serum glucose, potassium, magnesium, phosphate, bicarbonate), hepatic function, cardiac function, and evaluation of abnormal mental status.

Acute hypokalemic myopathy in alcoholics is distinguished from acute *alcoholic* myopathy by the absence of muscle cramps, pain, tenderness, and swelling. Proximal weakness may develop rapidly; CK levels are usually markedly increased. Potassium administration usually results in improved strength within a week. Severe hypokalemia occurs frequently during symptomatic alcohol withdrawal; losses from vomiting or diarrhea are most likely responsible.

Controversy exists about the contention that chronic alcoholic myopathy is independent of peripheral neuropathy. Most histologic changes considered characteristic of chronic alcoholic myopathy are equally characteristic of chronically denervated muscle. Most patients deemed to have chronic alcoholic myopathy also have peripheral neuropathy.

XVII. MYOGLOBINURIA[158, 277]

Myoglobin is a 17.5-kd protein found in skeletal muscle at a concentration of 4 mg/g.

The "normal" serum myoglobin concentration is about 20 ng/mL. The threshold serum concentration for renal excretion is 300 ng/mL. If the urine is grossly discolored (i.e., cola colored), the urine myoglobin concentration exceeds 250 µg/mL. Dipstick evaluation is positive for blood if the myoglobin concentration exceeds 500 ng/mL. This can be distinguished from hematuria by the absence of red cells on microscopic examination. Hemoglobinemia may produce pink serum; myoglobinemia is associated with clear serum. Immunochemical assays for myoglobin do not cross-react with hemoglobin.

Children and adults who are *not* susceptible to MH may have 10- to 100-fold increases in serum myoglobin following succinylcholine; repeated or intermittent administration is associated with more prominent increases in serum myoglobin.[278, 279] Children tend to have greater increases in serum myoglobin than adults following succinylcholine.[280] Administration of barbiturate, ketamine, or curare-like drugs before succinylcholine results in a less dramatic increase of serum myoglobin or CK than is seen after induction of anesthesia with halothane.[281, 282] Increases in serum myoglobin occur earlier after muscle injury than increases in CK. Peak levels of serum CK may not be observed until 12 to 24 hours after muscle injury. Life-threatening succinylcholine-induced hyperkalemia has been reported in children with undiagnosed myopathy; most of these children are boys younger than 11 years who have Duchenne's or Becker's muscular dystrophy. Gronert and Rosenberg estimate that unanticipated succinylcholine-induced hyperkalemia occurs in six children each year (one per 1 million pediatric anesthetics), with more than 50 per cent mortality.[283] Succinylcholine-induced hyperkalemia is also seen in conditions with upregulation of skeletal muscle acetylcholine receptors; this may occur several days after muscle denervation, burns, or massive soft tissue trauma.[284]

Rhabdomyolytic *crush syndrome* may be secondary to trauma (e.g., surviving trapped in a building collapsed by earthquake or explosion).[285] Trauma is often accompanied by hypovolemia and acidosis; the injured muscle sequesters a large volume of extracellular fluid following reperfusion, further aggravating hypovolemia. Compartment syndromes from bleeding or edema may exacerbate muscle and nerve ischemia. The combination of myoglobinuria, hypovolemia, acidosis, and hyperuricemia increases the risk of acute renal failure. Early, vigorous fluid resuscitation reduces the incidence of acute renal failure. Mannitol is recommended both for its osmotic diuretic effect and its ability to scavenge hydroxyl radicals produced after reperfusion of ischemic muscle.[286] Alkalinization is recommended to reduce precipitation of myoglobin acid hematin in renal tubules. Calcium deposition in injured muscle is associated with hypocalcemia. Hyperkalemia may develop from release of potassium from damaged muscle (100 mEq/kg). The combination of hyperkalemia and hypocalcemia may result in life-threatening arrhythmias; calcium administration is recommended only when arrhythmias are present. DIC may complicate rhabdomyolysis, regardless of its cause. Persistent disability is more often due to peripheral nerve injury than to rhabdomyolysis.

Most cases of myoglobinuria are associated with coma (pressure-induced muscle ischemia)[287] or exertion. Other factors associated with myoglobinuria include (1) membrane injury from drugs, toxins, or underlying myopathy (e.g., Becker's or Duchenne's muscular dystrophy), (2) ischemia or hypoxia, (3) metabolic defects causing abnormal utilization of glucose or fatty acids, and (4) elevated core (± ambient) temperature.

A specific enzyme abnormality is found in approximately 50 per cent of adults with recurrent exertional myoglobinuria.[158, 277] The incidence of exertional myoglobinuria is higher in males. CPT deficiency is the most frequently demonstrated enzyme defect in adults and children with recurrent myoglobinuria. CPT is essential for transport of long-chain fatty acyl-CoA from the cytosol into the mitochondrial matrix. Attacks of myoglobinuria may follow sustained, moderate exercise, fasting, fever, or emotional stress. The CK level is usually normal between attacks. Phosphorylase (PPL) deficiency (McArdle's disease) is associated with myoglobinuria; PPL activity is necessary for glycogenolysis. Myoglobinuria may follow brief, intense muscle exertion; exercise intolerance without myoglobinuria is also noted in PPL deficiency. CK level is often moderately elevated between attacks. Other glycolytic defects associated with myoglobinuria include (1) PPL b kinase deficiency, (2) phosphofructokinase (PFK) deficiency, (3) phosphoglycerate kinase (PGK) deficiency, (4) phosphoglycerate mutase (PGAM) deficiency, and (5) muscle LDH deficiency. Disorders of mitochondrial function associated with myoglobinuria include (1) CPT deficiency, (2) disorders of fatty acid oxidation, (3) tricarboxylic acid (Krebs) cycle enzyme defects (e.g., succinate dehydrogenase), and (4) respiratory chain disorders. Primary carnitine deficiency and myoadenylate (AMP) deaminase deficiency (MADD) are infrequently associated with myoglobinuria. Metabolic defects associated with myoglobinuria are characterized by autosomal-recessive inheritance; an exception is X-linked PGK deficiency. Muscle biopsy may demonstrate glycolytic defects, CPT deficiency, or RRF associated with mitochondrial disorders. Poels and colleagues performed in vitro contracture testing on six patients with unexplained recurrent myoglobinuria; five were MH susceptible. Only one of these patients had a history of anesthetic-associated myoglobinuria.[288]

Exertional heat stroke (EHS) is a common cause of rhabdomyolysis. Risk factors include lack of physical training and high ambient temperature and humidity. Mechanisms of acclimatization to heat include vasodilatation, enhanced heat loss with sweating, and sodium conservation. Physical training reduces, but does not eliminate, the risk of exertional heat stroke.[289] Persons with sickle cell trait may be at increased risk for EHS.[290] Figarella-Branger and colleagues performed contracture testing on 45 subjects with a history of EHS. Eleven were susceptible to MH; eight had equivocal results (susceptible to caffeine or halothane, but not both); twenty-six were MH negative. Muscle histology was normal in 10 of the 11 MH-susceptible subjects.[291] Heat stroke is relatively common and usually not familial; MH is rare and often is inherited. Studies have not demonstrated superior outcome with dantrolene therapy for heat stroke; one study demonstrated more rapid cooling in patients receiving dantrolene plus surface evaporative cooling.[292] Frequent MH susceptibility on contracture testing of subjects with previous EHS is an intriguing finding and usually is not associated with a family history of anesthetic-triggered MH.

One may observe nonexertional heat stroke in elderly persons exposed to high ambient temperatures. Significant contributing factors may include the use of medications that impair thermoregulation (e.g., phenothiazines or drugs with anticholinergic effects). Other conditions associated with hyperthermia and rhabdomyolysis include (1) uncontrolled exertion (e.g., seizures, agitation against restraints,[293] tetanus), (2) neuroleptic malignant syndrome,[294] (3) serotonin syndrome,[295] and (4) MH. Interestingly, myoglobinuria has been seen following frostbite; this probably represents a reperfusion injury.

Rhabdomyolysis has been reported following prolonged positioning—prone kneeling (knee-chest) and prone,[296] lateral decubitus, lithotomy and exaggerated lithotomy[297]—for surgery. Pressure-induced ischemia is most likely responsible for skin and muscle necrosis. Peripheral nerve injury may coexist with rhabdomyolysis.

XVIII. MALIGNANT HYPERTHERMIA AND DRUG-INDUCED TRISMUS

MH typically is a fulminant, life-threatening disease, also referred to as a *syndrome,* which occurs when a person with malignant hyperthermia susceptibility (MHS) trait is exposed to triggering factors, which include halogenated inhalational anesthetics, succinylcholine, and, rarely, stress. Classic MH is characterized by hypermetabolism, muscle rigidity, muscle injury, and increased sympathetic nervous system activity. Hypermetabolism, reflected by elevated carbon dioxide production, precedes the increase in body temperature. *Drug-induced trismus* is rigidity of the jaw muscles triggered by succinylcholine (with or without halogenated inhalational anesthetics), occurring as a separate self-limiting phenomenon or as part of MH. Human MHS is a pharmacogenic disorder.[221] An inherited autosomal-dominant gene probably accounts for 50 per cent of the cases. Codominance, incomplete expressivity or penetrance, recessive gene, or bi- or multifactorial inheritance accounts for the incomplete heritability.

Each case of MHS carries serious socioeconomic implications. The seriousness of the problem is underscored by two factors: (1) the mortality of MH is extremely high unless the patient is properly managed and (2) the incidence of MH is not insignificant. Since its recognition as a disease entity by Denborough and Lovell,[298] the mortality rate for MH has decreased from nearly 80 per cent to less than 10 per cent in 35 years. Obviously, the incidence and mortality rates depend on the criteria for diagnosis (i.e., was MH the correct diagnosis, or was a different life-threatening disorder—e.g., septic shock or hemolytic transfusion reaction—overlooked?). The prevalence of MHS trait cannot be precisely stated. It has been estimated to affect 1 of 10,000 to 100,000 in the patient population—toward 1 in 10,000 when the estimation was based on pediatric anesthesia experience and 1 in 50,000 when based on an adult population.[299, 300] It is much more prevalent in certain geographic areas, such as Wisconsin, where a few large, susceptible families reside. The decreasing incidence of MH and of clinical expression of MHS with age does not mean that MHS persons outgrow the trait. The statistics are influenced partly by the high prevalence of succinylcholine-induced trismus in children, which has been estimated to be as high as 1 per cent following a halothane and succinylcholine combination (see Drug-Induced Trismus).

A. CLINICAL FEATURES OF MALIGNANT HYPERTHERMIA

Practically every aspect of MH entails variations and controversies. This necessitates that the physician be familiar with the "typical fulminant case." Typically, the patient is a child or young adult. History and physical examination findings are usually normal. The patient may have a relatively benign musculoskeletal abnormality such as strabismus, kyphoscoliosis, hernia, hyperextensible joints, frequent cramps, or similar disorders. The incidence of these benign musculoskeletal conditions is probably similar in MH–susceptible persons and in the general population.[301] Patients with known anesthesia problems in the family may be very apprehensive, but most give a negative family history or only some vague difficulties with general anesthesia long ago. Preoperative laboratory reports are usually normal, except for the serum CK level, which may be elevated. In one version, the patient receives succinylcholine for intubation of the trachea following thiopental or halothane induction, or both, and immediately goes into rigid and hypermetabolic crisis with exaggerated fasciculation and trismus. In another version, succinylcholine is not used; generalized rigidity and hypermetabolic crisis follow halothane induction and are recognized early during surgery. In yet another version, the patient has some degree of trismus following succinylcholine administration. The anesthetist manages to intubate the trachea in spite of the trismus. Rigidity

and hypermetabolic crisis develop later. In the latter versions, tachycardia, hypertension, cardiac arrhythmia, resumed or enhanced breathing activity of the patient, and tight abdomen may be erroneously attributed to atropine or light anesthesia, or both. The anesthetist might have increased the halothane concentration before recognizing that halothane should be discontinued. Subsequently, it is noted that the patient is hot and that his or her color "does not look right." From this point on, the patient's condition deteriorates rapidly. Even with proper treatment, an advanced case of MH is frequently fatal. The most frequent causes of death are severe hyperkalemia, cardiac arrhythmia, cardiovascular collapse, hypoxia, cerebral edema, and DIC.[302]

From a clinical point of view, hypermetabolism of skeletal muscle is the key feature. The severity of each clinical sign depends on the degree of susceptibility, the triggering agent, and the stage of the crisis. During the crisis, the skeletal muscle feels hot and rigid. The chest may become so rigid that ventilation becomes difficult; however, *absence of rigidity does* not *preclude the diagnosis of MH.* Severe muscle injury and hypermetabolism can occur in the absence of muscle rigidity. An increase of core temperature 1°C every 5 minutes, or to 44°C in 1 to 2 hours, may be observed. Fever up to 46°C has been observed. Sweating is common; however, early or mild forms of MH may be afebrile. Because hypermetabolism is the main pathophysiologic feature, excessive thermogenesis and venous desaturation occur early. Arterial hypoxemia follows later, when severe venous blood desaturation, shunting, and cardiac decompensation ensue. Tachycardia, hypertension, and increased cardiac output are early compensatory reactions to excessive thermogenesis, oxygen consumption, and hypercarbia. Cardiac arrhythmia may follow later because of hyperkalemia, acidosis, and hyperthermia, but it may also occur early because of involvement of the cardiac muscle in the primary defect.[303] Ventricular premature beats, bigeminy, ventricular tachycardia, and fibrillation are common.

Carbon dioxide production parallels or exceeds oxygen consumption secondary to increased aerobic metabolism and bicarbonate buffering of elevated lactic acid levels. Metabolic rate may increase to 500 per cent of baseline;[304] surprisingly, this is far less than the more than 10-fold increase in metabolic rate associated with maximal aerobic exercise in untrained persons. In a severe case, the $PaCO_2$ value may increase severalfold, in spite of hyperventilation. The breathing circuit and the soda lime canister may become very hot, and the carbon dioxide absorbent is soon exhausted. Both conditions lead to further carbon dioxide and heat retention. Acidosis is both respiratory and metabolic and may reach moribund values.

Cyanosis, mottling of skin, and hypotension are late signs. With consumption coagulopathy (DIC), the injection and incision sites may ooze blood. Serum catecholamine levels are increased. Laboratory findings include myoglobinemia, myoglobinuria, and hemoconcentration. Serum CK and other muscle enzyme levels may increase thousandsfold. Severe hyperkalemia, hypocalcemia, and increased serum inorganic phosphate levels are common, but serum potassium and calcium concentrations typically fluctuate widely as the crisis progresses.

If the patient survives the acute fulminant episode, delayed sequelae may soon follow. The patient may awake from anesthesia slowly or may suffer permanent brain damage. Recurrent attacks of MH may happen up to 24 to 48 hours later. Fluctuating potassium and calcium concentrations may lead to recurrent cardiac arrhythmias. Acute renal failure may ensue. In addition DIC, thrombocytopenia, cerebral edema, pulmonary edema, myocardial infarction, and cerebral vascular accidents can also occur. Hyperglycemia and markedly increased blood concentration of catecholamines may be observed. Coma may be due to hypoxia, extreme hypercarbia, ischemia, or extreme hyperthermia.[305] Surviving patients may feel severe muscle aching and weakness for days or weeks and may notice muscle swelling followed by necrosis and wasting. Respiratory muscle failure from dantrolene therapy is rare; therapy with dantrolene may add to muscle weakness (see Section on Dantrolene).

Variations of this course are observed. Patients may present with an alarming family history of anesthetic mishaps. Babies (including one in the delivery room[306]) and patients as old as 78 years have had MH,[299] although the incidence is highest in the first three decades of life. Isolated rigidity of the jaw muscles, resulting in trismus and difficult intubation of the trachea, may be the only overt manifestation of MH or of muscle diseases related or unrelated to MHS (see Section on Drug-Induced Trismus). Patients with tachycardia resulting from anxiety or atropine premedication may not show a conspicuous increase in heart rate; a well-conditioned athlete may display hypermetabolism with an increase in heart rate to less than 100 bpm (only relative tachycardia). Postoperative CK elevation and myoglobinuria may be the only signs of MH or other mild forms of muscle disease. Clinical expression of susceptibility varies.[307] A patient may have an episode of MH despite a history of uneventful general anesthetics, even ones that included triggering agents.

B. PATHOGENESIS OF MALIGNANT HYPERTHERMIA

Figure 10–4 is a simplified scheme of muscle responses to the action potential of its cell membrane sarcolemma. Normally, the sarcolemma, the SR, and the mitochondria actively sequester and store calcium away from the sarcoplasma, to maintain the muscle in the resting state. A calcium concentration gradient of 10,000 times is maintained between the serum and the sarcoplasm.[308] When these biologic membranes are activated, free calcium is released into the sarcoplasm, especially from the SR, in processes of calcium-induced calcium release and depolarization-induced calcium release. Muscle contraction and intracellular catabolic processes ensue. Return of the muscle to the relaxed state and termination of the enhanced catabolic processes depend on calcium resequestration and clearance of the released calcium away from the sarcoplasm.[309] Sequestration of calcium requires consumption of energy (ATP), whereas calcium release does not.

The pathogenesis of MH has been investigated extensively. The syndrome is generally considered an idiosyncratic self-perpetuating hypercatabolic state precipitated by triggering factors such as anesthetic drugs and, rarely, stress. The main defect seems to be excessive release of calcium from the SR.[310] Point mutations in the ryanodine receptor (calcium release channel of the SR) gene have been demonstrated in some extended families as well as all MH (or porcine stress syndrome [PSS])–susceptible swine.[311] Ability of the SR to resequester calcium appears normal when examined in vitro without triggering agents;[312] during a fulminant MH episode, the sustained massive increase in sarcoplasmic calcium level overwhelms the capacity for SR

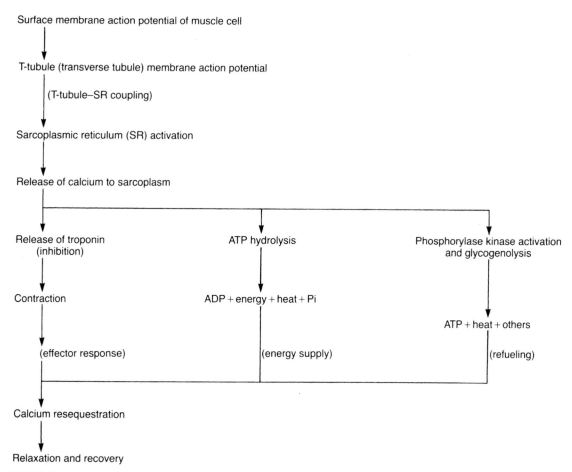

Surface membrane action potential of muscle cell

T-tubule (transverse tubule) membrane action potential

(T-tubule–SR coupling)

Sarcoplasmic reticulum (SR) activation

Release of calcium to sarcoplasm

| Release of troponin (inhibition) | ATP hydrolysis | Phosphorylase kinase activation and glycogenolysis |

Contraction   ADP + energy + heat + Pi

ATP + heat + others

(effector response)   (energy supply)   (refueling)

Calcium resequestration

Relaxation and recovery

FIGURE 10–4. Main events in EC coupling (action potential excitation to contraction) and recovery of skeletal muscle cell. Calcium is also released into the sarcoplasm to a lesser degree through the surface membrane and by the mitochondria.

active calcium reuptake to maintain the resting calcium level.[308, 309] The resultant excess calcium in the sarcoplasm, in turn, causes (1) persistent contracture of the myofibril; (2) excessive activation of ATPase and hydrolysis of ATP, resulting in depletion of ATP and creatine phosphate (CP); and (3) activation of ATP–regenerating mechanisms with glycogenolysis. It may, by "poisoning" mitochondrial function, secondarily cause uncoupling of oxidative phosphorylation. The preceding, i.e., sustained elevation of sarcoplasmic calcium and its pursuant effects, would explain most clinical features of MH, especially the rigidity, the hypermetabolic state, the muscle damage, and the severe electrolyte and acid-base imbalances. Secondary alpha-adrenergic stimulation seems to play an important role in the pathogenesis of MH and in the perpetuation of the catabolic process; intense cutaneous vasoconstriction reduces heat loss.[313]

The mechanism of MH just described is not without controversy. The relative importance of defects in SR, mitochondria, and sarcolemma has been disputed. Defects in calmodulin and adrenergic innervation of the muscle are also possible. Others have proposed that elevated intracellular free fatty acids or inositol trisphosphate (1,4,5-IP$_3$) enhance SR calcium release in MHS muscle.[314, 315] Serotonin receptor 2A subtype (5-HT$_{2A}$) agonists produce fulminant MH when given to *awake* MHS pigs; however, the 5-HT$_{2A}$ receptor antagonist ritanserin did not prevent or successfully treat halothane-induced MH. Interestingly, pigs premedicated with the neuroleptics azaperone and metomidate did not develop fulminant MH when given the 5-HT$_{2A}$ agonist 5-MeO-DMT.[316] MH without rigidity, in spite of presumed excessive myoplasmic calcium, is more difficult to explain than MH with rigidity. Ryan and colleagues suggest that increases of myoplasmic calcium levels to less than 1 µM are associated with hypermetabolism and only slight increases in muscle tone.[317] Microscopic examinations of the MHS muscle tissue may reveal the muscle damage but add little to the understanding of its pathogenesis.[318] Investigations of porcine MH play a key role in our understanding of human MHS. Besides the well-known pig models (Landrace, Pietrain, Poland, China), dogs, cats, and horses[319] have been observed occasionally to have MH.

C. DIAGNOSIS OF MALIGNANT HYPERTHERMIA

The tentative diagnosis of a fulminant case of MH should be made clinically, and treatment should be started without waiting for laboratory results or other confirmatory tests. Suggestive past anesthetic experience, muscle cramps and weakness, suspicious family history of anesthetic mishaps, unexplained myoglobinuria, elevated preoperative serum CK levels, history of anesthesia-induced CK elevation, abnormal muscle build, other musculoskeletal disorders such as strabismus, and a history of unexpected increases in temperature intraoperatively or early postoperatively should heighten suspicion. Laboratory tests supporting the working diagnosis and guiding the therapeutic measures are listed further in the section on Preplanned Therapeutic Regimen for Malignant Hyperthermia. These tests center around electrolyte, acid-base, blood gas, muscle enzyme, and myoglobin determinations.

Guidelines for a definite clinical diagnosis of less fulminant cases of MH are not available. None of the early signs of MH are pathognomonic. Conditions such as light anesthesia, thyroid storm, sepsis, pheochromocytoma, drug and pyrogen reactions, transfusion reactions, congenital or acquired resistance to succinylcholine, and other muscle diseases such as myotonic muscular dystrophy and disuse myopathy should be included in the differential diagnosis.[320] We suggest that central (or femoral) venous desaturation (especially when arterial hypoxemia or low cardiac output is absent), central or femoral venous hypercarbia, progressive or marked respiratory and metabolic respiratory acidosis, generalized muscle rigidity and warmth, myoglobinuria, progressive temperature increase, and marked hypermetabolism

with increased carbon dioxide production and respiratory drive are signs indicative of a working diagnosis of MH. Other signs—tachycardia, tachypnea, hypertension, cardiac arrhythmia, and unstable blood pressure—are less specific but serve as warning signs. In the presence of a positive personal or family history of MHS, MH should be seriously considered, even if the clinical signs are nonspecific. In routine anesthesia practice, without specific suspicion of MHS and therefore without invasive monitoring, sudden tachycardia and increased end-expiratory carbon dioxide value should prompt suspicion of MH. Larach and colleagues described a clinical grading scale that may be used to estimate the likelihood that an adverse anesthetic event was MH; the scale uses signs (e.g., rigidity, inappropriate tachycardia, cola-colored urine) and laboratory results (e.g., blood gas results, serum or urine myoglobin, CK, potassium), and points are assigned to each pathologic process (e.g., rigidity, muscle breakdown, respiratory acidosis).[321]

Because the diagnosis of MHS may have serious medical and social impact on a large number of people, this diagnosis should be made only with great care. Contracture testing of *living muscle strips* obtained by biopsy is the current standard for definite laboratory diagnosis of MHS.[302, 322–324] The Malignant Hyperthermia Association of the United States (MHAUS, P.O. Box 1069, Sherburne, NY 13460-1069), the Malignant Hyperthermia Association (of Canada), and the European Malignant Hyperthermia Group maintain a list of medical centers and experts throughout the countries where muscle biopsy and caffeine-halothane contracture tests are performed. Similar organizations exist in other parts of the world. Expert advice is available on muscle biopsy and on overall patient management.

It is the prevailing opinion of experts that muscle biopsy should be prescribed for high-risk families. In the past there were considerable problems with standardization of the technique and interpretation of the result, especially in equivocal cases. Great progress has been made toward solving these standardization problems. For example, the European MH Group adopted halothane contracture at 2 per cent v/v or less *and* a caffeine contracture at 2 mmol/L or less, as MHS (*undoubtedly* MH susceptible). *Neither* contracture constitutes MHN (*not* MH susceptible). All other results constitute MHE (*equivocal*); MHE patients are treated as MHS when they require anesthetic care. The MHE category would be subject to permanent review, to eventually reclassify to either the susceptible or nonsusceptible category.[325] The North American Malignant Hyperthermia (NAMH) Registry also established its own criteria in 1987.[326] Whatever the criteria for diagnosis, it should be stressed that contracture tests are performed on *living* muscle strips only. The experts should be consulted or the instructions obtained from authoritative sources followed *before* muscle biopsy is undertaken.

In 1990, the NAMH Registry reported the results of contracture tests in 183 control patients from 12 biopsy centers. Two mM caffeine produced ≥ 0.2 g contracture in 21 per cent of controls; 3 per cent halothane produced ≥ 0.7 g contracture in 15 per cent of controls. These are presumed to be false-positive test results.[327] Many experts recommend that both parents of an MHS patient be tested because of the possibility of a false-positive result and the fact that the condition is not uniformly autosomal dominant. A small number (fewer than 10 of several thousand) false-negative results have been reported using the European or North American testing protocols.[328, 329] It is recommended that patients who have survived a fulminant MH episode or whose anesthetic history is very suspicious for MH (e.g., hypermetabolism and muscle injury with or without masseter spasm, triggering agent administered) should be treated as MHS even with a negative contracture test. Diagnostic interpretation of a contracture test includes review of the clinical history. Diagnostic criteria must be very sensitive to avoid the potential catastrophe of giving triggering agents to a true MHS patient.

Alternative methods of diagnosis include testing calcium release from the SR, calcium uptake by SR, and calcium-related functions of the contractile system using chemically skinned single muscle fibers.[330] Unfortunately, muscle biopsy is a major procedure: all diagnostic tests require a high degree of expertise and the cost is considerable. Only relatively older children can undergo a biopsy procedure. Translation of equivocal results into clinical implications is difficult. Other tests, such as the ATP depletion test or SR calcium uptake using frozen muscle, are less valuable. A noninvasive test for MHS with high specificity is needed; in vivo 31P MR spectroscopy (MRS or NMR) has shown promise.[331, 332]

Serum CK values have been widely used to warn of MHS preoperatively, to diagnose MH episodes, and to follow up the progress of the attack. In general, the higher the CK values are, the worse the muscle damage has been and the more likely it is that MH or a related disease has occurred. However, CK values are nonspecific and imprecise. Absence of CK elevation alone does not rule out MHS, and its presence alone does not diagnose MHS or an MH episode. It has been suggested that the serum CK level be abandoned as a screening or diagnostic test of MHS.[333] Morphologic studies of human and porcine MHS muscle have revealed a variety of myopathic and neuropathic features,[318] some of which may be characteristic of related diseases, such as central core disease. None of them, however, is pathognomonic of MHS. Until triggered by stress or drugs, MHS muscle is usually normal in structure and function. For a review of the numerous diagnostic tests proposed for MHS see Ording[324] or Fletcher.[334]

D. MOLECULAR GENETICS AND MALIGNANT HYPERTHERMIA

In February 1990, two reports described DNA testing in several families in which autosomal-dominant transmission of the MH phenotype was documented over several generations.[335, 336] Individual MHS had been characterized by either contracture tests in at least 10 family members or well-documented MH episodes. These reports demonstrated very significant odds (e.g., greater than 1,000:1; logarithm of odds [*lod score*] >3) of linkage between inheritance of the MH phenotype and polymorphisms of the skeletal muscle ryanodine receptor (RYR1) gene; polymorphisms are alleles that differ in DNA base pair composition. The ryanodine receptor is a large homotetrameric protein that functions as the calcium release channel of the terminal cisternae of the SR.[311] The gene locus for RYR1 has been mapped to chromosome 19. In swine, the RYR1 gene is located on chromosome 6. A point mutation of the RYR1 gene (C to T, base pair 1843) is found in all MHS swine;[337] this results in substitution of cysteine for arginine at position 615 of the ryanodine receptor subunit. The porcine mutation is found in fewer than 5 per cent of families with MHS. Different RYR1 polymorphisms are strongly associated with MHS in several families; at least four point mutations of the RYR1 gene have been linked statistically with MHS.[338] Fletcher and coworkers reported a person with the porcine mutation who had 18 uneventful general anesthetics before an episode of masseter spasm not accompanied by hypermetabolism; they suggested that the presence of the point mutation is insufficient to explain the full clinical expression of MHS.[339] Several studies have described a lack of complete concordance between RYR1 polymorphisms linked with MHS and contracture test results.[340] Investigators have suggested that this discordance may be due to (1) false-positive contracture test results, (2) rare false-negative contracture results, or (3) insufficient sensitivity of testing for DNA polymorphisms to evaluate MHS (e.g., statistically linked polymorphism not truly causal; undescribed non-RYR1 mutation causal; inheritance not autosomal dominant). Several family studies have shown no linkage (i.e., significant recombination) between RYR1 polymorphisms and MHS, indicating genetic heterogeneity of human MHS. Loci on chromosome 7 and chromosome 3 have been statistically linked with MHS in single families.[341, 342] The locus on chromosome 7 is adjacent (not identical) to the gene for the alpha 2/delta subunit of the skeletal muscle dihydropyridine receptor.

DNA evaluation may be useful in selected families where RYR1 polymorphisms have demonstrated strong linkage with MHS. Subsequent family members who have the MHS-associated polymorphism may not require contracture testing; MHS may be assumed. MHN diagnosis by DNA testing is controversial; most experts would not feel confident diagnosing MHN when clearly abnormal contracture tests have been associated with absence of MHS-associated RYR1 polymorphisms.[343] Unlike porcine MH, the genetic heterogeneity of human MH precludes the use of DNA diagnosis in most persons whose history raises suspicion of MH.

E. DISEASES RELATED TO MALIGNANT HYPERTHERMIA

Numerous muscle diseases may be associated with MHS, and patients with these muscle diseases may contract MH when exposed to triggering agents; however, on reevaluation, strong association with MHS appears to exist only in the case of central core disease and King-Denborough syndrome.[344] Point mutations in the skeletal muscle RYR1 gene have been found in families with central core disease/MHS and in some families with only MHS. Islander and coworkers described a family whose daughter had central core disease; several close relatives *without* central core disease were given contracture tests that demonstrated MHS.[345] King-Denborough syndrome is a rare disorder first reported in males with short stature, myopathy, facial anomalies, cryptorchidism, pectus carinatum, thoracic kyphosis, and lumbar lordosis; affected girls have been described. Chitayat and colleagues reviewed 14 patients with King-Denborough syndrome; 12 patients had MH episodes.[346] Possible association exists, in roughly decreasing order, with Duchenne's muscular dystrophy, myoadenylate deaminase deficiency, the Schwartz-Jampel syndrome, Fukuyama's muscular dystrophy, Becker's muscular dystrophy, pectus excavatum,[347] periodic paralysis, myotonia congenita, SR ATPase deficiency syndrome, and mitochondrial myopathy. An association between MHS and SIDS[348] or neuroleptic malignant syndrome (NMS) has been discounted. Succinylcholine may cause rigidity in several muscle diseases, but that feature alone does not establish MHS in those patients. Whatever the degree of association with MHS, each of these diseases carries certain risks with certain drugs used in anesthesia. NMS bears a similarity to MH in several important clinical features. Caroff and coworkers reported a high incidence of positive response to the caffeine-halothane contracture test in seven patients with previous NMS;[349] recently, Bello and colleagues reported normal contracture tests in 29 of 32 patients with previous NMS.[350] The clinical manifestations of both diseases are drug induced. Nevertheless, considerable differences exist between them, especially in their heritability and response to succinylcholine (see Section on Neuroleptic Malignant Syndrome).

F. TREATMENT OF MALIGNANT HYPERTHERMIA

Because of the fulminant time course and the high mortality of MH, especially if treated late, it is imperative to have a regimen preplanned before MH occurs. Posters are available with diagnostic and therapeutic guidelines from MHAUS and other sources, as are telephone numbers for emergency and elective consultations. We suggest that updated copies of these posters be posted in strategic and conspicuous places. A local expert should personally direct the emergency treatment of every case, if possible. MHAUS has a telephone line (1-[800]-644-9737 [MH-HYPER]) open around the clock for referral to experts for consultations. A suggested plan for fulminant MH is described later. The plan can be modified for less fulminant cases. Care should be taken not to delay treatment; otherwise, even less fulminant cases might become disastrous. For a list of drugs to be avoided or discontinued, see Elective Anesthesia. If possible, have available a trigger-free anesthesia machine without halogenated anesthetics. Use this spare machine for elective anesthesia on MHS patients. When this is not practical, turn the vaporizer off and run oxygen flow at 10 L per minute. This results in a very low (e.g., fewer than 10 parts per million) residual halogenated anesthetic concentration within 5 minutes.[351] A small dose of droperidol or chlorpromazine may provide vasodilatation and stop shivering to facilitate cooling. Overcooling the patient should be avoided.

Several issues concerning drug therapy during an MH crisis deserve comment. First of all, *timely, effective therapy with dantrolene often eliminates the need for many other therapeutic measures.* In sporadic case reports *d*-tubocurarine has been causally linked to MH; however, it is difficult to understand why it could be harmful when other nondepolarizing neuromuscular relaxants are safe. In the MH crisis, nondepolarizing relaxants may not be helpful. Once triggered by inhalational anesthetics or succinylcholine, the rigid and hypermetabolic processes perpetuate themselves in the muscle, and the rigidity cannot be relieved by nondepolarizing neuromuscular block. If rigidity of MH coexists with normal neuromuscular transmission, the rigidity should be treated with dantrolene; the latter may be blocked with nondepolarizing neuromuscular relaxants if this seems clinically advisable (see Dantrolene).

Hypocalcemia during MH is thought to be due to calcium influx into the muscle cells. Supplying calcium may aggravate the intracellular calcium excess; however, cardiac arrest during MH crisis resulting from hyperkalemia has been successfully treated with calcium.[352] Perhaps, once the MH crisis is arrested by dantrolene, hypocalcemia and hyperkalemia can be corrected by calcium administration without compounding the intracellular calcium excess. The value of calcium channel blockers in MH crisis is unclear.[353, 354] The combination of dantrolene and verapamil may result in severe hyperkalemia, myocardial depression, heart block, or death.[355–357] Hyperkalemia has also been reported following dantrolene in an MHS patient taking diltiazem and metoprolol.[358] Cardiac glycosides may increase myoplasmic calcium levels, but MHS swine do not respond abnormally to digoxin.[359] The serum potassium concentration fluctuates markedly during and following MH crisis, as does the serum glucose concentration. Damage, stabilization, and recovery of muscle cells are associated with efflux and influx of large quantities of potassium. Renal failure may further derange electrolyte balance. During MH crisis, control of hyperkalemia may require infusion of glucose and insulin. During convalescence, a large quantity of potassium may be required to replace potassium loss caused by renal excretion and reentry into the recovering muscle cells. Alpha-adrenergic stimulation may aggravate the MH process by limiting transcutaneous heat loss; however, α-adrenergic agonists do not trigger MH in susceptible swine.[360] Adrenergic agonists may be used when indicated to maintain cardiac output and tissue perfusion during MH crises.

Arrhythmias usually respond to treatment of the episode with dantrolene and hyperventilation, resulting in cooling and resolution of acidosis and hyperkalemia. For control of cardiac arrhythmia, procainamide or lidocaine may be used. When cardiac arrhythmia occurs early in MH crisis, either may be combined with dantrolene therapy. Lidocaine was previously surrounded with controversy. Amide local anesthetics were previously thought to be harmful because lidocaine may enhance contracture in vitro by inhibiting calcium resequestration into the SR; however, reexamination has shown that lidocaine does not trigger MH in MHS swine, even when given in doses greater than the convulsive threshold;[361] all local anesthetics, including the amides, are acceptable for anesthetic purposes.[362, 363]

During convalescence, intensive care is necessary, usually for 1 or 2 days. MH crisis may occur, become aggravated, or recur postoperatively. Precautionary maintenance use of dantrolene therapy is recommended for at least 24 hours (see Dantrolene).

G. COUNSELING OF PATIENTS WITH MALIGNANT HYPERTHERMIA SUSCEPTIBILITY

Individuals suspected of or diagnosed as having MHS should be counseled on heritability of MHS, muscle biopsy and contracture tests, drugs or situations to be avoided, anesthesia precautions, lifestyle, availability of services from MHAUS, Medic Alert and similar associations, and the advisability of wearing a Medic Alert bracelet and carrying a warning card. There are no set rules on how extensive the counseling should be. Again, expert opinions can be sought from consultants. Persons with MHS who are careful plan ahead before traveling to parts of the world where awareness of the disease may be poor and where dantrolene may not be available. Two concerns that are often raised are the safety of nonprescription drugs and beverages containing caffeine and the use of amide local anesthetics for minor surgery and dental care. Sufficient evidence seems to have accumulated to indicate that both are safe.[362, 363] Another concern is the use of triggering agents in patients with negative contracture test results. Preliminary evidence seems to confirm its safety; however, findings are still inconclusive.[362, 364] It is important to realize that one uneventful anesthesia experience does not rule out MHS.

H. ELECTIVE ANESTHESIA FOR PATIENTS WITH MALIGNANT HYPERTHERMIA SUSCEPTIBILITY

Anesthesia may be required for patients with MHS, either for diagnostic muscle biopsy or for general surgical conditions. Local, regional, spinal, and epidural anesthesia are acceptable. For muscle biopsy, femoral and lateral femoral cutaneous nerves can be blocked.[363] Patients should be sedated. Addition of epinephrine or Neo-Synephrine to the local anesthetic is acceptable to improve motor block or decrease the risk of systemic toxicity. Sedation, neuroleptanalgesia, and general anesthesia with droperidol, promethazine, diazepam, midazolam, ketamine, propofol,[365] etomidate, various narcotics, narcotic antagonists, narcotic agonist-antagonists, various barbiturates, various nondepolarizing

neuromuscular blocking relaxants and nitrous oxide are safe. Residual neuromuscular block should be reversed. Anticholinergic agents are safe, but they may mask or aggravate tachycardia. Glucocorticoids are harmless. Ketamine does not trigger MH; its use may be associated with tachycardia and mild temperature elevation in normal persons.[366] Physostigmine seems safe. *Succinylcholine and all potent inhalational anesthetics (halothane, enflurane, isoflurane, sevoflurane, desflurane, ether, and so on) are to be avoided.*[367, 368] Aerating the system for 24 hours ensures a vapor-free anesthesia machine. An oxygen flow of 10 L per minute through the system for 5 to 10 minutes, especially if the rubber hose from the machine's fresh gas outlet is changed, makes it virtually vapor free.[351] Prophylactic use of dantrolene may be considered, but is usually unnecessary when any technique is employed that scrupulously avoids the use of triggering agents (see Dantrolene). Carr and coworkers reported a 0.46 per cent prevalence of probable MH reactions in 1082 MHS patients undergoing muscle biopsy; 97 per cent of these patients received general anesthesia using a nontriggering technique; all reactions occurred in the recovery room; dantrolene treatment resulted in prompt resolution of tachycardia, tachypnea, and hyperthermia.[369]

Monitoring should consist at least of ECG, blood pressure determinations, core $\pm$ axillary temperatures, pulse oximetry readings, and end-tidal carbon dioxide determinations. Liquid crystal display of skin temperature is inaccurate; in fulminant MH, cutaneous vasoconstriction may prevent skin temperature from increasing with core temperature. In addition, liquid crystal thermography may display falsely *elevated* skin temperature; one manufacturer's device displays a temperature 2.5°C higher than actual skin temperature, to "compensate" for the normal core–skin temperature gradient. This may result in factitious hyperthermia with cutaneous vasodilatation following anesthetic induction.[370] One should also observe skin color, pupils, muscle tone, jaw tension, status of the carbon dioxide absorbent, heart tones, breath sounds, and spontaneous breathing activity. End-expiratory carbon dioxide monitoring may provide an early clue to hypermetabolism, which is quite specific to the disease process. Depending on the nature of the surgery and the patient's general condition, one should consider urine output and central venous pressure determinations, a Swan-Ganz catheter, central venous oximetry, and an arterial line. Neuromuscular transmission, urine output, hematologic features, acid-base and electrolyte balance, and blood chemistry should be monitored as needed. Attention should be paid to muscle enzyme levels, myoglobinemia, and myoglobinuria.

General protective measures include relief of anxiety and prevention of emotional stress, hot ambient temperature, fever caused by infection, and muscle injury. Britt reported cases to illustrate that stress, alcohol, and cocaine, particularly in combination, may be capable of triggering or co-triggering MH reactions.[371] If the patient is pregnant, the effect of dantrolene on the fetus should be considered (see Dantrolene). Patients at risk for MH may be discharged as outpatients following careful observation in the recovery room for at least 4 hours; patients with evidence of hypermetabolism (e.g., unexplained tachypnea, tachycardia, or temperature elevation) should be evaluated appropriately; patients with suspected myoglobinuria should be admitted.

I. DRUG-INDUCED TRISMUS

Rigidity of the jaw muscles during anesthesia following injection of succinylcholine, with or without co-administration of halogenated inhalational anesthetics, is a serious matter.[372, 373] Studies indicate that trismus following succinylcholine administration occurs often in myotonia congenita, central core disease, and myotonia dystrophica. As a precursor of MH, it precedes other clinical manifestations of MH, either immediately or after some interval. The jaw muscles are rigid, but the rest of the body may be either rigid or flaccid. Some 0.3 to 1 per cent of all children induced with a halothane-succinylcholine combination may exhibit masseter muscle rigidity.[374–376] Trismus may be more common in children with strabismus.[374] Contracture test results for MHS can be positive in as many as 40 to 60 per cent of children with succinylcholine-induced trismus.[377] Lazzell and colleagues prospectively studied the incidence of masseter muscle rigidity in more than 5000 children; 4457 were induced with intravenous Pentothal. Not a single child induced with Pentothal had masseter muscle rigidity.[378] Lazzell suggested that masseter muscle rigidity following Pentothal induction is distinctly abnormal and should prompt follow-up investigation of MH susceptibility. Lazzell's

group found a 0.5 percent prevalence of masseter muscle rigidity in 607 children induced with halothane. Carroll and coworkers reported a prevalence of 2.8 per cent in a subgroup who had strabismus; no masseter muscle rigidity was observed in 586 children with strabismus (98 induced with halothane) in Lazzell's study. Obviously, 1 percent of children cannot all be susceptible to MH. To add to the confusion, an important observation was that succinylcholine routinely increases the jaw muscle tone of children "under" halothane anesthesia[379] or enflurane anesthesia.[380] The degree of masseter muscle rigidity should be considered. In a severe case, the jaw cannot be opened despite great effort; CK elevation and myoglobinuria follow; and the patient may have myalgia and weakness afterward. MH may be more likely in this case. Lesser degrees of rigidity may not be as significant. Sometimes poor relaxation of the jaw muscles can be attributed to inadequate neuromuscular block alone. The heritability of drug-induced trismus is not clear. In patients with negative MHS contracture test results, drug-induced trismus may be a separate disease entity. It is usually self-limited.

To be on the safe side, drug-induced trismus should tentatively be presumed to be MH and treated accordingly; however, consensus is lacking on how aggressively drug-induced trismus without other signs of MH should be handled.[381] Littleford and colleagues reported 57 children with masseter muscle rigidity (without generalized rigidity) in whom the halogenated anesthetic was continued. They did not observe fulminant MH or postoperative rhabdomyolytic renal failure.[376] They did observe marked increases in postoperative CK levels, some in excess of 50,000 IU/L. In addition, 25 per cent of these children had moderate temperature elevations postoperatively. Respiratory or moderate metabolic acidosis frequently was observed; respiratory acidosis was attributed to hypoventilation during spontaneous ventilation. In contrast, O'Flynn and coworkers reported onset of clinical MH (respiratory acidosis despite adequate ventilation and base deficit in excess of 8) in 5 of 70 children with masseter muscle rigidity referred for contracture testing; 59 per cent (41 of 70) had contracture test results consistent with MH susceptibility.[382] Following masseter muscle rigidity, anesthesia may be terminated and surgery cancelled, or one may continue the anesthetic using a nitrous oxide–narcotic–

intravenous hypnotic–nondepolarizing relaxant technique, as indicated. Most experts recommend that halogenated anesthetics be discontinued; monitoring must include capnography and continuous temperature monitoring. The urine must be examined for myoglobinuria. Serum CK should be checked, including a specimen drawn the following morning.

Rosenberg thinks that patients should definitely undergo muscle biopsy and contracture tests for MHS, except perhaps when MHS can be diagnosed without the test by unequivocal clinical manifestations or by a CK level greater than 20,000 IU/L after trismus.[372] Without a definitive diagnosis, the patient and all family members may have to be considered MH susceptible; however, the contracture test alone can cost $4000.[322] Muscle biopsy and rescheduling surgery and anesthesia are also costly and inconvenient. Contracture tests are not performed for children younger than 6 years or lighter than 20 kg. The psychological impact on the patient of coming back for the same surgery a second time and worrying about anesthesia death must also be considered. Furthermore, the patient may end up undergoing the same surgery next time, still without a definite diagnosis of MHS, or the contracture test result may be negative. In the worst scenario, the patient may then contract MH because triggering agents are given by mistake for lack of communication. Therefore, many anesthesiologists faced with a case of drug-induced trismus would search for other clues of MH and proceed with the surgery with trigger-free agents provided that excessive risk of MH appears unlikely and the trismus subsides. The pitfall then is that clinical manifestations of MH may occur later. It behooves the staff to be prepared to deal with MH at its worst. Prophylactic use of dantrolene may be considered but has not been proved beneficial.

A patient with drug-induced trismus should be observed very closely for at least 4 hours, whether the surgery is cancelled or proceeds. Patients with myoglobinuria or evidence of hypermetabolism (e.g., respiratory and/or metabolic acidosis associated with tachypnea, tachycardia, or hyperthermia) should be admitted as inpatients. Even patients without evidence of hypermetabolism should have serum CK drawn the next day, since CK levels may not peak until 12 to 24 hours after trismus. Follow-up after anesthesia should include counseling (see Counseling of Patients with Malignant Hyperthermia Susceptibility). According to preliminary data, patients with negative contracture test results may safely receive subsequent anesthesia, even with triggering agents.[362, 364, 383] We avoid succinylcholine since it is used for rapid control of the airway, and if trismus recurs rapid (endotracheal) intubation is not possible.

J. DANTROLENE: CLINICAL USE AND PHARMACOLOGY

The use of dantrolene for treatment of MH has dramatically reduced morbidity and mortality. Before dantrolene, reported mortality of acute MH usually exceeded 50 per cent; with dantrolene treatment, mortality of acute fulminant MH has been reduced to 10 per cent or less. Dantrolene sodium is a hydantoin derivative used orally in the treatment of chronic skeletal muscle spasticity associated with upper motor neuron diseases such as stroke, cerebral palsy, and spinal cord injury that can be painful or disabling or can interfere with nursing care. Prophylactic use of dantrolene against MH is controversial in terms of timing, dose, and necessity. An intravenous dose of 2 to 3 mg/kg given 10 to 30 minutes before anesthesia is often recommended. Oral administration of 5 mg/kg given in divided doses over 24 hours—the last dose no earlier than 4 hours before anesthesia—is also acceptable;[384] however, patients who have been proved to have MHS and who are scheduled for elective surgery usually do not require dantrolene prophylaxis. *Trigger-free anesthesia usually makes dantrolene prophylaxis unnecessary.* Kaplan has suggested that prophylactic dantrolene be considered for high-risk patients, including those with (1) a history of "stress-induced" MH, (2) renal insufficiency, (3) significant coronary artery disease or stenotic valvular disease, or (4) cerebrovascular disease.[385] For treatment of a clinical case of MH, dantrolene is titrated to effect. The starting dose is 2 to 3 mg/kg at a rate of 1 mg/kg per minute intravenously at the earliest possible time, once a definite working diagnosis is made. More than 10 mg/kg may be required initially; after that, the dantrolene is stopped for a few minutes to reassess the response. If indicated, the cycle of 1 mg/kg per minute may be started again. The usual dose requirement is 2.5 mg/kg,[386] but it ranges from 1 to

17 mg/kg.[387, 388] When severe rigidity is present, large doses of dantrolene may be required; decreased muscle perfusion may impede dantrolene delivery to its intended site of action. The same dose formulas apply to pediatric patients. Each intravenous dose of 1 mg/kg of dantrolene should be carried with ample fluid into a free-running intravenous line. The muscle-relaxing effect of dantrolene has immediate onset, and each dose produces most of its effects in 2 to 3 minutes and is fully effective in 5 to 10 minutes.[386, 389] Following effective treatment with dantrolene and relief of muscle rigidity and hypermetabolism, stabilization and improvement in the patient's general condition ensue rather dramatically. Lowering of temperature following dantrolene treatment is not specific or diagnostic for MH. After the crisis, a maintenance dose of dantrolene, 4 to 8 mg/kg per day (e.g., 1 to 2 mg/kg every 6 hours) in divided doses, is generally recommended for 1 to 3 days.

The serum half-life of dantrolene is 4 to 12 hours. Oral medication results in good absorption. Dantrolene crosses the placental barrier readily and can harm the fetus. Its use in pregnant women requires serious justification. Dantrolene before delivery may result in neonatal hypotonia. It is metabolized by oxidative and reductive enzymes in hepatic microsomes.

Dantrolene is supplied in relatively large (70-mL) bottles with 20 mg of drug each, to be dissolved in 60 mL of sterile water (without preservatives) supplied in separate bottles. Each bottle of 20 mg lyophilized dantrolene also contains 3 g of mannitol. It also has sodium hydroxide. Dantrolene is poorly soluble and requires shaking, a large volume of solvent, and high pH (9.5 when reconstituted) to dissolve. If reconstituted properly, it can be infused in spite of an appearance that is less than crystal clear. It is an irritant to tissue and requires a large, free-running intravenous line to avoid local tissue injury. To reduce venous irritation, maintenance doses of dantrolene can be given orally whenever the patient can tolerate taking it by mouth.

To formulate an adequate supply of intravenous dantrolene may take 60 to 70 bottles (20 mg/kg). At least a quarter of these (5 mg/kg) should be available immediately, another quarter in a few minutes, and the rest at a moment's notice. Some neighboring day surgical centers and suburban hospitals have worked out cost-sharing plans to supply dantrolene.

Therapeutic doses of dantrolene produce muscle weakness; however, even relatively excessive doses of dantrolene rarely cause respiratory paralysis. The ED_{75} for twitch depression is 2.5 mg/kg.[386] Dantrolene acts by direct muscle depression. Its effect on muscle strength is additive to that of nondepolarizing neuromuscular block.[255] It has no effective antidote but can be antagonized transiently by 4-aminopyridine, germine monoacetate, and anticholinesterase agents.[390] It is not antagonized by calcium in clinical doses. If respiratory function is compromised by dantrolene, ventilatory support, not pharmacologic intervention, is advised.

Dantrolene-induced muscle depression can be differentiated from nondepolarizing neuromuscular block. During nondepolarizing neuromuscular block, tetanic fade is observed; train-of-four also fades. During dantrolene-induced muscle depression, the tetanus is well-preserved. Neither tetanus nor train-of-four fades significantly. Successive action potentials in the tetanic train build up intracellular calcium concentration to sustain the tetanus. Since all physiologic activities are tetanic contractions of some sort they are relatively spared during dantrolene therapy.

Dantrolene has demonstrable but clinically insignificant effects on neuromuscular transmission. It depresses neurally evoked muscle force but not the corresponding EMG.[255] It does not interfere with reversal of coexisting nondepolarizing neuromuscular block. Its mechanism of action is mainly reduction of calcium release from the SR, which it does indirectly.[391] Complete blockade of calcium release is impossible; therefore, the effect of very large doses of dantrolene levels off.[386]

Dantrolene has also been used to treat NMS effectively (see Neuroleptic Malignant Syndrome). Its therapeutic effects in other muscle diseases outlined in this chapter are not clear. It may be effective for perioperative control of spasticity, but it may cause respiratory failure in patients with myotonic dystrophy.

Dantrolene is not an innocuous drug and is no substitute for vigilance against MH. Its side effects include muscle weakness (including dysphagia), local thrombophlebitis, transient dizziness, diplopia, dysarthria, and swelling of the tongue. Abnormal liver functions and skin rash may occur with *chronic* treatment.[353, 391]

The availability of intravenous preparations of dantrolene since 1979 has revolution-ized clinical management of MH; however, the mortality of MH has remained unaccept-ably high at 7 per cent. We should strive for survival without sequelae with vigilance, close monitoring, and early intervention.

K. PREPLANNED THERAPEUTIC REGIMEN FOR MALIGNANT HYPERTHERMIA

I. PREPAREDNESS
A. Sufficient supply of dantrolene sodium
B. Intravenous fluids in refrigerator, 5 L
C. Cooling devices and large supply of ice
D. Emergency MH drugs
  (1) Sodium bicarbonate, 12 ampules
  (2) Furosemide, 4×100-mg ampules
  (3) Mannitol, 4×12.5-g ampules
  (4) Dantrolene sodium, 36×20-mg bottles
  (5) Regular insulin, 1×100 U ampules
  (6) 50 per cent D/W, 50 mL
  (7) Procainamide, 1 g
E. Poster of therapeutic regimen and MHAUS Hotline, 1-(800)-MH-HYPER (644-9737).

II. ON WORKING DIAGNOSIS OF MALIGNANT HYPERTHERMIA TREATMENT
A. Discontinue all triggering agents, hyperventilate (e.g., 300 cc/kg per minute in adults) with 100 per cent oxygen at high fresh gas flow rates; advise the surgeon (immediately); request skilled assistance (help for mixing dantrolene, obtaining laboratory values, establishing invasive monitoring, cooling the patient); do not waste time changing the anesthesia machine.
B. Clinically reconfirm working diagnosis of MH, and give dantrolene sodium 2.5 mg/kg intravenously and then titrate to effect at 1 mg/kg per minute. Repeat doses of dantrolene should be given as long as rigidity, fever, acidosis, or tachycardia persist. More than 10 mg/kg may be required for successful initial therapy.
C. Therapy with bicarbonate should be guided by blood gas results. If such results are not promptly available, give 1 to 3 ampules of sodium bicarbonate, 1 to 2 mEq/kg in children, while sending for help.
D. Sedate, if appropriate, and treat with neuroleptics, narcotics, benzodiazepines, intravenous hypnotic

agents, and nondepolarizing relaxants if necessary.
E. Hydrate with refrigerated intravenous fluids and begin cooling via all immediately available accesses (e.g., open abdomen or nasogastric tube). Active cooling should stop when core temperature is reduced to 38°C, to avoid unintentional hypothermia.
F. Enhance monitoring and secure appropriate arterial and venous lines, urinary catheter, and nasogastric tube. Send blood samples for analysis for potassium level, serum myoglobin and CK, and coagulation studies.
G. Maintain urine output at 1 to 2 mL/kg per hour, for example, with mannitol, 0.25 g/kg intravenously (each bottle of dantrolene contains 3 g mannitol). Furosemide, 1 mg/kg intravenously, may be used for patients who cannot tolerate intravascular volume expansion.
H. Monitor and optimize acid-base balance and correct electrolyte abnormalities. If necessary, use glucose and insulin to treat hyperkalemia.
I. Control cardiac rhythm and cardiovascular parameters. For cardiac arrhythmia not responsive to dantrolene and hyperventilation, infuse procainamide, 200 mg at a rate of 25 to 50 mg per minute, and repeat as needed; if the QRS interval increases by 50 per cent, discontinue procainamide and recheck serum potassium. Lidocaine may be used to treat ventricular arrhythmias. *Do not give verapamil or diltiazem during therapy with dantrolene.*
J. Perform clotting and hemolytic studies to detect DIC, and treat accordingly.

III. LABORATORY TESTS TO BE CONSIDERED
A. Arterial and central or femoral venous blood gases, electrolytes (Ca^{2+}, K^+, Cl^-, phosphate), glucose, and osmolality determinations.
B. Muscle enzyme (CK) and muscle protein (myoglobinemia and myoglobinuria) determinations.
C. Hematologic parameters (hemolysis (e.g., Coombs' test), red cell count, platelet count and function, coagulation studies).
D. Other tests: blood cultures (infectious disease workup), serum catecholamines, thyroid hormone, and serum magnesium determinations.

IV. POSTOPERATIVE CARE
A. Continue intensive care (1 to 3 days), follow up on muscle damage, treat complications and sequelae. Care

should continue in an intensive care setting until hyperthermia, hypermetabolism, and acidosis have resolved with no evidence of recurrence.

B. Dantrolene sodium maintenance, intravenously or orally for at least 24 hours. Given the long half-life of dantrolene, intensive care should continue for at least 24 hours after the last dose of dantrolene.

V. **FOLLOW UP (CONSIDER CONSULTATIONS OR REFERRAL TO MH CENTER)**
   A. Patient and family counseling.
   B. Consider muscle biopsy and registration with Medic Alert Foundation.
   C. Refer patient and family to MHAUS (P.O. Box 1069, Sherburne, NY 13460-1069; phone (607) 674-7901).

XIX. NEUROLEPTIC MALIGNANT SYNDROME AND LETHAL CATATONIA

NMS is a rare but potentially fatal idiosyncratic reaction to antipsychotic neuroleptic drugs, including haloperidol, fluphenazine, clozapine, perphenazine, thiothixene, trifluoperazine, thioridazine, chlorpromazine, and others.[392–395] Droperidol, prochlorperazine (Compazine), promethazine (Phenergan), and metoclopramide have also been associated with NMS. Withdrawal of L-dopa in patients with Parkinson's disease may result in NMS.[396] *Lethal catatonia* is a hyperthermic exhaustion syndrome that may affect patients with schizophrenia or bipolar affective disorder; it closely resembles NMS but can develop without administration of neuroleptics. Both are characterized by rigidity, dyskinesia, rhabdomyolysis, autonomic dysfunction (hypertension, hypotension, tachycardia, tachypnea, diaphoresis, urinary incontinence), hyperthermia, and mental status changes, possibly including delirium, mutism, or stupor. Leukocytosis and serum CK elevations are often observed. The rigidity can develop into cogwheeling, posturing, and opisthotonos. Patients suspected to have NMS should be evaluated for CNS or systemic infection. Approximately 10 to 20 per cent of reported cases have been fatal, usually as a result of respiratory arrest, myoglobinuria with acute renal failure, or cardiovascular collapse.[392–394] Permanent neurologic sequelae may develop, including dementia and signs of parkinsonism or cerebellar dysfunction. NMS is not as fulminant as MH, and death comes more gradually.

Symptoms of NMS may occur on the day of neuroleptic therapy, or they may be delayed until several months of continuous therapy have ensued. Insidious onset of 24 to 72 hours is common, and the temperature often levels off at a plateau. Estimation of the prevalence varies, but it may be as great as 1.4 per cent.[393] Caroff and colleagues pooled data from 17 studies and obtained an overall prevalence of 0.2 percent.[396] Treatment of NMS is supportive therapy and prompt discontinuation of the offending neuroleptic. Recent experiences suggest that dantrolene sodium, L-dopa, and bromocriptine usually produce rapid relief.[393, 397] Dantrolene sodium relieves fever and normalizes CK levels, and bromocriptine (a dopamine agonist) relieves obtundation, rigidity, and tremulousness. If bromocriptine is effective, it should be continued for 10 days after resolution of symptoms, to prevent recrudescence. Scheftner and Shulman suggest that electroconvulsive therapy may be indicated if NMS fails to improve after 2 days' treatment with bromocriptine and/or dantrolene.[398] Electroconvulsive therapy (ECT) provided prompt cure of NMS in other reported cases.[399, 400]

The exact relationship between NMS and MH is not clear. Clinical evidence suggests that inhibition of central dopaminergic activity by the neuroleptic drugs leads to disturbed thermoregulation. Conflicting halothane contracture test results and fluphenazine contracture test results previously suggested that NMS was closely related to a hypermetabolic state in the skeletal muscle, as is MH.[401] Bello and coworkers recently reported normal contracture tests in 29 of 32 patients with previous NMS.[350] Patients receiving ECT for NMS have received succinylcholine safely without developing MH, although cardiac arrhythmias and hyperkalemia have been reported in the presence of severe rhabdomyolysis (e.g., CK above 5000 IU/L).[400–403] Anesthetic experience with NMS is scanty. Whether or not succinylcholine and inhalational anesthetics are contraindicated for patients with NMS is controversial.[404] There have been no case reports of MH in response to halogenated anesthetics or succinylcholine in patients with a history of NMS; NMS is not an inherited disorder. There is no reason to avoid using halogenated anesthetics in patients with a history of NMS but no personal or family history of MH. Muscle rigidity in MH is not relaxed by NDMRs but rigidity in NMS patients undergoing surgery is. Another difference between the two syndromes is that neuroleptic agents are acceptable for anesthetic management of MH patients but not of NMS patients. NMS has no clear genetic link.

XX. MYASTHENIC SYNDROMES

A. MYASTHENIA GRAVIS

Myasthenia gravis is characterized by fluctuating weakness that increases throughout the day. The weakness, not fatigue, is the principal complaint of the patient, and although weakness is exacerbated by exercise, patients may not make this connection. The muscles affected most commonly are the ocular muscles, which are involved initially in 40 per cent of patients (eventually in 85 per cent), causing both ptosis and diplopia. Weakness in the distribution of the cranial nerves is seen, with limitation of facial movement, and oropharyngeal involvement produces dysarthria, dysphagia, nasal regurgitation, and nasal speech. Limb and neck weakness are common, but only when cranial nerve muscles are already involved. Respiratory muscle weakness is less common and is seen almost exclusively during myasthenic crisis.[405]

Myasthenic patients have been classified by Osserman[405] as follows: group I, ocular disease only (20 per cent); group IIA, mild generalized symptoms (30 per cent); group IIB, moderate generalized symptoms with some bulbar symptoms (20 per cent); group III, acute, severe, presents in weeks to months with severe bulbar symptoms (11 per cent); group IV, late, severe cases with marked bulbar symptoms and severe generalized weakness (9 per cent).

The incidence is about 3 in 100,000 population. Between ages 10 and 40 years, it occurs three times as often in women as in men; the incidence is equal thereafter. Patients younger than 16 years account for 10 per cent of all cases. Pediatric cases can be divided as follows:

1. Neonatal transient—approximately 20 per cent of neonates born to myasthenic mothers have transient neonatal myasthenic symptoms. They require therapy for 1 to 2 months.

2. Neonatal persistent—onset is usually at 2 to 3 months of age. This is a rare form of the disease. Patients with neonatal onset frequently have no antibodies to acetylcholine receptors, and at least some may have a totally unrelated disease, so more care is required in diagnosis.

3. Juvenile—these cases are similar to the adult cases and can be grouped in the same manner.

Although respiratory insufficiency is rare, some patients require permanent tracheostomy and ventilation, usually at night. One must distinguish between patients who have bulbar symptoms alone and those with primary respiratory muscle weakness. Bulbar involvement with oropharyngeal weakness occurs in one third of patients as a presenting symptom and in two thirds of patients at some time in the disease process. Oropharyngeal weakness may make patients with normal respiratory reserve have difficulty in breathing. Secretions pool in the hypopharynx and cannot readily be swallowed or cleared. This produces obstruction—and, on occasion, aspiration. Those with primary respiratory symptoms have weakness of the respiratory muscles, making it difficult to clear secretions. A combination of both bulbar and primary respiratory weakness can lead to rapidly progressive respiratory failure, yet the patient may appear well-compensated until some slight change (e.g., a small dose of sedative, secretions, viral illness) starts the downhill course. It should not be forgotten that many nonanesthetic drugs, such as the "mycin" antibiotics, exacerbate the muscle weakness in these patients. These drugs must be avoided if possible, and if they are used, careful monitoring of respiratory function is required.[161] Patients in remission and those with mild forms of the disease are not truly "normal," and a myasthenic response to drugs, though it does not always occur, must be anticipated.

Although the causal event is unknown, approximately 85 per cent of patients have antibodies to human skeletal muscle acetylcholine receptors.[405] The antibodies produced vary greatly in specificity and action. Their clinical significance is just beginning to be understood.[406] The presence of antibody to receptor is highly specific for the disease (only 5 per cent of patients with Eaton-Lambert syndrome and 10 per cent of patients with amyotrophic lateral sclerosis exhibit positive results; virtually all other neurologic illnesses give negative results), although the absence of antibody does not rule out myasthenia. In one series, however, the false-positive results were all from patients who had anesthesia within 48 hours and were given muscle relaxants.[406] The cause for this remains unknown, but blood for antibody levels must not be obtained shortly after an anesthesia procedure. The antibody to the acetylcholine receptor is also found in patients with penicillamine-induced myasthenia gravis[407] and after bone marrow transplantation. The latter have an increased incidence of both the disease and antibody levels.[408] The antibody is not bound directly to the site that binds acetylcholine, but it is close to it and causes an increase in the rate of receptor destruction. The antibody may also directly reduce binding of acetylcholine to the receptor. A further mechanism would be complement binding to the receptor. It is likely that the reduction in binding of acetylcholine is not the major mechanism of action of the antibody, since antibody titers frequently do not correlate with the severity of the disease, even serial values in a single patient. Previously held theories—including excessive hydrolysis of acetylcholine and packets of acetylcholine containing subnormal quantities of acetylcholine at the nerve terminal—do not account for classic myasthenia gravis but may be responsible for rarer myasthenia-like syndromes.

The thymus gland is intimately involved in the disease process. This observation has led to the use of thymectomy as a therapeutic measure. Roughly 25 per cent of patients have remission (i.e., they can stop drug therapy completely). A total of 70 to 80 per cent improve after thymectomy. The improvement may occur rapidly, but maximum response may require several years.[409] The finding that antibody can be made by long-lived plasma cells in bone marrow and lymph nodes may explain the slow response to thymectomy.[410] Though the association of myasthenia and the thymus was discovered because some 30 to 50 per cent of patients with thymoma have myasthenia, patients with thymoma actually have a poorer response rate to thymectomy: only 25 per cent show improvement after tumor removal. Myasthenia may even first occur after the tumor is removed or become worse with surgery or radiation therapy, and there must be awareness of this possibility to prevent further complications.

The prevalence of other autoimmune diseases is high in these patients,[411] especially of rheumatoid arthritis and thyroid diseases. Hyperthyroidism is a common association. Seizures are also seen with a higher frequency than would be expected, which may in some way relate to the antibodies seen in the cerebrospinal fluid of mice with experimental autoimmune myasthenia gravis.

The diagnosis of myasthenia can be made by both the clinical symptoms and the characteristic EMG, which shows that by 2.5 seconds at least 10 per cent fade at 2 Hz and 50 per cent at 50 Hz.[412] Clinically, the observed weakness on repeated use shows improvement following the administration of an anticholinesterase agent such as edrophonium. Relatively small doses are used—1-, 3-, and 6-mg doses at 3-minute intervals. The response may be difficult to evaluate in patients with pure ocular weakness. A placebo, usually atropine to prevent cholinergic symptoms, is injected first, and the patient's strength is noted, looking at eye motion, speech, vital capacity, and grip strength; the patient is then retested after anticholinesterase administration. A small percentage of patients who do not show the characteristic improvement with anticholinesterase administration may require a curare test for diagnosis. The curare test, once very popular, is rarely used now. The drawbacks of curare testing are that it exacerbates the symptoms of myasthenia and may actually produce severe respiratory embarrassment. The maximum dose of d-tubocurarine given to the test is 0.03 mg/kg, one tenth the normal curarizing dose. It is drawn into a syringe and given in increments intravenously. As soon as there is an exaggeration of symptoms or the characteristic EMG (fade on repetitive nerve stimulation) is seen, the test is stopped. Aggravation of symptoms and onset of weakness before the maximum test dose is given is diagnostic of myasthenia. Preparation for assisting ventilation is mandatory, and anesthesiologists usually get involved at this point. Use of the curare test below a tourniquet was also employed, in a manner similar to a Bier block, using curare, 0.2 mg, instead of a local anesthetic. EMG is useful only if the tested muscle is involved. In some studies, 95 per cent of patients can be diagnosed if three muscle groups are tested. A nerve stimulator, even in the train-of-four mode, may not show fade in the muscles tested. Commonly, the weakness is proximal, the fade may be less than 20 per cent, and recovery may occur after the fourth twitch. If high rates of stimulation are used, post-tetanic facilitation occurs, but this is followed within 5 to 10 minutes by exhaustion with progressive weakness. Fade, even in affected muscles, may not be seen at less than 50 Hz.[413]

Therapy for the disease consists of giving anticholinesterase agents; the one most commonly used is oral pyridostigmine. Patients seem to prefer pyridostigmine to neostigmine or physostigmine, as its duration of action is longer and it does not cause as many side effects. Parenteral use of these agents requires care; the doses usually used to reverse neuromuscular block are much larger than those required to treat myasthenia and may well precipitate cholinergic crisis. The correct amount is 1/30 as much pyridostigmine; alternatively, 1/15 of the neostigmine oral dose can be given parenterally for the same effect. Thus, doses of 1 to 2 mg of pyridostigmine or 0.25 to 0.5 mg of neostigmine are frequently adequate. Ephedrine may also be used to increase the patient's sense of well-being and to potentiate the effects of the anticholinesterase; however, it is rarely used now. The course of the disease improves under medical treatment in 30 per cent of patients, whereas surgery improves the condition in almost 90 per cent of patients.[414] Surgery is being recommended for more and more of these patients, as documentation of its superiority and low morbidity and mortality makes it the logical choice.

The use of steroids in large doses has gained in popularity, but this does have a high rate of complications.[415] The myasthenia is frequently made worse initially (7 to 14 days), and the rates of cataracts and other steroid-related problems are high. The steroids are given in an attempt to decrease the antibody response to muscle acetylcholine receptors. At present, there is some question about whether steroid therapy, or for that matter remission after surgery, actually changes the myasthenia patient's response to muscle relaxants (see later discussion). Other immunosuppressive agents are being used with varying success. The most commonly used ones—cyclophosphamide, azathioprine, and cyclosporine—each produce remission and potentiation of the steroid effect but also carry risks. The effects of immunosuppressive therapy take longer to peak than the effects of steroids.[416] The sensitivity to muscle relaxants has not been systematically tested in any patient in remission, whether the remission

was spontaneous, after thymectomy, or drug induced. The results of testing would, of course, depend on the particular group of muscles chosen and might not reflect those we are most interested in clinically, such as the oropharyngeal muscles.

Plasmapheresis as a method of obtaining short-term improvement has shown promise, though it is time consuming and may deplete pseudocholinesterase and cause electrolyte abnormalities.[416–420] Its use every other day for five times per day improves symptoms in 3 to 14 days. One study showed that it significantly shortened the postoperative requirement for ventilation and intensive care stay.[421] The use of intravenous gamma globulin, 0.4 g/kg per day, produces results very much like those of plasmapheresis and last as long as 50 days.[416]

Myasthenic crisis is defined as an exacerbation of symptoms so severe that it involves the respiratory muscles. It may result directly from increased muscle weakness or it can be secondary to infection. Oropharyngeal weakness predisposes to respiratory infection. Increased secretions, respiratory infection, and muscle weakness produce a vicious cycle leading to respiratory failure. These symptoms may not satisfactorily respond to anticholinesterase therapy, and the patient may well need respirator support. Exacerbations of the disease occur spontaneously, and myasthenia patients may die unexpectedly and for no apparent reason. They must be watched closely.

Cholinergic crisis, which is sometimes difficult to distinguish from myasthenic crisis, is the result of overtreatment with anticholinesterase agents. It consists of worsening of the myasthenic syndrome, not just cholinergic symptoms of increased secretions and bradycardia (which could be easily treated with atropine). Since the individual muscle sensitivity to anticholinesterase agents varies, it is possible to overtreat some muscles while undertreating others. This is particularly common in patients with ocular myasthenia. The ocular muscles are relatively resistant to treatment with anticholinesterase agents, and to achieve adequate relief of ocular symptoms overtreatment of other muscle groups may occur, resulting in increased muscle weakness.

It has been recommended that these two crises be distinguished by the injection of edrophonium, to a maximum dose of 10 mg in an average 70-kg patient. If muscle strength improves, the patient is undertreated with anticholinesterase therapy. If no increase in muscle strength occurs or if respiratory distress becomes worse, the patient is probably in a cholinergic crisis. Respiratory support, if needed, should not await the anticholinesterase test. For patients with weak levator palpebrae and otherwise stable disease, surgery to shorten the levators works well. This decreases the need for anticholinesterase agents and indirectly makes cholinergic crisis less likely.

The published anesthetic experience in this disease is quite large and continues to grow. The reports frequently relate the use of the newest agents and demonstrate their safety; however, the vast majority of reports are of patients having thymectomy.[409, 422-26] Anesthesia for this procedure requires no muscle relaxation, but postoperative ventilatory assistance is common because myasthenic patients may have exacerbations of symptoms and may well develop myasthenic crises after any operative intervention. Postoperative ventilatory assistance may be required even for peripheral surgery. Experience with regional and local anesthesia[427] has indicated that, if possible, these techniques should be used; however, ester local anesthesia may prove more toxic to these patients. The anticholinesterase agents inhibit pseudocholinesterase and reduce hydrolysis of ester local anesthetic agents. Small doses, such as tetracaine in spinal anesthesia, would not be contraindicated.

An unresolved controversy is whether to maintain myasthenic patients on anticholinesterase therapy preoperatively, intraoperatively, and postoperatively.[423, 424, 427, 428] Patients who are dependent on anticholinesterase therapy for their well-being and who have more than just ocular symptoms would seem best treated with little break in their usual anticholinesterase therapy regimen. Thus, a patient who describes severe weakness on arising in the morning, has trouble with respiration before the first dose of anticholinesterase, and can barely swallow the pills should continue taking the drug, particularly if the operation is going to take place late in the morning or in the afternoon. Conversely, patients who have only mild symptoms can clearly do without their medication, especially if the operative procedure is to take place early in the day. Anticholinesterase agents complicate the anesthetic management, as they potentiate vagal responses and (as mentioned) decrease the metabolism of

ester local anesthetics. Relaxation may also be more difficult to produce. Anticholinesterase agents have also been seen to *increase* the duration and efficacy of narcotics. Preoperative anticholinesterase therapy should produce little problem for the anesthesiologist who understands the drug's action.

As mentioned earlier in this chapter, patients with little respiratory reserve tolerate any sedative premedication poorly. Therefore, myasthenic patients should be given little premedication, if any. Suggestions that patients be intentionally tired out so that muscle relaxation secondary to tiring will facilitate intubation seem unnecessary and in fact may lead to exhaustion, with prolonged muscle weakness.[429] Dantrolene did not work as an aid in muscle relaxation, and, in fact, myasthenic patients may be somewhat resistant to its muscle-relaxing effects.[430] The patient with an empty stomach may be given intravenous induction, which is deepened with an inhalational anesthetic. The patient is then intubated without the use of either nondepolarizing or depolarizing muscle relaxants. The potent inhalational agents cause relaxation in large doses, and isoflurane causes more depression of the twitch height than halothane at equal multiples of MAC.[431] If muscle relaxants are necessary intraoperatively, the smallest doses possible are given, remembering that myasthenic patients are exquisitely sensitive to nondepolarizing muscle relaxants. Recently, the intermediate-duration relaxants vecuronium[412, 432-434] and atracurium[435-437] have been used, with expected results: small doses produce good relaxation, and reversal was possible. There was, however, wide patient variation, and no arbitrarily selected dose would be either safe or adequate. As expected, the pharmacokinetics remain normal, so the dose needed per hour is related to the original sensitivity;[431] although, if the procedure can be performed with general anesthesia alone, it does not seem warranted to use muscle relaxants.[424] The use of succinylcholine for intubation has both advantages and disadvantages. The myasthenic patient is inherently less responsive to succinylcholine, and the ED_{90} may be greater than 1 mg/kg (as compared with 0.3 in normal healthy persons). Thus, larger doses are recommended to produce adequate block.[413] Anticholinesterase agents are also pseudocholinesterase antagonists, however, so the response to succinylcholine is somewhat unpredictable. In general, the normal intubating doses of succinylcholine are used when succinylcholine must be used in a myasthenic patient. In our experience, the usual intubating dose of succinylcholine produces adequate relaxation and apparently rapid recovery; however, careful study of neuromuscular transmission by EMG has shown disturbing results in a number of patients. Phase II block occurs frequently, even at 0.5 mg/kg, and recovery is slow.[413] We have seen some patients who recover to less than 60 per cent of normal and then maintain this degree of blockade for several hours after a single dose of succinylcholine. Succinylcholine is nevertheless not contraindicated in these patients, as long as the possibility of prolonged neuromuscular block is understood. The use of mivacurium is more complex. Since it is metabolized by pseudocholinesterase, patients taking anticholinesterase agents may recover slowly. Patients not taking these agents may benefit by the short duration of action. It must be remembered that sensitivity to the muscle relaxants varies and that the response to stimulating the ulnar nerve may not predict the degree of weakness of the accessory muscles of respiration— bulbar muscles and diaphragm. This may have been responsible for the appearance of respiratory failure, in spite of normal twitch, in a patient reported by Frazer.[438]

Several groups of investigators have attempted to predict which myasthenic patients will require postoperative ventilation.[422, 423, 425, 426, 439] At present, no criteria have been developed that uniformly distinguish patients who require long-term ventilation from those who do not. Radically different durations of ventilatory support seem to correlate more with the prejudices of the institution than with differences in patients. Some institutions keep most myasthenic patients intubated for 3 days or more, whereas others expect to extubate all patients in the operating room.[440] Certain findings do seem to warn of potential problems and are clearly more important for patients undergoing more physically demanding operations. Patients who have a preoperative vital capacity less than 2 L, an expiratory force less than 40 cm H_2O, and an inspiratory force less than 30 cm H_2O may be difficult to wean. Both inspiration and expiration should be measured, since the expiratory muscles are needed to clear secretions and may be weaker than the inspiratory muscles in many patients.[426] Other factors that alert to postoperative problems include duration of disease greater than 6 years and any intercurrent respiratory problems. A recent scoring system has been useful in transcervical thymectomy,[422] but it may not be as useful for transsternal thymectomy and may not be useful in all hands.[425, 426, 439, 441] It is of doubtful value for abdominal surgery.

Although our own prejudice is that bulbar symptoms are a poor prognostic sign, they have not been shown conclusively to affect the requirement for postoperative ventilation. Bulbar symptoms may[423, 425] or may not[422] contribute to the need for postoperative ventilatory support. Clearly, a larger percentage of patients undergoing major upper abdominal or thoracic surgery require respiratory support.

There is some question as to whether long-term use of anticholinesterase agents by patients who undergo bowel anastomoses may increase the risk of anastomotic leaks.[442] Because of this, it is suggested that patients who have bowel surgery not be given continuous anticholinesterase therapy in the postoperative period but rather, if necessary, be ventilated. Continuous anticholinergic therapy may be an alternative.

In spite of major improvements in their clinical symptoms, patients taking large doses of steroids may still have increased sensitivity to nondepolarizing muscle relaxants. One patient reported by Griggs showed an eightfold decrease in sensitivity to curare after adrenocorticotropic hormone therapy. Others have also seen normal responses after remission.[435] In contrast, Lake[443] reported one patient who underwent two successive operations, one 2 months and the other 4 months after the start of steroid therapy (good symptomatic improvement in myasthenia symptoms was reported). The patient remained exquisitely sensitive to small doses of *d*-tubocurarine. On one occasion, the patient required reversal 2 hours after the administration of 6 mg of curare. Others have reported abnormal sensitivity during remission[444] or even excessive sensitivity to "mycin" antibiotics after surgical remission.[417] We have seen a patient who had been treated with steroids for her myasthenia respond normally to pancuronium. Others have reported normal sensitivity to succinylcholine during remission.[445] A wide range of responses may thus be anticipated.

Regardless of preoperative management, postoperative anticholinesterase therapy should be based on the edrophonium test, since the requirements for anticholinesterase agents change in the postoperative period.[427, 428] Early extubation, if possible, seems warranted by the published case reports, though it must be understood that the patient may tire and require reintubation after many hours of apparently normal ventilation. Our personal practice is to allow a trial of spontaneous ventilation when the patient has an inspiratory force greater than -30 cm H_2O and a vital capacity of at least 15 mL/kg body weight. The patient is then allowed to maintain ventilation for 1 to 2 hours, during which time arterial blood gases are checked to ensure that there is no fatigue. In addition, vital capacity measurements and clinical assessment continue. Under these conditions, anticholinesterase therapy may be reinstituted and the patient may be extubated. Even then, it is mandatory that respiratory support be available immediately. We manage these patients in an intensive care unit. Those who do not meet these criteria preoperatively may still be able to support themselves postoperatively. In this case, we use their preoperative level as a goal. Such patients may be particularly difficult to wean, and multiple attempts may be necessary before they become independent of ventilatory assistance.

Occasionally, patients will maintain adequate vital capacity and adequate blood gas parameters with an endotracheal tube in place only to suffer rapid decompensation on extubation. We feel that these patients are predominantly the ones who have oropharyngeal weakness and are incapable of taking care of their own secretions and maintaining a patent airway. The response of such patients is difficult to predict. Only careful evaluation and constant vigilance allow them to be extubated safely.

Pregnancy is a stress to the myasthenic patient. The symptoms of the disease respond unpredictably to pregnancy, but the patient has a 30 per cent chance of getting worse during the puerperium and then returns to the prepregnant state of weakness immediately postpartum.[446–448] Maternal and fetal mortality rates are increased approximately fivefold by the disease. The use of regional anesthesia is preferred, but complications in the unprotected airway may result from weakness alone.[449] As mentioned earlier, 20 per cent of newborns of myasthenic mothers are myasthenic in the neonatal period. These infants require careful evaluation and respiratory support as well as anticholinesterase therapy when indicated.

In summary, the treatment of the myas-

thenic patient must be individualized to the preoperative severity of the disease. The use of regional or local anesthesia seems warranted whenever possible. General anesthesia can be performed safely. Postoperatively, patients must be carefully monitored and frequently evaluated, as changes in ventilatory status are unpredictable. Patients in remission may still be myasthenic in their response to drugs and stress. The use of anticholinesterase agents in the immediate preoperative and postoperative periods is still controversial.

B. EATON-LAMBERT SYNDROME

Patients with the Eaton-Lambert syndrome characteristically have weakness, usually in the proximal limb muscles, the lower muscles being more involved than the upper ones.[450] Rarely are bulbar or ocular muscles involved. Unlike in myasthenia gravis, strength increases with activity. Characteristically, this disease is thought of only as a neuromuscular disease, but recent reports have demonstrated a defect in the autonomic nervous system. Thus, on ECG, RR interval variability normally seen with respiration is decreased, and symptoms of constipation, dry mouth, urinary retention, and orthostatic hypotension are common.[451] This syndrome has been associated with carcinoma, most often of the bronchus, but patients have been observed with thoracic extensions of carcinoma of the prostate, breast, stomach, and rectum. One third of patients never have a tumor.[450] The degree of muscle weakness is not related to the severity of other systemic effects of the tumor, such as weight loss and muscle wasting. The carcinoma itself may not be obvious on examination and it may take as long as 2 years after the symptoms of muscle weakness develop before it is discovered. Removal of the tumor does not always affect the weakness.

There is reduced muscle response to single-nerve stimulus; however, using tetanic stimulation, muscle strength increases progressively as the frequency and duration of the stimulation are increased. This picture is the reverse of that seen in myasthenia gravis. Post-tetanic potentiation is marked. At the present time, the best evidence is that the number of quanta of acetylcholine released per nerve impulse is decreased, but the end-plate sensitivity is normal—again, unlike myasthenia gravis. The mechanism seems to be reduced access of calcium through voltage-operated calcium channels, with a reduction of the calcium-dependent exocytosis of acetylcholine packets through the presynaptic membrane.[452] Although as many as 5 per cent of these patients have antiacetylcholine receptor antibodies,[406] they are not thought responsible for the disease. The cause is also autoimmune: serum or IgG can transfer the disease to an animal model. An antibody to voltage-operated calcium channels has been demonstrated but does not account for all cases, and some patients with the antibody do not have the disease.[452] An antibody to a calcium channel–associated protein synaptogamin has also been demonstrated and may help our understanding of the mechanism. Some of these patients show improvement after corticosteroid and azathioprine administration, though there is concern about using the latter drug in a patient with a neoplasm.[450] Also, like autoimmune myasthenia gravis, plasmapheresis can be used acutely to treat the disease, and the same warnings about the effects of plasmapheresis apply here.

Patients are extremely sensitive to both nondepolarizing and depolarizing muscle relaxants, and the weakness that occurs after use of these agents may last many days. Other drugs that cause weakness include antiarrhythmics, procainamide, beta blockers, quinidine, calcium channel blockers, aminoglycoside antibiotics, magnesium, and iodine contrast. The response to anticholinesterase drugs is poor, but guanidine hydrochloride will produce marked improvement. Guanidine is used in doses of 10 to 35 mg/kg per day, but it has many toxic effects, including renal failure, bone marrow depression, atrial fibrillation, and hypotension. Experimentally, 3,4-diaminopyridine, which increases release of acetylcholine on nerve impulses, seems like the best agent.[452] Since many of these patients require anesthesia for biopsy and treatment of their primary malignancy, anesthesiologists are confronted with a patient who may need general anesthesia and muscle relaxation but who would suffer prolonged weakness from muscle relaxants. The use of an inhalational anesthetic would seem the wisest course; however, if adequate muscle relaxation cannot be provided by the inhalational anesthetic, short-acting muscle relaxants may be used, with the understanding that prolonged ventilatory assistance may be required. At the end of the procedure, the usual means for evaluating muscle relaxation can be used and anticholinesterase agents can be given to re-verse nondepolarizing block. The patients should then be tested for ventilatory adequacy. This should include a trial of spontaneous ventilation, to see if the patient requires ventilatory assistance. The usual means and criteria for extubation should be applied to these patients.

C. OTHER MYASTHENIA SYNDROMES

A rare patient has myasthenia-like symptoms, frequently from birth, that appear to be hereditary. All patients show fatigue, but not all respond to anticholinesterase treatment. The neuromuscular defect has been identified in several of these patients, whereas others still are not fully characterized. The best-documented is the absence of acetylcholine esterase at the end-plate. In the one patient found so far, this defect produced fluctuating ptosis, strabismus, slowed motor development, scoliosis, and reduced motor bulk. The patient has not responded to anticholinesterase therapy as might be predicted from the cause. Another, more common, form is a defect in acetylcholine mobilization, originally called *familial infantile myasthenia*. It is an autosomal recessive trait. Infants with this disease show fluctuating weakness with episodes of profound weakness and apnea, and death may occur after crying. The defect is decreased mobilization of acetylcholine after stimulation (i.e., after exercise). These patients respond well to anticholinesterase therapy. A third disorder called *slow-channel syndrome* is a dominant trait that can present at any age, with weakness and fatigability. The muscles most affected are those in the fingers and hands. As its name implies, it is caused by prolonged open time of the acetylcholine receptor channel. No therapy is currently available for this syndrome. There are also patients who exhibit reduced numbers of receptors, reduced affinity of the receptor for acetylcholine, and even an increase in the receptor's affinity for curare. No anesthetic experience is reported for any of these patients, but anesthesia would be expected to produce problems with the use of muscle relaxants, and the underlying weakness might well cause respiratory difficulty on its own.[450]

These rare syndromes are presented to alert readers to the possibility of unusual causes of myasthenia that might well increase the risk and change the therapy for the myasthenic patient who is assumed to be of the autoimmune type.[450]

REFERENCES

Muscular Dystrophies

1. Engel AG: Duchenne dystrophy. *In* Engel AG, Banker BQ (eds): Myology. New York, McGraw-Hill, 1986.
2. Fadic R, Sunada Y, Waclawik AJ, et al: Deficiency of a dystrophin-associated glycoprotein (adhalin) in a patient with muscular dystrophy and cardiomyopathy. N Engl J Med 334:362, 1996.
3. Thompson MW: The genetic transmission of muscle diseases. *In* Engel AG, Banker BQ (eds): Myology. New York, McGraw-Hill, 1986.
4. Bushby KM, Goodship JA, Nicholson LV, et al: Variability in clinical, genetic and protein abnormalities in manifesting carriers of Duchenne and Becker muscular dystrophy. Neuromuscul Disord 3:57, 1993.
5. Goedde HW, Christ I, Benkmann HG, et al: Creatine kinase isoenzyme patterns in Duchenne muscular dystrophy. Clin Genet 14:257, 1978.
6. Griggs RC, Mendell JR, Miller RG: The muscular dystrophies. *In* Evaluation and Treatment of Myopathies. Philadelphia, FA Davis, 1995.
7. Shapiro F, Sethna N, Colan S, et al: Spinal fusion in Duchenne muscular dystrophy: A multidisciplinary approach. J Muscle Nerve 15:604, 1992.
8. Chenard AA, Becane HM, Tertrain F, et al: arrhythmia in Duchenne muscular dystrophy: Prevalence, significance and prognosis. Neuromuscul Disord 3:201, 1993.
9. Jenkins JG, Bohn D, Edmonds JF, et al: Evaluation of pulmonary function in muscular dystrophy patients requiring spinal surgery. Crit Care Med 10:645, 1982.
10. Milne B, Rosales JK: Anaesthetic considerations in patients with muscular dystrophy undergoing spinal fusion and Harrington rod insertion. Can Anaesth Soc J 29:250, 1982.
11. Smith CL, Bush GH: Anaesthesia and progressive muscular dystrophy. Br J Anaesth 57:1113, 1985.
12. DiMarco AF, Kelling JS, DiMarco MS, et al: The effects of inspiratory resistive training on respiratory muscle function in patients with muscular dystrophy. Muscle Nerve 8:284, 1985.
13. Raphael JC, Chevret S, Chastang C, Bouvet F: Randomised trial of preventive nasal ventilation in Duchenne muscular dystrophy. French Multicentre Cooperative Group on Home Mechanical Ventilation Assistance in Duchenne de Boulogne Muscular Dystrophy. Lancet 343:1600, 1994.
14. Cobham IG, Davis HS: Anesthesia for muscular dystrophy patients. Anesth Analg 43:22, 1964.
15. Richards WC: Anaesthesia and serum creatine phosphokinase levels in patients with Duchenne's pseudohypertrophic muscular dystrophy. Anaesth Intensive Care 1:150, 1972.
16. Boba A: Fatal postanesthetic complications in two muscular dystrophic patients. J Pediatr Surg 5:71, 1970.
17. Genever EE: Suxamethonium-induced cardiac arrest in unsuspected pseudohypertrophic muscular dystrophy. Case report. Br J Anaesth 43:984, 1971.
18. Kepes ER, Martinez LR, Andrews CI, et al: Anesthetic problems in hereditary muscular abnormalities. Clinical Anesthesia Conference. NY State J Med 72:1051, 1972.
19. Miller ED Jr, Sanders DB, Rowlingson JC, et al: Anesthesia-induced rhabdomyolysis in a patient with Duchenne's muscular dystrophy. Anesthesiology 48:146, 1978.
20. Seay AR, Ziter FA, Thompson JA: Cardiac arrest during induction of anesthesia in Duchenne muscular dystrophy. J Pediatr 93:88, 1978.
21. Marchildon MB: Malignant hyperthermia. Current concepts. Arch Surg 117:349, 1982.
22. Oka S, Igarashi Y, Takagi A, et al: Malignant hyperpyrexia and Duchenne muscular dystrophy: A case report. Can Anaesth Soc J 29:627, 1982.
23. Smith CL, Bush GH: Anaesthesia and progressive muscular dystrophy. Br J Anaesth 57:1113, 1985.
24. Brownell AKW: Malignant hyperthermia: Relationship to other diseases. Br J Anaesth 60:303, 1988.
25. Ginsburg RS, Porterfield K, Lippmann M: Propofol: Bolus induction plus continuous infusion in a patient with Duchenne muscular dystrophy [letter]. Anesthesiology 75:376, 1991.
26. Maccani RM, Wedel DJ, Melton A, Gronert GA: Femoral and lateral femoral cutaneous nerve block for muscle biopsies in children. Paediatr Anaesth 5:223, 1995.
27. Reich DR, Neff J: Oral-surgical management of an odontogenic keratocyst in a patient with Duchenne muscular dystrophy. Pediatr Dent 3:343, 1981.
28. Sethna NF, Berde CB: Continuous subarachnoid analgesia in two adolescents with severe scoliosis and impaired pulmonary function. Reg Anesth 16:333, 1991.
29. Barohn RJ, Levine EJ, Olson JO, et al: Gastric hypomotility in Duchenne's muscular dystrophy. N Engl J Med 319:15, 1988.
30. Bush GH: Pharmacogenetics and anesthesia. Proc R Soc Med 61:171, 1968.
31. Wislicki L: Anaesthesia and postoperative complication in progressive muscular dystrophy. Anaesthesia 17:482, 1962.
32. Fairfield MC: Increased propofol requirements in a child with Duchenne muscular dystrophy [letter]. Anaesthesia 48:1013, 1993.
33. Bushby KM, Thambyayah M, Gardner-Medwin D: Prevalence and incidence of Becker muscular dystrophy. Lancet 337:1022, 1991.
34. Grimm T: Becker dystrophy. In Engel AG, Banker BQ (eds): Myology. New York, McGraw-Hill, 1986.
35. Chalkiadis GA, Branch KG: Cardiac arrest after isoflurane anaesthesia in a patient with Duchenne's muscular dystrophy. Anaesthesia 45:22, 1990.
36. Bush A, Dubowitz V: Fatal rhabdomyolysis complicating general anaesthesia in a child with Becker muscular dystrophy. Neuromuscul Disord 1:201, 1991.
37. Waters DD, Nutter DO, Hopkins LC, et al: Cardiac features of an unusual X-linked humeroperoneal neuromuscular disease. N Engl J Med 293:1017, 1975.
38. Emery AE: X-linked muscular dystrophy with early contractures and cardiomyopathy (Emery-Dreifuss type). Clin Genet 32:360, 1987.
39. Morrison P, Jago RH: Emery-Dreifuss muscular dystrophy. Anaesthesia 46:33, 1991.
40. Ras GJ, van Staden M, Schultz C, et al: Respiratory manifestations of rigid spine syndrome. Am J Respir Crit Care Med 150:540, 1994.

41. Kilburn KH, Eagan JT, Sicker HO: Cardiopulmonary insufficiency in myotonic and progressive muscular dystrophy. N Engl J Med 261:1089, 1959.

42. Dresner DL, Ali HH: Anaesthetic management of a patient with Facioscapulohumeral muscular dystrophy. Br J Anaesth 62:331, 1989.

43. Rowland LP, Eskenazi AN: Myasthenia gravis with features resembling muscular dystrophy. Neurology 6:667, 1956.

44. Ross RT: Ocular myopathy sensitive to curare. Brain 86:67, 1963.

45. Jacob JG, Varkey GP: Curare sensitivity in ocular myopathy. Can Anaesth Soc J 13:449, 1966.

46. Robertson JA: Ocular muscular dystrophy. A cause of curare sensitivity. Anaesthesia 39:251, 1984.

47. Landrum AL, Eggers GW: Oculopharyngeal dystrophy: An approach to anesthetic management. Anesth Analg 75:1043, 1992.

48. Banker BQ: Congenital muscular dystrophy. In Engel AG, Banker BQ (eds): Myology. New York, McGraw-Hill, 1986.

49. Fletcher R, Blennow G, Olsson A-K, et al: Malignant hyperthermia in a myopathic child. Prolonged postoperative course requiring dantrolene. Acta Anaesthesiol Scand 26:435, 1982.

Myotonias

50. Harper PS: Myotonic disorders. In Engel AG, Banker BQ (eds): Myology. New York, McGraw-Hill, 1986, pp. 1267–1296.

51. Ptacek LJ, Johnson KJ, Griggs RC: Mechanisms of disease: Genetics of the myotonic muscle disorders. N Engl J Med 328:482, 1993.

52. Denny-Brown D, Nevein S: The phenomenon of myotonia. Brain 64:1, 1941.

53. Landau W: Essential mechanism in myotonia: An electromyographic study. Neurology 2:369, 1952.

54. Orndahl G: Myotonic human musculature; stimulation with depolarizing agents. 1. Mechanical registration of the effects of acetylcholine and choline. Acta Med Scand 172:739, 1962. 2. Clinicopharmacologic study. Acta Med Scand 172:753, 1962.

55. Harley HG, Brook JD, Rundle SA, et al: Expansion of an unstable DNA region and phenotypic variation in myotonic dystrophy. Nature 355:545 1992.

56. Moorman JR, Coleman RE, Packer DL, et al: Cardiac involvement in myotonic muscular dystrophy. Medicine (Baltimore) 64:371, 1985.

57. Cannon PJ: The heart and lungs in myotonic muscular dystrophy. Am J Med 32:765, 1962.

58. Harris MN: Extradural analgesia and dystrophia myotonia [letter]. Anaesthesia 39:1032, 1984.

59. Grigg LE, Chan W, Mond HG, et al: Ventricular tachycardia and sudden death in myotonic dystrophy: Clinical, electrophysiologic and pathologic features. J Am Coll Cardiol 6:254, 1985.

60. Johnson ER, Abresch RT, Carter GT, et al: Profiles of neuromuscular diseases. Myotonic dystrophy. Am J Phys Med Rehab 74(5 Suppl):S104, 1995.

61. Meyers MB, Garash PG: Case history number 90: Cardiac decompensation during enflurane anesthesia in a patient with myotonia atrophica. Anesth Analg 55:433, 1976.

62. Begin R, Bureau MA, Lupien L, et al: Pathogenesis of respiratory insufficiency in myotonic dystrophy: The mechanical factors. Am Rev Respir Dis 125:312, 1982.

63. Nightingale P, Healy TE, McGuinness K: Dystrophia

64. Kilburn KH, Eagan JT, Heyman A: Cardiopulmonary insufficiency associated with myotonic dystrophy. Am J Med 26:929, 1959.

65. Coccagna G, Mantovani M, Parchi C, et al: Alveolar hypoventilation and hypersomnia in myotonic dystrophy. J Neurol Neurosurg Psychiatry 38:977, 1975.

66. Tsueda K, Shibutani K, Lefkowitz M: Postoperative ventilatory failure in an obese, myopathic woman with periodic somnolence: A case report. Anesth Analg 54:523, 1975.

67. de Backer M, Bergmann P, Perissino A, et al: Respiratory failure and cardiac disturbances in myotonic dystrophy. Eur J Intensive Care Med 2:63, 1976.

68. Pruzanski W, Profis A: Pulmonary disease in myotonic dystrophy. Ann Rev Respir Dis 91:874, 1965.

69. Blanloeil Y, Rochedreux A, Arnould JF, et al: Complications respiratories postoperatoires de la myotonie dystrophique (maladie de Steinert). Ann Fr Anesth Reanim 3:303, 1984.

70. Desnoyers Y: A propos de la dystrophie myotonique. Can Anaesth Soc J 16:377, 1969.

71. Dundee JW: Thiopentone in dystrophia myotonica. Curr Res Anesth 31:257, 1952.

72. Bourke TD, Zuck D: Thiopentone in dystrophica myotonia. Br J Anaesth 29:35, 1957.

73. Hewer CL: Correspondence. Br J Anaesth 29:180, 1957.

74. Gardy HH: Dystrophia myotonica in pregnancy. Report of a case. Obstet Gynecol 21:441, 1963.

75. Gilbertson A, Boulton TB: Anesthesia in difficult situations. 6. Influence of disease on the preoperative preparation and choice of anesthesia. Anaesthesia 22:607, 1967.

76. Watson BM: Pharmacogenetics. Anaesthesia 24:230, 1969.

77. Aldridge LM: Anaesthetic problems in myotonic dystrophy. A case report and review of the Aberdeen experience comprising 48 general anaesthetics in a further 16 patients. Br J Anaesth 57:1119, 1985.

78. Muller H, Punt-van Manen JA: Maxillo-facial deformities in patients with dystrophia myotonica and the anaesthetic implications. J Maxillofacial Surg 10:224, 1982.

79. Speedy H: Exaggerated physiological responses to propofol in myotonic dystrophy. Br J Anaesth 64:110, 1990.

80. Tzabar Y, Marshall R: Myotonia dystrophy and target controlled propofol infusion. Br J Anaesth 74:108, 1995.

81. Kaufman L: Anesthesia in dystrophia myotonica: A review of the hazards of anesthesia. Proc R Soc Med 53:183, 1959.

82. Hunter AR: Commenting on a paper by Kaufman. Proc R Soc Med 53:187, 1959.

83. Ravin M, Newmark Z, Saviello G: Myotonia dystrophica—an anesthetic hazard: Two case reports. Anesth Analg 54:216, 1975.

84. Haley FC: Anaesthesia in dystrophic myotonia. Can Anesth Soc J 9:270, 1962.

85. Johnson GW, Chadwick S, Eadsforth P, Hartopp I: Anaesthesia and myotonia [letter]. Br J Anaesth 75:113, 1995.

86. Bouly A, Nathan A, Feiss P: Propofol in myotonic dystrophy Anaesthesia 46:705, 1991.

87. Hakim CA, Thomlinson J: Myotonia congenita in pregnancy. J Obstet Gynaecol Br Cwlth 76:561, 1969.

88. Hook R, Anderson EF, Noto P: Anesthetic manage-

ment of a parturient with myotonia atrophica. Anesthesiology 43:689, 1975.

89. Wheeler AS, James FM: Local anesthesia for laparoscopy in a case of myotonia dystrophica. Anesthesiology 50:169, 1979.

90. Mitchell MM, Ali HH, Savarese JJ: Myotonia and neuromuscular blocking agents. Anesthesiology 49:44, 1978.

91. Stirt JA, Stone DJ, Weinberg G, et al: Atracurium in a child with myotonic dystrophy. Anesth Analg 64:369, 1985.

92. Boheimer N, Harris JW, Ward S: Neuromuscular blockade in dystrophia myotonica with atracurium besylate. Anaesthesia 40:872, 1985.

93. Dawson AD, Duncan BA: Dantrolene sodium and dystrophia myotonica [letter]. Anaesthesia 40:596, 1985.

94. Buzello W, Krieg N, Schlickewei A: Hazards of neostigmine in patients with neuromuscular disorders. Report of two cases. Br J Anaesth 54:529, 1982.

95. Punt van Manen JA, Muller H, Kalenda Z: Anaesthesie bei Dystrophia Myotonica mit Hilfe des Kapnogramm. Anaesthetist 33:348, 1984.

96. Kaufman J, Friedman JM, Sadowsky D, et al: Myotonic dystrophy: Surgical and anesthetic considerations during orthognathic surgery. J Oral Maxillofac Surg 41:667, 1983.

97. Paterson I: Generalized myotonia following suxamethonium. Br J Anaesth 34:340, 1962.

98. Phillips DC, Ellis FR, Exley KA, et al: Dantrolene sodium and dystrophia myotonica. Anaesthesia 39:568, 1984.

99. Suppan P: Althesin in dystrophia myotonica. Anaesthesia 30:95, 1975.

100. Cope DK, Miller JN: Local and spinal anesthesia for cesarean section in a patient with myotonic dystrophy. Anesth Analg 65:687, 1986.

101. Paterson RA, Tousignant M, Skene DS: Caesarean section for twins in a patient with myotonic dystrophy. Can Anaesth Soc J 32:418, 1985.

102. Bray RJ, Inkster JS: Anaesthesia in babies with congenital dystrophia myotonica. Anaesthesia 39:1007, 1984.

103. Anderson BJ, Brown TC: Congenital myotonic dystrophy in children—a review of ten years' experience. Anaesth Intensive Care 17:320, 1989.

104. Alexander C, Wolf S, Ghia JN: Caudal anesthesia for early onset myotonic dystrophy. Anesthesiology 55:597, 1981.

105. Russell SH, Hirsch NP: Anaesthesia and myotonia. Br J Anaesth 72:210, 1994.

106. Hoffman EP: Voltage-gated ion channelopathies: Inherited disorders caused by abnormal sodium, chloride, and calcium regulation in skeletal muscle. Annu Rev Med 46:431, 1995.

107. Griggs RC, Mendell JR, Miller RG: Periodic paralysis and myotonia. In Evaluation and Treatment of Myopathies. Philadelphia, FA Davis, 1995.

108. Reece IJ, Kennedy JA, Simpson JA, et al: Hypothermic cardiopulmonary bypass in paramyotonia congenita: A case report. Thorax 38:476, 1983.

109. Vita GM, Olckers A, Jedlicka AE, et al: Masseter muscle rigidity associated with glycine 1306–to–alanine mutation in the adult muscle sodium channel alpha-subunit gene. Anesthesiology 82:1097, 1995.

Family Periodic Paralysis

110. Robson NJ: Emergency surgery complicated by thyrotoxicosis and thyrotoxic periodic paralysis. Anaesthesia 40:27, 1985.

111. Bashford AC: Case report: Anaesthesia in familial hypokalaemic periodic paralysis. Anaesth Intensive Care 5:74, 1977.

112. Horton B: Anesthetic experiences in a family with hypokalemic familial periodic paralysis. Anesthesiology 47:308, 1977.

113. Melnick B, Chang JL, Larson CE, et al: Hypokalemic familial periodic paralysis. Anesthesiology 58:263, 1983.

114. Fozard JR: Anaesthesia and familial hypokalaemic periodic paralysis [letter]. Anaesthesia 38:293, 1983.

115. Rollman JE, Dickson CM: Anesthetic management of a patient with hypokalemic familial periodic paralysis for coronary artery bypass surgery. Anesthesiology 63:526, 1985.

116. Egan TJ, Klein R: Hyperkalemic familial periodic paralysis. Pediatrics 24:761, 1959.

117. Ashwood EM, Russell WJ, Burrow DD: Hyperkalaemic periodic paralysis and anaesthesia. Anaesthesia 47:579, 1992.

118. Paasuke RT, Brownell AK: Serum creatine kinase level as a screening test for susceptibility to malignant hyperthermia. JAMA 255:769, 1986.

Endocrine Myopathies

119. Kaminski HJ, Ruff RL: Endocrine myopathies. In Engel AG, Franzini-Armstrong C (eds): Myology. New York, McGraw-Hill, 1994.

120. Weiner P, Azgad Y, Weiner M: The effects of corticosteroids on inspiratory muscle performance in humans. Chest 104:1788, 1993.

121. Askari A, Vignos PJ, Moskowitz RW: Steroid myopathy in connective tissue disease. Am J Med 61:485, 1976.

122. Falduto MT, Czerwinski SM, Hickson RC: Glucocorticoid-induced muscle atrophy prevention by exercise in fast-twitch fibers. J Appl Physiol 69:1058, 1990.

123. Elia M, Carter A, Bacon S, et al: Clinical usefulness of urinary 3-methylhistidine excretion in indicating muscle protein breakdown. Br Med J Clin Res 282:351, 1981.

124. Griggs RC, Mendell JR, Miller RG: Myopathies of systemic disease. In Evaluation and Treatment of Myopathies. Philadelphia, FA Davis, 1995.

125. Durant NN, Briscoe JR, Katz RL: The effects of acute and chronic hydrocortisone treatment on neuromuscular blockade in the anesthetized cat. Anesthesiology 61:144, 1984.

126. Schwartz AE, Matteo RS, Ornstein E, et al: Acute steroid therapy does not alter nondepolarizing muscle relaxant effects in humans. Anesthesiology 65:326, 1986.

127. Robinson BJ, Lee E, Rees D, et al: Betamethasone-induced resistance to neuromuscular blockade: A comparison of atracurium and vecuronium in vitro. Anesth Analg 74:762, 1992.

128. Watling SM, Dasta JF: Prolonged paralysis in intensive care unit patients after the use of neuromuscular blocking agents: A review of the literature. Crit Care Med 22:884, 1994.

129. Segredo V, Caldwell J, Matthay MA, et al: Persistent paralysis in critically ill patients after long-term administration of vecuronium. N Engl J Med 327:524, 1992.

130. Rossiter A, Souney P, McGowan S, et al: Pancuronium-induced prolonged neuromuscular blockade. Crit Care Med 19:1583, 1991.

131. Gooch J, Suchyta MR, Balbierz JM, et al: Prolonged

paralysis after treatment with neuromuscular junction blocking agents. Crit Care Med 19:1125, 1991.

132. Lebrault C, Duvaldestin P, Henzel D, et al: Pharmacokinetics and pharmacodynamics of vecuronium in patients with cholestasis. Br J Anaesth 25:983, 1986.

133. Danon MJ, Carpenter S: Myopathy with thick filament loss following prolonged paralysis with vecuronium during steroid treatment. Muscle Nerve 14:1131, 1991.

134. Griffin D, Fairman N, Coursin D, et al: Acute myopathy during treatment of status asthmaticus with corticosteroids and steroidal muscle relaxants. Chest 102:510, 1992.

135. Douglass JA, Tuxen DV, Horne M, et al: Myopathy in severe asthma. Am Rev Respir Dis 146:517, 1992.

136. Kupfer Y, Namba T, Kaldawi E, et al: Prolonged weakness after longterm infusion of vecuronium. Ann Intern Med 117:484, 1992.

137. Zochodne DW, Bolton CF, Walls GA, et al: Critical illness polyneuropathy. Brain 110:818, 1987.

138. Hemming AE, Charlton S, Kelly P: Hyperkalemia, cardiac arrest, suxamethonium and intensive care [letter]. Anaesthesia 45:990, 1990.

139. Horton WA, Fergusson NV: Hyperkalemia and cardiac arrest after the use of suxamethonium in intensive care. Anaesthesia 43:890, 1988.

140. Meyer KC, Prielipp RC, Grossman JE, et al: Prolonged weakness after infusion of atracurium in two intensive care unit patients. Anesth Analg 78:772, 1994.

141. Sweatman MCM, Chambers L: Disordered oesophageal motility in thyrotoxic myopathy. Postgrad Med J 61:619, 1985.

142. Bennett WR, Huston DP: Rhabdomyolysis in thyroid storm. Am J Med 77:733, 1984.

143. Blessing W, Walsh JC: Myotonia precipitated by propranolol therapy. Lancet 1:73, 1977.

144. Shergy WJ, Caldwell DS: Polymyositis after propylthiouracil treatment for hyperthyroidism. Ann Rheum Dis 47:340, 1988.

145. Peters KR, Nance P, Wingard DW: Malignant hyperthyroidism or malignant hyperthermia? Anesth Analg 60:613, 1981.

146. Ambus T, Evans S, Smith NT: Thyrotoxicosis factitia in the anesthetized patient. Anesthesiology 81:254, 1994.

147. Takamori M, Gutmann L, Crosby TW, et al: Myasthenic syndromes in hypothyroidism: Electrophysiological study of neuromuscular transmission and muscle contraction in two patients. Arch Neurol 26:326, 1972.

148. Miller LR, Benumof JL, Alexander L, et al: Completely absent response to peripheral nerve stimulation in an acutely hypothyroid patient. Anesthesiology 71:779, 1989.

149. Riggs JE: Acute exertional rhabdomyolysis in hypothyroidism: The result of a reversible defect in glycogenolysis? Mil Med 155:171, 1990.

150. Martinez FJ, Bermudez-Gomez M, Celli BR: Hypothyroidism, a reversible cause of diaphragmatic dysfunction. Chest 96:1059, 1989.

151. Domm BM, Vassallo CL: Myxedema coma with respiratory failure. Am Rev Respir Dis 107:842, 1973.

152. Takita K, Goda Y, Kemmotsu O, et al: Secondary hyperparathyroidism shortens the action of vecuronium in patients with chronic renal failure. Can J Anaesth 42:395, 1995.

153. Kirita A, Iwasaki H, Fujita S, et al: Vecuronium-induced neuromuscular blockade in two patients with hyperparathyroidism and a patient with hypoparathyroidism. Masui 41:136, 1992.

154. Wooldridge TD, Bower JD, Nelson NC: Rhabdomyolysis, a complication of parathyroidectomy and calcium supplementation. JAMA 239:643, 1978.

155. Russell JA: Osteomalacic myopathy. Muscle Nerve 17:578, 1994.

156. DiMauro S, Tonin P, Servidei S: Metabolic myopathies. *In* LP Rowland, S DiMauro (eds): Myopathies. Amsterdam, Elsevier, 1992.

157. Muchler HC, Renz D, Ludecke DK: Anesthetic management of acromegaly. *In* Ludecke DK, Tolis G (eds): Growth Hormone, Growth Factors, and Acromegaly: Progress in Endocrine Research and Therapy, vol. 3. New York, Raven, 1987.

158. Penn AS: Myoglobinuria. *In* Engel AG, Franzini-Armstrong C (eds): Myology. New York, McGraw-Hill, 1994.

159. Singhal PC, Abramovici M, Venkatesan J: Rhabdomyolysis in the hyperosmolar state. Am J Med 88:9, 1990.

160. Buckingham BA, Roe TF, Yoon J-W: Rhabdomyolysis in diabetic ketoacidosis. Am J Dis Child 135:352, 1981.

161. Rainey RL, Estes PW, Neeley CL, et al: Myoglobinuria following diabetic acidosis. Arch Intern Med 111:564, 1963.

162. George R, Shiu MH: Hypophosphatemia after major hepatic resection. Surgery 111:281, 1992.

Glycogen Storage Diseases

163. DiMauro S, Mehler M, Arnold S, et al: Genetic heterogeneity of glycogen diseases. *In* Pathogenesis of Human Muscular Dystrophies. Proceedings, Fifth International Scientific Conference of the Muscular Dystrophy Association, Colorado, 1976. Amsterdam, Excerpta Medica, 1977.

164. Casson H: Anaesthesia for portacaval bypass in patients with metabolic disease. Br J Anaesth 47:969, 1975.

165. Cox JM: Anesthesia and glycogen storage disease. Anesthesiology 29:6, 1968.

166. Shenkman Z, Golub Y, Meretyk S, et al: Anaesthetic management of a patient with glycogen storage disease type 1b. Can J Anaesth 43:467, 1996.

167. Engel AG: Acid maltase deficiency. *In* Engel AG, Banker BQ (eds): Myology. New York, McGraw-Hill, 1986.

168. Kaplan R: Pompe's disease presenting for anesthesia. Anesthesiol Rev 7:21, 1980.

169. Gitlin MC, Jahr JS, Garth KL, Grogono AW: Uteroscopic removal of left ureteral lithiasis in a patient with acid maltase deficiency. Anesth Analg 76:662, 1993.

170. Brown BI: Debranching and branching enzyme deficiencies. *In* Engel AG, Banker BQ (eds): Myology. New York, McGraw-Hill, 1986.

171. DiMauro S, Bresolin N: Phosphorylase deficiency. *In* Engel AG, Banker BQ (eds): Myology. New York, McGraw-Hill, 1986.

172. Slonim AE, Goans PJ: Myopathy in McArdle's syndrome: Improvement with a high protein diet. N Engl J Med 312:355, 1985.

173. Layzer RB: McArdle's disease in the 1980s. N Engl J Med 312:370, 1985.

174. Rajah A, Bell CF: Atracurium and McArdle's disease. Anaesthesia 41:93, 1986.

175. Ryan JF, Papper EM: Malignant fever during and following anesthesia. Anesthesiology 32:196, 1970.
176. Tarui S: Glycolytic defects in muscle: Aspects of collaboration between basic science and clinical medicine. Muscle Nerve 18(Suppl. 3):S2–9, 1995.
177. Griggs RC, Mendell JR, Miller RG: Metabolic myopathies. *In* Evaluation and Treatment of Myopathies. Philadelphia, FA Davis, 1995.
178. Edelstein G, Hirshman CA: Hyperthermia and keto-acidosis during anesthesia in a child with glycogen-storage disease. Anesthesiology 52:90, 1980.

Blocks in Glycolysis

179. DiMauro S, Bresolin N: Newly recognized defects in distal glycolysis. *In* Engel AG, Banker BQ (eds): Myology. New York, McGraw-Hill, 1986.
180. Satoyoshi E, Kowa H: A new myopathy. Am Neurol Assoc Trans 90:46, 1965.
181. Tsujino S, Shanske S, Sakoda S, et al: Molecular genetic studies in muscle phosphoglycerate mutase (PGAM-M) deficiency. Muscle Nerve (Suppl 3):S50, 1995.
182. Kanno T, Maekawa M: Lactate dehydrogenase M subunit deficiencies: Clinical features, metabolic background and genetic heterogeneities. Muscle Nerve 18(Suppl 3):S54, 1995.

Myositis Ossificans Progressive

183. Banker BQ: Other inflammatory myopathies. *In* Engel AG, Banker BQ (eds): Myology. New York, McGraw-Hill, 1986.

Mitochondrial Myopathies

184. Griggs RD, Mendell JR, Miller RG: Mitochondrial myopathies. *In* Evaluation and Treatment of Myopathies. Philadelphia, FA Davis, 1995.
185. Morgan-Hughes JA: Mitochondrial diseases. *In* Engel AG, Franzini-Armstrong C (eds): Myology. New York, McGraw-Hill, 1994.
186. DiMauro S, Tonin P, Servidei S: Metabolic myopathies. *In* Rowland LP, DiMauro S (eds): Myopathies. Amsterdam, Elsevier, 1992.
187. Schon EA: Mitochondrial disorders in muscle. Curr Opin Neurol Neurosurg 6:19, 1993.
188. Poulton J, Morten KJ, Marchington D, et al: Duplications of mitochondrial DNA in Kearns-Sayre syndrome. Muscle Nerve 18(Suppl 3):S154, 1995.
189. Barohn RJ, Clanton T, Sahenk Z, et al: Recurrent respiratory insufficiency and depressed ventilatory drive complicating mitochondrial myopathies. Neurology 40:103, 1990.
190. Manni R, Piccolo G, Banfi P, et al: Respiratory patterns during sleep in mitochondrial myopathies with ophthalmoplegia. Eur Neurol 31:12, 1991.
191. James RH: Induction agent sensitivity and ophthalmoplegia plus. Anaesthesia 41:216, 1986.
192. James RH: Thiopentone and ophthalmoplegia plus. Anaesthesia 40:88, 1985.
193. Scarlato G, Bresolin N, Moroni I, et al: Multicenter trial with ubidecarenone: Treatment of 44 patients with mitochondrial myopathies. Rev Neurol (Paris) 147:542, 1991.
194. Fukuhara N: Clinicopathological features of MERRF. Muscle Nerve 18(Suppl 3):S90, 1995.
195. Goto Y-I: Clinical features of MELAS and mitochondrial DNA mutations. Muscle Nerve 18(Suppl 3):S107, 1995.
196. Grattan-Smith PJ, Shield LK, Hopkins IJ, et al: Acute respiratory failure precipitated by general anesthesia in Leigh's syndrome. J Child Neurol 5:137, 1990.

Defects of Oxidative Phosphorylation

197. Luft R, Ikkos G, Palmieri L, et al: A case of severe hypermetabolism of non-thyroid origin with a defect in maintenance of mitochondrial respiratory control: Correlated clinical biochemical and morphological study. J Clin Invest 41:1776, 1962.
198. Haydar NA, Conn HL Jr, Afifi A, et al: Severe hypermetabolism with primary abnormality of skeletal muscle mitochondria. Ann Intern Med 74:548, 1971.
199. Afifi AK, Ibrahim MZM, Bergman RA, et al: Non-pathologic features of hypermetabolic mitochondrial disease. J Neurol Sci 15:271, 1972.
200. Luft R: Personal communication, 1969.
201. van Wijngaarden GK, Bethlem J, Meijer AE, et al: Skeletal muscle disease with abnormal mitochondria. Brain 90:577, 1967.
202. Scholte HR, Busch HFM, Luyt-Houwen IEM, et al: Defects in oxidative phosphorylation. Biochemical investigations in skeletal muscle and expression of the lesion in other cells. J Inherit Metab Dis 10(Suppl):81, 1987.
203. Przyembel H: Therapy of mitochondrial disorders. J Inherit Metab Dis 10(Suppl):129, 1987.
204. Lauwers MH, Van Lersberghe C, Camu F: Inhalation anaesthesia and Kearns-Sayre syndrome. Anaesthesia 49:876, 1994.
205. Burns AM, Shelly MP: Anaesthesia for patients with mitochondrial myopathy. Anaesthesia 44:975, 1989.
206. Keyes MA, Van de Wiele B, Stead SW: Mitochondrial myopathies: An unusual cause of hypotonia in infants and children. Paediatr Anaesth 6:1, 1996.
207. Maslow A, Lisbon A: Anesthetic considerations in patients with mitochondrial dysfunction. Anesth Analg 76:884, 1993.
208. D'Ambra MN, Dedrick D, Savarese JJ: Kearns-Sayer syndrome and pancuronium-succinylcholine induced neuromuscular blockade. Anesthesiology 51:343, 1979.
209. Ohtani Y, Miike T, Ishitsu T, et al: A case of malignant hyperthermia with mitochondrial dysfunction. Brain Dev 7:249, 1985.

Lipid Myopathies

210. Engel AG, Angelini C: Carnitine deficiency of human skeletal muscle with associated lipid storage myopathy: A new syndrome. Science 179:899, 1973.
211. Engel AG: Carnitine deficiency syndromes and lipid storage myopathies. *In* Engel AG, Banker BQ (eds): Myology. New York, McGraw-Hill, 1986.
212. Cornelio F, Di Donato S, Testa D, et al: "Carnitine deficient" myopathy and cardiomyopathy with fatal outcome. Ital J Neurol Sci 1:95, 1980.
213. Beilin B, Shulman D, Schiffman Y: Anaesthesia in myopathy of carnitine deficiency [letter]. Anaesthesia 41:92, 1986.
214. Kurahashi K, Andoh T, Sato K, et al: Anesthesia in a patient with carnitine deficiency syndrome. Masul 42:1223, 1993.
215. Engel AG: Carnitine deficiency syndromes and lipid storage myopathies. *In* Engel AG, Banker BQ (eds): Myology. New York, McGraw-Hill, 1986.
216. Vianey-Liaud C, Divry P, Gregersen N, et al: The inborn errors of mitochondrial fatty acid oxidation. J Inherit Metab Dis 10(Suppl):159, 1987.

217. Cornelio F, DiDonato S, Peluchetti D, et al: Fatal cases of lipid storage myopathy with carnitine deficiency. J Neurol Neurosurg Psychiatry 40:170, 1977.
218. Bank WJ, DiMauro S, Bonilla E, et al: A disorder of muscle lipid metabolism and myoglobinuria: Absence of carnitine palmityl transferase. N Engl J Med 292:443, 1975.
219. DiMauro S, Papadimitriou A: Carnitine palmitoyl-transferase deficiency. *In* Engel AG, Banker BQ (eds): Myology. New York, McGraw-Hill, 1986.
220. Katsuya H, Misumi M, Ohtani Y, et al: Postanesthetic acute renal failure due to carnitine palmitoyl transferase deficiency. Anesthesiology 68:945, 1988.

Gongenital Myopathies

221. Griggs RC, Mendell JR, Miller RG: Congenital myopathies. *In* Evaluation and Treatment of Myopathies. Philadelphia, FA Davis, 1995.
222. Denborough MA, Bennett X, Anderson RM: Central core disease and malignant hyperpyrexia. Br Med J 1:272, 1973.
223. Paasuke RT, Brownell AK: Serum creatine kinase level as a screening test for susceptibility to malignant hyperthermia. JAMA 255:769, 1986.
224. Ording H, Ranklev E, Fletcher R: Investigation of malignant hyperthermia in Denmark and Sweden. Br J Anaesth 56:1183, 1984.
225. Brownell AKW: Malignant hyperthermia: Relationship to other diseases. Br J Anaesth 60:303, 1988.
226. Harriman DGF, Ellis FR: Central core disease and malignant hyperpyrexia [correspondence]. Br Med J 3:545, 1973.
227. Koch BM, Bertorini TE, Eng GD, et al: Severe multicore disease associated with reaction to anesthesia. Arch Neurol 42:1204, 1985.
228. Hopkins IJ, Lindsey JR, Ford FR: Nemaline myopathy: A long term clinico-pathological study of affected mother and daughter. Brain 89:299, 1966.
229. Cunliffe M, Burrows FA: Anaesthetic implications of nemaline rod myopathy. Can Anaesth Soc J 32:543, 1985.
230. Heard SO, Kaplan RF: Neuromuscular blockade in a patient with nemaline myopathy. Anesthesiology 59:588, 1986.
231. Asai T, Fujise K, Uchida M: Anaesthesia for cardiac surgery in children with nemaline myopathy. Anaesthesia 47:405, 1992.
232. Stackhouse R, Chelmow D, Dattel BJ: Anesthetic complications in a pregnant patient with nemaline myopathy. Anesth Analg 79:1195, 1994.
233. Quinn RD, Pae WE Jr, McGary SA, Wickey GS: Development of malignant hyperthermia during mitral valve replacement. Ann Thorac Surg 53:1114, 1992.
234. Price SR, Currie J: Anaesthesia for a child with centronuclear myopathy. Paediatr Anaesth 5:267, 1995.

Inflammatory Myopathies and "Overlap" Syndromes

235. Engel AG, Hohlfeld R, Banker BQ: Inflammatory myopathies: The polymyositis and dermatomyositis syndromes. *In* Engel AG, Franzini-Armstrong C (eds): Myology. New York, McGraw-Hill, 1994.
236. Hochberg MC, Feldman D, Stevens MB: Adult onset polymyositis/dermatomyositis: An analysis of clinical and laboratory features and survival in 76 patients with a review of the literature. Semin Arthritis Rheum 15:168, 1986.
237. Gottdiener JS, Sherber HS, Hawley RJ, et al: Cardiac manifestations in polymyositis. Am J Cardiol 41:1141, 1978.
238. Arsura EL, Greenberg AS: Adverse impact of pulmonary fibrosis on prognosis in polymyositis and dermatomyositis. Semin Arthritis Rheum 18:29, 1988.
239. Dalakas MC: How to diagnose and treat the inflammatory myopathies. Semin Neurol 14:137, 1994.
240. Caccamo DV, Keene CY, Durham J, et al: Fulminant rhabdomyolysis in a patient with dermatomyositis. Neurology 43:844, 1993.
241. Dalakas MC, Illa I, Dambrosia JM, et al: A controlled trial of high-dose intravenous immune globulin infusions as treatment for dermatomyositis. N Engl J Med 329:1993, 1993.
242. St. Guily JK, Perie S, Willig, T-N, et al: Swallowing disorders in muscular diseases: Functional assessment and indications of cricopharyngeal myotomy. ENT J 73:34, 1994.
243. Brown S, Shupak RC, Patel C, et al: Neuromuscular blockade in a patient with active dermatomyositis. Anesthesiology 77:1031, 1992.
244. Flusche G, Unger-Sargon J, Lambert DH: Prolonged neuromuscular paralysis with vecuronium in a patient with polymyositis. Anesth Analg 66:180, 1986.
245. Griggs RC, Mendell JR, Miller RG: Inflammatory myopathies. *In* Evaluation and Treatment of Myopathies. Philadelphia, FA Davis, 1995.

Infectious Diseases

246. Dalakas MC: Retrovirus-related muscle diseases. *In* Engel AG, Franzini-Armstrong C (eds): Myology. New York, McGraw-Hill, 1994.
247. Hays AP, Gamboa E: Acute viral myositis. *In* Engel AG, Franzini-Armstrong C (eds): Myology. New York, McGraw-Hill, 1994.
248. Brackmann T, Lang W: Case report of florid trichinosis in otorhinolarynglolgy. HNO 33:409, 1985.
249. Heinze J, Junginger W, Muller G, et al: Anaphylactic shock during excision of an intraosseous *Echinococcus granulosus* cyst. Anaesthetist 36:659, 1987.
250. Banker BQ: Other inflammatory myopathies. *In* Engel AG, Franzini-Armstrong C (eds): Myology. New York, McGraw-Hill, 1994.
251. Kohlschutter B, Baur H, Roth F: Suxamethonium-induced hyperkalaemia in patients with severe intra-abdominal infections. Br J Anaesth 48:557, 1976.
252. Horton WA, Fergusson NV: Hyperkalemia and cardiac arrest after the use of suxamethonium in intensive care. Anaesthesia 43:890, 1988.
253. Antognini JF: Splanchnic release of potassium after hemorrhage and succinylcholine in rabbits. Anesth Analg 78:687, 1994.
254. Khan TZ, Khan RM: Changes in serum potassium following succinylcholine in patients with infections. Anesth Analg 62:327, 1983.
255. Erttmann M, Havemann D: Treatment of gas gangrene: Results of a retrospective and prospective analysis of a traumatologic patient sample over 20 years. Unfallchir 95:471, 1992.
256. Roth F, Wuthrich H: The clinical importance of hyperkalemia following suxamethonium administration. Br J Anaesth 41:311, 1969.
257. Keusch GT, Deresiewicz RL: Cholera and other vibrioses. *In* Isselbacher KJ, Braunwald E, Wilson JD,

et al (eds): Harrison's Principles of Internal Medicine, 13th ed. New York, McGraw-Hill, 1994.

258. Schattner A, Hay E, Lifschitz-Mercer B, et al: Fulminant streptococcal myositis. Ann Emerg Med 18:320, 1989.

259. Clayton AJ, Peacocke JE, Ewan PE: Toxic shock syndrome in Canada. CMA J 126:776, 1982.

260. Graham DR, O'Brien M, Hayes JM, et al: Postoperative toxic shock syndrome. Clin Infect Dis 20:895, 1995.

Myopathy Due to Drugs or Toxins

261. Victor M, Sieb JP: Myopathies due to drugs, toxins and nutritional deficiency. In Engel AG, Franzini-Armstrong C (eds): Myology. New York, McGraw-Hill, 1994.

262. Pierce LR, Wysowski DK, Gross TP: Myopathy and rhabdomyolysis associated with lovastatin-gemfibrozil combination therapy. JAMA 264:71, 1990.

263. Corpier CL, Jones PH, Suki WN, et al: Rhabdomyolysis and renal injury with lovastatin use: Report of two cases in cardiac transplant recipients. JAMA 260:239, 1988.

264. von Moltke LL, Greenblatt DJ: Drugs in cardiac transplantation [letter]. N Engl J Med 334:401, 1996.

265. Smith PF, Eydelloth RS, Grossman SJ, et al: HMG-CoA reductase inhibitor–induced myopathy in the rat: Cyclosporine A interaction and mechanism studies. J Pharmacol Exp Ther 257:1225, 1991.

266. Kobashigawa JA, Katznelson S, Laks H, et al: Effect of pravastatin on outcomes after cardiac transplantation. N Engl J Med 333:621, 1995.

267. Kane MJ, Silverman LR, Rand JH, et al: Myonecrosis as a complication of the use of epsilon amino-caproic acid: A case report and review of the literature. Am J Med 85:861, 1988.

268. Karalliedde L, Senanayake N: Organophosphorus insecticide poisoning. Br J Anaesth 63:736, 1989.

269. Weeks DB, Ford D: Prolonged suxamethonium-induced neuromuscular block associated with organophosphate poisoning [letter]. Br J Anaesth 62:237, 1989.

270. Wallace JF: Disorder caused by venoms, bites, and stings. In Isselbacher KJ, Braunwald E, Wilson JD, et al (eds): Harrison's Principles of Internal Medicine, 13th ed. New York, McGraw-Hill, 1994.

271. Mastaglia FL: Toxic myopathies. In Rowland LP, DiMauro S (eds): Myopathies. Amsterdam, Elsevier, 1992.

272. Verny C, de Gennes C, Sebastien P, et al: Heart conduction disorders in long-term treatment with chloroquine. Two new cases. Presse Med 21:800, 1992.

273. Wright GD, Wilson C, Bell AL: D-Penicillamine induced polymyositis causing complete heart block. Clin Rheumatol 13:80, 1994.

274. Griggs RC, Mendell JR, Miller RG: Inflammatory myopathies. In Evaluation and Treatment of Myopathies. Philadelphia, FA Davis, 1995.

275. Roth D, Alarcon FJ, Fernandez JA, et al: Acute rhabdomyolysis associated with cocaine intoxication. N Engl J Med 319:673, 1988.

276. Warrian WG, Halikas JA, Crosby RD, et al: Observations on increased CPK levels in "asymptomatic" cocaine abusers. J Addict Dis 11:83, 1992.

Myoglobinuria

277. Tein I, DiMauro S, Rowland LP: Myoglobinuria. In Rowland LP, Di Mauro S (eds): Myopathies. Amsterdam, Elsevier, 1992.

278. Plotz J: [Letter]. Anesth Analg 67:798, 1988.

279. Airaksinen M, Tammisto T: Myoglobinuria after intermittent administration of succinylcholine during halothane anesthesia. Clin Pharmacol Ther 7:583, 1966.

280. Ryan JF, Kagen LJ, Hyman AI: Myoglobinemia after a single dose of succinylcholine. N Engl J Med 285:824, 1971.

281. Blanc VF, Vaillancourt G, Brisson G: Succinylcholine, fasciculations and myoglobinemia. Can Anaesth Soc J 33:178, 1986.

282. Harrington JF, Ford DJ, Striker TW: Myoglobinemia after succinylcholine in children undergoing halothane and non-halothane anesthesia. Anesthesiology 61:A431, 1984.

283. Rosenberg H, Gronert GA: Intractable cardiac arrest in children given succinylcholine. Anesthesiology 77:1054, 1992.

284. Martyn JAJ, White DA, Gronert GA, et al: Up- and down-regulation of skeletal muscle acetylcholine receptors: Effects on neuromuscular blockers. Anesthesiology 76:822, 1992.

285. Better OS, Stein JH: Early management of shock and prophylaxis of acute renal failure in traumatic rhabdomyolysis. N Engl J Med 322:825, 1990.

286. Odeh M: The role of reperfusion-induced injury in the pathogenesis of the crush syndrome. N Engl J Med 324:1417, 1991.

287. Owen CA, Mubarak SJ, Hargens AR, et al: Intramuscular pressures with limb compression. N Engl J Med 300:1169, 1979.

288. Poels PJE, Joosten EMG, Stadhouders Am, et al: In vitro contracture test for malignant hyperthermia in patients with unexplained recurrent rhabdomyolysis. J Neurol Sci 105:67, 1991.

289. Hurley JK: Severe rhabdomyolysis in well-conditioned athletes. Mil Med 154:244, 1989.

290. Kark JA, Posey DM, Schumacher HR, et al: Sickle-cell trait as a risk factor for sudden death in physical training. N Engl J Med 317:781, 1987.

291. Figarella-Branger D, Kozak-Ribbens G, Rodet L, et al: Pathological findings in 165 patients explored for malignant hyperthermia susceptibility. Neuromuscul Disord 3:553, 1993.

292. Channa AB, Seraj MA, Saddique AA, et al: Is dantrolene effective in heat stroke patients? Crit Care Med 18:290, 1990.

293. Mercieca J, Brown E: Acute renal failure due to rhabdomyolysis associated with use of a straitjacket in lysergide intoxication. Br Med J 288:1949, 1949.

294. Velamoor VR, Swamy GN, Parmar L-R, et al: Management of suspected neuroleptic malignant syndrome. Can J Psychiatry 40:545, 1995.

295. Sporer KA: The serotonin syndrome: Implicated drugs, pathophysiology and management. Drug Safety 13:94, 1995.

296. Ziser A, Friedhoff RJ, Rose SH: Prone position: Visceral hypoperfusion and rhabdomyolysis. Anesth Analg 82:412, 1996.

297. Targa L, Droghetti L, Caggese G, et al: Rhabdomyolysis and operating position. Anaesthesia 46:141, 1991.

Malignant Hyperthermia and Drug-Induced Trismus

298. Denborough MA, Lovell RRH: Anaesthetic deaths in a family. Lancet 2:45, 1960.

299. Britt BA, Kalow W: Malignant hyperthermia: A statistical review. Can Anaesth Soc 17:293, 1970.

300. Britt BA: Recent advances in malignant hyperthermia. Anesth Analg 54:841, 1972.
301. Ranklev E, Henriksson KG, Fletcher R, et al: Clinical and muscle biopsy findings in malignant hyperthermia susceptibility. Acta Neurol Scand 74:452, 1986.
302. Gronert GA: Malignant hyperthermia. Anesthesiology 53:395, 1980.
303. Roewer N, Greim C, Rumberger E, et al: Abnormal action potential responses to halothane in heart muscle isolated from malignant hyperthermia–susceptible pigs. Anesthesiology 82:947, 1995.
304. Gronert GA, Theye RA: Halothane-induced porcine malignant hyperthermia: Metabolic and hemodynamic changes. Anesthesiology 44:36, 1976.
305. Kochs E, Hoffman WE, Schulte am Esch J: Improvement of brain electrical activity during treatment of porcine malignant hyperthermia with dantrolene. Br J Anaesth 71:881, 1993.
306. Sewall K, Flowerdew RMM, Bromberger P: Severe muscular rigidity at birth: Malignant hyperthermia syndrome? Can Anaesth Soc J 27:279, 1908.
307. Nelson TE, Flewellen EH, Gloyna DF: Spectrum of susceptibility to malignant hyperthermia—diagnostic dilemma. Anesth Analg 62:545, 1983.
308. Nelson, TE: Skeletal muscle sarcoplasmic reticulum in the malignant hyperthermia syndrome. In Britt BA (ed): Malignant Hyperthermia. Boston, Martinus Nijhoff, 1987.
309. Britt BA: Aetiology and pathophysiology of malignant hyperthermia. In Britt BA (ed): Malignant Hyperthermia. Boston, Martinus Nijhoff, 1987.
310. Jaffe M, Savage N, Silove M: The biochemistry of malignant hyperthermia: Recent concepts. Int J Biochem 24:387, 1992.
311. MacLennan DH, Phillips MS: Malignant hyperthermia. Science 256:789, 1992.
312. Lopez JR, Gerardi A, Lopez MJ, et al: Effects of dantrolene on myoplasmic free (Ca + 2) measured in vivo in patients susceptible to malignant hyperthermia. Anesthesiology 76:711, 1992.
313. Gronert GA, Antognini JF: Malignant hyperthermia. In Miller RD (ed): Anesthesia. New York, Churchill Livingstone, 1994.
314. Fletcher JE, Tripolitis L, Rosenberg H, et al: Malignant hyperthermia: Halothane- and calcium-induced calcium release in skeletal muscle. Biochem Molec Biol 29:763, 1993.
315. Tonner PH, Scholz J, Richter A, et al: Alterations of inositol polyphosphates in skeletal muscle during porcine malignant hyperthermia. Br J Anaesth 75:467, 1995.
316. Loscher W, Gerdes C, Richter A: Lack of prophylactic or therapeutic efficacy of $5-HT_{2A}$ receptor antagonists in halothane-induced porcine malignant hyperthermia. Naunyn-Schmiedebergs Arch Pharmacol 350:365, 1994.
317. Ryan JF, Lopez JR, Sanchez VB, et al: Myoplasmic calcium changes precede metabolic and clinical signs of porcine malignant hyperthermia. Anesth Analg 79:1007, 1994.
318. Harriman DGF: Malignant hyperthermia myopathy—a critical review. Br J Anaesth 60:309, 1988.
319. Klein L, Rosenberg H: Malignant hyperthermia in animals other than swine. In Britt BA, (ed): Malignant Hyperthermia. Boston, Martinus Nijhoff, 1987.
320. Weglenski MR, Wedel DJ: Differential diagnosis of hyperthermia during anesthesia and clinical import. In Levitt RC (ed): Temperature regulation during anesthesia. Anesth Clin North Am 12:475, 1994.

321. Larach MG, Localio AR, Allen GC, et al: A clinical grading scale to predict malignant hyperthermia susceptibility. Anesthesiology 80:771, 1994.
322. Britt BA: Muscle assessment of malignant hyperthermia patients. In Britt BA (ed): Malignant Hyperthermia. Boston, Martinus Nijhoff, 1987.
323. European MH Group: Laboratory diagnosis of malignant hyperthermia susceptibility (MHS). Br J Anaesth 57:1038, 1985.
324. Ording H: Diagnosis of susceptibility to malignant hyperthermia in man. Br J Anaesth 60:287, 1988.
325. European MH Group: Laboratory diagnosis of malignant hyperthermia susceptibility (MHS). Br J Anaesth 57:1038, 1985.
326. North American Malignant Hyperthermia Group: Recommendations for Standardization of the Caffeine Halothane Contracture Test. Hershey, Pa, The North American Malignant Hyperthermia Registry, Department of Anesthesia, Pennsylvania State University College of Medicine, 1989.
327. Larach MG, Landis JR: False positive diagnosis of malignant hyperthermia susceptibility in control subjects using the North American caffeine halothane contracture test. Anesthesiology 73:A1013, 1990.
328. Isaacs H, Badenhorst M: False-negative results with muscle caffeine halothane contracture testing for malignant hyperthermia. Anesthesiology 79:5, 1993.
329. Wedel DJ, Nelson TE: Malignant hyperthermia—diagnostic dilemma: False-negative contracture responses with halothane and caffeine alone. Anesth Analg 78:787, 1994.
330. Kikuchi H, Matsui K, Morio M: Diagnosis of malignant hyperthermia in Japan by the skinned fibre test. In Britt BA (ed): Malignant Hyperthermia. Boston, Martinus Nijhoff, 1987.
331. Olgin J, Rosenberg H, Allen G, et al: A blinded comparison of noninvasive, in vivo phosphorous nuclear magnetic resonance spectroscopy and the in vitro halothane/caffeine contracture test in the evaluation of malignant hyperthermia susceptibility. Anesth Analg 72:36, 1991.
332. Payen JF, Bosson J-L, Bourdon L, et al: Improved noninvasive testing for malignant hyperthermia susceptibility from a combination of metabolites determined in vivo with P^{31}-magnetic resonance spectroscopy. Anesthesiology 78:848, 1993.
333. Paasuke RT, Brownell AKW: Serum creatine kinase level as a screening test for susceptibility to malignant hyperthermia. JAMA 255:769, 1986.
334. Fletcher JE: Current laboratory methods for the diagnosis of malignant hyperthermia susceptibility. Anesth Clin North Am 12:553, 1994.
335. McCarthy TV, Healy MS, Heffron JJA, et al: Localization of the malignant hyperthermia susceptibility locus to human chromosome 19q12-13.2. Nature 343:562, 1990.
336. MacLennanm DH, Duff C, Zorzato F, et al: Ryanodine receptor gene is a candidate gene for predisposition to malignant hyperthermia. Nature 343:559, 1990.
337. Fujii J, Otsu K, Zorzato F, et al: Identification of a mutation in porcine ryanodine receptor associated with malignant hyperthermia. Science 253:448, 1991.
338. Wallace AJ, Wooldridge W, Kingston HM, et al: Malignant hyperthermia—a large kindred linked to the RYR1 gene. Anaesthesia 51:16, 1996.
339. Fletcher JE, Tripolitis L, Hubert M, et al: Genotype and phenotype relationships for mutations in the

ryanodine receptor in patients referred for diagnosis of malignant hyperthermia. Br J Anaesth 75:307, 1995.

340. Serfas KD, Bose D, Patel L, et al: Comparison of segregation of the RYR1 C1840T mutation with segregation of the caffeine/halothane contracture test results for malignant hyperthermia susceptibility in a large Manitoba Mennonite family. Anesthesiology 84:322, 1996.

341. Sudbrak R, Procaccio V, Klausnitzer M, et al: Mapping of a further malignant hyperthermia susceptibility locus to chromosome 3q13.1. Am J Hum Genet 56:684, 1995.

342. Iles DE, Lehmann-Horn F, Scherer SW, et al: Localization of the gene encoding the alpha 2/delta-subunits of the L-type voltage-dependent calcium channel to chromosome 7q and analysis of the segregation of flanking markers in malignant hyperthermia susceptible families. Human Molec Genet 3:969, 1994.

343. Hopkins PM, Halsall PJ, Ellis FR: Diagnosing malignant hyperthermia susceptibility [editorial]. Anaesthesia 49:373, 1994.

344. Wedel DJ: Malignant hyperthermia and neuromuscular disease. Neuomuscul Disord 2:157, 1992.

345. Islander G, Henriksson KG, Ranklev-Twetman E: Malignant hyperthermia susceptibility without central core disease (CCD) in a family where CCD is diagnosed. Neuromuscul Disord 5:125, 1995.

346. Chitayat D, Hodgkinson KA, Ginsburg O, et al: King syndrome: A genetically heterogeneous phenotype due to congenital myopathies. Am J Med Genet 43:954, 1992.

347. Komatsu H, Enzan K, Suzuki M: A case of abortive malignant hyperthermia during funnel chest surgery. Masui 42:1053, 1993.

348. Ellis FR, Halsall PJ, Harriman DGF: Malignant hyperpyrexia and sudden infant death syndrome. Br J Anaesth 60:28, 1988.

349. Caroff SN, Rosenberg H, Fletcher JE, et al: Malignant hyperthermia susceptibility in neuroleptic malignant syndrome. Anesthesiology 67:20, 1987.

350. Bello N, Adnet P, Saulnier F, et al: Lack of sensitivity to per-anesthetic malignant hyperthermia in 32 patients who developed neuroleptic malignant syndrome. Ann Franc Anesth Reanim 13:663, 1994.

351. Beebe JJ, Sessler DI: Preparation of anesthesia machines for patients susceptible to malignant hyperthermia. Anesthesiology 69:395, 1988.

352. Murakawa M, Hatano Y, Magaribuchi T, et al: Should calcium administration be avoided in treatment of hyperkalemia in malignant hyperthermia? Anesth Analg 67:604, 1988.

353. Harrison GG: Dantrolene—dynamics and kinetics. Br J Anaesth 60:279, 1988.

354. Gallant EM, Foldes FF, Rempel WE, et al: Verapamil is not a therapeutic adjunct to dantrolene in porcine malignant hyperthermia. Anesth Analg 64:601, 1985.

355. Lynch C, Durbin CG, Fisher NA, et al: Effects of dantrolene and verapamil on atrioventricular conduction and cardiovascular performance in dogs. Anesth Analg 65:252, 1986.

356. Saltzman LS, Kates RA, Corke BL, et al: Hyperkalemia and cardiovascular collapse after verapamil and dantrolene administered in swine. Anesth Analg 63:473, 1984.

357. Rubin AS, Zablocki AD: Hyperkalemia, verapamil and dantrolene. Anesthesiology 66:246, 1982.

358. Yoganathan T, Casthely PA, Lamprou M: Dantro-

lene-induced hyperkalemia in a patient treated with diltiazem and metoprolol. J Cardiothorac Anesth 2:363, 1988.

359. Gronert GA, Ahern CP, Milde JH, et al: Effects of CO_2, calcium, digoxin, and potassium on cardiac and skeletal muscle metabolism in malignant hyperthermia susceptible swine. Anesthesiology 64:24, 1986.

360. Maccani RM, Wedel DJ, Hofer RE: Norepinephrine does not potentiate porcine malignant hyperthermia. Anesth Analg 82:790, 1996.

361. Wingard DW, Bobko S: Failure of lidocaine to trigger porcine malignant hyperthermia. Anesth Analg 58:99, 1989.

362. Brownell AKW: Counselling of malignant hyperthermia susceptible individuals. In Britt BA (ed): Malignant Hyperthermia. Boston, Martinus Nijhoff, 1987.

363. Berkowitz A, Rosenberg H: Femoral nerve block with mepivacaine for muscle biopsy in malignant hyperthermia patients. Anesthesiology 62:651, 1985.

364. Islander G, Ranklev-Twetman E: Evaluation of anaesthesias in malignant hyperthermia negative patients. Acta Anaesthesiol Scand 39:819, 1995.

365. McKenzie AJ, Couchman KG, Pollock N: Propofol is a "safe" anaesthetic agent in malignant hyperthermia susceptible patients. Anaesth Intensive Care 20:165, 1992.

366. Gronert GA: Malignant hyperthermia. In Engel AG, Franzini-Armstrong C (eds): Myology. New York, McGraw-Hill, 1994.

367. Otsuka H, Komura Y, Mayumi T, et al: Malignant hyperthermia during sevoflurane anesthesia in a child with central core disease. Anesthesiology 75:699, 1991.

368. Wedel DJ, Gammel SA, Milde JH, et al: Delayed onset of malignant hyperthermia induced by isoflurane and desflurane compared with halothane in susceptible swine. Anesthesiology 78:1138, 1993.

369. Carr AS, Lerman J, Cunliffe M, et al: Incidence of malignant hyperthermia reactions in 2,214 patients undergoing muscle biopsy. Can J Anaesth 42:281, 1995.

370. Marsh ML, Sessler DI: Failure of intraoperative liquid-crystal temperature monitoring. Anesth Analg 82:1102, 1996.

371. Britt BA: Combined anesthetic- and stress-induced malignant hyperthermia in two offspring of malignant hyperthermic-susceptible parents. Anesth Analg 67:393, 1988.

372. Rosenberg H: Trismus is not trivial (Editorial Views). Anesthesiology 67:453, 1987.

373. Donlon JV, Newfield P, Sreter F, et al: Implication of masseter spasm after succinylcholine. Anesthesiology 49:298, 1987.

374. Carroll JB: Increased incidence of masseter spasm in children with strabismus anesthetized with halothane and succinylcholine. Anesthesiology 67:559, 1987.

375. Schwartz L, Rockoff MA, Koka BV: Masseter spasm with anesthesia: Incidence and implications. Anesthesiology 61:772, 1984.

376. Littleford JA, Patel LR, Bose D, et al: Masseter muscle spasm in children: Implications of continuing the triggering anesthetic. Anesth Analg 72:151, 1991.

377. Ellis FR, Halsall PJ: Suxamethonium spasm. Br J Anaesth 56:381, 1984.

378. Lazzell VA, Carr AS, Lerman J, et al: The incidence of masseter muscle rigidity after succinylcholine in infants and children. Can J Anaesth 41:475, 1994.

379. Van Der Spek AFL, Fang WB, Ashton-Miller JA, et al: The effects of succinylcholine on mouth opening. Anesthesiology 67:459, 1987.
380. Van Der Spek AFL, Fang WB, Ashton-Miller JA, et al: Increased masticatory muscle stiffness during limb muscle flaccidity associated with succinylcholine administration. Anesthesiology 69:11, 1988.
381. Gronert GA: Management of patients in whom trismus occurs following succinylcholine. (Reply by Rosenberg, H.) Anesthesiology 68:653, 1988.
382. O'Flynn RP, Shutack JG, Rosenberg H, et al: Masseter muscle rigidity and malignant hyperthermia susceptibility in pediatric patients. Anesthesiology 80:1228, 1994.
383. Allen GC, Rosenberg H, Fletcher JE: Safety of general anesthesia in patients previously tested negative for malignant hyperthermia susceptibility. Anesthesiology 72:619, 1990.
384. Allen GC, Cattran CB, Peterson RG, et al: Plasma levels of dantrolene following oral administration in malignant hyperthermia susceptible patients. Anesthesiology 69:900, 1988.
385. Kaplan RF: Clinical controversies in malignant hyperthermia susceptibility. In Levitt RC (ed): Temperature regulation in anesthesia. Anesth Clin North Am 12:537, 1994.
386. Flewellen EH, Nelson TE, Jones WP, et al: Dantrolene dose response in awake man: Implications for management of malignant hyperthermia. Anesthesiology 59:275, 1983.
387. Blank JW, Boggs SD: Successful treatment of an episode of malignant hyperthermia using a large dose of dantrolene. J Clin Anesth 5:69, 1993.
388. DeRuyter ML, Wedel DJ, Berge KH: Hyperthermia requiring prolonged administration of high-dose dantrolene in the postoperative period. Anesth Analg 80:834, 1995.
389. Lee C: Personal communication, 1990.
390. Lee C, Durant NN, Au E et al: Reversal of dantrolene sodium–induced depression of skeletal muscle in the cat. Anesthesiology 54:61, 1981.
391. Britt BA: Dantrolene—an update. In Britt BA (ed): Malignant Hyperthermia, Boston, Martinus Nijhoff, 1987.

Neuroleptic Malignant Syndrome

392. Levenson JL: Neuroleptic malignant syndrome. Am J Psychiat 142:1137, 1985.
393. Pope HG Jr, Keck PE Jr, McElroy SL: Frequency and presentation of neuroleptic malignant syndrome in a large psychiatric hospital. Am J Psychiat 143:1227, 1986.
394. Bond WS: Detection and management of the neuroleptic malignant syndrome. Clin Pharm 3:302, 1984.
395. Weinberg S, Twersky RS: Neuroleptic malignant syndrome. Anesth Analg 62:848, 1983.
396. Caroff SN, Mann SC, Campbell EC: Hyperthermia and neuroleptic malignant syndrome. In Levitt RC (ed): Temperature regulation during anesthesia. Anesth Clin North Am 12:491, 1994.
397. Granato JE, Stern BJ, Ringel A, et al: Neuroleptic malignant syndrome: Successful treatment with dantrolene and bromocriptine. Ann Neurol 14:89, 1983.
398. Scheftner WA, Shulman RB: Treatment choice in neuroleptic malignant syndrome. Convuls Ther 8:267, 1992.
399. Jessee SS, Anderson GF: ECT in the neuroleptic malignant syndrome: Case report. J Clin Psychiatry 44:186, 1983.
400. Addonizio G, Susman VL: ECT as a treatment alternative for patients with symptoms of neuroleptic malignant syndrome. J Clin Psychiatry 48:102, 1987.
401. Caroff SN, Rosenberg H, Fletcher JE, et al: Malignant hyperthermia susceptibility in neuroleptic malignant syndrome. Anesthesiology 67:20, 1987.
402. George AL Jr, Wood CA: Succinylcholine-induced hyperkalemia complicating the neuroleptic malignant syndrome. Ann Intern Med 106:172, 1987.
403. Geiduschek J, Cohen SA, Khan A, et al: Repeated anesthesia for a patient with neuroleptic malignant syndrome. Anesthesiology 68:134, 1988.
404. Addonizio G, Susman V: Neuroleptic malignant syndrome and use of anesthetic agents. Am J Psychiatry 143:127, 1986.

Myasthenia Gravis

405. Engel AG: Acquired autoimmune myasthenia gravis. In Engel AG, Banker BQ (eds): Myology. New York, McGraw-Hill, 1986.
406. Howard FM Jr, Lennon VA, Finley J, et al: Clinical correlations of antibodies that bind, block, or modulate human acetylcholine receptors in myasthenia gravis. Ann NY Acad Sci 505:526, 1987.
407. Fried MJ, Protheroe DT: D-Penicillamine induced myasthenia gravis. Its relevance for the anaesthetist. Br J Anaesth 58:1191, 1986.
408. Lefvert AK, Bolme P, Hammarstrom L, et al: Bone marrow grafting selectively induces the production of acetylcholine receptor antibodies, immunoglobulins bearing related idiotypes, and antiidiotypic antibodies. Ann NY Acad Sci 505:825, 1987.
409. Girnar DS, Weinreich AI: Anesthesia for transcervical thymectomy in myasthenia gravis. Anesth Analg 55:13, 1976.
410. Fujii Y, Hashimoto J, Monden Y, et al: Specific activation of lymphocytes against acetylcholine receptor in the thymus in myasthenia gravis. J Immunol 136:887, 1986.
411. Rodriquez M, Gomez MR, Howard FM Jr, et al: Myasthenia gravis in children: Long-term follow-up. Ann Neurol 13:504, 1983.
412. Keens SJ, Desmond MJ, Utting JE: Carcinoid syndrome with myasthenia gravis. An unusual and interesting case. Anaesthesia 41:404, 1986.
413. Wainwright AP, Brodrick PM: Suxamethonium in myasthenia gravis. Anaesthesia 42:950, 1987.
414. Mulder DG, Herrmann C Jr, Keesey J, et al: Thymectomy for myasthenia gravis. Am J Surg 146:61, 1983.
415. Evoli A, Tonali P, Scoppetta C, et al: Myasthenia gravis in the elderly: Report of 37 cases. J Am Geriatr Soc 31:352, 1983.
416. Richman DP, Agius MA: Myasthenia gravis: Pathogenesis and treatment. Semin Neurol 14:106, 1994.
417. Olanow CW, Wechsler AS, roses AD: A prospective study of thymectomy and serum acetylcholine receptor antibodies in myasthenia gravis. Ann Surg 196:113, 1982.
418. Robinson CL: The role of surgery of the thymus for myasthenia gravis. Ann R Coll Surg (Engl) 65:145, 1983.
419. Lumley J: Prolongation of suxamethonium following plasma exchange. Br J Anaesth 52:1149, 1980.
420. Spence PA, Morin JE, Katz M: Role of plasmapheresis in preparing myasthenic patients for thymectomy: Initial results. Can J Surg 27:303, 1984.

421. d'Empaire G, Hoaglin DC, Perlo VP, et al: Effect of prethymectomy plasma exchange on postoperative respiratory function in myasthenia gravis. J Thorac Cardiovasc Surg 89:592, 1985.
422. Leventhal SR, Orkin FK, Hirsch RA: Prediction of the need for postoperative ventilation in myasthenia gravis. Anesthesiology 53:26, 1980.
423. Loach AB, Young AC, Spalding JMK, et al: Postoperative management after thymectomy. Br Med J 1:309, 1975.
424. Wahlin A, Havermark KG: Enflurane (Ethrane) anesthesia on patients with myasthenia gravis. Acta Anaesthesiol Belg 2:215, 1974.
425. Gracey DR, Divertie MB, Howard FM Jr, et al: Postoperative respiratory care after transsternal thymectomy in myasthenia gravis. A 3-year experience in 53 patients. Chest 86:67, 1984.
426. Younger DS, Braun NM, Jaretzki A III, et al: Myasthenia gravis: Determinants for independent ventilation after transsternal thymectomy. Neurology 34:336, 1984.
427. Greene LF, Ghosh MK, Howard FM Jr: Transurethral prostatic resection in patients with myasthenia gravis. J Urol 112:226, 1974.
428. Davies DW, Steward DJ: Myasthenia gravis in children and anesthetic management for thymectomy. Can Anaesth Soc J 20:253, 1973.
429. Dalal FY, Bennett EJ, Gregg WS: Congenital myasthenia gravis and minor surgical procedures. Anaesthesia 27:61, 1972.
430. Mora CT, Eisenkraft JB, Papatestas AE: Intravenous dantrolene in a patient with myasthenia gravis. Anesthesiology 64:371, 1986.
431. Nilsson E, Muller K: Neuromuscular effects of isoflurane in patients with myasthenia gravis. Acta Anaesthesiol Scan 34:126, 1990.
432. Hunter JM, Bell CF, Florence AM, et al: Vecuronium in the myasthenic patient. Anaesthesia 40:848, 1985.
433. Pelton CI: Vecuronium in myasthenia gravis [letter]. Anaesthesia 40:82, 1985.
434. Eisenkraft JB, Sawhney RK, Papatestas AE: Vecuronium in the myasthenic patient [letter]. Anaesthesia 41:666, 1986.
435. Vacanti CA, Ali HH, Schweiss JF, et al: The response of myasthenia gravis to atracurium. Anesthesiology 62:692, 1985.
436. Bell CF, Florence AM, Hunter JM, et al: Atracurium in the myasthenic patient. Anaesthesia 39:961, 1984.
437. Ward S, Wright DJ: Neuromuscular blockade in myasthenia gravis with atracurium besylate. Anaesthesia 39:51, 1984.
438. Frazer RS, Chalkiadis GA: Anaesthesia and undiagnosed myasthenia gravis. Anaesthesia Intensive Care. 23:114, 1995.
439. Eisenkraft JB, Papatestas AE, Kahn CH, et al: Predicting the need for postoperative mechanical ventilation in myasthenia gravis. Anesthesiology 65:79, 1986.
440. Saraiva PA, Lee JM, deAssis JL, et al: Association tiapride-ketamine dans l'anesthesie en vue d'une thymectomie transsternale dans la myasthenie grave. Ann Chir 39:391, 1985.
441. Grant RP, Jenkins LC: Prediction of the need for postoperative mechanical ventilation in myasthenia gravis: Thymectomy compared to other surgical procedures. Can Anaesth Soc J 29:112, 1982.
442. Bell CMA, Lewis CB: Effect of neostigmine on integrity of ileorectal anastomoses. Br Med J 3:587, 1968.
443. Lake CL: Curare sensitivity in steroid-treated myasthenia gravis: A case report. Anesth Analg 57:132, 1978.
444. Hunter JM, Bell CF, Florence AM, et al: Vecuronium in the myasthenic patient. Anaesthesia 40:848, 1985.
445. Abel M, Eisenkraft JB, Patel N: Response to suxamethonium in a myasthenic patient during remission. Anaesthesia 46:30, 1991.
446. Rolbin SH, Levinson G, Shnider SM, et al: Anesthetic considerations for myasthenia gravis and pregnancy. Anesth Analg 57:441, 1978.
447. Thoulon JM, Galopin G, Seffert P, et al: Myasthenie et grossesse. J Gynecol Obstet Biol Reprod 7:1395, 1978.
448. Coaldrake LA, Livinstone P: Myasthenia gravis in pregnancy. anaesth Intensive Care 11:254, 1983.
449. Lu CH, Liou CM, Chen YS, et al: Anesthetic management in myasthenic parturient. Ma Tsui Hsueh Tsa Chi Anaesthesiol Sin 30:193, 1992.

Myasthenic Syndromes

450. Engel AG: Myasthenic syndromes. *In* Engel AG, Banker BQ (eds): Myology. New York, McGraw-Hill, 1986.
451. Phillips LH: Autonomic nervous system abnormalities in Eaton-Lambert syndrome: Response to immunosuppressive therapy. Ann NY Acad Sci 505:780, 1987.
452. Sanders DB: Lambert-Eaton myasthenic syndrome: Pathogenesis and treatment. Semin Neurol 14:111, 1994.

Connective Tissue Diseases

John H. Eisele, Jr.

The connective tissue system is the extracellular framework of the body composed of structural elements—the fibers—set in a nonstructural matrix—the ground substance. Classification of diseases involving the fibers and their ground substance is not an easy division, since many variations of disturbances have to be considered. This chapter treats three groups of diseases primarily of connective tissue: (1) rheumatoid arthritis and associated or rheumatic disease; (2) the so-called collagen vascular diseases, which include systemic lupus erythematosus, scleroderma, dermatomyositis, periarteritis nodosa, and associated vasculitis syndromes; and (3) granulomatous diseases, namely, Wegener's granulomatosis, lethal midline granuloma, and sarcoidosis. The diseases are discussed in the preceding order and a few less known conditions are included. In covering the various pathologic manifestations, emphasis is placed on the cardiopulmonary system, the nervous system, and other areas of special concern in anesthesiology and surgery.

I. ANESTHETIC CONSIDERATIONS IN CONNECTIVE TISSUE DISEASES

There is no clearly established cause for these diseases and, with the exception of rheumatoid arthritis, the connective tissue disorders are truly uncommon. As a consequence, there is little reported experience on anesthetic management of these patients, except those with rheumatoid arthritis. Likewise, there is little information on the effects, if any, of the connective tissue disorders on anesthetic requirements or on drug kinetics or dynamics. For the practice of anesthesia, however, at least two considerations are very important. First, patients with connective tissue disease are often systemically and chronically ill. This means that anemia, hypovolemia, hypoproteinemia, and reduced ability to handle stress are common. Many of these patients have pulmonary manifestations of their disease, which present an added risk. Less frequently, there may be cardiac, vasomotor, renal, or gastrointestinal involvement. Second, and equally important to the anesthesiologist, is the drug treatment history. Most of the connective tissue diseases in their acute form are treated with corticosteroids. As a result, a history of some steroid medication is almost inevitable.

It is important to clarify some of the physiologic considerations of adrenal function because there are clinical reports as early as 1952[1] of patients who had previously taken steroids and who collapsed during or after operation. The finding that corticotropin (adrenocorticotropic hormone, ACTH) and the hormones of the adrenal gland (cortisol, corticosterone, aldosterone) could be suppressed by exogenous cortisone was put on firm scientific ground in 1965 after measurement of plasma corticotropin became possible (Table 11–1).[2] In patients receiving higher than physiologic doses of cortisone for at least a year, the following events occur:

1. During the first month after withdrawal, there is a tendency for depression of both ACTH and 17-hydroxycorticosteroid (17-OHCS) levels, which is evidence of both pituitary and adrenal hypofunction. Nevertheless, the normal physiologic circadian variation is present.

2. Through the second to fifth months, corticotropin levels rise to what would be considered greater than normal range, whereas 17-OHCS levels tend to remain low—evidence of hyperpituitarism and hypoadrenocorticism.

3. From 5 to 9 months, 17-OHCS levels are in the normal range, but only by virtue of continued high corticotropin levels.

4. After 9 months, there is no detectable difference in treated patients and untreated patients.

Roberts[3] referred to the difficulties in interpreting the many reports of postoperative adrenocortical failure. He pointed out that it was often difficult to discern whether the crisis resulted from inadequate corticotropin output, insufficient adrenal response because of glandular atrophy, or some other unrelated problem. There is a wide range of normal values for plasma 17-OHCS in healthy per-

TABLE 11–1

Normal Values for Adrenal Steroids		
Steroid	Daily Production	Plasma Concentration
Cortisol	20 mg	4–16 µg/100 ml
Corticosterone	5 mg	2 µg/100 ml
Aldosterone	0.25 mg	0.01 µg/100 ml

sons at any time of day, and there is circadian variation: early morning values are double those at evening. In studies by Oyama and colleagues[4] of surgical patients who were not receiving corticosteroids, premedication with atropine, pentobarbital, and morphine reduced the plasma 17-OHCS levels to less than control levels. Halothane and nitrous oxide anesthesia for 40 minutes before surgery was associated with a steady rise in plasma 17-OHCS (14 to 19 μg/dl), which continued to rise after the start of the operation. It is interesting that this rise did not occur when anesthesia was induced with thiopental. Oyama and Takiguichi also studied plasma ACTH levels in anesthesia and observed a transient but large increase during the first 20 minutes of halothane and nitrous oxide anesthesia and a second peak some 30 minutes after starting the operation.[5] It is noteworthy that spinal anesthesia prevents intraoperative and postoperative elevations in 17-OHCS levels.[6]

II. ANESTHETIC MANAGEMENT IN CONNECTIVE TISSUE DISEASES

Every patient taking long-term corticosteroid therapy should be considered abnormal. The question is whether the patient is sufficiently abnormal to require steroid support to withstand the stress of surgery. A clinical test for separating normal from abnormal responses and determining the degree of abnormality would be useful. Thorn's diagnostic test[7] of giving ACTH and measuring plasma 17-OHCS levels over the next hour is worthwhile, but it does not test the ACTH release mechanism. There are other tests for pituitary-adrenal function, but they are too complex and expensive for routine use. In clinical practice, then, we must realize that, although some patients on steroids are still capable of activating their pituitary-adrenal axis in response to stress, we cannot predict who they might be. We are left with an obligation to provide steroid coverage for these patients, regardless of the magnitude of the procedure, because adrenal insufficiency has even been reported after simple bunionectomy.[8] It is worthwhile to review the signs and symptoms of acute adrenal insufficiency, which include hypotension, restlessness, weakness, anorexia with nausea and abdominal pain, and frequently, hyperpyrexia, which may be extreme. When a patient is taking or has

taken steroids, prevention and treatment consist of intravenous hydrocortisone. A common approach is to give hydrocortisone, 100 mg intravenously, just before induction of anesthesia and to continue this dose every 8 hours for 1 to 3 days postoperatively. The following regimen is recommended by Plumpton[9]:

Day of operation and postoperative days 1 through 4: Give hydrocortisone, hemisuccinate or acetate, 100 mg intramuscularly, and every 6 hours thereafter, plus maintenance dose of steroid, if any.

Fourth postoperative day: Discontinue hydrocortisone, but continue maintenance dose of steroid, if any.

Other regimens have been used successfully, and, in general, they depend on the magnitude of the surgical procedure.

III. RHEUMATOID ARTHRITIS

A. GENERAL

Rheumatoid arthritis is a systemic disease that primarily affects connective tissue. Although lesions may be widespread, joint inflammation is the dominant clinical manifestation. The course is variable, but it tends to be chronic and progressive, leading to characteristic deformities and disabilities.

Unlike the collagen diseases, rheumatoid arthritis is far from uncommon. Its prevalence may be as high as 2 to 5 per cent of the population of men and women older than 55 years.[10] In socioeconomic terms, arthritis and rheumatism are second only to heart disease as causes of chronic limitation of activity. Women are affected three to five times as frequently as men, depending on age. The disease can begin at any age, but the most common age of onset is in the fourth decade. By contrast, juvenile rheumatoid arthritis, referred to as Still's disease, has its onset between 2 and 12 years and may be associated with fever, adenopathy, splenomegaly, and a morbilliform rash, but its pathologic appearance is indistinguishable from adult rheumatoid arthritis.

Regarding the etiology, attention has been focused on immunogenetics and autoimmune complexes, but the exact role of each of the many features of immunology remains unclear. Serologic abnormalities, such as the presence of macroglobulins in the plasma cells of diseased synovial membranes, suggest an antigenic stimulus in the articular area. A positive anti–gamma globulin agglutination test result is very common. Antibodies to tissue components are often found, for example, antinuclear and antithyroid antibodies; however, transfusion of these antibodies fails to cause the illness in normal volunteers.

B. PATHOLOGIC FEATURES

Proliferative inflammation of synovial tissue is the outstanding feature of rheumatoid arthritis. The synovial membrane is at first thickened by edema and cell infiltration and is later thrown into folds with hypertrophic villi. As the disease progresses, the synovial tissue grows from the margins onto the joint surface of the articular cartilage or invades the area between it and the bone. The development of granulation tissue, which eventually is converted into dense fibrous scar tissue, dominates the later stages of the disease. Erosion of both cartilage and bone can progress to total destruction of the joint with resultant subluxations, deformities, and contractures of periarticular tissue such as tendons and ligaments (Fig. 11–1).

C. CLINICAL PICTURE

The typical patient usually appears chronically ill, undernourished, and anemic; however, symptoms characteristically disappear for months or years. In most cases, the disease returns, each time in a more chronic form. Most adult cases are polyarticular, affecting the small joints of the hands and feet, usually symmetrically, producing swelling, pain, and limitation of motion. Unlike the collagen diseases or other rheumatic disorders, the disease process tends to persist in any given joint or joints.

Extraarticular manifestations are probably more common than was previously thought. The extent and frequency of visceral involvement in rheumatoid arthritis are difficult to determine because it is often noted only at necropsy. It has been suggested that nonarticular problems in rheumatoid arthritis, in particular vasculitis, are related in some way to steroid therapy. Regardless of their origin, awareness of cardiac, pulmonary, and hematopoietic changes is essential to the care of these patients.

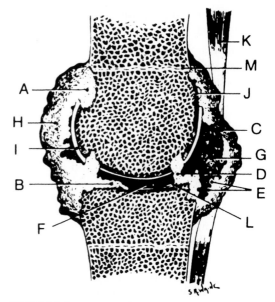

FIGURE 11–1. Diagram of changes in a synovial joint in rheumatoid arthritis. A, Invasion of subchondral bone. B, Erosion of articular cartilage (pannus). C, Fibrotic area. D, Fibrous adhesions. E, Multiple villi. Joint space: F, Narrowing. G, Loculated effusion. H, Laxity of thickened capsule and ligaments. I, Articular cartilage. J, Subchondral bone. K, Muscle. L, Fibrocartilage. M, Old epiphyseal plate.

According to Cathcart and Spodick,[11] the incidence of heart disease in patients with rheumatoid arthritis is 34.7 per cent, as compared with 14.7 per cent in a control group. The most frequent cardiac signs and symptoms are enlargement of the left ventricle, congestive heart failure, and angina pectoris.

Rheumatoid lung or other specific lung lesions in rheumatoid arthritis have been described extensively. Lung involvement, a diffuse infiltrate, produces restriction and thus loss of compliance. What has not been well appreciated is the loss of chest wall compliance that accompanies arthritis in the costovertebral and intervertebral joints. When diffuse interstitial fibrosis is present, there may be an associated oxygen diffusion problem in addition to loss of compliance, and, as a result, arterial PO_2 may be reduced more than is appreciated.

The severity of the lung involvement is usually in keeping with the degree of joint inflammation. In most cases, joint symptoms precede the pulmonary manifestations, but sometimes they appear at the time of recrudescence of joint symptoms and, on rare occasions, acute joint and pulmonary involvement appear simultaneously at the onset of the disease.[12] Pulmonary manifestations generally fall into three patterns:

1. Diffuse interstitial fibrosis can occur without any apparent explanation or related condition. This is perhaps the most common pulmonary lesion associated with rheumatoid arthritis.[13]

2. Granulomatous lesions can occur and, like subcutaneous nodules, can be hard to distinguish from infectious granulomas. They may be multiple or coalescent and produce a honeycombed x-ray picture.

3. Diffuse, large nodules have been described by Caplan in the lungs of coal miners with rheumatoid arthritis.[14] The nodules may represent altered tissue reactivity to silica particles.

Subcutaneous nodules may occur in 5 per cent of patients with rheumatoid arthritis, and they are usually found over the elbow or extensor aspect of finger joints, although they have also been found occasionally in striated muscle, peripheral nerve, heart, lung, uveal tract, and sclera. Lesions resembling subcutaneous nodules have been observed in cardiac valve leaflets and rings, myocardium, and endocardium, although their frequency is hard to estimate.

The most common renal problem associated with rheumatoid arthritis is amyloidosis, which has been found in as many as 20 per cent of autopsy specimens. If severe, this complication can, of course, reduce the excretion of any drugs administered.

In contrast to visceral involvement, the anemia of rheumatoid arthritis is a more constant clinical finding. About 25 per cent of patients with rheumatoid arthritis have normocytic hypochromic anemia, which has the characteristics of the anemia of chronic infection. This anemia is resistant to treatment with oral iron, and despite the rise in serum iron levels, intravenous iron increases the hemoglobin levels only slightly. Blood transfusions have correlated with some clinical improvement and with a decrease in the sedimentation rate.[15] The anemia seen in rheumatoid arthritis, however, is not usually severe, and if the hemoglobin level is less than 10 g, other causes should be sought.

D. TREATMENT

Basic principles of the treatment of this disease include rest, pain relief, maintenance of joint function, prevention and correction of deformities by orthopedic principles, and correction of any factors deleterious to the health of the patient. For analgesia, acetylsalicylate, phenylbutazone, and indomethacin have been used extensively. Gastric disturbance and occult gastrointestinal bleeding are always to be looked for in patients taking the first two drugs. It should be mentioned that sodium salicylate has a direct stimulant effect on metabolism and respiration. In normal humans, prolonged salicylate administration increases the sensitivity of the respiratory center to carbon dioxide.[16] Phenylbutazone has produced occasional bone marrow depression with leukopenia and agranulocytosis. Retention of sodium and water often occurs during the first 10 days of using this drug.

Numerous other compounds have been tried for the treatment of rheumatoid disorders, and today the most common, other than aspirin, are the nonsteroidal antiinflammatory drugs (NSAIDs). These drugs act as aspirin does, by cyclooxygenase inhibition, but they have less serious side effects. Frequently, they are used together with aspirin.

Gold salts have been used extensively in the treatment of rheumatoid arthritis, and there is evidence that these compounds can induce remission of the disease, especially if treatment is begun early. Dermatitis, stomatitis, renal damage, and bone marrow depression have limited the wide use of gold.

Systemic use of adrenal corticosteroids is effective in suppressing the disease, but there is nearly always a relapse when the drug is stopped. The dangers of inducing a hypoadrenocortical state are well-known; consequently, this drug is employed only after other methods of controlling the disease fail. In current practice, however, a large number of patients with rheumatoid arthritis are taking maintenance levels of steroids, and one must be continually on guard for peptic ulceration, aggravation of infection, fracture of long bones, and psychic disturbances.

IV. OTHER DISEASES WITH PATHOLOGIC SIMILARITIES TO RHEUMATOID ARTHRITIS

A. ANKYLOSING SPONDYLITIS

The discovery of the association of ankylosing spondylitis with a genetic marker—the HLA B27 antigen—has revealed that the disease is more common than was previously thought and that it is distributed equally between men and women.[17] It is pathologically indistinguishable from rheumatoid arthritis and is a chronic progressive disease of the sacroiliac and the synovial joints (apophyseal) of the spine, including the surrounding soft tissues. Bony bridges develop along the vertebrae, giving rise to ankylosis and the classic bamboo spine x-ray appearance. It differs from rheumatoid arthritis in that the disease is generally confined to the spine and hips, and the vertebral and sacroiliac changes produce characteristic (and diagnostic) x-ray pictures. Impaired rotation and limitation of bending of the spine can produce significant restriction of chest expansion. Most patients have restrictive ventilatory defects, and residual volume can be increased by fixation of the ribs in a position of inspiration. Eventually, ventilation becomes totally dependent on diaphragmatic function. Pulmonary, cardiovascular, and neurologic manifestations are relatively rare, though they are more common in long-standing disease.[18]

Scarring of the aorta and aortic valve cusps can lead to aortitis and aortic insufficiency, whereas involvement of the conduction tissue can lead to Stokes-Adams attacks and the need for a pacemaker.[19] Neurologic signs and symptoms can include spinal cord compression, the cauda equina syndrome, vertebrobasilar insufficiency, and peripheral nerve lesions. Patients with ankylosing spondylitis may experience atlantooccipital subluxation or dislocation from relatively minor trauma, which is of great concern to the anesthesiologist. Cricoarytenoid arthritis may also occur in these patients, and when coupled with cervical spine limitation and atlantooccipital fragility, it presents the most serious array of intubation and airway hazards imaginable.

B. REITER'S SYNDROME

This triad of nongonococcal urethritis, conjunctivitis, and subacute or chronic polyarthritis occurs mainly in young adult men. Mucocutaneous lesions are common. The arthritis dominates the clinical picture and usually lasts 3 to 4 months; it then undergoes spontaneous remission but recurrences are common. Most patients recover completely, but chronic arthritis and residual joint damage can occur. Antibiotics are not recom-

mended; however, success has been reported with azathioprine,[20] an antimetabolic agent.

C. SJÖGREN'S SYNDROME

Sjögren's syndrome is a chronic inflammatory disease marked by diminished lacrimal and salivary gland secretion resulting in a combination of keratoconjunctivitis sicca, xerostomia, and rheumatoid arthritis. The joint involvement has no distinguishing characteristics. More than 90 per cent of patients are women, and they exhibit features of severe oral and ocular dryness, often accompanied by parotitis and neck swelling caused by lymphoproliferation. The lack of lacrimal and salivary secretions, called the *siccalike syndrome*, is a benign condition treated with fluids and appropriate lubricants. Enlargement of the submandibular and parotid glands can produce serious problems in maintaining an airway and in visualizing the glottic opening (Fig. 11–2).

1. Anesthetic Management of Rheumatoid Arthritis and Associated Diseases

Because of the frequency of rheumatoid arthritis and associated diseases, the anesthesiologist is likely to see many patients undergoing surgery for corrective orthopedic

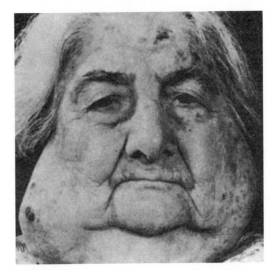

FIGURE 11–2. Massive enlargement of the parotids in an 82-year-old woman with Sjögren's syndrome. Swelling of the glands was first noted seven years before this photograph was obtained.

procedures and complications of corticosteroid therapy, as well as for the usual surgical causes.

Involvement of the cricoarytenoid joint may occur in as many as 26 per cent of patients with rheumatoid arthritis.[21] It can also be seen in patients with Reiter's syndrome or systemic lupus erythematosus. The symptoms of cricoarytenoid arthritis, in order of frequency, are fullness or tightness in the throat, a sensation of a foreign body in the throat, hoarseness or stridor, dysphagia, pain on swallowing, dyspnea, and pain radiating to the ears. Preoperative diagnosis can be made by direct laryngoscopy, whereupon the arytenoid mucosa may appear red and edematous or thick, rough, and irregular. The glottic opening may be narrowed, and the vocal cords, though normal in appearance, bow in the middle during inspiration. The degree of cricoarytenoid involvement is apparently related to the activity of the disease. An excellent review of the pathologic presentation of cricoarytenoid arthritis and its problems related to anesthesia was given by Phelps[22] (Fig. 11–3).

Many clinicians believe that, for these patients, regional anesthesia is safer than general anesthesia. When the operative site precludes a regional block, preoperative tracheostomy may have to be considered. Edelist, in his 1966 review,[23] states that the most common airway problem in patients with rheumatoid arthritis is a flexion deformity of the cervical spine, and he warns that the head and neck should be manipulated with great care during positioning and intubation, since cervical vertebral erosion and subluxation can occur, especially at the atlantoaxial joint (Fig. 11–4).

Arthritis and ankylosis of the temporomandibular joint may be the only airway problems in many patients with rheumatoid arthritis. If the mouth cannot be opened, nasal intubation or tracheostomy must be performed to ensure a patent airway during an-

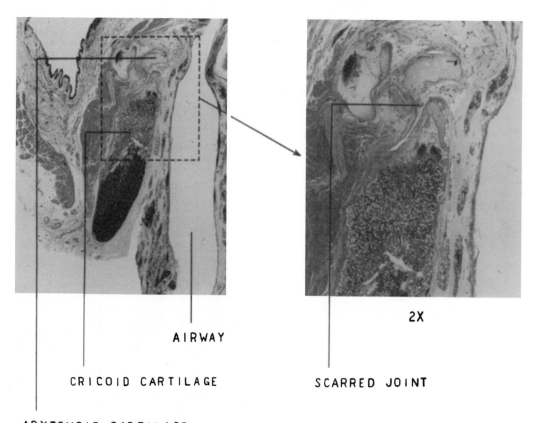

AIRWAY

CRICOID CARTILAGE

2X

SCARRED JOINT

ARYTENOID CARTILAGE

FIGURE 11–3. Coronal (frontal) section of the right half of the larynx from a 61-year-old Caucasian female with severe, generalized rheumatoid arthritis, revealing eburnation of the cartilages, marked fibrosis, and almost complete loss of the right cricoarytenoid joint. (Reprinted with permission from Phelps, J. A.: Laryngeal obstruction due to cricoarytenoid arthritis. Anesthesiology 27:518–522, 1966.)

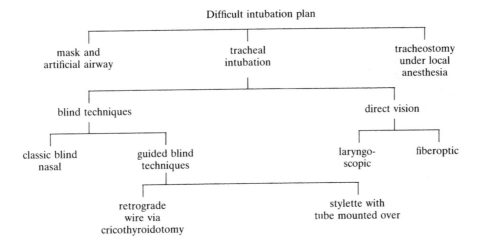

esthesia. Temporomandibular problems are common, and patients who have only partial limitation, tenderness, or crepitus of this joint usually do not have increased symptoms after extubation.[24] A most unusual case of severe cervical spondylosis in a man unable to lift his head off his chest, which precluded tracheostomy, and who also was unable to open his mouth, has been described by Munson and Cullen.[25] Intubation with the patient awake was cleverly performed without moving the patient by using a nasal endotracheal catheter and an oral wire hook to direct the tip of the catheter into the larynx (Figs. 11–5 and 11–6). Cervical osteotomy was then performed so that the head could be extended enough to permit the patient to open the mouth and so that the ulcers that had formed over the chin and sternum could heal. Thus, it is essential to have a clear plan of airway

management alternatives. The chart at the top of this page is an example of a difficult intubation plan.

It is necessary to assist or control ventilation during general anesthesia for patients who have rheumatoid lung changes and possibly costochondral involvement limiting chest wall expansion. Jenkins[26] states that chronic diffuse interstitial pulmonary fibrosis is the most serious pulmonary lesion of rheumatoid arthritis, and he warns that an unrecognized tuberculous lung is not unusual in patients with rheumatoid arthritis. Gardner and Holmes indicate that patients with rheumatoid arthritis are extremely sensitive to agents that depress respiratory function, and they question how efficiently these patients can mobilize drugs.[27] There is general agreement that patients with rheumatoid arthritis should not be left alone postopera-

FIGURE 11–4. *A,* Advanced rheumatoid arthritis of the cervical spine consisting of resorption of the dens (odontoid) and spinous processes *(black arrows),* ankylosis of the C2-C3 apophyseal joints, erosions at the joints of Luschka and adjacent end-plates *(white arrows),* moderate disc narrowing, anterior subluxation of C6-C7, and, finally, generalized demineralization. *B,* Typical "step ladder" subluxations and disc narrowing in advanced rheumatoid arthritis.

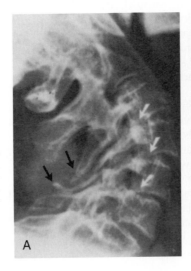 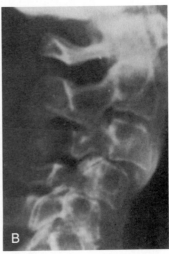

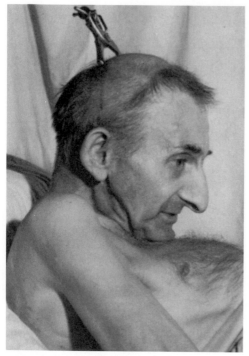

FIGURE 11–5. A 55-year-old man with a severe, fixed deformity of the cervical spine. Skin ulcerations developed over both mandible and sternum, and he could take nourishment only through a straw. A cervical osteotomy was performed to permit some neck extension.

To evaluate the operative risk and to determine the hazards attending the preoperative management of patients with rheumatoid arthritis the following checklist is recommended:

1. Examination of neck and jaw mobility
2. Indirect laryngoscopy (if arytenoid arthritis is suspected)
3. Chest x-ray film
4. Skeletal x-ray film (if there is spine limitation)
5. Pulmonary function tests
6. Blood gas analysis
7. Electrocardiography
8. Hemoglobin and sedimentation rate determinations
9. White blood cell and platelet counts
10. Urinalysis
11. Occult blood in stool
12. Creatinine clearance
13. Drug therapy history
14. Recent general anesthesia

The same general considerations should govern the management of the associated or

tively and that it is wise to carefully watch, and even assist, respiratory function.

Anemia in patients with rheumatoid arthritis can be a serious problem, and preoperative evaluation is imperative. Causes for anemia must be investigated, especially in taking drugs known sometimes to produce gastrointestinal bleeding. The presence of anemia may mean there is also hypovolemia and hypoproteinemia. Blood replacement should be planned for extensive operations. It is common practice today to have patients donate their own blood for autotransfusion in anticipation of major elective surgery, thus avoiding the risks associated with blood-borne diseases.

There is universal agreement that supplemental steroids should be given to patients currently taking corticosteroids, to those who have been on prolonged therapy within 1 year of surgery, and to those who have been on prolonged steroid therapy up to 2 years before surgery when evidence of hypocortisonism exists. For a detailed discussion of this aspect of management, the reader is referred to "Anesthetic Management in Connective Tissue Diseases" earlier in this chapter.

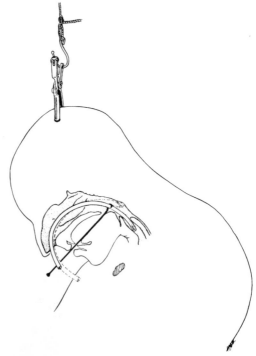

FIGURE 11–6. Drawing showing position of endotracheal catheter after anterior placement by wire "hook." (Reprinted with permission from Munson, E. S., and Cullen, S.C.: Endotracheal intubation in a patient with ankylosing spondylitis of the cervical spine. Anesthesiology 26:365, 1965.)

rheumatoid diseases. With ankylosing spondylitis, it is extremely important to determine the range of motion of the head and neck and the spine preoperatively. Spinal or epidural anesthesia may be difficult (if not impossible) if the intervertebral ligaments are calcified. Caudal anesthesia has been used successfully for hip surgery in ankylosing spondylitis,[28] but it is surely not appropriate for most patients. The authors recommended preoperative x-ray studies of the sacrum to exclude technical difficulties. Wittman and Ring[29] consider epidural or spinal block to be contraindicated because the ossification of interspinous ligaments and bony bridges make the placement of a needle very difficult, and there is a higher risk of causing a vertebral fracture, which can produce a severe neurologic deficit. In addition, if there is a complication with the block, such as intravenous injection, intubation has to be done emergently. They recommend intubation with the patient awake using fiberoptic laryngoscopy or a guidewire passed up from the cricothyroid membrane.[30] Extubation should be done only when the patient has fully regained laryngeal reflexes. From the anesthetic point of view, preoperative assessment, including indirect laryngoscopy and careful preparation for potential problems, should enable those patients to be managed safely. In severe cases of cervical spondylitis, one should consider sensory evoked potentials (SEPs) to monitor neurologic function if manipulation is anticipated, either for anesthesia or surgical positioning.

The greatest danger occurs when these patients present for surgical procedures unrelated to their condition and difficulties are not anticipated. Trivial procedures can end up in disaster; therefore, one should always be prepared with appropriate intubating equipment and a so-called difficult intubation plan.

In Sjögren's syndrome, it is appropriate to omit the use of drying agents, since the secretory glands are fibrosed. It would be helpful to employ a rebreathing system with added humidification to avoid excessive drying of the airways during endotracheal anesthesia.

V. COLLAGEN VASCULAR DISEASES

Today, the term *immune-complex diseases* has practically replaced the term *collagen* (or *collagen vascular*) *diseases* because of the character-istic pathologic feature of deposition of immune complexes in a specific organ or tissue, the most common sites being the glomerulus of the kidney and the blood vessel walls. The immune deposits are thought to arise from antigen-antibody complexes formed in the circulation, which once deposited activate a variety of potent mediators of inflammation such as complement proteins, leading to an influx of polymorphonuclear neutrophils and monocytes. These activated cells release toxic products of oxygen metabolism as well as proteases and other enzymes, ultimately causing tissue damage. Although the specific cause of these diseases is variable, they share a common pathophysiology. The clinical features of these diseases are quite diverse, ranging from mild cutaneous eruptions to severe organ involvement with pericarditis, glomerulonephritis, and vasculitis. The concept of collagen diseases was advanced years ago and it implied pathologic similarities in diseases of unknown cause that had common alterations in interfibrillary ground substance, proliferation of fibroblasts, a predominant mononuclear inflammatory reaction, and necrosis associated with production of fibrinoid material.

The following disorders listed in order of prevalence in the United States are generally considered collagen vascular diseases: systemic lupus erythematosus, scleroderma and scleredema, and dermatomyositis. Also in the classification of immune-complex diseases are the vasculitis syndromes: polyarteritis nodosa, thrombotic thrombocytopenic purpura, temporal or cranial arteritis, and Takayasu's arteritis. Thrombotic thrombocytopenic purpura is discussed in another chapter.

A. SYSTEMIC LUPUS ERYTHEMATOSUS

1. General

Systemic lupus erythematosus (SLE) has numerous manifestations associated with lesions of connective tissue in the vascular system, the dermis, and the serous and synovial membranes. The multitude of visceral manifestations that are often present in a complex pattern make the diagnosis difficult. Lupus is predominantly a disease of women of childbearing age. It appears to be more common than was previously thought and is more common among black Americans than white ones.

There are many serum protein abnormalities, including the factor that produces lupus erythematosus cells, and many abnormal serum gamma globulins, giving rise to the concept that lupus is an autoimmune disorder. The finding of abnormal serum antibodies can be helpful in the diagnosis, since lupus can imitate almost any other clinical entity. A genetic factor may play a role, leading to formation of excessive antibodies and impaired suppressor T cells. The incidence of lupus in homozygous twins is 70 per cent. With reduced T cells and decreased activity of complement, the body is unable to destroy the excessive antigen-antibody complexes that can precipitate in kidney tissues, leading to damage. Most of the reactions affect the small blood vessels, causing widespread vasculitis.

2. Clinical Picture

The general symptoms associated with this disease are usually fatigue, wasting, anorexia, and fever. The initial clinical picture is variable, though skin and joints are common sites of onset. A characteristic malar facial erythematous rash of butterfly shape is helpful but is present in fewer than half the cases (Fig. 11–7). Changes in pigmentation and telangiectasia and ulcerations can develop. Joint pain and swelling may resemble rheumatoid arthritis and obscure the diagnosis. Renal involvement occurs in 75 per cent of patients, and it produces glomerulonephritis that is often progressive and fatal. More than half of patients have involvement of the pericardium, endocardium, or myocardium. When fever and a pericardial friction rub are present, the disease resembles rheumatic fever.

Pleurisy accompanied by a small effusion is a common feature of lupus. There may be progressive dyspnea and cyanosis, but fine basilar rales may be the only finding. Pulmonary infiltrates, which appear in many cases, are frequently migratory, and on x-ray film they look like basal pneumonitis with focal atelectasis.[31] Sometimes there is a micronodular pattern resembling ground glass. Histologic changes of focal necrosis of alveolar walls may be similar to lesions seen in polyarteritis nodosa and rheumatoid arthritis.

Neurologic signs may include diverse mental and personal deterioration. Peripheral neuropathy, involving cranial and peripheral nerves, occurs in 10 per cent of cases. There can be a simple foot drop or a complex as-

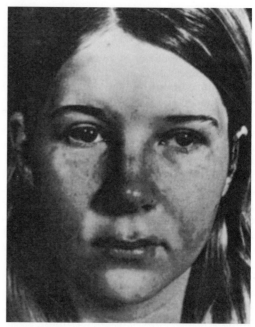

FIGURE 11–7. Facies of a 19-year-old girl with acute systemic lupus erythematosus. There is a classic butterfly eruption over the bridge of the nose and malar regions.

cending polyneuritis like Guillain-Barré syndrome. Grand mal seizures may occur in 20 per cent of cases.

The clinical course is marked by exacerbations and remissions extending over years. Spontaneous remissions are common, lasting months or even years. It is interesting that long-term administration of drugs such as hydralazine, isoniazid, para-aminosalicylic acid, procainamide, and others can induce the clinical lupus syndrome, including the serum antibodies. This suggests that there may be a host abnormality predisposing to abnormal immunologic reactivity. Judicious use of steroids in the majority of cases results in prolongation of life and a nearly normal existence.

When lupus occurs in pregnancy, fetal wastage increases and prematurity is also frequent. A large percentage of pregnant women with lupus have babies with congenital heart block; therefore a slow fetal heart rate during labor does not necessarily mean fetal distress.

3. Anesthetic Management

The cutaneous lesions (discoid lupus) can present as severe nasal and malar eruptions that make the fit of a face mask difficult during anesthesia. Intubation may be necessary for a good airway, and though this should not be a problem, there are rare reports of cricoarytenoid arthritis with a narrowed airway in SLE.[32]

The preparation of lupus patients for surgery may not be easy, since they are generally very sick, with fever and often pneumonitis and renal involvement. It is important that the anesthesiologist be aware of any and all related problems. In particular, the chest x-ray film should be studied, as well as the serum electrolytes and the blood count. Anemia is very common and occasionally a hemorrhagic disorder similar to thrombocytopenic purpura may develop. Occasionally, cryoglobulins have been noted as well as circulating anticoagulants associated with a prolongation of clotting times. Thus, a platelet count and bleeding and clotting time determinations are useful prior to surgery.

The clotting factors are also affected, but tests such as the partial thromboplastin time (PTT) can be falsely elevated because the lupus antibodies react with phospholipids used to determine the PTT. A more serious manifestation, though rare, is the reaction of antibodies with factors VIII, IX, and XII, which leads to bleeding. There is little or no correlation between the coagulation tests and clinical hemorrhage. Therefore, if the patient with lupus has clinical bleeding or petechial hemorrhages, spinal or epidural anesthesia is contraindicated. This is a special problem in obstetrical anesthesia, as SLE is more prevalent in women in their childbearing years.[33]

In the presence of advanced renal disease, the anesthesiologist must carefully consider the need to give drugs excreted principally by the kidneys. At the same time, it should be noted that hypotension during anesthesia can lead to reduced renal blood flow and, hence, reduced renal clearance. The perfusion threshold for the kidney in these patients may not be known, but the anesthesiologist should appreciate that there is less tolerance of hypotension.

Treatment with corticosteroids in this disease invariably is attempted at some time; therefore, adequate preoperative and intraoperative coverage must be considered.

B. SCLERODERMA (PROGRESSIVE SYSTEMIC SCLEROSIS)

1. General

Scleroderma causes widespread symmetric, leathery induration of the skin, followed by atrophy and pigmentation. The skin lesions are the external manifestation of a systemic disease, and the muscles, bones, mucous membranes, heart, lungs, intestinal tract, and other internal organs may be involved. Scleroderma occurs more often in women, and the usual onset is age 30 to 50 years. There is a local form of this disease, morphea, as well as the generalized form. Histologic diagnosis depends on an increase in otherwise normal collagen fibers. Later, there is atrophy of the epidermis, and in some cases calcification develops. The association of *c*alcinosis, *R*aynaud's phenomenon, *e*sophageal hypomotility, *s*clerodactyly, and *t*elangiectasias is known as the CREST syndrome.

Vasospastic phenomena are seen so commonly in this disease that it has led investigators to propose a hypersensitivity of autonomic nerves as an important causative factor. Studies have shown a greater increase in peripheral blood flow following intravenous procaine administration in these patients when compared with individuals without scleroderma. Coffman observed a 30 to 50 per cent decrease in blood flow to the subcutaneous tissues of the forearm in scleroderma.[34] Improving blood flow with dextran had no effect on the duration of local anesthesia, but using a bicarbonate infusion did normalize the time of local anesthetic effect, which suggests that tissue pH is reduced in scleroderma.[35]

In contrast, Henriksen and Kristensen[36] studied 10 patients with scleroderma and Raynaud's phenomenon, noting a significant reduction in finger blood pressure that was unaltered by sympathetic blockade, suggesting an increased flow resistance in the palmar arch and digital arteries not caused by augmented sympathetic vasoconstrictor activity.

2. Clinical Picture

In the classic form of scleroderma, the cutaneous changes pass through several stages. First, there is a brawny, nonpitting edema, which gives the hands, feet, and face a puffy white appearance with smoothing of the normal folds. Second, the skin becomes waxy, smooth, and tight so that it is fixed to the deeper structures. Over time, this may be more prominent on the fingers, back of the hands, and ankles. The face may become mask-like (Fig. 11–8). Weakness and loss of

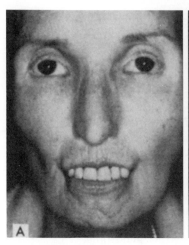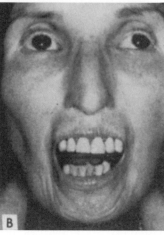

FIGURE 11–8. Typical facies of scleroderma; smoothness and loss of lines of expression are apparent. Oral aperture is markedly decreased.

weight are common, and fever and joint pains may also occur sometimes as prodromata.

Raynaud's phenomenon and sclerodactyly, often associated with esophageal involvement, may be present years before the skin changes. Scleroderma of the gastrointestinal tract is common. As the disease advances to the atrophic stage, the skin becomes thinner and adheres to the shrunken muscles. Joint movement may be progressively restricted until the patient resembles a living mummy.

Pulmonary complications occur in almost all cases of scleroderma. Ritchie[37] noted that 21 of 22 patients with scleroderma had abnormal lung function. Vital capacity and lung volumes are reduced because of replacement of lung by fibrous tissue and alterations in the elastic properties of the alveoli. Lung compliance is commonly reduced, to a degree out of proportion to the lung volume reduction. There is an increase in dead space from widening of the airways, which also reduces resistance, and the result is that these patients breathe at a faster rate to preserve normal alveolar ventilation. Impaired pulmonary diffusing capacity is common in scleroderma and, as with sarcoidosis, a lowered diffusing capacity may be present with minimal symptoms or alterations seen on x-ray films. Progressive generalized scleroderma may involve the chest wall and intercostal muscles without systemic involvement. Such a case resulted in death from respiratory failure. No pulmonary pathologic condition was found.[38] Another case report pointed out that respiratory failure may be a result of sclerodermatous involvement of the diaphragm.[39]

Pulmonary hypertension was seen in half of the patients with scleroderma studied by Sackner,[40] and is a major cause of death in these patients.[41] The degree of restrictive lung disease, diffusing capacity, and the appearance of the chest x-ray film correlate poorly with pulmonary artery pressures, indicating that this hypertension is another manifestation of a widespread vascular disturbance.[42]

Cardiac involvement or sclerodermatous heart disease can result from myocardial fibrosis and can lead to heart failure; however, it is rare. In patients with scleroderma and an associated myositis, however, myocarditis is common and is responsive to steroid therapy unless there is a conduction defect.[43] A study emphasizing 24-hour monitoring of the electrocardiogram indicated a high incidence of abnormalities attributed to scleroderma, though their significance was not determined.[44] Most cases of congestive heart failure are secondary to pulmonary hypertension. Left ventricular hypertrophy may occur as a result of scleroderma of the kidney with severe hypertension. Significant renal involvement is uniformly fatal, as the disease can affect the renal arteries, producing a pathologic picture indistinguishable from malignant nephrosclerosis.

Therapy in scleroderma has not had much effect in changing the clinical course, which finds almost 50 per cent of the patients dead in 2 years. In many, the disease is chronic and prolonged. Steroids have been used extensively with varying but not encouraging results.

C. SCLEREDEMA (SCLEREDEMA ADULTORUM OF BUSCHKE)

This is a rare condition that follows acute infection. It has a benign course and is characterized by brawny, nonpitting edema of the skin that may resemble that of scleroderma. It is a diffuse disease of collagen that usually develops a few weeks after infection, which is most frequently of streptococcal origin. There is sometimes a prodromal period of fever, malaise, and myalgia. Most cases occur in girls, and the neck is the first area to be involved, with subsequent spread to the face, chest, abdomen, and extremities. Involvement of the tongue and pharynx results in dysphagia, whereas chest wall changes may produce dyspnea. There is resolution of the edema in 6 to 18 months; however, the disease may remain for years.

Scleredema is differentiated from scleroderma in that the induration is more prominent in the superficial layers of the skin, and neither atrophy nor pigmentation develops. Hands and feet are rarely involved. Other conditions such as trichinosis, myxedema, and edema from cardiac or renal origin are distinguished by the associated manifestations.

1. Anesthetic Management of Scleroderma and Scleredema

Because of the gastrointestinal complications and, to some extent, the consequences of cutaneous calcification, it is not rare to see scleroderma patients undergoing surgery. Recorded anesthetic management of scleroderma is sparse; nonetheless, certain principles would seem evident.

Tightening of the skin around the mouth may produce severe jaw limitation, so it is important to determine how wide these patients can open their mouths, as intubation may require a nasal approach or a fiberoptic technique. Pulmonary problems are the rule in scleroderma; therefore, lung function studies should be performed preoperatively to determine the degree of restrictive disease. Blood gas analyses should also be performed. Evidence of pulmonary hypertension should be looked for on x-ray film, electrocardiograms, single-breath diffusion tests, and clinical auscultation for an accentuated pulmonic sound. Ventilation may be difficult in patients with scleroderma as a result of altered compliance; consequently, it is unwise to permit spontaneous breathing during anesthesia, particularly if the preoperative blood gas values were abnormal. It is important that these patients be observed with great care in the immediate postoperative period, as they may need ventilatory assistance, especially if narcotics are used.

Vasospastic phenomena in scleroderma are so common that one should consider the possible hemodynamic consequences after induction of anesthesia and its associated vasodilatation. Scleroderma patients may, in effect, have reduced circulating red cell volume (like some hypertensive patients, e.g., those with pheochromocytoma), and when the peripheral vascular bed opens, profound hypotension can develop. This situation can be anticipated and treated with a plasma expander if crystalloids are not sufficient.

Regional anesthesia may be considered preferable in scleroderma, especially in view of the frequent pulmonary problems. In this regard, the author warns against the prolonged effect of local anesthetics with epinephrine in patients with Raynaud's phenomenon. An axillary block with 1.5 per cent xylocaine with epinephrine 1:100,000 produced sensory deficits in the fingers for 24 hours in a patient with scleroderma.[45] This same patient was then tested with small (2-ml) subcutaneous injections on each side of the umbilicus. One side was anesthetized with 1 per cent xylocaine for 6 to 7 hours; the other side with 1 per cent xylocaine and 1:100,000 epinephrine for more than 10 hours. This surprising result on the anterior abdominal wall suggests that vasomotor instability was widespread, which counsels caution in the use of any local anesthetic in scleroderma, and in particular to avoid epinephrine. Regional anesthesia has been used successfully for cesarean section in a pregnant patient who had progressive scleroderma for 4 years.[46] One should be prepared, however, to manage a very difficult airway should the block fail. In a case report of pulmonary edema after cesarean section under general anesthesia,[47] the authors did not explain the mechanism but suggested placing a pulmonary artery catheter before induction of anesthesia, especially if there is pulmonary hypertension and cardiac or renal involvement, or both.

In patients with scleroderma and Raynaud's phenomenon, measurement of blood pressure can be difficult and findings have been misleading. Forearm blood flow is markedly reduced in these patients. Ultrasonic or Doppler blood pressure instruments may be necessary for monitoring, since arterial catheterization is not recommended because of the increased risk of severe ischemia to the hand.

Skin temperatures are generally reduced, and intramuscular temperature has been recorded to be 1.5°C lower than core temperature in this disease. For long surgical procedures warming the room and using warmed blankets are strongly recommended. Warm compresses may be especially helpful for locating veins in the extremities. A gas induction may be necessary when venous access is impossible. Pretreatment with antacids and histamine H_2 blockers should be considered in such cases because of poor gastric emptying and an uncertain airway, which argue against rapid-sequence induction.[48] Awake intubation in the head-up position is a safer approach.

D. DERMATOMYOSITIS (NEUROMYOSITIS, POLYMYOSITIS)

1. General

The hallmarks of dermatomyositis are edema, dermatitis, and inflammation of multiple muscles. The microscopic appearance of muscle and skin is not, however, pathognomonic. The skin, affected in 50 per cent of instances, shows atrophy of the epidermis, whereas the dermis is edematous and mucoid, and the connective tissue is condensed, fibrotic, and infiltrated with cells. The appearance resembles scleroderma, but systemic involvement is quite rare. The muscle fibers become vacuolated and degenerated. Calcinosis may eventually develop in the subcutaneous tissues, muscles, and fascia. The disease is rare, affects females more than males, and its usual onset is in the 40- to 50-year age range; however, it is the collagen vascular disorder most commonly seen in children. The familial occurrence of myositis and the presence of HLA-B8 antigen in many patients suggest a genetic disposition to the disease.

2. Clinical Picture

The onset is often heralded by a facial rash with edema and vague malaise. The rash spreads in a butterfly distribution as in lupus erythematosus, but it is more bluish. The eyelids may be swollen and show the heliotrope color caused by telangiectasis (Fig. 11–9). The dermal and muscle manifestations do not run

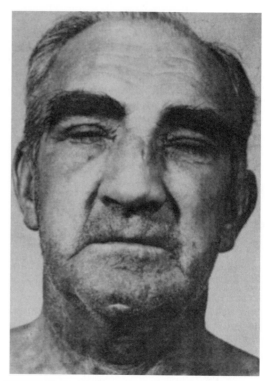

FIGURE 11–9. Classic skin rash in dermatomyositis. There is marked periorbital edema and erythema with facial edema, especially of the cheeks. Dusky erythema is also present on the neck, the sides of the forehead, and the "V" of the neck.

parallel. In 50 per cent of patients, rheumatic signs appear in conjunction with the muscle weakness. Muscle involvement is usually bilateral and symmetric, affecting the neck, shoulders, and pelvic muscles. Eventually, there is muscle wasting and stiffness, and fixation of the joints may occur. Diplopia, dyspnea, and impaired sphincter control may be seen. Isolated lung disease is very rare in this disorder; however, Hepper[49] reported three types of pulmonary involvement: (1) aspiration pneumonia related to weakness of the muscles involved in swallowing, (2) respiratory insufficiency caused by progressive weakening of the intercostal and diaphragm muscles, and (3) lung involvement from the connective tissue disease itself. It was described as a patchy infiltrative process throughout both lungs that responded favorably to steroid therapy. Intermittent fever, malaise, and anorexia are common, and the course progresses to death in about half of the patients. Those who survive 1 year may go into a long remission. Corticosteroids appear to be effective when used in large doses, especially in the early phase.

3. Anesthetic Management of Dermatomyositis

Since dermatomyositis is a systemic disease, the anesthesiologist should be concerned with anemia as well as intercurrent infection, which may be common in patients who have lost their ability to swallow. These patients do not have the tight skin—and thus the problems in opening the mouth—associated with scleroderma. Two case reports of this disease developing shortly after local anesthesia of the amide type for dental procedures are interesting.[50] It was speculated that in one case an immunoreactive process occurred in which the local anesthetic acted as a haptene. There are analogous reports of similar drugs triggering lupus erythematosus.

It seems reasonable that dermatomyositis patients should require less neuromuscular relaxant drug because of their diminished muscle mass. There is some evidence that they may have altered sensitivity to the muscle relaxants referred to by Wylie and Churchill-Davidson.[51] In examining ten patients with dermatomyositis, they found two who demonstrated a myasthenic response using a decamethonium test. This means that electromyographically recorded fasciculations were not blocked by decamethonium, which is the finding in myasthenia gravis. One of the two patients, however, had bronchogenic carcinoma, and it was not stated whether or not he had a neuropathy. Carcinomas of breast, ovary, lung, and stomach occur in as many as 15 per cent of patients with dermatomyositis, and carcinomatous neuropathies are more frequent in these tumors. This is significant in that patients with dermatomyositis may have an occult carcinoma associated with neuromuscular weakness and myasthenic responses. Although this complication of dermatomyositis may not be common, it should alert the anesthesiologist to give small test doses of relaxants if relaxation is required.

A review of the anesthetic management of a child demonstrated a careful evaluation of the hand muscle twitch response to succinylcholine (1 mg/kg intravenously). The child showed a contracture response similar to that seen following succinylcholine given to a patient with myotonic dystrophy. The twitch depression was associated with a rise in the baseline value, normal duration, and return to control of twitch tension with a normal (20 per cent) rise in serum potassium levels.[52]

In view of reports of respiratory impairment caused by either aspiration pneumonia or weakness of inspiratory muscles, it is imperative to determine ventilatory adequacy preoperatively. A vital capacity measurement, blood gas analysis, and chest film, coupled with a good clinical evaluation, dictates how these patients can best be managed during anesthesia and surgery. If the patient's ventilatory status before surgery is marginal with reduced vital capacity, he or she should not be permitted to breathe spontaneously, either during surgery or in the immediate postoperative period.

E. POLYARTERITIS NODOSA (PERIARTERITIS, NECROTIZING ANGIITIS)

1. General

Polyarteritis nodosa is characterized by widespread vascular lesions manifested in variable signs and symptoms from any organ, except that pulmonary arteries are not involved in the classic form. The presence of hepatitis B antigens and complement in blood vessel walls strongly suggests the role of immune phenomena in the pathogenesis of this disease. Diagnosis is made from an arterial biopsy specimen that demonstrates vasculitis without eosinophils, which are present in allergic vasculitis.

Unlike other collagen diseases, polyarteritis affects males three times more often than females. The lesions involve arteries of medium and small caliber, with necrosis, fibrinoid changes, and infiltration with leukocytes. Weakening and dilatation of the vessel wall can lead to hemorrhage. The vessels are typically involved segmentally. The lesions are common in the kidneys, heart, gastrointestinal tract, liver, lungs, adrenal glands, testes, brain, and peripheral nerves.

2. Clinical Picture

Many patients who develop polyarteritis already have chronic or acute respiratory infection, and the early symptoms are fever and tenderness of the extremities. Involvement of the alimentary tract, skin, joints, and peripheral nerves are the common early signs. Renal lesions are frequent, and they produce glomerulitis that leads to renal failure, whereas survivors develop renal hypertension. Abdominal pain resulting from arteritis of abdominal viscera and painful peripheral neuritis are common symptoms. There may be central nervous system involvement, manifested as subarachnoid hemorrhage, facial palsy, hemiplegia, and convulsions. The coronary vessels can be involved, producing myocardial infarction. Heart failure may be associated with severe hypertension, which is often present.

Pulmonary lesions of polyarteritis are common and interesting because they usually precede polyarteritis in other areas and can mimic asthma, pneumonia, or bronchitis. Focal lesions scattered throughout the lungs may suggest tuberculosis, sarcoidosis, or carcinomatosis. Unlike with other polyarteritis lesions, there is an eosinophilia, and sometimes nasal granulomata, making it difficult to differentiate from Wegener's granulomatosis. Rose and Spencer[53] found that lung lesions could precede generalized polyarteritis by years and that treatment with corticosteroids could lead to permanent control.

Other common manifestations of this disease include joint involvement, which is usually migratory and resembles that of rheumatic fever, and sometimes chronic deformation of joints that resembles rheumatoid arthritis. Skin lesions are found in 25 per cent of patients in the form of nodules that vary in size and are frequently tender.

The course of this disease is variable, but it is usually fatal when there is involvement of kidneys, lungs, or heart. Long remissions have occurred and are probably related to steroid therapy. Biopsy specimens have shown suppression of arterial inflammation within weeks after steroid treatment, which may require large doses.

F. TEMPORAL ARTERITIS AND TAKAYASU'S ARTERITIS

Temporal arteritis, also called *cranial* or *giant cell arteritis,* is an inflammation of medium-sized and large arteries. It is part of a generalized vascular disorder in which the carotid arterial system is so often involved that it is designated a separate clinical entity. The larger arteries are affected, particularly the temporal and occipital ones, but the disease is a panarteritis with inflammation starting in the adventitia and spreading into the media. It affects principally older people of both sexes equally. The clinical stages can be divided into (1) headache, (2) ocular complications, and (3) systemic complications. The eye manifestations can result from ophthalmoplegic or vascular lesions affecting the optic nerve and retina. Complete blindness is the most common end result. Systemic arteritis, with skin and visceral lesions, polyneuropathy, and muscle and joint involvement, may occur, although in most cases the disease subsides in 1 to 2 years. This disease is exquisitely sensitive to steroids, so all patients should be treated with steroids as soon as the diagnosis is made to prevent blindness.

Takayasu's arteritis, or pulseless disease, is a chronic occlusive panarteritis affecting all large and medium arteries. It occurs mainly in girls, especially Asian ones, and is progressive and frequently fatal. It characteristically affects the aorta, the proximal portions of its main branches, and sometimes the pulmonary arteries. Ischemia and neurovascular hypertension follow involvement of the renal arteries, and it may be the most important cause of renal hypertension in Asian children.

1. Anesthetic Management of Polyarteritis Nodosa and Cranial Arteritis

Patients with polyarteritis nodosa and cranial arteritis often come to surgery: a report from one hospital states that 10 of 12 patients with polyarteritis nodosa had abdominal operations.[54] The diagnosed patients are either very sick and hospitalized or are in remission and taking large doses of steroids. It is of interest that patients with polyarteritis nodosa and temporal arteritis have been observed who had acute pharyngeal edema in which the uvula and peripharyngeal areas were severely swollen.[55]

Hypertension is invariable with renal involvement, and it is important to try to maintain normal blood pressure, since the critical closing pressure in organs affected by arteritis is likely to be altered. This would mean that coronary and cerebral thrombosis are of major concern in allowing hypotension to occur. There are, however, no data to confirm or refute this precaution.

McGowan[56] reported a case of blindness occurring during general anesthesia in a 76-year-old man with active temporal arteritis. The patient had lost his vision in one eye just before admission with signs of laryngeal carcinoma. Temporal artery biopsy confirmed the diagnosis of the associated ocular lesion, and steroid treatment was started. Transient blindness in the "good eye" occurred 2 days before surgery for laryngectomy, which required 3½ hours. During the operation, the blood pressure fell from 160/90 to 120/70 mm Hg for 20 minutes. The subsequent blindness after anesthesia may or may not have been related to this; nonetheless, McGowan proposed that elective surgery be postponed until acute temporal arteritis subsides.

The frequent involvement of the lungs and the almost invariable kidney complications should alert the anesthesiologist to the problem of evaluating these patients before surgery. If there is a suggestion of pulmonary involvement, the degree of lung dysfunction, if any, should be determined by appropriate tests. Likewise, any degree of renal failure should be known preoperatively.

In Takayasu's arteritis, monitoring arterial pressure is usually the most important problem. Direct arterial exposure and cannulation may be required. In addition, pulmonary artery catheterization is recommended, and despite pulmonary artery disease in 50 per cent of these patients, the catheter can be inserted without difficulty.[57] Epidural anesthesia has also been suggested in these patients in order to reduce vascular resistance as well as cardiac afterload.[58]

VI. GRANULOMATOUS DISEASES

A. WEGENER'S GRANULOMATOSIS

Wegener's granulomatosis is one of a group of clinical and pathologic syndromes—a spectrum at one end of which are pure necrotizing and granulomatous lesions without arteritis and at the other pure arteritis without granulomatous reaction. Each disease has certain distinguishing features—population affected, distribution of vascular lesions, size of the vessels, and histologic features. Wegener's granulomatosis has a constant triad of necrotizing giant cell granulomatosis of the upper respiratory tract and lungs, widespread necrotizing vasculitis of the small arteries and veins, and focal glomerulonephritis. It affects both sexes, mostly between 20 and 40 years of age. Its onset is insidious, with purulent

rhinorrhea, epistaxis, nasal pain, or cough. As the process spreads, it leads to mucosal ulceration and destruction of cartilage and bone in the nose, palate, and orbit, as well as pulmonary congestion. Destructive lesions of the epiglottis are common, whereas the laryngeal wall may be thickened or fibrotic, resulting in narrowing of the lumen.[59] Subglottic involvement is most common in patients with an ulcerative or proliferative type of lesion.

Later, there is systemic involvement of skin and muscles, bone peripheral neuropathy, and almost always severe renal disease. It is differentiated from lethal midline granuloma by the histologic features of the latter. It also must be distinguished from tuberculosis, sarcoidosis, and mycotic infection. The appearance of the chest film in this disease is extremely varied, from increased vascular markings (vasculitis of pulmonary vessels), to patchy pneumonia, to diffuse miliary nodularity. One interesting manifestation is asymptomatic and clinically undetectable, circumscribed, nodular densities that simulate metastatic neoplasms.[60] They appear suddenly and may undergo central necrosis and cavitation. Pulmonary involvement that can look like carcinoma is similar in both forms of Wegener's disease, producing two major problems. The first is vasculitis with plasma cell infiltration of small pulmonary arteries and veins. This leads to lysis of leukocytes in the vessels with liberation of organelles, platelet aggregation, fibrin deposition, and necrosis with subsequent obstruction of the lumen. The resulting necrosis and cavitation lead to increased dead space and ventilation-perfusion abnormalities. Second, bronchi may be eroded with subsequent obstruction, leading to increased pulmonary shunting and arterial desaturation.

The clinical course is downhill and fatal. Although symptomatic control can be achieved with steroid therapy, death is merely delayed. Cytotoxic drugs are necessary to prevent renal involvement. Renal transplantation has been reported, but multisystem problems must be controlled.

B. LETHAL MIDLINE GRANULOMA

Lethal midline granuloma is a rare, invariably fatal disease resulting in destruction of the middle area of the face. It affects men more than women, and onset is most common between 30 and 50 years of age. Ulceration begins in the nose and progressively destroys bone, cartilage, and skin. The granuloma may replace the midface, nasopharynx, and oropharynx. Nasal congestion, rhinorrhea, or sinusitis may be present for years before other evidence of the disease appears. Later there may be interference with sight, and speech, and eventually airway problems. The average course is about 1 year, and death usually results from cachexia. The diagnosis must exclude neoplasms and the many infectious processes that produce ulcerations of the nose and upper respiratory tract. The absence of vasculitis distinguishes it from Wegener's granulomatosis. Corticosteroid or radiation therapy occasionally impedes the destructive process, and a favorable report has followed the use of methotrexate.

1. Anesthetic Management of Wegener's Granulomatosis and Lethal Midline Granuloma

The role of the anesthesiologist in these conditions can be very important, since establishment of a good airway may require careful advance planning because of possible structural abnormalities. One should not use the crash induction technique without knowing the exact involvement of the lesions, which may be hard to determine preoperatively. Preoperative indirect laryngoscopy can be important in assessing the airway. An often neglected role of the anesthesiologist can be the ability to spot or diagnose abnormalities when an ulceration or hole in the palate or pharynx may be the first sign of one of these diseases. Equipment for alternative methods, including tracheostomy, may be necessary.

The pulmonary infection in Wegener's granulomatosis can progress to widespread consolidation and present a formidable anesthetic risk, especially if arterial oxygen desaturation exists. Regional anesthesia and supplemental oxygen may be preferable in these cases, since there are likely to be infected granulomatous lesions throughout the upper airway. Even during regional anesthesia, however, supplemental oxygen should be administered. A thorough review of the multisystem effects of this disease and the anesthetic considerations has been done by

Lake.[61] In this review, she warns of the vasculitis in the coronary arteries, involvement of cardiac valves, fibrinous pericarditis, and conduction defects, in addition to the left ventricular hypertrophy associated with renal hypertension.

C. SARCOIDOSIS (BESNIER-BOECK DISEASE, SCHAUMANN'S DISEASE, OR UVEOPAROTID FEVER)

1. General

Sarcoidosis is a systemic granulomatous disease characterized by spontaneous and complete remissions in the early stages and by a slowly progressive course if the disease persists. The lung is the organ most often involved. Lymph node, liver, spleen, eye, and skin involvement is also common, but any tissue or organ can be affected, including the central nervous system and cranial nerves.

The epidemiology and cause of this disease have provoked a large number of interesting international studies. It occurs in almost all races and all regions of the world. The highest prevalence is in Sweden, but neighboring Finland has about the lowest. In the United States, there is a preponderance among blacks and those born in rural areas. Sarcoidosis occurs at all ages, with the greatest prevalence between 20 and 40 years, with a slightly higher rate among females. The production of sarcoid granuloma by a variety of stimuli, such as beryllium, zirconium, silica, quartz, talc, and so on, has led some to consider sarcoidosis as a host reaction pattern involving immune mechanisms. *Mycobacterium tuberculosis* and pine pollen have received extensive consideration as causative agents, but they have not received general acceptance. It is likely that there is no specific pathogen and that rather, the disease results from an abnormal immune response to many different antigens.

2. Pathologic Features

The first manifestation of the disease is an accumulation of mononuclear inflammatory cells, mostly helper T lymphocytes and mononuclear phagocytes, in affected organs. This is followed by the formation of granulomas. The epithelioid cell granuloma, or tubercle, is the cardinal feature of the tissue reaction in sarcoidosis. Unlike in tuberculosis, caseation and necrosis are rare, and healing takes place by fibrosis with dense scar formation that later contracts and becomes hyalinized. All organs and tissues may show evidence of the disease, and the constitutional symptoms are produced almost entirely by mechanical interference with organ function by the granulomas or scars. The extent of these functional impairments determines the seriousness of the disease.

3. Clinical Picture

One outstanding and important clinical feature of sarcoidosis is the disparity between the extensive involvement of organs and the mildness or absence of symptoms. Asymptomatic onset occurs most often in North America, whereas acute illness with fever, rash (erythema nodosum), arthralgia, and bilateral hilar adenopathy can be seen at the onset more often in Europe. In most cases, the symptoms subside in a few months, and complete clearing of the pulmonary changes occurs within 2 years and without specific therapy. If the disease persists, progressive involvement of lung or other organs may occur for years, and functional impairment of an organ is not rare. Only a small proportion of patients die of the disease.

Pulmonary changes, which develop in approximately 50 per cent of patients, are characterized by granulomatous infiltration of the alveolar walls, which are replaced by fibrous scar tissue. This reduces effective diffusing surface and, when extensive, can lead to dyspnea and oxygen desaturation. Nickerson[62] describes three distinct areas of pulmonary lesions: (1) pleural, often forming subpleural fibrous masses; (2) peribronchial, occurring as solitary lesions encircling small bronchioles; and (3) septal, occurring as solitary lesions in alveolar septa.

The most clearly recognizable sign of pulmonary sarcoidosis is the enlarged symmetric hilar adenopathy whose outer border casts smooth-contoured shadows on x-ray films. This can lead to extrinsic bronchial obstruction and distal atelectasis or infiltration of the bronchial mucosa, which causes asthma symptoms[63] and progresses to produce bronchial stenosis.

In a study of the mechanics of ventilation in sarcoidosis, Snider and Doctor[64] showed that 17 of 21 patients had compliance values below normal or at the low end of the normal range. Some of the low compliance values were observed in patients without x-ray evidence of parenchymal disease.

In general, total lung volume is usually diminished with pulmonary sarcoid infiltration, and the gas transfer factor (diffusing capacity) tends to fall earlier and to a greater degree. Johnson[65] found that the major change was in transfer of gas from alveoli to capillaries, whereas the alveolar capillary volume was less affected.

The upper airway can be involved by mucosal infiltrations of the nose, nasopharynx, tonsils, palate, and larynx.[66] All parts of the larynx have been involved, nearly always in association with other parts of the respiratory tract. Women seem to be afflicted in this area more than men. There are numerous case reports of lobulated swellings of the vocal cords, epiglottis, arytenoids, and aryepiglottic folds, necessitating tracheostomy.

Although the prevalence of granulomatous cardiac lesions in autopsy cases of sarcoidosis is 20 per cent,[67] this does not reflect the clinical picture. The most common cardiovascular complication of sarcoidosis is right ventricular enlargement. Svanborg[68] observed that 7 of 11 patients with moderate pulmonary fibrosis had elevated pulmonary artery pressures. Right ventricular failure, however, is no more common than it is with other pulmonary diseases.

Sarcoid lesions have occasionally been found in the valves, but more often in the myocardium, sometimes resulting in arrhythmias or heart block. Ventricular tachycardia is the abnormal rhythm most frequently reported, and sudden death has been recorded: autopsy revealed destruction of the conducting system by sarcoid lesions (Fig. 11–10).

Sarcoid lesions have been seen in every organ of the body, including the skin, but this condition is of particular interest when it affects the eyes. According to Scadding,[66] 14 per cent of his patients had symptomatic uveitis at some stage of this disease. It affects principally the anterior uveal tract, producing iridocyclitis, which is an indication for corticosteroid treatment.

The diagnosis of sarcoid is usually based on the clinical findings and the finding of a sarcoid granuloma in a tissue biopsy specimen (Kveim's test). Because the lung is so frequently involved, it is the most likely site

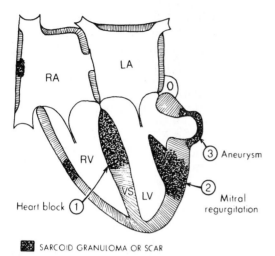

FIGURE 11-10. Diagram showing the most common sites of sarcoid granulomas or scars in the heart and the most frequent functional consequences of these lesions.

to biopsy, usually through a fiberoptic bronchoscope. An increased sedimentation rate and hypergammaglobulinemia are common, whereas hypercalcemia and hypercalciuria are present in about 25 per cent of cases. The differential diagnosis consists of berylliosis, lymphomas, and tuberculosis and must be made if corticosteroid therapy is considered necessary. Corticosteroid therapy is indicated for ocular, cardiac, and central nervous system lesions, progressive pulmonary parenchymal involvement, and persistent hypercalcemia.

4. Anesthetic Management of Sarcoidosis

The pulmonary pathologic appearance and, to a lesser degree, the cardiac involvement are major concerns for anesthesiologists. One important feature of pulmonary sarcoidosis is the discrepancy between the patient's symptoms and the pathologic changes that may be present. A case from the author's hospital can serve to demonstrate the problem. A 35-year-old man who came to the clinic with blurred vision caused by a detached retina was scheduled for immediate corrective eye surgery. He had a history of sarcoidosis, which was diagnosed 1 year earlier by chest x-ray studies (Fig. 11–11), and characteristic skin lesions. He had no pulmonary symptoms, and physical examination revealed slight tachypnea, bronchovesicular breath sounds with minimal

dry rales at the lung bases, cervical and axillary adenopathy, and a palpable spleen tip. Preoperative blood gas analysis showed an oxygen saturation of 90 per cent, $PaCO_2$ of 38 mm Hg, pH of 7.37, and a bicarbonate level of 22 mEq/L. Endotracheal anesthesia was maintained with halothane and nitrous oxide and oxygen, 40 per cent. Shortly after the start of surgery, cyanosis of the fingers and nail beds was noted, at which time oxygen was increased to 60 per cent and respiration was more vigorously assisted. After 10 minutes, an arterial blood gas analysis indicated an oxygen saturation of only 91 per cent, whereupon the nitrous oxide was discontinued. In this case, only the magnitude of pulmonary venous admixture can be appreciated and not its cause, whether poor oxygen diffusion or ventilation-perfusion discrepancy, as there was no obvious cardiac problem. It was unfortunate that there was no preoperative pulmonary function study, but the point is that a patient with asymptomatic lung disease whose oxygenation on air was marginal became worse during halothane anesthesia, inspiring 40 per cent to 60 per cent oxygen.

It is important to define the pulmonary function status before operation in patients

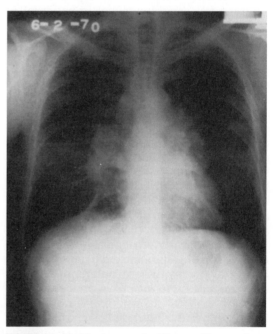

FIGURE 11-11. Chest x-ray of a 36-year-old man, showing characteristic hilar shadows and parenchymal infiltration of sarcoidosis. When seen preoperatively, he appeared asymptomatic.

with evidence of pulmonary sarcoidosis. In particular, if possible, the diffusing capacity should be determined. Diffusing capacity under halothane anesthesia was not significantly altered in 12 patients with normal awake diffusion capacities studied by Bergman.[70] It is not known, however, what might happen to the diffusing capacity under anesthesia in a patient with a diffusion impairment. Decreased lung compliance is common in pulmonary sarcoidosis and should be kept in mind before the administration of anesthetic. In addition to routine pulmonary function studies, diffusing capacity, and blood gas analysis, there should be a cardiac evaluation. In particular, evidence of pulmonary hypertension, right ventricular hypertrophy, and any arrhythmias should be sought. During anesthesia and surgery, electrocardiographic monitoring is essential, for if there is sarcoid heart disease, the most common abnormalities are ventricular tachycardia and sudden arrest. Laryngeal sarcoid lesions have been reported to occur in 5 per cent of patients, and its seriousness has been noted in a case report of an unusual airway complication.[71] Thirty-six hours after a very difficult intubation, a patient with sarcoidosis suffered severe airway obstruction from laryngeal edema and reduced cord movement. The medical records revealed noncaseating granulomas in previous biopsy specimens of nodular lesions in the proximal trachea. Treatment with dexamethasone and racemic epinephrine was successful.

Often, patients with sarcoidosis have been on long-term corticosteroid treatment, in which case preoperative and intraoperative coverage with additional steroids is essential.

REFERENCES

Connective Tissue Diseases—General

Harrison's Principles of Internal Medicine, 11th ed. New York, McGraw-Hill, 1987.

McCarty DJ (ed): Arthritis and Allied Conditions: A Textbook of Rheumatology, 10th ed. Philadelphia, Lea & Febiger, 1985.

Primer on Rheumatic Diseases, 8th ed. Atlanta, The Arthritis Foundation, 1983.

Sackner MA: Scleroderma. New York, Grune & Stratton, 1966.

Scadding JG, Mitchell DN: Sarcoidosis. London, Chapman and Hall, 1985.

Steroid Therapy

1. Fraser CG, Preuss FS, Bigford WD: Adrenal atrophy and irreversible shock associated with cortisone therapy. JAMA 149:1542–1543, 1952.
2. Haynes RC Jr, Murad F: Adrenocorticotropin hormone; adrenocortical steroids, their synthetic analogues; inhibitors of adrenocortical steroids biosynthesis. In Gilman AG, Goodman LS, Gilman A (eds): The Pharmacologic Basis of Therapeutics, 6th ed. New York, Macmillan, 1980, pp 1466–1496.
3. Roberts JC: Operative collapse after corticosteroid therapy—a survey. Surg Clin North Am 50:363–379, 1970.
4. Oyama T, Shibata S, Matsumoto F, et al: Effects of halothane anesthesia and surgery on adrenocortical function in man. Can Anaesth Soc J 15:258–266, 1968.
5. Oyama T, Takiguichi M: Plasma levels of ACTH and cortisol in man during halothane anesthesia and surgery. Anesth Analg 49:363–366, 1970.
6. Hume DM, Wittenstein GJ: The relationship of the hypothalamus to pituitary-adrenocortical function. Proceedings First Clinical ACTH Conference. Philadelphia, Blakiston, 1950, p 134.
7. Thorn GW: Clinical considerations in the use of corticosteroids. N Engl J Med 274:775–781, 1966.
8. Salassa RM, Bennet WA, Keating FR, et al: Postoperative adrenal cortical insufficiency. Occurrence in patients previously treated with cortisone. JAMA 152:1509–1515, 1953.
9. Plumpton FS, Besser GM, Cole PV: Corticosteroid treatment and surgery. The management of steroid cover. Anaesthesia 24:12–18, 1969.

Rheumatoid Arthritis and Ankylosing Spondylitis

10. Medsger TA Jr, Masi AT: Epidemiology of the rheumatic diseases. In McCarty DJ (ed): Arthritis and Allied Conditions: A Textbook of Rheumatology, 10th ed. Philadelphia, Lea & Febiger, 1985.
11. Cathcart ES, Spodick DH: Rheumatoid heart disease: A study of the incidence and nature of cardiac lesions in rheumatoid arthritis. N Engl J Med 266:959–964, 1962.
12. Rubin EH: Pulmonary lesions in rheumatoid disease with remarks on diffuse interstitial pulmonary fibrosis. Am J Med 19:569–582, 1955.
13. Lee FI, Brain AT: Chronic diffuse interstitial pulmonary fibrosis and rheumatoid arthritis. Lancet 2:693–695, 1962.
14. Caplan A: Certain unusual radiological appearances in chests of coal miners suffering from rheumatoid arthritis. Thorax 8:29–37, 1953.
15. Syndas DA: The anaemia of rheumatoid arthritis and its treatment with blood transfusions. Acta Rheumatol Scand 7:95, 1961.
16. Tenney SM, Miller RM: Respiratory and circulatory actions of salicylate. Am J Med 19:498–508, 1955.
17. Calin A, Fries JF: Striking prevalence of ankylosing spondylitis in "healthy" W27 positive males and females. N Engl J Med 293:835–839, 1975.
18. Sinclair JR, Mason RA: Ankylosing spondylitis. The case for awake intubation. Anaesthesia 39:3–11, 1984.
19. Murray GC, Persellin RH: Cervical fracture complicating ankylosing spondylitis. Am J Med 70:1033–1041, 1981.
20. Burns T, Marks S, Calin A: A double-blinded placebo-controlled cross over trial of azathioprine in refracting Reiter's syndrome. Arthritis Rheum 26:539–545, 1983.
21. Lofgren RH, Montgomery WW: Incidence of laryngeal involvement in rheumatoid arthritics. N Engl J Med 267:193–195, 1962.

22. Phelps JA: Laryngeal obstruction due to cricoarytenoid arthritis. Anesthesiology 27:518–522, 1966.
23. Edelist G: Principles of anesthetic management in rheumatoid arthritic patients. Anesth Analg 43:227–231, 1964.
24. Taylor RC, Way WL, Hendrixson R: Temporomandibular joint problems in relation to the administration of general anesthesia. J Oral Surg 26:327–329, 1968.
25. Munson ES, Cullen SC: Endotracheal intubation in a patient with ankylosing spondylitis of the cervical spine. Anesthesiology 26:365, 1965.
26. Jenkins LC, McGraw RW: Anaesthetic management of the patient with rheumatoid arthritis. Can Anaesth Soc J 16:407–415, 1969.
27. Gardner DL, Holmes F: Anaesthetic and postoperative hazards in rheumatoid arthritis. Br J Anaesth 33:258–264, 1961.
28. DeBoard JW, Ghia JN, Guildord WB: Caudal anesthesia in a patient with ankylosing spondylitis for hip surgery. Anesthesiology 54:164–166, 1981.
29. Wittman FW, Ring PA: Anaesthesia for hip replacement in ankylosing spondylitis. J R Soc Med 79(8):457–459, 1986.
30. Roberts KW: New use for Swan-Ganz introducer wire. Anesth Analg 61:67, 1981.

Systemic Lupus Erythematosus

31. Divertie MB: Lung involvement in the connective tissue disorders. Med Clin North Am 48:1015–1030, 1964.
32. Sourander LB, Pulkkinen K: Simultaneous occurrence of ankylosis of the cricoarytenoid joints with dyspnea and L.-E. syndrome in rheumatoid arthritis. Acta Rheum Scand 8:255–257, 1962.
33. Abouleish E: Obstetric anesthesia and systemic lupus erythematosus. Middle East J Anaesthesiol 9(5):435–446, 1988.

Scleroderma

34. Coffman JD: Skin blood flow in scleroderma. J Lab Clin Med 76:480–488, 1970.
35. Lewis ABH: Prolonged regional anesthesia in scleroderma. Can Anaesth Soc J 21:495–497, 1974.
36. Henriksen O, Kristensen JK: Reduced systolic blood pressure in fingers of patients with generalized scleroderma (acrosclerosis). Acta Dermatorener 61:531–534, 1981.
37. Ritchie B: Pulmonary function in scleroderma. Thorax 19:28–36, 1964.
38. Russell DC, Maloney A, Muir AL: Progressive generalized scleroderma: Respiratory failure from primary chest wall involvement. Thorax 36:219–220, 1981.
39. Iliffe GD, Pethgrew N: Hypoventilatory respiratory failure in generalized scleroderma. Br Med J 286:337–338, 1983.
40. Sackner MA: Scleroderma. New York, Grune & Stratton, 1966.
41. Salerni R, Rodman GP, Leon DF, et al: Pulmonary hypertension in the CREST syndrome variant of progressive systemic sclerosis (scleroderma). Ann Intern Med 86:394–399, 1977.
42. Ungerer RG, Tashkin DP, Furst D, et al: Prevalence and clinical correlates of pulmonary arterial hypertension in progressive systemic sclerosis. Am J Med 75:65–74, 1983.
43. West SG, Killian PJ, Lawles OJ: Association of myositis and myocarditis in progressive systemic sclerosis. Arthritis Rheum 24:662–667, 1981.

44. Clements PJ, Furst DE, Cabeen W, et al: The relationship of arrhythmias and conduction disturbances to other manifestations of cardiopulmonary disease in progressive systemic sclerosis (PSS). Am J Med 71:38–46, 1981.
45. Eisele JH, Reitan JA: Scleroderma, Raynaud's phenomena, and local anesthetics. Anesthesiology 34:386–387, 1971.
46. Thompson J, Conklin KA: Anesthetic management of a pregnant patient with scleroderma. Anesthesiology 59:68–71, 1983.
47. Younker D, Harrison B: Scleroderma and pregnancy. Br J Anaesth 57:1136–1139, 1985.
48. Smith GB, Shribman AJ: Anesthesia and severe skin disease. Anesthesia 39:443–455, 1984.

Dermatomyositis

49. Hepper NG, Ferguson RH, Howard FM Jr: Three types of pulmonary involvement in polymyositis. Med Clin North Am 48:1031–1042, 1964.
50. Rose T, Nothjungle J, Schlotz W: Familial occurrence of dermatomyositis and progressive scleroderma after injection of a local anesthetic for dental treatment. Eur J Pediatr 143:225–228, 1985.
51. Wylie WD, Churchill-Davidson HC: A Practice of Anesthesia, Chap 32. Chicago, Year Book, 1962.
52. Johns RA, Finlundt DA, Stirt JA: Anesthetic arrangement of a child with dermatomyositis. Can Anaesth Soc J 33:71–74, 1986.

Polyarteritis Nodosa and Vasculitis Syndromes

53. Rose GA, Spencer H: Polyarteritis nodosa. Q J Med 26:43–81, 1957.
54. Colton CL, Butler TJ: The surgical problem of polyarteritis nodosa. Br J Surg 54:393–396, 1967.
55. Martin TH: Pharyngeal edema associated with arteritis: A report of two cases. Can Med Assoc J 101:229–231, 1969.
56. McGowan BL: Active temporal arteritis. Am J Ophthalmol 64:455–457, 1967.
57. Warner MA, Hughes DR, Messick JM: Anesthetic management of a patient with pulseless disease. Anesth Analg 62:532–535, 1983.
58. Thornburn JR, James MFM: Anesthetic management of Takayasu's arteritis. Anaesthesia 41:734–738, 1986.

Wegener's Granulomatosis

59. Talerman A, Wright D: Laryngeal obstruction due to Wegener's granulomatosis. Arch Otolaryngol 56:376–379, 1972.
60. Blatt IM, Seltzer HS, Rubin P, et al: Fatal granulomatosis of the respiratory tract. Arch Otolaryngol 70:707–757, 1959.
61. Lake CL: Anesthesia and Wegener's granulomatosis: Case report and review of the literature. Anesth Analg 57:353–359, 1978.

Sarcoidosis

62. Nickerson DA: Boeck's sarcoid: A report of 6 cases in which autopsies were made. Arch Pathol 24:19–29, 1937.
63. Benedict EB, Castleman B: Sarcoidosis with bronchial involvement: Report of a case with bronchoscopic and pathological observations. N Engl J Med 224:186–189, 1941.

64. Snider GL, Doctor LR: The mechanics of ventilation in sarcoidosis. Am Rev Respir Dis 89:897–908, 1964.
65. Johnson RL Jr, Lawson WH, Wilcox WCN: Alveolar capillary block in sarcoidosis. Clin Res 9:196, 1967.
66. Scadding JG: Sarcoidosis, Chap. 13. London, Eyre and Spottiswoode, 1967.
67. Porter GH: Sarcoid heart disease. N Engl J Med 263:1350–1357, 1960.
68. Svanborg N: Studies on cardiopulmonary function in sarcoidosis. Acta Med Scand Suppl 366:1–130, 1961.
69. Chamovitz DL, Culley AW, Carlson KE: Cardiac sarcoidosis: Report of a case with paroxysmal ventricular tachycardia. JAMA 182:574–576, 1962.
70. Bergman NA: Pulmonary diffusing capacity and gas exchange during halothane anesthesia. Anesthesiology 32:317–324, 1970.
71. Wills MH, Harris MM: An unusual airway complication in sarcoidosis. Anesthesiology 66:554–555, 1987.

Skin and Bone Disorders

Brian L. Partridge

I. INTRODUCTION

This chapter presents uncommon diseases of skin and bone and their associated anesthetic considerations and problems. At the end of each disease presentation, management guidelines are listed that are intended to guide the reader in the safe conduct of anesthesia for these patients.

Anesthetic management for patients with skin diseases involves special measures to avoid skin trauma, special difficulties in maintenance of an airway, special challenges for monitoring, the frequent need for perioperative corticosteroid coverage, and difficulties associated with general debilitation. Anesthetic management considerations for the bone diseases are similar in that most of them involve the need for careful movement, transfer, and positioning of fracture-susceptible patients, difficulties in conduction anesthesia, airway and ventilatory difficulties associated with kyphoscoliosis or jaw and cervical spine immobility, and problems associated with concomitant congenital anomalies.

II. EPIDERMOLYSIS BULLOSA

Epidermolysis bullosa (EB) refers to a group of rare, hereditary mucocutaneous disorders (Table 12–1) whose common primary feature is the formation of blisters following even trivial trauma. Mucous membranes, particularly of the oropharynx and esophagus, may be involved. The basic defect is thought to be loss of intercellular bridges so that epidermal

cells separate with minor trauma. The numerous forms of EB have been divided into two major groups, *nonscarring* and *scarring*.[1]

Included in the nonscarring category are EB simplex, localized (Weber-Cockayne syndrome) or generalized (Koebner's); junctional EB (letalis); and localized absence of skin with blistering and nail dystrophy (Bart's syndrome). EB simplex types are inherited as an autosomal-dominant trait. Onset may occur from birth to adulthood. Blistering may be limited to the hands and feet (Weber-Cockayne syndrome) or may involve much of the skin surface (Koebner's) but rarely produces oral or nailbed lesions and heals without scarring. Incidence of the disease increases with warmer ambient temperatures (i.e., in summer months) and results from cytolysis of basal and suprabasal layers of the epidermis. Junctional EB, formerly described as *epidermolysis bullosa letalis,* is inherited as an autosomal-recessive trait. It is characterized by onset at birth of severe generalized blistering involving the skin, oral cavity, and esophagus. Moderate to severe refractory anemia is common. The majority of patients succumb within the first 2 years of life. Patients who survive infancy usually develop the complications associated with the scarring recessive dystrophic type. Large-dose systemic corticosteroid therapy during life-threatening periods may be useful and is frequently employed.[2, 3]

Included in the scarring category are dystrophic EB, autosomal-dominant (hyperplastic Cockayne's and Torraine's or albopapuloid Pasini's syndrome) EB, dystrophic EB, (autosomal-recessive; polydysplastic), and acquired EB (acquisita). Dominant dystrophic EB occurs in infancy. Blistering may be localized to the extremities or become generalized. Oral lesions, when present, are mild. Recessive dystrophic EB has its onset at birth or early infancy. Oropharyngeal, esophageal, and anal mucosal lesions present nutritional problems. Ocular and genitourinary involvement may occur. Chronic anemia may be present. Dystrophic recessive EB is a disease of stratified squamous epithelium. Laryngeal involvement with scarring and airway obstruction has been reported (the mucosa of the true vocal cords is stratified squamous epithelium),[4] and bronchial involvement is a theoretical possibility.[5] A review of the literature by Berryhill and colleagues found no reports of tracheal involvement.[6] Acquired EB occurs in adulthood without evidence of ge-

TABLE 12–1

The Group of Epidermolysis Bullosa Disorders

I.   Nonscarring
1. EB simplex
2. Localized (Weber-Cockayne syndrome)
3. Generalized (Koebner's syndrome)
4. Junctional EB (letalis)
5. Bart's syndrome

II.   Scarring
1. Dystrophic EB, autosomal-dominant hyperplastic Cockayne's and Torraine's (or albopapuloid Pasini's syndrome)
2. Dystrophic EB, autosomal-recessive (polydysplastic)
3. Acquired EB (acquisita)

netic disease, tends to be localized to the extremities, and has variable oropharyngeal involvement.

Treatment for all forms of EB is largely supportive and generally less than satisfactory. Local skin care, avoidance of mucosal and cutaneous trauma, control of secondary bacterial infections with appropriate antibiotics, and use of corticosteroid therapy during life-threatening periods constitute conventional conservative treatment. Surgery for most of these patients consists principally of dental restoration or superficial reconstructive operations to alleviate severe scarring. Intraabdominal and thoracic operations have been performed for the usual indications.

An association of EB with porphyria has been suggested.[7] Appropriate precautions (for example, avoiding thiopental) have frequently been suggested. Recently, this has been called into question,[8, 9] and patients who have been tested for porphyria have uniformly tested negative.[5, 8, 10] Nonetheless, since other induction agents such as propofol are available, avoidance of thiopental should be considered.

A. ANESTHETIC MANAGEMENT

Although EB includes a broad spectrum of disease with minimal to severe systemic involvement, general guidelines for the anesthetic and perioperative management of patients with this disease can be set forth:

1. Prevention of friction and trauma is essential since any friction or trauma can produce bullae. In particular, rubbing of the skin and mucosal surfaces must be avoided. When possible, patients should move *themselves* to and from the operating table; otherwise they must be transferred with great *care*. Use of a Surgilift is recommended.[3] Tape of any type should be avoided. Intravenous or arterial catheters may be sutured in place. Blood pressure cuffs, tourniquets, precordial and esophageal stethoscopes, esophageal or rectal temperature probes, and adhesive electrocardiography (ECG) electrodes should be used only when specifically indicated; when they are necessary, the skin and mucosal surfaces must be well protected by generous use of lubricant and/or lubricant-soaked gauze or cotton sponges. Needle electrodes have been

employed successfully, as have standard ECG pads from which the adhesive has been removed.[11] Monitoring in the recovery room should also be limited to essentials. Care must be exercised in establishing and securing intravenous cannulas (e.g., spraying with antiseptic skin preparation and wrapping with gauze). The eyes should be protected with an appropriate ophthalmic ointment and not taped shut.

2. Airway management may be extremely difficult. A general principle should be to avoid all airway manipulation whenever possible. Although laryngoscopy and endotracheal intubation have been performed in many patients without sequelae,[10, 12] life-threatening oropharyngeal bullae and hemorrhage have occurred.[13] Laryngeal scarring has been reported,[4, 14] but tracheal involvement has not. This may be attributable to the difference between the mucosa of the upper and lower airway.[6] In addition, 17 of 31 patients reported by James and Wark[12] had restricted mouth opening or gross dental problems that interfered with intubation, and the physicians were unable to intubate two of them.

If there is a clear airway and spontaneous ventilation and inhalation drugs are used, large fresh gas flows delivered by a mask held above the skin surfaces of the face and nose provide anesthesia while avoiding facial trauma. If tight mask fitting becomes necessary, the face must be protected by lubricant-soaked cotton or gauze sponges. Various types of head bags and boxes and insufflation techniques have also been used.[15, 16] Oropharyngeal and nasopharyngeal airways, as well as esophageal stethoscopes and temperature probes, should be avoided. Use of a laryngeal mask airway (LMA) is probably contraindicated.

If endotracheal intubation is necessary, a laryngoscope and a small endotracheal tube, both literally "dripping" with lubricant, should be used to minimize friction. A Macintosh laryngoscope blade is preferred to a Miller blade, to avoid trauma to the epiglottis. Under these controlled conditions, tracheal intubation may be a less threatening procedure than insertion of oral or nasal airways. In some patients tracheostomy may ultimately be required to secure the airway; however, tracheostomy may also produce subsequent airway management problems. A surgeon and equipment to perform tracheostomy should be at hand during the induction of anesthesia and postoperatively, during extubation. Extubation of the trachea requires the same gentleness as intubation. Oropharyngeal suctioning may prove life threatening. Postoperatively, patients must be closely observed for the development of airway obstruction.

3. Most patients will be taking or will have taken corticosteroid drugs at some time before surgery; therefore, appropriate perioperative therapy with corticosteroids is indicated.

4. Other associated disease states include general debilitation with malnutrition, electrolyte imbalance, and anemia. Congenital pyloric atresia, porphyria, amyloidosis, multiple myeloma, enteritis, diabetes mellitus, and hypercoagulable states are also reported.[17] Skin wounds may be secondarily infected, and sepsis may occur. These complications must be diagnosed and corrected before administration of anesthesia and surgery.

5. The use of potent inhalation drugs is discussed above. Isoflurane and sevoflurane have been used successfully, and all inhalation agents are probably acceptable.[18, 19] Intravenous barbiturate induction has been used satisfactorily; however, the possibility of associated porphyria must be remembered, so propofol is probably the induction drug of choice. Ketamine has been used intramuscularly and intravenously as the sole anesthetic drug.[20] Regardless of the type of anesthesia used, induction of anesthesia must be smooth and struggling must be avoided. Local anesthetic infiltration should be avoided because of the potential for skin sloughing. Dorne and coworkers report using spontaneous ventilation with Positive End-Expiratory Pressure (PEEP) applied via a Plexiglas box sealed around the patient's head with Vi Drapes.[19] End-tidal carbon dioxide values were not reported, and may have been quite high. Anesthesia with a propofol infusion and spontaneous ventilation would obviate a tight mask fit or intubation for many types of surgery.

6. Recently interest has been growing in the use of regional anesthetic techniques to avoid or minimize airway management difficulties. Spinal and continuous epidural anesthesia have been employed successfully,[11, 21] as have brachial plexus blockade[3, 8, 22] and block of the lateral femoral cutaneous nerve.[8]

7. All members of the medical team must be alerted to the special problems of these patients. Meticulous care in the operating room is wasted if the patient is mishandled in the postoperative period.

III. PEMPHIGUS AND PEMPHIGOID

Pemphigus comprises a group of mucocutaneous diseases, probably of autoimmune causes, that are characterized by bullous eruptions of the skin and mucous membranes. Various forms include pemphigus vulgaris, pemphigus vegetans, pemphigus foliaceus, pemphigus erythematosus (Senear-Usher syndrome), and Brazilian pemphigus foliaceus. Pemphigoid is considered a separate clinical entity although the two may coexist.[23] Differentiation is determined by histologic and immunologic tests.[23–25]

Pemphigus vulgaris, the most common form of the disease, occurs predominantly in Jewish or Mediterranean peoples, usually in the fourth to sixth decades of life, although occurrence from age 3 1/2 to 70 years has been reported. The tender, painful bullous eruptions and erosions are located within the epidermis and heal without scarring. Nikolsky's sign (separation of the epidermis with lateral finger pressure) is frequently present. Mucous membranes are commonly involved, and oral lesions may antedate cutaneous lesions by several months. Severe oropharyngeal lesions may interfere with adequate nutrition. Lesions of the pharynx and larynx may produce hoarseness. Nasal, vaginal, and anal mucosa may be affected. With extensive disease, electrolyte imbalance and hypoalbuminemia are common. Large-dose corticosteroid therapy has markedly reduced the mortality of untreated disease, which previously reached 90 per cent. Immunosuppressive drugs, methotrexate, cyclophosphamide, and azathioprine are used.[26] A hormonal component has been suggested by premenstrual exacerbations and remission after abdominal hysterectomy.[27, 28] Gold therapy has also been effective, and plasma exchange has been suggested for patients with acute exacerbations of the disease, as has oophorectomy and hormonal suppression.[29, 30] Other organ systems do not appear to be primarily involved, although there is a 5 to 6 per cent chance of internal malignancy.[27] Degeneration of the adrenal glands, pulmonary edema, pneumonia, atelectasis, and focal myocardial degeneration have been observed at autopsy in patients who died with fulminant pemphigus, and cardiac arrest has been reported.[29] Pemphigus vegetans differs from pemphigus vulgaris in that, with healing of the denuded skin and mucosa hypertrophic verrucoid granulations occur, occasionally with pustular areas (intraepidermal eosinophilic abscesses) at the periphery of these lesions. Otherwise, the clinical presentation and course closely resemble those of pemphigus vulgaris. Pulse steroid therapy with the addition of cyclophosphamide has been advocated to avoid the side effects of long-term steroids.[29]

Pemphigus foliaceus and pemphigus erythematosus are the less severe forms of the disease. The latter is a localized variant of the more generalized pemphigus foliaceus in which the seborrhea-like eruptions are confined primarily to the anterior chest and a "butterfly" distribution on the face. Brazilian pemphigus is a variant of pemphigus foliaceus that is endemic to south-central Brazil. In contrast to pemphigus vulgaris, oropharyngeal lesions are not frequently present.

Benign familial pemphigus (Hailey-Hailey disease) is a hereditary vesiculobullous eruption of recurrent lesions in intertriginous areas of the skin.[31] The disease is autosomal dominant and usually occurs early in adult life, becoming less severe with increasing age. Oropharyngeal lesions are unusual; when present, they call the diagnosis into question. Topical and systemic corticosteroids are the treatment of choice.

Pemphigoid is distinguished from pemphigus by virtue of the fact that the bullous eruptions occur subepidermally rather than intraepidermally.[32] Bullous pemphigoid is characterized by large, tense bullae occurring primarily in intertriginous areas. It can also involve oropharyngeal, esophageal, anal, and vaginal mucosa, although to a lesser extent than pemphigus. It is a disease of the elderly but has been documented in childhood.[33] The clinical course is one of exacerbations and remissions. Cicatricial pemphigoid (benign mucous membrane pemphigoid) is characterized by bullous eruptions that heal with scarring and involve principally the mucous membranes of the oropharynx, nasopharynx, conjunctiva, larynx, esophagus, genitalia, and anus. Intertriginous areas of the skin may be affected. Because of scarring, stenosis of the various mucosal orifices can result in airway, genitourinary, and gastrointestinal obstruction. Like pemphigus, there is a 5 to 6 per cent incidence of internal malignancy.[27] Therapy of pemphigus consists of corticosteroids, immunosuppressants (methotrexate, cyclophosphamide, and azathioprine), sulfapyridine, and sulfones. For reasons unknown, treatment of cicatricial pemphigoid is less than satisfactory.

Benign chronic bullous dermatosis of childhood affects children of preschool age, is characterized by large, tense bullae of the skin, and clinically resembles adult bullous pemphigoid. The disease does not persist into adult life and has a clinical course of exacerbations and remissions, spontaneous remission usually occurring within 2 to 3 years of onset. Therapy may include corticosteroids and sulfa drugs.

A. ANESTHETIC MANAGEMENT

Guidelines for the anesthetic management of patients with pemphigus or pemphigoid are as follows:

1. Airway management may be difficult because of cutaneous, oropharyngeal, and laryngeal involvement; therefore, the principles of airway management discussed under Epidermolysis Bullosa should be considered. Airway instrumentation should be avoided if at all possible. If necessary, endotracheal intubation with a small tube (tied rather than taped) is preferable to LMA.

2. Other disease states associated with pemphigus and pemphigoid include myasthenia gravis, systemic lupus erythematosus, rheumatoid arthritis, pernicious anemia,[34] and primary hepatic cirrhosis,[35] suggesting an autoimmune mechanism for the disease. In addition, increased levels of autoantibodies, complement, and immune complexes are found in these patients[36] and support the autoimmune hypothesis. Because each of these associated diseases has serious anesthetic management implications (e.g., muscle relaxants and myasthenia gravis), preanesthetic diagnosis of these conditions is extremely important. In addition, pemphigus is associated with increased frequency of malignancy, especially of the lymphoid and reticuloendothelial systems.[37, 38]

3. Potentially toxic bone marrow and hepatic effects of the drugs used for treatment dictate that preoperative laboratory evaluation of hematopoietic and hepatic functions be performed. Dapsone (sulfone) has also been implicated in causing a peripheral neuropathy.[39]

4. Because water and salt can be lost through the mucocutaneous lesions, degree of hydration and electrolyte balance should be assessed.

5. Many patients will have taken cortico-steroid drugs before surgery; therefore, appropriate perioperative therapy with cortico-steroids is indicated. Withholding steroids may be associated with exacerbation of the disease in the perioperative period.[36]

6. No particular anesthetic drug or technique is recommended. Local infiltration should be avoided because of the potential for skin sloughing. Airway management remains the principal concern. Only three cases of anesthetic management of this disease have been reported. In the first, continuous thoracic epidural anesthesia was supplemented with ketamine intravenously for cholecystectomy.[40] The patient had no complications. In both other case reports, intravenous ketamine and diazepam were employed with spontaneous ventilation.[36, 41] No reports of intubation of patients with pemphigus have appeared, although this author intubated without incident a patient with a history of pemphigus but no apparent disease.

IV. GENERALIZED INFLAMMATORY SKIN DISEASES

A series of severe generalized inflammatory skin diseases have been described, including erythema multiforme (EM), Stevens-Johnson syndrome (SJS), toxic epidermal necrolysis (TEN), and staphylococcal scalded-skin syndrome (SSSS). There has been considerable debate about which of these constitute separate entities, and a number of alternative nomenclatures have been proposed. Consensus seems to be developing that SJS is a severe form of EM but that EM, TEN, and SSSS are separate entities, through their presentations, causes, and symptoms overlap.[42, 43] Recently, however, an international group of dermatologists reviewed skin lesions of 200 patients and published a "consensus" classification of increasing body surface area (BSA) involvement. EM consists of lesions covering less than 10 per cent of BSA; SJS shows detachment of 10 per cent of body surface with widespread erythematous lesions; an overlap category of SJS–TEN consists of 10 to 30 per cent BSA involvement; and TEN is defined as greater than 30 per cent BSA involvement.[43] From an anesthesiologist's perspective, the importance of appropriate diagnosis lies in the different treatment (SSSS requires antibiotics, for instance) and mortality (low for SSSS but as high as 20 to 60 per cent for TEN).[44, 45] In this section, the pathophysiology of each condition is discussed separately, but anesthetic management is discussed for the group of syndromes as a whole.

A. ERYTHEMA MULTIFORME

EM describes a spectrum of acute inflammatory diseases ranging from EM minor, a mild illness, to EM major, a severe, life-threatening condition often known as *Stevens-Johnson syndrome*. Many precipitating factors have been implicated in EM, although in approximately half the cases no specific cause is found. Drug associations have been prominent and include barbiturates, sulfonamides (including sulfamethoxazole), penicillin, salicylates, antipyrine, phenytoin, hydralazine, digitalis, nonsteroidal antiinflammatory agents, and others. EM may be a manifestation of dermatomyositis, lupus erythematosus, polyarteritis nodosa, rheumatoid arthritis, or Wegener's granulomatosis. Viral, bacterial, fungal, and parasitic infections and malignancy have also been implicated. *Mycoplasma pneumoniae* may be present, or even the cause.[46, 47]

EM minor accounts for as many as 1 per cent of dermatologic outpatient visits. The disease rarely occurs in persons older than 50 years and typically is seasonal (spring and fall).[48] A mild prodrome of low-grade fever, malaise, arthralgia, and upper respiratory tract symptoms frequently heralds the characteristic rash. The rash is generally symmetric and present on the extensor surfaces of extremities, and it can involve palms, soles, oral mucosa, and conjunctiva. Lesions are characteristic and appear as circumscribed concentric rings of alternating pale and erythematous zones with a central dusky papule or vesicle; they are thus known as "targets" or "irises." Lesions appear in crops over a period of 2 to 3 days, last about a week, and then heal. Recurrences are common.[49] EM minor generally requires little treatment. Corticosteroid therapy may be necessary for short periods when cutaneous or mucosal involvement is extensive.

B. STEVENS-JOHNSON SYNDROME

SJS, the most severe form of EM, occurs infrequently, usually within the first three decades, and occurrence peaks in winter. The disease is an extremely serious one and has a 10 to 20 per cent mortality rate. Prodromal illness typically consists of fever, malaise, cough, sore throat, chest pain, vomiting, diarrhea, myalgia, and arthralgia. This is followed by explosive appearance of inflammatory bullous lesions of the skin and mucous membranes. The severe cutaneous lesions result in sloughing of the epithelium, leaving large denuded areas of skin. The severe mucosal lesions cause ulceration of the nose, oropharynx, larynx, trachea, and bronchi.[49] Oral lesions may interfere with adequate nutrition. The eyes are also commonly affected with conjunctivitis, corneal ulceration, anterior uveitis, or panophthalmitis. Bullae of visceral pleura have resulted in bronchiolar-alveolar-pleural fistulas and bilateral pneumothorax with subcutaneous emphysema.[50] Ulceration of the esophagus and colon has caused perforation and fatal gastrointestinal hemorrhage.[51] Anemia secondary to bleeding, infection, or poor nutrition is common. Acute atrial fibrillation has been reported,[52] and acute myocarditis has been found at autopsy. Inflammatory renal lesions may cause acute renal failure. SJS has a protracted clinical course of 2 to 7 weeks and recurrences in up to 20 per cent of cases. There is no specific therapy. Associated conditions such as the collagen diseases or infection should be treated. Any drugs associated with the disease should be discontinued. Corticosteroids should be administered until the lesion heals. Careful attention to fluid and electrolyte balance is imperative. Local skin care, ocular care, and oral hygiene are important. Secondary infections and pulmonary complications are the most common causes of death.

C. TOXIC EPIDERMAL NECROLYSIS

TEN (Lyell's disease) is a severe mucocutaneous disorder characterized by sudden onset of widespread erythema and detachment of epidermis. It is most frequently distinguished from EM by its sudden onset and mucous membrane involvement and greater surface area involvement.[43, 53, 54] The large majority of cases occur in adults. A prodrome of conjunctival irritation, skin tenderness, fever, malaise, and arthralgia may antedate onset of a morbilliform rash. The rash often becomes confluent within 24 hours and is accompa-

nied by diffuse erythema and vesiculation that can involve the entire skin surface.[55] Nikolsky's sign is present in the erythematous areas. Mucous membranes, including the oropharynx, tongue, esophagus, larynx, and tracheobronchial tree, may be severely involved and may result in esophageal and gastrointestinal hemorrhage and tracheitis with cicatricial healing of the mucosa. Hypovolemia, electrolyte imbalance, and albuminuria may proceed to hypoperfusion, renal failure, and pulmonary edema.[56] Hypovolemia, sepsis, and pulmonary insufficiency are the major causes of death.[45] Mortality may reach 20 to 45 per cent.[44]

Most often implicated as causal factors are drugs—barbiturates, sulfonamides, antibiotics, and hydantoins.[57, 58] In addition, pentazocine has been questionably implicated as producing this disease and reversible renal insufficiency.[59] Other diseases that have been associated with TEN include viral (especially herpes simplex),[47] bacterial (*Escherichia coli*), and fungal (pulmonary aspergillosis) infections. Vaccination and neoplastic disease have also been implicated.[60] An idiopathic form of the disease has been described that has a high mortality rate.[44] Histologic examination reveals selective necrosis (necrolysis) of the basal layers of the epidermis, which distinguishes this disease from other (full-thickness) necrotic skin maladies such as SSSS (see below).[55] Early skin biopsy is imperative for appropriate treatment, since corticosteroids are indicated for TEN but contraindicated for SSSS.

There is no specific therapy. Fluid and electrolyte balance must be maintained. Maintenance of urine output may protect the kidneys. Specific antibiotic therapy for identified pathogens is indicated. Skin care, oral hygiene, and ocular care are important. Early administration of large doses of corticosteroids appears to help. Plasmapheresis has been suggested as therapy for TEN, but its efficacy is unproved.[45] Improvement in survival in the past 20 years is due primarily to advances in the control of infection and other supportive care.[44, 45] Care of TEN patients in a specialized burn intensive care unit (ICU) is appropriate and may improve survival. A major difference between patients with TEN and those with severe burns is that in TEN mucosal involvement often antedates skin necrolysis by several days, exacerbating the fluid deficits on presentation.

D. STAPHYLOCOCCAL SCALDED-SKIN SYNDROME

SSSS (Ritter's disease) is a mucocutaneous disorder ranging from localized bullous impetigo to widespread epidermolysis and superficial desquamation.[61] The cause has been identified as group 2 *Staphylococcus aureus*, and the disease is now recognized as being distinct from TEN. The syndrome may overlap with toxic shock syndrome.[53]

SSSS occurs primarily in neonates and children, but since 1972 it has been reported with increasing frequency in adults, and especially in immunocompromised persons.[62–64] A prodrome of purulent conjunctivitis, otitis media, occult nasopharyngeal infection, and, classically, cutaneous tenderness antedates onset of a scarlatiniform rash. Nikolsky's sign may or may not be present. Large flaccid bullae then appear, with separation of the epidermis and superficial desquamation. Necrolysis does not occur.[55] Mucosal involvement is rare, and healing usually occurs within 5 to 7 days.

Therapy includes penicillinase-resistant antistaphylococcal antibiotics, skin care, hydration, and maintenance of electrolyte balance. Routine corticosteroid therapy is contraindicated because of the bacterial cause. Mortality is 2 to 3 per cent.[64, 65]

E. ANESTHETIC MANAGEMENT

Guidelines for the anesthetic management of patients with EM, SJS, TEN, or SSSS are as follows:

1. The patient with EM minor usually presents no major problems for the anesthesiologist. Patients with SJS or TEN, however, present a significant challenge. Because many of the anesthetic considerations for these diseases are similar to those of epidermolysis bullosa, the reader is additionally referred to that section.

2. Care must be taken in transferring patients to the operating room, particularly if they have large areas of skin involvement. Minimal preoperative sedation allows patients to move and position themselves. An alternative is to employ a Surgilift, which allows gentle transfer of the patient both pre- and postoperatively.

3. If significant oropharyngeal and laryngeal edema is present, tracheostomy should be considered before administration of anesthesia. Placement of endotracheal tubes, oral or nasopharyngeal airways, and esophageal stethoscopes or temperature probes may result in hemorrhagic bullae that can rupture and severely compromise the airway. If a mask is used, the face should be protected by lubricated cotton or gauze sponges. In SSSS, mucosal involvement is rare; however, since the potential for traumatic bulla formation exists, airway manipulation should be gentle.

4. The possible occurrence of visceral pleural blebs and pneumothorax suggests that positive-pressure ventilation should be avoided if possible.

5. When possible, use of disposable equipment is recommended. The frequent presence of *Mycoplasma pneumoniae* and other pulmonary pathogens, particularly in EM, necessitates careful decontamination and isolation of anesthesia equipment. Because SSSS is a bacterial infection, equipment must be carefully sterilized and clothing changed to prevent spreading infection to other patients (e.g., epidemic impetigo). Possible viral causes mandate careful application of universal precautions.

6. The skin should be protected from blood pressure cuffs and precordial stethoscopes.

7. Because of the potential for dysrhythmias and myocarditis, five-lead ECG monitoring is recommended; however, care must be used in placing and removing electrodes.

8. Use of a cooling blanket is recommended because of the frequency of febrile episodes. The axilla is a convenient, and generally atraumatic, site for monitoring temperature.

9. Ocular involvement is common in TEN—and to a lesser degree in EM. Antibiotic or antiseptic eye drops may be required hourly. Artificial tears are recommended, even for short procedures. Survivors of TEN frequently suffer permanently from sicca syndrome and inadequate tear formation.[44]

10. The state of hydration and electrolyte balance must be assessed and appropriately corrected. Fluid deficits may be massive in patients with EM or TEN. As with burn patients, nitrogen balance is critical, and continuation of nasogastric feedings until the start of surgery may be worthwhile despite the increased risk associated with a full stomach.

11. Most patients with EM or TEN will be taking or will have taken corticosteroids sometime before surgery; therefore, appropriate perioperative therapy with corticoste-

roids is indicated. Corticosteroids are contra-indicated for patients with SSSS.

12. No specific anesthetic drugs or techniques are recommended. Local anesthetic infiltration and regional anesthesia may be used, depending on the condition of the skin overlying the site of entry and the presence of systemic infection. Barbiturates should be used with caution because of their association as a precipitating factor for EM and TEN. Propofol has not been implicated. In patients with renal insufficiency, potentially nephrotoxic drugs (sevoflurane, enflurane)[59] and drugs eliminated via the kidney (metocurine, and, to a lesser extent, curare and pancuronium) should be used with caution or avoided. Use of an LMA (if there is no oropharyngeal involvement) or regional anesthesia may obviate muscle relaxants. Ketamine has been used intramuscularly and intravenously as the sole anesthetic, with success.[66]

V. BEHÇET'S DISEASE

Behçet's disease, originally described in 1937 as a symptom triad of recurring iritis, ulceration of the mouth, and ulceration of the genitalia, is now recognized to involve additional organ systems, including the skin, central nervous system, heart, any part of the vasculature, lungs, and joints.[67] Fibrinolysis is altered in some patients. Possible causes of the disease include viral, parasitic, and bacterial infections; defective fibrinolytic activity; and, most recently, identified an autoimmune mechanism.[68] Males are affected much more often than females.[69] The disease is most common in Japan and in the Mideast and eastern Mediterranean. Mean age of onset is in the third decade, although patients as young as 12 have been reported.[70] Although there is an association with HLA-B5, HLA-DRw5, and especially HLA-B51, occurrence in family members is rare.[68] A previously reported association with HLA-B27 was probably due to misdiagnosis of chronic inflammatory bowel disease.[69] Several systems of diagnostic criteria have been proposed for the disease; the most accepted one divides criteria into major (oral, genital, ocular, and skin lesions) and minor ones (gastrointestinal, cardiovascular, and central nervous system lesions; thrombophlebitis; arthritis; family history). The diagnosis of Behçet's disease is based on the presence of three major criteria or a combination of two major and two minor ones.[71] Unfortu-nately, no diagnostic test is available. Presenting symptoms may be as diverse as endocarditis,[70] intestinal ulcerations, renal infarction,[72] or pseudotumor cerebri resulting from sinus thrombosis.[73]

The disease may involve any large or small artery, vein, or organ, in unpredictable combinations.[67] Oral, genital, or ocular lesions are the most common initial manifestations of the disease and may antedate other symptoms by several years. The mucosal lesions are recurrent, painful, 2- to 10-mm diameter ulcers that have a yellowish necrotic base, may be shallow or deep, and last 7 to 14 days. The aphthous oral ulcerations ("canker sores") may involve the lips, gums, tongue, mucosa, tonsils, and larynx and can interfere with adequate nutrition. Healing usually occurs without scarring, but severe oropharyngeal scarring has been reported.[72] Ocular manifestations include iridocyclitis, hypopyon (pus in the anterior chamber), optic atrophy, choroiditis, and relapsing conjunctivitis.[73, 74] Blindness may result. Skin lesions include papules, vesicles, pustules, pyoderma, folliculitis, acne, furuncles, abscesses, and erythema nodosum–like lesions. Nonspecific inflammatory reactivity to any scratches or intracutaneous lesions is characteristic and has even been proposed as a diagnostic test.

The central nervous system can be affected in many ways, including hemiparesis, quadriparesis, dementia, ataxia, meningitis, seizures, pseudobulbar palsy, spinal cord lesions, cauda equina syndrome, hyperreflexia, sinus thrombosis, and coma.[73, 74] These symptoms may resolve and then recur. Cardiovascular manifestations include pericarditis, valvular vegetations, recurrent thrombophlebitis, superior and inferior vena cava obstruction, and arterial aneurysms.[74–77] Pulmonary vasculitis, pulmonary aneurysms, hemoptysis, and obstructive airway disease have been reported, as has pulmonary artery thrombosis.[67, 78–81] Vascular lesions may result in renal infarction.[81]

The natural history of Behçet's disease is one of recurrent exacerbations and remissions with gradual overall deterioration. Arthritis is usually recurrent and limited to the large joints, and it generally does not cause deformities or roentgenographic changes. Small joints such as those of the fingers are usually spared. The arthritis is usually accompanied by low-grade fever. Relative inhibition of the fibrinolytic system can be demonstrated in patients during periods of thrombophlebitis;

however, this defect returns to normal during periods of remission. Intestinal ulceration may require surgery, but 80 per cent of patients have recurrences within a few years.[82]

Treatment for Behçet's disease has included administration of systemic and topical corticosteroids, immunosuppressant drugs (cyclophosphamide), and fibrinolytic drugs (streptokinase, streptodornase), but the results have been generally unsatisfactory and the treatment does not appear to alter the natural history of the disease.[69, 72] Absorption of orally administered drugs may be impaired.[83] Because aneurysms may occur at the site of arterial punctures, and thrombosis may occur at the site of venous punctures after injection of contrast material, arteriography and venography should be avoided in favor of computed tomography (CT) and magnetic resonance imaging (MRI) scanning.[67]

A. ANESTHETIC MANAGEMENT

Guidelines for the anesthetic management of patients with Behcet's disease are as follows:

1. Scarring from recurrent ulceration of the oropharyngeal and nasopharyngeal mucosa (though not the usual circumstance) can result in complete obliteration of the nasopharynx and extreme difficulty in endotracheal intubation.[74] In such instances, while the patient is awake the trachea should be intubated with the aid of nebulized topical anesthesia and/or sedation. Fiberoptic bronchoscopic intubation or tracheostomy may be necessary. No reports of use of LMA have been published, but the LMA may be contraindicated in cases of oropharyngeal lesions.

2. Organ systems that may be involved—the skin, the cardiovascular and pulmonary systems, the kidneys, and the joints—need careful preoperative evaluation. A careful preoperative neurologic examination should also be performed. Chest films should be obtained for all patients, regardless of age, and followed up with MRI or CT if indicated.[81]

3. Needle punctures should be kept to a minimum because of the diffuse inflammatory skin changes and pyoderma that can occur. Regional nerve blocks (glossopharyngeal and superior laryngeal) for awake intubation are thus relatively contraindicated. Potential sites for injections or intravenous catheters must be inspected closely for signs of early infection.

4. Autonomic hyperreflexia resulting in acute severe hypertension is a potential problem in patients with spinal cord or renal artery involvement.[84]

5. If the airway can be secured, no particular anesthetic technique is recommended. The advantages of regional anesthesia must be weighed carefully against subsequent central nervous system complications that may develop during the natural course of the disease. Use of succinylcholine in patients with neurologic involvement may result in sudden hyperkalemia and cardiac dysrhythmias.[85] Oral premedication may be ineffective owing to decreased absorption.[67]

VI. PSORIASIS

Psoriasis is a chronic skin disease characterized by accelerated epidermal turnover and epidermal hyperplasia. The disease appears to have both genetic and environmental etiologic components.[86] The initial appearance is often associated with superficial cutaneous trauma (a burn, cut, or scratch) and exposure to low humidity, chemical injury, and drugs (corticosteroids). Sites of skin involvement are usually the sacral region, elbows, knees, and scalp. The palms, soles, oral mucosa, and entire integument are occasionally affected. The cutaneous lesions of psoriasis consist of hypertrophic dermal papillae and epidermis, which form thick, loosely adherent scales of increased vascularity. Arthritis and hyperuricemia are associated with psoriasis. Psoriatic erythroderma, a more fulminant form of the disease, is characterized by involvement of the entire skin, fever, leukocytosis, and prostration. Blood flow to the psoriatic plaques is increased.[87] High-output congestive heart failure has been reported as a result of greatly increased cutaneous blood flow.[88]

In 20 to 50 per cent of patients, the psoriatic lesions are culture positive for *Staphylococcus aureus*[89, 90]; however, most of these patients do not have clinical pyoderma. The carriage rate for *S. aureus* on the skin of the normal population is less than 10 per cent. In one report an epidemic of staphylococcal wound infection was traced to an anesthetist with psoriasis who was an *S. aureus* carrier.[91]

Treatment includes low-dose ultraviolet light, topical tars, psoralen, anthralin, methotrexate, hydroxyurea, and topical steroids.[92]

A. ANESTHETIC MANAGEMENT

Guidelines for the anesthetic management of patients with psoriasis are as follows:

1. Specific measures should be taken to avoid any type of trauma to the skin, particularly in the areas of existing psoriatic lesions. Likewise, tape should be used on skin surfaces only when necessary. Intravenous catheters may be sutured in place or wrapped with web roll.

2. Because of the increased presence of *S. aureus* in psoriatic lesions, these areas should be avoided as administration sites for regional anesthesia or intravenous cannulas.

3. In patients with psoriatic erythroderma, evaluation of the cardiovascular system for undiagnosed high-output congestive heart failure is recommended.

4. Apart from the first three recommendations, there appears to be no contraindication to any particular technique or drug.

VII. NEUROFIBROMATOSIS

Neurofibromatosis of von Recklinghausen is an autosomal dominant disease (incidence 1 in 3000 births) in which the skin, nervous system, bones, endocrine glands, and sometimes other organs are the sites of a variety of congenital abnormalities, tumors, and hamartomas.[93, 94]

Clinical diagnosis in most patients is based on the presence of spots of cutaneous hyperpigmentation (*cafe au lait* spots or nevi) and cutaneous and subcutaneous tumors (neurofibromas). A presumptive diagnosis of the disease is made by the presence of five or more *cafe au lait* nevi each larger than 1.5 cm in one dimension. Freckling in the axillary folds is particularly characteristic. Neurofibromas may affect all areas of the skin, including genitals, palms, and soles. The neurofibromas may be soft or hard and may coalesce to form large plexiform neurofibromas. These tumors are thought to derive from the neurilemmal sheath (Schwann cells) or fibrocytes of peripheral nerve coverings, and may be painful.[94, 95]

Central nervous system involvement is common in neurofibromatosis; in one series the prevalence was as high as 66 per cent. There is also an increased incidence of meningiomas, schwannomas, and gliomas. Both malignant and benign spinal cord lesions are seen, and nerve root tumors are common.[94] The cranial nerves are often affected by the neurofibromas. Acoustic neuromas may produce deafness and other symptoms of cerebellopontine angle tumors. Involvement of the optic nerve may result in visual impairment. Cranial nerves V and X may also be affected.[94, 95] Fibromatous growth near the pituitary gland or hypothalamus can produce a variety of endocrine abnormalities, including stunted growth and precocious sexual development.[93] Mental retardation is not uncommon. Fibromas of the spinal cord can mimic cord transection. Intrathoracic fibromas and meningocele have been reported.[94, 96, 97]

Pharyngeal and laryngeal neurofibromatosis have occurred, resulting in airway obstruction, dyspnea, dysphonia, dysphagia, and, occasionally, the need for tracheostomy.[98] Respiratory distress in a child of an affected parent should suggest this possibility.[97, 99] In neurofibromatosis patients between 35 and 60 years of age, there can be as much as 20 per cent incidence of interstitial lung disease (fibrosing alveolitis). Pulmonary involvement may result in hypoxemia from ventilation-perfusion and diffusion abnormalities. Cor pulmonale, progressive respiratory failure, and death may occur.[100]

Visceral hypertrophy may result from plexiform neuromas of the autonomic nervous system. Pheochromocytoma occurs in as many as 1 per cent of patients. Involvement of the genitourinary system can result in obstruction and uremia. In obstetric patients, obstructed labor from neurofibromas preventing vaginal delivery has been reported.[101]

In children, hypertension associated with neurofibromatosis is generally due to renal artery stenosis, whereas in adults it is generally due to pheochromocytoma.[93]

Subperiosteal fibromas can produce bone resorption and cyst formation, with resultant fracture. Abnormalities of the vertebral column such as scoliosis or kyphoscoliosis are common.[102] Prolonged neuromuscular block in response to administration of succinylcholine, *d*-tubocurarine, and pancuronium has been reported in three patients, respectively.[103, 104]

Quality of life of patients with neurofibromatosis may be greatly altered: mean age at death is 43 years, according to one study.[105] Malignancies are usually the cause of death and often include sarcomatous degeneration or tumors in the spinal cord.[106, 107] Many patients with this disease require surgery for cosmetic reasons or for excision of malignancy. Nerve decompression for paresthesias or pain may be required. Obstructive uropathy, renal artery stenosis, and pheochromocytoma require surgery. Reduction of pathologic fractures is sometimes necessary.

A. ANESTHETIC MANAGEMENT

Guidelines for the anesthetic management of patients with neurofibromatosis are as follows:

1. Because of possible laryngeal involvement, meticulous preoperative evaluation of the airway is important, including CT, MRI, or indirect laryngoscopy if necessary. Instability of the cervical spine and compression by occult tumor have been reported.[108] Awake fiberoptic bronchoscopic intubation or tracheostomy may be necessary if an LMA is not appropriate for the surgery and regional anesthesia cannot be utilized.

2. A careful history of pulmonary complaints and exercise tolerance is essential. Preoperative pulmonary evaluation is indicated for patients with kyphoscoliosis or chronic lung disease and includes chest radiograph, arterial blood gases, and static and dynamic lung volumes and gas flow rates. Intraoperatively, frequent blood gas analysis may be necessary. A preoperative ECG is necessary for patients with severe kyphoscoliosis.

3. Examination of the back for deformities is essential when regional anesthesia is considered. Additionally, the anesthetist should consider the implications of the natural history of the disease, which includes the development of neurologic abnormalities. Asymptomatic intraspinal neurofibromas can make identification and entry into the epidural or subarachnoid space difficult or impossible, as can the occurrence of sacrolumbar meningoceles.[109]

4. Careful positioning and padding of pressure areas is important.

5. Preoperative determination of urinary catecholamine levels is recommended for all patients because of the association of pheochromocytoma. Appropriate drugs to treat a hypertensive crisis should be readily available.

6. Evaluation of pituitary function may be indicated.

7. No particular anesthetic drug or technique is recommended. In patients with spi-

nal cord lesions above the midthoracic level, autonomic hyperreflexia is a potential complication.[84] In patients with muscle atrophy, avoidance of succinylcholine is recommended.[110] The reports of prolonged neuromuscular block following succinylcholine, *d*-tubocurarine, and pancuronium dictate use of a nerve stimulator for evaluation of neuromuscular function. Regional anesthesia (including both subarachnoid and Bier blocks) has been used successfully, as has epidural anesthesia for a laboring patient.[107, 111]

VIII. ERYTHEMA NODOSUM

The primary manifestation of erythema nodosum (EN) is the appearance of inflammatory cutaneous nodules on the extremities. The disease occurs most often between 15 and 30 years of age, affects females more than males (by a ratio of 3:1), and is felt to be a hypersensitivity response to a variety of antigens.[112, 113] Numerous antigens have been proposed, including infections such as streptococcosis, tuberculosis, brucellosis, shigellosis,[114] leptospirosis,[115] toxoplasmosis, coccidioidomycosis, psittacosis,[116] Q fever,[117] and viruses; drugs (particularly antibiotics, but also including sulfonamides, oral contraceptives, phenytoin, and salicylates); and enteropathies. Behçet's syndrome has also been implicated, as has sarcoidosis.[113, 116] In fact, in one series 5 of 20 patients who presented with EN were shown to have sarcoid by subsequent biopsy.[118] Sarcoid should be strongly suspected when adenopathy is present. One case report describes EN resulting from lymphoma.[119]

The clinical presentation includes a prodrome of fever, malaise, arthralgia, pain, and gastrointestinal disturbances. The nodules, which are multiple, bilateral, extremely tender, red, and slightly elevated, occur over the extensor surfaces of the limbs, particularly the lower extremities. In patients with joint involvement, effusion, swelling, and tenderness usually occur, although crippling arthritis is rare. Knees, ankles, wrists, fingers, elbows, shoulders, and hips may be involved. Over a 2- to 3-week period the color changes from red to purple, resembling a bruise, and then to yellow green. Ulceration of the nodules is rare, and healing occurs without a scar.[112] No mucosal involvement is reported. Biopsy of the nodules fails to show noncaseating granulomas, even when sarcoid is present.[118] Laboratory findings include accelerated erythrocyte sedimentation rate (77 per cent of patients), increased antistreptolysin O titer (11 per cent) abnormal chest roentgenogram (15 per cent), and positive tuberculosis screen (PPD) (50 per cent).[113] Erythema nodosum is a self-limited disease that resolve 3 to 5 weeks after onset. Any mortality is due to the associated underlying disease.

Treatment is directed at the cause, when known. Thus, appropriate antibiotics are indicated for bacterial, fungal, and viral infections. Known associated drugs should be discontinued. Bed rest, wet dressings to areas of nodule formation, and administration of salicylates or nonsteroidal drugs (if these were not the cause) are important. Corticosteroids should be avoided if the cause is unknown. Potassium iodide has also been used.

A. ANESTHETIC MANAGEMENT

Guidelines for the anesthetic management of patients with erythema nodosum are as follows:

1. Because of the possible infectious cause of the disease (including tuberculosis), careful cleansing of all anesthesia equipment and use of airway filters is mandatory. If possible, disposable equipment should be used.

2. A chest film should be examined for signs of hilar adenopathy suggesting sarcoidosis; if these are present, pulmonary function tests are appropriate.

3. Corticosteroids, unless specifically indicated, should be avoided because of the possibility of an underlying infection.

4. If arthritis is present, careful evaluation of the airway is important. Care in positioning of the patient is necessary.

5. No particular anesthetic drug or technique is recommended.

IX. MASTOCYTOSIS

Mastocytosis is a disease of abnormal accumulation of mast cells in various organs of the body. Five variants of mastocytosis exist: urticaria pigmentosa, systemic mastocytosis, solitary mastocytoma, telangiectasia macularis eruptiva persistans, and diffuse cutaneous mastocytosis.[120] Most commonly the mast cell proliferation occurs in the skin, appears as multiple reddish brown or yellow macules,

papules, or nodules, and is identified as urticaria pigmentosa.[121, 122] Isolated dermal infiltrates (mastocytomas) can occur and are amenable to excision. Vesiculation and bulla formation in the skin are seen in lesions of children younger than 2 years. Urticaria pigmentosa was formerly thought to be a benign disorder of little consequence to the anesthesiologist, but severe intraoperative hypotension was recently reported in a patient with previously asymptomatic disease, and multiple severe hypotensive episodes have been seen in patients after aspirin administration.[120, 123] Systemic mastocytosis involves multiple organs, including bone, liver, spleen, lymph nodes, gastrointestinal tract, and skin. Mast cell leukemia can be a malignant form of this disease. More than 50 per cent of patients may have liver involvement, with increased liver enzymes (GGTP, alkaline phosphatase) and hypoprothrombinemia, which may be pronounced.[124] Cirrhosis is not seen, but partial fibrosis is common and may lead to portal hypertension, ascites, and even death.[124, 125] Patients whose disease is limited to cutaneous involvement have the best prognosis.[126]

The attacks associated with mastocytosis are thought to result from non–IgE-mediated mast cell activation.[127] The pathophysiology of the disease is related to the substances that are stored in the mast cell, namely histamine, heparin, and prostaglandin D_2. Release of these substances can cause urticaria, pruritus, flushing, headache, abdominal cramps, vomiting, diarrhea, febrile episodes, or grand mal seizures. Systemic vascular dilatation can result in hypotension, tachycardia, dizziness, syncope, and cardiovascular collapse that may be profound and intractable; however, bronchospasm is unusual. Histamine release was formerly thought to be responsible for the symptoms described above, but the questionable ability of H_1- and H_2-blocking agents to prevent attacks has led to speculation that prostaglandin D_2, also present in increased quantities in these patients, is the true culprit.[125, 127, 128] Stimuli that may produce these signs and symptoms include mechanical irritation of the lesion, psychological stress, temperature change, alcohol consumption, vomiting, exercise, and histamine-releasing drugs.[121] Systemic heparin release may be responsible for the occasional hemorrhagic diathesis observed in patients with or without systemic mastocytosis.[129]

The development of mast cell leukemia results in severe anemia and thrombocytopenia and is rapidly fatal. Hepatosplenomegaly occurs as a result of accumulation of mast cells in the liver and spleen. Hepatic involvement and gastrointestinal malabsorption result in decreased synthesis of coagulation factors. Diffuse lymphadenopathy may occur. Bone lesions can be osteoporotic or osteosclerotic. They are painful; commonly involve the pelvis, ribs, vertebrae, skull, and long bones; and may result in pathologic fractures. Lung tumors and pulmonary eosinophilic granuloma have been reported. Pulmonary function, however, is usually normal.[130]

Because there is no specific treatment for mastocytosis, therapy is directed toward relief of symptoms. Corticosteroids, adrenocorticotropin (ACTH), antihistamines, and antimetabolites have been used, with varying results. H_1- and H_2-blocking agents (chlorpheniramine and cimetidine or ranitidine) have been advocated by some as prophylaxis, but their efficacy is debatable.[127, 128, 131, 132] Similarly, prostaglandin inhibitors (aspirin, indomethacin) have been recommended,[127, 128] but may themselves result in severe hypotension.[123] Cromolyn sodium, is also employed, for its ability to inhibit mast cell degranulation.[131] From an anesthetic standpoint, use of H_2 blockers is warranted because of a possible association with gastric hypersecretion. Beta$_2$-adrenergic stimulants have proved useful in the treatment of chronic urticaria. Local irradiation for bone pain is also sometimes helpful.[129]

Patients with mastocytosis may present for gastrointestinal surgery, splenectomy, thoracotomy, and pulmonary resection, excision of isolated cutaneous lesions, or reduction of pathologic fractures resulting from the disease.

A. ANESTHETIC MANAGEMENT OF PATIENTS WITH MASTOCYTOSIS

1. In patients who have unexplained episodes of pruritus, urticaria, flushing, dizziness, and syncope, this disease must be suspected.

2. Preoperative laboratory data should include hemogram, platelet count, liver enzymes, and evaluation of coagulation, including prothrombin and partial thromboplastin times (PT/PTT) and bleeding time. Platelet transfusion, vitamin K, or fresh-frozen plasma may be necessary. Serum electrolyte values should be determined in patients with gastrointestinal disturbances. Volume status should be ascertained.

3. Appropriate perioperative corticosteroid coverage is indicated for patients taking corticosteroids.

4. When bones are involved, movement and positioning of the patient must be done with care because of the potential for fracture.

5. Preoperative H_1- and H_2-blocking agents are recommended, but their efficacy is controversial. Preoperative aspirin therapy to inhibit production of prostaglandin D_2 has also been advocated but remains unproved; indeed, aspirin has been implicated in some instances of mast cell degranulation.[123]

6. No specific anesthetic drugs or techniques are recommended, owing to insufficient data for these patients. The prime concern is avoidance of histamine release. Histamine release can occur spontaneously or from psychological, chemical, or physical stimuli. Therefore, adequate premedication is important to reduce anxiety and produce sedation, and an antihistamine drug may be used as part of the premedication. Occasionally, however, an antihistamine drug precipitates release of histamine. Use of histamine-releasing drugs such as morphine, codeine, metocurine, curare, atracurium, atropine, and dextran should be avoided. Sodium thiopental[133] and pancuronium[134] have also been implicated in histamine release. A histamine reaction has been reported with the use of an intravenous regional block of the upper extremity using lidocaine.[121] Inhalational anesthetics do not appear to release histamine. Adequate depth of anesthesia is important, and potent inhalational agents may inhibit mast cell degranulation. Epidural anesthesia has been used successfully but carries some risk of exacerbating hypotension.[124]

7. Rubbing of the skin should be minimized.

8. Fluctuations in temperature should be avoided. Use of a forced-air blanket is recommended.

9. Consideration should be given to premedication with acetaminophen and an antihistamine before transfusion. Transfusion reactions that are minor in normal patients may be life threatening in patients with mastocytosis.

10. Appropriate drug therapy to treat sudden intraoperative hypotension, including

catecholamines, antihistamines, bronchodilators, and intravenous fluids, should be immediately available. Epinephrine infusion is often necessary if profound hypotension occurs and should be initiated early in therapy.

11. Although involvement of oral mucosa may occur, bulla formation has not been reported. Therefore, airway management should not be unusually difficult.

X. MALIGNANT ATROPHIC PAPULOSIS

Malignant atrophic papulosis (Degos' syndrome) is a rare, almost always fatal, multisystem disease noted for characteristic skin lesions and infarctions of the gastrointestinal tract and central nervous system.[135] The heart, pericardium, lungs, pleura, eyes, and kidneys may also be involved. The vascular lesion is thought to be thromboangiitis obliterans, whose cause is unknown.[136] Previously thought to be uniformly fatal, the disease is increasingly seen to have a cutaneous variant associated with prolonged survival.[137] Histologic findings include lymphocytic infiltrations around and in the walls of venules and arterioles with varying degrees of necrotizing vasculitis. Antiphospholipid antibodies are often present.[138] Hyperkeratosis and dermal acid mucopolysaccharide deposits are common.[137, 139] Blood fibrinolytic activity may be impaired and platelet agregation decreased.[140]

The skin lesions appear as porcelain white papules, 2 to 5 mm in size with a telangiectatic rim,[138] which subsequently form an atrophic scar.[141] In one study, the wedge-shaped skin infarctions previously thought to be characteristic of malignant atrophic papulosis were found in only 3 of 27 biopsy specimens, and these were from older, scarred lesions.[139] Gastrointestinal tract involvement usually results in perforation of the gut, peritonitis, and death. Lung and pleural involvement can result in pleuritis and pleural effusion with subsequent severe restrictive pulmonary disease. Constrictive pericarditis with calcification can also occur.[142] Progressive central nervous system infarctions can result in cerebral edema, increased intracranial pressure, and uncal herniation as well as spastic paralysis.[141, 143] Although malignant atrophic papulosis was once thought to be uniformly fatal, the severity of the disease and its course are variable. Patients ranging from 10 to 54 years of age have been reported.

Survival after diagnosis may be longer than 14 years with treatment with aspirin and dipyridamole.[138] Nonetheless, the disease is frequently fatal within 2 to 3 years of systemic involvement.[141] ACTH, hydrocortisone, vitamin K, antiinflammatory steroids, phenylbutazone, antistreptococcal vaccines, sulfonamides, and antibiotics have been employed, without success.[138] The cause of the disease is not known, but several case reports of familial clusters suggest a hereditary basis or longitudinal transmission.[144, 145] The role of a hypercoagulable state and of circulating immune complexes are debated.[140, 146–148]

The patient with malignant atrophic papulosis usually presents as a surgical emergency with a perforated viscus and peritonitis. In some instances pulmonary decortication or pericardiectomy may be necessary.

A. ANESTHETIC MANAGEMENT OF PATIENTS WITH MALIGNANT ATROPHIC PAPULOSIS

1. Careful preoperative assessment of volume status is essential. Because of frequent peritonitis, large volumes of intravenous fluid may be required for adequate perioperative fluid resuscitation. Invasive cardiovascular monitoring may be necessary.

2. Because of potential pleural or pericardial involvement, these patients require special attention to the preoperative evaluation of pulmonary and cardiac function. Chest radiography and ECG are essential.

3. Bleeding time should be ascertained.

4. Similar skin lesions are sometimes seen in systemic lupus erythematosus, and this disease should be considered in the differential diagnosis.[148]

5. Corticosteroids may exacerbate gastrointestinal complications of the disease and are relatively contraindicated.[146]

6. A careful preoperative nervous system examination is essential to document any deficits. With extensive central nervous system involvement cerebral edema may occur, and, subsequently, increased intracranial pressure. Under these circumstances, anesthetic drugs and techniques that decrease intracranial pressure (barbiturates, narcotics, hyperventilation) should be used. Otherwise, no particular anesthetic drug or technique is recommended.

XI. ECTODERMAL DYSPLASIAS

The ectodermal dysplasias (EDs) are a heterogeneous collection of more than 100 syndromes of congenital abnormalities having in common diffuse and nonprogressive defects in tissues of ectodermal origin.[149] The most common ED is a sex-linked recessive disorder, but other inheritance patterns, including autosomal dominant and autosomal recessive, are seen. Variable penetrance makes genetic counseling difficult. Hereditary anhidrotic or hypohidrotic ED is a disorder characterized by ectodermal atrophy during development and subsequent malformations. Absent or decreased numbers of sweat glands result in hypohidrosis or anhidrosis and altered thermoregulation. Hypotrichosis (decreased amount of hair) and anodontia (absence of teeth) are characteristic.[150, 151] Maxilla and mandible may be underdeveloped.[152, 153] Lacrimation may be decreased or absent. An associated entodermal defect may result in absence of seromucous glands throughout the respiratory tract; this defect may result in frequent respiratory tract infections. Ocular manifestations are common, including strabismus, ptosis, and nystagmus.[154] Infection is common, as is anemia resulting from thymic dysplasia and decreased stem cell elements.[155-157] Digestive tract abnormalities may include achalasia, malrotation of the bowel, omphalocoele, and anal atresia.[158, 159] Recurrent unexplained (and occasionally fatal) fever in infants and children may result from this disease.[160, 161]

Autosomal-dominant ED syndromes include ectodactyly ED with cleft lip (EEC syndrome) and Rapp-Hodgkin hypohidrotic ED. In addition to the features common to ED, EEC and Rapp-Hodgkin ED are characterized by unilateral or bilateral cleft lip and palate, ectodactyly (lobster-claw deformities of the hands or feet), and growth abnormalities. Abnormalities of the auditory canals and hypospadias may also be present.[152, 162] Patients with ED frequently come to the operating room for strabismus, dental, bowel surgery.

A. ANESTHETIC MANAGEMENT OF PATIENTS WITH ED

1. The anesthesiologist should expect that airway management, including adequate mask fit and tracheal intubation, may be difficult because of the dental, maxillary, and mandibular abnormalities, especially in patients with cleft lip and palate. Appropriate alternative preparations should be made in advance. Particular care must be taken not to dislodge hypoplastic teeth.

2. Hyperthermia may be a problem, owing to decreased thermoregulation. The patient's temperature should be monitored continuously and the environment kept cool. A cooling blanket or forced-air blanket should be available for use if necessary. In patients with hypohidrosis, use of anticholinergic drugs such as atropine, scopolamine, or glycopyrrolate with premedication should be avoided; atropine or glycopyrrolate used with an anticholinesterase to reverse a nondepolarizing neuromuscular block could, theoretically, create additional heat loss problems. Theoretically, if a vagolytic drug must be given, as for example in pediatric cases, glycopyrrolate would be preferred. Intraoperative hyperthermia must be distinguished from malignant hyperthermia.

3. It is essential to use an ophthalmic ointment and to tape the patient's eyes closed because of decreased lacrimation.

4. Humidification of inspired gases is recommended because of associated decreased or absent respiratory tract mucous glands. Vigorous postoperative pulmonary care is necessary.

5. Hypospadias may make placement of Foley catheters difficult or impossible. Urologic consultation should be sought preoperatively.

6. No particular anesthetic technique is recommended.

XII. FABRY'S DISEASE

Fabry's disease (angiokeratoma corporis diffusum) is a sex-linked disorder characterized by a deficiency of α-galactosidase A that results in widespread deposition of the neural glycosphingolipid ceramide trihexoside in the vasculature of multiple organ systems, including skin, mucous membranes, eyes, brain, heart, liver, and kidneys. Life expectancy is significantly reduced. Heterozygotes (female carriers) of the disease generally do not show overt symptoms. Exceptions to this rule occur[163] presumably are due to mosaicism and inactivation of one X chromosome. Such persons may manifest cardiac, renal, or cutaneous symptoms or signs.[164, 165]

The cutaneous lesions (angiokeratomas) are ectasias of small vessels in the dermis and are found principally in the scrotal, sacral, and umbilical areas, thighs, and oral mucosa, with sparing of the face, scalp, palms, and soles. Acroparesthesias (burning pains of the hands and feet) are a cardinal symptom[166] and are not usually relieved by analgesics.[167] Recently, success was reported with carbamazepine, phenytoin, and low-dose morphine infusion.[168] Hypohidrosis and hypotrichosis (loss of hair) are also features of this disease. Acute febrile episodes have been triggered by exercise, temperature change, fatigue, and stress.[163]

Ocular symptoms include corneal opacities, lens involvement, and tortuosity of conjunctival and retinal vessels and central retinal artery occlusion.[169, 170] Central nervous system involvement causes presenile dementia, vertigo, myoclonic seizures, and pontine hemorrhages.[171] Cerebrovascular accidents often occur early in adult life. Cardiac involvement includes hypertension, angina pectoris, myocardial infarction,[172] and valvular disease (mitral insufficiency).[173] Accelerated atrioventricular conduction and paroxysmal atrial tachycardia have been reported.[174] Renal damage, frequently the most serious complication of the disease, results in proteinuria, edema, renal failure, uremia, and hypertension and may occur in childhood.[175, 176]

No specific therapy corrects the biochemical defect of the disease. Cardiac and renal failure must be treated symptomatically. Amiodarone has been shown to be helpful. Paresthesias and pain of the extremities have been controlled with oral administration of phenytoin and carbamazepine,[164] and by small doses of morphine.[168] Renal transplantation has also improved symptoms.[167, 177] Most males die between 40 and 50 years of age from renal failure or cerebrovascular accident. In females the course appears to be more benign, although cardiomegaly and subsequent cardiac failure have been reported.[165] A short PR interval and giant negative T waves may be diagnostic.[172, 178, 179] Hemodialysis is poorly tolerated because of concomitant cardiac dysfunction, and dialysis graft survival is poor, perhaps owing to the disease process itself. Kidney transplantation has been tried, with variable results, in an effort to reverse the progressive renal failure. Patients often have a stormy postoperative course, probably as a result of their systemic disease, and there is a high rate of posttransplant mortality.[180]

Nonetheless, at least 25 long-term survivors are reported.[178]

A. ANESTHETIC MANAGEMENT OF PATIENTS WITH FABRY'S DISEASE

1. Preoperative evaluation of cardiovascular and renal function is necessary. Recent onset of peripheral edema or weight gain suggests either cardiac or renal failure. Angina pectoris is indicative of coronary artery involvement resulting in insufficient myocardial oxygen supply and possible impending myocardial infarction. Cardiomegaly and ventricular hypertrophy may be demonstrated by chest roentgenogram and ECG. In particular, short PR intervals (≤ 0.10 second) and giant negative T waves are diagnostic. Laboratory tests include blood urea nitrogen (BUN), serum creatinine, and electrolytes, and the presence of albuminuria may indicate significant renal impairment.

2. Because of central and peripheral nervous system involvement, any preoperative neurologic deficit should be well-documented. Careful consideration should be given before using regional anesthesia techniques.

3. Moderate premedication is indicated to reduce preoperative stress and the possibility of febrile reactions.

4. Temperature should be carefully monitored.

5. In patients receiving hemodialysis, volume status and electrolytes must be checked preoperatively and the usual care taken of dialysis graft or shunt sites.

6. Ocular manifestations are common, and the eyes should be protected with ophthalmic ointment and taping.

7. No particular anesthetic technique is recommended, although peripheral regional blocks are relatively contraindicated. Lesions of the mouth are not sufficiently extensive to cause difficulty during airway instrumentation. If coronary artery disease is present, appropriate management to prevent large changes in blood pressure and heart rate is, of course, necessary. For patients with renal disease avoidance of potentially nephrotoxic drugs, such as sevoflurane and enflurane, is recommended.[181]

8. Stable environmental temperatures are recommended because of possible precipi-

tation of extremity pain and acute febrile episodes in the presence of hypohidrosis. Avoidance of anticholinergic drugs is also recommended if hypohidrosis exists.

9. Postoperative pain control with patient-controlled analgesia and a low background infusion of morphine may prevent acroparesthesias.

XIII. INCONTINENTIA PIGMENTI

Incontinentia pigmenti (Bloch-Sulzberger syndrome) is a hereditary disease that consists of dermatologic, neurologic, skeletal, ocular, and dental defects. Inheritance is either by an autosomal-dominant gene or by a sex-linked dominant gene, both of which are almost always lethal in males. Female patients are therefore far more common than males (37:1). The second X chromosome is thought to be protective. When males survive with the disease, Klinefelter's syndrome (karyotype XXY) or another genetic condition that provided a second X chromosome must be suspected.[182] If the disease is not present from birth onset occurs within 2 weeks in 90 per cent of cases.[183, 184]

Skin involvement, the most visible but least compromising organ disease, is manifested by erythematous, vesicular trunk and extremity eruptions, followed by verrucous lesions and finally by irregular macules that have streaks and splashes of brown to slate-gray pigmentation.[185] These skin lesions gradually resolve and are usually absent by adulthood. They are replaced by atrophic, hypopigmented lesions. These white, nontanning streaks (achromic lesions) occur mostly on the extremities.[185–187] Focal alopecia is common.

Central nervous system involvement includes motor and psychomotor retardation, diplegic, hemiplegic, or tetraplegic spastic paralysis, and seizures. Microcephaly, hydrocephalus, and cortical atrophy are reported.[183, 188, 189]

Ocular manifestations include strabismus, cataracts, retinitis proliferans, retrolental fibroplasia (even in the absence of oxygen therapy), chorioretinitis, metastatic ophthalmitis, uveitis, retinal detachment, optic nerve atrophy, and foveal hypoplasia.[185] Blindness usually results.

Skeletal abnormalities, although infrequent, include skull deformities, dwarfism, spina bifida, cleft lip or cleft palate, and chondrodys-

trophy. Mandibular growth appears normal. Partial anodontia and pegged (conical) deformity of the teeth are characteristic. Recently, focal absence of sweating has been reported, which appears to be a common feature.[186] This and other morphologic similarities have led to the suggestion that incontinentia pigmenti and anhidrotic ectodermal dysplasia, both X-linked recessive conditions, may share a genetic basis.[187]

A. ANESTHETIC MANAGEMENT OF PATIENTS WITH INCONTINENTIA PIGMENTI

1. Despite numerous physical abnormalities, technical difficulties relating to the administration of anesthesia have not been reported. Because of the dental abnormalities, airway instrumentation must be performed gently. Since mandibular development is normal, laryngoscopy and tracheal intubation should not be unusually difficult.

2. Care must be taken when positioning the head. Pressure must be minimized because of the tendency for alopecia. In addition, if macrocephaly is present, special padding may be required to place the head in a neutral position.

3. Autonomic hyperreflexia (mass reflex), which can result in acute severe hypertension, has not been reported in this disease; however, this complication remains a potential problem in patients with spinal cord involvement.[84]

4. No particular anesthetic technique is recommended. With central nervous system involvement and spastic paralysis, succinylcholine should be used with caution or avoided because of the potential for serum potassium increases and dysrhythmias. Any preoperative neurologic or ocular deficit should be well documented and considered before using regional anesthesia.

XIV. HEREDITARY ANGIONEUROTIC EDEMA

Hereditary angioneurotic edema (HANE) is a fairly rare, genetically determined disorder of the complement cascade, kinin, and fibrinolytic systems. Transmission is autosomal dominant. The disease is characterized by an abnormally low plasma level of esterase inhibitor (in 85 per cent of patients) or nonfunctional C_1-esterase inhibitor (in 15 per cent of patients). The fibrinolytic system may also be abnormal. One report lists the incidence of HANE at 1 in 10,000 persons.[190]

The syndrome usually presents as brawny, nonpitting edema, erythema of the extremities, abdominal pain, diarrhea, and facial or laryngeal edema. The latter is a frequent cause of death in patients with HANE and, when it occurs, carries 20 to 30 per cent mortality. The precise sequence of events during attacks is not fully elucidated. It appears that minor trauma activates the complement system, the first component of the system, C_1, being converted to C_5-esterase. Lack of C_1-esterase inhibitor results in runaway activation of the complement system with release of vasoactive peptides and lysis of cell membranes resulting in edema.

Acute development of circumscribed areas of edema is common. Attacks of edema may be spontaneous; more commonly, they follow trauma (as minor as that caused to the fingers by typing), stress, pregnancy, menses, temperature extremes, or surgery. Swelling can occur anywhere but is seen most often on the skin of the face and extremities, the gastrointestinal mucosa, and the upper airway. Deaths due to upper airway edema have been reported during dental anesthesia—local and general. Increasingly, abdominal pain mimicking acute abdomen and resulting from sequestration of fluid in the peritoneal cavity and abdominal wall has been recognized in these patients.[191, 192] Life-threatening hypovolemia may ensue, requiring massive fluid replacement.[192]

Treatment of HANE includes inhibitors of plasminogen-activating factors with such agents as ε-aminocaproic acid, tranexemic acid, and, most recently, with androgens and modified androgens. Danazol has been employed for both long- and short-term prophylaxis and appears to be treatment of choice; it apparently acts by increasing synthesis of C_1-esterase inhibitor. Unlike allergic angioedema, acute attacks of HANE may not respond to the usual therapy of steroids, catecholamines, or antihistamines, although epinephrine is nonetheless usually recommended.[193] Most useful for short-term prophylaxis is fresh-frozen plasma, which is recommended preoperatively; its effects can be seen in 20 minutes and last up to 3 or 4 days.[194]

A. ANESTHETIC MANAGEMENT OF PATIENTS WITH HANE

1. Careful preparation is essential. Transport teams, operative staff, and postoperative staff must all be apprised of the significant risks faced by patients with HANE, especially with respect to possible airway edema.

2. Preoperative treatment for 2 weeks with danazol has been recommended.[190] Doses must be individualized, but often doses of 200 to 300 mg per day appear to prevent acute attacks. Fresh-frozen plasma should be given 24 hours before surgery (2 to 4 U has been recommended for adults).[190, 193, 194, 195] Additional fresh-frozen plasma should be available but may not act in time to help if acute airway obstruction occurs. Partially purified C_1-esterase inhibitor has been suggested in place of fresh-frozen plasma because of a lower hepatitis risk,[196] but its cost is high and it is not routinely available.

3. If general anesthesia is required, no specific anesthetic drugs are recommended. Thiopental and succinylcholine have been employed successfully for induction and intubation, followed by nitrous oxide and enflurane.[190] Transtracheal jet ventilation has been employed successfully,[197] but the risk of tension pneumothorax because inspired gases cannot escape a potentially edematous airway must be remembered. Regional anesthesia has been advocated for parturients.[198]

XV. OSTEOPOROSIS, OSTEOMALACIA, AND OSTEOPETROSIS

Osteoporosis is a disorder in which the overall quantity of bone substance is reduced without alteration of the bone's normal shape, composition, or morphology.[199, 200] Osteoporosis occurs most frequently in elderly patients as a result of progressive bone loss after age 40 years.[201] Withdrawal of estrogen at menopause in women is the most common precipitating factor, but the disease affects men as well. Women with small frames, light weight, and European ancestry are at greatest risk.[202, 203] Osteoporosis may occur in the setting of hyperthyroidism, hyperparathyroidism, Cushing's syndrome, diabetes mellitus, acromegaly, malabsorption, malnutrition, or alcoholism.[202, 204] Long-term corticosteroid therapy can also be a causal factor.

The pathophysiology appears to be an imbalance between bone resorption and formation.[201] Osteoblast activity (bone formation) is at its peak in adolescence. Osteoblast and osteoclast (bone resorption) activity are nearly equal in middle age, maximum bone density occurring at age 30 to 40 years. Thereafter, bone density decreases by approximately 2 per cent per year.[205] As a result of the loss of bone substance, bones fracture more readily. Fractures may occur at any site, with minimal trauma. The most common fracture sites include vertebral bodies (with vertebral column compression), the neck of the femur, the distal radius, the proximal humerus, and the pelvis. Annual cost of hip fractures alone in the United States exceeds 5.2 billion.[206] Vertebral fractures are usually wedge or crush fractures. Bone pain is a frequent symptom but usually subsides after 1 to 2 months.[207] Severe kyphosis is not uncommon. Significant neurologic sequelae are rare, although symptoms of sciatica are not uncommon. Osteolytic vertebral body metastasis from cancer may present in identical fashion and must be excluded.

Treatment is less than satisfactory because long-term results fail to show an increase in bone density. Drugs that have been used in therapy include systemic and tissue-specific estrogens, anabolic steroids, parathyroid hormone, vitamin D, calcium, calcitonin, diphosphonates, and sodium fluoride. Patients may require surgical stabilization of fractures, but immobilization, other than local splinting, should be kept to a minimum since it exacerbates the condition. Osteoporosis may be prevented by developing greater bone mass before menopause through calcium supplementation and exercise.[208]

Osteomalacia is a metabolic bone disorder in which normal bone is replaced by nonmineralized osteoid tissue. The resultant soft, pliable bones are easily deformed or fractured. Causal factors include vitamin D deficiency (caused by malabsorption, abnormal liver and/or kidney metabolism, inadequate exposure to sunlight), Fanconi's syndrome, hypocalcemia, hypophosphatemia, hypophosphatasia, tumors, renal failure, and aluminum toxicity.[209–211] Major symptoms include bone pain and tenderness and muscle weakness. Paresthesias, muscle cramps, and tetany may occur as a result of severe associated hypocalcemia. Scoliosis and kyphosis may be present. Roentgenographic signs include a nonspecific decrease in radiodensity of bone and pseudofracture (Looser's zone). Therapy includes provision of adequate nutrition, calcium, phosphate, vitamin D, and exposure to sunlight; correction of abnormalities of the gastrointestinal and biliary tracts, if present; removal of tumors, if present; and renal transplantation if renal failure occurs.[212] Unlike osteoporosis, the response of osteomalacia to treatment is usually good. Previously incapacitated patients may become asymptomatic in 2 or 3 months. If osteoporosis is also present, however, skeletal recovery may not be complete, and the risk of fracture remains.

The osteopetroses (abnormally dense bone) are now recognized as a group of hereditary disorders characterized by various combinations of bone sclerosis and modeling defects resulting in brittle bone.[213] Inheritance can be autosomal dominant or recessive. Before bone marrow transplantation, the infantile recessive form of the disease was uniformly fatal.[214] Currently, the osteopetroses are classified into four major categories: (1) osteosclerosis (hard, dense bone), (2) craniotubular dysplasia, (3) craniotubular hyperostoses and hypertrophy of bone, and (4) miscellaneous sclerosing and hyperostotic disorders.[215] Knowledge of the variable degrees of bone fragility, muscle weakness, scoliosis, and cranial, facial bone, and mandibular (micro- or macrognathia) involvement is important. In sclerosteosis, progressive overgrowth of the skull may cause increased intracranial pressure. Sudden death from brain stem herniation through the foramen magnum has been reported in adults.[216]

A. ANESTHETIC MANAGEMENT OF PATIENTS WITH OSTEOPOROSIS, OSTEOMALACIA, OR OSTEOPETROSIS

1. All elderly patients of European descent must be considered at risk for osteoporosis. Because of their age, a careful search for intercurrent medical problems must be made.

2. Because of the greatly increased risk of bone fracture, these patients must be moved and positioned carefully. Padding of all pressure areas is recommended.

3. Knowledge of any existing metabolic or endocrine disorders and their anesthetic im-

plications in these patients before surgery is important.

4. If kyphoscoliosis is present, evaluation of the patient's pulmonary function is recommended.

5. The cervical spine should be carefully evaluated and range of painless motion ascertained. Any preoperative neurologic deficit should be well documented.

6. In patients with sclerostenosis, the potential for increased intracranial pressure must be remembered, and anesthetic techniques that either decrease—or at least do not increase—intracranial pressure should be considered.

7. Patients with osteoporosis frequently undergo open reduction of femoral fractures. Morbidity and mortality in these patients have been reduced by early operation and mobilization.[217, 218] Careful attention must be paid to associated medical conditions, and especially to pulmonary function because of the risk of pneumonia in these patients.

8. Except for persons with sclerosteosis, no particular anesthetic drugs or techniques are recommended. The choice of anesthetic technique depends on the operative site and concurrent disease states. The presence of vertebral compression may make the use of regional techniques (e.g., subarachnoid, epidural) difficult. Nonetheless, many anesthesiologists prefer regional anesthesia for reduction of hip fractures because of less blood loss and decreased incidence of pulmonary embolism.

XVI. OSTEOGENESIS IMPERFECTA

Osteogenesis imperfecta (OI) is a rare autosomal dominant disease whose incidence is approximately 1 in 30,000 live births.[219] Although the disease is a generalized connective tissue disorder that affects many organs, it is considered primarily a dwarfing syndrome. The primary bone lesion is absence of normal ossification of the endochondral bone, resulting in very fragile bones. Classically, two major clinical types are recognized: (1) osteogenesis imperfecta congenita (fetal type), in which skeletal fractures with resulting deformities occur in utero and thus are present at birth, and (2) osteogenesis imperfecta tarda, in which skeletal fractures and deformities occur after birth.[220, 221] The tarda form of OI usually presents in childhood with blue

scleras, multiple fractures after trivial trauma, dwarfing syndrome with bowing of the femurs and scoliosis, and progressive otosclerosis and deafness.[221-223] Of particular interest to anesthesiologists is the fact that mandibular fractures occur more frequently in these patients than in the normal population although facial bone fractures do not.[224]

Other abnormalities associated with OI include hyperthermia, hyperhidrosis, platelet dysfunction resulting in easy bruising and bleeding,[225] kyphoscoliosis, cor pulmonale, congenital heart disease, valvular heart disease,[226] joint laxity, and thin skin. Fragile teeth are particularly susceptible to caries.[227, 228] Hyperthermia and hyperhidrosis appear to be secondary to either an abnormal central nervous system temperature-regulating mechanism or abnormal cellular energy metabolism,[225] but malignant hyperthermia has been reported in three patients[229] and moderate to severe metabolic acidosis was seen on induction in each of five patients in one series.[230] Platelet dysfunction is caused by decreased release of platelet factor III and platelet adhesiveness; this may be due to immature platelets[225] since the platelet count is normal. Kyphoscoliosis may cause significant mechanical pulmonary disease resulting in cor pulmonale.[226] Additional thoracic deformities may include pectus carinatum and pectus excavatum. Cardiac lesions include patent ductus arteriosus, atrial septal defect, ventricular septal defect, and mitral or aortic insufficiency.[226, 227] Usually, valvular stenosis occurs only after bacterial endocarditis.[226] Cleft palate and hydrocephalus may accompany OI.[228] Central retinal artery occlusion and resultant blindness have been reported following controlled hypotension with the patient in the prone position and the dependent eye resting on towels.[231] This presumably resulted from continued extrinsic pressure on the eye and low perfusion.

A. ANESTHETIC MANAGEMENT OF PATIENTS WITH OI

1. When moving the patient to and from the operating table or turning and positioning the patient, care must be exercised to avoid fractures. Padding of all pressure areas is recommended. Padding of blood pressure cuffs with web roll is necessary because fractures have occurred from the compression of the

cuff.[232] Care must be taken when tourniquets are applied to facilitate intravenous cannulation.

2. If airway management requires the use of a face mask or laryngoscopy and tracheal intubation, caution must be exercised to avoid mandibular and facial bone fractures. Care should be taken to avoid extension of the neck and possible fracture of the brittle cervical spine. Padding may be built up under the back and shoulders in patients with hydrocephalus and resulting macrocephaly.

3. Bleeding time and coagulation profile should be checked preoperatively. Unusual bleeding may require platelet transfusion.

4. Careful examination must be made for concomitant pulmonary or cardiac disease. Pulmonary function testing is indicated if the patient has significant kyphoscoliosis or evidence of thoracic cage deformities.

5. Intraoperative hyperthermia without muscle rigidity and malignant hyperpyrexia (MH) have been reported in patients with OI undergoing general anesthesia.[229, 234] In addition, OI patients may be susceptible to metabolic acidosis upon induction, even in the absence of recognizable temperature or carbon dioxide changes.[230] Until further data are available, OI patients must be considered at risk for intraoperative hyperthermia, and possibly MH. Elective surgery should be postponed if an OI patient is febrile. Preoperative creatine phosphokinase (CPK) levels may identify patients at particular risk for MH. Because hypermetabolism may contribute to intraoperative hyperthermia, a cool environment is recommended. Continuous temperature monitoring and avoidance of known MH-triggering drugs are recommended, as are end-tidal carbon dioxide monitoring and blood gas monitoring. Mechanisms for cooling and treatment of MH (e.g., dantrolene and sodium bicarbonate) must be readily available. Use of a forced-air or heating/cooling blanket is recommended.

6. Central retinal artery occlusion following controlled hypotension in a prone patient with OI has been reported.[231] Special care must be taken for prone positioning of patients with OI, to avoid any extrinsic pressure on the eyes. A standard T cutout foam headrest is recommended. Frequent observation for extrinsic pressure is necessary.

7. No particular anesthetic technique is recommended. Ketamine has been used successfully both intramuscularly and intravenously to obviate intubation or positive-pressure

ventilation, and total intravenous anesthesia has been advocated.[232, 233] Both regional and general anesthetics with endotracheal intubation have been successfully accomplished.[221, 222, 225] Enflurane and isoflurane are preferred to halothane because of the possible risk of MH, as presumably, are sevoflurane and desflurane. (Note that all halogenated anesthetics have been associated with MH.) Succinylcholine should be avoided, both as a possible trigger for MH and because any fasciculations may result in bone fractures. Anticholinergics should also be avoided, if possible, because of possible exacerbation of hyperthermia. Use of an LMA may obviate muscle relaxants if intubation is necessary for the procedure and may place less pressure on the eyes than a mask would.

XVII. DWARFISM

Dwarfism has a variety of presentations: more than 55 distinct syndromes, with many subtypes, have been described. Many cases of dwarfism have not yet been classified. Patients with these syndromes are placed into one of two major categories: (1) those with disproportionate short stature ("dwarfs") and (2) those with proportionate short stature ("midgets"). Further subdivision is made according to the abnormal development of bone and/or cartilage (osteochondrodysplasias) or malformations of individual bones (dysostoses). The distinction is made between involvement of the appendicular skeleton (short limbs) and the axial skeleton (short trunk); the prefix *spondylo-* refers to spine involvement. Classification according to the roentgenographic evidence of bone involvement (epiphyseal, metaphyseal, or diaphyseal) is also used. Rhizomelic (proximal segment), mesomelic (middle segment), and acromelic (distal segment) shortening describes the affected segments of long bones. A further distinction is made according to mode of inheritance; for example, X linked versus autosomal.[235]

The cause for most of the skeletal dysplasias is unknown. Known causative factors include nutritional disorders, chromosome aberrations, primary metabolic abnormalities, and endocrine, hematologic, neurologic, renal, gastrointestinal, and cardiopulmonary disorders.[236, 237] Diagnosis is based primarily upon clinical and roentgenographic findings. Except for a few syndromes (e.g., mucopolysaccharidoses, hypophosphatasia, mucolipidoses, and hypercalciuria), biochemical procedures are of little value in the diagnosis. Diagnosis is frequently made by fetal ultrasonography.[238]

Major abnormalities that may be present in patients with dwarfism and of which the anesthesiologist should be aware include the following (each abnormality is discussed in greater detail below): (1) atlantoaxial instability, (2) spinal stenosis, (3) airway and facial and dental abnormalities, (4) thoracic dystrophy, (5) pectus carinatum, (6) scoliosis, kyphosis, and lordosis, (7) congenital cardiac disease, (8) hydrocephaly, (9) mental retardation, (10) seizure disorders, and (11) compression of the trachea during head flexion. Dwarfed patients may require anesthesia for surgical correction of many of these abnormalities, and especially for scoliosis.[239, 240] Surgery for perforated ulcers and for coronary artery disease has also been reported.[241, 242]

1. Atlantoaxial instability can result from a normal, hypoplastic, aplastic, or detached odontoid process and varying degrees of ligamentous laxity. Dwarfing syndromes in which odontoid dysgenesis[236, 237, 243, 244] has been found include spondyloephiphyseal dysplasia tarda, spondyloepiphyseal dysplasia congenital, achondroplasia, pseudo-achondroplasia, pseudo-Morquio's syndrome (non–keratin-secreting), multiple epiphyseal dysplasia congenital, Morquio's mucopolysaccharidosis, metatrophic dwarfism, spondylometaphyseal dysplasia (Murdock's), spondylometaphyseal dysplasia (Kozlowski's), metaphyseal chondrodysplasia (McKusick's, cartilage-hair hypoplasia), and Kneist dwarfism. The classic signs of atlantoaxial instability are progressive weakness, hypotonia, neuromuscular disturbances (spasticity, clonus, hyperreflexia, Babinski's sign), paraplegia, quadriplegia, and (on occasion) sudden death. *Transection of the cervical cord and resultant death following endotracheal intubation have been reported.*[245] An evaluation of the atlantoaxial joint should be made in the dwarf who exhibits any of the following: dwarfism of the osteochondrodystrophy group, a disproportionately short trunk, roentgenographic vertebral body involvement, congenital slipped epiphyses, or decreasing physical endurance.[236] Currently, the recommended treatment is surgical fusion.[246, 247]

2. Spinal stenosis describes a syndrome that results from a spinal canal so narrowed that the contents of the canal completely fill the available space.[248] Symptoms and signs of spinal cord and nerve root compression result; for example, weakness, paralysis, and cauda equina syndrome. High cervical cord compression due to stenosis of the foramen magnum may occur. Treatment is decompression laminectomy or decompression of the foramen magnum. Spinal stenosis most often occurs in achondroplastic dwarfism but may also occur in Morquio's syndrome and diastrophic dwarfism. Surgery is not without risk, however: in a series of 27 patients, two suffered cervical cord infarctions.[249] In patients with cervical spondylosis, even mild sedation may unmask underlying neurologic deficits[250] or relax the muscles holding the head in a position of minimal spinal compromise, with the same effect.

3. Airway management difficulty may result from hypoplasia of the mandible or micrognathia, cleft palate, and cleft lip. Hypoplastic mandible is associated with the following dwarfing syndromes:[236, 237] acrocephalopolysyndactyly type II (Carpenter's syndrome), idiopathic hypercalcemic syndrome, mesomelia (Langer's syndrome), metaphyseal chondrodysplasia (Jansen's disease), *cri du chat* syndrome, antimongolism, oculomandibulodyscephaly (Hallermann-Streiff syndrome), ring-4 chromosome syndrome, trisomy 22, and craniocarpotarsal dystrophy (Freeman-Sheldon syndrome, whistling face syndrome). Anesthesia given to an achrondoplastic dwarf in the sitting position has been followed by massive tongue swelling from lingual vein thrombosis.[249] Postoperative airway obstruction and sleep apnea have been reported, as has subglottic stenosis.[249, 241]

4. Thoracic dystrophy is a deformity of the trunk characterized by a small, narrow, contracted chest cage, marked shortening of the ribs, thoracic lordosis, and segmentation defects of the vertebrae. The dwarfing syndromes involving lethal thoracic dystrophy include thanatophoric dwarfism, achondrogenesis, and short rib, thoracic dystrophy polydactyly syndrome (Majewski's syndrome, Salvino-Noonan syndrome). With these syndromes death occurs in the newborn period. A second group denoted as surviving thoracic dystrophy includes asphyxiating thoracic dystrophy (Jeune's syndrome),[251] metatrophic dwarfism, chondroectodermal dysplasia (Ellis-van Creveld syndrome), and spondylothoracic dysplasia. Affected infants

are plagued with ventilatory problems from birth, frequent pneumonia, and high mortality; however, several of the second group have survived and often present serious management problems because of spinal curves and decreased ventilatory capacity.[246] Such patients may have multiple organ failure or dysfunction, including end-stage renal failure, hepatic fibrosis, and cardiac dysfunction.[251] Jeune's syndrome is inherited as an autosomal-recessive disease. More than 100 cases have been reported. The most seriously affected persons have pulmonary hypoplasia in addition to chest wall deformities, causing severe restriction to ventilation. Patients are prone to pneumothorax during positive-pressure ventilation because of the high peak inspiratory pressure required.

5. Scoliosis and kyphoscoliosis occur frequently and vary from mild to severe. The short trunk causes severe crowding of the normal-sized abdominal viscera and general congestion of the thoracic and abdominal contents. Hydronephrosis may occur. Severe scoliosis compounds these problems. As a result, pulmonary and cardiovascular function in the dwarf can be severely impaired.[246, 252] Kyphosis and lordosis may progress to produce spinal cord compression. These conditions may require surgery for correction or stabilization.

6. Congenital cardiac disease (patent ductus arteriosus, atrial septal defects, coarctation of the aorta) is associated with thanatophoric dwarfism and achondrogenesis. Spondylometaphyseal dysplasia is associated with mitral valve prolapse.[244] Large atrial septal defects may be seen with chondroectodermal dysplasia (Ellis–van Creveld syndrome).[237] Acquired cardiac disease also occurs, of course.[242]

7. Central nervous system involvement can include mental retardation, hydrocephaly, and seizure disorders.[235, 237, 244]

A. ANESTHETIC MANAGEMENT OF PATIENTS WITH DWARFING SYNDROMES

1. Stability of the atlantoaxial joint should be evaluated by history, neurologic examination, and appropriate lateral flexion and extension roentgenographic views of the cervical spine. CT and MRI may be necessary. If atlantoaxial instability is present, procedures to ensure protection of the spinal cord must be used.[253] Cervical spine extension is generally maintained in symptomatic patients. Efforts should be made to keep this position during induction and maintenance of anesthesia. Application of cervical stabilizing devices such as a halo collar should be considered.[254] Care should be taken with sedative medications, since they may unmask neurologic deficits or reduce the patient's ability to maintain the head position that minimizes spinal compression.[250] Intubation with an LMA, fiberoptic bronchoscope, or Bullard or Upsher layrngoscope may reduce the need for neck movement or extension.

2. Regional anesthesia (subarachnoid and epidural) has been used successfully in dwarfs, without apparent neurologic sequelae; however, because of the potential for development of neurologic problems due to spinal stenosis and vertebral misalignment, regional anesthesia should be reserved for patients for whom there is a specific indication and for whom the immediate advantages of regional techniques outweigh those of alternatives.[255, 256] Any preoperative neurologic deficit should be well documented.

3. Careful evaluation of the patient's airway must be made to assess the ease or difficulty with which tracheal intubation could be performed, if necessary. Appropriate equipment (fiberoptic bronchoscope) must be available for tracheal intubation of a patient with a "difficult airway."[257] The possibility of tracheal compression with head flexion must be recognized, and tracheal stenosis has been reported.[249, 252, 258] Appropriate endotracheal tube size will probably be 0.5 to 1 mm smaller than would be predicted for the patient's age.[249, 255] Recently, a laryngeal mask has been successfully employed for surgery.[259]

4. Ventilatory problems may occur in patients with thoracic dystrophy, pectus carinatum,[244] or vertebral misalignment. These patients may need mechanical ventilatory assistance and may be difficult to wean from it.

5. Cardiac defects, mental retardation, hydrocephaly, or seizures must be considered in the design of the anesthetic technique to be used.[258]

6. Autonomic hyperreflexia is a potential problem for patients who have spinal cord lesions resulting from spinal stenosis or vertebral misalignment.[260] Appropriate drugs (alpha- and beta-blockers, vasodilators) must be immediately available.

7. For patients with thoracic dystrophy,

care must be taken to keep peak airway pressures as low as possible, to prevent barotrauma.

8. Somatosensory evoked potentials have been suggested for scoliosis surgery.[240]

9. No particular anesthetic drug appears to be contraindicated for patients with dwarfing syndromes. A patient with both acute intermittent porphyria and achondroplastic dwarfism has been reported.[256] One patient anesthetized with sevoflurane and nitrous oxide exhibited interoperative hypertension, but its significance was unknown and may have been related to autonomic hyperreflexia as described above.[241]

XVIII. CRANIOFACIAL AND MANDIBULOFACIAL DYSOSTOSES

Several syndromes that are characterized by abnormalities of the skull, facial bones, and mandible frequently are not associated with dwarfism. Most affected patients are children.

Apert's syndrome (acrocephalosyndactyly) is characterized by craniosynostosis, high forehead, flat bridge of the nose, maxillary hypoplasia, relative mandibular prognathism, synostosis of the cervical spine, visceral malformations, and congenital heart defects.[261–263] Cruzon's disease is characterized by craniosynostosis, maxillary hypoplasia, relative mandibular prognathism, and a prominent nose ("parrot beak"). Increased intracranial pressure has been observed in these patients.[262] Goldenhar's syndrome (oculoauriculovertebral dysplasia) is characterized by eye and ear abnormalities, micrognathia, maxillary hypoplasia, cleft or high-arched palate, synostosis of the cervical spine, and congenital heart defects.[261, 264] Treacher Collins syndrome (Franceschetti-Zwahlen-Klein syndrome) is characterized by antimongoloid obliquity of the palpebral fissures, coloboma, microphthalmia, choanal atresia, hypoplasia of the zygoma, maxillary, and mandibular bones, deafness, congenital heart defects, and occasionally dwarfism.[261, 265]

François' syndrome is intermediate between mandibulofacial and craniofacial dysostosis.[266] It is notable for microphthalmos, milky cataracts, severe frontal bossing, and mandibular hypoplasia with forward dislocation of the mandibular joint. Anesthesia has not been reported for patients with this syndrome, but difficulty with intubation would be anticipated.

Pierre Robin syndrome is characterized by severe micrognathia, cleft palate, and glossoptosis (tongue forced back into the airway channel), resulting in life-threatening airway obstruction. Respiratory distress and cyanosis occur most frequently when the infant is placed supine and are generally relieved when the infant is placed prone or on one side. Nasoesophageal intubation has been effective in attenuating the respiratory distress.[267] As the child grows older, the glossoptosis decreases and the respiratory distress resolves, owing to relatively faster growth of the mandible.

Meckel's syndrome consists of microcephaly, cleft palate, cleft tongue and epiglottis, micrognathia, congenital heart defects, and renal abnormalities. It is usually fatal in infancy as a result of renal insufficiency.[268] Osteodysplasty (Melnick-Needles syndrome) is characterized by exophthalmos, full cheeks, micrognathia, and misalignment of the teeth. Hanhart's syndrome is characterized by micrognathia and a variety of limb abnormalities. Aglossia adactylia consists of a small tongue or none, micrognathia, and variable limb abnormalities. Oral-facial-digital syndrome is characterized by hypoplasia of the nasal alae, micrognathia, lobate tongue, cleft lip, and a high-arched cleft palate.[268]

Hemifacial microsomia is characterized by unilateral facial involvement. One side of the mandible may be hypoplastic or absent.[261] The mouth and face show marked asymmetry. Hypoplasia or agenesis of the lung may occur on the affected side.[261] In addition, patients with severe hydrocephalus occasionally present to the operating room for reduction cranioplasty.

A. ANESTHETIC MANAGEMENT OF PATIENTS WITH VARIOUS CRANIOFACIAL DYSOSTOSES

1. The necessity for careful evaluation of the airway is usually very obvious on simple observation of the patient. Hypoplasia of the maxillary bones (midface) may make mask fitting difficult. Micrognathia with a receding chin can make visualization of the larynx impossible during attempted direct laryngoscopy. Temporomandibular joint dysfunction

may prevent wide opening of the jaws. Cervical vertebral synostosis may prevent flexion or extension of the neck, and choanal atresia or hypoplasia may prevent blind nasotracheal intubation.

Methods for tracheal intubation may include conventional awake intubation, the use of the fiberoptic bronchoscope or the optical stylet, direct palpation of the epiglottis followed by "blind" oro- or nasotracheal intubation, and transtracheal retrograde passage of a guidewire into the oropharynx. More recently, availability of the LMA has allowed an additional approach: placement of the LMA, even in the lateral position, and then fiberoptic intubation through the LMA. Care should be taken with sedative medications since they may unmask neurologic deficits or reduce the patient's ability to maintain the head position, which minimizes spinal compression.[269]

2. Patients must be evaluated for abnormalities of the heart, lungs, and other visceral organs.

3. Patients with craniosynostoses may also have increased intracranial pressure.[262, 270]

4. No particular anesthetic drugs are recommended. Techniques that allow spontaneous ventilation by the patient until the anesthetist is certain that the airway can be managed (with a mask or LMA if necessary) are recommended. Only then, if at all, should muscle relaxants be used to facilitate tracheal intubation.[261] Awake oral or blind nasotracheal (when the nares are patent) intubation is a viable alternative, except when it interferes with the operative field. The surgeon and tracheostomy equipment should be present during induction of anesthesia. Tracheostomy with local anesthesia may be necessary before the induction of anesthesia.

5. During surgery for repair of cranial synostoses, the endotracheal tube should be secured by suturing it to the teeth or gums to prevent extubation during manipulation of the head.

6. Sudden loss of cerebrospinal fluid may be associated with intractable hypertension.[264]

XIX. PAGET'S DISEASE

Paget's disease (osteitis deformans) is a metabolic disorder of unknown cause characterized by excessively rapid remodeling of bone.[271] The disease may occur in as many as 2 to 8 per cent of the population of Britain older than 55.[272] Three phases are recognized

in this remodeling process. First, intense resorption of existing bone is produced by increased osteoclast activity. Second, deposition of new bone occurs by increased osteoblast activity. Third, as bone resorption begins to decrease, continued bone formation results in sclerotic areas of bones (the roentgenographic "cotton wool" appearance), which are weak and fracture easily. Most patients present with bone pain and fractures at involved sites. Areas most frequently affected include the pelvis, femurs, skull, tibias, and vertebrae. The jaw is sometimes also affected.[273] Symptoms and signs of spinal cord compression can result from vertebral fracture, atlantoaxial instability,[273] or basilar invagination of the skull. Hydrocephalic dementia[274] and death from cerebellar tonsillar herniation[275] secondary to basilar invagination of the skull have occurred. Hearing loss is common. Severe kyphosis may be present. Dental extraction may be more difficult than in unaffected patients and associated with postextraction bleeding and slow healing.[272]

Cardiac output may be greatly increased owing to the increased vascularity of the affected areas of bone, and high-output congestive heart failure may result. Arteriovenous anastomotic shunting does not appear to be the cause of the increased cardiac output.[276] With treatment and resolution of Paget's disease, cardiac output may return to normal.[277] Treatment has included large doses of salicylates and corticosteroids for short periods (side effects have precluded long-term use of these drugs). Calcitonin, mithramycin, and diphosphonates are also used.

A. ANESTHETIC MANAGEMENT OF PATIENTS WITH PAGET'S DISEASE

1. Careful moving and positioning of the patient are required because fractures may occur with even mild trauma. Padding of all pressure areas is recommended.

2. Preoperative evaluation of atlantoaxial stability is recommended. If instability is found, extreme care must be used to maintain a neutral position of the cervical spine, particularly if laryngoscopy and tracheal intubation are performed.

3. In patients with kyphosis, pulmonary function should be evaluated. Patients with decreased pulmonary reserve may require

postoperative mechanical ventilatory assistance.

4. The cardiovascular system should be evaluated for high-output congestive heart failure. If heart failure is present, elective operations should be postponed until the failure can be corrected.

5. No particular anesthetic drug or technique is recommended. The presence of vertebral compression may make the use of regional (e.g., subarachnoid or epidural) techniques difficult. General anesthesia has been proposed for dental extraction because of the greater difficulty encountered with the procedure and the increased risk of postextraction bleeding.[272]

6. Autonomic hyperreflexia is a potential complication in patients with spinal cord injury.[278]

7. Appropriate perioperative corticosteroid coverage is recommended for those who took corticosteroids preoperatively.

8. Platelet function should be evaluated by bleeding time estimation in patients taking salicylates.

XX. FIBROUS DYSPLASIA

Fibrous dysplasia is a disorder of unknown cause characterized by expanding fibroosseous lesions in bone. The three major types are (1) monostotic (single bone involvement), (2) polyostotic (multiple bone involvement), and (3) Albright's syndrome (multiple bone involvement, cutaneous pigmentation, endocrine dysfunction, and precocious puberty in females).[279, 280] The major skeletal defect in fibrous dysplasia is weakened structural integrity, and fractures are frequently produced by mild trauma. Clinical features include pain, fracture, deformity, and an enlarging mass. A painful lesion signals impending fracture, enlargement of the fibroosseous mass, or a malignant change, which is rare. Craniofacial involvement with grotesque facial deformity is not uncommon.[281–285] Spine involvement, although unusual, includes vertebral collapse or an expanding fibroosseous mass.[279, 286] Weakness, spasticity, and paralysis may result. Associated endocrine dysfunction includes acromegaly, hyperparathyroidism, hyperthyroidism, and Cushing's syndrome.[281, 287] Treatment is symptomatic; for example, fracture reduction and stabilization, reconstruction of deformity, and treatment of endocrine dysfunction.

A. ANESTHETIC MANAGEMENT OF PATIENTS WITH FIBROUS DYSPLASIA

1. Careful movement, turning, and positioning of the patient are required because fractures occur with even mild trauma. Padding of all pressure areas is recommended. Laryngoscopy and tracheal intubation must be performed gently, to avoid mandibular fracture.

2. With extensive maxillomandibular involvement, airway management may prove to be difficult. Direct laryngoscopy may be impossible. Indirect laryngoscopy is recommended to evaluate the epiglottis and laryngeal inlet. Awake blind nasotracheal intubation, fiberoptic laryngoscopy, or use of an intubating bronchoscope may be necessary.[282, 285] Tracheostomy may be required.

3. Any existing endocrine disorder must be evaluated preoperatively and the anesthetic implications considered.

4. No particular anesthetic technique is recommended. In patients with spinal cord injury, regional anesthesia (subarachnoid, epidural, or regional nerve block) should be used with extreme caution. Any preoperative neurologic deficit should be well-documented. Intraligamental injection of local anesthetics has been recommended over standard intraoral nerve blocks, since the latter may be ineffective if fibrous overgrowth has "barricaded" the nerves.[288]

5. Autonomic hyperreflexia is a potential complication in patients with spinal cord lesions.[84]

REFERENCES

Epidermolysis Bullosa

1. Bauer EA, Briggaman RA: The mechanobullous diseases (epidermolysis bullosa). *In* Fitzpatrick TB (ed): Dermatology in General Medicine, 2nd ed. New York, McGraw-Hill, 1979.
2. Smith GB, Schribman AJ: Anesthesia and severe skin disease. Anaesthesia 39:443, 1984.
3. Kelly RE, Koff HD, Rothaus KO, et al: Brachial plexus anesthesia in eight patients with recessive dystrophic epidermolysis bullosa. Anesth Analg 66:1318, 1987.
4. Cohen SR, Landing BH, Isaacs H: Epidermolysis bullosa associated with laryngeal stenosis. Ann Otol Rhinol Laryngol 87:25, 1978.
5. Tomlinson AA: Recessive dystrophic epidermolysis bullosa. Anaesthesia 38:485, 1983.
6. Berryhill RE, Benumof JL, Saidman LJ, et al: Anes-

thetic management of emergency cesarean section in a patient with epidermolysis bullosa dystrophica polydysplastica. Anesth Analg 57:281, 1977.

7. Marshall BE: A comment on epidermolysis bullosa and its anesthetic management for dental operations. Br J Anesth 35:724, 1963.

8. Kaplan R, Strauch B: Regional anesthesia in a child with epidermolysis bullosa. Anesthesiology 67:262, 1987.

9. Spargo PM, Smith GB: Epidermolysis bullosa and porphyria. Anesth Analg 67:297, 1988.

10. Reddy ARR, Wong WHW: Epidermolysis bullosa, a review of anaesthetic problems and case reports. Can Anaesth Soc J 19:536, 1972.

11. Broster T, Placek R, Eggers GWN Jr: Epidermolysis bullosa: Anesthetic management for cesarean section. Anesth Analg 66:341, 1987.

12. James I, Wark H: Airway management during anesthesia in patients with epidermolysis bullosa dystrophica. Anesthesiology 56:323, 1982.

13. Pratilar V, Biezumski A: Epidermolysis bullosa manifested and treated during anesthesia. Anesthesiology 45:581, 1975.

14. Ramadass T, Thangavelu TA: Epidermolysis bullosa and its ENT manifestations. J Laryngol Otol 92:441, 1978.

15. Petty WC, Gunther RC: Anesthesia for nonfacial surgery in polydysplastic epidermolysis bullosa (dystrophic). Anesth Analg 49:246, 1970.

16. Fisk GC, Kern IB: Anesthesia for eosophagoscopy in a child with epidermolysis bullosa—a case report. Anaesth Intensive Care 1:297, 1973.

17. Tio TH, Waardenberg PJ, Vermeullen HJ: Blood coagulation in epidermolysis bullosa hereditaria. Arch Dermatol 88:76, 1963.

18. Yasui Y, Yamamoto Y, Sodeyama O, et al: Anesthesia in a patient with epidermolysis bullosa. Masui 44:260, 1995.

19. Dorne R, Tassaux D, Ravat F, et al: Surgery for epidermolysis bullosa in children: value of the association of inhalation anesthesia and locoregional anesthesia. Ann Fr Anesth Reanim 113:425, 1994.

20. LoVerne SR, Oropollo AT: Ketamine anesthesia in dermolytic bullous disease (epidermolysis bullosa). Anesth Analg 56:398, 1977.

21. Farber NE, Todd RJ, Turco G: Spinal anesesthesia in a patient with epidermolysis bullosa. Anesthesiology 83:1364, 1995.

22. Rowlingson JC, Rosenblum SM: Successful regional anesthesia in a patient with epidermolysis bullosa. Regional Anesth 8:81, 1983.

Pemphigus and Pemphigoid

23. Jordan RE: Pemphigus. *In* Fitzpatrick TB (ed): Dermatology in General Medicine, 2nd ed. New York, McGraw-Hill, 1979.

24. Ide A, Hashimoto T, Tanaka M, Nishikawa T: Detection of autoantibodies against bullous pemphigoid and pemphigus antigens by an enzyme-linked immunosorbent assay using the bacterial recombinant proteins. Exp Dermatol 4:112, 1995.

25. Matsubara K, Kanauchi H, Tanaka T, Imamura S: Coexistence of pemphigus and bullous pemphigoid. J Dermatol 22:68, 1995.

26. Lever WF, Schaumburg-Lever G: Immunosuppressants and prednisone in pemphigus vulgaris. Arch Dermatol 113:1236, 1977.

27. Morioka S, Sakuma M, Ogawa H: The incidence of internal malignancies in autoimmune blistering diseases: Pemphigus and bullous pemphigoid in Japan. Dermatology 189 (Suppl 1):82, 1994.

28. Cotterill JA, Barker DJ, Millard LG, et al: Plasma exchange in the treatment of pemphigus vulgaris. Br J Dermatol 98:243, 1978.

29. Chryssomallis F, Dimitriades A, Chaidemenos GC, et al: Steroid-pulse therapy in pemphigus vulgaris long term follow-up. Int J Dermatol 34:438, 1995.

30. James MP, Williams RM: Benign familial pemphigus—premenstrual exacerbation suppressed by goserelin and oophorectomy. Clin Exp Dermatol 20:54, 1995.

31. Lever WF: Familial benign pemphigus. *In* Fitzpatrick TB (ed): Dermatology in General Medicine, 2nd ed. New York, McGraw-Hill, 1979.

32. Jordan RE: Bullous pemphigoid, cicatricial pemphigoid and chronic bullous dermatosis of childhood. *In* Fitzpatrick TB (ed): Dermatology in General Medicine, 2nd ed. New York, McGraw-Hill, 1979.

33. Piamphongsant T: Bullous pemphigoid in childhood: Report of three cases and a review of literature. Int J Dermatol 16:126, 1977.

34. Obasi OE, Savin JA: Pemphigoid and pernicious anemia. Br Med J 2:1458, 1977.

35. Hamilton DV, McKenzie AW: Bullous pemphigoid and primary biliary cirrhosis. Br J Dermatol 99:447, 1978.

36. Lavie CJ, Thomas MA, Fondak AA: The perioperative management of the patient with pemphigus vulgaris and villous adenoma. Cutis 34:180, 1984.

37. Krain LS, Bierman SM: Pemphigus vulgaris and internal malignancy. Cancer 33:1091, 1974.

38. Naysmith A, Hancock BW: Hodgkin's disease and pemphigus. Br J Dermatol 94:696, 1976.

39. Epstein FW, Bohn M: Dapsone-induced peripheral neuropathy. Arch Dermatol 112:1761, 1976.

40. Jeyaram C, Torda TA: Anesthetic management of cholecystectomy in a patient with buccal pemphigus. Anesthesiology 40:600, 1975.

41. Vatashky E, Aronson JB: Pemphigus vulgaris: Anaesthesia in the traumatised patient. Anaesthesia 37:1195, 1982.

Generalized Inflammatory Skin Diseases

42. Goldstein SM, Wintroub BW, Elias PM, et al: Toxic epidermal necrolysis. Arch Dermatol 123:1153, 1987.

43. Roujeau JC: The spectrum of Stevens-Johnson syndrome and toxic epidermal necrolysis: A clinical classification. J Invest Dermatol 102:28S, 1994.

44. Revuz J, Penso D, Roujeau J-C, et al: Toxic epidermal necrolysis. Arch Dermatol 123:1160, 1987.

45. Revuz J, Roujeau J-C, Guillaume J-C, et al: Treatment of toxic epidermal necrolysis. Arch Dermatol 123:1156, 1987.

46. Adunsky A, Steiner ZP, Eframian A, et al: Stevens-Johnson syndrome associated with *Mycoplasma pneumoniae* infection. Cutis 40:123, 1987.

47. Rasmussen JE: Erythema multiforme, Stevens-Johnson Syndrome and toxic epidermal necrolysis. Dermatol Nurs 7:37, 1995.

48. Elias PM, Fritsch OP: Erythema multiforme. *In* Fitzpatrick TB (ed): Dermatology in General Medicine, 2nd ed. New York, McGraw-Hill, 1979.

49. Chanda JJ, Callen JP: Erythema multiforme and the Stevens-Johnson syndrome. South Med J 71:566, 1978.

50. Broadbent RV: Stevens-Johnson disease presenting with pneumothorax. Rocky Mountain Med J 64:69, 1967.

51. Cucchiara RF, Dawson B: Anesthesia in Stevens-Johnson syndrome: Report of a case. Anesthesiology 35:537, 1971.

52. Schartum S: Stevens-Johnson syndrome with cardiac involvement. Acta Med Scand 179:729, 1966.

53. Sluysmans T, DeBont B, Cornu G: Acute epidermal necrolysis or Lyell syndrome. Eur J Pediatr 146:199, 1987.

54. Guillaume J-C, Roujeau J-C, Revus J, et al: The culprit drugs in 87 cases of toxic epidermal necrolysis (Lyell's syndrome). Arch Dermatol 123:1166, 1987.

55. Lyell A: Toxic epidermal necrolysis (the scalded skin syndrome): A reappraisal. Br J Dermatol 100:69, 1979.

56. Krumlovsky FA, Del Greco F, Herdson PB, et al: Renal disease associated with toxic epidermal necrolysis (Lyell's disease). Am J Med 57:817, 1974.

57. Stuttgen G: Toxic epidermal necrolysis provoked by barbiturates. Br J Dermatol 88:291, 1973.

58. Pollack MA, Burk PG, Nathanson G: Mucocutaneous eruptions due to antiepileptic drug therapy in children. Ann Neurol 5:262, 1979.

59. Hunter JA, Davison AM: Toxic epidermal necrolysis associated with pentazocine therapy and severe reversible renal failure. Br J Dermatol 88:287, 1973.

60. Fritsch OP, Elias PM: Toxic epidermal necrolysis. *In* Fitzpatrick TB (ed): Dermatology in General Medicine, 2nd ed. New York, McGraw-Hill, 1979.

61. Melish ME, Glasgow LA: Staphylococcal scalded skin syndrome. The expanded clinical syndrome. J Pediatr 78:958, 1971.

62. Elias PM, Fritsch P, Epstein EH: Staphylococcal scalded skin syndrome. Clinical features, pathogenesis and recent microbiological and biochemical developments. Arch Dermatol 113:207, 1977.

63. Alcalay J, Sandbank M, David M: Bullous impetigo and localized scalded skin syndrome in the elderly. Isr J Med Sci 23:300, 1987.

64. Blanc M-F, Janier M: Staphylococcies exfoliantes (SSSS) de l'adulte. Ann Dermatol Venereol 113:833, 1986.

65. Elias PM, Fritsch PO: Staphylococcal scalded-skin syndrome. *In* Fitzpatrick TB (ed): Dermatology in General Medicine, 2nd ed. New York, McGraw-Hill, 1979.

66. Cucchiara RF, Dawson B: Anesthesia in Stevens-Johnson syndrome: Report of a case. Anesthesiology 35:537, 1971.

Behçet's Disease

67. Tunaci A, Berkmen YM, Gokmen E: Thoracic involvement in Behçet's disease: Pathologic, clinical, and imaging features. Am J Roentgenol 164:51, 1995.

68. Inoue C, Itoh R, Kawa Y, Mizoguchi M: Pathogenesis of mucocutaneous lesions in Behçet's disease. J Dermatol 21:474 1994.

69. Jorizzo JL: Behçet's disease. Neurol Clin 5:427, 1987.

70. Nakata Y, Awazu M, Kojima Y, et al: Behçet's disease presenting with a right atrial vegetation. Pediatr Cardiol 16:150, 1995.

71. Mason RM, Barnes CG: Behçet's syndrome with arthritis. Ann Rheum Dis 28:95, 1969.

72. Turner ME: Anesthetic difficulties associated with Behçet's syndrome. Br J Anaesth 44:100, 1972.

73. Fujikado T, Imagawa K: Dural sinus thrombosis in Behçet's disease—a case report. Jpn J Opthamol 38:411, 1995.

74. Chajeh T, Fainarn M: Behçet's disease. Report of 41 cases and a review of the literature. Medicine 54:179, 1975.

75. Kozin F, Haughton V, Bernhard GC: Neuro-Behçet's disease: Two cases and neuroradiologic findings. Neurology 27:1148, 1977.

76. Roguin N, Haim S, Reshef R, et al: Cardiac involvement and superior vena caval obstruction in Behçet's disease. Thorax 33:375, 1978.

77. Hamza M: Large artery involvement in Behçet's disease. J Rheumatol 14:554, 1987.

78. Cadman EC, Lundberg UB, Mitchell MS: Pulmonary manifestations in Behçet's syndrome. Arch Intern Med 136:944, 1976.

79. Powderly WG, Lombard MG, Murray FE, et al: Oesophageal ulceration in Behçet's disease presenting with haemorrhage. Ir J Med Sci 156:193, 1987.

80. Ahonen AV, Stenius-Aarniala BSM, Viljanen BC, et al: Obstructive lung disease in Behçet's syndrome. Scand J Respir Dis 59:44, 1978.

81. Puckette TC, Jolles H, Proto AV: Magnetic resonance imaging confirmation of pulmonary artery aneurysm in Behçet's disease. J Thorac Imaging 9:172, 1994.

82. Lida M, Kobayashi H, Matsumoto T, et al: Postoperative recurrence in patients with intestinal Behçet's disease. Dis Colon Rectum 37:16, 1994.

83. Chaleby K, El-Yazigi A, Atiyeh M: Decreased drug absorption in a patient with Behçet's syndrome. Clin Chem 33:1679, 1987.

84. Basta JW, Niedjadlik K, Pallares V: Autonomic hyperreflexia: Intraoperative control with pentolinium tartrate. Br J Anesth 49:1087, 1977.

85. Cooperman LH: Succinylcholine-induced hyperkalemia in neuromuscular disease. JAMA 213:1867, 1970.

Psoriasis

86. Farber EM, VanScott EJ: Psoriasis. *In* Fitzpatrick TB (ed): Dermatology in General Medicine, 2nd ed. New York, McGraw-Hill, 1979.

87. Krogstad AL, Swanbeck G, Wallin BG: Axon-reflex–mediated vasodilatation in the psoriatic plaque? J Invest Dermatol 104:872, 1995.

88. Fox RH, Shuster S, Williams R: Cardiovascular, metabolic and thermoregulatory disturbances in patients with erythrodermic skin diseases. Br Med J 1:619, 1965.

89. Raza A, Maiback HI, Mandel A: Bacterial flora in psoriasis. Br J Dermatol 95:603, 1976.

90. Marples RR, Heaton CL, Kligman AM: *Staphylococcus aureus* in psoriasis. Arch Dermatol 107:568, 1973.

91. Payne RW: Severe outbreak of surgical sepsis due to *Staphylococcus aureus* of unusual type and origin. Br Med J 4:17, 1967.

92. Yamamoto T, Yokozeki H, Katayama I, Nushioka K: Uveitis in patients with generalized pustular psoriasis. Br J Dermatol 132:1023, 1995.

Neurofibromatosis

93. Wander JV, Das Gupta TK: Neurofibromatosis. Curr Probl Surg 14:11, 1977.

94. Roos KL, Muckway M: Neurofibromatosis. Dermatol Clin 13:105, 1995.

95. Krohel GB, Rosenberg PN, Wright JE, et al: Localized orbital neurofibromas. Am J Ophthalmol 100:458, 1985.

96. Leech RW: Intrathoracic meningocele and vertebral

anomalies in a case of neurofibromatosis. Surg Neurol 9:55, 1978.

97. Abel M: Emergency medicine and anesthesiology aspects of neurofibromatosis in childhood. Anasth Intensivther Notfallmed 20:76, 1985.

98. Chang-lo M: Laryngeal involvement in von Recklinghausen's disease: A case report and review of the literature. Laryngoscope 87:435, 1977.

99. Cohen SR, Landing BH, Isaacs H: Neurofibroma of the larynx in a child. Ann Otol Rhinol Laryngol 87:29, 1978.

100. Sagel SS, Forrest JV, Askin FB: Interstitial lung disease in neurofibromatosis. South Med J 68:647, 1975.

101. Griffits ML, Theron EJ: Obstructed labor from pelvic neurofibroma. South Afr Med J 53:781, 1978.

102. Chaglassian JH, Riseborogh EJ, Hall JE: Neurofibromatous scoliosis. J Bone Joint Surg 58A:695, 1976.

103. Magbagbeola JAO: Abnormal responses to muscle relaxants in patients with von Recklinghausen's disease. Br J Anaesth 42:710, 1970.

104. Yamasha M: Anaesthetic considerations in von Recklinghausen's disease (multiple neurofibromatosis). Abnormal response to muscle relaxants. Anaesthetist 26:317, 1977.

105. Imaizumi Y: Mortality of neurofibromatosis in Japan, 1968–1992. J Dermatol 22:191, 1995.

106. Elster AD: Occult spinal tumors in neurofibromatosis: Implications for screening. Am J Roentgenol 165:956, 1995.

107. Dounas M, Mercier FJ, Lhuissier C, Benhamou D: Epidural analgesia for labour in a parturient with neurofibromatosis. Can J Anaesth 42:420, 1995.

108. Haddad FS, Williams RL, Bentley G: The cervical spine in neurofibromatosis. Br J Hosp Med 53:318, 1995.

109. Drevelengas A, Kalaitzoglou I: Giant lumbar meningocele in a patient with neurofibromatosis. Neuroradiology 37:195, 1995.

110. Cooperman LH: Succinylcholine-induced hyperkalemia in neuromuscular disease. JAMA 213:1967, 1970.

111. Fisher MM: Anesthetic difficulties in neurofibromatosis. Anaesthesia 30:648, 1975.

Erythema Nodosum

112. de Moragas JM: Panniculitis (erythema nodosum). *In* Fitzpatrick TB (ed): Dermatology in General Medicine, 2nd ed. New York, McGraw-Hill, 1979.

113. Puavilai S, Sakuntabhai A, Sriprachaya-Anunt S, et al: Etiology of erythema nodosum. J Med Assoc Thai 78:72, 1995.

114. Tami LF: Erythema nodosum associated with *Shigella* colitis. Arch Dermatol 5:590, 1985.

115. Buckler JMH: Leptospirosis presenting with erythema nodosum. Arch Dis Child 52:418, 1977.

116. Longmore HJA: Toxoplasmosis and erythema nodosum. Br Med J 1:490, 1977.

117. Conget I, Mallolas J, Mensa J, et al: Erythema nodosum and Q fever. Arch Dermatol 123:867, 1987.

118. Andonopoulos AP, Asimakopoulos G, Mallioris C, et al: The diagnostic value of gastrocnemius muscle biopsy in sarcoidosis presenting with erythema nodosum and hilar adenopathy. Clin Rheumatol 6:192, 1987.

119. Matsuoka LY: Neoplastic erythema nodosum. J Am Acad Dermatol 32:361, 1995.

Mastocytosis

120. Kovenblat PE, Wedner HJ, White MP, et al: Systemic mastocytosis. Arch Intern Med 144:2249, 1984.

121. Rosenbaum KJ, Strobel GE: Anesthetic considerations in mastocytosis. Anesthesiology 38:398, 1973.

122. Koitabashi T, Takino Y: Anesthetic management of a patient with urticaria pigmentosa. Masui 44:279, 1995.

123. Butterfield JH, Kao PC, Klee GC, Yocum MW: Aspirin idiosyncrasy in systemic mast cell disease: A new look at mediator release during aspirin desensitization. Mayo Clin Proc 70:481, 1995.

124. Mican JM, Di Bisceglie AM, Fong TL, et al: Hepatic involvement in mastocytosis: Clinicopathologic correlations in 41 cases. Hepatology 22:1163, 1995.

125. Fonga-Djimi HS, Gottrand F, Bonnevalle M, Farriaux JP: A fatal case of portal hypertension complicating systemic mastocytosis in an adolescent. Eur J Pediatr 154:819, 1995.

126. Gruchalla RS: Southwestern Internal Medicine Conference: Mastocytosis: Developments during the past decade. Am J Med Sci 309:328, 1995.

127. Scott HW, Parris WCV, Sandidge PC, et al: Hazards in operative management of patients with systemic mastocytosis. Ann Surg 197:507, 1983.

128. Parris WCV, Scott HW, Smith BE: Anesthetic management of systemic mastocytosis: Experience with 42 cases. Anesth Analg 65:5117, 1986.

129. Parker F, Odland GF: The mastocytosis syndrome. *In* Fitzpatrick TB (ed): Dermatology in General Medicine, 2nd ed. New York, McGraw-Hill, 1979.

130. Wyre HW, Henrichs WD: Systemic mastocytosis and pulmonary eosinophilic granuloma. JAMA 239:856, 1978.

131. Freiri M, Alling DW, Metcalfe DD: Comparison of the therapeutic efficacy of cromolyn sodium with that of combined chlorpheniramine and cimetidine in systemic mastocytosis. Am J Med 78:9, 1985.

132. Hosking MP, Warner MA: Sudden intraoperative hypotension in a patient with asymptomatic urticaria pigmentosa. Anesth Analg 66:344, 1987.

133. Brown TP: Thiopentone anaphylaxis—case report. Anaesth Intens Care 3:257, 1975.

134. Buckland RW, Avery RF: Histamine release following pancuronium: A case report. Br J Anaesth 45:518, 1973.

Malignant Atrophic Papulosis

135. Black M: Malignant atrophic papulosis (Degos' disease). Int J Dermatol 15:405, 1976.

136. Snow JL, Muller SA: Degos' syndrome: Malignant atrophic papulosis. Semin Dermatol 14:99, 1995.

137. Schwayder TA: Scaly papules with atrophy. Arch Dermatol 122:93, 1986.

138. Ashershon RA, Cervera R: Antiphospholipid syndromes. J Invest Dermatol 100:21S. 1993.

139. Su WPD, Schroeter AL, Lee DA, et al: Clinical and histologic findings in Degos' syndrome (malignant atrophic papulosis). Cutis 35:131, 1985.

140. Vasques-Doval FJ, Ruiz de Erenchun F, Paramo JA, Quintanilla E: Malignant atrophic papulosis. A report of two cases with altered fibrinolysis and platelet function. Clin Exp Dermatol 18:441, 1993.

141. Christensen HK, Thonsen K, Vejlsgaard GL: Lymphomatoid papulosis: A follow-up study of 41 patients. Semin Dermatol 13:197, 1994.

142. Pierce RN, Smith GJW: Intrathoracic manifestations

of Degos' disease (malignant atrophic papulosis). Chest 73:79, 1978.

143. Horner F, Myers G, Stumpf D, et al: Malignant atrophic papulosis (Kohlmeier-Degos' disease) in childhood. Neurology 26:317, 1976.

144. Habbema L, Kisch LS, Starink TM: Familial malignant atrophic papulosis (Degos' disease)—additional evidence for heredity and a benign course. Br J Dermatol 114:134, 1986.

145. Kisch LS, Bruynzeel DP: Six cases of malignant atrophic papulosis (Degos' disease) occurring in one family. Br J Dermatol 111:469, 1984.

146. Tribble K, Archer ME, Jorizzo JL, et al: Malignant atrophic papulosis: Absence of circulating immune complexes or vasculitis. J Am Acad Dermatol 15:365, 1986.

147. Molenaar WM, Rosman JB, Donker AJM, et al: The pathology and pathogenesis of malignant atrophic papulosis (Degos' disease). Pathol Res Pract 182:98, 1987.

148. Doutre MS, Beylot C, Bioulac P, et al: Skin lesion resembling malignant atrophic papulosis in lupus erythematosus. Dermatology 175:45, 1987.

Ectodermal Dysplasias

149. Solomon LM, Keuer EJ: The ectodermal dysplasias. Arch Dermatol 116:1295, 1980.

150. Parent P, Castel Y, Guillet G, et al: Le syndrome EEC. Ann Pediatr (Paris) 34:293, 1987.

151. Burgdorf WHC, Alper JC, Goldsmith LA: Genodermatoses. J Am Acad Dermatol 16:1045, 1987.

152. Guha PK, Kishore V, Singh G, et al: Anhidrotic ectodermal dysplasia. J Acad Pediatr India 35:236, 1987.

153. Rapp RS, Hodgkin WE: Anhidrotic ectodermal dysplasia: Autosomal dominant inheritance with palate and lip anomalies. J Med Genet 5:269, 1968.

154. Young TL, Ziylan S, Schaffer DB: The ophthalmologic manifestations of the cardio-facio-cutaneous syndrome. J Pediatr Ophthalmol Strabismus 30:48, 1993.

155. Brooks EG, Klimpel GR, Vaidya, SE, et al: Thymic hypoplasia and T-cell deficiency in ectodermal dysplasia: Case report and review of the literature. Clin Immunol Immunopathol 7:44, 1994.

156. Lynch SA, de Berker D, Lehmann AR, et al: Trichothiodystrophy with sideroblastic anaemia and developmental delay. Arch Dis Child 73:249, 1995.

157. Piletta PA, Calza AM, Masouye I, et al: Hypohidrotic ectodermal dysplasia with recurrent otitis and sebaceous gland hypertrophy of the face. Dermatology 19:355, 1995.

158. Shimohashi N, Furukawa M, Yamaguchi H, et al: Ectodermal dysplasia syndrome in siblings with true keloids, stenosis of the esophagus after operations for congenital achalasia and renovascular hypertension due to stenosis of renal artery. Intern Med 34:406, 1995.

159. De Smet L, Fryns JP: Anal atresia and abdominal wall defect as unusual symptoms in EEC syndrome. Genet Couns 6:127, 1995.

160. Ramchander V, Jankey N, Ramkissoon R, et al: Anhidrotic ectodermal dysplasia in an infant presenting with pyrexia of unknown origin. Clin Pediatr 17:50, 1978.

161. Bernstein ML, Weakley-Jones B: ''Sudden infant death'' associated with hypohidrotic ectodermal dysplasia. J Ky Med Assoc 85:191, 1987.

162. Myer CM, III: The role of an otolaryngologist in the care of ectodermal dysplasia. Pediatr Dermatol 4:34, 1987.

Fabry's Disease

163. Paller AS: Metabolic disorders characterized by angiokeratomas and neurologic dysfunction. Neurol Clin 5:441, 1987.

164. Paller AS: Vascular disorders. Dermatol Clin 5:239, 1987.

165. Yokoyama A, Yamazoe M, Shibata A: A case of heterozygous Fabry's disease with a short PR interval and giant negative T waves. Br Heart J 57:296, 1987.

166. Jansen W, Lentner A, Genzel I: Capillary changes in angiokeratoma corporis diffusum Fabry. J Dermatol Sci 7:68, 1994.

167. Frost A, Spaeth GL: Alpha-galactosidase A deficiency: Fabry's disease (angiokeratoma corporis diffusum universale). In Fitzpatrick TB (ed): Dermatology in General Medicine, 2nd ed. New York, McGraw-Hill, 1979.

168. Gordon KE, Ludman MD, Finley GA: Successful treatment of painful crises of Fabry disease with low dose morphine. Pediatr Neurol 12:250, 1995.

169. Zadnik K: Fabry's disease. J Am Optomet Assoc 58:87, 1987.

170. Andersen MV, Dahl H, Fledelius H, Nielsen NV: Central retinal artery occlusion in a patient with Fabry's disease documented by scanning laser ophthalmoscopy. Acta Ophthalmol (Copenh) 72:635, 1994.

171. Taaffe A: Angiokeratoma corporis diffusum: The evolution of a disease entity. Postgrad Med J 53:78, 1977.

172. Ferrans VJ, Hibbs RG, Burda CD: The heart in Fabry's disease. Am J Cardiol 24:95, 1969.

173. Desnick RJ, Blieden LC, Sharp HL, et al: Cardiac valvular anomalies in Fabry disease. Circulation 54:818, 1976.

174. Rowe JW, Caralis DG: Accelerated atrioventricular conduction in Fabry's disease. Angiology 29:562, 1978.

175. Ko YH, Kim HJ, Roh YS, et al: Atypical Fabry's disease. An oligosymptomatic variant. Arch Pathol Lab Med 120:86, 1996.

176. Hiraizumi Y, Kanoh M, Shigematsu H, et al: A case of Fabry's disease with granulomatous interstitial nephritis. Nippon Jinzo Gakkai Shi 37:655, 1995.

177. Friedlaender MM, Kopolovic J, Rubinger D, et al: Renal biopsy in Fabry's disease eight years after successful renal transplantation. Clin Nephrol 27:206, 1987.

178. Tamura T, Murayama K, Hayashi R, et al: Two cases of women with Fabry's disease detected by electrocardiographic abnormalities. Nippon-Naika-Gakkai-Zasshi 75:1123, 1987.

179. Whyte MP: Electrocardiographic PR interval in Fabry's disease. N Engl J Med 294:342, 1976.

180. Maizel SE, Simmons RL, Kjellstrand C, et al: Ten-year survival experience in renal transplantation for Fabry's disease. Transplant Proc 13:57, 1981.

181. Eichhorn JH, Hedley-Whyte J, Steinman TI, et al: Renal failure following enflurane anesthesia. Anesthesiology 45:557, 1976.

Incontinentia Pigmenti

182. Ormerod AD, White MI, McKay E, et al: Incontinentia pigmenti in a boy with Klinefelter's syndrome. J Med Genet 24:439, 1987.

183. Carney RG: Incontinentia pigmenti, a world statistical analysis. Arch Dermatol 112:535, 1976.
184. Goldberg MF, Custis PH: Retinal and other manifestations of incontinentia pigmenti (Bloch-Sulzberger syndrome). Ophthalmology 100:1645, 1993.
185. Sahn EE, Davidson LS: Incontinentia pigmenti: Three cases with unusual features. J Am Acad Dermatol 31:852, 1994.
186. Moss C, Ince P: Anhidrotic and achromians lesions in incontinentia pigmenti. Br J Dermatol 116:839, 1987.
187. Kuster W, Happle R: Neurocutaneous disorders in children. Curr Opin Pediatr 5:436, 1993.
188. Takematsu H, Sato S, Igarashi M, et al: Incontinentia pigmenti achromians (Ito). Arch Dermatol 119:391, 1983.
189. Kegel MF: Dominant disorders with multiple organ involvement. Dermatol Clin 5:205, 1987.

Hereditary Angioneurotic Edema

190. Poppers PJ: Anaesthetic implications of hereditary angioneurotic oedema. Can J Anaesth 1:76, 1987.
191. Talavera A, Larraona JL, Ramos JL, et al: Hereditary angioedema: An infrequent cause of abdominal pain with ascites. Am J Gastroenterol 90:471, 1995.
192. Cohen N, Sharonm A, Golik A, et al: Hereditary angioneurotic edema with severe hypovolemic shock. J Clin Gastroenterol 6:237, 1993.
193. Abada RP, Owens WD: Hereditary angioneurotic edema, an anesthetic dilemma. Anesthesiology 46:428, 1977.
194. Jaffe CJ, Atkinson JP, Gelfand JA, et al: Hereditary angioedema; the use of fresh frozen plasma for prophylaxis in patients undergoing oral surgery. J Allergy Clin Immunol 55:386, 1975.
195. Gibbs PS, LoSasso AM, Moorthy SS, et al: The anesthetic and perioperative management of a patient with documented hereditary angioneurotic edema. Anesth Analg 56:571, 1977.
196. Gadek JE, Hosea SW, Gelfand JA, et al: Replacement therapy in hereditary angioedema; successful treatment of acute episodes of angioedema with partly purified C1 inhibitor. N Engl J Med 302:542, 1980.
197. Baraka A, Sibai AN, Azar IA, Zaytoun G: Transtracheal jet ventilation in an adult patient with severe hereditary angioneurotic edema. Middle East J Anesthesiol 12:171, 1993.
198. Cox M, Holdcroft A: Hereditary angioneurotic oedema: Current management in pregnancy. Anaesthesia 50:547, 1995.

Osteoporosis, Osteomalacia, and Osteopetrosis

199. Marcus R: Clinical review 76: The nature of osteoporosis. J Clin Endocrinol Metab 81:1, 1996.
200. Chalmers GL: Disorders of bone. Practitioner 220:711, 1978.
201. Lindsay R: The menopause and osteoporosis. Obstet Gynecol 87:16S, 1996.
202. Gandy S, Payne R: Back pain in the elderly: Updated diagnosis and management. Geriatrics 41:59, 1986.
203. Bauer RL, Deyo RA: Low risk of vertebral fracture in Mexican-American women. Arch Intern Med 147:1437, 1987.
204. Wheeler M: Osteoporosis. Med Clin North Am 60:1213, 1976.

205. Kalu DN: Evolution of the pathogenesis of postmenopausal bone loss. Bone 17:135S, 1995.
206. Zohman GL, Lieberman JR: Perioperative aspects of hip fracture. Guidelines for intervention that will impact prevalence and outcome. Am J Orthop 24:666, 1995.
207. Khairi MRA, Johnson CC: What we know and don't know about bone loss in the elderly. Geriatrics 33:67, 1978.
208. Seeman E, Tsalamandris C, Bass S, Pearce G: Present and future of osteoporosis therapy. Bone 17:23S, 1995.
209. Heaf JG, Joffe P, Ptodenphant J, et al: Noninvasive diagnosis of uremic osteodystrophy: Uses and limitations. Am J Nephrol 7:203, 1987.
210. Clarke BL, Wynne AG, Wilson DM, Fitzpatrick LA: Osteomalacia associated with adult Fanconi's syndrome: Clinical and diagnostic features. Clin Endocrinol (Oxf) 43:479, 1995.
211. Hewison M: Tumor-induced osteomalacia. Curr Opin Rheumatol 6:340, 1994.
212. Frame B, Parfitt AM: Osteomalacia: Current concepts. Ann Intern Med 89:966, 1978.
213. Stalder H, von Hochstetter A, Schreiber A: Valgus tibial osteotomy in a patient with benign dominant osteopetrosis (Albers-Schoenberg disease). A case report. Int Orthoped 18:304, 1994.
214. Scott MC: Osteopetrosis ("marble bone" disease). Am Fam Physician 47:175, 1993.
215. Beighton P, Horan F, Hamersma H: A review of osteopetroses. Postgrad Med J 53:507, 1977.
216. Beighton P, Durr L, Hamersma H: The clinical features of sclerosteosis. Ann Intern Med 84:393, 1975.
217. Keever JE, Rockwood CA: Early mobilization of the severely injured patient. In Zander HT (ed): Anesthesia for Orthopaedic Surgery. Philadelphia, FA Davis, 1980.
218. Stehling L: Anesthetic considerations for the patient with a fractured hip. In Zander HT (ed): Anesthesia for Orthopaedic Surgery. Philadelphia, FA Davis, 1980.

Osteogenesis Imperfecta

219. Bailey JA II: Disproportionate Short Stature: Diagnosis and Management. Philadelphia, WB Saunders, 1973, pp. 223–231.
220. Marion MJ, Gannon FH, Fallon MD, et al: Skeletal dysplasia in perinatal lethal osteogenesis imperfecta. A complex disorder of endochondral and intramembranous ossification. Clin Orthop 293:327, 1993.
221. Cunningham AJ, Donnelly M, Comerford J: Osteogenesis imperfecta: Anesthetic management of a patient for cesarean section: A case report. Anesthesiology 61:91, 1984.
222. Libman RH: Anesthetic considerations for the patient with osteogenesis imperfecta. Clin Orthop 159:123, 1981.
223. Allanson JE, Hall JG: Obstetric and gynecologic problems in women with chondrodystrophies. Obstet Gynecol 67:74, 1986.
224. Bergstrom L: Osteogenesis imperfecta: Otologic and maxillofacial aspects. Laryngoscope 87 (Suppl 6):1, 1977.
225. Solomons CC, Nillar EA: Osteogenesis imperfecta—new perspectives. Clin Orthop 96:299, 1973.
226. Stein D, Kloster FE: Valvular heart disease in osteogenesis imperfecta. Am Heart J 94:637, 1977.
227. Shoenfeld Y, Fried A, Ehrenfeld NE: Osteogenesis

imperfecta: Review of the literature with presentation of 29 cases. Am J Dis Child 129:679, 1975.

228. McCarthy-Sauer AR, Joyce TH III: Management of a patient with osteogenesis imperfecta: A case study. Am Assoc Nurse Anesth J 49:580, 1981.

229. Rampton AJ, Kelly DA, Shanahan EC, et al: Occurrence of malignant hyperpyrexia in a patient with osteogenesis imperfecta. Br J Anaesth 56:1443, 1984.

230. Sadat-Ali M, Sankaran-Kutty M, Adu-Gyamfi Y: Metabolic acidosis in osteogenesis imperfecta. Eur J Pediatr 145:324, 1986.

231. Bradish CF, Flowers M: Central retinal artery occlusion in association with osteogenesis imperfecta. Spine 12:193, 1987.

232. Oliverio RN: Anesthetic management of intramedullary nailing in osteogenesis imperfecta: Report of a case. Anesth Analg 52:232, 1973.

233. Baines D: Total intravenous anesthesia for patients with osteogenesis imperfecta. Paediatr Anaesth 5:144, 1995.

234. Solomons CC, Myers DN: Hyperthermia of osteogenesis imperfecta and its relationship to malignant hyperthermia. *In* Gordon RA, Britt BA, Kalow W (eds): Malignant Hyperthermia. Springfield, IL, Charles C Thomas, 1971.

Dwarfism

235. Sillence DO, Rimonin DL, Lachman R: Neonatal dwarfism. Pediatr Clin North Am 25:453, 1978.

236. Bailey JA II: Disproportionate Short Stature: Diagnosis and Management. Philadelphia, WB Saunders, 1973, pp. 13–25, 35–56.

237. Rimonin DL: The chondrodystrophies. Adv Hum Genet 5:1, 1975.

238. Berkowitz ID, Raja SN, Bender KS, Kopits SE: Dwarfs: Pathophysiology and anesthetic implications. Anesthesiology 73:739, 1990.

239. Lin HJ, Sue GY, Berkowitz ID, et al: Microdontia with severe microcephaly and short stature in two brothers: Osteodysplastic primordial dwarfism with dental findings. Am J Med Genet 58:136, 1995.

240. Roberts W, Henson LC: Anesthesia for scoliosis: Dwarfism and congenitally absent odontoid process. AANA J 63:332, 1995.

241. Shiraishi N, Takakuwa K, Yamamoto N, et al: Anesthetic management of Seckel syndrome: A case report. Masui 44:735, 1995.

242. Balaguer JM, Perry D, Crowley J, Moran JM: Coronary artery bypass grafting in an achondroplastic dwarf. Texas Heart Inst J 22:258, 1995.

243. Gulati DR, Ront D: Atlantoaxial dislocation with quadriparesis in achondroplasia. J Neurosurg 40:394, 1974.

244. Benson KT, Dozier NJ, Goto H, et al: Anesthesia for cesarean section in a patient with spondylometepiphyseal dysplasia. Anesthesiology 63:548, 1985.

245. Brill CB, Rose JS, Godniolow L, et al: Spastic quadriparesis due to C1-C2 subluxation in Hurler syndrome. J Pediatr 92:441, 1978.

246. Goldberg MJ: Orthopedic aspects of bone dysplasias. Orthop Clin North Am 7:445, 1976.

247. Lipson SJ: Dysplasia of the odontoid process in Morquio's syndrome causing quadriparesis. J Bone Joint Surg 59A:340, 1977.

248. Kopits SE: Orthopedic complications of dwarfism. Clin Orthop 114:153, 1976.

249. Mayhew JF, Katz J, Miner M, et al: Anesthesia for the achondroplastic dwarf. Can Anaesth Soc J 33:216, 1986.

250. Miller RA, Crosby G, Sundaram P: Exacerbated spinal neurologic deficit during sedation of a patient with cervical spondylosis. Anesthesiology 67:844, 1987.

251. Borland LM: Anesthesia for children with Jeune's syndrome (asphyxiating thoracic dystrophy). Anesthesiology 66:86, 1987.

252. Hope EOS, Farebrother MJB, Bainbridge D: Some aspects of respiratory function in three siblings with Morquio-Brailsford disease. Thorax 28:335, 1973.

253. Jones AEP, Croley TF: Morquio syndrome and anesthesia. Anesthesiology 51:261, 1979.

254. Birkinshaw KJ: Anesthesia in a patient with unstable neck: Morquio's syndrome. Anesthesia 30:46, 1975.

255. Waltz LF, Finerman G, Wyatt GM: Anesthesia for dwarfs and other patients of pathological small stature. Can Anaesth Soc J 22:703, 1975.

256. Bancroft GH, Lauria JI: Ketamine induction for cesarean section in a patient with acute intermittent porphyria and achondroplastic dwarfism. Anesthesiology 59:143, 1983.

257. Ravindran R, Stoops CM: Anaesthetic management of a patient with Hallermann-Streiff syndrome. Anesth Analg 58:254, 1979.

258. Sjøgren P, Pedersen T, Steinmetz S: Mucopolysaccharidoses and anaesthetic risks. Acta Anaesthesiol Scand 31:214, 1987.

259. Theroux MC, Kettrick RG, Khine HH: Laryngeal mask airway and fiberoptic endoscopy in an infant with Schwartz-Jampel syndrome. Anesthesiology 82:605, 1995.

260. Basta JW, Niejadlik K, Pallares V: Autonomic hyperreflexia: Intraoperative control with pentolinium tartrate. Br J Anaesth 49:1087, 1977.

Craniofacial and Mandibulofacial Dysostoses

261. Gravenstein JS: Congenital malformation. *In* Saidman LJ, Moya F (eds): Complications of Anesthesia. Springfield, IL, Charles C Thomas, 1970.

262. Cohen MM Jr: Craniofacial dysostoses. Birth Defects 11:145, 1975.

263. Whitaker LA, Bartlett SP: The craniofacial dysostoses: Guidelines for management of the symmetric and asymmetric deformities. Clin Plast Surg 14:73, 1987.

264. Feingold M, Baum J: Goldenhar's syndrome. Am J Dis Child 132:136, 1978.

265. Sklar GS, King BD: Endotracheal intubation and Treacher Collins syndrome. Anesthesiology 44:247, 1976.

266. van Balen ATM: François' syndrome. Ophthal Paediatr Gen 6:59, 1985.

267. Gershanik JJ, Nervez C: Nasoesophageal intubation in the Pierre Robin syndrome. Clin Pediatr 15:173, 1976.

268. Goldberg MJ, Ampola MG: Birth defect syndromes in which orthopedic problems may be overlooked. Orthop Clin North Am 7:411, 1976.

269. Miller RA, Crosby G, Sundram P: Exacerbated spinal neurological deficit during sedation of a patient with cervical spondylosis. Anesthesiology 67:844, 1987.

270. Parsons DP, Samuels SI, Steinberg G, et al: Reduction cranioplasty and severe hypotension. Anesthesiology 68:145, 1988.

Paget's Disease

271. Krane SM: Paget's disease of bone. Clin Orthop 127:24, 1977.
272. Sofaer JA: Dental extractions in Paget's disease of bone. Int J Oral Surg 13:79, 1984.
273. Brown HP, La Rocca H, Wickstrom JK: Paget's disease of the atlas and axis. J Bone Joint Surg 53A:1441, 1971.
274. Goldhammer Y, Braham J, Kosary IZ: Hydrocephalic dementia in Paget's disease of the skull: Treatment by ventriculoatrial shunt. Neurology 29:513, 1979.
275. Epstein BS, Epstein JA: The association of cerebellar tonsillar herniation with basilar impression incident to Paget's disease. Am J Roentgenol 107:535, 1969.
276. Rhodes BA, Greyson ND, Hamilton CR, et al: Absence of anatomic arteriovenous shunts in Paget's disease of bone. N Engl J Med 287:686, 1972.
277. Woodhouse NJY, Crosbie WA, Mohamedally SM: Cardiac output in Paget's disease: Response to long-term salmon calcitonin therapy. Br Med J 4:686, 1975.
278. Basta JW, Niejadlik K, Pallares V: Autonomic hyperreflexia: Intraoperative control with pentolinium tartrate. Br J Anaesth 49:1087, 1977.

Fibrous Dysplasia

279. Grabias SL, Campbell CJ: Fibrous dysplasia. Orthop Clin North Am 8:771, 1977.
280. Albright F, Butler A, Hampton A, et al: Syndrome characterized by osteitis fibrosa disseminata, areas of pigmentation and endocrine dysfunction, with precocious puberty in females. Report of five cases. N Engl J Med 216:727, 1937.
281. Caudill R, Saltzman D, Guarm S, et al: Possible relationship of primary hyperparathyroidism and fibrous dysplasia: Report of case. J Oral Surg 35:483, 1977.
282. Kunder JP, Pan AK: Congenital fibro-osseous dysplasia of jaws ("hippopotamus face"), an anesthetic problem. Br J Anaesth 51:465, 1979.
283. De Iure F, Campanacci L: Clinical and radiographic progression of fibrous dysplasia: Cystic change or sarcoma? Description of a clinical case and review of the literature. Chir Organi Mov 80:85, 1995.
284. Hansen-Knarhoi M, Poole MD: Preoperative difficulties in differentiating intraosseous meningiomas and fibrous dysplasia around the orbital apex. J Craniomaxillofac Surg 22:226, 1994.
285. Strauss EJ, Poplak TM, Braude BM: Anaesthetic management of a difficult intubation. S Afr Med J 68:414, 1985.
286. Montoya G, Evart CM, Dohn DF: Polyostotic fibrous dysplasia and spinal cord compressions. J Neurosurg 29:102, 1968.
287. Dal Cin P, Sciot R, Speleman F, et al: Chromosome aberrations in fibrous dysplasia. Cancer Genet Cytogenet 77:114, 1994.
288. Kourie J, Zenon D: Intraligamental analgesia in monostotic fibrous dysplasia—a case report. Diastema 14:18, 1986.

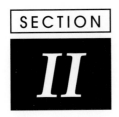

SECTION

II

Uncommon Diseases and Problems by Type of Patient

The Pregnant Patient and the Uncommon Disorders of Pregnancy

Laurence S. Reisner
David R. Gambling

I. INTRODUCTION

The pregnant patient is really two patients—the mother and the fetus. Of concern to the anesthetist is the well-being of both patients as well as the anatomic and physiologic attachment between the two. Conditions and situations that are uncommon to the average anesthetist, that might adversely affect the patient–attachment–patient complex, consist of a whole host of pharmacologic considerations, unusual maladies of the uteroplacental complex, fetal demise, critical illness in the mother, high-order gestations, and advanced maternal age. In this chapter we consider all these obstetric entities and their anesthesiologic implications.

II. PHARMACOLOGIC CONSIDERATIONS FOR SURGERY DURING PREGNANCY

A. GENERAL PHARMACOLOGIC CONSIDERATIONS AND TERATOGENICITY, WITH SPECIAL EMPHASIS ON NITROUS OXIDE

The need for anesthesia and nonobstetric surgery during pregnancy occurs in 1.5 to 2.0 per cent of all pregnancies.[1] Anesthetists and surgeons alike are concerned with the possible effects of this trespass on the developing fetus. The hazards to the fetus may come from teratogenic effects of drugs administered in the perioperative period, including anesthetic agents, from premature labor, from alterations in uteroplacental blood flow, and from maternal hypoxia or acidosis or both. Since organogenesis occurs during the first trimester of pregnancy, it is commonly advised that any but truly emergent surgery be postponed until later in pregnancy, to avoid potential teratogenicity and intrauterine fetal death. Premature labor is more likely in the third trimester. Although the risks to the fetus are quite real, careful management should minimize the potential for fetal harm.

One of the major concerns, among patients and physicians alike faced with the possibility of surgery during gestation, is what effect the anesthetic and adjuvant drugs will have on the developing fetus. Virtually every drug that anesthesiologists employ can be found to be teratogenic in some species under some circumstances at some particular point in time during gestation. Numerous individual studies and reviews fill the literature with information on this subject.[2–7] Several principles of teratology need to be kept in mind when this information is considered.[1] First, the specificity of the substance could be quite broad or limited to an effect in a single species. Second, the dose of the agent that reaches the conceptus determines the degree of teratogenic effect, if any, that will be manifested. This, in turn, depends on the factors that govern placental transfer (e.g., some of the neuromuscular-blocking agents are teratogenic to chick embryos when directly injected but when injected into a pregnant woman cross the placenta in such minuscule amounts as to be no hazard in the clinical setting.[8]) Finally, the stage of embryogenesis at which exposure takes place is crucial. For instance, a specific drug may either kill the blastocyst or allow it to develop entirely normally if exposure occurs during the first 2 weeks of gestation because the cells are totipotential at this point. If given after 12 weeks only organ size—or perhaps brain development—may be affected, as organogenesis is complete.

Teratogenicity can result from a number of mechanisms (Table 13–1) that lead to excessive cell death, reduced proliferation, decreased cellular interactions, impaired morphogenic movements, reduced biosynthesis, or mechanical cellular disruption. The ultimate change is lack of cells. To establish proof of teratogenicity one must look at both retrospective and prospective evidence. Prospectively, confirmatory animal studies need to be undertaken, realizing that the population size may need to be enormous to prove teratogenicity. Retrospectively, there should be a demonstrable increase in an anomaly beginning at the time of the drug's introduction. The

TABLE 13–1

Mechanisms of Teratogenicity

Altered membrane characteristics
Chromosomal nondysjunction
Depletion of energy sources
Enzyme inhibition
Interference with substrate precursors
Mutation
Osmolar imbalance

exposure should have occurred at the appropriate time in fetal development, and a dose-response curve might be evident. The teratogenic potential of anesthetic agents and the adjunctive drugs used as premedicants have been thoroughly reviewed in several authoritative sources.[9–12] It is clear that we have not been able to recommend a "best" anesthetic agent for these applications because none has as yet been definitely identified as a human teratogen. Nitrous oxide, however, has come under scrutiny owing to its ability to inhibit the function of methionine synthase.[13]

Although nitrous oxide has a long record of safety when used in general anesthesia for obstetrics and is used as an analgesic during labor, concerns have developed over its demonstrated ability to oxidize cob(I)alamin (vitamin B_{12}) and thus inhibit methionine synthase activity. This activity is a key link in the synthesis of S-adenosylmethionine and in the tetrahydrofolic acid cycle. Ultimately, DNA production, myelin deposition, and other folate and methylation process–dependent reactions might be affected. This may be of particular concern when nitrous oxide is administered for a nonobstetric operation in a pregnant woman. In a study employing human lymphoblasts exposed to nitrous oxide, Boss demonstrated decreased methionine and serine synthesis.[14] He found that purine synthesis was more rapidly reduced in the absence of folate than in its presence. The authors conclude that cobalamin inactivation decreases purine synthesis by both trapping methylfolate and reducing intracellular methionine synthesis. Fassoulaki and coworkers found that nitrous oxide did not impair the ability of rat liver to repair hepatic injury induced by hypoxia and halothane. They hypothesize that, although DNA production has been shown to be impaired by nitrous oxide in humans, it may not be seriously impaired.[15] Vina evaluated the influence of nitrous oxide on methionine, S-adenosylmethionine, and other amino acids in rats.[16] Nitrous oxide administration caused a significant reduction in methionine production and several other amino acids and reduced the concentration of S-adenosylmethionine in the brain and the liver. The administration of methionine did not reverse any of the amino acid changes but did increase the concentration of methionine and S-adenosylmethionine in liver and brain. There was no evidence of disturbance to the liver glutathione pool. These authors and others[17] note that, while methionine syn-

thase inactivation occurs with nitrous oxide, prophylaxis with methionine, folic acid, and vitamin B_{12} is feasible but has yet to prove clinically effective. A study comparing nitrous oxide administration to isoflurane inhalation in rats demonstrated that, although there was an increase in anomalies with nitrous oxide, this effect was reversed if isoflurane was administered simultaneously. This suggests that nitrous oxide exerts its effect by some mechanism other than methionine synthase inhibition.[18] Therefore, although the evidence is inconclusive, nitrous oxide should probably be avoided during the first trimester of pregnancy.

Studies that have attempted to identify a relationship between anesthesia for surgery and congenital malformations have been unable to do so.[11, 19] Duncan and coworkers have shown in a large epidemiologic study, utilizing matched controls, that there is no increase in the incidence of congenital anomalies associated with surgery during pregnancy.[20] Although such evidence is encouraging, it cannot be assumed that some potential for teratogenicity does not exist. It is therefore prudent to postpone elective surgical procedures until after pregnancy or, if that is not possible, until after the first trimester. It is of more than parenthetic interest that many women who present for elective surgery may be in an early phase of gestation and not yet aware of it. It behooves the surgeon and the anesthetist to make this determination before proceeding with surgery in sexually active women of childbearing age.

B. REVERSAL OF MATERNAL MUSCLE RELAXANTS WITH NEOSTIGMINE AND GLYCOPYRROLATE VERSUS ATROPINE

Agents and techniques that have been widely used and evaluated should be employed when administering an anesthetic to a patient during pregnancy. Barbiturates, narcotics, halothane, isoflurane, and muscle relaxants are all examples of such agents. Concern has been expressed about the reversal of muscle relaxants with neostigmine and glycopyrrolate. A recent case report illustrates a phenomenon the authors have observed as well (i.e., onset of fetal bradycardia following use of this combination).[21] Both drugs are quite polar and should cross the placenta to only a very limited degree; however, in this case report it was noted that the fetal bradycardia did not occur when a neostigmine and atropine combination was used. Those authors suggest that neostigmine may cross the placenta to a greater degree than glycopyrrolate, thus inducing bradycardia. Because atropine does cross the placenta, it is more effective at protecting the fetus from the potent muscarinic effects of neostigmine.

C. REGIONAL ANESTHESIA

When circumstances warrant, regional anesthesia may be preferred. Spinal anesthesia offers the least fetal drug transfer for the degree of anesthesia achieved;[22] therefore, if premature labor and delivery follow the operation, the neonate may not have to deal with the systemic effects of the agent. Hypotension, aortocaval compression, and maternal hypoxia and acidosis need to be avoided or treated promptly. Other forms of regional anesthesia, such as epidural anesthesia or brachial plexus block, do yield higher local anesthetic blood levels and thus more placental transfer. There has been no association with teratogenic effects in humans from reasonable levels of local anesthetics, and recent animal studies tend to confirm the human observations. Fujinaga and Mazze have demonstrated the lack of teratogenicity of a long-term lidocaine infusion in the rat model.[23]

D. MATERNAL LACTATION

A final consideration for drug transfer to the infant is in the postpartum period. Nearly all substances given to the mother are secreted in breast milk. There is some transfer of opioids and their metabolites to the infant. Greater neonatal neurobehavioral depression has been reported when postoperative analgesia is provided with meperidine than with morphine, presumably owing to the presence of normeperidine in breast milk.[24] This consideration should be given to the lactating mother (particularly if she chooses not to have her infant exposed) and regional (spinal) anesthesia used whenever applicable.

E. TOCOLYTICS

Some obstetricians use tocolytics such as magnesium sulfate, ritodrine, and terbutaline

in the immediate postoperative period to prevent preterm labor. It is therefore appropriate for anesthesiologists to be aware of their side effects.[25] Magnesium sulfate, popular in the treatment of preeclampsia, is also effective at suppressing uterine contractions. Magnesium appears to uncouple the excitation-contraction sequence in smooth muscle, decrease the frequency of action potentials, and relax the contractile elements in uterine muscle.[26] It appears to be effective in the same dose range as that used for the prevention of convulsions; therefore, the same precautions must be observed (e.g., monitor respiratory rate, deep tendon reflexes, and urine output). Magnesium also has an effect at the neuromuscular junction, principally inhibition of release of acetylcholine, and it therefore potentiates all of the neuromuscular-blocking agents. This effect can be reversed partially by administration of calcium.

Beta-adrenergic agonists are a popular and efficacious method of suppressing premature labor. Although many have been and are employed (isoxsuprine, terbutaline, ritodrine), only ritodrine (Yutopar) carries FDA approval for this application. The beta-2 mechanism of action is mediated by coupling of the drug to the receptor, which leads to activation of adenyl cyclase and by some mechanism as yet unknown increases the sequestration of intracellular calcium and results in smooth muscle relaxation.[27] Unfortunately, these drugs all produce significant beta-1 and beta-2 systemic effects, including vasodilatation, tachycardia, and hypotension. This has been managed with aggressive volume replacement; however, the use of terbutaline and ritodrine, especially in the presence of concomitant steroid administration, has led to maternal pulmonary edema.[28] The mechanism is unknown and does not appear to be cardiogenic. Additional cardiac complications such as myocardial ischemia and myocardial infarction have been reported. Isoxsuprine appears to have the lowest incidence of major cardiac problems. Pulmonary edema and dysrhythmias have been reported in association with the administration of anesthesia.[29]

Hypokalemia, which may persist after the drug has been discontinued, has also been reported.[30] Aggressive potassium replacement is not recommended, however, as this condition generally regresses in a short time. Hyperglycemia and other metabolic changes associated with beta-adrenergic activity may be seen. Obviously, careful monitoring of cardiac performance and fluid and electrolyte status is mandatory. Withdrawal of the drug may be necessary if adverse symptoms persist. If anesthesia becomes necessary, it is optimal to allow for a period of abstinence from the drug before induction, but this is not always possible. It would be wise to choose a technique that does not exaggerate the cardiovascular effects of the drugs and that avoids catecholamine interaction leading to the production of arrhythmias.

Finally, the major common obstetric anesthetic principles for providing appropriate care for the pregnant patient who requires surgery must be observed. Attention must be paid to the maternal physiologic adjustments and their influence on anesthetic techniques to provide maximum maternal and fetal safety. Endotracheal intubation should be considered for all patients beyond 20 weeks' gestation because the alterations produced by pregnancy on the gastrointestinal system place the patient at higher risk for regurgitation or aspiration. Adequate uteroplacental perfusion must be maintained by avoiding or treating hypotension and aortocaval compression. Drugs and techniques that have a good record of fetal safety must be selected. The anesthesiologist must provide surveillance of fetal well-being by observing fetal heart rate and uterine activity whenever possible with the fetal monitor. Finally, appropriate maternal monitoring (e.g., pulse oximetry, anesthetic and respiratory gas analysis) must be utilized to provide optimal fetal *and* maternal environments.

III. HYDATIDIFORM MOLE

A. THE DISEASE

Hydatidiform mole and choriocarcinoma are the components of the disease entity known as *gestational trophoblastic disease*. Choriocarcinoma is a rare tumor, occurring either de novo from germinal epithelium in the ovary or embryonic rests or, more commonly, following either a normal or a molar pregnancy.[31] Hydatidiform mole is a benign neoplasm in which part or all of the chorionic villi are converted into a mass of clear, grape-like vesicles. Usually no fetus or embryo is present, but there have been occasional reports of a mole coexisting with a fetus.[32] Varying degrees of trophoblastic proliferation take place. The incidence of molar pregnancy ranges from 1 in 2500 live births in the United States to 1 in 173 in the Philippines.[33] The diagnosis is suspected when a fetal heartbeat is not detectable by Doppler ultrasound at the end of the first or the beginning of the second trimester of pregnancy. A presumptive diagnosis may be rendered if serum or urine human chorionic gonadotropin (HCG) levels are found to be elevated beyond that expected for the stage of gestation. Confirmation of the diagnosis is made by an ultrasound study.[34] Complicated moles are classified into three groups. *Retained mole* refers to persistent molar tissue in the uterine cavity after evacuation. An *invasive mole* is one whose villi have penetrated into the uterine wall. A *metastatic mole* is one that has spread via the venous system to extrauterine sites, and this is a far more serious lesion. Eighty per cent of molar pregnancies are discovered between 12 and 18 weeks' gestation and are uncomplicated.

B. PATHOPHYSIOLOGY

The patient with a molar pregnancy may have no symptoms at all. The lesion is discovered either because her physician has a high index of suspicion or at a routine ultrasound examination. While traditionally the common clinical presentation involved a patient during the second trimester of pregnancy with significant vaginal bleeding, a uterus that was larger than appropriate for the stage of gestation, symptoms of severe preeclampsia (25 per cent), and perhaps hyperemesis, a recent study indicates that vaginal bleeding is the only common finding (84 per cent) and that excessive uterine size and preeclampsia are quite infrequent findings.[35] These authors note that this is due to the earlier diagnosis achieved when ultrasound, rather than a clinical constellation, is used. Currently, the median gestational age at diagnosis is 12 weeks rather than 16 weeks.

The human placenta contains two thyrotropic substances, HCG and molar thyrotropin, which when elaborated by patients with trophoblastic disease can lead to hyperthyroidism. Thyroid function test results are elevated in a large proportion of patients, but only a few demonstrate clinical signs of thyrotoxicosis.[36] This overactivity is cured by evacuation of the molar material. Trophoblastic embolization occurs in 2 per cent or less of cases, and, while often fatal, has responded favorably to chemotherapeutic agents and aggressive pulmonary therapeutic management.[37, 38]

C. THERAPY

The initial treatment of molar pregnancy is evacuation of the uterine contents. This may be accomplished by dilation of the cervix followed by sharp curettage for patients with a small uterus. The most common method of emptying the uterus today, however, is suction curettage. Under some circumstances (e.g., a very large uterus) hysterotomy with uterine evacuation or hysterectomy may be performed. Nonsurgical evacuation of the uterus using oxytoxic agents or prostaglandins has been recommended by some authors.[39] Regardless of the mode of uterine evacuation, the patient is followed carefully for persistence of trophoblastic tissue by sensitive HCG assays. Persistent trophoblastic disease is usually treated by chemotherapy with methotrexate and/or actinomycin D. Certain patients deemed at high risk may receive chemoprophylaxis.

D. ANESTHETIC CONSIDERATIONS

The patient who presents for evacuation of a molar pregnancy requires assessment and consideration of the following variables:

1. Blood volume may be depleted owing to vaginal bleeding. Anemia may be masked by hemoconcentration secondary to preeclampsia or dehydration. Since blood loss may be substantial at surgery, deficits should be corrected and additional blood and blood products made available. Hemorrhage may occur at the time of dilatation or during the evacuation. Postevacuation bleeding may occur as the result of uterine perforation, cervical laceration, or uterine atony. Intravenous lines of adequate caliber and number should be placed. Central venous pressure monitoring is occasionally indicated.

2. Fluid and electrolyte status should be assessed, particularly if hyperemesis is present.

3. If preeclampsia exists, blood pressure and volume should be under control before surgery. Severe preeclampsia is a far more difficult management problem and is identified by the presence of (1) blood pressure of 160/110 mm Hg or greater, (2) proteinuria of 5 g per day or greater, (3) oliguria (400 ml of urine output or less per day), (4) cerebral or visual symptoms, and (5) pulmonary edema or cyanosis. The presence of coagulopathy or persistent and severe epigastric pain are accepted by many as evidence of severe preeclampsia. Appropriate monitoring (e.g., central venous catheter, pulmonary artery catheter, and/or arterial line) and pharmacologic therapy should be instituted, as for other preeclampsia patients.

4. The potential for hyperthyroidism needs to be evaluated by thyroid function tests, and specific therapeutic agents such as iodine, steroids, adrenergic-blocking agents, and antithyroid drugs must be readily available when indicated. Some investigators advocate spinal anesthesia for molar evacuation in the presence of trophoblastic hyperthyroidism, to control sympathetic activity and avoid the arrhythmogenic complications associated with beta-2 agonist tocolysis and halogenated anesthetics.[40]

5. Uterine relaxation further increases blood loss; therefore, the inhalation anesthetics, all of which relax uterine muscle, should be used in low concentrations, if at all.[41]

6. Oxytocin, usually as an infusion, will be required before, during, and after curettage. It should be remembered that an intravenous bolus of 10 U or more, or rapid infusion of a highly concentrated solution, will result in hypotension that lasts 3 to 5 minutes.[42] On occasion, the surgeon will request increased uterine contractility. A pressor effect may be seen in 22 to 48 per cent of patients after Ergotrate administration.[43] Dangerous levels of hypertension have been observed after intravenous administration, and it is therefore recommended principally for intramuscular use. It should not be used in combination with a vasopressor or in patients who have signs and symptoms of preeclampsia.

The anesthetic management for evacuation of a molar pregnancy is based on the degree of symptoms and the physiologic alterations. On some occasions, regional anesthesia is acceptable if the uterus is small and hypovolemia is not present. Appropriate monitoring and preparation for blood loss, extended surgical procedures, metabolic derangements, and hypertensive crises are among the requisite considerations for a safe intraoperative course.

IV. PLACENTA ACCRETA, INCRETA, PERCRETA

A. THE DISEASE

Placenta accreta is abnormal adherence of the placenta to the uterine wall owing to an absent, scanty, or faulty decidua basalis. In contrast to normal placentation, in which the chorionic villi implant into the decidua, the chorionic villi are attached directly to uterine musculature. *Placenta increta* refers to the situation in which the chorionic villi have penetrated the uterine muscle, and *placenta percreta* refers to the condition in which the villi have penetrated through the serosa of the uterine wall and may actually invade other organs, most often the bladder. Placenta accreta is the most common form and usually is a diagnosis made after delivery, when the placenta refuses to separate from the uterine wall. The incidence of placenta accreta has most recently been found to be approximately 1 in 10,000 deliveries.[44] This rate is consistent with those reported in the past.[45, 46] The incidence of placenta accreta, increta, and percreta increases significantly with the presence of placenta previa and is substantially increased with presence of a uterine scar from previous cesarean section. Clark and coworkers found that patients with placenta previa but no history of cesarean section had an incidence of placenta accreta of approximately 5 per cent.[47] The presence of placenta previa and one prior cesarean section led to placenta accreta in 24 per cent of patients. The likelihood of accreta increased with each subsequent cesarean section: it occurred 67 per cent of the time in women who had placenta previa and four or more cesarean sections. An antenatal diagnosis can be made in patients at risk using ultrasound, color Doppler imaging,[48] magnetic resonance imaging (MRI),[49] and maternal serum α-fetoprotein levels, which are significantly elevated in 45 per cent of patients with placenta accreta.[50] Early diagnosis allows time to develop a management plan and to perform surgery on an elective, rather than an emergent, basis.

B. PATHOPHYSIOLOGY AND TREATMENT

The diagnosis after a vaginal delivery is recognized when the placenta fails to separate from the uterine wall. This is because the placenta has implanted in uterine muscle or scar tissue rather than in decidua basalis. Obstetric management may include an attempt to manually remove the placenta, curettage, or leaving the placenta in situ and treating the patient with antibiotics[51] and/or methotrexate.[52] The options at cesarean delivery are the same and often include a plan for elective hysterectomy. The major risk with attempted manual removal is that severe, uncontrollable hemorrhage may necessitate emergency hypogastric (internal iliac) artery ligation[53] and/or hysterectomy under less than optimal conditions. Indeed, abnormal placentation is the leading cause of obstetric hysterectomy.[54, 55] Hemorrhage occurs because the usual hemostatic mechanisms of the uterus are not present due to the absence of the decidua and implantation in fibrous scar tissue. Placenta percreta adds the risk of invasion of abdominal organs, most frequently the bladder, and may even result in antenatal intraabdominal hemorrhage.[56] The treatment of choice for placenta percreta invading the bladder is usually cesarean delivery by classical incision, leaving the placenta in situ, followed by immediate hysterectomy.[57] This is often a very complex procedure because of organ invasion, and massive bleeding may occur very rapidly. One recent case report describes predelivery insertion of ureteral stents after induction of general anesthesia when a diagnosis of bladder invasion by placental percreta had been established antenatally.[58] The stents assisted with the surgical approach and protected the ureters, which are often difficult to identify. Abnormal placentation may also become a problem in the first and second trimesters of pregnancy, causing significant bleeding during pregnancy termination procedures.[59, 60]

Maternal mortality is approximately 6 per cent for women treated surgically and even higher among those receiving alternative treatment.[61, 62] The primary problem is massive hemorrhage and the associated complications of coagulopathy and massive volume replacement. Obstetric hemorrhage remains a leading cause of maternal death.[63] Another cause of maternal death associated with placenta accreta is pulmonary embolization of trophoblastic tissue.[64]

C. ANESTHETIC AND MANAGEMENT CONSIDERATIONS

There are two circumstances under which anesthetists encounter patients with abnormal placentation. One is as an emergency situation, when the diagnosis was not previously suspected. This situation requires rapid assessment of the degree of hemorrhage and blood loss and establishment of appropriate monitors and vascular access to allow for rapid volume replacement and to provide a suitable anesthetic for surgical control of the bleeding without further compromising the patient. If continuous regional anesthesia was previously established it may be continued if the patient is hemodynamically stable. Otherwise, an appropriate general anesthetic will be required with minimal use of volatile agents, as they have the potential to decrease uterine tone and increase blood loss. While advance preparation for the particular patient may not have taken place, protocols for the management of obstetric hemorrhage should be established in labor and delivery suites that include mechanisms for rapidly obtaining blood and blood products and for gaining the assistance of additional skilled personnel.

The second situation is when placenta accreta, increta, or percreta is diagnosed antenatally. A planned elective cesarean delivery or cesarean section with hysterectomy allows ample time for preparation. The need for hysterectomy must be anticipated even if invasion is not considered deep by imaging techniques. The following issues should be considered:

1. Blood and blood products will be required. The patient may donate several units of blood during her pregnancy. These can be fractionated into red blood cells and fresh-frozen plasma or cryoprecipitate. Red cells should be stored as frozen cells, with the exception of those units donated in the few weeks before the planned procedure. The frozen cells will have to be thawed and washed in advance of their anticipated need. The number of units varies with the type of procedure anticipated and the condition of the patient. It should be made clear to the patient that additional banked blood products may become necessary and additional designated donor products may be desired. Discussion with blood bank personnel should emphasize the rapidity with which hemorrhage can occur, so that they will be prepared to procure products in a timely manner.

2. Monitoring needs will again vary, depending on the planned procedure. The authors have found that an arterial catheter is extremely useful for these cases and either routinely place a radial artery catheter or use one of the axillary artery sheaths, as discussed below, for pressure monitoring and blood gas sampling. The base excess is very useful for assessing adequacy of perfusion. Central venous monitoring is recommended for patients with placenta percreta, as blood loss is substantial and rapid with dissection of the bladder plane.

3. Vascular access should include a minimum of two large-bore catheters. The authors utilize a 7 French rapid-infusion line (Rapid Infusion Catheter Exchange Set, Arrow International Inc., Reading, Pa.) in the arm as well as an 8.5 French Cordis introducer placed in the internal jugular vein when managing patients with placenta increta or percreta. These catheters are connected to a rapid-infusion roller pump (like that used during liver transplant surgery; COBE Perfusion System, Lakewood, Colo.) so that volume losses can be corrected instantly. This approach adds significantly to the cost of care, but the reduction in morbidity and mortality justifies the effort.

4. Reduction in the uterine blood supply is often used to decrease blood loss. One method previously mentioned is ligation of the hypogastric arteries. This is difficult to perform as a prophylactic measure at the time of cesarean hysterectomy; therefore, at the authors' institution an interventional radiologist places an introducer sheath into each axillary artery and inserts balloon catheters into each internal iliac artery. The balloons are then inflated as soon as the infant is delivered, as a measure to reduce blood loss when caring for patients with placenta percreta. One of the sheaths has a side port from which arterial pressure can be monitored and blood samples obtained. The procedure is performed before surgery in the radiology suite with local anesthesia, and patients occasionally require gentle sedation and/or systemic analgesia.

5. The anesthesia of choice in the authors' institution is usually continuous lumbar epidural anesthesia. This allows for the customary obstetric interactions: the mother can see her baby; postoperative analgesia may be provided; and the significant other may be present in the operating room for the delivery portion of the procedure. The combined spi-

nal-epidural anesthesia technique may also have utility for this operation, providing rapid onset of anesthesia with the option for continuing neuraxial blockade later. Occasionally, general anesthesia has been induced later, when the anesthesiologist believed that hemodynamic stability would be compromised with reinjection of the epidural catheter. A multiinstitutional review of obstetric hysterectomies has revealed that the use of epidural anesthesia was not associated with poorer outcomes.[65] No patient who received continuous epidural anesthesia required induction of general anesthesia. Others disagree and recommend avoiding regional anesthesia for hysterectomy with placenta percreta but note its acceptability with placenta accreta.[66]

Placenta previa with abnormal placentation over a uterine scar and adherence and invasion through the uterine wall has become much more common than it was in the past. Early diagnosis, supplemented with a carefully designed management plan utilizing resources of multiple disciplines, may significantly reduce the morbidity and mortality of this entity.

V. INTRAUTERINE FETAL DEMISE

A. THE CONDITION

Intrauterine fetal demise is a situation frequently encountered by obstetricians around the world but is not frequently a management issue for anesthesiologists. The causes are legion, but the most frequent ones are missed abortion, febrile illness, syphilis, diabetes mellitus, preeclampsia, hypertension, renal disease, Rh incompatibility, and indeterminate causes.[67] Common difficulties that may be encountered are an extremely emotional patient and coagulopathy if the dead fetus remains in utero longer than 4 to 5 weeks. The coagulopathy may present principally as fibrinolysis or as disseminated intravascular coagulation.[68] The precise mechanisms remain unclear but are assumed to be related to the release of tissue thromboplastin from the fetal-placental unit into the circulation with activation of the extrinsic pathway of coagulation.[69] Fibrinogen levels are commonly followed in cases of intrauterine fetal demise as an indicator of coagulopathy. Hypo-

fibrinogenemia has been observed in 10 per cent of cases of fetal demise within 4 weeks of the terminal event and in 20 per cent after 4 weeks.[70] The coagulation changes have become much less of a clinical problem owing to early ultrasound diagnosis of the condition. Management of intrauterine fetal demise in the United States in the first trimester is usually vacuum curettage; in the second trimester it is either dilation and evacuation of the uterus (D&E) or prostaglandin E_2 suppository induction; in the third trimester it is either prostaglandin E_2 induction or oxytocin infusion.

B. ANESTHETIC CONSIDERATIONS

1. Anesthesia may be required for evacuation of the uterus. Unless coagulopathy exists, either general or regional anesthesia may be utilized. If coagulopathy is present, the nature of the defect will need to be determined and treated appropriately. Bleeding at uterine evacuation may be increased significantly.

2. Some patients desire epidural analgesia during induction and infusion techniques for emptying the uterus. Again, there are no additional concerns, except for assessment of the coagulation system. If there is significant coagulopathy, regional anesthesia is best avoided.

3. Although administered in suppository form, the prostaglandins are not without side effects. Nausea, vomiting, diarrhea, tachycardia, tachypnea, decreased blood pressure, increased cardiac output, and hyperpyrexia have all been observed with prostaglandin E_2 suppositories. The constellation of pyrexia, hypotension, and tachycardia resembles endotoxin-mediated shock and may create a diagnostic and therapeutic dilemma.[71]

VI. THE CRITICALLY ILL OBSTETRIC PATIENT

Thankfully, critically ill obstetric patients are not encountered frequently, but they can present a challenge to the anesthesiologist, especially during the acute phase of the condition. Most critically ill pregnant women are transferred to tertiary care centers to be managed by perinatologists, intensivists, obstetric anesthesiologists, and other specialist team

TABLE 13–2

Monitoring and Therapeutic Support During Transfer of the Critically Ill Parturient

Measure	(%)*
ECG	100
Pulse oximetry	80
Intraarterial pressure	93
Central venous pressure	75
Mechanical ventilation	68
PEEP	3.3
Drug infusions (>1)	72

*Percentage of all patients in this study who required transfer to another hospital for management of a critical illness.
Modified from Donnelly JA, Smith EA, Runcie CJ: Transfer of the critically ill obstetric patient. Int J Obstet Anesth 4:45, 1995.

members; however, transfer of the patient from the community is not without its own problems.[72] The parturient must be appropriately prepared for transport and all necessary monitors and therapeutic equipment taken along (Table 13–2). Monitors' battery life should be checked before leaving and temperature and urine output monitored during transfer. Heat loss may be a problem, and urine output will help gauge the adequacy of fluid resuscitation. It is essential to stabilize the patient's condition to make the transfer safe, and a short delay while this is undertaken is acceptable.

Critical maternal illness can be caused by obstetric and nonobstetric conditions (Table 13–3). The clinical considerations include initial resuscitation and management of the underlying disorder. For example, for an eclampsia patient, initial resuscitation involves airway management and seizure con-

TABLE 13–3

Examples of Critical Maternal Illness or Injury

Obstetric Conditions	Nonobstetric Conditions
Preeclampsia/eclampsia	Acute respiratory failure
Obstetric hemorrhage	Cardiac disease
Sepsis	Central nervous system
HELLP syndrome	disorders
Fatty liver of pregnancy	Autoimmune disease
Amniotic fluid embolism	Endocrine disorders
	Acute surgical emergencies and trauma

trol. Subsequent therapy addresses blood pressure control, pulmonary edema, fluid balance, coagulation status, and preparation for delivery of the fetus. Obstetric hemorrhage may be associated with life-threatening hypovolemia and obtundation. Again, initial resuscitation involves airway management, oxygen therapy, and rapid IV fluid and blood therapy. Definitive treatment depends on the source of the hemorrhage (e.g., abruption, placenta previa, accreta, uterine atony, uterine inversion, and/or the presence of disseminated intravascular coagulation).

Three principal factors that confound the management of the critically ill pregnant woman are the altered physiology of pregnancy, difficulty in cardiopulmonary resuscitation of a pregnant mother, and the well-being of the fetus. When a pregnant woman is in a critical condition, both mother and baby are at high risk for significant morbidity and mortality. After an initial period of medical treatment to stabilize the condition of the mother, the baby may require expeditious delivery (if mature enough to survive in an extrauterine environment). In extreme situations the fetus may need to be delivered regardless of gestation, to save at least one life.

In general, the anesthesiologist must remember that hypovolemia and shock are contraindications to regional anesthetic techniques. In addition, an obtunded parturient is often unable to maintain and protect her airway, so immediate orotracheal intubation may be necessary. As a result of the physiologic changes of pregnancy and increased risk for hypoxemia, the airway should be secured by an experienced anesthesiologist. The impact of anesthetic induction agents and positive-pressure ventilation on a hypovolemic patient should be remembered and two large-bore IV cannulas should be in place, with inotropic agents (e.g., ephedrine, dopamine) readily available. Avoidance of aortocaval compression is especially important in these patients. Following delivery, they are usually cared for in an intensive care unit. Obstetric anesthesiologists often play a role in postpartum medical management, working closely with the intensivist. A recent review of critical care in pregnant patients serves to remind intensivists of the issues involved and is recommended reading.[73] Motor vehicle accidents and crush injuries represent severe forms of surgical trauma and create unique problems for emergency medical personnel.[74] An estimated 6 per cent of pregnant patients suffer traumatic injuries, and trauma is the leading nonobstetric cause of maternal death.[75]

VII. CARDIAC ARREST AND CARDIOPULMONARY RESUSCITATION DURING PREGNANCY

A. CAUSES OF CARDIAC ARREST

Cardiopulmonary failure in pregnancy is uncommon, which is all the more reason for obstetric units to have written protocols in place and to review the process with regular mock "codes" that involve personnel from nursing, obstetrics and anesthesiology. The causes of cardiopulmonary arrest in pregnancy are numerous (Table 13–4). Myocardial

---

TABLE 13–4

Causes of Cardiopulmonary Arrest in Pregnancy

1. Airway misadventure. Failed airway management is a major cause of death in pregnant patients; cannot ventilate by mask, cannot conventionally intubate rescue options, such as insertion of laryngeal mask airway, combitube, or transtracheal airway, must be begun to provide adequate ventilation and oxygenation.
2. Hemorrhage.
3. Local anesthetic toxicity, especially bupivacaine.
4. Total spinal block and respiratory arrest from intraspinal opioids.
5. Cardiac disease. May be an expression of primary myocardial, pericardial, or valve disorders. Pregnant patients can also present with complex congenital heart disease involving shunts and dysrhythmias. Attention must be paid to the possibility of complications associated with anticoagulant therapy, antiarrhythmic drugs, or infection.
6. Illicit drug use (cocaine and "crack" cocaine cause myocardial ischemia in young pregnant women).
7. Drug error (a number of drugs used in obstetrics have the potential for severe cardiopulmonary side effects when given in excessive doses (e.g., magnesium, prostaglandin F_2-alpha, ergometrine, terbutaline[29]).
8. Septic shock.
9. Anaphylaxis.
10. Trauma.
11. Cerebral lesions.
12. Malignant hyperthermia.

---

infarction (MI) is rare in pregnancy but carries high mortality (20 to 40 per cent), especially in the third trimester. Today we see more parturients of advanced age (over 35 years), who are at greater risk for MI (see below).[76, 77] An unusual risk factor for MI during pregnancy is coronary artery aneurysm associated with Kawasaki's disease, which presents at a younger age. Kawasaki's disease is a form of vasculitis of unknown cause that is characterized by mucosal inflammation, peripheral edema, skin rash, and cervical lymphadenopathy. Coronary aneurysms occur in 20 per cent, and occasionally they are giant aneurysms (larger than 8 mm diameter). It is likely that the number of pregnancies in patients with a history of Kawasaki's disease will increase.[78]

B. MANAGEMENT OF CARDIAC ARREST

Cardiac arrest is a rare event in pregnancy (~ 1 in 30,000),[79, 80] but the incidence may be on the increase as the obstetric population gets older and advances in medicine and surgery have produced a new population of high-risk parturients. Cardiac arrest is the final common pathway of many pathologic processes, and, although the initial resuscitation will be the same, definitive treatment will depend on the cause. The use of cardiopulmonary resuscitation (CPR) in the general population has led to improved survival, but resuscitation of the parturient is complicated by anatomic and physiologic changes of pregnancy. These changes significantly decrease the cardiovascular and pulmonary reserve and place mother and fetus at increased risk. The pregnant patient has altered airway anatomy. The larynx lies farther anterior and cephalad. The mucosa of the upper airway is more vascular, edematous, and friable. Consequently, failed intubation is more common in pregnancy.[81]

- Oxygen consumption is increased by 20 per cent late in pregnancy, secondary to the metabolic requirements of the fetus, uterus, placenta, and breast tissue. Consequently, an apneic pregnant patient becomes hypoxemic much faster than a nonpregnant woman.
- Functional residual capacity is decreased at term as a result of cephalad elevation of the diaphragm, which contributes to

the rapid reductions in maternal oxygen tensions in arterial and venous blood during apnea. Chest wall compliance is reduced, thus hindering the ability to mechanically ventilate the lungs during CPR. Maternal brain damage is likely after 4 to 6 minutes of sustained cardiac arrest.[82] A delay of 6 to 9 minutes may lead to irreversible brain damage in the mother.[83] As described below in the section on respiratory failure, fetal oxygen reserve is about 2 minutes. Clinically, the fetus may survive undamaged for slightly longer, but most intact survivors are delivered within 5 minutes of maternal arrest (see Perimortem Cesarean).

- Hyperventilation, with an increase in minute ventilation of 45 per cent at term, is a response to the increased demands for oxygen and the increase in carbon dioxide production. There is an increase in renal excretion of bicarbonate, to compensate for the resultant chronic respiratory alkalosis. This leads to a lower serum bicarbonate level, mild metabolic acidosis, and reduced buffering capacity.
- Cardiac output increases throughout pregnancy to 50 per cent of prepregnancy values at term, and further increases are seen during labor and delivery. Blood volume is increased by 45 per cent of prepregnancy values, and there is physiologic anemia.
- Aortocaval compression by the gravid uterus in a supine gravida compromises blood flow to the uterus and kidneys and significantly reduces venous return. This in turn reduces cardiac output and can cause hypotension and bradycardia. Maternal hypoxia, hypotension, and lactic acidosis can result in uterine artery vasoconstriction and fetal acidosis.

Cardiopulmonary resuscitation can be successful if adequate cardiac output is achieved through chest compressions, but even in the best circumstances CPR can generate only 30 per cent of the cardiac output.[84] Closed chest massage produces artificial circulation by phasic fluctuations in intrathoracic pressure.[85] Forward flow occurs after a pressure gradient develops between the arterial and venous systems, with the heart acting as a passive conduit. Competent venous valves are required to prevent retrograde flow. The benefits of closed-chest compressions decline when CPR extends beyond 15 minutes[86] and

will not be successful unless extreme left uterine displacement is used. Exogenous adrenergic agonists are essential elements in ensuring the success of CPR by increasing aortic diastolic pressure and venous return and preventing collapse of the carotid arteries.[87] If resuscitation has not been successful within 4 minutes of maternal cardiac arrest, a perimortem cesarean section provides the best chance of maternal and fetal survival.[88, 89] Delivery of the baby (at more than 20 weeks' gestation) and placenta reduces maternal oxygen consumption, aortocaval compression, and production of carbon dioxide and hydrogen ions by the uteroplacental unit. A recent case report describing successful resuscitation during pregnancy reconfirms these points, emphasizing that emptying the uterus is more effective than displacing it, in terms of maximizing venous return—and, thus, preload and stroke volume.[90] It must be remembered that CPR has the ability to cause injury to the liver and uterus, hemothorax, and hemoperitoneum. Standard advanced cardiac life support (ACLS) resuscitation algorithms and defibrillation guidelines are applicable to the pregnant patient. Most resuscitation drugs cross the placenta, but concern about fetal effects is secondary to achieving successful maternal resuscitation. In general terms, if the mother's condition is bad, the fetus' is worse, and what benefits the mother will, in turn, benefit the fetus.

In centers where experienced surgeons are available, open-chest cardiac massage may offer the only chance of maternal survival when external cardiac massage has failed after 15 minutes. Direct heart massage generates greater cardiac output with less reduction in coronary and cerebral perfusion;[91] however, its effectiveness in pregnancy is not well described and the risk of substantial blood loss is great.

Cardiopulmonary bypass may be life saving, where available, in situations of severe ventilation-perfusion mismatch or when prolonged resuscitation is needed. An example of the latter would be when normal cardiac rhythm cannot be restored, as with hypothermia and local anesthetic cardiotoxicity.

VIII. RESPIRATORY FAILURE IN PREGNANCY

Respiratory failure in pregnancy is characterized by severe maternal and fetal hypox-

TABLE 13–5

Causes of Respiratory Failure in Pregnancy

Pulmonary embolism (thrombus, amniotic fluid, air)
ARDS (from septicemia or pneumonia)
Aspiration of gastric contents
Asthma
Beta-adrenergic tocolysis
Pneumothorax/pneumomediastinum
Extrapulmonary causes (e.g., upper airway obstruction, central nervous system disorders, respiratory muscle weakness)

emia and/or hypercarbia, acid-base disturbances, possible hemodynamic consequences, and impaired nutrition to the fetus.[92] The causes of respiratory failure include some conditions that are unique to pregnancy, such as amniotic fluid embolism, and others that are not, such as adult respiratory distress syndrome (ARDS) from systemic sepsis (Table 13–5). Respiratory failure from various causes accounts for 30 to 35 per cent of maternal deaths.

Most causes of respiratory failure in pregnancy are characterized by problems associated with hypoxemia. Chronic hypoxemia in pregnancy is associated with intrauterine growth retardation or fetal death. Adequate delivery of oxygen from the maternal circulation via the placenta and umbilical vessels is also critical to fetal well-being in the face of acute hypoxemia. Increasing the oxygen gradient across the placenta by providing maternal hyperoxia is essential for providing increased oxygen transfer to the fetus.[93] One example of hypoxemic respiratory failure is ARDS, which can result from multiple causes. The syndrome is characterized by an accumulation of excess lung water secondary to increased microvascular permeability mediated by neutrophils, proinflammatory mediators, and activation of the complement cascade.[92] It is diagnosed on the basis of x-ray evidence of pulmonary edema, exclusion of cardiac failure, and severe hypoxemia despite an F_IO_2 greater than 0.5 and positive end-expiratory pressure (PEEP). These patients' mortality ranges from 30 to 70 per cent and is higher with multiorgan system failure. If gestation is at or near term, delivery may aid subsequent maternal management as her metabolic demands and related cardiorespiratory "overdrive" will be removed.

Causes of hypercarbic ventilatory failure

include severe asthma and extrapulmonary factors (Table 13–5). Acute severe asthma requires rapid and intensive management, including early hospital admission and aggressive management of ventilation in an intensive care setting.[94] A serious problem may occur if the decision to delay mechanical ventilation is made without considering the normal range for arterial blood gases in pregnancy. A P_{CO_2} of 38 to 40 mm Hg, which is normal for the nonpregnant state, may signal the need for urgent intervention in a pregnant woman. A decision to provide supportive ventilation must take into account coexisting hypoxemia, tachypnea, metabolic acidosis, and maternal fatigue (Table 13–6). In pregnancy, a drop in maternal P_aO_2 can lead to significant and rapid fetal deterioration, since the fetus operates on the steep portion of the oxygen dissociation curve. It is likely, however, that maternal arterial oxygen content is more important than P_aO_2 in providing sufficient oxygen to the fetus. The oxygen content of uterine arterial blood and maternal cardiac output are critical determinants of oxygen delivery to the fetus. Oxygen tension, hemoglobin concentration, oxyhemoglobin saturation, and blood flow are all determinants of oxygen content. When considering the oxygen status of fetal blood a number of points must be remembered:[95]

1. Umbilical vein blood is oxygenated relative to umbilical arterial blood.

2. Since as a gas exchanger, the placenta is coupled in parallel with fetal tissues, only 50 per cent of blood is oxygenated during one circulation (as compared with adult lungs, which are coupled in series with tissues).

3. Despite lower oxygen tension in the umbilical vein as compared with maternal values, umbilical artery and vein oxygen concentrations are similar to maternal values

TABLE 13–6

Indications for Maternal Tracheal Intubation and Mechanical Ventilation

Maternal exhaustion
Reduced level of consciousness
Hypercarbia (P_{CO_2} > 38 mm Hg)
Hypoxemia (P_{O_2} < 60 mm Hg)
Acidemia (pH < 7.35)
Hemodynamic instability (hypotension, dysrhythmias)
Peak expiratory flow rate < 70 L/min
Pneumothorax (clinically significant)

because fetal hemoglobin has a steeper oxy-hemoglobin saturation curve with a shift to the left.

4. The fetus copes with hypoxemia by increasing cardiac output and redistributing blood flow to vital organs, but in a term fetus oxygen stores only last about 2 minutes after complete interruption of maternal oxygen supply.

Therapy for respiratory failure includes oxygenation, tracheal intubation, and ventilatory, hemodynamic and nutritional support. Pharmacologic therapy consists of direct airway delivery of aerosolized beta-2 agonists, corticosteroids, and cromolyn sodium. This route of administration minimizes systemic absorption and reduces their impact on the fetus and uterus. As stated in the discussion on CPR, these drugs should not be withheld because of concerns about fetal effects; the well-being of the mother comes first, and her welfare is inextricably linked to that of the passenger. Ventilator settings are similar to those for nonpregnant patients. The aim is to keep the F_1O_2 below 50%, use PEEP if the P_aO_2 falls below 60 to 65 mm Hg, and maintain P_aCO_2 at 30 to 32 mm Hg, in keeping with normal pregnancy values.

IX. HIGH-ORDER MULTIPLE GESTATIONS

Multiple gestations, including twins and triplets, have increased in some parts of the United States by 250 per cent over the last 4 years. This has been a result of increased numbers of women conceiving by artificial reproductive techniques, such as ovulation induction and gamete or embryo transfers.[96, 97] High-order multiple gestation is defined as multiple gestations greater than three (i.e., quadruplets, quintuplets, etc.), and these pose unique obstetric problems that are of concern to anesthesiologists.[98] Maternal and neonatal morbidity and mortality risks are greater than for singleton gestations.[99] Maternal complications include pregnancy-induced hypertension and gestational diabetes. Maternal problems may also arise as a result of infection, antepartum hemorrhage, or tocolytic therapy.[99] Premature labor and intrauterine growth retardation are frequent causes of neonatal morbidity and demise in multiple pregnancies. Other fetal concerns include abnormal presentations, umbilical cord pro-

lapse, congenital anomalies, interfetal transfusions, and early placental separation.

The normal physiologic changes of pregnancy are exaggerated: increases in blood volume, red cell mass, and cardiac output are substantial. There is a potential for a greater than normal decrease in functional residual capacity (FRC) in these patients, which is important when preparing for cesarean delivery under general anesthesia or placing a central venous catheter in the Trendelenburg position. They very rapidly become hypoxemic after brief periods of apnea and do not tolerate position changes that have an adverse effect on FRC. Two large-bore IV cannulas should be in situ and blood products available if required. Early placement of an epidural catheter for labor and delivery is recommended since fetal manipulation may be necessary at the time of delivery. Since this may be time consuming and general anesthesia may cause significant neonatal cardiorespiratory depression, general anesthesia should be avoided if at all possible. If cesarean delivery is planned, spinal or epidural anesthesia would be preferable to general anesthesia because parental involvement in the birth can occur, the (often premature) fetus is exposed to fewer drugs, and the risks of uterine atony, acid aspiration, and airway management problems are significantly reduced. There are some drawbacks to regional anesthesia, however: (1) these women may have subjective dyspnea that worsens with a high sensory block; (2) the risk of hypotension is increased; and (3) there may be technical difficulties with the block from exaggerated lumbar lordosis. Despite the type of anesthetic, before induction of anesthesia (regional or general) all women receive 30 ml of a nonparticulate antacid by mouth, 10 mg IV metoclopramide, and oxygen by face mask, and leftward uterine displacement is ensured. Postpartum hemorrhage from uterine atony is increased, so the anesthesiologist should be prepared to administer IV fluids rapidly and have oxytocin, ergometrine, and prostaglandin $F_{2\alpha}$ readily available.

X. ADVANCED MATERNAL AGE

As a result of social and demographic changes in today's society and technological advances in the treatment of infertility, the number of women older than age 35 who become pregnant has increased over the last decade. In addition, between 1976 and 1986, the rate of first births in women aged 40 years or more doubled.[100] Women over age 35 are more susceptible to numerous complications of pregnancy than their younger counterparts.[101, 102] Complications due to diabetes and hypertensive disorders are seen more frequently in women over age 35 than in those in the 20- to 25-year range. Advanced maternal age is more likely to be associated with cardiovascular (including coronary artery disease), neurologic, connective tissue, renal, and pulmonary disorders, in addition to cancer and alcoholism. There is increased risk of fetal demise in older women, which may be due to failure of the uterine vasculature to adapt to the increased hemodynamic demands of pregnancy. Anesthetic considerations are the same as for any parturient, but these patients must be considered at high risk owing to the increased likelihood of peripartum morbidity. A predelivery anesthetic consultation is important to rule out any coexisting medical or surgical conditions, to order appropriate tests (e.g., ECG, pulmonary function tests), to allay patient anxiety, and to discuss analgesic and anesthetic options. The anesthetic considerations depend on the presence of coexisting medical or obstetric complications and can be modified according to the situation. Of concern would be the interpretation of ECG changes during cesarean section[103] and the risk of pulmonary edema in an older woman with preeclampsia or chronic hypertension or in those receiving beta-adrenergic tocolysis.[104] There is increased risk of cesarean delivery in these women, and it has been postulated that this is the result of intercurrent disease, dysfunctional labor, fetal distress, and malpresentations.[105] Others, however, have suggested that the obstetrician is more likely to intervene with cesarean birth because the fetus at risk is often viewed as a "precious baby," in part because there is less chance for a future pregnancy.[106]

REFERENCES

Introduction; Pharmacologic Considerations for Surgery During Pregnancy

1. Brodsky JB, Cohen EM, Brown BW, et al: Surgery during pregnancy and fetal outcome. Am J Obstet Gynecol 138:1165, 1980.
2. Adamsons K, Joelsson I: The effects of pharmacologic agents upon the fetus and newborn. Am J Obstet Gynecol 96:437, 1966.
3. Sutherland JM, Light IJ: The effects of drugs upon the developing fetus. Pediatr Clin North Am 12:781, 1965.
4. Bussard DA, Stoelting RK, Peterson C, et al: Fetal changes in hamsters anesthetized with nitrous oxide and halothane. Anesthesiology 41:275, 1974.
5. Pope WDB, Halsey MJ, Lansdown ABG, et al: Fetotoxicity in rats following chronic exposure to halothane, nitrous oxide, or methoxyflurane. Anesthesiology 48:11, 1978.
6. Smith RF, Bowman RE, Katz J: Behavioral effects of exposure to halothane during early development in the rat. Anesthesiology 49:319, 1978.
7. Smith BE, Gaub ML, Moya F: Investigations into the teratogenic effects of anesthetic agents: The fluorinated agents. Anesthesiology 26:260, 1965.
8. Drachman DB, Coulombre AJ: Experimental clubfoot and arthrogryposis multiplex congenita. Lancet 2:523, 1962.
9. Pedersen H, Finster M: Anesthetic risk in the pregnant surgical patient. Anesthesiology 51:439, 1979.
10. Levinson G, Shnider SM: Anesthesia for surgery during pregnancy. In Shnider SM, Levinson G (eds): Anesthesia for Obstetrics, 3rd ed. Baltimore, Williams & Wilkins, 1993.
11. Shnider SM, Webster GM: Maternal and fetal hazards of surgery during pregnancy. Am J Obstet Gynecol 92:891, 1965.
12. Leicht CH: Anesthesia for the pregnant patient undergoing nonobstetric surgery. Anesth Clin North Am 8:131, 1990.
13. Nunn JF: Clinical aspects of the interaction between nitrous oxide and vitamin B_{12}. Br J Anaesth 59:3, 1987.
14. Boss GR: Cobalamin inactivation decreases purine and methionine synthesis in cultured lymphoblasts. J Clin Invest 76:213, 1985.
15. Fassoulaki A, Eger EI, Johnson BH, et al: Nitrous oxide, too, is hepatotoxic in rats. Anesth Analg 63:1076, 1984.
16. Vina JR, Davis DW, Hawkins RA: The influence of nitrous oxide on methionine, S-adenosylmethionine, and other amino acids. Anesthesiology 64:490, 1986.
17. O'Sullivan H, Jennings F, Ward K, et al: Megaloblastic bone marrow changes after repeated nitrous oxide anaesthesia. Br J Anaesth 58:1469, 1986.
18. Fujinaga M, Baden JM, Yhap EO, Mazze RI: Reproductive and teratogenic effects of nitrous oxide, isoflurane, and their combination in Sprague-Dawley rats. Anesthesiology, 67:960, 1987.
19. Smith BE: Fetal prognosis after anesthesia during gestation. Anesth Analg 42:521, 1963.
20. Duncan PG, Pope WDB, Cohen MM, Greer N: Fetal risk of anesthesia and surgery during pregnancy. Anesthesiology 64:790, 1986.
21. Clark RB, Brown MA, Lattin DL: Neostigmine, atropine, and glycopyrrolate: Does neostigmine cross the placenta? Anesthesiology 84:450, 1996.
22. Kuhnert BR, Philipson EH, Pimental R, et al: Lidocaine disposition in mother, fetus, and neonate after spinal anesthesia. Anesth Analg 65:139, 1986.
23. Fujinaga M, Mazze RI: Reproductive and teratogenic effects of lidocaine in Sprague-Dawley rats. Anesthesiology 65:626, 1986.
24. Wittels B, Scott DT, Sinatra RS: Exogenous opioids in human breast milk and acute neonatal neurobehavior: a preliminary study. Anesthesiology 73:864, 1990.
25. Caritis SN, Edelstone DI, Mueller-Heubach E: Phar-

macologic inhibition of preterm labor. Am J Obstet Gynecol 133:557, 1979.

26. Kumar D, Zourlas PA, Barnes AC: In vitro and in vivo effects of magnesium sulfate on human uterine contractility. Am J Obstet Gynecol 86:1036, 1963.

27. Steer MI, Atlas D, Levitski A: Interelations between beta-adrenergic receptors, adenylate cyclase, and calcium. N Engl J Med 292:409, 1975.

28. Katz M: Severe cardiovascular complications associated with beta-sympathomimetic tocolysis and their prevention. West J Med 134:528, 1981.

29. Ravindran R, Viegas OJ, Padilla LM: Anesthetic considerations in pregnant patients receiving terbutaline therapy. Anesth Analg 59:391, 1980.

30. Hurlbert BJ, Edelman JD, David K: Serum potassium levels during and after terbutaline. Anesth Analg 60:723, 1981.

Hydatidiform Mole

31. Hertig AT, Mansell H: Atlas of Tumor Pathology, Fasc. 33. Tumors of the Female Sex Organs. Part I. Hydatidiform Mole and Choriocarcinoma. Washington, DC, Armed Forces Institute of Pathology, 1956.

32. Rubino SM: Diagnosis of an intact hydatidiform mole with co-existent fetus by amniography. Obstet Gynecol 46:364, 1975.

33. Goldstein DP: Surgery of moles and choriocarcinoma. In Barber HRK, Graber EA (eds): Surgical Disease in Pregnancy. Philadelphia, WB Saunders, 1974.

34. Baird AM: The ultrasound diagnosis of hydatidiform mole. Clin Radiol 8:637, 1977.

35. Soto-Wright V, Bernstein M, Goldstein DP, Berkowitz RS: The changing clinical presentation of complete molar pregnancy. Obstet Gynecol 86:775, 1995.

36. Bruun T, Kristoffersen K: Thyroid function during pregnancy with reference to hydatidiform mole and hyperemesis. Acta Endocrinol 88:383, 1978.

37. Lipp RG, Kendschi JD, Shmitz R: Death from pulmonary embolism associated with hydatidiform mole. Am J Obstet Gynecol 83:1644, 1962.

38. Natonson R, Shapiro BA, Harrison RA, et al: Massive trophoblastic embolization and PEEP therapy. Anesthesiology 51:469, 1979.

39. Southern EM: Evacuation of the uterus in benign gestational trophoblastic disease with prostaglandins. In Karim SM (ed): Obstetric and Gynaecologic Use of Prostaglandins. Lancaster, England, MTP Press, 1976.

40. Solak M, Akturk G: Spinal anesthesia in a patient with hyperthyroidism due to hydatidiform mole. Anesth Analg 77:851, 1993.

41. Munson ES, Embro WJ: Enflurane, isoflurane, and halothane and isolated uterine muscle. Anesthesiology 46:11, 1977.

42. Weis FR, Peak I: Effects of oxytocin on blood pressure during anesthesia. Anesthesiology 40:189, 1974.

43. Abouleish E: Postpartum hypertension and convulsion after oxytocic drugs. Anesth Analg 55:813, 1976.

Placenta Accreta, Increta, Percreta

44. Makhseed M, El-Tomi N, Moussa M: A retrospective analysis of pathological placental implantation—site and penetration. Int J Gynecol Obstet 47:127, 1994.

45. Breen JL, Neubecker R, Gregori CA, et al: Placenta accreta, increta, and percreta. Obstet Gynecol 49:43, 1977.

46. Neckestein LN, Masserman JSH, Garite TJ: Placenta accreta: A problem of increasing clinical significance. Obstet Gynecol 69:480, 1987.

47. Clark SL, Koonings PP, Phelan JP: Placenta previa/accreta and prior cesarean section. Obstet Gynecol 66:89, 1985.

48. Rosemond RL, Kepple DM: Transvaginal color Doppler sonography in the diagnosis of placenta accreta. Obstet Gynecol 80:508, 1992.

49. Thorp JM, Councell RB, Sandridge DA, Wiest HH: Antepartum diagnosis of placenta previa percreta by magnetic resonance imaging. Obstet Gynecol 80:506, 1992.

50. Zelop C, Nadel A, Frigoletto FD Jr, et al: Placenta accreta/increta/percreta: A cause of elevated maternal serum α-fetoprotein. Obstet Gynecol 80:693, 1992.

51. Komulainen MJ, Vayrynen MA, Kauko ML, Saarikoski S: Two cases of placenta accreta managed conservatively. Eur J Obstet Gynecol Reprod Biol 62:135, 1995.

52. Legro RS, Price FV, Hill LM, Caritis SN: Nonsurgical management of placenta percreta: A case report. Obstet Gynecol 83:847, 1994.

53. Peraskevaides E, Noelke L, Afrasiabi M: Internal iliac artery ligation (IIAL) in obstetrics and gynaecology. Eur J Obstet Gynecol Reprod Biol 5:73, 1993.

54. Zelop CM, Harlow BL, Frigoletto FD, et al: Emergency peripartum hysterectomy. Am J Obstet Gynecol 168:1443, 1993.

55. Stanco LM, Schrimmer DB, Paul RH, et al: Emergency peripartum hysterectomy and associated risk factors. Am J Obstet Gynecol 168:879, 1993.

56. Archer GE, Furlong LA: Acute abdomen caused by placenta percreta in the second trimester. Am J Obstet Gynecol 157:146, 1987.

57. Sanders RR: Placenta praevia percreta invading the urinary bladder. Aust N Z J Obstet Gynaecol 32:375, 1992.

58. Hunter T, Kleiman S: Anaesthesia for Caesarean hysterectomy in a patient with a preoperative diagnosis of placenta percreta with invasion of the urinary bladder. Can J Anaesth 43:246, 1996.

59. Ecker JL, Sorem KA, Soodak L, et al: Placenta increta complicating a first-trimester abortion. A case report. J Reprod Med 37:893, 1992.

60. Rashbaum WK, Gates EJ, Jones J, et al: Placenta accreta encountered during dilation and evacuation in the second trimester. Obstet Gynecol 85:701, 1995.

61. Fox H: Placenta accreta, 1945–1969. Obstet Gynecol Surv 27:475, 1972.

62. Chattopadhyay SK, Kharif H, Sherbeeni MM: Placenta previa and accreta after previous cesarean section. Eur J Obstet Gynecol Reprod Biol 52:151, 1993.

63. Rochat RW, Koonin LM, Atrash HK, Jewett JF: Maternal mortality in the United States: Report from the Maternal Mortality Collaborative. Obstet Gynecol 72:91, 1988.

64. Rashid AM, Moir CL, Butt JC: Sudden death following cesarean section for placenta previa and accreta. Am J Forensic Med Pathol 15:32, 1994.

65. Chestnut DH, Dewan DM, Redick LF, et al: Anesthetic management for obstetric hysterectomy: A multi-institutional study. Anesthesiology 70:607, 1989.

66. Acario T, Greene M, Ostheimer GW, et al: Risks of placenta previa/accreta in patients with previous cesarean deliveries, abstracted. Anesthesiology 69:A659, 1988.

Intrauterine Fetal Demise

67. Kuhn W, Rath W: International colloquy on the management of intrauterine fetal death. Int J Gynaecol 25:185, 1987.
68. Romero R, Copel JA, Hobbins JC: Intrauterine fetal demise and hemostatic failure: The fetal death syndrome. Clin Obstet Gynecol 28:24, 1985.
69. Weiner AE, Reid DE, Roby CC, Diamond LK: Coagulation defects with intrauterine death from Rh isosensitization. Am J Obstet Gynecol 60:1015, 1950.
70. Parasnis H, Raje B, Hinduja IN: Relevance of plasma fibrinogen estimation in obstetric complications. J Postgrad Med 38:183, 1992.
71. Hughes WA, Hughes SC: Hemodynamic effects of prostaglandin E$_2$. Anesthesiology 70:723, 1989.

The Critically Ill Obstetric Patient

72. Donnelly JA, Smith EA, Runcie CJ: Transfer of the critically ill obstetric patient: Experience of a specialist team and guidelines for the non-specialist. Int J Obstet Anesth 4:45, 1995.
73. Lapinsky SE, Kruczynski K, Slutsky AS: Critical care in the pregnant patient. Am J Respir Crit Care Med 152:427, 1995.
74. Schoenfeld A, Warchaizer S, Royburt M, et al: Crush injury in pregnancy: An unusual experience in obstetrics. Obstet Gynecol 86:655, 1995.
75. Rozycki GS, Champion HR, Drass MJ: Traumatic injuries in the pregnant patient. Hosp Physician July: 20, 1989.

Cardiac Arrest and Cardiopulmonary Resuscitation During Pregnancy

76. Verkaaik APK, Visser W, Deckers JW, Lotgering FK: Multiple coronary artery dissections in a woman at term. Br J Anaesth 71:301, 1993.
77. Donnelly S, McKenna P, McGing P, Sugrue D: Myocardial infarction during pregnancy. Br J Obstet Gynaecol 100:781, 1993.
78. Alam S, Sakura S, Kosaka Y: Anaesthetic management for Caesarean section in a patient with Kawasaki disease. Can J Anaesth 42:1024, 1995.
79. Rees GAD, Willis BA: Resuscitation in late pregnancy. Anaesthesia 43:347, 1988.
80. Oates S, Williams GL, Rees GAD: Cardiopulmonary resuscitation in late pregnancy. Br Med J 297:404, 1988.
81. Rosen M: Difficult and failed intubation in obstetrics. In Latto IP, Rosen M (eds): Difficulties in Tracheal Intubation. London, Balliere, 1985.
82. American Heart Association: Textbook of Advanced Cardiac Life Support. Dallas, American Heart Association, 1987.
83. Weber CE: Postmortem cesarean section: Review of the literature and case reports. Am J Obstet Gynecol 110:158, 1971.
84. Gonik B: Intensive care monitoring of the critically ill pregnant patient. In Creasy RK, Resnik R (eds): Maternal-Fetal Medicine: Principles and Practice. Philadelphia, WB Saunders, 1989.
85. Peters J, Ihle J: Mechanics of the circulation during cardiopulmonary resuscitation: pathophysiology and techniques. Intensive Care Med 16:11, 1990.
86. Krause GS, Kumar K, White BC: Ischemia, resuscitation and reperfusion. Am Heart J 11:768, 1986.
87. Brown CG, Werman HA: Adrenergic agonists during cardiopulmonary resuscitation. Resuscitation 19:1, 1990.
88. Katz VL, Dotters DJ, Droegemueller W: Perimortem cesarean delivery. Obstet Gynecol 68:571, 1986.
89. American Heart Association Subcommittee on Emergency Cardiac Care: Guidelines for Cardiopulmonary Resuscitation and Emergency Cardiac Care. JAMA 268:2172, 1992.
90. O'Connor RL, Sevarino FB: Cardiopulmonary arrest in the pregnant patient: A report of a successful resuscitation. J Clin Anesth 6:66, 1994.
91. Bayne CG, Josing W: Reversal of inadequate cardiac output and perfusion during CPR by open-chest cardiac massage. Am J Emerg Med 2:138, 1984.

Respiratory Failure in Pregnancy

92. Hollingsworth HM, Irwin RS: Acute respiratory failure in pregnancy. Clin Chest Med 13:723, 1992.
93. Bassell GM, Marx GF: Optimization of fetal oxygenation. Int J Obstet Anesth 4:238, 1995.
94. Clark SL and the National Asthma Education Program Working Group on Asthma and Pregnancy: Asthma in pregnancy. Obstet Gynecol 82:1036, 1993.
95. Siggard-Andersen O, Huch R: The oxygen status of fetal blood. Acta Anaesth Scand 39:129, 1995.

High-Order Multiple Gestations

96. Collins MS, Bleyl JA: Seventy-one quadruplet pregnancies: Management and outcome. Am J Obstet Gynecol 162:1384, 1990.
97. Lipitz S, Frenkel Y, Watts C, et al: High order multifetal gestation—management and outcome. Obstet Gynecol 76:215, 1990.
98. Craft JB, Levinson G, Shnider S: Anesthetic considerations in cesarean section for quadruplets. Can Anesth Soc J 25:236, 1978.
99. Crosby ET, Elliot RD: Anaesthesia for Caesarean section in a parturient with quintuplet gestation, pulmonary oedema and thrombocytopenia. Can J Anaesth 35:417, 1988.

Advanced Maternal Age

100. National Center for Health Statistics, Ventura SJ: Trends and variations in first births to older women, 1970–86. Vital and health statistics. Series 21. No. 47. DHHS publication no. (PHS) 89–1925. Washington, DC: U.S. Government Printing Office, 1989.
101. Cunningham FG, Leveno KJ: Childbearing among older women—the message is cautiously optimistic [editorial]. N Engl J Med 333:1002, 1995.
102. Fretts RC, Schmittdiel J, McLean FH, et al: Increased maternal age and the risk of fetal death. N Engl J Med 333:953, 1995.
103. Burton A, Camann W: Electrocardiographic changes during cesarean section: A review. Int J Obstet Anesth 5:47, 1996.
104. Tatara T, Morisaki H, Shimada M, et al: Pulmonary edema after long-term beta-adrenergic therapy and cesarean section. Anesth Analg 81:417, 1995.
105. Lehmann DK, Chism J: Pregnancy outcome in medically complicated and uncomplicated patients aged 40 years and older. Am J Obstet Gynecol 157:738, 1987.
106. O'Reilly-Green C, Cohen WR: Pregnancy in women aged 40 and older. Obstet Gynecol Clin North Am 20:313, 1993.

Uncommon Malformation Syndromes of Infants and Pediatric Patients

David D. Frankville

I. INTRODUCTION

This chapter focuses on the numerous malformation syndromes, most of which become apparent during infancy and childhood. Some malformation syndromes are lethal during infancy or childhood and are seen only by pediatric anesthesiologists; however, most anesthesiologists periodically anesthetize children with malformation syndromes. Appendix 14–1, which is an essential and major component of this chapter, is intended to serve as a quick reference for those infrequent but regular encounters with children with known malformation syndromes. The remainder of the chapter is intended to present a systematic approach to the anesthetic management of children with malformations (Fig. 14–1).

A Child with a Malformation
    One or more major malformations
    Three or more minor malformations

            Search for other malformations,
            anomalies, or disorders of
            importance to the anesthesiologist
                Growth anomalies
                Mental deficiency
                Airway malformations
                Chest and cardiac malformations
                Brain and neuromuscular anomalies
                Skeletal malformations
                Renal failure or insufficiency
                Endocrine and hematologic disorders

Malformations consistent with known
syndrome, sequence, or association
    Literature search for anesthetic implications

            Unknown pattern of malformations
                Repeat evaluation for other malforma-
                tions, anomalies, or disorders of impor-
                tance to the anesthesiologist

FIGURE 14–1. General approach to a child with a malformation. Major malformations may be thought of as those that alter the ability of an organ or organ system to perform its usual functional tasks. Minor malformations may be thought of as those that do not result in functional impairment. A single isolated minor malformation is rarely associated with a major malformation. Three or more minor malformations seldom occur without an associated major malformation. Malformations of importance to the anesthesiologist are those that mandate alteration of the anesthetic plan.

Some of the syndromes included in Appendix 14–1 will have few, if any, significant anesthetic implications; however, knowing that there are no major anesthetic implications can be of tremendous value to the clinician. The reader should be aware that, because these syndromes are rare, there is usually a lack of published information on which to base anesthetic management. Epidemiologic information such as incidence and genetic transmission will not be presented. Knowing how rare are the odds of encountering a child with a rare malformation is of little use when that child is waiting for you in the preoperative area.

A. MALFORMATIONS

A *malformation* is defined as poor tissue formation. Malformation is contrasted with *deformation*, which is a result of mechanical forces causing altered morphogenesis in utero. Malformation is also distinct from *disruption*, in which the fetus is subjected to a destructive problem in utero, such as placental vascular insufficiency or infection. The underlying cause of a malformation is a single localized anomaly such as a chromosome defect or the effects of a teratogen. A *malformation syndrome* is a recurring pattern of malformation defects. For example, Down's syndrome is a collection of malformations that includes flat facies, slanted palpebral fissures, small ears, mental deficiency, hypotonia, cardiac defects, and other anomalies. The cause is trisomy 21. Most malformation syndromes are thought to be caused by a single unifying anomaly or defect. A *malformation sequence* is defined as several malformations that can be explained on the basis of a single problem that sequentially causes the malformation of other tissues. For example, the Robin sequence is the result of mandibular hypoplasia prior to week 9 in utero. This results in posterior displacement of the tongue, which then impairs closure of the posterior palatal shelves. The result is the Robin sequence, consisting of micrognathia, glossoptosis, and cleft soft palate. An *association* is an assortment of malformations, usually involving more than one organ system, that does not demonstrate a familial pattern of occurrence. For the purposes of this chapter, the term *malformation syndrome* is intended to include malformation syndromes, malformation sequences, and malformation associations.

Numerous malformation syndromes have

been described[1] and nearly 300 are included in Appendix 14–1. Most malformations that comprise these syndromes are of little or no significance to the anesthesiologist. Examples of these are scalp and facial hair patterning, hypertelorism, inner epicanthal folds, cleft lip, hypodontia, clinodactyly, hypogonadism, and many others. Malformations that are important to the anesthesiologist include airway malformations, cardiopulmonary malformations, central nervous system malformations, neuromuscular anomalies, skeletal malformations, renal malformations leading to renal dysfunction, and endocrine and hematologic anomalies associated with malformation syndromes (Table 14–1). Each of these malformations that may concern the anesthesiologist is covered later in this chapter.

Many infants and children who present for surgery with malformations will not be categorized as having a particular syndrome. These children with their unusual appearances may provide the anesthesiologist with an unpleasant surprise. In this situation, the child should be examined for each of the malformations of concern to the anesthesiologist. The presence of one obvious malformation should trigger a thorough search for others. If three or more minor malformations are found, there is a high likelihood that the child has a malformation syndrome or a major malformation. Minor malformations include anomalies of the dermal ridge patterns, eyes, mouth, ears, fingers, toes, hair, and genitalia. Inconsequential malformations should not lead to complacency. For example, children with a facial malformation as the predominant feature also have a surprisingly high incidence of associated cardiac malformations.

B. GROWTH AND MENTAL DEFICIENCY

Growth deficiency and mental deficiency are not malformations; however, they are in-cluded in this discussion because of the frequency with which they are associated with malformation syndromes. Of these two, mental deficiency presents the more difficult problem to the anesthesiologist. Children (and adults) with mental deficiency or a severe behavioral disorder require anesthesia for procedures that are usually done without anesthesia. In addition, the manner in which anesthesia is induced must often be modified to circumvent the inability or unwillingness of the patient to cooperate. This becomes especially difficult as these children become young adults, with the size and strength to match. It is not uncommon to approach these older children or young adults with alternative induction techniques, as if they were young children.

Growth deficiency is perhaps the most common feature of malformation syndromes. While it is not at all specific, when present, it should not be ignored as an indication of a significant underlying disorder. Major organ system failure should be ruled out before disregarding the small size of a child.

Endocrine disorders, hematologic disorders, and malignancies are also not usually considered malformations; however, they are frequently associated with some malformation syndromes, and a brief discussion of these associations is included in this chapter.

II. AIRWAY MALFORMATIONS

Airway malformations are obviously important to the anesthesiologist. Some airway malformations can lead to a variety of debilitating disease states, including chronic airway obstruction, chronic aspiration, chronic pulmonary infections, and chronic respiratory insufficiency. Airway malformations can also cause difficulty with bag and mask ventilation or laryngoscopy and endotracheal intu-

TABLE 14–1

Malformations Important to Anesthesiologists

Airway malformations	Choanal atresia, micrognathia, microstomia, macroglossia, anomalies of the larynx or trachea, cervical spine anomalies
Cardiopulmonary malformations	Small thoracic cage with or without pulmonary hypoplasia, cardiac malformations, anomalies of the blood vessels
Central nervous system and neuromuscular anomalies	Major brain defects, encephalocele, hydrocephalus, hypotonia, hypertonia
Miscellaneous	Endocrine disorders, hematologic disorders, malignancies
Renal anomalies	Renal insufficiency
Skeletal anomalies	Vertebral anomalies, joint laxity, joint contractures, bone fragility

bation. Abnormal tracheal structures or tracheal fistulas can make ventilation during anesthesia difficult. Problematic airway malformations, and the syndromes with which they might be associated, are presented in Table 14–2. The addition of any of the more common pediatric airway problems, such as enlarged tonsils or active respiratory infections, can further complicate the airway management of these children.

Some airway malformations are not readily apparent by simple physical examination. This is particularly true for malformations of the larynx and trachea. In general, when confronted with a child who has an unfamiliar syndrome, it is prudent to consult a reference such as this to determine the likelihood of encountering these types of airway malformations.

The general goals of preoperative airway assessment—to determine the ease with which ventilation or endotracheal intubation can be accomplished—are the same for both children and adults. In actual practice, it may be difficult to evaluate the airway of infants and children because they may not cooperate; however, most children can usually be cajoled into opening their mouth and extending their neck so the examiner can assess tongue size and neck extension. The hyomental distance can be assessed by viewing the child in profile and by palpating the structures themselves. Sternal retraction, stridor, or mouth breathing may indicate upper airway obstruction. The pediatric airway examination remains more subjective than the adult airway examination because there are no fully tested age- or size-adjusted parameters for infants and children that predict difficulty with mask ventilation or endotracheal intubation.

A. CHOANAL ATRESIA

Choanal atresia or stenosis is often diagnosed by the inability to pass a suction catheter through the posterior nose. Bone tissue is the cause of obstruction in the vast majority of cases. In infants, respiratory distress will occur if both nostrils are obstructed. In this situation, the mouth must be kept open to prevent total upper airway obstruction. Surgical correction or tracheotomy may be required. Even after surgical correction, the nares may remain obstructed until the soft tissue swelling has subsided. Unilateral obstruction may be manifested as chronic nasal

discharge from that nostril. Careful examination for associated airway malformations that would make laryngoscopy difficult should be performed before induction of anesthesia.

Craniosynostosis malformations such as Antley-Bixler syndrome, Apert's syndrome (acrocephalosyndactyly), Crouzon's syndrome (craniofacial dysostosis), Pfeiffer's syndrome (Pfeiffer-type acrocephalosyndactyly), and Saethre-Chotzen syndrome represent a group with a relatively high incidence of choanal atresia. This is not surprising, as these syndromes represent a group in which the bony growth of the head and face is abnormal. Airway obstruction can be severe in Treacher Collins syndrome (Franceschetti-Klein syndrome), Antley-Bixler syndrome, Crouzon's syndrome, and Marshall-Smith syndrome. Patients with Treacher Collins syndrome or Marshall-Smith syndrome present a particularly difficult problem, as both have anatomic features that make both ventilation and laryngoscopy difficult.

B. MICROGNATHIA

Micrognathia is a possible component of more than 25 per cent of all human malformation syndromes. Micrognathia alone, unless quite severe, causes only moderate additional difficulty when a laryngoscopy is performed. In children with severe micrognathia, as can occur with the Robin sequence, Treacher Collins syndrome, facioauriculovertebral spectrum (Goldenhar's syndrome), or trisomy 18 (among others), it may be nearly impossible to visualize the vocal cords with a laryngoscope. When additional airway malformations are present, the level of suspicion that direct laryngoscopy may not be easy or successful must be raised and the anesthetic technique modified to take that into consideration. Table 14–3 lists malformation syndromes associated with multiple (three or more) airway malformations. Of those syndromes listed in Table 14–3, Goldenhar's syndrome and Treacher Collins syndrome are notorious for presenting multiple, particularly difficult airway management problems; however, Table 14–3 is not intended to be an all-inclusive list of difficult airways in pediatrics. Note that the Robin sequence is not included, because it is not associated with multiple airway malformations.

Micrognathia is thought to be a result of reduced movement of the mandible in utero.

Text continued on page 488

TABLE 14-2

Airway Malformations and Associated Syndromes

Choanal Atresia or Stenosis	Micrognathia	Microstomia	Macroglossia	Anomalies of the Larynx and/or Trachea	Cervical Spine Anomalies
Antley-Bixler syndrome (multisynostotic osteodysgenesis, trapezoidcephaly–multiple synostosis)	13q– syndrome	Distal arthrogryposis syndrome	Athyrotic hypothyroidism sequence (hypothyroidism sequence)	Camptomelic dysplasia	Aarskog's syndrome
Apert's syndrome (acrocephalosyndactyly)	18p– syndrome	Freeman-Sheldon syndrome (whistling face syndrome)	Beckwith-Wiedemann syndrome (exomphalos-macroglossia-gigantism)	Cerebrocostomandibular syndrome	Achondroplasia
CHARGE association	4p– syndrome (#4 short arm deletion)	Hallermann-Streiff syndrome (oculomandibulodyscephaly with hypotrichosis syndrome)	Generalized gangliosidosis syndrome, type I (severe infantile type, Caffey pseudo-Hurler syndrome, familial neurovisceral lipidosis)	CHARGE association	Alcohol effects (fetal alcohol syndrome)
Crouzon's syndrome (craniofacial dysostosis)	5p– syndrome (cri-du-chat, partial deletion of short arm of chromosome 5)	Hecht's syndrome (trismus pseudocamptodactyly syndrome)	Hunter's syndrome (mucopolysaccharidosis II)	Chondrodysplasia punctata (Conradi-Hünermann syndrome)	Amyoplasia congenita disruptive sequence (classic arthrogryposis)
de Lange syndrome (Cornelia de Lange, Brachmann-de Lange)	9p– syndrome (9p monosomy)	Oromandibular-limb hypogenesis spectrum (Moebius syndrome, Charlie M. syndrome, facial-limb disruptive spectrum)	Hurler's syndrome (mucopolysaccharidosis I H)	Diastrophic dysplasia (diastrophic nanism syndrome)	Beals' syndrome (Beals' contractural arachnodactyly syndrome)
Di George sequence	Achondrogenesis, type II (Langer-Saldino achondrogenesis, hypochondrogenesis)	Otopalatodigital syndrome, type I (Taybi's syndrome)	Killian/Teschler-Nicola syndrome (Pallister's mosaic syndrome, tetrasomy, 12p)	Di George sequence	Camptomelic dysplasia
Early amnion rupture sequence	Alcohol effects (fetal alcohol syndrome)	Pena-Shokeir phenotype (fetal akinesia/hypokinesia sequence)	Robinow syndrome (fetal face syndrome)		Diastrophic dysplasia (diastrophic nanism syndrome)

Lenz-Majewski hyperostosis syndrome	Aminopterin effects	Popliteal pterygium syndrome (faciogenitopopliteal syndrome)	Scheie's syndrome, (mucopolysaccharidosis I S)	Fabry's syndrome (Anderson-Fabry disease, angiokeratoma corporis diffusum)	Dyggve-Melchior-Clausen syndrome
Marshall-Smith syndrome	Amyoplasia congenita disruptive sequence (classic arthrogryposis)	Rapp-Hodgkin ectodermal dysplasia syndrome (hypohidrotic ectodermal dysplasia, autosomal-dominant type)	Schinzel-Giedion syndrome	Facioauriculovertebral spectrum (hemifacial microsomia, Goldenhar's syndrome)	Escobar's syndrome (multiple pterygium syndrome)
Oral-facial-digital syndrome (OFD syndrome, type I)	Aniridia–Wilms' tumor association	Ruvalcaba's syndrome	Triploidy and diploid-triploid mixoploidy syndrome	Fraser's syndrome (cryptophthalmos syndrome)	Facioauriculovertebral spectrum (hemifacial microsomia, Goldenhar's syndrome)
Pfeiffer's syndrome (Pfeiffer-type acrocephalosyndactyly)	Beals' syndrome (Beals' contractural arachnodactyly syndrome)	Treacher Collins syndrome, (Franceschetti-Klein syndrome)	Trisomy 21 (Down's syndrome)	Frontometaphyseal dysplasia	Fragile X syndrome (Martin-Bell, marker X syndrome)
Saethre-Chotzen syndrome	Bloom syndrome	Trisomy 18 syndrome	Trisomy 4p syndrome (trisomy of the short arm of chromosome 4)	Larsen's syndrome	Frontometaphyseal dysplasia
Schinzel-Giedion syndrome	Camptomelic dysplasia	Valproate effects		Marshall-Smith syndrome	Gorlin's syndrome (basal cell nevus syndrome)
Treacher Collins syndrome (Franceschetti-Klein syndrome)	Cat-eye syndrome (coloboma of iris-anal atresia)			Maternal phenylketonuria (PKU) fetal effects	Jarcho-Levin syndrome (spondylothoracic dysplasia)
Triploidy and diploid-triploid mixoploidy syndrome	Cerebrocostomandibular syndrome			Meckel-Gruber syndrome (dysencephalia splanchnocystica)	Klippel-Feil sequence
Trisomy 18 syndrome	Cerebrooculofacioskeletal (COFS) syndrome			Meningomyelocele, anencephaly, iniencephaly sequences	Kozlowski's spondylometaphyseal dysplasia (Kozlowski's spondylometaphyseal chondrodysplasia)

Table continued on following page

TABLE 14-2

Airway Malformations and Associated Syndromes (Continued)

Choanal Atresia or Stenosis	Micrognathia	Microstomia	Macroglossia	Anomalies of the Larynx and/or Trachea	Cervical Spine Anomalies
	CHARGE association			Miller's syndrome (postaxial acrofacial dysostosis syndrome)	Larsen's syndrome
	Chondrodysplasia punctata (Conradi-Hünermann syndrome)			Multiple neuroma syndrome (multiple endocrine neoplasia, type 2b)	Lethal multiple pterygium syndrome
	Cohen's syndrome			Nager's syndrome (Nager's acrofacial dysostosis syndrome)	Maroteaux-Lamy mucopolysaccharidosis syndrome, (mucopolysaccharidosis VI)
	de Lange syndrome (Cornelia de Lange, Brachmann-de Lange)			Opitz syndrome (hypertelorism-hypospadias, Optiz-Frias, G syndrome, BBB syndrome)	Maternal PKU fetal effects
	Diastrophic dysplasia (diastrophic nanism syndrome)			Pachyonychia congenita syndrome	Meningomyelocele, anencephaly, iniencephaly sequences
	Dubovitz syndrome			Pallister-Hall syndrome	Morquio's syndrome (mucopolysaccharidosis IV, types A and B)
	Escobar's syndrome (multiple pterygium syndrome)			Robin sequence (Pierre Robin syndrome)	Mucopolysaccharidosis VII (Sly's syndrome, β-glucuronidase deficiency)
	Facioauriculovertebral spectrum (hemifacial microsomia, Goldenhar's syndrome)			Short rib–polydactyly syndrome, Majewski's type (short rib syndrome, type II)	Murcs' association

Femoral
hypoplasia–unusual
facies syndrome

Fibrochondrogenesis

Frontometaphyseal
dysplasia

Hajdu-Cheney
syndrome (Cheney's
syndrome,
acroosteolysis
syndrome,
arthrodentoosteodysplasia)

Hallermann-Streiff
syndrome
(oculomandibulodyscephaly
with hypotrichosis
syndrome)

Hurler-Scheie
compound
syndrome
(mucopolysaccharidosis
I H/S)

Killian/Teschler-Nicola
syndrome (Pallister's
mosaic syndrome,
tetrasomy 12p)

Langer's mesomelic
dysplasia
(homozygous
Leri-Weill
dyschondrosteosis
syndrome)

Langer-Giedion
syndrome
(trichorhinophalangeal
syndrome with
exostosis)

Shprintzen's syndrome
(velocardiofacial
syndrome)

Treacher Collins
syndrome
(Franceschetti-Klein
syndrome)

Trisomy 18 syndrome

Trisomy 21 (Down's
syndrome)

VATER association

Pallister-Hall syndrome

Rubinstein-Taybi
syndrome

Spondyloepiphyseal
dysplasia tarda
(X-linked
spondyloepiphyseal
dysplasia)

Trisomy 18 syndrome

Trisomy 21 (Down's
syndrome)

Turner's syndrome
(XO)

Table continued on following page

TABLE 14-2

Airway Malformations and Associated Syndromes (Continued)

Choanal Atresia or Stenosis	Micrognathia	Microstomia	Macroglossia	Anomalies of the Larynx and/or Trachea	Cervical Spine Anomalies
	Lenz-Majewski hyperostosis syndrome				
	Lethal multiple pterygium syndrome				
	Marshall-Smith syndrome				
	Maternal PKU fetal effects				
	Meckel-Gruber syndrome (dysencephalia splanchnocystica)				
	Melnick-Needles syndrome				
	Metaphyseal chondrodysplasia, Jansen type (metaphyseal dysostosis, Jansen type)				
	Miller's syndrome (postaxial acrofacial dysostosis syndrome)				
	Miller-Dieker syndrome (lissencephaly syndrome)				
	Moebius sequence				
	Mohr's syndrome (OFD syndrome, type II)				
	Murcs' association				
	Nager's syndrome (Nager's acrofacial dysostosis syndrome)				
	Neu-Laxova syndrome				
	Noonan's syndrome (Turner-like syndrome)				

Oral-facial-digital
  syndrome (OFD
  syndrome, type I)
Oromandibular-limb
  hypogenesis
  spectrum (Moebius
  syndrome, Charlie M.
  syndrome, facial-limb
  disruptive spectrum)
Otopalatodigital
  syndrome, type II
Pallister-Hall syndrome
Pena-Shokeir
  phenotype (fetal
  akinesia-hypokinesia
  sequence)
Progeria syndrome
  (Hutchinson-Gilford
  syndrome)
Pyknodysostosis
  (Toulouse-Lautrec
  disease)
Radial aplasia-
  thrombocytopenia
  syndrome (TAR
  syndrome)
Retinoic acid
  embryopathy
  (Accutane
  embryopathy)
Roberts-SC
  phocomelia
  syndrome
  (pseudothalidomide
  syndrome)
Robin sequence (Pierre
  Robin syndrome)
Robinow's syndrome
  (fetal face
  syndrome)
Rubinstein-Taybi
  syndrome
Russell-Silver syndrome
  (Silver's syndrome)

Table continued on following page

TABLE 14–2

Airway Malformations and Associated Syndromes (Continued)

Choanal Atresia or Stenosis	Micrognathia	Microstomia	Macroglossia	Anomalies of the Larynx and/or Trachea	Cervical Spine Anomalies
	Schwartz-Jampel syndrome (chondrodystrophica myotonia)				
	Seckel's syndrome				
	Shprintzen's syndrome (velocardiofacial syndrome)				
	Smith-Lemli-Opitz syndrome				
	Stickler's syndrome (hereditary arthroophthalmopathy)				
	Treacher Collins syndrome (Franceschetti-Klein syndrome)				
	Trichorhinophalangeal syndrome				
	Trimethadione effects (fetal trimethadione syndrome, tridione syndrome)				
	Triploidy and diploid-triploid mixoploidy syndrome				
	Trisomy 13 syndrome				
	Trisomy 18 syndrome				
	Trisomy 8 syndrome (trisomy 8/normal mosaicism)				
	Trisomy 9 mosaic syndrome				
	Turner's syndrome (XO)				
	Weaver's syndrome				

TABLE 14-3

Malformation Syndromes Associated with Multiple Airway Malformations of Importance to Anesthesiologists

	Choanal Atresia	Micrognathia	Microstomia	Macroglossia	Abnormal Larynx (L), Trachea (T), or Tracheoesophageal Fistula (TEF)	Cervical Spine
Camptomelic dysplasia		X			T	Vertebral anomalies
CHARGE association	X	X			TEF	
Diastrophic dysplasia (diastrophic nanism syndrome)		X			L	Odontoid hypoplasia
Facioauriculovertebral spectrum (hemifacial microsomia, Goldenhar's syndrome)		X			L	Vertebral fusion
Frontometaphyseal dysplasia		X			T	Vertebral anomalies
Marshall-Smith syndrome	X	X			L	
Maternal PKU fetal effects		X			TEF	Vertebral anomalies
Pallister-Hall syndrome		X			L	Vertebral anomalies
Treacher Collins syndrome (mandibulofacial dysostosis, Franceschetti-Klein syndrome)	X	X	X		L	
Triploidy and diploid-triploid mixoploidy syndrome	X	X		X		
Trisomy 21 (Down's syndrome)				X	TEF	Odontoid hypoplasia
Trisomy 18 syndrome	X	X	X		TEF	Vertebral fusion

This reduced movement can be secondary to physical limitation, myopathy, or central nervous system anomalies. With this in mind, it is not surprising that limited mandibular opening is associated with micrognathia.

In infants, the diagnosis of micrognathia can be made by viewing the profile. This is usually a very subjective assessment. While the tongue often appears to be large and in the way, in most cases it is normal in size but displaced by the small mandible. In the Pierre-Robin syndrome, one of the better-known uncommon malformations of importance to the anesthesiologist, micrognathia is a temporary condition in which the mandible will eventually grow to normal size. Once the patient is past infancy, laryngoscopy is not as difficult a task, because the child has "grown out of it."

C. MICROSTOMIA

Microstomia is a relatively uncommon airway malformation as compared with micrognathia (see Table 14–2). When mild, it is a minor obstacle to laryngoscopy. When it is severe, or when combined with micrognathia, macroglossia, or poor neck extension, direct laryngoscopy may be impossible. When the oral aperture is very small, it may even be difficult to insert fiberoptic intubating guides, laryngeal mask airways, or even oral airways. Skill with blind intubation techniques, fiberoptic bronchoscopy, light wand techniques, or the Bullard laryngoscope can be helpful in this situation. Syndromes associated with severe microstomia include trisomy 18, Hallermann-Streiff syndrome (oculomandibulodyscephaly with hypotrichosis syndrome), and Treacher Collins syndrome. Patients with trisomy 18 or Treacher Collins syndrome may be in the unfortunate situation of having both a small mouth and choanal atresia. Microstomia may be distinguished from micrognathia or limited mouth opening; however, the implications for the anesthesiologist remain the same.

Hecht's syndrome (trismus-pseudocamptodactyly syndrome) is an unusual condition in which the mouth is not particularly small but mouth opening is severely limited by trismus. The trismus is not due to increased muscle tone, but rather to the length of the muscle itself. For this reason, muscle relaxants are of no use, and considering the potential difficulties with laryngoscopy, spontaneous ventilation should be maintained if at all possible. On occasion, patients with distal arthrogryposis syndrome may also suffer from trismus.

Freeman-Sheldon syndrome (whistling face syndrome) is characterized by fibrotic contractures of the facial muscles resulting in a "whistling" appearance. The contractures make laryngoscopy and intubation difficult, particularly if other facial and neck muscles are involved. Because the underlying defect is thought to be a myopathy, there has been some discussion about a possible association with malignant hyperthermia. It has been postulated that the gene responsible for malignant hyperthermia may be linked to or be located near the gene responsible for myopathy.

D. MACROGLOSSIA

Macroglossia is also a relatively uncommon malformation as compared with micrognathia. Children with micrognathia are often thought to have macroglossia; however, this is usually an artifact of trying to enclose a normal-sized tongue within a small space. For the practicing anesthesiologist the clinical problems associated with each are similar. The two general categories of malformations that are most frequently associated with macroglossia are chromosomal malformation syndromes and storage disorder syndromes.

Chromosomal malformation syndromes that feature macroglossia include trisomy 21, trisomy 4p syndrome (trisomy of the short arm of chromosome 4), and triploidy and diploid-triploid mixoploidy syndrome. Trisomy 21 is the condition most frequently associated with macroglossia. Fortunately, in this situation it rarely prevents successful laryngoscopy.

Storage disorders that feature macroglossia include generalized gangliosidosis syndrome type I (severe infantile type, Caffey's pseudo-Hurler's syndrome, familial neurovisceral lipidosis), Hurler's syndrome (mucopolysaccharidosis IH), and Scheie's syndrome (mucopolysaccharidosis IS). In these situations the accumulation of mucopolysaccharides in the tissue of the tongue accounts for the enlargement.

Perhaps the best-known uncommon syndrome associated with macroglossia is Beckwith-Wiedemann syndrome (exophthalmos-macroglossia-gigantism). In the infant, the tongue may be large enough to cause nearly complete airway obstruction. Partial glossectomy may be required in some cases. This is usually deferred until after the newborn period. Laryngoscopy is usually successful, but the anesthesiologist should be prepared for the worst.

E. LARYNGEAL AND TRACHEAL MALFORMATIONS

The best-known laryngeal or tracheal malformation is tracheoesophageal fistula and esophageal atresia. The anesthetic management of this malformation is well documented in most standard pediatric anesthesia textbooks. Other less common laryngeal-tracheal malformations are listed in Table 14–4.

The fact that the larynx or trachea cannot be viewed directly at routine preoperative physical examination is disconcerting; however, almost all of the syndromes known to be associated with laryngeal or tracheal malformations also have associated facial malformations that should give warning to the anesthesiologist. The Di George sequence is the only malformation syndrome that has no external manifestations to warn of the internal anomalies. Many of the syndromes associated with laryngeal or tracheal malformations also have associated micrognathia, and many also have a facial malformation as the predominant feature. Malformation syndromes with laryngeal or tracheal malformations also have associated cervical spine anomalies a large part of the time. What may be surprising, but of great importance to the anesthesiologist, is that the majority of syndromes with laryngeal

---

TABLE 14–4

Tracheal, Laryngeal, and Bronchial Anomalies Important to Anesthesiologists

Tracheoesophageal fistula
Laryngeal or tracheal stenosis
Laryngeal webbing
Laryngeal cleft
Dysplastic tracheal cartilage or rings
Tracheal calcifications
Small or rudimentary epiglottis
Absence of the right or left lung
Tracheal or laryngeal obstruction by tumor or other tissue
Infolding or easily displaced arytenoids
Short trachea

---

or tracheal malformations can also involve cardiovascular malformations. These include Pallister-Hall syndrome, Shprintzen's syndrome (velocardiofacial syndrome), CHARGE association, VATER association, Di George sequence, and trisomy 18 syndrome. For this reason, evaluation of any child with known laryngeal or tracheal anomalies should include a thorough examination directed at detecting cardiovascular defects. It is also interesting to note that none of the syndromes that can present with laryngeal or tracheal malformations are associated with renal malformations severe enough to cause renal failure.

Laryngeal web describes a condition of the vocal cords or arytenoids being joined by a web of membranous tissue.[2] The symptoms are proportionate to the degree of obstruction. In infants whose obstruction is not severe, stridor is the most common sign. As the tissue bridge may be relatively thick, division of the web is best left to the surgeon. In extreme cases, rigid bronchoscopy could be used to relieve total or nearly total airway obstruction. Shprintzen's syndrome (velocardiofacial syndrome) is one of the few syndromes associated with laryngeal webbing.

More common than obstruction by laryngeal webbing is obstruction from a tumor or deposits of abnormal tissue. Laryngeal or tracheal obstruction caused by tumor is a feature of two of the hamartosis syndromes: multiple neuroma syndrome and the Peutz-Jeghers syndrome. Obstruction caused by deposits of abnormal tissue occurs in chondrodysplasia punctata (calcium deposits), pachyonychia congenita syndrome (leukokeratosis), and Fabry's syndrome (ceramide trihexoside deposits).

A short trachea or shorter than normal distance between the vocal cords and the carina has been associated with a number of malformation syndromes. In particular, this anomaly is seen with some regularity in the Di George sequence, some skeletal dysplasias, congenital rubella, and syndromes with associated cardiac malformations. A combination of short tracheal rings and fewer tracheal rings accounts for this malformation. The implication is that the usual formulas for positioning the tip of the endotracheal tube may result in endobronchial intubation.

F. CERVICAL SPINE ANOMALIES

Cervical spine anomalies important to the anesthesiologist include those that reduce cervical spine mobility, allow cervical spine sub-luxation, or are associated with spinal cord or nerve compression. Cervical spine immobility can result from either a bony anomaly or muscle contracture. Cervical spine subluxa-tion and rigidity are the two of the most difficult anomalies for the anesthesiologist to manage.

Osteochondrodysplasias, including dia-strophic dysplasia, Dyggve-Melchior-Clau-sen syndrome, Kozlowski's spondylometa-physeal dysplasia, spondyloepiphyseal dys-plasia tarda, camptomelic dysplasia, and frontometaphyseal dysplasia, are frequently associated with cervical spine anomalies. Odontoid hypoplasia is the most common anomaly in this group. Children with glyco-gen storage disorders also have a relatively high rate of cervical spine malformations. As in the osteochondrodysplasias, odontoid hy-poplasia is the most frequently encountered anomaly.

Cervical spine subluxation most often in-volves the alanto-occipital joint. Syndromes associated with cervical spine subluxation or instability are listed in Table 14–5. Of the mal-formation syndromes listed, trisomy 21 is en-countered most often by the anesthesiologist. The anesthetic management of children with trisomy 21 can be considered a model for all children with cervical spine subluxation malformations, including those in the catego-ries of osteochondrodysplasias and glycogen storage disorder.

In children with trisomy 21, cervical spine instability or subluxation, as evidenced by abnormal radiographs or even symptoms of cord compression, is present up to 20 per cent of time. This high prevalence of cervical spine lesions has led some authors to recommend radiography before elective surgery for all children with trisomy 21; however, a recent review of practice in North America suggests that this recommendation is not widely fol-lowed. It does seem reasonable to obtain cer-vical spine radiographs of children with symptoms of cord compression and to avoid any unnecessary twisting, extension, or posi-tioning of the head when anesthetizing any child with trisomy 21. Children determined to be at substantial risk for cervical cord com-pression during intubation may benefit from fiberoptic-guided intubation (bronchoscope, fiberoptic laryngoscope blades) or the light wand. The author is not aware of any cases of spinal cord damage that were solely the result of laryngoscopy.

Without adequate cervical spine mobility, and particularly when combined with other airway anomalies, direct laryngoscopy can be exceedingly difficult. Klippel-Feil sequence and the facioauriculovertebral spectrum (first and second branchial arch syndrome, ocu-loauricular vertebral dysplasia, hemifacial mi-crosomia, Goldenhar's syndrome) are the two malformation syndromes most often associ-ated with reduced cervical spine mobility. Most authors have advocated using fiberoptic intubation techniques, though other devices, such as the light wand or the Bullard laryngo-scope, should also be effective. Blind intuba-tion techniques have not been utilized to the same extent since physicians have become more skilled with fiberoptic laryngoscopy.

III. CHEST AND CARDIAC MALFORMATIONS

Two categories of malformations of the chest and thorax are particularly important to the anesthesiologist. These are anomalies of the chest cavity with pulmonary hypoplasia, and malformations of the heart and great ves-sels. Tracheoesophageal fistula is discussed in the previous section on airway malforma-tions. The majority of infants with a small chest cavity and pulmonary hypoplasia have extremely limited life expectancy, and most anesthesiologists will not encounter them. Close to 50 malformation syndromes, how-ever, have a high incidence of associated car-diovascular anomalies, and nearly 50 more are distinctly, but less often, associated. This means that cardiovascular anomalies are as-sociated with approximately one third of all human malformation syndromes.

A. SMALL CHEST CAVITY AND PULMONARY HYPOPLASIA

Table 14–6 lists the malformation syn-dromes that are associated with a small tho-racic cavity, and possibly pulmonary hypo-plasia. A small thoracic cavity and pulmonary hypoplasia are frequently linked because a small chest cavity does not allow for normal development and growth of the lungs, which occurs relatively late in gestation. This is the same situation that occurs with diaphrag-matic hernia, when the intrusion of abdomi-nal contents into the chest cavity prevents

TABLE 14–5

Syndromes Associated with Cervical Spine Subluxation or Rigidity

Subluxation	Rigidity
Diastrophic dysplasia (diastrophic nanism syndrome)	Escobar's syndrome (multiple pterygium syndrome)
Dyggve-Melchior-Clausen syndrome	Facioauriculovertebral spectrum (hemifacial microsomia, Goldenhar's syndrome)
Kozlowski's spondylometaphyseal dysplasia (Kozlowski's spondylometaphyseal chondrodysplasia)	Gorlin's syndrome (basal cell nevus syndrome)
Maroteaux-Lamy mucopolysaccharidosis syndrome (mucopolysaccharidosis VI)	Klippel-Feil sequence
Morquio's syndrome (mucopolysaccharidosis IV, types A and B)	Trisomy 18 syndrome
Mucopolysaccharidosis VII (Sly's syndrome, β-glucuronidase deficiency)	Murcs' association
Trisomy 21 (Down's syndrome)	

TABLE 14–6

Malformation Syndromes Associated with a Small Chest Cavity, with or without Pulmonary Hypoplasia

Syndrome	Category
Achondrogenesis, type II (Langer-Saldino achondrogenesis, hypochondrogenesis)	Osteochondrodysplasias
Achondroplasia	Osteochondrodysplasias
Achondrogenesis, types Ia and Ib	Osteochondrodysplasias
Apert's syndrome (acrocephalosyndactyly)	Craniosynostosis
Camptomelic dysplasia	Osteochondrodysplasias
Cerebrocostomandibular syndrome	Miscellaneous
Chondroectodermal dysplasia (Ellis–van Creveld syndrome)	Osteochondrodysplasias
Cleidocranial dysostosis	Osteochondrodysplasia with osteopetrosis
Diastrophic dysplasia (diastrophic nanism syndrome)	Osteochondrodysplasias
Early amnion rupture sequence	Miscellaneous
Fibrochondrogenesis	Osteochondrodysplasias
Hypophosphatasia	Osteochondrodysplasias
Jarcho-Levin syndrome (spondylothoracic dysplasia)	Miscellaneous
Jeune's thoracic dystrophy	Osteochondrodysplasias
Lethal multiple pterygium syndrome	Brain or neuromuscular defects
Meckel-Gruber syndrome (dysencephalia splanchnocystica)	Brain or neuromuscular defects
Melnick-Needles syndrome	Miscellaneous
Metaphyseal chondrodysplasia, Jansen type (metaphyseal dysostosis, Jansen type)	Osteochondrodysplasias
Metatrophic dysplasia (metatrophic dwarfism syndrome)	Osteochondrodysplasias
Oligohydramnios sequence (Potter's syndrome)	Miscellaneous
Osteogenesis imperfecta syndrome, type II (osteogenesis imperfecta congenita, Vrolik's disease)	Connective tissue disorder
Otopalatodigital syndrome, type II	Characterized by facial defect
Pallister-Hall syndrome	Brain or neuromuscular defects
Pena-Shokeir phenotype (fetal akinesia-hypokinesia sequence)	Brain or neuromuscular defects
Progeria syndrome (Hutchinson-Gilford syndrome)	Miscellaneous
Proteus syndrome	Hamartosis
Pseudoachondroplastic spondyloepiphyseal dysplasia (SED)	Osteochondrodysplasias
Short rib–polydactyly syndrome, Majewski type (short rib syndrome, type II)	Osteochondrodysplasias
Short rib–polydactyly syndrome, non-Majewski type (short rib syndrome, type I)	Osteochondrodysplasias
Thanatophoric dysplasia	Osteochondrodysplasias
Trisomy 9 mosaic syndrome	Chromosomal

normal lung development. If the condition is not lethal early in infancy, these children will suffer chronic respiratory tract infections. As might be expected, almost all children with a small chest cavity also have vertebral or rib anomalies.

Surprisingly, the number of syndromes associated with *both* a small chest cavity *and* cardiovascular malformations is relatively small (Table 14–7). The most severe of these include chondroectodermal dysplasia (Ellis–van Creveld syndrome), Pallister-Hall syndrome, Apert's syndrome (acrocephalosyndactyly), lethal multiple pterygium syndrome, and Meckel-Gruber syndrome (dysencephalia splanchnocystica), each of which may have both pulmonary hypoplasia and a cardiac defect.

There are several syndromes that are associated with both a small chest and significant airway malformations. These include short rib–polydactyly syndrome (hypoplasia of epiglottis and larynx), lethal multiple pterygium syndrome (micrognathia and chin-to-sternum flexion contractures), cerebrocostomandibular syndrome (severe micrognathia and abnormal tracheal rings), Pallister-Hall syndrome (micrognathia, laryngeal cleft, dysplastic tracheal cartilage, cervical spine anomalies), camptomelic dysplasia (micrognathia, cervical spine anomalies, tracheobronchomalacia), and diastrophic dysplasia (micrognathia, odontoid hypoplasia with subluxation, laryngotracheal stenosis).

The majority of malformation syndromes that are associated with a small chest cavity, with or without pulmonary hypoplasia, fall into the general category of the osteochondrodysplasias. Note that, even with the small

stature seen with the osteochondrodysplasias, there is disproportionate reduction in the size of the thorax.

The anesthetic management of infants or children with a small chest cavity depends entirely on the severity of the pulmonary hypoplasia and on any other significant malformations that may be present. It is the immaturity or absence of adequate normal lung that leads to respiratory insufficiency or chronic pulmonary infections, and the anesthesiologist can do little to correct this situation. The hypoplastic lung will not seem to inflate properly, and excessive airway pressures can lead to pneumothorax. Gas exchange is impaired because of the reduced surface area of the lung. Children with chronic pulmonary infections may require removal of abnormal bronchial segments.

B. CARDIOVASCULAR MALFORMATIONS

Cardiovascular malformations are obviously important to the anesthesiologist. After the central nervous system, the cardiovascular system is the one most affected by anesthetic drugs. A discussion of the anesthetic management for every possible cardiovascular malformation is beyond the scope of this chapter; however, because cardiovascular malformations are so important to the anesthesiologist who must anesthetize children with malformation syndromes, two topics will be discussed. These are (1) identifying which malformation syndromes are likely to present with a cardiovascular defect, and (2) what to do if a cardiac malformation is suspected but the urgency of the surgical procedure leaves no time for proper preoperative evaluation.

1. Cardiac Defects and Associated Malformation Syndromes

Table 14–8 lists syndromes that are frequently or occasionally associated with cardiovascular malformations. Both lists are quite extensive. Some of the malformation syndromes listed in Table 14–8 occur often enough to link them to specific cardiovascular defects. Examples of these include the association between trisomy 21 and endocardial

---

TABLE 14–7

Malformation Syndromes Associated with Both a Small Chest and Cardiovascular Malformations

Chondroectodermal dysplasia (Ellis–van Creveld syndrome)
Pallister-Hall syndrome
Short rib–polydactyly syndrome, non-Majewski type (short rib syndrome, type I)
Trisomy 9 mosaic syndrome
Apert's syndrome (acrocephalosyndactyly)
Camptomelic dysplasia
Lethal multiple pterygium syndrome
Meckel-Gruber syndrome (dysencephalia splanchnocystica)
Thanatophoric dysplasia

cushion defects or Turner's syndrome and coarctation of the aorta. Many malformation syndromes associated with cardiac malformations do not have a known association with specific cardiac anomalies.

Chromosomal malformation syndromes are frequently associated with cardiovascular malformations (see Table 14–8). Of the 24 chromosomal malformation syndromes listed in Appendix 14–1, 14 are frequently associated with cardiovascular anomalies and another three are occasionally associated. The two major exceptions are those children that have XXY (Klinefelter's) syndrome, and XYY syndrome. Because of the high incidence of associated cardiac malformations, any child with a known chromosomal malformation syndrome should be evaluated for cardiac defects before surgery. Ideally, this should include a physical examination with particular attention to the weight, pulses, and blood pressure measurements in all extremities, skin color and perfusion, auscultation of the heart, and noninvasive measurement of the SpO_2. If any of these are abnormal, cardiac echocardiography is indicated. The types of cardiac defects seen with chromosomal malformation syndromes vary greatly and are not limited to atrioventricular canal–type defects.

Connective tissue malformation syndromes are associated with fairly specific types of cardiovascular anomalies. These are generally valvular or vessel wall anomalies. Examples include osteogenesis imperfecta syndrome type I (vessel fragility, mitral valve prolapse), Beals' syndrome (mitral valve prolapse), Ehlers-Danlos syndrome (fragile blood vessels, valvular prolapse, vessel dilatation), homocystinuria syndrome (medial weakness of the arteries with intimal hyperplasia leading to irregular vessel lumens and excessive vascular thrombosis), and Marfan's syndrome (ascending aortic dilatation or dissection, aortic valve insufficiency, aneurysms of other great vessels, mitral valve prolapse).

Another category of malformation syndromes with a strong association with valvular defects are the storage disorder malformation syndromes. Examples of these include Hurler's syndrome (cardiac failure secondary to coronary vascular narrowing or valvular disease), Morquio's syndrome (aortic valve insufficiency), pseudo-Hurler's polydystrophy syndrome (aortic valve disease), Scheie's syndrome (aortic valve disease), Hurler-Scheie compound syndrome (mitral valve prolapse), Maroteaux-Lamy mucopolysac-

charidosis syndrome (valvular heart disease), and mucopolysaccharidosis VII (valvular heart disease). In addition to the valvular anomalies, some of the syndromes in the storage disorder group may involve a severe cardiomyopathy in the absence of valvular disease. This is secondary to accumulation of metabolic materials in the cardiac tissue. These syndromes are Hunter's syndrome and Leroy I-cell syndrome.

Environmental agent malformations are frequently associated with cardiac defects. These include the effects of maternal exposure to alcohol, retinoic acid, rubella, valproate, hydantoin, trimethadione, and warfarin. No specific cardiovascular malformations are associated with the general group of environmental agent exposure malformations.

In addition to an association with cardiac defects, some hamartosis malformation syndromes are also susceptible to acquired cardiac defects from the accumulation of hamartoma in the heart. They can invade and disrupt the cardiac chambers, muscle walls, and even the conduction system. The best known of these are neurofibromatosis and tuberous sclerosis.

An interesting association exists between cardiac defects and syndromes characterized by facial or craniofacial defects. The cardiac defects are only occasional occurrences in these two groups of malformation syndromes; however, because head, face, and cardiac malformations are not commonly thought to be associated with each other, the unwary anesthesiologist may be taken by surprise. There are no specific cardiac anomalies that are closely associated with these groups. Severe airway malformations do occur in children with facial and craniofacial malformations. Examples of syndromes that may include both airway and cardiac malformations include Fraser's, Larsen's, Miller's, Nager's, Opitz', Roberts-SC phocomelia syndrome, Shprintzen's, Stickler's, Treacher Collins, Antley-Bixler, and Apert's syndromes. Anesthetizing a child with both cardiac and airway malformations is challenging for even the most skilled anesthesiologists.

2. Anesthetic Management of a Child with a Suspected Cardiac Defect

If a child with a malformation syndrome requires emergency surgery and there is no

TABLE 14-8

Syndromes Associated with Cardiovascular Malformations

Frequently Associated	Occasionally Associated
Brain or neuromuscular defects	Brain or neuromuscular defects
Miller-Dieker syndrome (lissencephaly syndrome)	Cohen's syndrome
Pallister-Hall syndrome	Lethal multiple pterygium syndrome
Steinert's myotonic dystrophy syndrome (Steinert's syndrome, dystrophia myotonica)	Meckel-Gruber syndrome (dysencephalia splanchnocystica)
Zellweger's syndrome (cerebrohepatorenal syndrome)	Neu-Laxova syndrome
Characterized by facial defect	Schinzel-Giedion syndrome
Noonan syndrome (Turner-like syndrome)	Characterized by facial defect
Shprintzen syndrome (velocardiofacial syndrome)	Blepharophimosis syndrome (familial blepharophimosis syndrome)
Williams syndrome	Coffin-Lowry syndrome
Chromosomal	FG syndrome
Trisomy 21, Down's syndrome	Fraser's syndrome (cryptophtalamos syndrome)
Turner syndrome (XO)	Hays-Wells syndrome of ectodermal dysplasia (ankyloblepharon-ectodermal dysplasia-clefting syndrome, AEC syndrome)
13q – syndrome	Larsen syndrome
18q – syndrome	Miller's syndrome (postaxial acrofacial dysostosis syndrome)
4p – syndrome (short arm deletion of chromosome 4)	Nager's syndrome (Nager's acrofacial dysostosis syndrome)
9p – syndrome (9p monosomy)	Opitz syndrome (hypertelorism-hypospadius, Opitz-Frias, G syndrome, BBB syndrome)
Cat-eye syndrome (coloboma of iris–anal atresia)	Roberts-SC phocomelia syndrome (pseudothalidomide syndrome, hypomelia-hypertrichosis-facial hemangioma syndrome)
Partial trisomy 10q syndrome	Robinow's syndrome (fetal face syndrome)
Triploidy and diploid-triploid mixoploidy syndrome	Ruvalcaba's syndrome
Trisomy 13 syndrome	Smith-Lemli-Opitz syndrome
Trisomy 18 syndrome	Stickler's syndrome (hereditary arthroopthalmopathy)
Trisomy 4p syndrome (trisomy of the short arm of chromosome 4)	Townes' syndrome
Trisomy 9 mosaic syndrome	Treacher Collins syndrome (mandibulofacial dysostosis, Franceschetti-Klein syndrome)
XXXXX (penta X syndrome)	Waardenburg's syndrome types I and II
Connective tissue disorder	Chromosomal
Beals' syndrome (Beals' contractural arachnodactyly syndrome)	5p – syndrome (cri du chat, partial deletion of short arm of chromosome 5)
Ehlers-Danlos syndrome	Trisomy 9p syndrome
Homocystinuria syndrome	XXXY and XXXXY syndromes
Marfan's syndrome	Connective tissue disorder
Environmental agents	Osteogenesis imperfecta syndrome, type I (autosomal-dominant osteogenesis imperfecta, Lobstein's disease)
Alcohol effects (fetal alcohol syndrome)	Craniosynostosis
Maternal PKU fetal effects	Antley-Bixler syndrome (multisynostotic trapezoidcephaly–multiple synostosis)
Retinoic acid embryopathy (Accutane embryopathy)	Apert's syndrome (acrocephalosyndactyly)
Rubella exposure effects	Baller-Gerold syndrome (craniosynostosis–radial aplasia syndrome)
Valproate effects	Carpenter's syndrome
Growth deficiency	Saethre-Chotzen syndrome
Mulibrey nanism syndrome (perheentupa syndrome)	
Rubinstein-Taybi syndrome	
Hamartosis	
Multiple lentigines syndrome (LEOPARD syndrome)	

Limb defects
  Aase's syndrome
  CHILD syndrome
  Holt-Oram syndrome (cardiac-limb defect)
  Radial aplasia–thrombocytopenia syndrome (TAR syndrome)
Miscellaneous
  Arteriohepatic dysplasia (Alagille's syndrome)
  CHARGE association
  Di George sequence
  Kartagener's syndrome
  Laterality sequences (Ivemark's syndrome, polysplenia syndrome, asplenia syndrome)
  VATER association
Osteochondrodysplasias
  Chondroectodermal dysplasia (Ellis–van Creveld syndrome)
  Geleophysic dysplasia
  Short rib–polydactyly syndrome, non-Majewski type (short rib syndrome, type I)
Storage disorders
  Hunter's syndrome (mucopolysaccharidosis II)
  Hurler's syndrome (mucopolysaccharidosis I H)
  Leroy's I-cell syndrome (mucolipidosis II)
  Morquio's syndrome (mucopolysaccharidosis IV, types A and B)
  Pseudo-Hurler's polydystrophy syndrome (mucolipidosis III)
  Scheie's syndrome (mucopolysaccharidosis I S)

Environmental agents
  Hydantoin effects (fetal dilantin syndrome, fetal hydantoin sequence)
  Trimethadione effects (fetal trimethadione syndrome, tridione syndrome)
  Warfarin effects (warfarin embryopathy, fetal warfarin syndrome)
Growth deficiency
  de Lange syndrome (Cornelia de Lange, Brachmann–de Lange)
Hamartosis
  Goltz's syndrome
  Linear sebaceous nevus sequence (nevus sebaceus of Jadassohn)
  Neurofibromatosis syndrome
  Sturge-Weber sequence
  Tuberous sclerosis syndrome (adenoma sebaceum)
Limb defects
  Fanconi's pancytopenia syndrome
Miscellaneous
  Bardet-Biedl syndrome
  Coffin-Siris syndrome
  Fabry's syndrome (Anderson-Fabry disease, angiokeratoma corporis diffusum)
  Facioauriculovertebral spectrum (first and second branchial arch syndrome, oculoauricular–vertebral dysplasia, hemifacial microsomia, Goldenhar's syndrome)
  Klippel-Feil sequence
Osteochondrodysplasias
  Camptomelic dysplasia
  Thanatophoric dysplasia
Other skeletal dysplasias
  Langer's mesomelic dysplasia (homozygous Leri-Weill dyschondrosteosis syndrome)
  Weill-Marchesani syndrome (brachydactyly-spherophakia syndrome)
Overgrowth
  Beckwith-Wiedemann syndrome (exomphalos-macroglossia-gigantism)
  Fragile X syndrome (Martin-Bell, marker X syndrome)
Storage disorders
  Hurler-Scheie compound syndrome (mucopolysaccharidosis I H/S)
  Maroteaux-Lamy mucopolysaccharidosis syndrome (mucopolysaccharidosis VI)
  Mucopolysaccharidosis VII (Sly's syndrome, β-glucuronidase deficiency)

time for a thorough cardiac evaluation, the anesthesiologist is placed in a difficult position. My approach is to search quickly for evidence of cardiac failure, hypoxemia, or dysrhythmias. These are the primary manifestations of cardiovascular disease.

Cardiac failure occurs when the heart is unable to pump enough blood to the body to meet systemic demands. This usually occurs when either systemic cardiac output is reduced or cardiac output is diverted away from the systemic circulation. Reduction of cardiac output is caused by the well-known mechanisms of bradycardia, reduced preload, increased afterload, or reduced contractility. Diversion of cardiac output occurs when there is a left-to-right shunt through either a ventricular septal defect or a large systemic arterial-pulmonary arterial connection (such as a patent ductus or a large surgical shunt). Cardiac failure may be secondary to a combination of both reduction and diversion of cardiac output.

Table 14–9 lists some of the signs and symptoms of cardiac failure. The most important of these is failure to thrive or low weight. While this is a very nonspecific sign, it usually indicates the presence of some systemic disorder. If there is a concern that the child has a cardiac defect, it must be assumed that the failure to thrive is secondary to cardiac disease. This occurs because the cardiovascular system is able to pump enough blood to keep the child alive but not enough to sustain adequate growth. A parent's account of a child's exercise tolerance is usually very subjective and less useful than knowing the child's weight.

If cardiac failure is diagnosed and the cardiac malformation causing it is not known,

it is reasonable to initiate empiric therapy. Specifically, (1) optimize the heart rate by treating any dysrhythmias; (2) optimize the preload with blood or intravenous fluids; (3) improve contractility with β-adrenergic drugs; and (4) minimize the impact of anesthetic drugs on any of the above. Many anesthesiologists are reluctant to use β-adrenergic drugs; however, in the presence of cardiac failure secondary to a cardiac malformation, these drugs support the cardiovascular system until more information is obtained.

This therapy successfully treats cardiac failure in the majority of cases; however, the cardiac output may still be diverted away from the systemic circulation by left-to-right shunting through a patent ductus, a ventricular septal defect, or an overly large systemic-pulmonary artery shunt. The diversion of cardiac output that occurs with excessive left-right shunting can be minimized by avoiding excessive FIO_2, respiratory alkalosis, and hypocarbia.

In this era of noninvasive SpO_2 measurement, diagnosis of hypoxemia is relatively easy. Table 14–9 summarizes some of the clinical signs and symptoms of chronic hypoxemia. Chronic hypoxemia is a systemic disorder. All of the major organ systems are injured to some extent. Just as with cardiac failure, the inability to grow is an important marker for significant chronic hypoxemia. Decreased exercise tolerance is an important but more subjective finding. Determining whether the hypoxemia is secondary to cardiac malformations or acute or chronic pulmonary disease can be difficult. Auscultation is helpful in differentiating the two as lung disease should have characteristic pulmonary findings.

If hypoxemia secondary to cardiac malfor-

TABLE 14–9

Manifestations of Cardiac Failure, Hypoxemia, and Dysrhythmias

Cardiac Failure	Hypoxemia	Dysrhythmias
Decreased weight or failure to thrive	Cyanosis or low SpO_2 reading	Episodic congestive heart failure
Decreased exercise tolerance	Decreased weight or failure to thrive	Palpitations
Pale or ashen color	Decreased exercise tolerance	Syncope
Diaphoresis	Polycythemia	Decreased exercise tolerance
Cardiomegaly	Surgical scar	Surgical scar
Wheezing, retractions, and rales	Unexpected hypoxemia during surgery	Dysrhythmias during surgery
Hepatomegaly or peripheral edema		
Hypoxemia		
Surgical scar		
Unexpected hypotension during surgery		

sure of the defect depends on the structures contained within. An anterior encephalocele may present as a mass in the nose causing airway obstruction, continuous nasal discharge, or recurrent meningitis. The basal encephalocele may contain the hypothalamus or other major structures. This may preclude surgical closure. The posterior encephalocele is associated with hydrocephalus and blindness. In addition, normal positioning of the head for laryngoscopy may be impossible if the occipital mass is large.[3]

Only a few malformation syndromes are associated with encephaloceles, and most of them are also associated with major structural brain defects and, thus, with very limited life expectancy. The two environmental agent exposures that lead to encephalocele are the hyperthermia-induced spectrum of defects and the early amnion rupture sequence, which almost always results in a stillbirth. The only two malformation syndromes associated with encephalocele in which survival past infancy is likely are Roberts-SC phocomelia syndrome (pseudothalidomide syndrome, hypomelia-hypertrichosis–facial hemangioma syndrome), and facioauriculo vertebral spectrum (first and second branchial arch syndrome, oculoauricular vertebral dysplasia, hemifacial microsomia, Goldenhar's syndrome).

C. HYDROCEPHALUS

Hydrocephalus is associated with over 30 malformation syndromes (see Table 14–10). Many are chromosomal malformation syndromes, or brain or neuromuscular defect syndromes of which hydrocephalus is just one of many structural brain defects. Hydrocephalus is a feature of the osteochondrodysplasias, occurring as a result of bony compression that prevents free flow of cerebrospinal fluid. Some of the craniosynostosis syndromes are associated with hydrocephalus for the same reason. Examples of these include achondroplasia, acrodysostosis, Antley-Bixler syndrome, Apert's syndrome, and Pfeiffer's syndrome.

Hydrocephalus can be a feature of the hamartosis and storage disorder syndromes when tumor or unusual tissue overgrowth obstructs flow of cerebrospinal fluid. This can occur in tuberous sclerosis and neurofibromatosis syndromes. The anesthetic management of children and adults with hydrocephalus is described in most anesthesia textbooks and will not be discussed here.

D. HYPOTONIA AND HYPERTONIA

Many malformation syndromes are characterized by abnormal muscle tone. Some malformations can be traced to abnormal movement or muscle tone during a critical part of development. Examples of this are reduced fetal movement, leading to joint contractures, and lack of diaphragmatic movement, leading to pulmonary hypoplasia. Malformation syndromes associated with hypotonia and hypertonia are listed in Table 14–11. Some syndromes may exhibit both hypotonia and hypertonia or begin with hypertonia which then progresses to hypotonia.

Hypotonia is more common than hypertonia. As alluded to earlier, lack of movement during development may be the cause of structural malformations. Because of this, hypotonia is frequently associated with other limb and skeletal malformations. Hypotonia may be due to a central nervous system defect, a defect of the neuromuscular junction, or a defect of the muscle itself. In addition, hypotonia may not be secondary to a malformation at all, but could instead be the result of a nutritional or metabolic disorder.

Hypotonia is associated with a wide variety of malformation syndromes. It is obviously a feature of many of the syndromes that fall into the brain or neuromuscular defect category; however, even within this category, hypotonia is the direct result of severe structural brain defects in only a few situations. These are the cerebrooculofacioskeletal (COFS) syndrome, Miller-Dieker syndrome, and Zellweger's syndrome. In most cases, muscle weakness is a clinical finding only, though it may be quite severe and debilitating. In most of the malformation syndromes presented in Table 14–11, hypotonia is thought to be secondary to central nervous system anomalies that are not apparent as major structural brain defects. In some categories, such as connective tissue disorders, hamartosis, and storage disorders, weakness is thought to be secondary to the muscle itself. It is surprising to note the number of malformation syndromes characterized by facial defects that are associated with hypotonia.

On occasion, the hypotonia is most severe during infancy, leading to problems with res-

TABLE 14–11

Malformation Syndromes Associated with Hypotonia and Hypertonia

Hypotonia

Category	Syndromes
Brain or neuromuscular defects	Angelman's syndrome (happy puppet syndrome) Cerebrooculofacioskeletal (COFS) syndrome Killian/Teschler-Nicola syndrome (Pallister's mosaic syndrome, tetrasomy 12p) Lowe's syndrome (oculocerebrorenal syndrome) Marinesco-Sjögren syndrome Miller-Dieker syndrome (lissencephaly syndrome) Pena-Shokeir phenotype (fetal akinesia/hypokinesia sequence) Prader-Willi syndrome Zellweger's syndrome (cerebrohepatorenal syndrome)
Characterized by facial defect	Blepharophimosis syndrome (familial blepharophimosis syndrome) Coffin-Lowry syndrome FG syndrome Langer-Giedion syndrome (trichorhinophalangeal syndrome with exostosis) Shprintzen's syndrome (velocardiofacial syndrome) Stickler's syndrome (hereditary arthroopthalmopathy) Trichorhinophalangeal syndrome Williams syndrome
Chromosomal	Trisomy 21 (Down's syndrome) 18q− syndrome 4p− syndrome (chromosome 4 short arm deletion)

Hypertonia

Category	Syndromes
Brain or neuromuscular defects	Menkes' syndrome, (Menkes' kinky hair syndrome) Schinzel-Giedion syndrome Sjögren-Larsson syndrome X-linked hydrocephalus syndrome Freeman-Sheldon syndrome (whistling face syndrome) Schwartz-Jampel syndrome (chondrodystrophica myotonia) Steinert's myotonic dystrophy syndrome (Steinert's syndrome, dystrophia myotonica) Oculodentodigital syndrome (oculodentodigital dysplasia) Smith-Lemli-Opitz syndrome
Characterized by facial defect	
Chromosomal	Trisomy 13 syndrome Trisomy 18 syndrome Trisomy 4p syndrome (trisomy of the short arm of chromosome 4)
Connective tissue disorder	Homocystinuria syndrome
Environmental agents	Iodine deficiency effects (endemic cretinism)
Growth deficiency	de Lange syndrome (Cornelia de Lange, Brachmann-de Lange) De Sanctis-Cacchione syndrome (xerodermic idiocy syndrome)
Hamartosis	Incontinentia pigmenti syndrome (Bloch-Sulzberger syndrome) Sturge-Weber sequence
Overgrowth	Weaver's syndrome
Skin dysplasias	Xeroderma pigmentosa syndrome

Category	Syndromes	Storage disorders
		Hunter's syndrome (mucopolysaccharidosis II)
Connective tissue disorder	5p− syndrome (cri-du-chat, partial deletion of chromosome 5 short arm) 9p− syndrome (9p monosomy) Trisomy 13 syndrome Trisomy 20p syndrome XXXY and XXXXY syndromes Camurati-Englemann syndrome (progressive diaphyseal dysplasia) Marfan's syndrome Osteogenesis imperfecta syndrome, type II (osteogenesis imperfecta congenita, Vrolik's disease)	
Environmental agents	Aminopterin effects Hyperthermia-induced spectrum of defects	
Growth deficiency	Johanson-Blizzard syndrome Mulibrey nanism syndrome (perheentupa syndrome)	
Hamartosis	Multiple neuroma syndrome (multiple endocrine neoplasia, type 2b) Proteus syndrome Ruvalcaba-Myhre syndrome	
Miscellaneous	Börjeson-Forssman-Lehmann syndrome Coffin-Siris syndrome Fabry's syndrome (Anderson-Fabry disease, angiokeratoma corporis diffusum) Rieger's syndrome	
Osteochondrodysplasias	Achondroplasia Frontometaphyseal dysplasia Hajdu-Cheney syndrome, (Cheney's syndrome, acroosteolysis syndrome, arthrodentoosteo dysplasia) Hypophosphatasia Pseudo-vitamin D-deficiency rickets Thanatophoric dysplasia	
Overgrowth	Fragile X syndrome (Martin-Bell, marker X syndrome) Marshall-Smith syndrome Weaver's syndrome	
Storage disorders	Generalized gangliosidosis syndrome, type I (severe infantile type, Caffey's pseudo-Hurler's syndrome, familial neurovisceral lipidosis)	

piratory infections and feeding, but with time it becomes less severe and may even be absent during late childhood or adulthood. With other malformation syndromes, the exact opposite may occur. For this reason, it is important to evaluate muscle strength each time an anesthetic is to be administered.

In a few cases malformation syndromes may display both hypotonia and multiple airway malformations. Examples of these include Pena-Shokeir phenotype, frontometaphyseal dysplasia, and Marshall-Smith syndrome. Close to half of those malformation syndromes that are associated with hypotonia are also associated with cardiac defects. Many of these are from the chromosomal malformations category.

The principal anesthetic consideration for infants and children with hypotonia is the use of muscle relaxants. The decision to use muscle relaxants is usually based on the severity and cause of the hypotonia. Children with central nervous system anomalies usually require normal, or only slightly reduced, doses of muscle relaxants for laryngoscopy or surgery. On the other hand, the dosage of muscle relaxants is usually reduced, or may not even be required, for children with hypotonia caused by neuromuscular anomalies.

Reliance on the nerve stimulator alone to monitor neuromuscular function in children with hypotonia is a common error. This is because muscle weakness caused by central nervous system defects or muscle defects are not monitored by the nerve stimulator. The nerve stimulator indicates when muscle relaxants have taken effect; however, it cannot be used alone to determine if there is enough muscle strength to sustain ventilation and prevent aspiration at the end of surgery. Even when muscle relaxants are not used, infants and children with severe muscle weakness may be unable to sustain adequate ventilation postoperatively.

Severe hypotonia is also associated with difficulty swallowing and with gagging and coughing. This leads to difficulty feeding and to chronic respiratory infections. On occasion, a gastrostomy or feeding tube is inserted to ensure adequate calorie intake or fundoplication may be performed in an attempt to minimize aspiration.

Patients with hypotonia need to be positioned carefully for anesthesia and surgery because hypotonia is frequently associated with both joint laxity and joint contractures. Only two malformation syndromes are associated with both hypotonia and cervical spine compression or subluxation—trisomy 21 and achondroplasia. This is to be expected, as bone and ligament anomalies rather than nerve and muscle anomalies lie behind the propensity toward cervical spine subluxation.

Hypertonia is defined as a state of increased muscle tone. This is different from myotonia, which is delayed relaxation of a muscle after contraction. Hypertonia is relatively uncommon as compared with hypotonia. While there are several causes for hypotonia, hypertonia seems always to be secondary to central nervous system anomalies. Table 14–11 lists those syndromes that are associated with hypertonia. In the majority, the hypertonia is a manifestation of central nervous system defects present at birth. In the remaining few, the hypertonia is a consequence of central nervous system damage that occurred after birth as part of the malformation syndrome. Examples of these include Menkes' syndrome (widespread arterial elongation and tortuosity secondary to defective copper metabolism), homocystinuria syndrome (medial weakness of the great arteries with intimal hyperplasia leading to irregular vessel lumens and excessive vascular thrombosis), and Sturge-Weber sequence (brain hemangioma).

The anesthetic considerations for children with hypertonia are relatively few. Positioning of patients with spasticity may be difficult. Since the cause of the increased muscle tone is almost always the central nervous system, the usual doses of muscle relaxants are effective in providing suitable conditions for laryngoscopy and surgery. I reserve succinylcholine for dire emergencies because of the reported association between succinylcholine administration, central nervous system injury, and hyperkalemia.

An effort should be made to distinguish clearly between hypertonia and myotonia. This is because of the unusual anesthetic considerations of children with myotonia, particularly in regard to the use of succinylcholine. There are only three malformation syndromes in Appendix 14–1 that are associated with myotonia. These are the Schwartz-Jampel syndrome (chondrodystrophica myotonia), Freeman-Sheldon syndrome (whistling face syndrome), and Steinert's myotonic dystrophy syndrome (Steinert's syndrome, dystrophia myotonica). The anesthetic management of patients with these and other types of myotonia is discussed elsewhere in this text.

V. SKELETAL MALFORMATIONS

The skeletal malformations important to anesthesiologists are joint contractures, joint laxity, vertebral malformations, and fragile bones. Many malformation syndromes are associated with other limb or skeletal malformations; however, these are not included in this section. Table 14–12 lists malformation syndromes that are associated with skeletal anomalies of importance to the anesthesiologist.

A. JOINT CONTRACTURES

Malformation syndromes associated with joint contractures usually fall into one of two broad categories. The first is joint contractures secondary to central nervous system anomalies that result in reduced movement. This accounts for the large number of chromosomal malformation syndromes and major brain defect malformation syndromes associated with contractures. The second is abnormal formation of bone or cartilage. This also limits movement, which ultimately results in joint contracture.

Joint contractures cause two problems for anesthesiologists. First, placement of intravenous catheters and arterial lines is made difficult, and positioning for laryngoscopy may also be hindered. Second, finding an acceptable position for surgery may be almost impossible. Muscle relaxants do not improve mobility of the limbs. The urge to force the limbs must be resisted.

B. JOINT LAXITY

Joint laxity is also a relatively common malformation. There does not appear to be a unifying theme associated with joint laxity. The syndromes most often associated with it are trisomy 21, Ehlers-Danlos syndrome, and Marfan's syndrome. In trisomy 21, the concern is about laxity of the cervical spine and possible subluxation with neck extension. This topic was covered earlier in the airway malformation section. With Ehlers-Danlos and Marfan's syndromes, the joint laxity makes it easy to hyperextend the extremities when the patient is anesthetized.

C. VERTEBRAL ANOMALIES

There are several anesthetic considerations for infants and children with vertebral anomalies. Table 14–13 is a list of the types of vertebral anomalies that can occur. Obviously important is how anomalies of the cervical spine alter our ability to perform laryngoscopy. This is discussed earlier in this chapter. Malformations of the spine may also affect our ability to perform regional anesthesia. Last, malformations of the spine may affect the functioning of other organ systems, in particular the pulmonary system and the spinal cord.

Vertebral malformations are most often associated with the skeletal dysplasias, and in particular the osteochondrodysplasias.[4] Nearly all types of vertebral anomalies are seen with the osteochondrodysplasias. Aside from the obvious impact on the height of the patient, these anomalies can also complicate provision of regional anesthesia. Positioning may be difficult if spinal mobility is reduced. Inserting the needle into the proper site may be difficult if there are bony anomalies; however, vertebral anomalies may only make neuroaxial anesthesia more difficult: they do not preclude its use. Special note should be made of those malformation syndromes associated with vertebral anomalies that lead to spinal cord or nerve root compression. These are achondroplasia, acrodysostosis, Klippel-Feil sequence, neurofibromatosis syndrome, occult spinal dysraphism sequence, progeria syndrome, and thanatophoric dysplasia. Distichiasis-lymphedema syndrome is associated with epidural cysts. Some of the hamartosis syndromes may be associated with nerve compression or even spinal cord vascular anomalies (von Hippel–Lindau syndrome).

D. FRAGILE BONES

While bone fragility would not seem to be an important anesthetic consideration, those who have heard a snap or a crunch during positioning of an anesthetized patient know its importance. Several syndromes are associated with fragile bones, usually secondary to abnormal bone development. These syndromes are listed in Table 14–12. Anesthetic care of these patients is obvious.

Text continued on page 512

TABLE 14–12

Malformation Syndromes Associated with Skeletal Anomalies Important to Anesthesiologists

Category	Joint Contractures	Joint Laxity	Vertebral Anomalies	Fragile Bones
Brain or neuromuscular defects	Cerebrooculofacio-skeletal (COFS) syndrome; Distal arthrogryposis syndrome; Hecht's syndrome (trismus-pseudocamptodactyly syndrome); Killian/Teschler–Nicola syndrome (Pallister's mosaic syndrome, tetrasomy 12p); Lethal multiple pterygium syndrome; Neu-Laxova syndrome; Pallister-Hall syndrome; Pena-Shokeir phenotype (fetal akinesia/hypokinesia sequence); Schwartz-Jampel syndrome (chondrodystrophica myotonia); X-linked hydrocephalus syndrome	Menkes' syndrome (Menkes' kinky hair syndrome); Schinzel-Giedion syndrome; Sjögren-Larsson syndrome; X-linked hydrocephalus syndrome	Cohen's syndrome; Freeman-Sheldon syndrome (whistling face syndrome); Pallister-Hall syndrome	
Characterized by facial defect	Zellweger's syndrome (cerebrohepatorenal syndrome); FG syndrome; Mietens' syndrome	Oculodentodigital syndrome (oculodentodigital dysplasia); Smith-Lemli-Opitz syndrome	Coffin-Lowry syndrome; FG syndrome; Noonan's syndrome (Turner-like syndrome); Otopalatodigital syndrome, type I (Taybi's syndrome); Robinow's syndrome (fetal face syndrome); Ruvalcaba's syndrome; Stickler's syndrome (hereditary arthroophthalmopathy)	
Chromosomal		Trisomy 13 syndrome; Trisomy 18 syndrome; Trisomy 4p syndrome (trisomy of the short arm of chromosome 4)	Partial trisomy 10q syndrome; Trisomy 20p syndrome	
Connective tissue disorder		Homocystinuria syndrome		Homocystinuria syndrome; Osteogenesis imperfecta syndrome, type I (autosomal-dominant osteogenesis imperfecta, Lobstein's disease); Osteogenesis imperfecta syndrome, type II (osteogenesis imperfecta congenita, Vrolik's disease)
Environmental agents		Iodine deficiency effects (endemic cretinism)		
Growth deficiency		de Lange syndrome (Cornelia de Lange, Brachmann-de Lange); De Sanctis-Cacchione syndrome (xerodermic idiocy syndrome)		
Hamartosis			Schwartz-Jampel syndrome (chondrodystrophic amyotonia)	Maffucci's syndrome; Osteochondromatosis syndrome (Ollier's disease, enchondromatosis)
Osteochondrodysplasia with osteopetrosis				Cleidocranial dysostosis; Osteopetrosis: autosomal-recessive-lethal (severe osteopetrosis, mild form termed Albers-Schönberg syndrome); Pyknodysostosis (Toulouse-Lautrec disease)
Osteochondro-dysplasias				Achondrogenesis, type II (Langer-Saldino achondrogenesis, hypochondrogenesis); Hajdu-Cheney syndrome (Cheney's syndrome, acroosteolysis syndrome, arthrodentoosteo-dysplasia); Hypophosphatasia; Pseudo-vitamin D–deficiency rickets
Other skeletal dysplasias				Langer's mesomelic dysplasia (homozygous Leri-Weill dyschondroosteosis syndrome)

Left-hand list:

Category	Syndrome
Hamartosis	Otopalatodigital syndrome, Type II
	Ruvalcaba's syndrome
Overgrowth	Stickler's syndrome (hereditary arthroophthalmopathy)
Skin dysplasias	
Storage disorders	
Chromosomal	Partial trisomy 10q syndrome
	Triploidy and diploid-triploid mixoploidy syndrome
	Trisomy 13 syndrome
	Trisomy 18 syndrome
	Trisomy 4p syndrome (trisomy of the short arm of chromosome 4)
	Trisomy 8 syndrome (trisomy 8/normal mosaicism)
Connective tissue disorder	Trisomy 9 mosaic syndrome
	XXXY and XXXXY syndromes
	Beals' syndrome (Beals' contractural arachnodactyly syndrome)
	Fibrodysplasia ossificans progressiva syndrome
Craniosynostosis	Antley-Bixler syndrome (multisynostotic osteodysgenesis, trapezoidcephaly/multiple synostosis)
	Apert's syndrome (acrocephalosyndactyly)
	Greig's cephalopolysyndactyly syndrome
	Saethre-Chotzen syndrome
Environmental agents	Alcohol effects (fetal alcohol syndrome)
	Hyperthermia-induced spectrum of defects
Growth deficiency	de Lange syndrome (Cornelia de Lange, Brachmann-de Lange)

Right-hand list:

Category	Syndrome
Hamartosis	Incontinentia pigmenti syndrome (Bloch-Sulzberger syndrome)
	Sturge-Weber sequence
Overgrowth	Weaver's syndrome
Skin dysplasias	Xeroderma pigmentosum syndrome
Storage disorders	Hunter's syndrome (mucopolysaccharidosis II)
	Trisomy 8 syndrome (trisomy 8/normal mosaicism)
Connective tissue disorder	Beals' syndrome (Beals' contractural arachnodactyly syndrome)
	Marfan's syndrome
	Osteogenesis imperfecta syndrome, type II (osteogenesis imperfecta congenita, Vrolik's disease)
Craniosynostosis	Baller-Gerold syndrome (craniosynostosis-radial aplasia syndrome)
	Saethre-Chotzen syndrome
Environmental agents	Hyperthermia-induced spectrum of defects
	Valproate effects
Growth deficiency	Hallermann-Streiff syndrome (oculomandibulodyscephaly with hypotrichosis syndrome)
Hamartosis	Goltz's syndrome
	Neurofibromatosis syndrome
Limb defects	Child's syndrome
	Escobar's syndrome (multiple pterygium syndrome)
	Femoral hypoplasia-unusual facies syndrome
	Holt-Oram syndrome (cardiac-limb defect)
	Poland's anomaly
Miscellaneous	Arteriohepatic dysplasia (Alagille's syndrome)
	Börjeson-Forssman-Lehmann syndrome
	Caudal dysplasia sequence (caudal regression syndrome)
	Cerebrocostomandibular syndrome

Table continued on following page

TABLE 14-12

Malformation Syndromes Associated with Skeletal Anomalies Important to Anesthesiologists *(Continued)*

	Joint Contractures	Joint Laxity	Vertebral Anomalies	Fragile Bones
Limb defects	Amyoplasia congenita disruptive sequence (classic arthrogryposis, arthrogryposis multiplex congenita, myodystrophia fetalis deformans, multiple congenital articular rigidities, congenital arthromyodysplasia, myophagism congenita)		Cockayne's syndrome	
	CHILD syndrome		Coffin-Siris syndrome	
	Escobar's syndrome (multiple pterygium syndrome)		Distichiasis-lymphedema syndrome	
	Femoral hypoplasia–unusual facies syndrome		Exstrophy of cloaca sequence	
	Popliteal pterygium syndrome (faciogenitopopliteal syndrome)		Facioauriculovertebral spectrum (first and second branchial arch syndrome, oculoauricular vertebral dysplasia, hemifacial microsomia, Goldenhar's syndrome)	
Miscellaneous	Caudal dysplasia sequence (caudal regression syndrome)		Jarcho-Levin syndrome (spondylothoracic dysplasia)	
	Cockayne's syndrome		Klippel-Feil sequence	
	Jarcho-Levin syndrome (spondylothoracic dysplasia)		Melnick-Needles syndrome	
	Oligohydramnios sequence (Potter's syndrome)		Meningomyelocele, anencephaly, iniencephaly sequences	
Osteochondrodysplasia with osteopetrosis	Lenz-Majewski hyperostosis syndrome		Murcs' association	
Osteochondrodysplasias	Achondroplasia		Occult spinal dysraphism sequence (tethered cord malformation sequence)	
	Acromesomelic dysplasia (acromesomelic dwarfism)		Progeria syndrome (Hutchinson-Gilford syndrome)	
	Chondrodysplasia punctata (Conradi-Hünermann syndrome)		Rokitansky's sequence	
	Diastrophic dysplasia (diastrophic nanism syndrome)		Sirenomelia sequence	
	Dyggve-Melchior-Clausen syndrome		VATER association	

Osteochondrodysplasias

Achondrogenesis, type II (Langer-Saldino achondrogenesis, hypochondrogenesis)
Achondroplasia
Achondrogenesis, types Ia and Ib
Acromesomelic dysplasia (acromesomelic dwarfism)
Atelosteogenesis (giant cell chondrodysplasia)

Camptomelic dysplasia

Dyggve-Melchior-Clausen syndrome

Fibrochondrogenesis

Frontometaphyseal dysplasia

Hajdu-Cheney syndrome (Cheney's syndrome, acroosteolysis syndrome, arthrodentoosteodysplasia)
Hypochondroplasia

Jeune's thoracic dystrophy

Kniest's dysplasia

Kozlowski's spondylometaphyseal dysplasia (Kozlowski's spondylometaphyseal chondrodysplasia)
Metaphyseal chondrodysplasia, McKusick type (cartilage-hair hypoplasia syndrome)

Fibrochondrogenesis

Geleophysic dysplasia
Hypochondroplasia

Kniest's dysplasia

Kozlowski's spondylometaphyseal dysplasia (Kozlowski's spondylometaphyseal chondrodysplasia)
Metaphyseal chondrodysplasia, Schmid type (metaphyseal dysplasia, Schmid type)
Metaphyseal chondrodysplasia, Jansen type (metaphyseal dysostosis, Jansen type)
Metaphyseal chondrodysplasia, McKusick type (cartilage-hair hypoplasia syndrome)
Metatrophic dysplasia (metatrophic dwarfism syndrome)
Multiple epiphyseal dysplasia

Pseudoachondroplastic spondyloepiphyseal dysplasia (SED)
Pyle's metaphyseal dysplasia (Pyle's disease)
Rhizomelic chondrodysplasia punctata syndrome (chondrodysplasia punctata, rhizomelic type)
Spondyloepiphyseal dysplasia tarda (X-linked spondyloepiphyseal dysplasia)
Spondyloepiphyseal dysplasia congenita

Table continued on following page

TABLE 14–12

Malformation Syndromes Associated with Skeletal Anomalies Important to Anesthesiologists (Continued)

	Joint Contractures	Joint Laxity	Vertebral Anomalies	Fragile Bones
Other skeletal dysplasias	Leri-Weill dyschondrosteosis		Metatrophic dysplasia (metatrophic dwarfism syndrome)	
	Multiple exostoses syndrome (diaphyseal aclasis, external chondromatosis syndrome)		Multiple epiphyseal dysplasia	
	Multiple synostosis syndrome (symphalangism syndrome)		Pseudoachondroplastic spondyloepiphyseal dysplasia (SED)	
	Nail-patella syndrome (hereditary osteoonychodysplasia)		Pyle's metaphyseal dysplasia (Pyle's disease)	
	Weill-Marchesani syndrome (brachydactyly-spherophakia syndrome)		Rhizomelic chondrodysplasia punctata syndrome (chondrodysplasia punctata, rhizomelic type)	
			Short rib-polydactyly syndrome, non-Majewski type (short rib syndrome, type I)	
			Spondyloepiphiseal dysplasia tarda (X-linked spondyloepiphyseal dysplasia)	
			Thanatophoric dysplasia	
Other skeletal dysplasias			Acrodysostosis	
			Langer's mesomelic dysplasia (homozygous Leri-Weill dyschondrosteosis syndrome)	
			Multiple synostosis syndrome (symphalangism syndrome)	
			Nail-patella syndrome (hereditary osteoonychodysplasia)	
Overgrowth	Weaver's syndrome			
Skin dysplasias	Senter's syndrome			
Storage disorders	Generalized gangliosidosis syndrome, type I (severe infantile type, Caffey's pseudo-Hurler's syndrome, familial neurovisceral lipidosis)			
	Hunter's syndrome (mucopolysaccharidosis II)			
	Hurler's syndrome (mucopolysaccharidosis I H)			
	Hurler-Scheie compound syndrome (mucopolysaccharidosis I H/S)			
	Leroy I-cell syndrome (mucolipidosis II)			

Storage disorders

Generalized gangliosidosis syndrome, type I (severe infantile type, Caffey's pseudo-Hurler's syndrome, familial neurovisceral lipidosis)

Hurler's syndrome (mucopolysaccharidosis I H)

Leroy I-cell syndrome (mucolipidosis II)

Maroteaux-Lamy mucopolysaccharidosis syndrome (mucopolysaccharidosis VI)

Morquio's syndrome (mucopolysaccharidosis IV, types A and B)

Mucopolysaccharidosis VII (Sly's syndrome, β-glucuronidase deficiency)

Pseudo-Hurler's polydystrophy syndrome (mucolipidosis III)

Sanfilippo's syndrome (mucopolysaccharidosis III, types A, B, C, and D)

Maroteaux-Lamy mucopolysaccharidosis syndrome (mucopolysaccharidosis VI)

Morquio's syndrome (mucopolysaccharidosis IV, types A and B)

Mucopolysaccharidosis VII (Sly's syndrome, β-glucuronidase deficiency)

Pseudo-Hurler's polydystrophy syndrome (mucolipidosis III)

Sanfilippo's syndrome (mucopolysaccharidosis III, types A, B, C, and D)

Scheie's syndrome (mucopolysaccharidosis I S)

TABLE 14–13

Vertebral Malformations Important to Anesthesiologists

Hemivertebrae
Fused vertebrae
Scoliosis
Bifid vertebrae
Extra vertebrae
Spina bifida occulta
Kyphosis
Osteoporosis
Subluxation of the atlantooccipital joint
Platyspondyly
Incomplete ossification
Posterior vertebral hypoplasia
Narrow caudal space

TABLE 14–14

Some Renal System Anomalies

Renal agenesis, bilateral or unilateral
Ectopic kidney
Cystic kidneys
Renal dysplasia
Horseshoe kidney
Hypospadias
Cryptorchidism
Hydrocele
Duplicate urinary collection system
Ureterovesical obstruction
Ureteropelvic obstruction
Exstrophy
Ureteroceles
Ureteropelvic duplications
Posterior uretheral valves
Renal vascular anomalies
Wilms' tumor

VI. RENAL MALFORMATIONS

Many malformation syndromes are associated with renal anomalies; however, they are rarely the most obvious malformation and are rarely the first malformation diagnosed. From the anesthesiologist's viewpoint, a child with a renal malformation usually presents for surgery with a low probability of having other major malformations that are undiagnosed. The vast majority of renal malformations are of little importance to the anesthesiologist as long as renal function is maintained (Table 14–14).

TABLE 14–15

Malformation Syndromes Associated with Renal Dysfunction

Syndrome	Category	Urinary System Disorder
Arteriohepatic dysplasia (Alagille's syndrome)	Miscellaneous	Decreased creatinine clearance
Bardet-Biedl syndrome	Miscellaneous	Renal anomalies, hypertension, occasional diabetes insipidus
Caudal dysplasia sequence (caudal regression syndrome)	Miscellaneous	Renal anomalies or agenesis
Early urethral obstruction sequence	Miscellaneous	Urethral obstruction leading to renal dysplasia and abdominal muscle deficiency
Fabry's syndrome (Anderson-Fabry disease, angiokeratoma corporis diffusum)	Miscellaneous	Ceramide trihexoside accumulation leading to progressive renal insufficiency
Jeune's thoracic dystrophy	Osteochondrodysplasias	Renal anomalies leading to progressive renal insufficiency
Lowe's syndrome (oculocerebrorenal syndrome)	Brain or neuromuscular defects	Renal tubular dysfunction
Nail-patella syndrome (hereditary osteoonychodysplasia)	Other skeletal dysplasias	Renal anomalies (but renal failure rare in childhood)
Neu-Laxova syndrome	Brain or neuromuscular defects	Occasional renal agenesis
Occult spinal dysraphism sequence (tethered cord malformation sequence)	Miscellaneous	Urinary tract obstruction secondary to nerve root injury
Williams syndrome	Characterized by facial defect	Occasional renal anomalies and/or degenerative disease
Zellweger's syndrome, (cerebrohepatorenal syndrome)	Brain or neuromuscular defects	Lack of dihydroxyacetone phosphate acyltransferase, renal anomalies

Table 14–15 lists malformation syndromes associated with malformations severe enough to lead to renal insufficiency. There does not seem to be any particular group of malformation syndromes that are frequently associated with renal malformations severe enough to cause renal insufficiency. There are several anesthetic considerations for children with renal failure. These are the pharmacokinetics of anesthetic drugs, changes in fluid and electrolyte balance, anemia, altered platelet function, nutrition, muscle weakness, infection, and poor growth. These topics are all covered in standard anesthesia texts.

VII. ENDOCRINE AND HEMATOLOGIC DISORDERS

Malformation syndromes that are associated with selected endocrine conditions are listed in Table 14–16. While these endocrine disorders are not malformations, they are important to anesthesiologists. The endocrine disorders considered important include diabetes mellitus, hypoglycemia with fasting, diabetes insipidus, adrenal hypoplasia, pituitary dysfunction, hypothalamic dysfunction, hyperthyroidism, hypothyroidism, hypercalcemia, and hypocalcemia.

Hypoglycemia with fasting has been de-

TABLE 14–16

Malformation Syndromes Associated with Certain Endocrine Disorders

Malformation Syndrome	Endocrine Disorder
Achondroplasia	Abnormal GTT
Albright's hereditary osteodystrophy (pseudohypoparathyroidism, pseudopseudohypoparathyroidism)	Hypothyroidism, hypocalcemia
Arteriohepatic dysplasia (Alagille's syndrome)	Hypothyroidism
Athyrotic hypothyroidism sequence (hypothryoidism sequence)	Frequently hypothyroidism, hypercalcemia
Bardet-Biedl syndrome	Diabetes insipidus
Beckwith-Wiedemann syndrome (exomphalos-macroglossia-gigantism)	Hypoglycemia
Berardinelli's lipodystrophy syndrome (generalized lipodystrophy)	Frequent diabetes
De Sanctis-Cacchione syndrome (xerodermic idiocy syndrome)	Hypothalamic dysfunction
Di George sequence	Hypocalcemia
Hypophosphatasia	Hypocalcemia
Iodine deficiency effects (endemic cretinism)	Hypothyroidism
Johanson-Blizzard syndrome	Frequently hypothyroidism
Kenny's syndrome	Hypocalcemia
McCune-Albright syndrome (osteitis fibrosa cystica)	Hyperthyroidism, diabetes
Metaphyseal chondrodysplasia, Jansen type (metaphyseal dysostosis, Jansen type)	Hypercalcemia
Osteopetrosis: autosomal-recessive–lethal (severe osteopetrosis, mild form termed *Albers-Schönberg syndrome*)	Hypocalcemia
Pallister-Hall syndrome	Hypopituitarism
Prader-Willi syndrome	Diabetes
Pseudo–vitamin D–deficiency rickets	Hypocalcemia
Rubella effects	Hypopituitarism, diabetes
Russell-Silver syndrome (Silver's syndrome)	Hypoglycemia
Ruvalcaba-Myhre syndrome	Diabetes
Septooptic dysplasia sequence	Hypopituitarism
Sotos' syndrome (cerebral gigantism)	Diabetes
Steinert's myotonic dystrophy syndrome (Steinert's syndrome, dystrophia myotonica)	Diabetes
Triploidy and diploid-triploid mixoploidy syndrome	Adrenal hypoplasia
Trisomy 21 (Down's syndrome)	Hypothyroidism, hyperthyroidism
Tuberous sclerosis syndrome (adenoma sebaceum)	Hypothyroidism
Turner's syndrome (XO)	Hypothyroidism, diabetes
Werner's syndrome	Frequent diabetes, hyperthyroidism, adrenal atrophy
Williams syndrome	Hypercalcemia
XXY (Klinefelter's) syndrome	Diabetes

TABLE 14-17

Malformation Syndromes Associated with Hematologic Defects

Malformation Syndrome	Category	Hematologic Defect
13q– syndrome	Chromosomal	Malignancies
18p– syndrome	Chromosomal	Immune deficiency
18q– syndrome	Chromosomal	Immune deficiency
Aase's syndrome	Limb defects	Frequent anemia
Aniridia–Wilms' tumor association	Chromosomal	Malignancies
Ataxia-telangiectasia syndrome (Louis-Bar syndrome)	Brain or neuromuscular defects	Malignancies, immune deficiency
Beckwith-Wiedemann syndrome (exomphalos-macroglossia-gigantism)	Overgrowth	Malignancies
Bloom syndrome	Growth deficiency	Immune deficiency, malignancies
Chédiak-Higashi syndrome	Miscellaneous	Frequent anemia, thrombocytopenia, malignancies
Cohen's syndrome	Brain or neuromuscular defects	Immune deficiency
De Sanctis–Cacchione syndrome (xerodermic idiocy syndrome)	Growth deficiency	Malignancies
Dyskeratosis congenita syndrome	Hamartosis	Immune deficiency, frequent anemia, thrombocytopenia, malignancies
Fabry's syndrome (Anderson-Fabry disease, angiokeratoma corporis diffusum)	Miscellaneous	Anemia
Fanconi's pancytopenia syndrome	Limb defects	Frequent anemia, thrombocytopenia, malignancies
Gardner's syndrome	Hamartosis	Malignancies
Gorlin's syndrome (basal cell nevus syndrome)	Hamartosis	Malignancies
Hypophosphatasia	Osteochondrodysplasias	Anemia
Kartagener's syndrome	Miscellaneous	Immune deficiency
Kenny's syndrome	Osteochondrodysplasias	Anemia
Langer-Giedion syndrome (trichorhinophalangeal syndrome with exostosis)	Characterized by facial defect	Anemia
Linear sebaceous nevus sequence (nevus sebaceus of Jadassohn)	Hamartosis	Malignancy
Maffucci's syndrome	Hamartosis	Malignancy

Syndrome	Category	
Metaphyseal chondrodysplasia, McKusick type (cartilage-hair hypoplasia syndrome)	Osteochondrodysplasias	Anemia
Multiple exostoses syndrome (diaphyseal aclasis, external chondromatosis syndrome)	Other skeletal dysplasias	Malignancy
Multiple neuroma syndrome (multiple endocrine neoplasia, type 2b)	Hamartosis	Malignancy
Neurocutaneous melanosis sequence	Hamartosis	Malignancy
Neurofibromatosis syndrome	Hamartosis	Malignancy
Osteochondromatosis syndrome (Ollier's disease, enchondromatosis)	Hamartosis	Malignancy
Osteopetrosis: autosomal-recessive-lethal (severe osteopetrosis, mild form termed *Albers-Schönberg syndrome*)	Osteochondrodysplasia with osteopetrosis	Frequent anemia, thrombocytopenia
Peutz-Jeghers syndrome	Hamartosis	Frequent anemia, malignancy
Radial aplasia–thrombocytopenia syndrome (TAR syndrome)	Limb defects	Frequent anemia, thrombocytopenia
Roberts-SC phocomelia syndrome (pseudothalidomide syndrome, hypomelia-hypertrichosis–facial hemangioma syndrome)	Characterized by facial defect	Thrombocytopenia
Rothmund-Thomson syndrome (poikiloderma congenitale syndrome)	Miscellaneous	Malignancy
Rubella effects	Environmental agents	Anemia, thrombocytopenia
Schwachman's syndrome (metaphyseal chondrodysplasia with pancreatic insufficiency and neutropenia)	Osteochondrodysplasias	Immune deficiency, anemia, thrombocytopenia, malignancy
Sotos syndrome (cerebral gigantism)	Overgrowth	Malignancy
Trisomy 13 syndrome	Chromosomal	Thrombocytopenia
Trisomy 18 syndrome	Chromosomal	Thrombocytopenia
Trisomy 21 (Down's syndrome)	Chromosomal	Malignancy
Trisomy 8 syndrome (trisomy 8/normal mosaicism)	Chromosomal	Anemia
Tuberous sclerosis syndrome (adenoma sebaceum)	Hamartosis	Malignancy
Von Hippel-Lindau syndrome (retinal angiomas, cerebellar hemangioblastoma)	Hamartosis	Malignancy
Werner's syndrome	Miscellaneous	Malignancy
Xeroderma pigmentosasyndrome	Skin dysplasias	Malignancy

scribed in the Russell-Silver syndrome. These children appear to be at risk until about 3 years of age. About one third to half of those with Beckwith-Wiedemann syndrome also have persistent hypoglycemia until about 4 months of age. Therapy with hydrocortisone analogs has been effective for children with Beckwith-Wiedemann syndrome. Diabetes mellitus is frequently seen in Berardinelli's lipodystrophy syndrome and Werner's syndrome. Berardinelli's lipodystrophy syndrome is thought to be due to an unidentified inborn error of metabolism. The result is an insulin-resistant nonketotic hyperglycemia, hyperglucagonemia, and hyperlipidemia. Survival to adulthood has not been reported. Werner's syndrome results in a senile appearance beginning in late childhood. Loss of subcutaneous fat, fibrous subcutaneous tissue, cataracts, sparse gray hair, and early loss of teeth contribute to the appearance of an elderly adult. Muscle hypoplasia, osteoporosis, and arteriosclerosis are all accelerated. Werner's syndrome is also associated with adrenal atrophy.

Bardet-Biedl syndrome is unique in its occasional association with diabetes insipidus. De Sanctis–Cacchione syndrome, Pallister-Hall syndrome, rubella exposure effects, and septooptic dysplasia sequence all involve anomalies of hypothalamic-pituitary axis function.

Malformation syndromes associated with abnormalities of the hematologic system are listed in Table 14–17. Hematologic anomalies may be as obvious as anemia or thrombocytopenia or as subtle as immune deficiency leading to increased risk of infection. Interestingly, several malformation syndromes are associated with the propensity to develop malignancies. Perhaps the best-known of these associations is leukemia and trisomy 21.

Several malformation syndromes are frequently associated with anemia. These are Aase's syndrome, Chédiak-Higashi syndrome, dyskeratosis congenita syndrome, Fanconi's pancytopenia syndrome, osteopetrosis: autosomal-recessive–lethal, Peutz-Jeghers syndrome, and radial aplasia–thrombocytopenia syndrome. The anemia related to these syndromes is caused by a wide variety of mechanisms. Thrombocytopenia occurs without anemia in Roberts-SC phocomelia syndrome, trisomy 13 syndrome, and trisomy 18 syndrome.

Hamartosis malformation syndromes are frequently associated with a propensity to develop malignancies. This is not surprising, as hamartomas are abnormal mixtures of tissue elements. Some of the hamartoma malformation syndromes and their associated malignancies are von Hippel–Lindau syndrome and pheochromocytoma, tuberous sclerosis and astrocytoma, neurocutaneous melanosis and melanomas, and Gardner's syndrome and colon cancer. It may be difficult to distinguish hamartomas from malignant tumors, as both are liable to have clinical manifestations.

Children with a propensity toward anemia should have a preoperative hematocrit study. Preoperative platelet counting should probably also be performed if that particular malformation syndrome is associated with thrombocytopenia, although it would be reasonable to obtain platelet counts only for patients who exhibit clinical evidence of abnormal hemostasis. Children with demonstrated immunodeficiency should be treated as all patients are who are immunosuppressed. Children with a propensity to develop malignancies may have disease manifestations from either the malformation syndrome itself or from a new malignancy.

REFERENCES

1. Jones AE, Pelton DA: An index of syndromes and their anaesthetic implications. Can Anaesth Soc J 23(2):207, 1976.
2. Capistrano-Baruh E, Wenig B, Steinberg L, et al: Laryngeal web: A cause of difficult endotracheal intubation. Anesthesiology 57(2):123, 1982.
3. Creighton RE, Relton JE, Meridy HW: Anaesthesia for occipital encephalocoele. Can Anaesth Soc J 21(4):403, 1974.
4. Berkowitz ID, Raja SN, Bender KS, et al: Dwarfs: Pathophysiology and anesthetic implications [see Comments]. Anesthesiology 73(4):739, 1990.
5. Kalla GN, Fening E, Obiaya MO: Anaesthetic management of achondroplasia. Br J Anaesth 58(1):117, 1986.
6. Mayhew JF, Katz J, Miner M, et al: Anaesthesia for the achondroplastic dwarf. Can Anaesth Soc J 33(2):216, 1986.
7. Honda N, Konno K, Itohda Y, et al: Malignant hyperthermia and althesin. Can Anaesth Soc J 24(4):514, 1977.
8. Hopkins PM, Ellis FR, Halsall PJ: Hypermetabolism in arthrogryposis multiplex congenita. Anaesthesia 46(5):374, 1991.
9. Oberoi GS, Kaul HL, Gill IS, et al: Anaesthesia in arthrogryposis multiplex congenita: Case report. Can J Anaesth 34(3(Pt 1)):288, 1987.
10. Quance DR: Anaesthetic management of an obstetrical patient with arthrogryposis multiplex congenita. Can J Anaesth 35(6):612, 1988.

11. Jotterand V, Boisjoly HM, Harnois C, et al: 11p13 deletion, Wilms' tumour, and aniridia: Unusual genetic, non-ocular and ocular features of three cases. Br J Ophthalmol 74(9):568, 1990.

12. Nargozian C: Apert syndrome. Anesthetic management. Clin Plast Surg 18(2):227, 1991.

13. Bawle E, Quigg MH: Ectopia lentis and aortic root dilatation in congenital contractural arachnodactyly. Am J Med Genet 42(1):19, 1992.

14. Gurkowski MA, Rasch DK: Anesthetic considerations for Beckwith-Wiedemann syndrome. Anesthesiology 70(4):711, 1989.

15. Suan C, Ojeda R, Garcia-Perla JL, et al: Anaesthesia and the Beckwith-Wiedemann syndrome. Paediatr Anaesth 6(3):231, 1996.

16. Tobias JD, Lowe S, Holcomb GW: Anesthetic considerations of an infant with Beckwith-Wiedemann syndrome. J Clin Anesth 4(6):484, 1992.

17. Stack CG, Wyse RK: Incidence and management of airway problems in the CHARGE Association. Anaesthesia 46(7):582, 1991.

18. Ulsoy H, Erciyes N, Ovali E, et al: Anesthesia in Chediak-Higashi syndrome—case report. Middle East J Anesthesiol 13(1):101, 1995.

19. Cook S: Cockayne's syndrome. Another cause of difficult intubation. Anaesthesia 37(11):1104, 1982.

20. Wooldridge WJ, Dearlove OR, Khan AA: Anaesthesia for Cockayne syndrome. Three case reports. Anaesthesia 51(5):478, 1996.

21. Sargent WW: Anesthetic management of a patient with Cornelia de Lange syndrome [letter]. Anesthesiology 74(6):1162, 1991.

22. Takeshita T, Akita S, Kawahara M: Anesthetic management of a patient with Cornelia de Lange syndrome. Anesth Prog 34(2):63, 1987.

23. Veall GR: An unusual complication of Cornelia de Lange syndrome. Anaesthesia 49(5):409, 1994.

24. Flashburg MH, Dunbar BS, August G, et al: Anesthesia for surgery in an infant with DiGeorge syndrome. Anesthesiology 58(5):479, 1983.

25. Mizushima A, Satoyoshi M: Anaesthetic problems in a child with ectrodactyly, ectodermal dysplasia and cleft lip/palate. The EEC syndrome. Anaesthesia 47(2):137, 1992.

26. Dolan P, Sisko F, Riley E: Anesthetic considerations for Ehlers-Danlos syndrome. Anesthesiology 52(3):266, 1980.

27. Kuzma PJ, Calkins MD, Kline MD, et al: The anesthetic management of patients with multiple pterygium syndrome. Anesth Analg 83(2):430, 1996.

28. Cooper CM, Murray-Wilson A: Retrograde intubation. Management of a 4.8-kg, 5-month infant. Anaesthesia 42(11):1197, 1987.

29. Madan R, Trikha A, Venkataraman RK, et al: Goldenhar's syndrome: An analysis of anaesthetic management. A retrospective study of seventeen cases [published erratum appears in Anaesthesia 45(5):424, 1990; see Comments]. Anaesthesia 45(1):49, 1990.

30. Scholtes JL, Veyckemans F, Van Obbergh L, et al: Neonatal anaesthetic management of a patient with Goldenhar's syndrome with hydrocephalus. Anaesth Intensive Care 15(3):338, 1987.

31. Joel M, Rosales JK: Fanconi syndrome and anesthesia. Anesthesiology 55(4):455, 1981.

32. Casamassimo PS, McIlvaine WB, Hagerman R, et al: General anesthesia and fragile X syndrome: Report of a case. Anesth Prog 32(3):104, 1985.

33. Jagtap SR, Malde AD, Pantvaidya SH: Anaesthetic considerations in a patient with Fraser syndrome [see Comments]. Anaesthesia 50(1):39, 1995.

34. Duggar RG Jr, DeMars PD, Bolton VE: Whistling face syndrome: General anesthesia and early postoperative caudal analgesia. Anesthesiology 70(3):545, 1989.

35. Jones R, Dolcourt JL: Muscle rigidity following halothane anesthesia in two patients with Freeman-Sheldon syndrome [see Comments]. Anesthesiology 77(3):599, 1992.

36. Laishley RS, Roy WL: Freeman-Sheldon syndrome: Report of three cases and the anaesthetic implications. Can Anaesth Soc J 33(3 Pt 1):388, 1986.

37. Mayhew JF: Anesthesia for children with Freeman-Sheldon syndrome [letter; see Comment]. Anesthesiology 78(2):408, 1993.

38. Mehta Y, Schou H: The anaesthetic management of an infant with frontometaphyseal dysplasia (Gorlin-Cohen syndrome). Acta Anaesthesiol Scand 32(6):505, 1988.

39. Marquez X, Roxas RS: Induction of anesthesia in an infant with frontonasal dysplasia and meningoencephalocele: A case report. Anesth Analg 56(5):736, 1977.

40. Pappas MT, Katz J, Finestone SC: Problems in anesthetic and airway management with Gardner's syndrome—report of a case. Anesth Analg 50(3):340, 1971.

41. Ezri T, Szmuk P, Soroker D: Anaesthesia for Golz-Gorlin syndrome [letter]. Anaesthesia 49(9):833, 1994.

42. Holzman RS: Airway involvement and anesthetic management in Goltz's syndrome. J Clin Anesth 3(5):422, 1991.

43. Yoshizumi J, Vaughan RS, Jasani B: Pregnancy associated with Gorlin's syndrome. Anaesthesia 45(12):1046, 1990.

44. Cohen MM Jr.: Hallermann-Streiff syndrome: A review [see Comments]. Am J Med Genet 41(4):488, 1991.

45. Ravindran R, Stoops CM: Anesthetic management of a patient with Hallermann-Streiff syndrome. Anesth Analg 58(3):254, 1979.

46. Browder FH, Lew D, Shahbazian TS: Anesthetic management of a patient with Dutch-Kentucky syndrome. Anesthesiology 65(2):218, 1986.

47. Mercuri LG: The Hecht, Beals, and Wilson syndrome: Report of case. J Oral Surg 39(1):53, 1981.

48. Teng RJ, Ho MM, Wang PJ, et al: Trismus-pseudocamptodactyly syndrome: Report of one case. Acta Paediatr Sin 35(2):144, 1994.

49. Vaghadia H, Blackstock D: Anaesthetic implications of the trismus pseudocamptodactyly (Dutch-Kentucky or Hecht Beals) syndrome. Can J Anaesth 35(1):80, 1988.

50. Crooke JW, Towers JF, Taylor WH: Management of patients with homocystinuria requiring surgery under general anaesthesia. A case report. Br J Anaesth 43(1):96, 1971.

51. Grover VK, Malhotra SK, Kaushik S: Anaesthesia and homocystinuria [letter]. Anaesthesia 34(9):913, 1979.

52. Koblin DD: Homocystinuria and administration of nitrous oxide [letter; see Comment]. J Clin Anesth 7(2):176, 1995.

53. Lowe S, Johnson DA, Tobias JD: Anesthetic implications of the child with homocystinuria [see Comments]. J Clin Anesth 6(2):142, 1994.

54. Parris WC, Quimby CW, Jr.: Anesthetic considerations for the patient with homocystinuria. Anesth Analg 61(8):708, 1982.

55. Herrick IA, Rhine EJ: The mucopolysaccharidoses and anaesthesia: A report of clinical experience. Can J Anaesth 35(1):67, 1988.

56. Kreidstein A, Boorin MR, Crespi P, et al: Delayed awakening from general anaesthesia in a patient with Hunter syndrome. Can J Anaesth 41(5 Pt 1):423, 1994.

57. Belani KG, Krivit W, Carpenter BL, et al: Children with mucopolysaccharidosis: Perioperative care, morbidity, mortality, and new findings. J Pediatr Surg 28(3):403, 1993.

58. Walker RW, Darowski M, Morris P, et al: Anaesthesia and mucopolysaccharidoses. A review of airway problems in children. Anaesthesia 49(12):1078, 1994.

59. Sjögren P, Pedersen T: Anaesthetic problems in Hurler-Scheie syndrome. Report of two cases. Acta Anaesthesiol Scand 30(6):484, 1986.

60. Borland LM: Anesthesia for children with Jeune's syndrome (asphyxiating thoracic dystrophy). Anesthesiology 66(1):86, 1987.

61. Ho AM, Friedland MJ: Kartagener's syndrome: Anesthetic considerations. Anesthesiology 77(2):386, 1992.

62. Janke EL, Fletcher JE, Lewis IH: Anaesthetic management of the Kenny-Caffey syndrome using the laryngeal mask. Paediatr Anaesth 6(3):235, 1996.

63. Daum RE, Jones DJ: Fibreoptic intubation in Klippel-Feil syndrome. Anaesthesia 43(1):18, 1988.

64. Dresner MR, Maclean AR: Anaesthesia for caesarean section in a patient with Klippel-Feil syndrome. The use of a microspinal catheter. Anaesthesia 50(9):807, 1995.

65. Naguib M, Farag H, Ibrahim Ae-W: Anaesthetic considerations in Klippel-Feil syndrome. Can Anaesth Soc J 33(1):66, 1986.

66. de Leon-Casasola OA, Lema MJ: Anesthesia for patients with Sturge-Weber disease and Klippel-Trenaunay syndrome. J Clin Anesth 3(5):409, 1991.

67. de Leon-Casasola OA, Lema MJ: Epidural anesthesia in patients with Klippel-Trenaunay syndrome [letter; see Comment]. Anesth Analg 74(3):470, 1992.

68. Gaiser RR, Cheek TG, Gutsche BB: Major conduction anesthesia in a patient with Klippel-Trenaunay syndrome. J Clin Anesth 7(4):316, 1995.

69. Lauder GR, Sumner E: Larsen's syndrome: Anaesthetic implications. Six case reports. Paediatr Anaesth 5(2):133, 1995.

70. Stevenson GW, Hall SC, Palmieri J: Anesthetic considerations for patients with Larsen's syndrome. Anesthesiology 75(1): 142, 1991.

71. Langer RA, Yook I, Capan LM: Anesthetic considerations in McCune-Albright syndrome: case report with literature review. Anesth Analg 80(6):1236, 1995.

72. Tobias JD: Anaesthetic considerations in the child with Menkes' syndrome. Can J Anaesth 39(7):712, 1992.

73. Richards M: Miller's syndrome. Anaesthetic management of postaxial acrofacial dysostosis. Anaesthesia 42(8):871, 1987.

74. Stevenson GW, Hall SC, Bauer BS, et al: Anaesthetic management of Miller's syndrome. Can J Anaesth 38(8):1046, 1991.

75. Krajcirik WJ, Azar I, Opperman S, et al: Anesthetic management of a patient with Moebius syndrome. Anesth Analg 64(3):371, 1985.

76. Beighton P, Craig J: Atlanto-axial subluxation in the Morquio syndrome. Report of a case. J Bone Joint Surg 55B(3):478, 1973.

77. Birkinshaw KJ: Anaesthesia in a patient with an unstable neck. Morquio's syndrome. Anaesthesia 30(1):46, 1975.

78. Jones AE, Croley TF: Morquio syndrome and anesthesia. Anesthesiology 51(3):261, 1979.

79. Rodrigo MR, Cheng CH, Tai YT, et al: "Leopard" syndrome. Anaesthesia 45(1):30, 1990.

80. Walker JS, Dorian RS, Marsh NJ: Anesthetic management of a child with Nager's syndrome [letter]. Anesth Analg 79(5):1025, 1994.

81. Dounas M, Mercier FJ, Lhuissier C, et al: Epidural analgesia for labour in a parturient with neurofibromatosis. Can J Anaesth 42(5 Pt 1):420, 1995.

82. Fisher MM: Anaesthetic difficulties in neurofibromatosis. Anaesthesia 30(5):648, 1975.

83. Halper J, Factor SM: Coronary lesions in neurofibromatosis associated with vasospasm and myocardial infarction. Am Heart J 108(2):420, 1984.

84. Naguib M, Al-Rajeh SM, Abdulatif M, et al: The response of a patient with von Recklinghausen's disease to succinylcholine and atracurium. Middle East J Anaesthesiol 9(5):429, 1988.

85. Richardson MG, Setty GK, Rawoof SA: Responses to nondepolarizing neuromuscular blockers and succinylcholine in von Recklinghausen neurofibromatosis. Anesth Analg 82(2):382, 1996.

86. Yong-Hing K, Kalamchi A, MacEwen GD: Cervical spine abnormalities in neurofibromatosis. J Bone Joint Surg 61A(5):695, 1979.

87. Campbell AM, Bousfield JD: Anaesthesia in a patient with Noonan's syndrome and cardiomyopathy. Anaesthesia 47(2):131, 1992.

88. Dadabhoy ZP, Winnie AP: Regional anesthesia for cesarean section in a parturient with Noonan's syndrome. Anesthesiology 68(4):636, 1988.

89. Schwartz N, Eisenkraft JB: Anesthetic management of a child with Noonan's syndrome and idiopathic hypertrophic subaortic stenosis. Anesth Analg 74(3):464, 1992.

90. Bolsin SN, Gillbe C: Opitz-Frias syndrome. A case with potentially hazardous anaesthetic implications. Anaesthesia 40(12):1189, 1985.

91. Cunningham AJ, Donnelly M, Comerford J: Osteogenesis imperfecta: Anesthetic management of a patient for cesarean section: A case report. Anesthesiology 61(1):91, 1984.

92. Peluso A, Cerullo M: Malignant hyperthermia susceptibility in patients with osteogenesis imperfecta [letter]. Paediatr Anaesth 5(6):398, 1995.

93. Rampton AJ, Kelly DA, Shanahan EC, et al: Occurrence of malignant hyperpyrexia in a patient with osteogenesis imperfecta. Br J Anaesth 56(12):1443, 1984.

94. Barros F: Caudal block in a child with osteogenesis imperfecta, type II [letter]. Paediatr Anaesth 5(3):202, 1995.

95. Clark JR, Smith LJ, Kendall BE, et al: Unexpected brainstem compression following routine surgery in a child with oto-palato-digital syndrome. Anaesthesia 50(7):641, 1995.

96. Mackenzie JW: Anaesthesia and the Prader-Willi syndrome. J R Soc Med 84(4):239, 1991.

97. Mayhew JF, Taylor B: Anaesthetic considerations in the Prader-Willi syndrome [letter]. Can Anaesth Soc J 30(5):565, 1983.

98. Milliken RA, Weintraub DM: Cardiac abnormalities during anesthesia in a child with Prader-Willi syndrome. Anesthesiology 43(5):590, 1975.

99. Palmer SK, Atlee JL: Anesthetic management of the Prader-Willi syndrome. Anesthesiology 44(2):161, 1976.

100. Sloan TB, Kaye CI: Rumination risk of aspiration of gastric contents in the Prader-Willi syndrome. Anesth Analg 73(4):492, 1991.

101. Yamashita M, Koishi K, Yamaya R, et al: Anaesthetic considerations in the Prader-Willi syndrome: report of four cases. Can Anaesth Soc J 30(2):179, 1983.

102. Chapin JW, Kahre J: Progeria and anesthesia. Anesth Analg 58(5):424, 1979.

103. Pennant JH, Harris MF: Anaesthesia for Proteus syndrome. Anaesthesia 46(2):126, 1991.

104. Chadd GD, Crane DL, Phillips RM, et al: Extubation and reintubation guided by the laryngeal mask airway in a child with the Pierre Robin syndrome [see Comments]. Anesthesiology 76(4):640, 1992.

105. Lapidot A, Rezvani F, Terrefe D, et al: A new functional approach to the surgical management of Pierre Robin syndrome: Experimental and clinical report. Laryngoscope 86(7):979, 1976.

106. Rasch DK, Browder F, Barr M, et al: Anaesthesia for Treacher Collins and Pierre Robin syndromes: A report of three cases. Can Anaesth Soc J 33(3 Pt 1):364, 1986.

107. Macdonald I, Dearlove OR: Anaesthesia and Robinow syndrome [letter]. Anaesthesia 50(12):1097, 1995.

108. Critchley LA, Gin T, Stuart JC: Anaesthesia in an infant with Rubinstein-Taybi syndrome. Anaesthesia 50(1):37, 1995.

109. Stirt JA: Anesthetic problems in Rubinstein-Taybi syndrome. Anesth Analg 60(7):534, 1981.

110. Dinner M, Goldin EZ, Ward R, et al: Russell-Silver syndrome: Anesthetic implications. Anesth Analg 78(6):1197, 1994.

111. Wrigley MW: Inadvertent dural puncture during caudal anaesthesia for Saethre-Chotzen syndrome [letter]. Anaesthesia 46(8):705, 1991.

112. Myles PS, Westhorpe RN: A patient with Sanfilippo syndrome and pseudocholinesterase deficiency, further complicated by post-tonsillectomy haemorrhage [see Comments]. Anaesth Intensive Care 17(1):86, 1989.

113. Ray S, Rubin AP: Anaesthesia in a child with Schwartz-Jampel syndrome. Anaesthesia 49(7):600, 1994.

114. Sherlock DA, McNicol LR: Anaesthesia and septo-optic dysplasia. Implications of missed diagnosis in the peri-operative period. Anaesthesia 42(12):1302, 1987.

115. Haji-Michael PG, Hatch DL: Smith-Lemli-Opitz syndrome and malignant hyperthermia [letter; see Comment]. Anesth Analg 83(1):200, 1996.

116. Petersen WC, Crouch ER, Jr.: Anesthesia-induced rigidity, unrelated to succinylcholine, associated with Smith-Lemli-Opitz syndrome and malignant hyperthermia. Anesth Analg 80(3):606, 1995.

117. Suresh D: Posterior spinal fusion in Sotos' syndrome. Br J Anaesth 66(6):728, 1991.

118. Boheimer N, Harris JW, Ward S: Neuromuscular blockade in dystrophia myotonica with atracurium besylate. Anaesthesia 40(9):872, 1985.

119. Bray RJ, Inkster JS: Anaesthesia in babies with congenital dystrophia myotonica. Anaesthesia 39(10):1007, 1984.

120. Buzello W, Krieg N, Schlickewei A: Hazards of neostigmine in patients with neuromuscular disorders. Report of two cases. Br J Anaesth 54(5):529, 1982.

121. Dalal FY, Bennett EJ, Raj PP, et al: Dystrophia myotonica: A multisystem disease. Can Anaesth Soc J 19(4):436, 1972.

122. Diefenbach C, Lynch J, Abel M, et al: Vecuronium for muscle relaxation in patients with dystrophia myotonica. Anesth Analg 76(4):872, 1993.

123. Nightingale P, Healy TE, McGuinness K: Dystrophia myotonica and atracurium. A case report. Br J Anaesth 57(11):1131, 1985.

124. Phillips DC, Ellis FR, Exley KA, et al: Dantrolene sodium and dystrophia myotonica. Anaesthesia 39(6):568, 1984.

125. Aldridge LM: An unusual cause of upper airways obstruction [letter]. Anaesthesia 42(11):1239, 1987.

126. Batra RK, Gulaya V, Madan R, et al: Anaesthesia and the Sturge-Weber syndrome. Can J Anaesth 41(2):133, 1994.

127. Brown RE Jr, Vollers JM, Rader GR, et al: Nasotracheal intubation in a child with Treacher Collins syndrome using the Bullard intubating laryngoscope. J Clin Anesth 5(6):492, 1993.

128. Ebata T, Nishiki S, Masuda A, et al: Anaesthesia for Treacher Collins syndrome using a laryngeal mask airway. Can J Anaesth 38(8):1043, 1991.

129. Inada T, Fujise K, Tachibana K, et al: Orotracheal intubation through the laryngeal mask airway in paediatric patients with Treacher Collins syndrome [see Comments]. Paediatr Anaesth 5(2):129, 1995.

130. Kovac AL: Use of the Augustine stylet anticipating difficult tracheal intubation in Treacher Collins syndrome. J Clin Anesth 4(5):409, 1992.

131. MacLennan FM, Robertson GS: Ketamine for induction and intubation in Treacher Collins syndrome. Anaesthesia 36(2):196, 1981.

132. Mayhew JF: Anaesthesia for Treacher Collins syndrome [letter]. Can J Anaesth 34(3(Pt 1)):328, 1987.

133. Roa NL, Moss KS: Treacher Collins syndrome with sleep apnea: Anesthetic considerations. Anesthesiology 60(1):71, 1984.

134. Sklar GS, King BD: Endotracheal intubation and Treacher Collins syndrome. Anesthesiology 44(3):247, 1976.

135. Martlew RA, Sharples A: Anaesthesia in a child with Patau's syndrome. Anaesthesia 50(11):980, 1995.

136. Pollard RC, Beasley JM: Anaesthesia for patients with trisomy 13 (Patau's syndrome). Paediatr Anaesth 6(2):151, 1996.

137. Harley EH, Collins MD: Neurologic sequelae secondary to atlantoaxial instability in Down syndrome. Implications in otolaryngologic surgery. Arch Otolaryngol Head Neck Surg 120(2):159, 1994.

138. Kobel M, Creighton RE, Steward DJ: Anaesthetic considerations in Down's syndrome: Experience with 100 patients and a review of the literature. Can Anaesth Soc J 29(6):593, 1982.

139. Litman RS, Zerngast BA, Perkins FM: Preoperative evaluation of the cervical spine in children with trisomy-21: Results of a questionnaire study. Paediatr Anaesth 5(6):355, 1995.

140. Mitchell V, Howard R, Facer E: Down's syndrome and anaesthesia. Paediatr Anaesth 5(6):379, 1995.

141. Moore RA, McNicholas KW, Warran SP: Atlantoaxial subluxation with symptomatic spinal cord compression in a child with Down's syndrome. Anesth Analg 66(1):89, 1987.

142. Lee JJ, Imrie M, Taylor V: Anaesthesia and tuberous sclerosis. Br J Anaesth 73(3):421, 1994.

143. Tsukui A, Noguchi R, Honda T, et al: Aortic aneurysm in a four-year-old child with tuberous sclerosis. Paediatr Anaesth 5(1):67, 1995.

144. Divekar VM, Kothari MD, Kamdar BM: Anaesthesia in Turner's syndrome. Can Anaesth Soc J 30(4):417, 1983.

145. Joffe D, Robbins R, Benjamin A: Caesarean section and phaeochromocytoma resection in a patient with Von Hippel Lindau disease. Can J Anaesth 40(9):870, 1993.

146. Matthews AJ, Halshaw J: Epidural anaesthesia in von Hippel-Lindau disease. Management of childbirth and anaesthesia for caesarean section. Anaesthesia 41(8):853, 1986.

147. Turner DR, Downing JW: Anaesthetic problems associated with Weaver's syndrome. Br J Anaesth 57(12):1260, 1985.

148. Mammi I, Iles DE, Smeets D, et al: Anesthesiologic problems in Williams syndrome: The CACNL2A locus is not involved. Hum Genet 98(3):317, 1996.

149. Patel J, Harrison MJ: Williams syndrome: Masseter spasm during anaesthesia [see Comments]. Anaesthesia 46(2):115, 1991.

150. Meyer RJ: Awake blind nasal intubation in a patient with xeroderma pigmentosum. Anaesth Intensive Care 10(1):64, 1982.

Appendix 14–1: Alphabetical Listing of Malformation Syndromes

Syndrome	Category	Anesthetic Considerations
13q − syndrome	Chromosomal	Growth deficiency, mental deficiency, ocular anomalies, micrognathia, cardiac defects, focal lumbar agenesis, predisposition to retinoblastoma
18p − syndrome	Chromosomal	Growth deficiency, mental deficiency, IgA absence or deficiency, micrognathia, joint laxity
18q − syndrome	Chromosomal	Growth deficiency, mental deficiency, deafness, hypotonia, poor coordination, cardiac defects, immune deficiency
4p − syndrome (4p deletion)	Chromosomal	Facial anomalies, severe growth deficiency, micrognathia, hypotonia, seizures, cardiac defects, respiratory infections
5p − syndrome (cri-du-chat, partial deletion of 5p)	Chromosomal	Characteristic mewing cry during infancy, mental deficiency, growth deficiency, micrognathia, vertebral anomalies, hypotonia, microcephaly and/or facial asymmetry, cardiac defects
9p − syndrome (9p monosomy)	Chromosomal	Mental deficiency, micrognathia, cardiac defects, seizures, hypotonia, craniostenosis
Aarskog's syndrome	Characterized by facial defect	Facial anomalies, cervical vertebral anomalies
Aase's syndrome	Limb defects	Anemia, cardiac anomalies
Accutane embryopathy	See Retinoic acid embryopathy	
Achondrogenesis, type II (Langer-Saldino achondrogenesis, hypochondrogenesis)	Osteochondrodysplasias	Early lethal disorder; large calvarium, facial anomalies, micrognathia, vertebral anomalies, small chest cavity, fractures
Achondroplasia[4–6]	Osteochondrodysplasias	Vertebral anomalies leading to cord and nerve root compression or hydrocephalus, mild muscle weakness, abnormal glucose tolerance test, moderately small chest, chronic respiratory infections
Achondrogenesis, types Ia and Ib	Osteochondrodysplasias	Early lethal disorder; facial anomalies, micrognathia, severe micromelia, fragile bones, small thorax, vertebral anomalies
Acroosteolysis syndrome	See Hajdu-Cheney syndrome	
Acrocephalosyndactyly	See Apert's syndrome	
Acrodysostosis	Other skeletal dysplasias	Growth deficiency, mental deficiency, facial anomalies, limb anomalies, vertebral anomalies or collapse, hydrocephalus
Acromesomelic dwarfism	See Acromesomelic dysplasia	
Acromesomelic dysplasia (acromesomelic dwarfism)	Osteochondrodysplasias	Kyphosis, joint contractures
Adams-Oliver syndrome	Limb defects	Dermal anomalies
Adenoma sebaceum	See Tuberous sclerosis syndrome	
AEC syndrome	See Hays-Wells syndrome of ectodermal dysplasia	

Syndrome	Category	Anesthetic Considerations
Aglossia-adactyly syndrome	See Oromandibular–limb hypogenesis spectrum	
Alagille's syndrome	See Arteriohepatic dysplasia	
Albers-Schönberg syndrome	See Osteopetrosis: autosomal-recessive–lethal	
Albright's hereditary osteodystrophy (pseudohypoparathyroidism, pseudopseudohypoparathyroidism)	Other skeletal dysplasias	Growth deficiency, mental deficiency, facial anomalies, variable hypocalcemia and hypophosphatemia, hypothyroid, ocular anomalies
Alcohol effects (fetal alcohol syndrome)	Environmental agents	Growth deficiency, mild mental deficiency, facial anomalies, cardiac anomalies, occasional micrognathia, occasional cervical vertebral anomalies, occasional meningomyelocele or hydrocephalus
Aminopterin effects	Environmental agents	Growth deficiency, facial anomalies, micrognathia, occasional hypotonia, joint laxity, occasional dextrocardia, small chest cavity
Amyoplasia congenita disruptive sequence (classic arthrogryposis, arthrogryposis multiplex congenita, myodystrophia fetalis deformans, multiple congenital articular rigidities, congenital arthromyodysplasia, myophagism congenita)[7–10]	Limb defects	Facial anomalies, micrognathia, torticollis, multiple flexion contractures, stiff spine
Anderson-Fabry disease	See Fabry's syndrome	
Angelman's syndrome (happy puppet syndrome)	Brain or neuromuscular defects	Mental deficiency, growth deficiency, paroxysms of inappropriate laughter, facial anomalies, ataxia, seizures, hypotonia
Angiokeratoma corporis diffusum	See Fabry's syndrome	
Aniridia–Wilms' tumor association[11]	Chromosomal	Growth deficiency, mental deficiency, micrognathia, Wilms' tumor in 50%, glaucoma
Ankyloblepharon–ectodermal dysplasia–clefting syndrome	See Hays-Wells syndrome of ectodermal dysplasia	
Antley-Bixler syndrome (multisynostotic osteodysgenesis, trapezoidcephaly–multiple synostosis)	Craniosynostosis	Facial anomalies, choanal atresia, upper airway obstruction causing apnea, limb anomalies, hydrocephalus, occasional cardiac anomalies, occasional renal anomalies
Apert's syndrome (acrocephalosyndactyly)[12]	Craniosynostosis	Variable mental deficiency, facial anomalies, limb anomalies, choanal atresia, atrophy of pulmonary arteries, cardiac anomalies, hydrocephalus
Arteriohepatic dysplasia (Alagille's syndrome)	Miscellaneous	Growth deficiency, facial anomalies, peripheral pulmonary stenosis, vertebral anomalies, cholestasis, decreased creatinine clearance, occasional mild mental deficiency, other cardiac anomalies, hypothyroid
Artrodentoosteodysplasia	See Hajdu-Cheney syndrome	
Arthrogryposis multiplex congenita	See Amyoplasia congenita disruptive sequence	
Asplenia syndrome	See Laterality sequences	

Syndrome	Category	Anesthetic Considerations
Ataxia-telangiectasia syndrome (Louis-Bar syndrome)	Brain or neuromuscular defects	Growth deficiency, progressive ataxia, mental deficiency, posterior spinal cord dysfunction, telangiectasia, chronic respiratory infections, thymic hypoplasia, immunoglobulin deficiency, predisposition to malignancy
Atelosteogenesis (giant cell chondrodysplasia)	Osteochondrodysplasias	Early lethal disorder; vertebral anomalies, facial anomalies
Athyrotic hypothyroidism sequence (hypothryoidism sequence)	Miscellaneous	Myxedema, decreased activity, feeding difficulties, macroglossia, hypothyroidism, hypercalcemia
Autosomal-dominant osteogenesis imperfecta	See Osteogenesis imperfecta syndrome, type I	
Baller-Gerold syndrome (craniosynostosis–radial aplasia syndrome)	Craniosynostosis	Facial anomalies, limb anomalies, occasional vertebral anomalies, occasional cardiac anomalies
Bardet-Biedl syndrome	Miscellaneous	Obesity, mental deficiency, renal anomalies and hypertension, cardiac anomalies, occasional diabetes insipidus, ocular anomalies, spinocerebellar degeneration
Basal cell nevus syndrome	See Gorlin's syndrome	
BBB syndrome	See Opitz syndrome	
Beals' auriculo-osteodysplasia syndrome	Other skeletal dysplasias	Growth deficiency, limb anomalies, joint laxity
Beals' contractural arachnodactyly syndrome	See Beals' syndrome	
Beals' syndrome (Beals' contractural arachnodactyly syndrome)[13]	Connective tissue disorder	Joint stiffness, kyphoscoliosis, mitral valve prolapse, micrognathia, short neck, cardiac anomalies
Beckwith-Wiedemann syndrome (exomphalos-macroglossia-gigantism)[14–16]	Overgrowth	Variable mental deficiency, macroglossia, facial anomalies, renal anomalies, fetal adrenocortical cytomegaly, neonatal polycythemia, hypoglycemia in early infancy, predisposition to malignancy, cardiac anomalies
Berardinelli's lipodystrophy syndrome (generalized lipodystrophy)	Miscellaneous	Mental deficiency, accelerated growth with excess glycogen and lack of adipose tissue, hepatomegaly, hyperlipemia, hyperglucagonemia, insulin-resistant nonketotic hyperglycemia, occasional cardiomegaly
Blepharophimosis syndrome (familial blepharophimosis syndrome)	Characterized by facial defect	Facial anomalies, hypotonia, occasional cardiac anomalies, occasional mental deficiency
Bloch-Sulzberger syndrome	See Incontinentia pigmenti syndrome	
Bloom's syndrome	Growth deficiency	Occasional mild mental deficiency, facial anomalies, micrognathia, immunoglobulin deficiency, predisposition to malignancy
Börjeson-Forssman-Lehmann syndrome	Miscellaneous	Growth deficiency, mental deficiency, facial anomalies, vertebral anomalies, brain anomalies, supraspinal hypotonia
Brachmann-de Lange	See De Lange syndrome	
Brachydactyly syndrome, type E	Other skeletal dysplasias	Growth deficiency, limb anomalies
Brachydactyly-spherophakia syndrome	See Weill-Marchesani syndrome	
Branchiootorenal (BOR) syndrome	See Melnick-Fraser syndrome	
Caffey pseudo-Hurler's syndrome	See Generalized gangliosidosis syndrome, type I	

Syndrome	Category	Anesthetic Considerations
Camptomelic dysplasia	Osteochondrodysplasias	Generally an early lethal disorder; brain anomalies, facial anomalies, micrognathia, cervical spine anomalies, vertebral anomalies, small chest cavity, tracheobronchiomalacia, cardiac anomalies, hydrocephalus
Camurati-Englemann syndrome (progressive diaphyseal dysplasia)	Connective tissue disorder	Hypotonia
Cardiac-limb defect	See Holt-Oram syndrome	
Carpenter's syndrome	Craniosynostosis	Mental deficiency, facial anomalies, limb anomalies, joint laxity, occasional cardiac anomalies
Cartilage–hair hypoplasia syndrome	See Metaphyseal chondrodysplasia, McKusick type	
Cat-eye syndrome, (coloboma of iris–anal atresia)	Chromosomal	Mild mental deficiency, renal anomalies, micrognathia, joint laxity, cardiac defects
Caudal dysplasia sequence (caudal regression syndrome)	Miscellaneous	Vertebral anomalies, including sacral and lumbar hypoplasia, distal spinal cord anomalies, joint contractures, renal anomalies or agenesis, meningomyelocele
Caudal regression syndrome	See Caudal dysplasia sequence	
Cerebellar hemangioblastoma	See von Hippel–Lindau syndrome	
Cerebral gigantism	See Sotos' syndrome	
Cerebrocostomandibular syndrome	Miscellaneous	Mental deficiency, growth deficiency, severe micrognathia, small thorax, vertebral anomalies, chronic respiratory infections, abnormal tracheal rings
Cerebrohepatorenal syndrome	See Zellweger's syndrome	
Cerebrooculofacioskeletal (COFS) syndrome	Brain or neuromuscular defects	Growth deficiency leading to death in early childhood, brain anomalies, muscle weakness, facial anomalies, micrognathia, ocular anomalies, joint contractures
CHARGE association[17]	Miscellaneous	Colobomatous malformation, cardiac anomalies, choanal atresia, growth deficiency, mental deficiency, micrognathia, genital hypoplasia, tracheoesophageal fistula, ear anomalies
Charlie M. syndrome	See Oromandibular– limb hypogenesis spectrum	
Chédiak-Higashi syndrome[18]	Miscellaneous	Partial albinism, pancytopenia, mental deficiency, seizures, peripheral neuropathy, predisposition to malignancy, anemia, thrombocytopenia
Cheney's syndrome	See Hajdu-Cheney syndrome	
CHILD syndrome	Limb defects	Unilateral hypomelia, unilateral dermal anomalies, unilateral vertebral anomalies, cardiac anomalies, occasional cranial nerve and brain anomalies, mild mental deficiency
Chondrodysplasia punctata (Conradi-Hünermann syndrome)	Osteochondrodysplasias	Facial anomalies, joint stiffness, dermal anomalies, micrognathia, tracheal calcifications with tracheal stenosis
Chondrodysplasia punctata, rhizomelic type	See Rhizomelic chondrodysplasia punctata syndrome	

Syndrome	Category	Anesthetic Considerations
Chondrodystrophica myotonia	See Schwartz-Jampel syndrome	
Chondroectodermal dysplasia (Ellis–van Creveld syndrome)	Osteochondrodysplasias	Facial anomalies, cardiac anomalies, small thorax, occasional mental deficiency
Classic arthrogryposis	See Amyoplasia congenita disruptive sequence	
Cleidocranial dysostosis	Osteochondrodysplasia with osteopetrosis	Facial anomalies, complete aplasia of the clavicle with associated muscle defects, vertebral anomalies, narrow thorax, fragile bones
Clouston's syndrome	Skin dysplasias	Dermal anomalies
Cockayne's syndrome[19, 20]	Miscellaneous	Growth deficiency, loss of adipose tissue, muscle weakness, joint contractures, mental deficiency, facial anomalies, vertebral anomalies, hepatomegaly, hypertension
Coffin-Lowry syndrome	Characterized by facial defect	Growth deficiency, mental deficiency, occasional cardiac anomalies, muscle weakness, vertebral anomalies, mitral insufficiency, joint laxity
Coffin-Siris syndrome	Miscellaneous	Growth deficiency, facial anomalies, mental deficiency, muscle weakness, occasional cardiac anomalies, occasional vertebral anomalies, brain anomalies, chronic respiratory infections
Cohen's syndrome	Brain or neuromuscular defects	Truncal obesity, mental deficiency, muscle weakness, facial anomalies, ocular anomalies, open mouth with prominent incisors, micrognathia, occasional mitral valve prolapse, occasional leukopenia, joint laxity, vertebral anomalies
Coloboma of iris–anal atresia	See Cat-eye syndrome	
Congenital arthromyodysplasia	See Amyoplasia congenita disruptive sequence	
Conradi-Hünermann syndrome	See Chondrodysplasia punctata	
Cornelia de Lange	See De Lange syndrome	
Craniofacial dysostosis	See Crouzon's syndrome	
Craniometaphyseal dysplasia	Osteochondrodysplasias	Craniofacial hyperostosis, compression of cranial nerves and brain
Craniosynostosis–radial aplasia syndrome	See Baller-Gerold syndrome	
Cri-du-chat	See 5p− syndrome	
Crouzon's syndrome (craniofacial dysostosis)	Craniosynostosis	Facial anomalies, mental deficiency, seizures, upper airway obstruction, choanal atresia, occasional ocular anomalies
Cryptophthalmos syndrome	See Fraser syndrome	
de Lange syndrome (Cornelia de Lange, Brachmann-de Lange)[21–23]	Growth deficiency	Mild mental deficiency, seizures, hypertonia, joint contractures, facial anomalies, micrognathia, choanal atresia, perioral cyanosis, occasional cardiac anomalies
De Sanctis–Cacchione syndrome (xerodermic idiocy syndrome)	Growth deficiency	Mental deficiency, brain anomalies, seizures, spasticity, hypothalamic dysfunction, xeroderma pigmentosa
Diaphyseal aclasis	See Multiple exostoses syndrome	
Diastrophic dysplasia (diastrophic nanism syndrome)	Osteochondrodysplasias	Vertebral anomalies, occasional micrognathia, odontoid hypoplasia with subluxation, small thorax, joint laxity, joint contractures, laryngotracheal stenosis

Syndrome	Category	Anesthetic Considerations
Diastrophic nanism syndrome	See Diastrophic dysplasia	
Di George sequence[24]	Miscellaneous	Hypoplasia or aplasia of the thymus, hypocalcemia secondary to parathyroid hypoplasia, seizures, cardiac anomalies, occasional choanal atresia, diaphragmatic hernia, tracheoesophageal fistula, short trachea
Dilantin effects	See Hydantoin effects	
Distal arthrogryposis syndrome	Brain or neuromuscular defects	Joint contractures, clenched hands, joint laxity, occasional trismus
Distichiasis-lymphedema syndrome	Miscellaneous	Epidural spinal cysts, other vertebral anomalies
Donohue's syndrome	See Leprechaunism syndrome	
Dubowitz's syndrome	Growth deficiency	Variable mental deficiency, facial anomalies, micrognathia
Dyggve-Melchior-Clausen syndrome	Osteochondrodysplasias	Mental deficiency, vertebral anomalies, joint stiffness, atlantoaxial instability due to odontoid hypoplasia
Dysencephalia splanchnocystica	See Meckel-Gruber syndrome	
Dyskeratosis congenita syndrome	Hamartosis	Dermal anomalies, pancytopenia, esophageal, urethral, ureteral, anal strictures, tracheoesophageal fistula, predisposition to malignancy, anemia, immune deficiency, thrombocytopenia
Dystrophia myotonica	See Steinert's myotonic dystrophy syndrome	
Early amnion rupture sequence	Miscellaneous	Facial anomalies, choanal atresia, limb anomalies, encephalocele, abdominal and thoracic wall defects
Early urethral obstruction sequence	Miscellaneous	Urethral obstruction leading to renal dysplasia, abdominal muscle deficiency, and iliac vessel compression
Ectrodactyly–ectodermal dysplasia–clefting syndrome (EEC syndrome)[25]	Characterized by facial defect	Facial, ocular, and limb anomalies, occasional renal anomalies
EEC syndrome	See Ectrodactyly–ectodermal dysplasia–clefting syndrome	
Ehlers-Danlos syndrome[26]	Connective tissue disorder	Joint laxity, fragile blood vessels, delayed wound healing, mitral valve prolapse, other valvular prolapse and vessel dilatation, other cardiac anomalies, occasional mental deficiency, glaucoma
Ellis–van Creveld syndrome	See Chondroectodermal dysplasia	
Enchondromatosis	See Osteochondromatosis syndrome	
Endemic cretinism	See Iodine deficiency effects	
Escobar's syndrome, (multiple pterygium syndrome)[27]	Limb defects	Facial anomalies, severe micrognathia, cervical spine fusion, joint contractures, joint laxity, other vertebral anomalies
Exomphalos-macroglossia-gigantism	See Beckwith-Wiedemann syndrome	
Exstrophy of cloaca sequence	Miscellaneous	Vertebral anomalies, hydromyelia
External chondromatosis syndrome	See Multiple exostoses syndrome	

Syndrome	Category	Anesthetic Considerations
Fabry's syndrome (Anderson-Fabry disease, angiokeratoma corporis diffusum)	Miscellaneous	Ceramide trihexoside accumulation, progressive renal insufficiency, seizures, hemiplegia, glycolipid infiltration of the heart, hypotonia, airway obstruction secondary to ceramide trihexoside in the airway epithelium, anemia from chronic blood loss
Facial-limb disruptive spectrum	See Oromandibular–limb hypogenesis spectrum	
Facioauriculovertebral spectrum (first and second branchial arch syndrome, oculoauricular vertebral dysplasia, hemifacial microsomia, Goldenhar's syndrome)[28–30]	Miscellaneous	Cervical spine fusion, ocular anomalies, hemifacial micrognathia, laryngeal anomalies, auricular anomalies, cardiac anomalies, variable mental deficiency, encephalocele, occasional renal anomalies, glaucoma
Faciogenitopopliteal syndrome	See Popliteal pterygium syndrome	
Familial blepharophimosis syndrome	See Blepharophimosis syndrome	
Familial neurovisceral lipidosis	See Generalized gangliosidosis syndrome, type I	
Fanconi's pancytopenia syndrome[31]	Limb defects	Mental deficiency, facial anomalies, joint laxity, renal anomalies, pancytopenia, occasional cardiac anomalies, predisposition to malignancy
Femoral hypoplasia–unusual facies syndrome	Limb defects	Small lower limbs, joint contractures, facial anomalies, micrognathia, vertebral anomalies
Fetal akinesia–hypokinesia sequence	See Pena-Shokeir phenotype	
Fetal face syndrome	See Robinow's syndrome	
Fetal trimethadione syndrome	See Trimethadione effects	
FG syndrome	Characterized by facial defect	Mental deficiency, muscle weakness, joint contractures, seizures, facial anomalies, occasional cardiac anomalies, vertebral anomalies
Fibrochondrogenesis	Osteochondrodysplasias	Early lethal disorder; facial anomalies, micrognathia, vertebral anomalies, small chest cavity, joint contractures
Fibrodysplasia ossificans progressiva syndrome	Connective tissue disorder	Severe immobilization, pain
First and second branchial arch syndrome	See facioauriculovertebral spectrum	
Fragile X syndrome (Martin-Bell, marker X syndrome)[32]	Overgrowth	Mild mental deficiency, facial anomalies, occasional muscle weakness, mitral valve prolapse, torticollis, mild connective tissue dysplasia, joint laxity
Franceschetti-Klein syndrome	See Treacher Collins syndrome	
Fraser's syndrome (cryptophthalamos syndrome)[33]	Characterized by facial defect	Facial anomalies, auricular anomalies, mental deficiency, laryngeal stenosis or atresia, renal anomalies, occasional cardiac anomalies
Freeman-Sheldon syndrome (whistling face syndrome)[34–37]	Brain or neuromuscular defects	Increased muscle tone, whistling facies causing microstomia, vertebral anomalies, myotonia, possible malignant hyperthermia risk
Frontometaphyseal dysplasia (Gorlin-Cohen syndrome)[38]	Osteochondrodysplasias	Facial anomalies, micrognathia, cervical vertebral anomalies, muscle weakness, mental deficiency, subglottic tracheal narrowing

Syndrome	Category	Anesthetic Considerations
Frontonasal dysplasia sequence (median cleft face syndrome)[39]	Characterized by facial defect	Facial anomalies, including completely divided nostrils, deficit in midline frontal bone, occasional mental deficiency
G syndrome	See under Opitz syndrome	
Gardner's syndrome[40]	Hamartosis	Polyposis of colon, occasional other hamartomasa, predisposition to malignancy
Geleophysic dysplasia	Osteochondrodysplasias	Facial anomalies, progressive thickening of heart valves leading to cardiac failure during childhood, joint contractures
Generalized gangliosidosis syndrome, type I (severe infantile type, Caffey's pseudo-Hurler's syndrome, familial neurovisceral lipidosis)	Storage disorders	Early lethal disorder, growth deficiency, mental deficiency, muscle weakness, facial anomalies, prominent maxilla and mild macroglossia, some joint limitation, vertebral anomalies, hepatomegaly
Generalized lipodystrophy	See Berardinelli's lipodystrophy syndrome	
Giant cell chondrodysplasia	See Atelosteogenesis	
Glossopalatine ankylosis syndrome	See Oromandibular–limb hypogenesis spectrum	
β-Glucuronidase deficiency	See Mucopolysaccharidosis VII	
Goldenhar's syndrome	See Facioauriculovertebral spectrum	
Goltz's syndrome[41, 42]	Hamartosis	Dermal anomalies, ocular anomalies, occasional mental deficiency, joint laxity, occasional cardiac anomalies, vertebral anomalies
Goniodysgenesis	See Rieger's eye malformation sequence	
Gorlin's syndrome (basal cell nevus syndrome)[41–43]	Hamartosis	Variable mental deficiency, facial anomalies, mandibular cysts, hydrocephalus, vertebral anomalies (including cervical spine fusion), dermal anomalies, predisposition to malignancy, glaucoma
Grebe's syndrome	Limb defects	Severe limb deficiency; otherwise normal
Greig's cephalopolysyndactyly syndrome	Craniosynostosis	Facial anomalies, limb anomalies, hydrocephalus, joint contractures
Hajdu-Cheney syndrome (Cheney's syndrome, acroosteolysis syndrome, arthrodentoosteodysplasia)	Osteochondrodysplasias	Facial anomalies, micrognathia, vertebral anomalies, fragile bones, muscle weakness
Hallermann-Streiff syndrome (oculomandibulodyscephaly with hypotrichosis syndrome)[44, 45]	Growth deficiency	Facial anomalies, micrognathia, small mouth, vertebral anomalies, occasional mental deficiency, ocular anomalies, chronic respiratory infections, glaucoma
Happy puppet syndrome	See Angelman's syndrome	
Hard ± E syndrome	See Warburg's syndrome	
Hays-Wells syndrome of ectodermal dysplasia (ankyloblepharon–ectodermal dysplasia–clefting syndrome, AEC syndrome)	Characterized by facial defect	Facial, limb, auricular, and occasional cardiac anomalies
Hecht's syndrome (trismus pseudocamptodactyly syndrome, Dutch-Kentucky)[46–49]	Brain or neuromuscular defects	Severely limited mouth opening secondary to trismus (muscle relaxants do not relieve the trismus), joint contractures
Hemifacial microsomia	See Facioauriculovertebral spectrum	

Syndrome	Category	Anesthetic Considerations
Hereditary arthroopthalmopathy	See Stickler's syndrome	
Hereditary osteoonychodysplasia	See Nail-patella syndrome	
Hereditary hemorrhagic telangiectasia	See Osler's hemorrhagic telangiectasia syndrome	
Holoprosencephaly sequence	Miscellaneous	Early lethal disorder; severe brain anomalies, cyclopia, incomplete midline facial development
Holt-Oram syndrome (cardiac–limb defect)	Limb defects	Upper limb and shoulder girdle defects, cardiac anomalies, hypoplasia of distal blood vessels, occasional vertebral anomalies
Homocystinuria syndrome[50-54]	Connective tissue disorder	Mental deficiency, ocular anomalies, osteoporosis, medial weakness of the great arteries with intimal hyperplasia leading to irregular vessel lumens and excessive vascular thrombosis; venipuncture may cause thrombosis, thromboembolic disease
Homozygous Leri-Weill dyschondrosteosis syndrome	See Langer's mesomelic dysplasia	
Hunter's syndrome (mucopolysaccharidosis II)[55, 56]	Storage disorders	Growth deficiency, mental deficiency, facial anomalies, macroglossia, airway obstruction, joint stiffness, hepatosplenomegaly, eventual development of congestive heart failure, seizures, hypertonia, hydrocephalus
Hurler's syndrome (mucopolysaccharidosis I H)[55, 57, 58]	Storage disorders	Growth deficiency, mental deficiency, facial anomalies, macroglossia, joint stiffness, cardiac failure secondary to coronary vascular narrowing or valvular disease, chronic respiratory infections, hepatosplenomegaly, hydrocephalus
Hurler-Scheie compound syndrome (mucopolysaccharidosis I H/S)[59]	Storage disorders	Growth deficiency, mental deficiency, micrognathia, moderate joint stiffness, occasional cardiac valve disease, occasional hepatosplenomegaly
Hutchinson-Gilford syndrome	See Progeria	
Hydantoin effects (fetal dilantin syndrome, fetal hydantoin sequence)	Environmental agents	Growth deficiency, variable mental deficiency, facial anomalies, occasional cardiac anomalies, joint laxity
Hypertelorism-hypospadias	See Opitz syndrome	
Hyperthermia-induced spectrum of defects	Environmental agents	Mental deficiency, muscle weakness, encephalocele, ocular anomalies, micrognathia, facial anomalies, joint contractures, vertebral anomalies
Hypochondrogenesis	See Achondrogenesis, type II	
Hypochondroplasia	Osteochondrodysplasias	Caudal narrowing of spine, vertebral anomalies, occasional mental deficiency, joint contractures
Hypoglossia-hypodactyly syndrome	See Oromandibular–limb hypogenesis spectrum	
Hypohidrotic ectodermal dysplasia syndrome	Skin dysplasias	Thin and hypoplastic skin, hypoplasia or absence of sweat glands, hyperthermia secondary to inability to sweat
Hypohidrotic ectodermal dysplasia–autosomal dominant type	See Rapp-Hodgkin ectodermal dysplasia syndrome	
Hypomelia–hypertrichosis–facial hemangioma syndrome	See Roberts-SC phocomelia syndrome	

Syndrome	Category	Anesthetic Considerations
Hypophosphatasia	Osteochondrodysplasias	Alkaline phosphatase deficiency, fragile bones, small chest cavity, muscle weakness, seizures, hypercalcemia, anemia
Hypothryoidism sequence	See Athyrotic hypothyroidism sequence	
Incontinentia pigmenti syndrome (Bloch-Sulzberger syndrome)	Hamartosis	Dermal anomalies, occasional mental deficiency, hydrocephalus, hypertonia, ocular anomalies, vertebral anomalies
Iodine deficiency effects (endemic cretinism)	Environmental agents	Mental deficiency, hypertonia, hypothyroidism
Ivemark syndrome	See Laterality sequences	
Jarcho-Levin syndrome (spondylothoracic dysplasia)	Miscellaneous	Facial anomalies, short neck, small thorax, multiple vertebral anomalies, occasional anal and urethral atresia, chronic respiratory infections
Jeune's thoracic dystrophy[60]	Osteochondrodysplasias	Early lethal disorder; small chest cavity with pulmonary hypoplasia, renal anomalies leading to progressive renal insufficiency, vertebral anomalies
Johanson-Blizzard syndrome	Growth deficiency	Hypothyroidism, hypotonia, facial anomalies, variable mental deficiency, pancreatic insufficiency
Jugular lymphatic obstruction sequence	Miscellaneous	Peripheral lymphedema
Kartagener's syndrome[61]	Miscellaneous	Situs inversus, other cardiac anomalies, frontal sinus anomalies, thick tenacious mucus, IgA deficiency, chronic respiratory infections, occasional asplenia
Kenny's syndrome[62]	Osteochondrodysplasias	Ocular anomalies, anemia, transient hypocalcemia secondary to hyperparathyroidism
Killian/Teschler-Nicola syndrome (Pallister's mosaic syndrome, tetrasomy 12p)	Brain or neuromuscular defects	Mental deficiency, seizures, muscle weakness, facial anomalies, occasional macroglossia, occasional micrognathia, joint contractures, joint laxity
Klinefelter's syndrome	See XXY syndrome	
Klippel-Feil sequence[63–65]	Miscellaneous	Fused cervical vertebrae, torticollis, spinal cord anomalies, cardiac anomalies, renal anomalies
Klippel-Trenaunay-Weber syndrome[66–68]	Hamartosis	Hemangiomas, limb anomalies, facial anomalies, occasional mental deficiency, growth deficiency, intravascular clotting anomaly, glaucoma
Kniest's dysplasia	Osteochondrodysplasias	Facial anomalies, joint stiffness, vertebral anomalies
Kozlowski's spondylometaphyseal chondrodysplasia	See Kozlowski's spondylometaphyseal dysplasia	
Kozlowski's spondylometaphyseal dysplasia (Kozlowski's spondylometaphyseal chondrodysplasia)	Osteochondrodysplasias	Vertebral anomalies, odontoid hypoplasia, joint stiffness
Lacrimoauriculodentodigital syndrome	See Levy-Hollister syndrome	
Langer's mesomelic dysplasia (homozygous Leri-Weill dyschondrosteosis syndrome)	Other skeletal dysplasias	Micrognathia, limb anomalies, occasional cardiac anomalies, tendency toward fractures
Langer-Giedion syndrome (trichorhinophalangeal syndrome with exostosis)	Characterized by facial defect	Growth deficiency, mental deficiency, facial anomalies, micrognathia, limb anomalies, muscle weakness, chronic respiratory infections, occasional cardiac anomalies, anemia

Syndrome	Category	Anesthetic Considerations
Langer-Saldino achondrogenesis	See Achondrogenesis, type II	
Larsen's syndrome[69, 70]	Characterized by facial defect	Facial anomalies, limb anomalies, mobile and infolding arytenoid cartilage, occasional cervical spine anomalies, occasional cardiac anomalies, joint laxity
Laterality sequences (Ivemark's syndrome, polysplenia syndrome, asplenia syndrome)	Miscellaneous	Severe cardiac anomalies, polysplenia or asplenia
Lenz-Majewski hyperostosis syndrome	Osteochrondrodysplasia with osteopetrosis	Mental deficiency, facial anomalies, choanal atresia, micrognathia, dermal anomalies
LEOPARD syndrome	See Multiple lentigines syndrome	
Leprechaunism syndrome (Donohue's syndrome)	Miscellaneous	Growth deficiency, mental deficiency, facial anomalies, lack of cellular response to insulin, hyperglycemia, hyperinsulinemia, dermal anomalies, chronic respiratory infections, hypoglycemia following prolonged fasting
Leri-Weill dyschondrosteosis	Other skeletal dysplasias	Limb anomalies, joint laxity and contractures
Leri-Weill homozygous dyschondrosteosis syndrome	See under Langer's mesomelic dysplasia	
Leroy I-cell syndrome (mucolipidosis II)	Storage disorders	Growth deficiency, mental deficiency, facial anomalies, hypertrophy of alveolar ridges, moderate joint limitation, congestive heart failure
Lethal multiple pterygium syndrome	Brain or neuromuscular defects	Early lethal disorder; facial anomalies, micrognathia, flexion, contractures (including chin to sternum), small chest cavity, cardiac hypoplasia, pulmonary hypoplasia
Levy-Hollister syndrome (lacrimoauriculodentodigital syndrome)	Limb defects	Facial anomalies, hearing loss
Linear sebaceous nevus sequence (nevus sebaceus of Jadassohn)	Hamartosis	Dermal anomalies, hydrocephalus, seizures, mental deficiency, ocular anomalies, cardiac anomalies, renal anomalies, predisposition to malignancy
Lip pit–cleft lip syndrome	See Van der Woude's syndrome	
Lissencephaly syndrome	See Miller-Dieker syndrome	
Lobstein's disease	See Osteogenesis imperfecta syndrome, type I	
Louis-Bar syndrome	See Ataxia-telangiectasia syndrome	
Lowe's syndrome (oculocerebrorenal syndrome)	Brain or neuromuscular defects	Muscle weakness, joint laxity, mental deficiency, growth deficiency, renal tubular dysfunction, seizures, glaucoma
Maffucci's syndrome	Hamartosis	Limb anomalies, hemangiomas, predisposition to malignancy, fractures
Mandibulofacial dysostosis	See Treacher Collins syndrome	
Marfan's syndrome	Connective tissue disorder	Muscle weakness, joint laxity, vertebral anomalies, ocular anomalies, ascending aortic dilatation or dissection, aortic valve insufficiency, aneurysms of other great vessels, mitral valve prolapse, tendency to spontaneous pneumothorax, vertebral anomalies

Syndrome	Category	Anesthetic Considerations
Marinesco-Sjögren syndrome	Brain or neuromuscular defects	Growth deficiency, mental deficiency, hypotonia, ocular anomalies
Marker X syndrome	See Fragile X syndrome	
Maroteaux-Lamy mucopolysaccharidosis syndrome (mucopolysaccharidosis VI)	Storage disorders	Growth deficiency, vertebral anomalies, odontoid hypoplasia, hepatospenomegaly, occasional macroglossia, occasional valvular heart disease, hydrocephalus, joint contractures
Marshall syndrome	Characterized by facial defect	Facial anomalies, protruding upper incisors, ocular anomalies, deafness, occasional mental deficiency
Marshall-Smith syndrome	Overgrowth	Mental deficiency, muscle weakness, micrognathia, small mandibular ramus, choanal atresia, rudimentary epiglottis, upper airway obstruction, brain anomalies, chronic respiratory infections
Martin-Bell	See Fragile X syndrome	
Maternal phenylketonuria (PKU) fetal effects	Environmental agents	Mental deficiency, increased muscle tone, growth deficiency, facial anomalies, micrognathia, cardiac anomalies, vertebral anomalies, esophageal atresia, tracheoesophageal fistula
McCune-Albright syndrome (osteitis fibrosa cystica)[71]	Hamartosis	Fibrous dysplasia, dermal anomalies, hyperthyroidism, hyperparathyroidism, Cushing's syndrome, diabetes, acromegaly, cranial nerve compression
Meckel-Gruber syndrome (dysencephalia splanchnocystica)	Brain or neuromuscular defects	Early lethal disorder; brain anomalies, encephalocele, hydrocephalus, micrognathia, facial anomalies, renal anomalies, lobulated tongue, cleft epiglottis, cardiac anomalies, pulmonary hypoplasia
Median cleft face syndrome	See Frontonasal dysplasia sequence	
Melnick-Fraser syndrome (branchiootorenal (BOR) syndrome)	Characterized by facial defect	Hearing loss, facial anomalies, auricular anomalies, renal anomalies
Melnick-Needles syndrome	Miscellaneous	Facial anomalies, small chest cavity, micrognathia, occasional pulmonary hypertension, joint laxity, vertebral anomalies
Meningomyelocele, anencephaly, iniencephaly sequences	Miscellaneous	Defective neural tube closure, severe brain anomalies, hydrocephalus, facial anomalies, diaphragmatic defects, vertebral anomalies, hypoplasia of the heart and/or lungs, cervical spine anomalies, short trachea
Menkes' kinky hair syndrome[72]	See Menkes' syndrome	
Menkes' syndrome (Menkes' kinky hair syndrome)	Brain or neuromuscular defects	Severe brain anomalies, seizures, hypertonia, dermal anomalies, widespread arterial elongation and tortuosity secondary to copper metabolism defect
Mesodermal dysgenesis of the iris	See Rieger's eye malformation sequence	
Metaphyseal chondrodysplasia, Schmid type (metaphyseal dysplasia, Schmid type)	Osteochondrodysplasias	Growth deficiency
Metaphyseal chondrodysplasia with pancreatic insufficiency and neutropenia	See Schwachman's syndrome	
Metaphyseal chondrodysplasia, Jansen type (metaphyseal dysostosis, Jansen type)	Osteochondrodysplasias	Facial anomalies, micrognathia, hypercalcemia, small thorax, joint contractures

Syndrome	Category	Anesthetic Considerations
Metaphyseal chondrodysplasia, McKusick type (cartilage–hair hypoplasia syndrome)	Osteochondrodysplasias	Vertebral anomalies, joint contractures, diminished T-cell response, anemia, intestinal malabsorption
Metaphyseal dysostosis, Jansen type	See Metaphyseal chondrodysplasia, Jansen type	
Metaphyseal dysplasia, Schmid type	See Metaphyseal chondrodysplasia, Schmid type	
Metatrophic dwarfism syndrome	See Metatrophic dysplasia	
Metatrophic dysplasia (metatrophic dwarfism syndrome)	Osteochondrodysplasias	Small thorax, vertebral anomalies, joint laxity and contractures
Methyl mercury effects	Environmental agents	Growth deficiency, mental deficiency,
Mietens' syndrome	Characterized by facial defect	Mild mental deficiency, facial anomalies, elbow flexion contracture, occasional vascular anomalies
Miller's syndrome (postaxial acrofacial dysostosis syndrome)[73, 74]	Characterized by facial defect	Facial anomalies, auricular anomalies, micrognathia, upper airway hypoplasia, limb anomalies, occasional cardiac anomalies
Miller-Dieker syndrome (lissencephaly syndrome)	Brain or neuromuscular defects	Brain anomalies, severe mental deficiency, hypotonia, seizures, facial anomalies, cardiac anomalies, death usually during infancy
Moebius' sequence[75]	Characterized by facial defect	Sixth and seventh nerve palsy, brain anomalies, micrognathia, chronic aspiration, occasional mental deficiency
Moebius' syndrome	See Oromandibular–limb hypogenesis spectrum	
Mohr's syndrome (OFD syndrome, type II)	Characterized by facial defect	Deafness, facial anomalies, hypoplasia of maxilla and mandible
Morquio's syndrome (mucopolysaccharidosis IV, types A and B)[55, 76–78]	Storage disorders	Growth deficiency, vertebral anomalies, odontoid hypoplasia, joint contractures and laxity, aortic valve insufficiency, hepatomegaly
Mucolipidosis II	See Leroy I-cell syndrome	
Mucolipidosis III	See Pseudo-Hurler's polydystrophy syndrome	
Mucopolysaccharidosis I H	See Hurler's syndrome	
Mucopolysaccharidosis I H/S	See Hurler-Scheie compound syndrome	
Mucopolysaccharidosis I S	See Scheie's syndrome	
Mucopolysaccharidosis II	See Hunter's syndrome	
Mucopolysaccharidosis III, types A, B, C, and D	See Sanfilippo's syndrome	
Mucopolysaccharidosis IV, types A and B	See Morquio's syndrome	
Mucopolysaccharidosis VI	See Maroteaux-Lamy mucopolysaccharidosis syndrome	
Mucopolysaccharidosis VII (Sly's syndrome, β-glucuronidase deficiency)	Storage disorders	Growth deficiency, mental deficiency, hydrocephalus, hepatosplenomegaly, occasional vertebral anomalies, occasional odontoid hypoplasia, valvular heart disease, joint contractures
Mulibrey nanism syndrome (Perheentupa syndrome)	Growth deficiency	Facial anomalies, hepatomegaly, onset of pericardial constriction during infancy, muscle weakness
Multiple congenital articular rigidities	See Amyoplasia congenita disruptive sequence	

Syndrome	Category	Anesthetic Considerations
Multiple endocrine neoplasia, type 2b	See Multiple neuroma syndrome	
Multiple epiphyseal dysplasia	Osteochondrodysplasias	Joint stiffness, vertebral anomalies
Multiple exostoses syndrome (diaphyseal aclasis, external chondromatosis syndrome)	Other skeletal dysplasias	Limb anomalies, predisposition to malignancy
Multiple lentigines syndrome (LEOPARD syndrome)[79]	Hamartosis	Lentigines, ECG abnormalities, ocular hypertelorism, pulmonic stenosis, abnormalities of genitalia, growth retardation, deafness, other cardiac anomalies, occasional mental deficiency
Multiple neuroma syndrome (multiple endocrine neoplasia, type 2b)	Hamartosis	Neuromas from mouth to rectum, thyroid carcinoma, pheochromocytoma, marfanoid habitus, parathyroid hypoplasia, laryngeal anomalies, muscle weakness, hypertension
Multiple pterygium syndrome	See Escobar's syndrome	
Multiple synostosis syndrome (symphalangism syndrome)	Other skeletal dysplasias	Facial anomalies, limb anomalies, vertebral anomalies, auricular anomalies
Multisynostotic osteodysgenesis	See Antley-Bixler syndrome	
Murcs' association	Miscellaneous	Cervical and thoracic vertebral anomalies, renal anomalies, limb anomalies, occasional micrognathia
Myodystrophia fetalis deformans	See Amyoplasia congenita disruptive sequence	
Myophagism congenita	See Amyoplasia congenita disruptive sequence	
Nager's acrofacial dysostosis syndrome	See Nager syndrome	
Nager's syndrome, (Nager's acrofacial dysostosis syndrome)[80]	Characterized by facial defect	Facial anomalies, auricular anomalies, severe micrognathia, upper airway hypoplasia, limb anomalies, occasional cardiac anomalies
Nail-patella syndrome (hereditary osteoonychodysplasia)	Other skeletal dysplasias	Limb anomalies, renal anomalies but renal failure rare in childhood, occasional vertebral anomalies, occasional mental deficiency, limited joint mobility
Neu-Laxova syndrome	Brain or neuromuscular defects	Early lethal disorder; encephalocele, hydrocephalus, growth deficiency, brain anomalies, facial anomalies, micrognathia, cardiac anomalies, occasional renal agenesis
Neurocutaneous melanosis sequence	Hamartosis	Melanosis of skin and CNS, seizures, hydrocephalus
Neurofibromatosis syndrome[81-86]	Hamartosis	Dermal anomalies, subcutaneous tumors, brain anomalies, vertebral anomalies, nerve compression, predisposition to malignancy, variable mental deficiency, occasional cardiac anomalies, occasional hypertension
Nevus sebaceus of Jadassohn	See Linear sebaceous nevus sequence	
Noonan's syndrome (Turner-like syndrome)[87-89]	Characterized by facial defect	Variable mental deficiency, facial anomalies, micrognathia, pectus excavatum, vertebral anomalies, cardiac anomalies, reports of malignant hyperthermia
Occult spinal dysraphism sequence (tethered cord malformation sequence)	Miscellaneous	Cord tethering, compression of sacral nerve roots, sacral vertebral anomalies, urinary obstruction secondary to nerve root injury
Oculocerebrorenal syndrome	See Lowe's syndrome	

Syndrome	Category	Anesthetic Considerations
Oculoauricular vertebral dysplasia	See Facioauriculovertebral spectrum	
Oculodentodigital dysplasia	See Oculodentodigital syndrome	
Oculodentodigital syndrome (oculodentodigital dysplasia)	Characterized by facial defect	Ocular anomalies, facial anomalies, hand and feet anomalies, hypertonia, joint laxity, glaucoma
Oculomandibulodyscephaly with hypotrichosis syndrome	See Hallermann-Streiff syndrome	
OFD syndrome, type I	See Oral-facial-digital syndrome	
OFD syndrome, type II	See Mohr's syndrome	
Oligohydramnios sequence (Potter's syndrome)	Miscellaneous	Pulmonary hypoplasia, facial anomalies, joint contractures and laxity
Ollier's disease	See Osteochondromatosis syndrome	
Opitz syndrome (hypertelorism-hypospadias, Opitz-Frias, G syndrome, BBB syndrome)[90]	Characterized by facial defect	Mental deficiency, facial anomalies, occasional cardiac anomalies, laryngotracheal cleft, malformation of the larynx, tracheoesophageal fistula, high carina, pulmonary hypoplasia, renal anomalies, chronic respiratory infections
Opitz-Frias syndrome	See Opitz syndrome	
Oral-facial-digital syndrome (OFD syndrome, type I)	Characterized by facial defect	Irregular clefts in alveolar ridge, facial anomalies, mental deficiency, choanal atresia, micrognathia, seizures, hydrocephalus, renal anomalies
Oromandibular–limb hypogenesis spectrum (hypoglossia-hypodactyly syndrome, aglossia-adactyly syndrome, glossopalatine ankylosis syndrome, Moebius' syndrome, Charlie M. syndrome, facial-limb disruptive spectrum)[75]	Miscellaneous	Micrognathia, microstomia, cranial nerve palsies, limb anomalies, brain anomalies
Osler's hemorrhagic telangiectasia syndrome (hereditary hemorrhagic telangiectasia)	Hamartosis	Telangiectases of the skin, mucosa, and organs, arteriovenous fistula of the lung, cirrhosis, aneurysms, brain vascular anomalies, epistaxes
Osteitis fibrosa cystica	See McCune-Albright syndrome	
Osteochondromatosis syndrome (Ollier's disease, enchondromatosis)	Hamartosis	Limb anomalies, fragile bones, predisposition to malignancy
Osteogenesis imperfecta congenita	See Osteogenesis imperfecta syndrome, type II	
Osteogenesis imperfecta syndrome, type I (autosomal-dominant osteogenesis imperfecta, Lobstein's disease)[91–93]	Connective tissue disorder	Growth deficiency, vertebral anomalies, joint laxity, fragile bones, vessel fragility and/or thrombocytopenia, mitral valve prolapse
Osteogenesis imperfecta syndrome, type II (osteogenesis imperfecta congenita, Vrolik's disease)[94]	Connective tissue disorder	Early lethal disorder; growth deficiency, vertebral anomalies, fragile bones, small thorax, hydrocephalus, muscle weakness
Osteopetrosis: autosomal-recessive–lethal (severe osteopetrosis, mild form termed Albers-Schönberg syndrome)	Osteochrondrodysplasia with osteopetrosis	Dense fragile bones, marrow compression causing pancytopenia, compression of cranial nerves and brain, hydrocephalus, hypocalcemia, limited life span
Otopalatodigital syndrome, type I (Taybi's syndrome)[95]	Characterized by facial defect	Mild mental deficiency, growth deficiency, facial anomalies, microstomia, vertebral anomalies, joint laxity

Syndrome	Category	Anesthetic Considerations
Otopalatodigital syndrome, type II	Characterized by facial defect	Growth deficiency, facial anomalies, micrognathia, limb anomalies, vertebral anomalies, small thorax, joint contractures and laxity
Pachydermoperiostosis syndrome	Skin dysplasias	Dermal anomalies, keloids
Pachyonychia congenita syndrome	Skin dysplasias	Dermal anomalies, leukokeratosis of mouth and tongue, laryngeal obstruction
Pallister's mosaic syndrome	See Killian/Teschler-Nicola syndrome	
Pallister-Hall syndrome	Brain or neuromuscular defects	Early lethal disorder; hypothalamic hamartoblastoma, hypopituitarism, other brain anomalies, micrognathia, laryngeal cleft, dysplastic tracheal cartilage, absent lung, abnormal lung lobulation, cardiac anomalies, cervical spine and vertebral anomalies
Partial trisomy 10q syndrome	Chromosomal	Prenatal growth deficiency, mental deficiency, cardiac defects, occasional vertebral malformations
Pena-Shokier phenotype (fetal akinesia hypokinesia sequence)	Brain or neuromuscular defects	Growth deficiency, facial anomalies, micrognathia, multiple ankylosis, microstomia, pulmonary hypoplasia, muscle weakness, joint contractures
Penta X syndrome	See XXXXX syndrome	
Perheentupa syndrome	See Mulibrey nanism syndrome	
Peutz-Jeghers syndrome	Hamartosis	Anemia secondary to polyposis, bronchial polyposis
Pfeiffer's syndrome (Pfeiffer-type acrocephalosyndactyly)	Craniosynostosis	Facial anomalies, limb anomalies, choanal atresia, hydrocephalus
Pfeiffer-type acrocephalosyndactyly	See Pfeiffer's syndrome	
Pierre Robin syndrome	See Robin's sequence	
Poikiloderma congenitale syndrome	See Rothmund-Thomson syndrome	
Poland anomaly	Limb defects	Unilateral defect of pectoralis major muscle, occasional vertebral anomalies, occasional renal anomalies
Polysplenia syndrome	See Laterality sequences	
Popliteal pterygium syndrome (faciogenitopopliteal syndrome)	Limb defects	Popliteal web, occasional vertebral anomalies, occasional webbing across mouth or eyelids
Postaxial acrofacial dysostosis syndrome	See Miller's syndrome	
Potter's syndrome	See Oligohydramnios sequence	
Prader-Willi syndrome[96-101]	Brain or neuromuscular defects	Obesity, facial anomalies, mental deficiency, muscle weakness, occasional seizures, occasional diabetes
Progeria (Hutchinson-Gilford syndrome)[102]	Miscellaneous	Growth deficiency, loss of adipose tissue, skeletal hypoplasia and dysplasia, facial anomalies, micrognathia, generalized artherosclerosis appearing as early as age 5 years
Progressive diaphyseal dysplasia	See Camurati-Englemann syndrome	
Proteus' syndrome[103]	Hamartosis	Asymmetric overgrowth, dermal anomalies, ocular anomalies, occasional mental deficiency, cystic lung malformations, muscle weakness
Pseudo-Hurler's polydystrophy syndrome (mucolipidosis III)	Storage disorders	Growth deficiency, mental deficiency, vertebral anomalies, facial anomalies, joint stiffness, aortic valve disease
Pseudo–vitamin D–deficiency rickets	Osteochondrodysplasias	Muscle weakness, seizures, brittle bones, hypocalcemia, natural history similar to vitamine D–deficiency rickets

Syndrome	Category	Anesthetic Considerations
Pseudoachondroplastic spondyloepiphyseal dysplasia (SED)	Osteochondrodysplasias	Vertebral anomalies, small thorax, joint laxity
Pseudohypoparathyroidism	See Albright hereditary osteodystrophy	
Pseudopseudohypoparathyroidism	See Albright hereditary osteodystrophy	
Pseudothalidomide syndrome	See Roberts-SC phocomelia syndrome	
Pyknodysostosis (Toulouse-Lautrec disease)	Osteochrondrodysplasia with osteopetrosis	Osteosclerosis, facial anomalies, occasional mental deficiency, mandibular fractures, micrognathia, fragile bones
Pyle's disease	See Pyle's metaphyseal dysplasia	
Pyle's metaphyseal dysplasia (Pyle's disease)	Osteochondrodysplasias	Facial anomalies, muscle weakness, joint pain
Radial aplasia–thrombocytopenia syndrome (TAR syndrome)	Limb defects	Severe thrombocytopenia, leukemoid granulocytosis, anemia, cardiac anomalies, facial anomalies, micrognathia, occasional mental deficiency, vertebral anomalies, renal anomalies
Rapp-Hodgkin ectodermal dysplasia syndrome (hypohidrotic ectodermal dysplasia, autosomal dominant type)	Skin dysplasias	Variable growth deficiency, microstomia, hyperthermia secondary to inability to sweat
Retinal angiomas	See von Hippel–Lindau syndrome	
Retinoic acid embryopathy (accutane embryopathy)	Environmental agents	Facial anomalies, micrognathia, cardiac anomalies, hydrocephalus
Rhizomelic chondrodysplasia punctata syndrome (chondrodysplasia punctata, rhizomelic type)	Osteochondrodysplasias	Mental deficiency, spasticity, facial anomalies, vertebral anomalies, death secondary to respiratory insufficiency during infancy
Rieger eye malformation sequence (mesodermal dysgenesis of the iris, goniodysgenesis)	Miscellaneous	Glaucoma
Rieger's syndrome	Miscellaneous	Glaucoma
Roberts-SC phocomelia syndrome (pseudothalidomide syndrome, hypomelia–hypertrichosis–facial hemangioma syndrome)	Characterized by facial defect	Mental deficiency, growth deficiency, facial anomalies, micrognathia, midfacial hemangioma, encephalocele, hydrocephalus, auricular anomalies, hypomelia, occasional cardiac and renal anomalies, occasional thrombocytopenia
Robin's sequence (Pierre Robin syndrome)[104–106]	Characterized by facial defect	Severe micrognathia, cleft soft palate, laryngeal anomalies, mandibular growth ``catches up'' during infancy and childhood
Robinow's syndrome (fetal face syndrome)[107]	Characterized by facial defect	Facial anomalies, micrognathia, macroglossia, cleft lip/palate, vertebral anomalies, seizures, occasional cardiac anomalies
Rokitansky's sequence	Miscellaneous	Renal anomalies, vertebral anomalies
Rothmund-Thomson syndrome (poikiloderma congenitale syndrome)	Miscellaneous	Poikiloderma, growth deficiency, dermal anomalies, mental deficiency, growth hormone deficiency, predisposition to malignancy
Rubella exposure effects	Environmental agents	Deafness, growth deficiency, mental deficiency, ocular anomalies, cardiac anomalies, intimal thickening of the large arteries, thrombocytopenia, anemia, occasional renal anomalies, occasional diabetes, occasional hypopituitarism

Syndrome	Category	Anesthetic Considerations
Rubinstein-Taybi syndrome[108, 109]	Growth deficiency	Mild mental deficiency, facial anomalies, microcephaly, occasional micrognathia, cervical spine anomalies, vertebral anomalies, cardiac anomalies, chronic respiratory infections, renal anomalies
Russell-Silver syndrome (Silver's syndrome)[110]	Growth deficiency	Skeletal asymmetry, facial anomalies, micrognathia, café-au-lait spots, hyperhydrosis, hypoglycemia during early childhood
Ruvalcaba's syndrome	Characterized by facial defect	Growth deficiency, mental deficiency, facial anomalies, microstomia, limb anomalies, vertebral anomalies, occasional cardiac anomalies
Ruvalcaba-Myhre syndrome	Hamartosis	Severe muscle weakness, variable mental deficiency, dermal anomalies, diabetes
Saethre-Chotzen syndrome[111]	Craniosynostosis	Facial anomalies, choanal atresia, limb anomalies, occasional increased intracranial pressure, and occasional vertebral, renal, and cardiac anomalies
Sanfilippo's syndrome (mucopolysaccharidosis III, types A, B, C, and D)[55, 112]	Storage disorders	Growth deficiency, mental deficiency, mild cardiac dysfunction, chronic respiratory infections
Scheie's syndrome (mucopolysaccharidosis I S)	Storage disorders	Joint stiffness, aortic valve disease, occasional macroglossia, occasional mental deficiency
Schinzel-Giedion syndrome	Brain or neuromuscular defects	Mental deficiency, seizures, spasticity, facial anomalies, choanal atresia, occasional macroglossia, early lethal disorder, occasional cardiac anomalies
Schwachman syndrome (metaphyseal chondrodysplasia with pancreatic insufficiency and neutropenia)	Osteochondrodysplasias	Exocrine pancreatic insufficiency, leukopenia, anemia, thrombocytopenia, immunoglobulin deficiency, predisposition to malignancy
Schwartz-Jampel syndrome (chondrodystrophica myotonia)[113]	Brain or neuromuscular defects	Myotonia, muscle weakness, micrognathia, vertebral anomalies, occasional mental deficiency
Sclerosteosis	Osteochondrodysplasia with osteopetrosis	Facial anomalies, compression of cranial nerves and brain
Seckel's syndrome	Growth deficiency	Mental deficiency, facial anomalies, micrognathia, joint laxity
SED	See Pseudoachondroplastic spondyloepiphyseal dysplasia	
Senter's syndrome	Skin dysplasias	Growth deficiency, dermal anomalies
Septooptic dysplasia sequence[114]	Miscellaneous	Ocular anomalies (including hypoplasia of the optic nerve), secondary hypopituitarism
Severe osteopetrosis	See Osteopetrosis: autosomal-recessive–lethal	
Short rib syndrome, type I	See Short rib–polydactyly syndrome, non-Majewski type	
Short rib syndrome, type II	See Short rib–polydactyly syndrome, Majewski type	
Short rib–polydactyly syndrome, Majewski type (short rib syndrome, type II)	Osteochondrodysplasias	Early lethal disorder; facial anomalies, small chest cavity, hypoplasia of epiglottis and larynx, renal anomalies, brain anomalies
Short rib–polydactyly syndrome, non-Majewski type (short rib syndrome, type I)	Osteochondrodysplasias	Early lethal disoder; small chest cavity, cardiac anomalies, vertebral anomalies

Syndrome	Category	Anesthetic Considerations
Shprintzen's syndrome (velocardiofacial syndrome)	Characterized by facial defect	Mild mental deficiency, growth deficiency, auricular anomalies, facial anomalies, micrognathia, muscle weakness, cardiac anomalies, occasional Robin sequence, occasional laryngeal web, obstructive apnea
Silver's syndrome	See Russell-Silver syndrome	
Sirenomelia sequence	Miscellaneous	Vertebral anomalies, renal anomalies, limb anomalies, hyperthermia secondary to reduced surface area
Sjögren-Larsson syndrome	Brain or neuromuscular defects	Mental deficiency, spasticity, ichthyosis
Sly's syndrome	See Mucopolysaccharidosis VII	
Smith-Lemli-Opitz syndrome[115, 116]	Characterized by facial defect	Mental deficiency, hypertonia, facial anomalies, micrognathia, occasional seizures, cardiac anomalies, and renal anomalies
Sotos' syndrome (cerebral gigantism)[117]	Overgrowth	Mental deficiency, facial anomalies, seizures, abnormal glucose tolerance test, predisposition to malignancy
Spondyloepiphyseal dysplasia tarda (X-linked spondyloepiphyseal dysplasia)	Osteochondrodysplasias	Vertebral anomalies, cervical spine anomalies, joint stiffness
Spondyloepiphyseal dysplasia congenita	Osteochondrodysplasias	Facial anomalies, ocular anomalies, vertebral anomalies, muscle weakness, joint stiffness, hypotonia
Spondylothoracic dysplasia	See Jarcho-Levin syndrome	
Steinert's myotonic dystrophy syndrome (Steinert's syndrome, dystrophia myotonica)[118–124]	Brain or neuromuscular defects	Myotonia, muscle weakness, cardiac conduction defects, occasional mental deficiency, occasional diabetes
Steinert's syndrome	See Steinert's myotonic dystrophy syndrome	
Stickler's syndrome (hereditary arthroopthalmopathy)	Characterized by facial defect	Facial anomalies, micrognathia, Robin sequence, mitral valve prolapse
Sturge-Weber sequence[66, 125, 126]	Hamartosis	Facial hemangioma, variable mental deficiency, seizures, brain hemangioma, cardiac anomalies, hypertonia
Symphalangism syndrome	See Multiple synostosis syndrome	
TAR syndrome	See Radial aplasia–thrombocytopenia syndrome	
Taybi's syndrome	See Otopalatodigital syndrome, type I	
TDO syndrome	See Trichodentoosseous syndrome	
Tethered cord malformation sequence	See Occult spinal dysraphism sequence	
Tetrasomy 12p	See Killian/Teschler-Nicola syndrome	
Thanatophoric dysplasia	Osteochondrodysplasias	Early lethal disorder; muscle weakness, facial anomalies, small chest cavity, vertebral anomalies (including narrow caudal space), brain anomalies, hydrocephalus, cardiac anomalies
Toulouse-Lautrec disease	See Pyknodysostosis	
Townes' syndrome	Characterized by facial defect	Auricular anomalies, thumb anomalies, renal anomalies, occasional cardiac anomalies
Trapezoidcephaly–multiple synostosis	See Antley-Bixler syndrome	

Syndrome	Category	Anesthetic Considerations
Treacher Collins syndrome (mandibulofacial dysostosis, Franceschetti-Klein syndrome)[106, 127–134]	Characterized by facial defect	Facial anomalies, auricular anomalies, choanal atresia, severe micrognathia, microstomia, upper airway hypoplasia, occasional cardiac anomalies
Trichodentoosseous syndrome (TDO syndrome)	Skin dysplasias	Occasional craniosysostosis
Trichorhinophalangeal syndrome	Characterized by facial defect	Growth deficiency, facial anomalies, micrognathia, limb anomalies, hypotonia, chronic respiratory infections
Trichorhinophalangeal syndrome with exostosis	See Langer-Giedion syndrome	
Tridione syndrome	See Trimethadione effects	
Trimethadione effects (fetal trimethadione syndrome, tridione syndrome)	Environmental agents	Mental deficiency, growth deficiency, facial anomalies, micrognathia, cardiac anomalies, vertebral anomalies, renal anomalies, joint laxity
Triploidy and diploid-triploid mixoploidy syndrome	Chromosomal	Growth deficiency, asymmetric growth, micrognathia, choanal atresia, macroglossia, cardiac defects, adrenal hypoplasia, brain anomalies, hydrocephalus
Trismus pseudocamptodactyly syndrome	See Hecht's syndrome	
Trisomy 13 syndrome[135, 136]	Chromosomal	Early lethal disorder; facial anomalies, brain anomalies, hydrocephalus, seizures, hypotonia, hypertonia, severe mental deficiency, micrognathia, apneic spells, cardiac anomalies, thrombocytopenia
Trisomy 18 syndrome	Chromosomal	Early lethal disorder; mental deficiency, hypoplasia of skeletal muscle, microstomia, micrognathia, choanal atresia, numerous cardiac defects, possible absence of right lung, tracheoesophageal fistula, brain anomalies, hydrocephalus, thrombocytopenia
Trisomy 20p syndrome	Chromosomal	Mental deficiency, hypotonia, hydrocephalus, vertebral defects, occasional cardiac defects
Trisomy 21 (Down's syndrome)[137–141]	Chromosomal	Mild mental deficiency, cardiac defects, muscle weakness, macroglossia, joint laxity, odontoid hypoplasia, tracheoesophageal fistula, predisposition to malignancy, hypothyroidism, hyperthyroidism
Trisomy 4p syndrome (trisomy of the short arm of chromosome 4)	Chromosomal	Growth deficiency, severe mental deficiency, hypertonia followed by hypotonia, seizures, macroglossia, occasional cardiac defects, respiratory infections, joint contractures
Trisomy 8 syndrome (trisomy 8/normal mosaicism)	Chromosomal	Mental deficiency, micrognathia, occasional vetebral anomaly, anemia
Trisomy 9 mosaic syndrome	Chromosomal	Early lethal disorder; auricular anomalies, severe mental deficiency, growth deficiency, micrognathia, cardiac defects, small thorax, renal defects
Trisomy 9p syndrome	Chromosomal	Growth deficiency, severe mental deficiency, hydrocephalus, occasional micrognathia, occasional cardiac defects
Tuberous sclerosis syndrome (adenoma sebaceum)[142, 143]	Hamartosis	Brain anomalies, seizures, variable mental deficiency, dermal anomalies, renal anomalies, sublingual fibromas, angiomas of heart and lungs, cardiac hamartomas, predisposition to malignancy

Syndrome	Category	Anesthetic Considerations
Turner syndrome (XO)[144]	Chromosomal	Growth deficiency, micrognathia, short neck, cardiac anomalies, occasional hypertension, hypothyroid, occasional diabetes
Turner-like syndrome	See Noonan's syndrome	
Valproate effects	Environmental agents	Facial anomalies, small mouth, cardiac anomalies, meningomyelocele
Van der Woude's syndrome (lip pit–cleft lip syndrome)	Characterized by facial defect	None described
Varicella effects	Environmental agents	Mental deficiency, seizures, growth deficiency, limb anomalies
VATER association	Miscellaneous	Vertebral anomalies, cardiac anomalies, tracheoesophageal fistula, esophageal atresia, limb anomalies, renal anomalies
Velocardiofacial syndrome	See Shprintzen's syndrome	
Vitamin D–resistant rickets	See X-linked hypophosphatemic rickets	
Von Hippel–Lindau syndrome (retinal angiomas, cerebellar hemangioblastoma)[145,146]	Hamartosis	Angiomas of eyes and cerebellum or spinal cord, multiple cysts of pancreas and kidneys, pheochromocytoma, predisposition to malignancy
Vrolik's disease	See Osteogenesis imperfecta syndrome, type II	
Waardenburg's syndrome, types I and II	Characterized by facial defect	Facial anomalies, deafness, partial albinism, occasional cardiac and vertebral anomalies
Warburg's syndrome (hard ± E syndrome)	Brain or neuromuscular defects	Severe brain anomalies, encephalocele, hydrocephalus, ocular anomalies
Warfarin effects (warfarin embryopathy, fetal warfarin syndrome)	Environmental agents	Upper airway obstruction in infancy from nasal hypoplasia, mental deficiency, occasional hydrocephalus, occasional cardiac anomalies
Weaver's syndrome[147]	Overgrowth	Hypertonia, joint contractures, facial anomalies, relative micrognathia, occasional brain anomalies
Weill-Marchesani syndrome (brachydactyly-spherophakia syndrome)	Other skeletal dysplasias	Growth deficiency, facial anomalies, limb anomalies, occasional cardiac anomalies
Werner's syndrome	Miscellaneous	Growth deficiency, early senile appearance, fibrous subcutaneous tissue with thin dermis, atherosclerosis, osteoporosis, retinal degeneration, hepatic atrophy, adrenal atrophy, frequent diabetes, predisposition to malignancy and organic brain syndrome
Whistling face syndrome	See Freeman-Sheldon syndrome	
Williams syndrome[148, 149]	Characterized by facial defect	Mental deficiency, ``cocktail party'' personality, facial anomalies, cardiac anomalies, peripheral arterial stenosis, occasional renal anomalies and/or degenerative disease, hypotonia, hypercalcemia, hypertension
X-linked hydrocephalus syndrome	Brain or neuromuscular defects	Hydrocephalus, mental deficiency, spasticity, brain anomalies, hydrocephalus
X-linked hypophosphatemic rickets (vitamin D–resistant rickets)	Osteochondrodysplasias	Hypophosphatemia, brittle bones
X-linked spondyloepiphyseal dysplasia	See Spondyloepiphyseal dysplasia tarda (X-linked spondyloepiphyseal dysplasia)	

Syndrome	Category	Anesthetic Considerations
Xeroderma pigmentosa syndrome[150]	Skin dysplasias	Sensitivity to sunlight, dermal anomalies, predisposition to malignancy, progressive neurological abnormalities
Xerodermic idiocy syndrome	See De Sanctis-Cacchione syndrome	
XXXX syndrome	Chromosomal	Mental deficiency
XXXXX (penta X syndrome)	Chromosomal	Mental deficiency, growth deficiency, cardiac defects
XXXY and XXXXY syndromes	Chromosomal	Growth deficiency, mental deficiency, short neck, occasional cardiac defect, hypotonia, joint contractures and laxity
XXY syndrome (Klinefelter's)	Chromosomal	Mild mental deficiency, tremor, diabetes, chronic bronchitis, behavior problems, obesity as adults
XYY syndrome	Chromosomal	Incidence of 1:840 newborn males; tall stature, behavior problems, poor fine motor coordination, ECG showing prolonged PR interval
Zellweger's syndrome (cerebrohepatorenal syndrome)	Brain or neuromuscular defects	Lack of dihydroxyacetone phosphate acyltransferase, growth deficiency, muscle weakness, chronic respiratory infections, brain anomalies, facial anomalies, hepatomegaly with dysgenesis, cardiac anomalies, renal anomalies

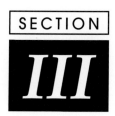
Uncommon Multisystemic Diseases and Anesthetic Problems

Uncommon Problems Related to Cancer

D. Edward Supkis, Jr.
Joseph Varon

I. INTRODUCTION

Enhanced anesthesiology and critical care capabilities have contributed substantially to improved survival of cancer, the second leading cause of death in the United States.[1] Anesthesia may be needed on a short-term basis for minor procedures or on a long-term basis for multiple-dose aggressive surgical antineoplastic therapy.[2] In addition, practicing anesthesiologists need to master the pre- and postoperative management of cancer patients, as many of them undergo major exploratory cancer surgery and are admitted to postanesthesia care units or critical care units.

Patients with a malignancy can come to the operating room for treatment of their primary neoplasm (typically surgical resection) or for another disease process totally unrelated to their cancer. It is well known that neoplasms produce alterations in the patient's homeostasis via mechanical and nonmechanical properties of the tumor.[2, 3] As described below, airway management may be one of the major mechanical challenges in a cancer patient, particularly those with head and neck cancers.[4] Additionally, some types of tumors (e.g., pheochromocytoma) may secrete a series of substances that may interfere with the anesthetic management of the patient.[5]

This chapter describes different types of cancer patients likely to need and benefit from anesthesia as well as postanesthetic care. Clinical judgment regarding appropriate use of anesthesia services is required in all patient populations, and the decision to offer technological support to cancer patients should be individualized. A review of selected oncologic disorders and complications of cancer that could potentially interfere with the anesthetic management of these patients follows.

II. PREOPERATIVE EVALUATION OF THE CANCER PATIENT

The preoperative evaluation of the cancer patient often reveals significant intercurrent disease that requires corrective medical intervention before elective surgery. The challenge to the anesthesiologist: optimizing the patient's physical status before surgery using appropriately prescribed testing and timely therapeutic interventions. In the preanesthetic patient interview, the anesthesiologist should obtain a pertinent medical history that is as comprehensive as the astute interview of any surgical patient, with important emphases, including questions about pre-existing conditions, previous surgery and anesthesia, medication, allergies, family history, and a complete review of organ systems. It is vitally important to assess the effects of cancer and cancer therapies on the patient. The appropriate use of laboratory and diagnostic tests as well as additional consultations will have an impact on the choice and management of anesthesia.

III. AIRWAY ASSESSMENT AND MANAGEMENT

Airways in patients with cancer of the head and neck usually present difficulties.[4] They can be troublesome to ventilate, regardless of the technical problems encountered in performing direct laryngoscopy.[6] Moreover, the vigilant anesthesiologist will remember that a patient whose cancer is elsewhere than in the head and neck area may have a difficult airway.

Over time a cancer patient will have the same identity but a different airway. Head and neck cancer patients *do* differ in presentation over time; clearly, such patients need to be evaluated every time they come to surgery, particularly for the anesthesiologist's ability to secure the airway. It is not uncommon for a patient undergoing initial surgical resection to have a very easy airway and, yet, when at a staged reconstructive procedure may be impossible to mask-ventilate and may require other types of ventilation.[7, 8] Placement of endotracheal tube by direct laryngoscopy in such patients could be either very difficult or quite easy. The forces exerted during direct laryngoscopy may damage previous reconstructive efforts. The physician who anticipates a real danger of damaging reconstructive efforts should proceed with awake fiberoptic intubation. With cancers of the head and neck, it is better to proceed with awake fiberoptic intubation in a sedate, well-"topicalized" patient than to struggle with direct laryngoscopy in an anesthetized, apneic patient. At the University of Texas, M. D. Anderson Cancer Center, anesthesiologists strongly favor awake, sedate, fiberoptic intubation, when a difficult airway is anticipated.

The anesthesiologist evaluating an airway should, as in any other patient, review systemic diseases and any history of intubations and perform a thorough physical examination of the airway.[9] More important aspects of the airway evaluation of the cancer patient include changes in the patient's voice.[10] A coarse, scratchy voice suggests a glottic tumor. A muffled voice suggests a supraglottic tumor.[11] Cancer patients with sleep apnea may have a vollecular mass.[10–12] Such difficulties impede mask ventilation and endotracheal intubation.[12] It is important to thoroughly evaluate a patient who is not able to breathe in the supine position. A patient who cannot breathe in a lateral or prone position may have a pharyngeal or anterior mediastinal mass. If such a patient undergoes routine induction of anesthesia, the tumor mass may well lead to severe airway obstruction.[10–12]

Patients who have received preoperative radiation therapy are especially difficult to evaluate. Radiation causes fibrosis of tissues within the field of exposure.[13] A patient with a base-of-the-tongue or floor-of-the-mouth lesion may have a normal Mallinpati classification, may be able to extend the head well, and may possess a normal mental hyoid distance, yet, the anesthesiologist may find direct laryngoscopy in such a patient to be impossible. During laryngoscopy, the tongue is depressed into the submandibular space and the space may be rendered noncompliant by postradiation fibrosis. Therefore, it is very important to palpate the submandibular space; such space can be filled with tumors or hematomas or abscesses.[14] It is important that this space be compliant as well as large enough to accept the tongue during conventional laryngoscopy.

Patients with cancer of the head and neck present some unique airway management problems that must be addressed in a manner that is not precisely delineated by the American Society of Anesthesiologists difficult airway algorithm.[6] Specific problems are described below.

A. SPECIAL ASSESSMENT CONSIDERATIONS

1. Head and Neck Tumors

The prudent anesthesiologist examining a head and neck tumor patient knows that patient may be at increased risk for uncontrolled hemorrhage and/or tumor aspiration. If the head and neck surgeon did not perform indirect laryngoscopy, the anesthesiologist should

do so; indirect laryngoscopy may reveal a friable and easily bleeding tumor that requires awake but sedated tracheostomy performed under local anesthesia.[15] If the anesthesiologist attempts an awake, sedated fiberoptic intubation, he may well encounter bleeding, preventing adequate visualization of the airway through the fiberoptic scope. And, such patients face increased risk of uncontrolled hemorrhage or tumor aspiration.[16] In certain volatile situations, it is not uncommon to lose control of the airway and resort to emergency transtracheal jet ventilation and tracheostomy.

2. Previous Surgery

Commonly, a patient presents initially with an easy airway and then, as a result of surgery, develops a difficult one. During such surgery, the patient's normal anatomic landmarks may be resected. Postoperatively, fibrosis limits mobility of the entire airway. Patients undergoing staged reconstructive procedures will often have a tracheostomy during their initial resection. If the patient did not receive a tracheostomy during initial resection, then the patient should undergo awake fiberoptic laryngoscopy for a staged reconstruction.[8]

3. Radiation Therapy

Radiation therapy causes fibrosis in the radiation field.[18] During laryngoscopy, the base of the tongue is displaced into the submandibular space. If the mental hyoid distance is too short to accept the base of the tongue during laryngoscopy, the patient will exhibit the appearance of an anterior larynx. The same condition may be observed in a patient who has received radiation therapy: the larynx will appear to be anterior, despite a normal mental hyoid distance, because the submandibular space is fibrosed, noncompliant, and will not accept the base of the tongue being displaced into the submandibular space.[8]

B. TECHNIQUES FOR AWAKE AIRWAY MANAGEMENT

Patients with cancer who undergo awake, sedate, fiberoptic intubation require little sedation and good topicalization. The alert anesthesiologist recognizes that his patient must be sedate but in meaningful contact with his surroundings.[17] Additionally, the prudent anesthesiologist will administer a drying agent such as glycopyrrolate to the airway before the topical anesthetic.[18] Before instrumentation of the nose, he will administer a vasoconstrictor, such as neosynephrine, 1/4 per cent nasal spray applied to the nasal mucosa. Nerve blocks and transtracheal blocks are relatively contraindicated for patients with cancer of the head and neck owing to the theoretical possibility of direct extension of tumor secondary to trauma from the needle passing through tumor.[19] Normal anatomy is distorted by tumor growth, distorting the vessels and nerves. A thrombocytopenic patient may hemorrhage. The best method of anesthetizing the airway is through topical techniques such as spraying the airway with a high-powered sprayer with 4 per cent lidocaine.[17] Another equally effective technique is "spray as you go."[18, 20] This is a technique utilizing 4 per cent lidocaine sprayed through the suction channel with the fiberoptic scope as one proceeds down the airway.[18, 19] Other authors provide detailed descriptions of other recognized techniques of fiberoptic intubation.[10, 17]

C. CANCER PATIENTS WITH ACUTE AIRWAY COMPROMISE

Patients with cancer with compromised airway receive a tracheostomy performed under local anesthesia.[8] These patients, because of hypoxemia and hypocarbia, are not sedated. A drying agent such as glycopyrrolate, along with constant suctioning of oral secretions, may improve their respiratory status. Patients who have tumor infringing on the upper airway typically are unable to swallow and to clear their oral secretions.

1. Transtracheal Jet Ventilation

Transtracheal jet ventilation can be useful in a patient with cancer and a difficult airway.[21] In a patient with thyroid cancer or other head and neck cancers, the cricothyroid membrane may be obliterated. The trachea may be displaced off the midline, making transtracheal jet ventilation more difficult to

perform. It is vital that the transtracheal jet ventilation catheter be within the lumen of the trachea before initiation of the ventilation. Jet ventilation through a jet stylet is extremely useful. The jet ventilation "buys time" for changing endotracheal tubes from a single-lumen one to a double-lumen tube.

D. EXTUBATION OF THE TRACHEA

After completion of the surgery, the patient's airway should be reevaluated with the recognition that there may have been a surgically induced anatomic change in the patient's airway. The anesthesiologist should recognize that the reconstructive procedures performed may make mask ventilation impossible along with direct laryngoscopy. And, surgical manipulation in the head and neck region may cause edema formation in the larynx and other portions of the airway.[15] Moreover, neck dissections can cause disruption of the recurrent laryngeal nerve, resulting in vocal cord paralysis.[22] This can also occur in resections of thyroid and parathyroid glands.

The anesthesiologist considering extubation at the end of the surgical procedure must review all extubation criteria (e.g., awake and complete reversal of the muscle relaxants) and must have a patient with an adequate airway. If the anesthesiologist has doubts about the status of the patient's airway, he can extubate the patient over a jet stylet. If extubation proceeds without difficulty, the anesthesiologist can leave the jet stylet in the patient and take the patient to the recovery room. The stylet is usually removed after the anesthesiologist is satisfied that the patient will not encounter airway difficulty.

The stylet can ordinarily be left in place in the trachea in the postanesthetic care unit for 30 to 60 minutes postoperatively, without complications. If the airway becomes obstructed, it should be a straightforward task to initiate jet ventilation via the stylet and a small endotracheal tube advanced over the stylet into the trachea. If there is any doubt, the patient should be kept intubated and sedated and taken to the surgical intensive care unit and placed in a head-up position, allowing 12 to 24 hours for airway edema to resolve or conduct a tracheostomy at the end of the procedure.

IV. SPECIFIC MEDICAL CONDITIONS IMPORTANT TO ANESTHESIOLOGISTS

Anesthesiologists must be aware of the following medical conditions complicating some neoplasms.

A. CARDIAC TAMPONADE

Cardiac tamponade is a life-threatening condition caused by an increase in the pericardial pressure resulting in limitation of ventricular diastolic filling and decreased stroke volume and cardiac output.[23] This condition is common in some types of malignancies, including metastatic tumors of the pericardium, primary pericardial tumors, and encasement of the heart by other types of tumors, and it can also be an effect of radiation and chemotherapy.[24]

Primary tumors of the pericardium producing tamponade are rare; metastatic tumors of the pericardium more often produce tamponade.[24, 25] These tumors cause tamponade by producing either effusions or constriction. Among the neoplasms more likely to result in cardiac tamponade are those of lungs, breasts, lymphoma, leukemia, and melanoma, accounting for 80 per cent of metastatic causes of cardiac tamponade.[24] While a primary pericardial tumor is rare, the pericardium is the most frequent site of injury from radiation therapy for other types of tumors.[25] The latent period between radiation therapy and the onset of clinical pericardial disease may be years.[26] Therefore, the anesthesiologist must be aware of the potential for injury to the pericardium.

The anesthesiologist must be astute to recognize early tamponade. The symptoms of cardiac tamponade are often nonspecific but often include the sensation of fullness in the chest, pericardial or interscapular pain, apprehension, dyspnea, and orthopnea.[23] On physical examination, the anesthesiologist may find altered mental status, hypotension, tachycardia, a narrow arterial pulse pressure, diminished heart tones with diminished apical impulses, tachypnea, oliguria, and diaphoresis.[27] Classic signs include pulsus paradoxus, Ewart's sign (dullness at the angle of the left scapula), and Kussmaul's sign (neck veins that bulge on inspiration).[23, 29]

On chest radiographs, a large, globular heart also known as the "water-bottle" configuration may be found; however, if the patient has less than 250 ml of pericardial fluid, the cardiac silhouette may be normal.[28] In most cases, the lung fields are clear unless the patient has primary or metastatic pulmonary disease. Pleural effusions in these patients are also common associated findings. Electrocardiographic signs include sinus tachycardia, low-voltage QRS, and, in some instances, "electrical alternans" (which results from the heart's oscillating in the full pericardial sack).[29] Changes of the QRS complex are specific for pericardial effusion.

In the operating room, the postanesthesia care unit, or the intensive care unit, echocardiography makes a quick and definite diagnosis of tamponade. Two-dimensional echocardiography is more sensitive than M-mode. The classic findings include the following: a prolonged diastolic collapse or inversion of the right atrial free wall and diastolic collapse of the right ventricular free wall.[30] Effusions as small as 30 ml are detected early by echocardiography.

Another useful tool in the operating room and intensive care unit is the pulmonary artery catheter. In patients with tamponade, elevated pulmonary capillary wedge pressure and filling pressures may reveal a prominent X descent with no significant Y descent, a finding known as the "square root" sign.[23] In addition, patients may likely have decreased stroke volume, systemic arterial pressure, and mixed venous oxygen saturation. Equalization of all pressures in diastole has also been observed as a common sign.[31]

The management of a cancer patient with pericardial tamponade depends on the urgency of the situation.[32] If a patient is hemodynamically compromised, therapeutic pericardiocentesis needs to be performed immediately. Two-dimensional echocardiography–guided pericardiocentesis is successful in 95 per cent of the cases with no major complications.[33] It is important to recognize that reaccumulation of fluid is most likely to occur in malignant effusions but may be prevented with chemical sclerosis (i.e., tetracycline), radiation therapy, or surgery (i.e., pleuropericardial window or pericardiectomy).

B. MYOCARDIAL TISSUE INJURY
(See Chapter 4)

Cancer patients receive a series of chemotherapeutic agents that can adversely affect the heart.[34–38] Anthracycline antibiotics (i.e., Adriamycin, doxorubicin, daunorubicin), for example, may impair contractility.[39] Patients receiving mitoxantrone in total doses larger than 140 mg/m^2 can suffer congestive heart failure and anthracycline-induced cardiomyopathy. Another agent known to cause myocardial tissue injury is cyclophosphamide.[40] A cyclophosphamide dose range of more than 120 mg/kg over 2 days can result in severe congestive heart failure and hemorrhagic myocarditis, pericarditis, and necrosis. Patients receiving busulfan in conventional oral daily doses may suffer endocardial fibrosis and signs and symptoms of constrictive cardiomyopathy.[41] Patients with preexisting cardiac disease receiving interferon in conventional doses may have exacerbations of their underlying illness. More recently, the use of mitomycin for extended periods has been shown to produce myocardial damage.[42] It is well-known that radiation causes a dose-dependent endocardial and myocardial fibrosis that can result in restrictive cardiomyopathy.[43]

The preoperative and anesthetic assessment of patients who have received the previously described chemotherapeutic agents or radiation therapy to the mediastinum requires two-dimensional echocardiography or scintigraphy.[23] Such studies permit precise measurement of the left ventricular ejection fraction and detection of regional and global myocardial dysfunction. Where congestive failure is discovered, the treatment is the same as for congestive failure of any other cause. There is no unique specific therapy directed at radiation or chemotherapy-induced myocardial damage.

In addition to the previously described antineoplastic side effects, anthracycline antibiotics can cause dysrhythmia unrelated to the cumulative dose.[23, 44] Such dysrhythmias may occur hours or even days after administration. Commonly observed dysrhythmias include supraventricular tachycardia, complete heart block, and ventricular tachycardia. In addition, doxorubicin may prolong the QT interval.[45] In recent years, practitioners have observed that taxol, when given in combination with cisplatin, can produce ventricular tachycardia.[46]

C. NEUROLOGIC COMPLICATIONS

Preoperatively, operatively, and postoperatively, altered mental status is probably one of the most common central nervous system presentations for cancer patients.[23] The anesthesiologist caring for patients with altered mental status needs to consider the differential diagnosis described below. If alternatives can be excluded and the patient has not received excessive narcotic or analgesic agents, then the patient should be treated presumptively for sepsis.[47] Altered mental status is a reliable though nonspecific sign of sepsis, which carries a high mortality rate in cancer patients.

1. Specific Causes of Altered Mental Status

a. Intracranial Mass Lesions

A history of headache, nausea, vomiting, or seizure activity with clinical evidence of papilledema or other signs of raised intracranial pressure suggests the presence of a intracranial mass lesion.[48] A moderate increase of intracranial pressure alone is tolerated relatively well; however, when intracranial pressure becomes critical, the brain shifts in the direction of least resistance, with the result of herniation through the tentorium or foramen magnum.

b. CNS Tumors (Primary)

Primary tumors of the central nervous system may present with focal neurologic signs, depending on the location.[49]

c. CNS Tumors (Secondary, Metastatic)

Secondary or metastatic tumors in the central nervous system present in approximately 15 to 30 per cent of patients with new-onset seizures.[50] Malignancies associated with cerebral metastasis include the breast, lung, kidney, and melanoma.

d. Bleeding

In patients with acute promyelocytic leukemia or those with some types of brain metastasis or relatively low platelet counts, cerebral hemorrhage may be a presenting sign.[23] These patients may need acute evacuation of blood in the operating room. In patients with a fluctuating level of consciousness, the presence of a subdural hematoma needs to be considered.[51]

e. Abscess

Thirty per cent of central nervous system infections in cancer patients are produced by brain abscesses.[23, 52] These entities usually present with fever, headache, drowsiness, confusion, and seizures. Clinically, intracranial hypertension and neurologic deficits are late signs.[53] They are most often seen in patients with leukemia or head and neck tumors.

f. Metabolic or Vascular Disease

Other causes of altered mental status in cancer patients include leptomeningeal metastasis, other types of cerebral vascular accidents, and metabolic encephalopathies. In a cancer patient who presents with lethargy, weakness, somnolence, agitation, psychosis, and focal generalized seizures, a metabolic workup should be considered.[23] On the other hand, the lack of focal neurologic signs may suggest a metabolic encephalopathy. Examples of metabolic encephalopathies include hypercalcemia, hyponatremia, hypomagnesemia, hypoglycemia, and uremia.

Two conditions that deserve special attention in a cancer patient with altered mental status are leukostasis and meningitis. Patients with hyperleukocytosis (arbitrarily defined as a peripheral white blood cell count of more than $100,000/mm^3$) may present with blurred vision, dizziness, ataxia, stupor, or intracranial hemorrhage.[54] Hemorrhage may result from leukostatic plugging of the arterioles and capillaries resulting in endothelial cell damage, capillary leaks, and small vessel disruption.[23] In addition, these patients may present with a hyperviscosity syndrome in which excessive elevations of serum paraproteins or the leukostasis can result in elevated serum viscosity, sludging, and decreased perfusion of the microcirculation with stasis.[55] The hyperviscosity syndrome can affect any organ system; however, characteristic clinical findings occur in the lungs and the central nervous system.

On the other hand, meningitis is probably the most frequently encountered central nervous system infection in patients with cancer.[23] The infection is encountered more often in patients with impaired cell-mediated immunity, and it is typically caused by *Crypto-coccus neoformans* or *Listeria monocytogenes*.[56, 57] Such patients present with fever, headache, and altered mental status. All cancer patients with a fever and altered mental status should undergo lumbar puncture preceded by head computed tomography (CT).[23] This is particularly important when placement of an epidural catheter is being considered.

The anesthetic evaluation of the central nervous system in cancer patients consists of a history, physical examination, and a careful neurologic evaluation emphasizing lateralizing signs and evidence of increased intracranial pressure. The authors recommend that the preoperative laboratory data include SaO_2, serum electrolytes (including calcium, magnesium, and phosphorous), glucose, and renal and hepatic function tests. In patients with a history of multiple myeloma or other paraprotein-producing tumors, the determination of serum viscosity is essential. Head CT is the diagnostic test of choice for patients with mass lesions, midline shifts, intracranial hemorrhage, or hydrocephalus.[58] Where available, magnetic resonance imaging (MRI) is a sensitive test to detect intracerebral metastasis and to differentiate between vascular and tumor-related masses.[59] As previously indicated, lumbar puncture is most useful in the diagnosis of meningeal carcinomatosis, central nervous system leukemia, and central nervous system infections.

D. PULMONARY COMPLICATIONS

Cancer patients often suffer pulmonary complications. Seventy-five to ninety per cent of pulmonary complications are secondary to infection. The cancer patient can suffer infectious complications secondary to chemotherapy (e.g., bleomycin), thoracic radiation, or multiple pulmonary resections.[23, 60]

Pulmonary complications are a significant problem; respiratory failure in cancer patients that requires assisted mechanical ventilation is associated with a 75 per cent mortality rate.[61-63] The anesthesiologist must consider multiple issues in evaluating the potential for pulmonary complications in the cancer patient. The cancer patient requires a full physical examination, adequate preoperative pulmonary function tests, and chest radiography.

In patients with systemic cancer, the differential diagnosis of pulmonary infiltrates seen on a routine chest radiograph is extensive;

there are many causes for such infiltrates.[64-67] A localized infiltrate, confined to a lobe or a segment in a patient with a compatible history, most frequently represents a bacterial process. On the other hand, diffuse bilateral infiltrates are usually suggestive of opportunistic infections, treatment-induced lung injury, or lymphagitic spread of the carcinoma. Additionally, the anesthesiologist should consider fluid overload when evaluating patients with bilateral infiltrates, particularly those who have gained weight rapidly.

For patients who have recently undergone bone marrow transplantation, pulmonary infiltrates may represent a life-threatening infection, generally occurring within the first 100 days after transplant.[62] Within the first 30 days, the most common pathogens for pneumonia are bacteria and fungus. On the other hand, interstitial pneumonia in a patient after bone marrow transplantation is a predominant problem occurring some 30 to 100 days after a transplant. This syndrome consists of dyspnea, hypoxemia, and diffuse bilateral infiltrates. Cytomegalovirus pneumonia accounts for the majority of interstitial pneumonitides.[68] The incidence of cytomegalovirus infection appears to be related to the loss of immunity during pretransplant conditioning and to the development of graft-versus-host disease. These are important considerations when a bone marrow transplant recipient requires elective or urgent surgery.

As discussed earlier, leukostasis can obstruct flow in small vessels. Leukostasis in the lungs is a consequence of the intravascular accumulation of immature rigid myeloblasts, observed principally in acute myelogenous leukemia and chronic myelogenous leukemia patients in blast phase.[69, 70] Vascular stasis results in local hypoxemia. The release of intercellular enzymes leads to vascular and pulmonary parenchymal damage manifested clinically by progressive dyspnea. These patients usually have a white blood cell count greater than 150,000 cells per cubic millimeter. Hypoxemia develops as a result of impaired pulmonary gas exchange; *however,* it is important for the anesthesiologist to realize that spuriously low values for a PaO_2 may be consistently obtained because of the large number of blasts consuming oxygen within the arterial blood gas specimen itself.[23, 71] The longer the interval between the collection and the analysis of the arterial blood gas, the lower the measure of PaO_2. This may make the assessment of gas exchange very difficult

in the operating room. Thus, pulse oximetry may be of special benefit in following the adequacy of arterial oxygenation in these patients.[23]

Cancer patients can also present with yet another type of pulmonary lesion: treatment-induced lung injury. A large number of chemotherapeutic agents can produce pulmonary toxicity—acutely or belatedly, years after therapy.[72] Commonly used agents with known pulmonary toxicity include alkylating agents (i.e., cyclophosphamide, chlorambucil, melphalan, busulfan).[73-78] Other medications, such as antimetabolites (i.e., methotrexate, azathioprine), antitumor antibiotics (i.e., bleomycin, mitomycin), and alkaloids (i.e., vincristine) may produce pulmonary toxicity.[79-84] Chemotherapy-induced lung injury may manifest itself as noncardiogenic pulmonary edema, chronic pneumonitis and fibrosis, and hypersensitivity pneumonitis.[85]

Radiation-induced lung toxicity is a clinical syndrome of dyspnea, cough, and fever in association with indistinct, hazy pulmonary infiltrates that may progress to lobar consolidation following treatment with ionizing radiation.[86] The likelihood of developing radiation-induced lung injury is influenced by a number of variables, including the total radiation dose, fractionation of doses, volume of lung irradiated, and a history of radiation or chemotherapy.[87] The pathophysiologic effects of radiation on the lung include a direct effect of ionizing particles on the alveolar structure as well as the generation of high-energy oxidant-free radicals in excess of what normal enzyme systems can remove. In addition, the release of vasoactive substances such as histamine and bradykinin may affect the capillary permeability and pulmonary vascular resistance, with ensuing pulmonary damage. It has been estimated that 5 to 15 per cent of patients undergoing radiation therapy will develop radiation pneumonitis, symptoms of which may occur within 1 to 6 months after completion of thoracic radiation.[86, 87]

E. GASTROINTESTINAL COMPLICATIONS

Gastrointestinal complications are common in cancer patients. Indeed, gastrointestinal hemorrhage occurs in a large number of patients with neoplasms. The most common cause is hemorrhagic gastritis (32 to 48 per cent) followed by peptic ulcer disease.[23] Only

12 to 18 per cent of bleeding occurs from the tumor itself. This tumor bleeding is most often seen in gastrointestinal lymphomas.[88] Less common causes of gastrointestinal tract hemorrhage include esophageal varices, Mallory-Weiss tears, *Candida* esophagitis, and enteritis. The careful anesthesiologist must consider all these factors when performing a preoperative assessment of a patient with cancer and ought further to realize that lymphomas are the most common malignancies to perforate during chemotherapy and to require urgent surgical treatment.

The anesthesiologist evaluating the cancer patient with gastrointestinal complications considers many issues similar to those of the normal patient population with upper gastrointestinal hemorrhage and hollow viscus perforation. One must keep in mind, however, the unique status of the cancer patient.

Cancer patients with gastrointestinal hemorrhage commonly suffer from thrombocytopenia as a result of immunosuppression. They are usually poor surgical candidates. They present to surgery when medical management fails them. This implies that they have been massively transfused. In most cancer institutions, blood products are irradiated on arrival at the blood bank. Radiation of red cells causes a decrease in red cell life and a rise in extracellular potassium levels in the unit of packed red blood cells. Transfusion-related hyperkalemia is quite common in these patients.[89] When patients arrive in the operating room, they must undergo rapid-sequence induction. The physician may often see effects of succinylcholine-induced hyperkalemia (i.e., peak T waves, dysrhythmias, cardiac arrest).[90, 91] For this reason, it is usually prudent to perform rapid-sequence induction of anesthesia with high-dose, short-acting, nondepolarizing muscle relaxants.[92] Most of the time, these patients remain intubated postoperatively because of the debilitating condition; prolonged muscle relaxant block is not a consideration. Patients with upper gastrointestinal hemorrhages can be thrombocytopenic owing to chemotherapeutic treatment of their primary cancers. These patients need to receive aggressive platelet transfusion therapy.

Cancer patients presenting to the operating room with a perforated hollow viscus are usually much more ill than the general population. Having received chemotherapeutic agents, they can be pancytopenic.[93] As a result, when they perforate a hollow viscus,

they are unable to mount an adequate immune response. Their white count is extremely low, owing to the marrow suppressive effects of most chemotherapeutic agents. They are unable to mount a febrile response. These patients usually present to the operating room in shock from sepsis and require aggressive fluid therapy and pharmacologic support of their hemodynamics. Invasive hemodynamic monitoring should be placed before surgical resection. Minimum monitoring for these patients is an invasive arterial line, central venous pressure monitoring, and, most likely, pulmonary artery catheterization.

F. METABOLIC DERANGEMENTS

Many cancer patients develop metabolic abnormalities secondary to tumor products (such as hormones or locally acting substances) or from tumor destruction by antineoplastic therapy.[23] The following list contains examples of potential complications that patients may have before, during, or after anesthesia related to metabolic abnormalities.

1. Hypercalcemia

Ten per cent of cancer patients suffer from hypercalcemia, the most common metabolic abnormality of cancer patients.[23, 94] It may occur with or without bone metastasis. Some malignancies are associated with the tendency to develop hypercalcemia.[95]

Breast cancer is associated with hypercalcemia in 27 to 35 per cent of patients.[96] The mechanisms for the development of this disorder include widespread osteolytic metastasis, production of parathyroid hormone–like hormone, and prostaglandin E_2 (PgE_2) following hormone therapy with estrogens or antiestrogens (humoral, osteoclast-activating factor and coexisting primary hyperthyroidism). Lung cancer is associated with hypercalcemia in 12.5 to 35 per cent of patients.[97] And, hypercalcemia is seen in patients with squamous cell carcinoma and rarely seen with small cell carcinoma.[98] It may occur early or late, with or without bone metastasis. The mechanisms of production include osteoclast-activating factor, transforming growth factor alpha, interleukin-1, and tumor necrosis factor.[99] Other neoplasms associated with hypercalcemia include multiple myeloma (prevalence 20 to 40 per cent of patients), lymphoma, head and neck malignancies, and renal and ovarian carcinomas, among others.[23, 94]

The clinical presentation of cancer patients with hypercalcemia depends on the degree of the disturbance and is affected by concurrent illness or debility, age, and other associated metabolic disturbances. In general, hypercalcemia of malignancy usually has rapid onset.[94] The neuromuscular manifestations that often predominate include lethargy, confusion, and coma (occurring when serum calcium level is higher than 13 mg/dl).[23] Hallucinations and psychosis, weakness, and decreased deep tendon reflexes are also common. Cardiovascular manifestations include increased cardiac contractility. Dysrhythmias present a special problem for these patients if they require an anesthetic procedure.[100] Polyuria and polydypsia with dehydration, decreased glomerular filtration, loss of urine-concentrating ability, and renal insufficiency may occur in some of these patients. They require careful monitoring of inputs and outputs.

The anesthesiologist confronted with this problem needs to act quickly, as hypercalcemia is often fatal if left untreated, especially when symptomatic or when the serum calcium level is higher than 13 mg/dl.[23] The treatment goals include promoting urinary calcium excretion, enhancing bone absorption, and reducing entry of calcium into the extracellular fluid compartment.[101] The authors suggest hydration in an attempt to restore intravascular volume and to increase urine output. We initially start 5 to 8 L of normal saline intravenously over the first 24 hours when the patient is on the floor and then provide adequate intravenous fluids to maintain a urine output of 3 to 4 L per day.

The same principles of hypercalcemia treatment apply when the patient is in the operating room. It is important to monitor electrolytes during normal saline infusion and to monitor urine output and cardiac status to avoid fluid overload. The use of loop diuretics (i.e., furosemide) promotes calciuresis by blocking calcium absorption in the ascending loop of Henle and augmenting the calciuretic effect of normal saline.[102–104] The recommended dose is 40 to 80 mg intravenously, which should be given *after adequate hydration has been provided.*

Symptomatic hypercalcemia can also be treated with mitomycin (usual dose is 25 μg/

kg intravenously over 6 hours), disodium etidronate (7.5 μg/kg per day in 250 ml of normal saline infused over 6 hours for 3 to 4 days), glucocorticoids (i.e., prednisone 1 to 2 μg/kg per day), and calcitonin (4 to 8 IU/kg intramuscular or subcutaneous q6h).[94, 95, 105] For patients who present with acute renal insufficiency or who cannot be treated with normal saline, hemodialysis may be indicated. Importantly, appropriate patients require antineoplastic therapy; this therapy is the most effective means of achieving long-term correction of cancer-related hypercalcemia.[94]

2. Tumor Lysis Syndrome

Another complication seen frequently in cancer patients is tumor lysis syndrome.[106] Chemotherapy induces rapid tumor cell lysis in patients with a large malignant cell burden in an exquisitely sensitive tumor.[107–109] This typically occurs with Burkitt's lymphoma, non-Hodgkin's lymphomas, acute lymphoblastic and non-lymphoblastic leukemias, and chronic myelogenous leukemia.[106–110] In addition, it may also occur continuously in patients with lymphomas and leukemia following treatment with chemotherapy, radiation, glucocorticoids, tamoxifen, or interferon. The clinical manifestations of this syndrome are related to the metabolic abnormalities.

For patients suspected to have tumor lysis syndrome or who are receiving chemotherapeutic agents likely to induce the syndrome, prevention is the mainstay of treatment.[23, 106] To prevent the development of acute renal failure, patients who are to undergo treatment for malignancies should receive vigorous intravenous hydration, often with diuretics or renal doses of dopamine to ensure adequate urine output.[23] Alkalization of the urine during the first 1 to 2 days of cytotoxic therapy, in an attempt to increase to the solubility of uric acid, is recommended, as is use of allopurinol to decrease the formation of uric acid.

3. Syndrome of Inappropriate Antidiuretic Hormone Secretion

Another metabolic abnormality in patients with cancer is syndrome of inappropriate antidiuretic hormone secretion (SIADH), which occurs in 1 to 2 per cent of cancer patients.[23, 111–115] It is most often seen with small cell carcinoma of the lung as well as those suffering from prostatic, pancreatic, and bladder cancer. Its management may be difficult and requires a good understanding of sodium metabolism.[114]

The SIADH is a state of euvolemic hyponatremia caused by excessive secretion of ADH. The secretion of ADH is independent of normal osmotic or hemodynamic stimuli. Moreover, secretion of excessive ADH may be ectopic or by the posterior pituitary. Because free water cannot be excreted normally in this syndrome, persistent ADH secretion causes water retention, hyponatremia, and progressive expansion of intracellular and extracellular fluid.[116–118] The expanded extracellular fluid stimulates natriuresis with an isotonic loss of the extracellular fluid, bringing the extracellular compartment back to its baseline.

There are several causes of this syndrome. Among the most important are the use of some anesthetic agents, positive-pressure ventilation, surgical stress, central nervous systems neoplasms, meningitis, brain abscesses, and intracranial hemorrhage. Other commonly seen causes include pulmonary diseases such as pneumonia, tuberculosis, bronchiectasis, chronic obstructive pulmonary disease, and status *asthmaticus*. Some drugs—vasopressin, chlorpropamide, carbamazepine, oxytocin, vincristine, vinblastine, cyclophosphamide, phenothiziancs, tricyclic antidepressant agents, narcotics, monoamine oxidase inhibitors—can also induce SIADH.[116] In addition, ectopic ADH production occurs with carcinoma of the lung, duodenum, and pancreas and with thymoma, lymphoma, hepatoma, carcinoid tumors, and Ewing's sarcoma. The anesthesiologist must not forget that stress, pain, or nausea can precipitate SIADH.

The astute clinician will realize that when mild to moderate mental status changes or lethargy is present the patient may have SIADH. However, if the hyponatremia is severe or of rapid onset, seizures and coma may occur. The anesthesiologist should evaluate the patient for evidence of euvolemia, and the laboratory evaluation should include serum sodium, urine osmolality, and plasma osmolality. A diagnosis of SIADH is made if the serum sodium value is no greater than 130 mmol/L, urinary sodium at least 30 mmol/L, and serum osmolality below 280 mOsm/kg.

Therapy for this disorder must be individualized. It is important to treat the underlying disease and to restrict fluids to no more than 500 to 800 ml per day.[117, 118] This may be difficult in the operating room or in the postoperative care unit; therefore, the practitioner ought to make an attempt to decrease the free water intake.

It is important to distinguish acute-onset (less than 2 to 3 days) from chronic hyponatremia and to determine the presence or absence of neurologic symptoms.[116] Symptomatic acute hyponatremia may be treated with isotonic or hypertonic (3 per cent saline solution) combined with a loop diuretic.[118–123] Furosemide or torsemides are usually added. This treatment is aimed at increasing the serum sodium by no more than 1 mmol/L per hour to a maximum safe increase of 10 to 12 mmol/day.[117]

Infusion of isotonic saline alone seems to be reasonable, but since isotonic saline is hypertonic relative to the patient's plasma, the patient with SIADH can excrete the infused sodium in a more concentrated form than it was given.[111] Then net effect can be further retention of free water and aggravation of hyponatremia.

In chronic hyponatremia with minimal symptoms the anesthesiologist should correct the sodium more slowly, at approximately 0.5 mmol per hour, to avoid central pontine myelinolysis, which can result from aggressive sodium replacement and cause permanent neurologic impairment or death.[111–120] Fluid balances should be measured every 4 to 8 hours, until the serum sodium level is 125 mmol/L or is corrected halfway to normal. Oral demeclocycline, 300 to 600 mg twice a day, may be useful for patients with chronic SIADH.[119–123]

V. CANCER-RELATED PAIN

Cancer patients often experience chronic pain, especially those with advanced disease.[124] A summary of 54 reports suggests that, overall for cancer patients the prevalence of chronic pain is 51 per cent.[125] In patients with advanced terminal cancer, the incidence of pain increases to 74 per cent. Cancer-associated pain seems to affect all cultures similarly.[126] Reports from India, Thailand, Vietnam, and the Philippines reflect similar prevalences of cancer-related pain.[127–130]

The pain of cancer is classified as moderate

to severe in 40 to 50 per cent of cases and severe to excruciating in 25 to 30 per cent.[125] Many factors affect the prevalence of cancer pain. The primary type of tumor affects the incidence of pain. Patients with cancer of the pancreas, liver, or biliary tract report the highest incidences of pain, whereas those with lymphomas and leukemia report the lowest incidences.

Patients with cancer experience many different types of pain, which can be acute or chronic. Pain can be directly associated with advancement of the cancer or with its treatment.[131] The patient with cancer-associated pain can have a preexisting chronic pain syndrome with superimposed cancer-related pain. It is not uncommon to find a patient with cancer-related pain who has a history of drug addiction, and it is very common for dying patients to have cancer-related pain.

The management of cancer pain usually begins with treatment of the underlying cancer and may proceed to neuroablative procedures.[125, 132, 133] Pharmacologic management of cancer-related pain usually commences with nonnarcotic analgesics such as nonsteroidal antiinflammatory drugs (NSAIDs). If the pain persists, narcotic agonist and antagonist drugs are added. If this pain still persists, potent opioid analgesics are utilized.[125] At each step of pain control, adjuvants or adjuvant therapy (e.g., amitriptyline) can be added. If the pain persists despite opioid treatment, a variety of nerve block procedures are often utilized.[134]

When a patient with cancer-related pain presents to the operating theater, the anesthesiologist ought to know what type of pain the patient is experiencing and, just as important, how much and what type of medication the patient is taking. If the patient is in the early stages of pain treatment, receiving, for example, NSAIDs, with or without adjuvant therapy, the anesthetic management is the same as for other patients receiving like therapy.[124]

Patients with moderate to severe pain syndromes controlled with oral opioids, with or without adjuvant therapy, have much tolerance for narcotics and benzodiazepines.[135] Before bringing these patients to the operating room, the physician ought to understand the patient's basal narcotic requirement. It is also important to obtain an accurate history of narcotic use in the previous 24 hours. Most patients who require cancer therapy tend to underestimate their narcotic use, resulting in

TABLE 15–1

Oral Opioid Conversion Factors

From Oral	To Oral Morphine (Multiply by)
Methadone	1.5
Hydromorphone	4
Meperidine	0.1
Levorphanol	7.5
Codeine	0.15
Oxycodone	1
Hydrocodone	0.15
Oxymorphone (rectal)	5

underestimation of their basal narcotic requirements.[124, 126, 127]

Once the 24-hour oral morphine requirement is known, the total dose is divided by 2 for incomplete cross tolerance. To convert oral morphine equivalent to parenteral morphine equivalent, the one morphine equivalent is divided by 3 (Table 15–1).[136] This gives the total parenteral dose of morphine per 24 hours. This dose of morphine is then given via patient-controlled analgesia pump over 24 hours.

Patients with severe cancer-related pain who require parenteral narcotics, with or without adjuvant therapy, are very difficult to treat in the operating theater. It is imperative that these patients keep taking their chronic infusions of narcotics. If the infusions of narcotics are abruptly stopped, the patient may undergo narcotic withdrawals during the operative procedure. This withdrawal is a classic narcotic withdrawal (hypertension, tachycardia, and diaphoresis).[137–139] To prevent this, the anesthesiologist should continue the patient's narcotic infusions at the same rate as existed on arrival in the operating room. The physician then administers additional narcotics as necessary. Narcotic-dependent patients are tolerant to narcotics, and an increased dose of narcotics and benzodiazepines will be necessary to achieve effects comparable to a given dose in a narcotic-naive patient.

REFERENCES

1. Jessup JM, McGinnis LS, Steele GD Jr, et al: The national cancer data base. Report on colon cancer. Cancer 78:918–926, 1996.
2. Mihalo RM, Cagle CK, Cronau LH Jr, et al: Preanesthetic evaluation of the cancer patient. Cancer Bull 47:8–12, 1995.

3. Hasan N, Mandhan P: Respiratory obstruction caused by lipoma of the esophagus. J Pediatr Surg 29:1565–1566, 1994.

4. Supkis DE, Dougherty TB, Nguyen DT, et al: Anesthetic management of the patient undergoing head and neck cancer surgery. Cancer Bull 47:19–23, 1995.

5. Dougherty TB, Cronau LH: Anesthetic implications for surgical patients with endocrine tumors. Cancer Bull 47:24–30, 1995.

6. Varon J, Fromm RE: Special techniques. In Varon J (ed): Practical Guide to the Care of the Critically Ill Patient. St. Louis, Mosby-Year Book, 1994, pp. 321–339.

7. El-Ganzouri AR, McCarthy RJ, Tuman KJ, et al: Preoperative airway assessment: Predictive value of a multivariate risk index. Anesth Analg 82:1197–1204, 1996.

8. Benumof JL, Scheller MS: The importance of transtracheal jet ventilation in the management of the difficult airway. Anesthesiology 71:769–778, 1989.

9. Stehling LC: Management of the airway. In Barash PG, Cullen BF, Stoeling RK (ed): Clinical Anesthesia, ed 2. Philadelphia, J. B. Lippincott, 1992, pp. 685–708.

10. Ninane V: Endoscopic management of acute respiratory failure related to tracheobronchial malignancies. Support Care Cancer 3:418–421, 1995.

11. Robie DK, Gursoy MH, Pokorny WJ: Mediastinal tumors—airway obstruction and management. Semin Pediatr Surg 3:259–266, 1994.

12. Mackie AM, Watson CB: Anaesthesia and mediastinal masses. A case report and review of the literature. Anaesthesia 39:899–903, 1984.

13. Koka A, Macklis RM: Trends in radiation oncology: A review for the nononcologist. Cleve Clin J Med 62:254–258, 1995.

14. Scamman FL: Anesthesia for surgery of head and neck tumors. In Thawley SE, Panje WR (eds): Comprehensive Management of Head and Neck Tumors. Philadelphia, WB Saunders, 1987, pp. 25–41.

15. Donham RT: Anesthesia complications in head and neck surgery. In Eisele DW (ed): Complications in Head and Neck Surgery. St. Louis, Mosby-Year Book, 1993, pp. 3–25.

16. Weymuller EA: Complications of intubations and emergency airway management. In Eisele DW (ed): Complications in Head and Neck Surgery. St Louis, Mosby-Year Book, 1993, pp. 323–332.

17. Benumof JL: Management of the difficult adult airway: With special emphasis on awake tracheal intubation. Anesthesiology 75:1087–1110, 1991.

18. Heindl WP: Anesthesia procedures for bronchoscopic intubation in a comparative study. Anasth Intensivther Notfallmed 24:81–87, 1989.

19. Ermanni M, Russi E: Experiences with fiberoptic bronchoscopic intubation. Prax Klin Pneumol 39:93–95, 1985.

20. Ovassapian A: Fiberoptic Airway Endoscopy in Anesthesia and Critical Care. New York, Raven, 1990, pp. 135–148.

21. Howland WS, Carlon GC, Goldiner PL, et al: High-frequency jet ventilation during thoracic surgical procedures. Anesthesiology 67:1009–1012, 1987.

22. Ezril T, Szmuk P, Shklar B, et al: Adult respiratory distress syndrome after radical neck dissection. Cancer J Anaesth 40:658–663, 1993.

23. Santos L, Curioso C, Martinez JG, et al: Oncologic critical care. In Varon J (ed): Practice Guide to the Care of the Critically Ill Patient. St. Louis, Mosby-Year Book, 1995, pp. 223–250.

24. Markman M: Common complications and emergencies associated with cancer and its therapy. Cleve Clin J Med 61:105–114, 1994.

25. Mani S, Duffy TP: Pericardial tamponade in chronic myelomonocytic leukemia. Chest 106:967–970, 1994.

26. Mittal S, Berko B, Bavaria J, et al: Radiation-induced cardiovascular dysfunction. Am J Cardiol 78:114–115, 1996.

27. Rodgers KG: Cardiovascular shock. Emerg Med Clin North Am 13:793–810, 1995.

28. Fadouach S, Azouzi L, Mehadji BA, et al: Cardiac tamponade disclosing neoplasm: Apropos of 23 cases. Arch Mal Coeur Vaiss 87:1333–1338, 1994.

29. Chong HH, Plotnick GD: Pericardial effusion and tamponade: Evaluation, imaging modalities, and management. Compr Ther 21:378–385, 1995.

30. Fowler NO: Cardiac tamponade. A clinical or an echocardiographic diagnosis? Circulation 87:1738–1741, 1993.

31. Teplinsky K: Pericardial involvement in critical illness. In Hall J, Schmidt GA, Wood LDH (eds): Principles of Critical Care. New York, McGraw-Hill, 1992, pp. 1525–1541.

32. Vaitkus PT, Herrmann HC, LeWinter MM: Treatment of malignant pericardial effusion. JAMA 272:59–64, 1994.

33. Callahan JA, Seward JB, Nishimura RA, et al: Two-dimensional echocardiographically guided pericardiocentesis: Experience in 117 consecutive patients. Am J Cardiol 55:476–479, 1985.

34. Lahtinen R, Kuikka J, Nousianinen T, et al: Cardiotoxicity of epirubicin and doxorubicin: A double-blind randomized study. Eur J Haematol 46:301–305, 1991.

35. Drzewoski J, Kasznicki J: Cardiotoxicity of antineoplastic drugs. Acta Haematol Pol 23:79–86, 1992.

36. Lekakis J, Vassilopoulos N, Psichoyiou H, et al: Doxorubicin cardiotoxicity detected by indium 111 myosin-specific imaging. Eur J Nucl Med 18:225–226, 1991.

37. Forbes JF: Long-term effects of adjuvant chemotherapy in breast cancer. Acta Oncol 31:243–250, 1992.

38. Fountzilas G, Afthonidis D, Geleris P, et al: Cardiotoxicity evaluation in patients treated with a mitoxantrone combination as adjuvant chemotherapy for breast cancer. Anticancer Res 12:231–234, 1992.

39. Weesner KM, Bledsoe M, Chauvenet A, et al: Exercise echocardiography in the detection of anthracycline cardiotoxicity. Cancer 68:435–438, 1991.

40. Lewkow LM, Hooker JL, Movahed A: Cardiac complications of intensive dose mitoxantrone and cyclophosphamide with autologous bone marrow transplantation in metastatic breast cancer. Int J Cardiol 34:273–276, 1992.

41. Solley GO, Maldonado JE, Gleich GJ, et al: Endomyocardiopathy with eosinophilia. Mayo Clin Proc 51:697–708, 1976.

42. Verweij J: Mitomycins. Cancer Chemother Biol Response Modif 16:48–56, 1996.

43. Stewart JR, Fajardo LF, Gillette SM, et al: Radiation injury to the heart. Int J Radiat Oncol Biol Phys 31:1205–1211, 1995.

44. Steinherz LJ, Steinherz PG, Tan CT, et al: Cardiac toxicity 4 to 20 years after completing anthracycline therapy. JAMA 266:1672–1677, 1991.

45. Burrows FA, Hickey PR, Colan S: Perioperative complications in patients with anthracycline chemotherapeutic agents. Can Anaesth Soc J 32:149–157, 1985.

46. Cortes JE, Pazdur R: Docetaxel. J Clin Oncol 13:2643–2655, 1995.
47. Pimentel L: Medical complications of oncologic disease. Emerg Med Clin North Am 11:407–419, 1993.
48. Fromm RE, Varon J: Neurologic disorders. *In* Varon J (ed): Practical Guide to the Care of the Critically Ill Patient. St. Louis, Mosby-Year Book, 1994, pp. 202–215.
49. Ferreri AJ, Reni M, Villa E: Primary central nervous system lymphoma in immunocompetent patients. Cancer Treat Rev 21:416–446, 1995.
50. Clouston PD, DeAngelis LM, Posner JB: The spectrum of neurological disease in patients with systemic cancer. Ann Neurol 31:268–273, 1992.
51. Knekt P, Reunanen A, Aho K, et al: Risk factors for a subarachnoid hemorrhage in a longitudinal population study. J Clin Epidemiol 44:933–939, 1991.
52. Pruitt AA: Central nervous system infections in cancer patients. Neurol Clin 9:867–888, 1991.
53. Bleck TP, Smith MC, Pierre-Louis SJC, et al: Neurologic complications of critical medical illness. Crit Care Med 21:98–103, 1993.
54. Murray JC, Dorfman SR, Brandt ML, et al: Renal venous thrombosis complicating acute myeloid leukemia with hyperleukocytosis. J Pediatr Hematol Oncol 18:327–330, 1996.
55. Hashimoto T: Hyperviscosity syndrome in patients with immunoproliferative disorder. Nippon Naika Gakkai Zasshi 84:1096–1099, 1995.
56. Pruitt A: Central nervous system infections in cancer patients. Neurol Clin 9:867–888, 1991.
57. Sculier JP: Indications for intensive care in the management of infections in cancer patients. Cancer Treat Res 79:233–244, 1995.
58. Kothari RU, Brott T, Broderick JP, et al: The ABCs of measuring intracerebral hemorrhage volumes. Stroke 27:1304–1305, 1996.
59. Pickuth D, Leutloff U: Computed tomography and magnetic resonance imaging findings in primitive neuroectodermal tumours in adults. Br J Radiol 69:1–5, 1996.
60. Varon J: Acute respiratory distress syndrome in the postoperative cancer patient. Cancer Bull 47:38–42, 1995.
61. Epner DE, White P, Krasnoff M, et al: Outcome of mechanical ventilation for adults with hematologic malignancy. J Investig Med 44:254–260, 1996.
62. Randle CJ Jr, Frankel LR, Amylon MD: Identifying early predictors of mortality in pediatric patients with acute leukemia and pneumonia. Chest 109:457–461, 1996.
63. Dumont P, Wihlm JM, Hentz JG, et al: Respiratory complications after surgical treatment of esophageal cancer. A study of 309 patients according to the type of resection. Eur J Cardiothorac Surg 9:539–543, 1995.
64. Williams DM, Krick JA, Remington JS: Pulmonary infection in the compromised host: part I. Am Rev Respir Dis 114:359–394, 1976.
65. Lombara CM, Churg A, Winokur S: Pulmonary veno-occlusive disease following therapy for malignant neoplasms. Chest 92:871–876, 1987.
66. Meysman M, Schoors DF, Reynaert H, et al: Respiratory failure with diffuse patchy lung infiltrates: An unusual presentation of squamous cell carcinoma. Thorax 49:1271–1272, 1994.
67. Schwarer AP, Hughes JM, Trotman-Dickenson B, et al: A chronic pulmonary syndrome associated with graft-versus-host disease after allogeneic marrow transplantation. Transplantation 54:1002–1008, 1991.
68. Schmidt GM, Horak DA, Niland JC, et al: A randomized, controlled trail of prophylactic ganciclovir for cytomegalovirus pulmonary infection in recipients of allogeneic bone marrow transplants; The City of Hope-Stanford-Syntx CMV Study Group. N Engl J Med 324:1005–1011, 1991.
69. Reichart E, Gerard H, Boerkmann P: Trypsin-induced leukostasis: Granulocyte migration in airspaces. C R Acad Sci III 319:371–375, 1996.
70. Hidou M, Caramella JP, Deletang D, et al: Postoperative pulmonary leukostasis responsible for fatal respiratory distress. Ann Fr Anesth Reanim 9:390–392, 1990.
71. Gartrell K, Rosenstrauch W: Hypoxaemia in patients with hyperleukocytosis: True or spurious, and clinical implications. Leuk Res 17:915–919, 1993.
72. Creaven PJ, Mihich E: The clinical toxicity of anticancer drugs and its prediction. Semin Oncol 4:147–163, 1977.
73. Leupold W, Ronisch P, Hahn B: The effect of radio and chemotherapy on lung function in children with malignant diseases. Pneumologie 44:1213–1216, 1990.
74. Cooper JA Jr, White DA, Matthay RA: Drug-induced pulmonary disease. Part 1: Cytotoxic drugs. Am Rev Respir Dis 133:321–340, 1986.
75. Jost LM: Overdose with melphalan (Alkerran): Symptoms and treatment. A review. Onkologie 13:96–101, 1990.
76. Van der Lelie H, Baars JW, Rodenhuis S, et al: Hemolytic uremic syndrome after high-dose chemotherapy with autologous stem cell support. Cancer 76:2338–2342, 1995.
77. Friedman HS, Bigner SH, Bigner DD: Cyclophosphamide therapy of medulloblastoma: From the laboratory to the clinic and back again (and again and again). J Neurooncol 24:103–108, 1995.
78. Gockerman JP: Drug-induced interstitial lung diseases. Clin Chest Med 3:521–536, 1982.
79. McCullough B, Collins JF, Johansen WG Jr, et al: Bleomycin-induced diffuse interstitial pulmonary fibrosis in baboons. J Clin Inves 61:79–88, 1978.
80. Chung F: Cancer, chemotherapy and anaesthesia. Can Anaesth Soc J 29:364–371, 1982.
81. Seiden MV, Elias A, Ayash L, et al: Pulmonary toxicity associated with high dose chemotherapy in the treatment of solid tumors with autologous marrow transplant: An analysis of four chemotherapy regimens. Bone Marrow Transplant 10:57–63, 1992.
82. Bourguet J, Bourdiniere J, Subileau C, et al: Respiratory changes during treatment with bleomycin. Ann Otolaryngol Chir Cervicofac 90:169–183, 1973.
83. Fraser RS, Paré JAP, Fraser RG, et al: Pulmonary disease caused by drugs, poisons, and inhaled toxic gases and aerosols. *In* Fraser RS, Paré JAP, Fraser RG, et al (eds): Synopsis of Diseases of the Chest, ed 2. Philadelphia, WB Saunders, 1994, pp. 753–780.
84. Gregory SA, Grippi MA: The clinical diagnosis of drug-induced pulmonary disorders. J Thorac Imaging 6:8–18, 1991.
85. Rosenow EC III, Myers JL, Swensen SJ, et al: Drug-induced pulmonary disease. An update. Chest 102:239–250, 1992.
86. Rubin P: Radiation toxicology: Quantitative radiation pathology for predicting effects. Cancer 39:729–736, 1977.
87. Gregor A: Radiotherapy of lung cancer. Ann Oncol 6:37–41, 1995.
88. Tissot E: Role of surgery in gastrointestinal lymphomas. Schweiz Med Wochenschr 126:836–840, 1996.

89. Schneider SM, Distelhorst CW: Chemotherapy-induced emergencies. Semin Oncol 16:572–578, 1989.

90. Gronert GA, Theye RA: Pathophysiology of hyperkalemia induced by succinylcholine. Anesthesiology 43:89–96, 1975.

91. Davidson JE: Neuromuscular blockade. Focus Crit Care 18:512–520, 1991.

92. Jones RM: Neuromuscular transmission and its blockade. Pharmacology, monitoring and physiology updated. Anaesthesia 40:964–976, 1985.

93. Johnson SA, Prentice AG, Phillips MJ: Treatment of acute leukaemia with early intensive induction therapy. Acta Oncol 27:527–534, 1988.

94. Ralston SH: Pathogenesis and management of cancer associated hypercalcaemia. Cancer Surv 21:179–196, 1994.

95. Walls J, Bundred N, Howell A: Hypercalcemia and bone resorption in malignancy. Clin Orthop 312:51–63, 1995.

96. Neskovic-Konstantinovic Z, Mitrovic L, Petrovic J, et al: Treatment of tumour-induced hypercalcaemia in advanced breast cancer patients with three different doses of disodium pamidronate adapted to the initial level of calcaemia. Support Care Cancer 3:422–424, 1995.

97. Galvez Valdovinos R, Gamez Garcia P, Diaz Hellin Gude V: Hypercalcemia and bronchogenic carcinoma. Arch Bronconeumol 31:489–490, 1995.

98. Raue F: Epidemiological aspects of hypercalcemia of malignancy. Recent Results Cancer Res 137:99–106, 1994.

99. Asamura H, Nakayama H, Kondo H, et al: AFP-producing squamous cell carcinoma of the lung in an adolescent. Jpn J Clin Oncol 26:103–106, 1996.

100. Ritch P: Treatment of calcium-related hypercalcemia. Semin Oncol 2:26–33, 1990.

101. Silverman P, Distelhorst CW: Metabolic emergencies in clinical oncology. Semin Oncol 16:471–489, 1989.

102. Davies M, Thomas P: Decision-making in surgery: The surgical management of a raised serum calcium. Br J Hosp Med 53:330–333, 1995.

103. Harvey HA: The management of hypercalcemia of malignancy. Support Care Cancer 3:123–129, 1995.

104. Chisholm MA, Mulloy AL, Taylor AT: Acute management of cancer-related hypercalcemia. Ann Pharmacother 30:507–513, 1996.

105. Raue F, Pecherstorfer M: Drug therapy of hypercalcemia due to malignancy. Recent Results Cancer Res 137:138–160, 1994.

106. Fleming DR, Doukas MA: Acute tumor lysis syndrome in hematologic malignancies. Leuk Lymphoma 8:315–318, 1992.

107. Van der Hoven B, Thunnissen PL, Sizoo W: Tumour lysis syndrome in haematological malignances. Neth J Med 40:31–35, 1992.

108. Jones DP, Mahmoud H, Chesney RW: Tumor lysis syndrome: Pathogenesis and management. Pediatr Nephrol 9:206–212, 1995.

109. Drakos P, Bar-Ziv J, Catane R: Tumor lysis syndrome in nonhematologic malignancies. Report of a case and review of the literature. Am J Clin Oncol 17:502–505, 1994.

110. Sondheimer JH, Migdal SD: Toxic nephropathies. Crit Care Clin 3:883–907, 1987.

111. Sorensen JB, Andersen MK, Hansen HH: Syndrome of inappropriate secretion of antidiuretic hormone (SIADH) in malignant disease. J Intern Med 238:97–110, 1995.

112. Haycock GB: The syndrome of inappropriate secretion of antidiuretic hormone. Pediatr Nephrol 9:375–381, 1995.

113. Spigset O, Hedenmalm K: Hyponatraemia and the syndrome of inappropriate antidiuretic hormone secretion (SIADH) induced by psychotropic drugs. Drug Safety 12:209–225, 1995.

114. Arieff AI: Central nervous system manifestation of disordered sodium metabolism. Clin Endocrinol Metab 13:269–294, 1984.

115. Rodriguez Cuartero A, Gonzalez Martinez F: Inappropriate ADH secretion syndrome. Ann Med Interna 13:127–129, 1996.

116. Anderson RJ, Chung HM, Kluge R, et al: Hyponatremia: A prospective analysis of its epidemiology and the pathogenetic role of vasopressin. Ann Intern Med 102:164–168, 1985.

117. Ayus JC, Arieff AI: Pathogenesis and prevention of hyponatremic encephalopathy. Endocrinol Metab Clin North Am 22:425–446, 1993.

118. Gross PA, Pehrisch H, Rascher W, et al: Pathogenesis of clinical hyponatremia: Observations of vasopressin and fluid intake in 100 hyponatremic medical patients. Eur J Clin Invest 17:123–129, 1987.

119. Ayus JC, Krothapalli RK, Arieff AI: Treatment of symptomatic hyponatremia and its relation to brain damage: A prospective study. N Engl J Med 317:1190–1195, 1987.

120. Ayus JC, Arieff AI: Pathogenesis and prevention of hyponatremic encephalopathy. Endocrinol Metab Clin North Am 22:425–446, 1993.

121. Ayus JC, Varon J: Pathogenesis and prevention of hyponatremic encephalopathy. (Patogénesis y prevención de la encefalopatía hiponatrémica). Nefrol Latinoam 2:193–206, 1995.

122. Ayus JC, Varon J, Fraser CL: Pathogenesis and management of hyponatremic encephalopathy. Curr Opin Crit Care 1:452–459, 1995.

123. Kinzie BJ: Management of the syndrome of inappropriate secretion of antidiuretic hormone. Clin Pharmacol 6:625–633, 1987.

124. Kelly JB, Payne R: Pain syndromes in the cancer patient. Neurol Clin 4:937–953, 1991.

125. American Society of Anesthesiologists Task Force on Pain Management, Cancer Pain Section: Practice guidelines for cancer pain management. Anesthesiology 84:1243–1257, 1996.

126. Grossman SA, Sheidler VR, Swedeen K, et al: Correlation of patient and caregiver ratings of cancer pain. J Pain Symptom Management 6:53–57, 1991.

127. Holder KA, Dougherty TB, Porche VH, et al: Postoperative pain management. Cancer Bull 47:43–51, 1995.

128. Ahles TA, Blanchard EB, Ruckdeschel JC: The multidimensional nature of cancer-related pain. Pain 17:277–288, 1983.

129. Todd KH, Samaroo N, Hoffman JR: Ethnicity as a risk factor for inadequate emergency department analgesia. JAMA 269:1537–1539, 1993.

130. Portenoy RK: Cancer pain: Epidemiology and syndromes. Cancer 63:2298–2307, 1989.

131. Foley KM: The treatment of cancer pain. N Engl J Med 313:84–95, 1985.

132. Jacox A, Carr DB, Payne R: New clinical-practice guidelines for the management of pain in patients with cancer. N Engl J Med 330:651–655, 1994.

133. Pagni CA: Role of neurosurgery in cancer pain: Re-evaluation of old methods and new trends. *In* Benedetti C, Chapman CR, Moricca GM (eds): Advances in Pain Research and Therapy, Vol 7. New York, Raven Press, 1984, pp. 603–629.

134. Raj PP: Prognostic and therapeutic local anesthetic block. *In* Cousins MJ, Bridenbaugh PO (eds): Neural Blockade in Clinical Anesthesia and Management of Pain, ed 2. Philadelphia, J.B. Lippincott, 1988, pp. 899–933.
135. Hansen J, Ginman C, Hartvig P, et al: Clinical evaluation of oral methadone in treatment of cancer pain. Acta Anaesth Scand Suppl 74:124–127, 1982.
136. Ferrer-Brechner T: Rational management of cancer pain. *In* Raj PP (ed): Practical Management of Pain. St. Louis, Mosby-Year Book, 1986, pp. 312–336.
137. Portenoy RK: Tolerance to opioid analgesics: Clinical aspects. Cancer Surv 21:49–65, 1994.
138. Farrell M: Opiate withdrawal. Addiction 89:1471–1475, 1994.
139. Foley KM: Opioids. Neurol Clin 11:503–522, 1993.

Uncommon Poisoning, Envenomation, and Intoxication

William C. Wilson
Randall Goskowicz

2. Lacrimators (Tear Gas, Pepper Spray, Mace)

3. Nerve Agents

F. INHALED DRUGS OF ABUSE

1. Solvents (Gasoline, Cleaning Solvents, Glue, Freon)

2. Tetrahydrocannabinol

3. Cocaine

IV. TOXIC INGESTIONS (POISONING)

A. MEDICATIONS ASSOCIATED WITH OVERDOSE AND TOXICITY

1. Acetaminophen

2. Aspirin

3. Antihistamines

4. Digoxin

5. Lithium

6. Theophylline

7. Tricyclic Antidepressants

B. NONINFECTIOUS FOOD POISONING

1. Poisonous Plants

a. Anticholinergic Alkaloids

b. Curare and Other Plant-Derived Neuromuscular Blocking Drugs

c. Ergot Poisoning and Lysergic Acid Diethylamide

d. Hemlock (*Conium maculatum*)

e. Mescaline

f. Mushrooms

i. Cyclopeptide Group

ii. Ibotenic Group

iii. Coprine Group

iv. Muscarine Group

v. Psilocybin Group

vi. Monomethyl Group

g. Strychnine

2. Ingested Marine Animal–Derived Toxins: Pelagic Poisoning

a. Fugu Poisoning

b. Ciguatera

c. Paralytic Shellfish Poisoning

C. INSECTICIDES

1. Anticholinesterase Drugs

a. Organophosphates (Irreversible Anticholinesterases)

b. Carbamates (Reversible Anticholinesterases)

2. Chlorinated Hydrocarbon Insecticides

3. Paraquat

D. ORGANIC SOLVENTS AND HYDROCARBONS

1. Alcohols

a. Ethyl Alcohol (Ethanol)

b. Ethylene Glycol

c. Isopropyl Alcohol (Isopropanol)

d. Methyl Alcohol (Methanol)

2. Alcohol-Free Distilled Hydrocarbons

a. Petroleum-Based Distilled Hydrocarbons

b. Nonpetroleum Distilled Hydrocarbons

E. HEAVY METALS

1. Antimony

2. Arsenic

3. Iron

4. Lead

5. Mercury

6. Phosphorus

7. Thallium

F. LYE

V. ANIMAL BITES, STINGS, AND ENVENOMATIONS

A. DOMESTICATED ANIMALS AND HUMANS

B. VENOMOUS REPTILES, PRINCIPALLY SNAKES

1. Identification of North American Venomous Snakes

2. Venom Toxicity

3. Families of Venomous Snakes (North American Emphasis)

a. Elapidae

i. Cobras (Africa, India, Asia)

ii. Coral Snakes (North and South America)

b. Crotalidae (Pit Vipers)

i. Rattlesnakes

ii. Cottonmouth (Water Moccasin)

iii. Copperhead

c. Hydrophidae (Venomous Sea Snakes, Indo-Pacific Region)

All substances are poisons; there is none which is not a poison. The right dose differentiates a poison from a remedy.

PARACELSUS[1]

I. INTRODUCTION

This chapter has been entirely rewritten for the current edition. New sections on toxic gases, vapors, poisonings, envenomations, chemotherapy, and radiation exposure have been added to provide an authoritative concise reference for intraoperative care of patients acutely afflicted with these uncommon problems. Section headings on drug abuse have been pared down because most anesthesiologists are aware of the pharmacologic implications of opiate and sedative hypnotic abuse. Emphasis is placed on identifying the life-saving therapy and anesthetic implications of each category.

In Section II we review the general approach to early diagnosis and detoxification for patients who have received a toxic exposure. Sections III, IV, and V cover toxic exposures that typically occur through inhalation (gases and vapors), ingestion (poisons), and percutaneously via envenomation (bites and stings), respectively. Sections VI and VII review the anesthetic implications of chemotherapeutics and radiation therapy.

II. GENERAL APPROACH TO PATIENTS EXPOSED TO A TOXIC SUBSTANCE

Although basic supportive care is the foundation of management for toxic exposures, several specific therapies and antidotes are available, but they must be administered early if toxicity is to be minimized. Thus, the search for an early, precise diagnosis of the poison, toxin, or venom that afflicts the patient must begin immediately after institution of the *ABCs* of life-saving therapy and supportive care. Once a tentative diagnosis is arrived at, specific corroborative blood levels should be drawn and therapy initiated. Utilization of resources (e.g., a poison control center) is recommended, to verify that the most recent advances in therapy for specific rare toxic exposures are employed. Finally, anyone who encounters a toxic exposure that has epidemic implications must notify public health officials.

A. DISCOVERING DIAGNOSTIC CLUES TO THE TOXIC AGENT

Clues to the source of toxic exposure are obtained from the history, physical examination, laboratory data, and knowledge of several autonomic syndromes associated with each type of intoxication. While sections III through VII detail the anesthetic implications of uncommon exposures, this section helps to focus on the "detective work" that should proceed simultaneously with the provision of supportive care.

1. History

If the patient is able to provide information about the specific drugs, foods, or animals involved in the toxic exposure, specific therapy can be employed sooner. Information on the source of toxic exposure may help both the patient and other potential victims. Family, friends, apartment managers, and colleagues at work are all useful resources. The paramedic who brings the patient to the hospital can often provide useful clues about the surroundings at the scene. The physician should always review the drugs that arrive with the patient and consider calling the pharmacist listed on the containers to determine which other drugs were prescribed. Asking a family member to go quickly through the trash at the patient's home can also yield useful information. For envenomations, it is good to ask the patient or family to bring in the carcass of the snake or other animal that bit or stung the patient.

2. Physical Examination

The physical examination should always include the vital signs and neurologic status. The vital signs—pulse, blood pressure (BP), respiration, and temperature—are critical (temperature measurements are frequently overlooked in adults, and BP measurements are commonly omitted in pediatric cases). Altered mental status should trigger verification from family members about the patient's normal neurologic status and previous episodes of altered mental status. The motor and sensory examination, including deep tendon reflexes, muscle tone (flaccid versus rigid), and abnormal muscle movements such as clonus, tremor, or seizures, should be noted. Pupil size and reactivity as well as the presence of disconjugate gaze or nystagmus are important findings. Pupils are small with narcotic intoxication and large with anticholinergic intoxication. Nystagmus occurs with phencyclidine (PCP) intoxication, just as with its related compound, ketamine. Skin color, temperature, and moisture content afford clues to the relative sympathetic (versus parasympathetic) tone induced by the toxic exposure. Ability to control bowel and bladder functions and the presence or absence of bowel sounds are other important clues to diagnosis.

3. Laboratory Studies

Critical laboratory tests that should be obtained for all patients with altered mental status or toxic exposure to substance(s) unknown include arterial blood gases, serum electrolytes, blood sugar, measured serum osmolality, urinalysis, electrocardiogram (ECG), and appropriate radiographs. Calculation of the anion and osmolar gaps are critical for accurate diagnosis of poisoning or overdose. For envenomations and other exposures that cause thrombocytopenia or coagulopathy, blood should be typed and cross-matched, and platelet counts and coagulation studies should be obtained. Also, an envenomating animal's carcass (e.g., dead snake, scorpion) should be examined and kept for definitive identification. Vomitus, pills, and leftover pieces of fish and mushrooms should likewise be saved for toxicologic analysis and definitive diagnosis. Patients who are scheduled for an operation following chemotherapy and radiation exposure should have specific samples sent to the laboratory related to the organ(s) at risk (see Sections VI, VII). With a focused history, physical examination, and routine laboratory tests, a tentative diagnosis can be reached relatively quickly and specific drug levels measured or toxicology samples sent for testing. Drug screening tests (as currently available) are not endorsed because they take too long (2 to 3 days) to provide useful information when the patient is at greatest risk.

4. Autonomic Syndromes

Many of the toxic compounds described in this chapter affect the autonomic nervous system, producing syndromes of diagnostic and therapeutic significance. The autonomic nervous system is composed of two competing systems, sympathetic and parasympathetic. The sympathetic nervous system (SNS) nerve cells arise from the thoracolumbar portions of the spinal cord (Fig. 16–1), whereas the parasympathetic nervous system (PNS) cells arise in the craniosacral portion of the spinal cord (Fig. 16–2).[2] The cells of origin for both the SNS and PNS give off myelinated preganglionic fibers that form synapses at nicotinic ganglia using acetylcholine as the neurotransmitter. The SNS ganglia reside close to

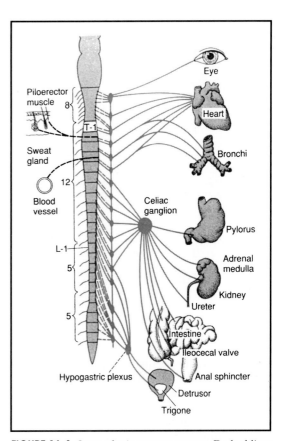

FIGURE 16–1. Sympathetic nervous system. Dashed lines represent postganglionic fibers in the gray rami leading to the spinal nerves for distribution to blood vessels, sweat glands, and piloerector muscles. The solid lines joining the thoracolumbar spinal cord with the various organs represent the postganglionic connection between the aforementioned ganglia and the innervated organ. For the adrenal medulla there is no synapse at the celiac ganglion. Instead, the fibers continue all the way to the adrenal gland, and the nicotinic ganglion is located there. The postganglionic effector organ is the adrenal medulla, which itself secretes norepinephrine and epinephrine. (From Guyton AC: Textbook of Medical Physiology, ed 8. Philadelphia, W.B. Saunders, 1991.)

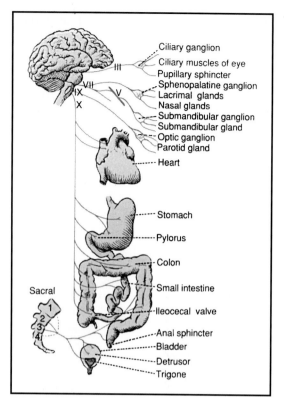

FIGURE 16–2. Parasympathetic nervous system. The solid line represents the preganglionic fibers emanating from the cranial and sacral nuclei as they proceed to the innervated organs. Note that the tenth cranial nerve (the vagus) is responsible for the entire thoracic and abdominal parasympathetic innervation. Approximately 75 per cent of all parasympathetic innervation is derived from the vagus nerve. The sacral nerves, chiefly the second through the fourth, provide the parasympathetic innervation to the anal sphincter, detrusor muscle of the bladder, and urinary sphincter. (From Guyton AC: Textbook of Medical Physiology, ed 8. Philadelphia, W.B. Saunders, 1991.)

the spinal column (an exception being the adrenal gland). In contrast, the ganglia for PNS fibers reside near or in the organ they innervate.

The postganglionic fibers of the SNS secrete norepinephrine at the receptor of the organ innervated (except at the sweat glands, piloerector muscles, and a few blood vessels, where acetylcholine is the neurotransmitter). In the PNS, acetylcholine is secreted at the "muscarinic" receptors of all the organs it innervates. The term *muscarinic* is derived from muscarine, a poison in mushrooms that activates only muscarinic receptors (not nicotinic ones). In contrast, nicotine stimulates only nicotinic receptors, whereas, acetylcholine stimulates both muscarinic and nicotinic

receptors. Beside the ganglia for both SNS and PNS, nicotinic receptors are found at the neuromuscular junctions of skeletal muscle. Muscarinic receptors are found in all effector cells stimulated by postganglionic fibers of the PNS, but also in the postganglionic fibers of the SNS innervating sweat glands, the piloerector muscles, and a few blood vessels (Fig. 16–3).

Increased sympathetic tone causes increased heart rate and blood pressure, dilated pupils, diaphoresis, bronchodilatation, decreased bowel sounds, decreased detrusor tone, increased urinary and anal sphincter tone, and release of epinephrine and norepinephrine from the adrenal medulla (fight-or-flight response to an acute stressor).

Increased parasympathetic tone leads to bradycardia and hypotension, constricted pupils, bronchoconstriction, increased peristaltic activity of the bowels, increased detrusor tone, and relaxed urethral and anal sphincter tone. However, the skin is also diaphoretic with stimulation of the PNS because acetylcholine is the neurotransmitter at the end-organ for all cholinergic systems, including the sweat glands of the skin (Table 16–1, and Figure 16–3). PNS stimulation also promotes diarrhea and copious secretions from the glands in the mouth and bronchial tree.

Antisympathetic (sympatholytic) drugs tend to decrease endogenous sympathetic tone without causing a completely cholinergic-dominated presentation. Opiates are a good example of this category of drug. The systemic administration of opiates results in miosis, dry skin, decreased bowel sounds, and urine retention.

Parasympatholytic (anticholinergic) drugs such as atropine cause an opposite response, including increased heart rate and blood pressure, dry, flushed skin, and decreased bowel sounds. If two patients present after ingesting unknown drugs, both with hypertension, tachycardia, agitation, and dilated pupils, but one patient has sweaty skin and the second one has dry and flushed skin, certain toxic drugs are implicated. The first patient's symptoms are consistent with a sympathomimetic syndrome, having all the features of high sympathetic tone that would follow cocaine or amphetamine injection. The second patient, who has all the same features but dry skin, manifests a parasympatholytic (anticholinergic) syndrome like that occurring with an atropine or tricyclic antidepressant (TCA) overdose. Anticholinergic symptoms should

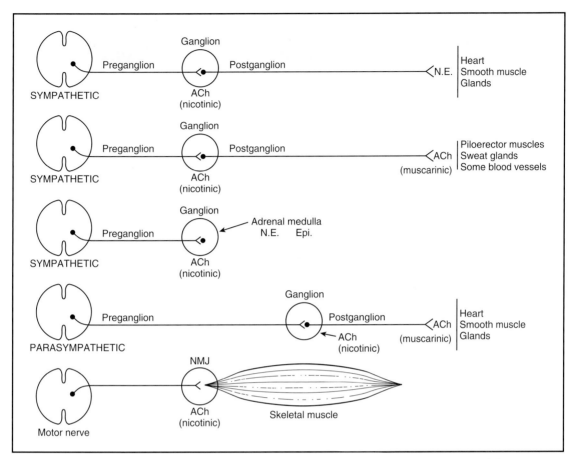

FIGURE 16–3. Schematic diagram of nicotinic and muscarinic sites in the autonomic nervous system and the neuromuscular junction. Acetylcholine is released as the neurotransmitter at the preganglionic fibers (nicotinic receptor type) of both the sympathetic and parasympathetic nervous systems and at the neuromuscular junction. Additionally, in the parasympathetic nervous system acetylcholine is also released as the neurotransmitter at all postganglionic sites (muscarinic receptor type) for all organs innervated. Whereas, the sympathetic nervous system releases norepinephrine at most postganglionic sites. At the adrenal medulla, both epinephrine and norepinephrine are released in large quantities into the systemic circulation. (The adrenal medulla is a giant postganglionic secreting gland.) Interestingly, at sweat glands, piloerector muscles, and a few blood vessels acetylcholine is the neurotransmitter released by the sympathetic system at these postganglionic (muscarinic) nerves. (Modified from Moss J, Craigo PA: The autonomic nervous system. In Miller RD [ed]: Anesthesia, ed 4. New York, Churchill Livingstone, 1994.)

prompt immediate consideration of intoxication with anticholinergic drugs (atropine, herbal teas [belladonna], TCA). Overdose involving TCAs should lead to immediate review of the ECG because clinically significant TCA overdose causes widening of the QRS, and can cause ventricular tachydysrhythmias, including *torsades de pointes.*

When a patient presents with pinpoint pupils and a history of intravenous drug abuse, one should consider heroin. If the heart rate is slow, bowel sounds depressed, and the pupils small, this would be supportive; however, other drugs that cause miotic pupils should also be considered, including clonidine and phenothiazines. Clonidine is a centrally act-

ing antihypertensive (α_2 agonist) that causes a decrease in sympathetic outflow and can mimic narcotic overdose by producing miosis, apnea, and coma. Clonidine does not respond to naloxone (even to large doses), and this can help to separate the two toxicities. Although phenothiazines cause some anticholinergic symptoms they also have potent alpha-blocking effects and can cause the pupils to be small, especially when ingested in large quantities or by small children. Small pupils associated with diaphoresis, salivation, and hyperactive bowel sounds should bring up the possibility of cholinesterase inhibitors like those in insecticides (organophosphates, carbamates).

TABLE 16–1

Autonomic Effects on Various Organs of Interest to Anesthesiologists

Organ	Effects of Stimulation	
	Sympathetic	Parasympathetic
Eye		
Pupil	Dilatation	Constriction
Ciliary muscle	Relaxation (far vision)	Constriction (near vision)
Glands		
Nasal	Vasoconstriction and slight secretion	Stimulation of copious secretion
Lacrimal		(containing many enzymes for
Parotid		enzyme-secreting glands)
Submandibular		
Gastric		
Pancreatic		
Sweat glands	Copious sweating (cholinergic)	Sweating palms
Apocrine	Thick, odoriferous secretion	None
Heart	Increased rate	Slowed rate
Muscle	Increased force of contraction	Decreased contractility
		(especially of atria)
Coronary vessels	Dilatation (β_2), constriction (α)	Dilatation
Lungs		
Bronchi	Dilatation	Constriction
Blood vessels	Mild constriction	? Dilatation
Gut		
Lumen	Decreased peristalsis & tone	Increased peristalsis & tone
Sphincter	Increased tone (usually)	Relaxation (most times)
Liver	Glucose release	Slight glycogen synthesis
Gallbladder, bile ducts	Relaxation	Contraction
Kidney	Decreased urine output & renin secretion	None
Bladder		
Detrusor	Relaxation (slight)	Contraction
Trigone	Contraction	Relaxation
Systemic arterioles		
Abdominal viscera	Constriction	None
Muscle	Constriction (α adrenergic)	None
	Dilatation (β_2 adrenergic)	
	Dilatation (cholinergic)	
Skin	Constriction	None
Coagulation	Increased	None
Basal metabolism	Increased (up to 100%)	None
Glucose	Increased	None
Lipids	Increased	None
Adrenal glands	Increased secretion (norepinephrine, epinephrine)	None
Brain	Increased mental activity	None
Muscles		
Piloerector	Contraction	None
Skeletal	Increased glycogenolysis	None
	Increased strength	

Modified from Guyton AC: Textbook of Medical Physiology, ed 8. Philadelphia, WB Saunders, 1991.

B. DECONTAMINATION PRINCIPLES

The decontamination recommendations provided here are based on the premise that care is occurring primarily in an operating room (OR) rather than an emergency room, the sole reason for admission to which was care of the overdose. Many patients that are seen in the OR have sustained trauma. The usual considerations for these patients still pertain (e.g., full stomach, cervical spine precautions); however, increasing numbers of trauma admissions are associated with drug intoxications and ingestion of multiple drugs, and overdose should be suspected in many of these patients.

1. Internal Bowel Decontamination

Internal decontamination refers to methods of decreasing or eliminating the toxic exposure by cleansing the gastrointestinal tract (by emesis, gastric lavage) or the blood (hemoperfusion, hemodialysis) of the toxins. Certain methods, such as giving ipecac or awake gastric lavage, may be appropriate for use at home or in the emergency ward, respectively. However, in the OR, time may not allow for awake gastric emptying and lavage before induction because of associated injuries or other reasons for operation.

a. Induced Emesis

Ipecac is mentioned only to be condemned for perianesthetic use. Although it can be used to induce emesis, the amount of drug removed from the stomach depends on the interval between ingestion of the toxin and ipecac administration. Ipecac is good for children at home if the parent can give it immediately after the ingestion; however, ipecac has no place in the OR for several reasons. First, after an hour or so, ipecac is of almost no use because much of the drug has been absorbed. Second, patients who are vomiting before induction of anesthesia are at increased risk for aspiration. Third, if the patient is vomiting when charcoal should be started, that could delay therapy. Fourth, corrosive materials and hydrocarbons may cause more harm if emesis is induced. Finally, if the patient is becoming comatose or has obtunded mental status, this is a poor time to induce vomiting, regardless of whether or not the patient is to undergo an operation.

b. Gastric Lavage

Gastric lavage has variable efficacy, depending on the interval since ingestion. If the procedure can be done within a few minutes of ingestion, a significant amount of material can be retrieved[3]; however, if several hours have elapsed since ingestion, very little material usually is returned. The other problem with lavage is that the amount, size, and configuration of material are important considerations. For example, if the material ingested becomes a solid concretion of pills that have not yet dissolved (as with iron overdose), gastric lavage does not yield much return (plain films of the abdomen can help identify this). If the material is a liquid or slurry, however, a significant amount can be returned. An advantage of gastric lavage over induced emesis is that one does not have to wait for the patient to begin vomiting. Another advantage of lavage is that the patient does not need to be awake or cooperative. A gastric tube should always be placed after intubation of any patient who presents to the OR with risk factors for intoxication. The tube should be lavaged until clear.

c. Activated Charcoal

Charcoal is probably best administered through the nasogastric tube already in place, and previously used for gastric lavage. Charcoal does not remove all toxins. Particularly, it does not absorb iron, sodium, lithium, potassium, bromide, borate, or mineral acids and alkalis. Charcoal does absorb cyanide, but it takes a large amount of material (Table 16–2).

Use of cathartics with charcoal is controversial because they promote dehydration and electrolyte disturbances. Cathartics in excessive doses may also cause the charcoal to pass through too quickly to absorb a sufficient quantity of drug; however, cathartics help to prevent charcoal from becoming stuck in the bowel (causing obstruction, the so-called charcoal briquette syndrome).[4] Additionally, cathartics can be used to purge items not easily removed with lavage (e.g., slow-release pills and tablet concretions).

d. Whole-Bowel Irrigation

Whole-bowel irrigation uses a balanced polyethylene glycol (PEG) electrolyte solution such as GoLYTELY. The result is similar to that of gut cleansing for bowel surgery. With PEG solutions there is no net fluid or electrolyte loss or gain. PEG solutions are also beneficial for purging the gastrointestinal tract of drugs that form concretions (such as iron tablets) or of slow-release tablets such as theophylline and other enteric-coated drugs. PEG

TABLE 16–2

Toxic Substances That Bind to Activated Charcoal

Acetaminophen	Dichloroethane	Nortriptyline
Acetylcysteine	Diethylaniline	Opiates
N-Acetylcysteine	Diethylene dioxide	Paraquat
Aconitine	Digitoxin	Parathion
Alcohol	Digoxin	Phencyclidine
Aminophylline	Diphenhydramine	Phenothiazine
Amitriptyline	Diphenoxylate	Phenylbutazone
Amphetamines	Disopyramide	Phenylpropanolamine
Arsenic	Doxepin	Phenytoin
Aspirin	Doxycycline	Pindolol
Atenolol	Estriol	Piroxicam
Atropine	Ethchlorvynol	Primaquine
Barbiturates	Ethylene dichloride	Propoxyphene
Belladonna alkaloids	Ethylene glycol	Pyridine
Benzene	Flecainide	Quinidine
Camphor	Glutethimide	Quinine
Carbamazepine	Imipramine	Salicylates
Carbaryl	Indomethacin	Sotalol
Carbon disulfide	Iodine	Strychnine
Carbon tetrachloride	Isoniazid	Sulfanilamide
Chloroquine	Kerosene	Tetrachlorethane
Chlorpheniramine	Malathion	Tetracycline
Chlorpromazine	Melanamic acid	Theophylline
Chlorpropamide	Meprobamate	Tilidine
Cimetidine	Mercuric chloride	Tolbutamide
Cocaine	Methotrexate	Tolfenamic acid
Colchicine	Methyl salicylate	Tricyclic antidepressants
Dapsone	Mexiletine	Trimethoprim
Desipramine	Nadolol	Valproic acid
Diazepam	Nicotine	Yohimbine

solutions are administered through a gastric tube at a rate of about 1 to 2 L per hour (for children 100 to 200 ml per hour) and are continued until the rectal effluent is clear. In the OR the patient should have a rectal tube placed to facilitate collection of rectal effluent.

2. Blood-Cleansing Techniques of Internal Decontamination

Supportive care is the guiding principle of treatment for patients who are able to breathe off, pass in the urine, or hepatically metabolize the toxic compounds. However, drugs that are not immediately metabolized to nontoxic forms by the liver, not excreted by the kidneys, or not exhaled quickly before causing injury should be removed with a blood-cleansing technique.

a. General Concepts and Definitions

Invasive blood-cleansing techniques should be considered for patients whose normal route of elimination is impaired (e.g., renal failure in a patient with lithium intoxication). Blood-cleansing techniques are also beneficial for patients who have ingested a known lethal dose of a toxin (e.g., *Amanita phalloides*) or has a measured lethal blood level of a drug (e.g., massive theophylline overdose with levels over 100 mg/L) and is very likely to suffer seizures.

For blood-cleansing systems to be beneficial, clearance of the drug by the blood-cleansing technique employed (hemoperfusion or hemodialysis) must be high and the volume of distribution low. The clearance is expressed as the number of milliliters of blood that are being cleared of the substance per unit of time. When the volume of distribution of the toxin is small, the toxin is confined mainly to the vascular space. If the poison has a large volume of distribution (several times the volume of body water), this suggests that the drug is out in the tissues and will not be removed quickly by the usual techniques of blood cleansing. Even though there may be very high clearance of a drug, if there is a very large volume of distribution the result will be minimal drug or toxin removal.

b. Hemodialysis

Hemodialysis is the procedure most frequently used to remove toxins from the blood. Dialysis requires that the patient be "instrumented" with a large-bore catheter and be "anticoagulated" during the procedure. Hemodialysis is ideal for small water-soluble drugs such as aspirin, alcohols, and other drugs that easily come across the water-based dialysate and then are removed from the body.

c. Hemoperfusion

Drugs that are larger or less water soluble or are highly protein bound are not going to move across the dialysis membrane into the dialysate, so in this case a procedure known as *hemoperfusion* should be used (Table 16–3). In hemoperfusion, the blood passes directly through a column containing charcoal, and toxins are absorbed directly by the charcoal as the blood passes through. Hemoperfusion is employed for many large drugs that are protein bound and not water soluble. Hemo-

perfusion is not a good choice for drugs that are poorly absorbed by charcoal (e.g., lithium and iron). Both hemodialysis and hemoperfusion are invasive blood-cleansing techniques that should be used only when necessary.

d. Noninvasive Blood-Cleansing Techniques

Less invasive blood-cleansing procedures are useful in some patients, including the administration of repeated doses of activated charcoal and forced diuresis with manipulation of the urine pH.

i. The Gut as a Dialysis Membrane

Repeated gut decontamination with a slurry of charcoal allows use of the gut as the dialysis membrane. This is effective for drugs (e.g., theophylline) that are bound by charcoal, have a low volume of distribution (confined to the intravascular space), and are not highly protein bound because such drugs readily cross back and forth between the gut wall capillaries and the charcoal inside the gut lumen (see Table 16–2). Although use of the gut seems less invasive, it can produce significant electrolyte and fluid problems because large amounts of charcoal, and often cathartics, are given to stimulate constant passage of the slurry. Some patients may produce 8 to 9 L of stool per day, resulting in severe electrolyte and fluid disturbances.

ii. Forced Diuresis and Urinary pH Manipulation

Digitoxin, in contrast to digoxin, has a small volume of distribution, and urinary excretion can be markedly enhanced by forced volume diuresis and pH manipulation. Unfortunately, forced diuresis is ineffective for most poisons and carries a risk of fluid imbalance. However, alkalinization of the urine by altering the pH may enhance elimination of some drugs, including salicylates and phenobarbital. These drugs are weak acids and tend to remain disassociated in the urine. In fact, urine flow needs to be increased only very little. Rather, the urinary pH needs to be alkalinized. For drug elimination to be enhanced in this way, the drug obviously needs to be one that is excreted principally in urine. Drugs like PCP and vecuronium are eliminated from the body principally via the biliary system. Only a very small percentage of

---

TABLE 16–3

Drugs That Can Be Removed by Hemoperfusion or Hemodialysis

Better Removal Procedure

Hemoperfusion	Hemodialysis
Acetaminophen	*Amanita phalloides*
N-Acetylprocainamide	(also removed well
Atropine	by hemoperfusion)
Barbiturates	Aminoglycosides
Cocaine	Arsenic
Digoxin	Aspirin
Glutethimide	Borates
Malathion	Bromide
Meprobamate	Ethanol
Methotrexate	Ethylene glycol
Muscarine	Fluoride
Paraquat	Iron
Parathion	Isoniazid (INH)
Penicillin	Isopropanol
Phenol	Lead
Phenylbutazone	Lithium
Phosphorus	Mercury
Procainamide	Methanol
Propoxyphene	Methyl salicylate
Quinidine	Penicillins
Theophylline	Potassium
Tricyclic antidepressants	

the total PCP is eliminated through the kidneys. Thus, even doubling or tripling the amount of PCP excretion in the urine would not have a significant impact on overall elimination. Elimination of some drugs, including PCP and amphetamines, is enhanced by urine acidification; however, acidification is to be avoided because this increases the potential for kidney damage as a result of rhabdomyolysis, a common problem in poisoning victims.

3. External Decontamination

External decontamination is aimed at halting secondary (downstream) contamination. Decontamination of clothing, as well as the external surface of the patient's body and hair, is an important first step for victims who are externally exposed to hazardous materials. External decontamination not only protects the patient from further injury from caustic compounds but also prevents secondary contamination of others, including health care workers.

There are two criteria for determining whether a hazardous material poses a risk for secondary contamination: the material must be both (1) acutely toxic (or have a potential for significant long-term effects) and (2) likely to be carried on the skin, hair, or clothing in quantities sufficient to cause a hazard downstream (e.g., ambulance and hospital personnel). Some agents may be toxic if inhaled from the victim's exhaled breath (e.g., the potent military neurotoxin VX). However, the vast majority of agents are not toxic in this manner (e.g., carbon monoxide exhaled by a victim dissipates into the environment without being toxic to health care workers). Liquids and solvents, especially oily and water-insoluble ones, are likely to remain on the victim's clothing and may pose a significant hazard for downstream contamination. Decontamination at the scene reduces the risk of secondary contamination. However, some chemicals remain secondary contamination hazards even after a complete water flush (among them compounds such as pesticides that are intrinsically very oily and those such as parathion that are dissolved in oily substances). Protective gear should be worn by workers who are decontaminating or managing the patient at the scene and at the hospital. The gear should cover all of the skin and clothing of the rescue worker. Occasionally, completely encapsulated suits (with self-contained breathing apparatus) are necessary, as for dealing with potent neurotoxins.

III. INHALED TOXIC GASES AND VAPORS

Sections III through V are organized according to the method of toxic exposure because discovery of the mechanism is an important first step in determining precisely what toxin is affecting the patient. Furthermore, once the particular toxin, poison, or venom type is identified, early application of specific therapy may proceed. In this regard, some drugs (e.g., cocaine, marijuana, cyanide) can enter the circulation via several routes, so its discussion under the *Inhaled* category is partly arbitrary.

A. OXYGEN TOXICITY

Although oxygen is essential for aerobic existence, in high concentrations or following administration of certain drugs oxygen becomes toxic. Oxygen toxicity can be relegated to the three major areas: precipitation of seizures, pulmonary injury, and retrolental fibroplasia.

1. Oxygen-Induced Seizures

Oxygen applied at partial pressures in excess of 2 atmospheres can result in seizures. This limits the concentration of oxygen that should be administered to patients as hyperbaric therapy for conditions other than carbon monoxide intoxication. The mechanism of seizure induction is not known but is thought to be associated with oxygen-induced decrement in the inhibitory neurotransmitter, gamma-aminobutyric acid (GABA). Indeed, GABA concentrations in the brain have been documented to decrease just before initiation of a seizure.[5] Both the concentration of brain tissue GABA and brain P_{O_2} are related to the seizure threshold. The changes in GABA concentration may be related to oxygen radical–induced decrements in sulfhydryl-containing enzymes.

2. Oxygen-Induced Pulmonary Toxicity

The partial pressure of oxygen is higher in the lungs than in any other area of the body, making the lungs the organs most vulnerable to oxygen toxicity. That pulmonary oxygen toxicity occurs is firmly established; however, the exact toxic levels in humans are not known because experimental subjects cannot ethically be exposed to toxic oxygen concentrations. Both oxygen concentration and duration of exposure appear to be important variables. Pulmonary tissue Po_2 is determined directly by the inhaled oxygen tension; thus, hypoxemia does not protect against oxygen toxicity.[6]

Reactive oxygen species are the most likely culprits in pulmonary oxygen toxicity. Molecular oxygen is a powerful oxidizing agent, and multiple reactive oxygen species occur in nature because the electrical ground state of molecular oxygen predisposes it to a univalent pathway of reduction. Oxidation-reduction reactions involved in the univalent pathway produce many highly reactive—and potentially toxic—intermediates. Superoxide, hydrogen peroxide (H_2O_2), and the hydroxyl radical are some of the best-understood toxic, reactive intermediates. Superoxide (O_2) is formed when one electron is added to molecular oxygen. Superoxide then undergoes a dismutation reaction (catalyzed by superoxide dismutase) to yield H_2O_2. The H_2O_2 formed is further reduced via either another dismutase reaction (catalyzed by catalase) or directly by glutathione (catalyzed by glutathione peroxidase) to form H_2O.[7]

In mammalian species, well over 90 per cent of respired oxygen is reduced via a series of linked electron-carrying enzymes in mitochondria, producing water without discharging harmful intermediates.[8] Some reactive oxygen species, however, are produced endogenously in mammalian systems by numerous mechanisms, including leakage from mitochondria during oxidative phosphorylation, microbial defense by phagocytic cells, and chemical reactions involving oxidant enzymes.[9–11] Important exogenous sources of reactive oxygen species are sunlight, ionizing radiation, air pollutants (i.e., nitrogen dioxide) and toxins (i.e., Paraquat).[12, 13] Normally, an elaborate array of extracellular and cytoplasmic antioxidant defense mechanisms protect the cells from oxidant injury (including catalase, superoxide dismutase, and glutathi-

one peroxidase); however, when production of toxic oxygen species exceeds clearance, cell damage can result.

Considerable evidence has accumulated that implicates oxidant-mediated injury in the pathophysiology of a great variety of pulmonary diseases and insults. For example, oxidant-mediated injury has been associated with such diverse conditions as the adult respiratory distress syndrome (ARDS),[14] pulmonary oxygen toxicity,[15, 16] endotoxic lung injury,[17, 18] emphysema, immune-complex alveolitis,[19] aspiration pneumonia,[20] interstitial lung disease,[21, 22] and ischemia-reperfusion–mediated lung injury.[23–28]

Oxygen radical activation of the arachidonic acid cascade can lead to synthesis of leukotrienes and thromboxanes, which may further mediate pulmonary leukosequestration and increase endothelial permeability.[29, 30] In addition, oxygen free radicals are thought to moderate an interleukin 2–induced rise in thromboxane B_2, increased production of H_2O_2 by neutrophils, and increased pulmonary microvascular permeability.[31] Moreover, oxygen free radicals produced by activated neutrophils entrapped in the lungs can damage the vascular barrier directly.[32, 33]

The dose-toxicity curve for humans is only approximate because it varies according to (1) barometric pressure, (2) FIO$_2$, (3) level of antioxidant exposure (i.e., to drugs like bleomycin), (4) integrity of the normal endogenous antioxidant defense system (outlined above), and (5) whether or not reperfusion is occurring after an anoxic period. Toxicity begins after 6 hours' exposure to 200 to 500 per cent oxygen (2 to 5 atmospheres), more than 12 hours' exposure to 100 per cent oxygen, more than 24 hours' exposure to 80 per cent oxygen, or more than 36 hours' exposure to 60 per cent oxygen.[34]

Symptoms of oxygen toxicity begin with substernal pain (thought to be due to irritation at the carina) that may be accompanied by coughing.[35] Symptoms continue to include severe coughing, acute lung injury, and ARDS. Care at this time is supportive: restriction of oxidizing drugs and limiting FIO$_2$. Administration of antioxidant vitamins E and C may have a role as well.

3. Retrolental Fibroplasia

Retrolental fibroplasia, also known as *retinopathy of prematurity* (ROP), occurs in premature neonates, and the incidence is inversely related to birth weight. The pathogenesis is unknown, but, in contrast to early theories blaming only oxygen concentration, the cause is now considered multifactorial. The concentration of oxygen in the atmosphere around the eye and the concentration of antioxidants (like vitamin E) may play a more important role than the inhaled oxygen tension or blood oxygen tension. Indeed, ROP occurs in premature infants who are not given oxygen supplementation, and in premature infants with cyanotic heart disease.[36] Furthermore, vitamin E supplementation decreases the incidence of ROP.[37] Thus, prophylactic intramuscular vitamin E is usually administered to premature infants until the retinal vasculature matures (around 44 to 46 weeks after conception). ROP is associated with apnea episodes until 46 weeks after conception as well.

Premature infants who require anesthesia for procedures should have the FIO_2 limited, so that the PaO_2 does not exceed 100 mm Hg. The intraarterial blood sampling site or transcutaneous oxygen sensor must be located above the ductus arteriosus, to prevent erroneous underestimation of the oxygen tension at the eyes. Vitamin E supplementation should be encouraged as well.

B. CARBON DIOXIDE ABSORBENT TOXICITY

The two absorbents in most common use are soda lime and barium hydroxide lime. The reader is referred to the texts by Dorsch and Dorsch[38] and Ehrenwerth and Eisenkraft[39] for a definitive discussion of these agents. Toxicity of carbon dioxide absorber systems has been noted in several contexts. First, there are several reports of inhalation of fine absorber dust resulting in bronchial irritation with bronchospasm.[40] These instances have been managed by supportive therapy and by redesigning absorber systems to avoid contaminating the inspiratory limb of the circle system with dust.

Carbon dioxide absorbents are known to react with volatile anesthetic agents to produce both carbon monoxide and various toxic compounds. In the first case, carbon monoxide elaboration is more common with barium than with soda absorbers, when the absorber is dry (usually when high flow rates are used), and when the absorber's temperature is elevated. Carbon monoxide production is

more common with some agents than others (desflurane more than enflurane, which is more than isoflurane, which is much more than either halothane or sevoflurane).[41] Overall, the incidence of toxicity is considered to be rather low, and only supportive care is indicated.[42]

The production of toxic compounds from the interaction of sevoflurane with absorber material is under investigation. The culprit toxin appears to be PIFE, a vinyl ether referred to as *compound A.* In rats, this compound has been shown to have a median lethal dose (LD_{50}) value of 300 ppm, with renal injury, hepatic injury, and cerebral injury at concentrations of 50, 350, and 400 ppm, respectively.[43] It is likely that the LD_{50} decreases with longer exposure. These concentrations are similar to those attainable in humans with low-flow systems. Frink found a mean concentration of 20 ppm, and a peak of 61 ppm was noted in one patient.[44] There are no data on the toxicity of compound A in humans.[45] Studies have noted that several predisposing factors increase the production of compound A, including the use of dry absorbent, the use of barium as opposed to soda lime, increased absorber heat, and higher sevoflurane concentrations. It appears that the capacity of absorbent to both generate and break down compound A may result in marked fluctuation of net output.[46] No clear syndrome of compound A toxicity has been described for humans; however, extrapolations from rat data suggest that renal toxicity should be manifested initially, and only following exposure to high concentrations.

C. TOXIC GASES ASSOCIATED WITH COMBUSTION

1. Carbon Monoxide

Carbon monoxide (CO) is an odorless, colorless, nonirritating gaseous product of incomplete combustion that typically emanates from stoves, furnaces, and automobile exhaust. In 1865, Claude Bernard accurately deduced that CO and oxygen competitively bind to the same site on hemoglobin molecules. J. S. Haldane and J. G. Priestly discovered in 1935 that CO binds to hemoglobin more than 200 times more tightly than does oxygen. When a patient is exposed to carbon monoxide at 0.1 per cent concentration for more than an hour, approximately 50 per cent of the hemoglobin becomes occupied with carboxyhemoglobin (COHb). Interestingly, patients can survive anemia of 50 per cent (i.e., a hemoglobin value 6 to 7 g/dl); however, 50 per cent carboxyhemoglobinemia is fatal to most patients (owing to neurologic and cardiac ischemia). Indeed, when CO binds to hemoglobin (Fig. 16–4) it alters the other heme-binding sites, inhibiting release of oxygen from hemoglobin peripherally (leftward shift in the oxyhemoglobin dissociation curve). Furthermore, factors other than sim-

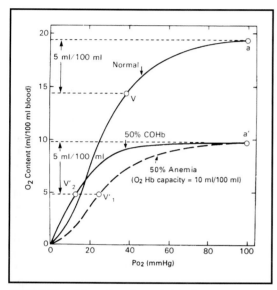

FIGURE 16–4. Normal oxyhemoglobin dissociation curve and curves for the cases of 50 per cent anemia and of 50 per cent carboxyhemoglobinemia. These figures demonstrate that the normal oxyhemoglobin dissociation curve results in an arterial oxygen content close to 20 ml per 100 ml of blood. The mixed venous oxygen content is three fourths the arterial value, normally resulting in just under 15 ml of oxygen per 100 ml of blood. In the case of 50 per cent anemia, the arterial content begins at approximately 10 ml of oxygen per 100 ml of blood. Because the patient will still consume approximately 5 ml of oxygen per 100 ml of blood, the mixed venous blood in the patient with 50 per cent anemia decreases to 5 ml of oxygen per 100 ml of blood. The P_vO_2 is approximately half of normal, or around 20 mm Hg, instead of 40 mm Hg. In contrast, with 50 per cent carboxyhemoglobin concentration, the mixed venous oxygen content (P_vO_2) will be much lower still (in the range of 10 mm Hg). Thus, there is a requirement for a far greater drop in PO_2 in order to deliver the same volume of oxygen in the case of carboxyhemoglobinemia (from point a' to point v'_2) than with a simple anemia of the same magnitude (from point a' to point v'_1). (From Bartlett D Jr: Effects of Carbon Monoxide in Human Physiologic Processes. Proceeding of the Conference on Health Effects of Air Pollution. Serial 93–15. Washington, D.C., US Government Printing Office, November 1973, pp 103–126.)

ple hypoxia contribute to carbon monoxide poisoning. CO inhibits cytochrome C oxidase and impairs metabolism at the mitochondrial level. Portions of the brain that are most sensitive to carbon monoxide injury include the higher metabolizing areas such as the basal ganglia, hippocampus, and cerebral cortex, although carbon monoxide can also cause injury to white matter portions of the brain.[47]

Clinically, symptoms are variable, depending on the quantity of inhaled CO. Intoxication can be insidious, and many patients die in their sleep. Most patients complain of headache, leading to vertigo, impaired vision, drowsiness, and coma. Mild shortness of breath and exertional dyspnea also occur. Cardiovascular manifestations include tachycardia, dysrhythmias, angina, and hypotension.

Diagnosis. Cherry-red color of the skin belies the true degree of oxyhemoglobin saturation. Similarly, pulse oximetry yields a spuriously high saturation value. Indeed, Barker and colleagues found that dogs administered CO had measured saturations greater than 90 per cent in the presence of 70 per cent COHb.[48] Furthermore, Gonzalez and coworkers corroborated the experimental dog laboratory data in a case report of human smoke inhalation victims.[49] One such patient had a COHb value of 32 per cent, pulse oximeter saturation of 96 per cent, and a cooximeter saturation of 66.1 per cent; the other had a COHb of 22.7 per cent, a pulse oximeter saturation of 99 per cent, and a cooximeter value of 77.0 per cent. Therefore, patients with smoke inhalation injuries should have both their COHb level and oxygen saturation quantified with arterial blood gas sample, using a cooximeter for measurement.

Treatment. Treatment includes immediate administration of 100 per cent oxygen and determination of COHb level. If the COHb level is above 0.5 per cent the patient will benefit from hyperbaric therapy as well. COHb levels below 20 per cent usually do not result in any neurologic impairment; however, levels greater than 30 per cent are associated with metabolic acidosis and neurologic compromise. If any neurologic symptoms arise, these patients should be treated with hyperoxia and hyperbaric therapy. CO is not a cumulative poison and, thus, is reversibly liberated in the presence of hyperoxia, especially at increased atmospheric pressures. The recovery half time, in terms of blood COHb in resting adults breathing room air at one atmosphere, is 320 minutes. When oxygen is administered, the time decreases to 80 minutes. Further reductions can occur with hyperbaric therapy with pure oxygen. Therefore, current recommendations are 2.5 to 3 atmospheres for 90 to 120 minutes with one or more treatments, followed by additional treatment, if necessary, for victims with neurologic impairment, regardless of the blood COHb level (Table 16–4).

2. Phosgene

Phosgene gas is colorless, heavier-than-air, mildly pungent, and toxic. It was used with tremendous lethality in World War I and was then retired from use as an antipersonnel agent. It is now a principal precursor in industrial synthesis and processing and a prominent breakdown product of a number of chemical compounds, including paint removers and dry-cleaning fluid.[50] The accidental release of 25 tons of methylisocyanate in Bhopal, India in 1984 resulted in the formation of phosgene and cyanide that killed several thousand people.[51] Phosgene is one of the principal lethal components of smoke in typical structure fires and is a primary concern in treating smoke inhalation victims (see section on Smoke Inhalation). The toxicity from phosgene results from its hydrolysis in the water phase of mucous membranes, producing hydrochloric acid and carbon dioxide. The slow speed of this reaction enables the agent to be breathed deeply into the respiratory tree before damage to the nasal and oral mucosa becomes apparent to the victim and

limits inhalation. Severe bronchial and pulmonary necrosis may occur as a result of hydrochloric acid damage. In addition, phosgene reacts directly with proteins, vitamins, and intermediate metabolites and results in cytotoxic and enzymatic poisoning. The full clinical picture may develop over several minutes to several days, with hemolysis, hypovolemia, hypotension, respiratory distress, and hepatic and renal damage. Anesthetic considerations include careful monitoring for evidence of toxicity during the latent period of this agent and appropriate supportive therapy after exposure.

3. Nitrogen Dioxide (Smog)

The nitrogen oxides include nitric oxide (NO), nitrous oxide (N_2O), nitrogen dioxide (NO_2), and others. The most common routes of exposure to these agents are from cigarette smoking, smog, therapeutic exposure, industrial accidents, and agricultural silos.[52] In trace amounts NO and N_2O are not toxic; however, NO_2 is extremely hazardous when inhaled. Additionally, both NO and N_2O can degrade to highly lethal NO_2. The pathologic effects of NO_2 follow exposure to mucosal water to form acids that directly damage the respiratory mucosa. In addition, NO_2 directly oxidizes lecithin in pulmonary surfactant and oxidizes unsaturated fatty acids, resulting in free radical damage and cytotoxicity. Because the nitrogen oxides are relatively insoluble in water and undergo conversion to acid slowly, they are inhaled into the lungs before their irritant effects on the nasal mucosa are noted. When high concentrations are inhaled, pulmonary edema, bronchorrhea, inflammatory constriction, and exudative bronchial necrosis may occur.[53] The clinical effects of toxicity are divided into three discrete phases in a waxing and waning pattern that can last several months. Prominent systemic effects, including hypotension (a direct effect of nitrate exposure), metabolic acidosis (both nitrous and lactic acidosis), and methemoglobinemia (from the avid binding of NO to hemoglobin), are noted. The progressive, remitting nature of this presentation is very characteristic and may present after exposure to nitrogen dioxide in a silo or in a fire.

The therapeutic use of NO as a selective pulmonary vasodilator has provoked concern over the toxic effects of the nitrogen oxides. The concentrations administered are typically

TABLE 16–4

Carboxyhemoglobin Half-Life for Various Fractional Inhaled Oxygen Concentrations and Atmospheric Pressures		
Atmospheres/ Pressure (mm Hg)	FIo$_2$	Approximate Half-Life (hr)
1 (760)	0.21	5
1 (760)	1.0	1
0.8 (600)	0.21	7
0.8 (600)	1.0	1.5
3 (2280)	1.0	0.33

From Shapiro BA, Peruzzi WT: Respiratory care. In Miller RD (ed): Anesthesia, ed 4. New York, Churchill Livingstone, 1994, p. 2432.

FIo$_2$ = Fractional inhaled oxygen concentration.

in the 10- to 80-ppm range, as compared with concentrations of 1000 ppm in inhaled cigarette smoke. By providing monitored low concentrations and flowing the gas mixture through a baralyme filter to remove NO_2, the toxic potential of therapeutic NO may be limited.[54] Additionally, the propensity of NO to convert to N_2O is limited by the avoidance of high FIo_2.

Anesthetic implications of a patient's exposure to nitrogen oxides is primarily supportive. Steroids may help limit inflammation. Bronchodilators, pressors, and supportive therapy for methemoglobinemia and acidosis are indicated.[55, 56] The long-term effects of exposure and the relapsing nature of toxicity require a high degree of vigilance for manifestations of exposure, even several months after exposure.

D. TOXIC GASES OF INDUSTRY

1. Methylbromide

Methylbromide, a hydrogenated hydrocarbon, is typically used as a fumigant gas insecticide. It is colorless and, except in high concentrations, odorless. Patients at highest risk for exposure to this toxic agent are homeless persons and burglars who crawl into homes that are being fumigated. Symptoms include pulmonary edema, hemorrhage, and pneumonitis. Early signs of methylbromide poisoning include headache, dizziness, nausea, and ataxia. Respiratory symptoms may occur 4 to 12 hours after exposure, followed by tremulousness, convulsions, and coma. Treatment is supportive and should include dimercaprol (BAL) and acetylcysteine because these agents can react with unbound methylbromide. Additionally, anticonvulsants (including barbiturates and benzodiazepines) are used to control seizures.

2. Chlorine

Chlorine poisoning occurs in industrial accidents, with swimming pool chlorinators, and when household bleach is mixed with a strong acid. Accidental injection of bleach by intravenous drug abusers has been described and has not yet been associated with any apparent clinical sequelae.[57]

Chlorine gas reacts with water to form hydrochloric and hypochlorous acids. All three compounds are toxic to skin, eyes, mucosal surfaces, and respiratory epithelium. Because chlorine gas is very water soluble, irritation manifests immediately upon contact with the nasal mucosa and attenuates further exposure by forcing the victim to escape the fumes, limiting pulmonary exposure. Most high-concentration exposures occur when the means of escape is limited. When exposure is significant, immediate irritation of the respiratory tree is manifested in coughing, bronchospasm, and chest pain. If chlorine exposure is sufficient, hyperchloremic metabolic acidosis may ensue.[58] Treatment is supportive and consists of topical irrigation of exposed skin surfaces, standard bronchodilator therapy, and corticosteroids. Severe pulmonary injury may result in pulmonary edema requiring mechanical ventilation with PEEP.[59]

A related hazard to chlorine gas is chloramine gas, which is produced by mixing bleach and ammonia.[60] Chloramine, which is poorly water soluble, is delivered to the distal airways in larger amounts than chlorine and reacts with water to produce ammonia and hypochlorous acid, resulting in pneumonitis. Presentation and management are essentially the same as for chlorine gas poisoning.

3. Cyanide

Although anesthesiologists most often encounter cyanide toxicity during nitroprusside therapy, cyanide compounds are found in many forms throughout industry, providing multiple opportunities for toxic exposure. Hydrogen cyanide (prussic acid) is used as a fumigant in cargo ships and buildings and to sterilize soils. Because of its ability to form complexes with metals, cyanide has many industrial applications, including metallurgy, electroplating, and metal cleaning.

a. Cyanide Poisoning

Cyanides are ubiquitous in nature, and many poisonings are related to ingestion of plant products. Free hydrocyanic acid is found in leaves, barks, and seeds of many plants, including apple, pear, cassava, and lima beans. Small amounts of cyanide are normally metabolized by binding endogenous thiosulfate to form thiocyanate and then are excreted via the kidneys. Konzo is a tropical neuropathy associated with ingestion of cassava beans in the absence of adequate thiosulfate. Cyanide is rapidly absorbed from the stomach, lungs, and mucosal surfaces and through unbroken skin. It inhibits mitochondrial utilization of oxygen and is bound within cells to cytochrome enzymes that contain iron.[61] Within 5 minutes of cyanide ingestion acute symptoms develop, and death may occur within 20 minutes.

b. Nitroprusside-Induced Cyanide Toxicity

Cyanide toxicity can occur in the OR or surgical ICU in patients who have received large amounts of sodium nitroprusside (in high concentrations and/or after prolonged administration). Indeed, nitroprusside contains 44 per cent cyanide by weight on a molar basis. Cyanide toxicity can occur when more than 2 μg/kg per minute of nitroprusside is used. The first sign of cyanide toxicity in critically ill patients may be increased mixed venous saturation with bright red venous blood (secondary to inability to utilize oxygen peripherally) and concurrent lactic acidosis. Symptoms in nonanesthetized patients include headache, faintness, vertigo, seizures, and coma. Respiratory symptoms include dyspnea and a burning sensation in the throat and mouth. Cyanosis may be absent in the early stages of poisoning; however, as cyanide toxicity progresses and respiration is depressed, cyanosis develops. Patients may also manifest weakness leading to paralysis. Cardiovascular signs include dysrhythmias and hypotension. Additionally the patient's exhaled breath may smell like almonds.

c. Treatment of Cyanide Toxicity

The acute treatment of cyanide toxicity typically includes administration of commercially prepared cyanide antidote (sodium thiosulfate and sodium nitrite); however, oxygen administration is a critical first consideration to anyone diagnosed with cyanide toxicity and can enhance specific treatment as well.[62] The goal of specific therapy is to draw the intracellular cyanide back into the circulation where it can be detoxified and excreted. Cyanide antidote kits contain both amyl nitrite ampules and sodium nitrite for the production of methemoglobinemia. Methemoglobin produced by either of these nitrites binds free cyanide as cyanmethemoglobin. An empiric recipe for amyl nitrite therapy includes inhalation from an ampule for 30 seconds of

each minute using a new ampule every 3 minutes. This produces a methemoglobin concentration around 5 per cent in the average 70-kg adult. In addition, sodium nitrite can be administered intravenously to produce methemoglobin in higher concentrations; however, intravenous nitrite dosage must be calculated carefully to minimize overdose, which can result in toxic levels of methemoglobin. Methemoglobin itself can cause dyspnea, acidosis, seizures, coma, and dysrhythmias. Other drugs that cause methemoglobinemia are listed in Table 16–5.

Additionally, sodium thiosulfate may be administered, producing thiocyanate molecules (via the naturally occurring enzyme rhodanase). Thiocyanate is excreted in the kidneys; however, thiocyanate is itself toxic when produced in supranormal amounts, causing tinnitus, miosis, hyperreflexia, and impaired iodine uptake, among other problems. Thiocyanate excretion can be enhanced with urinary pH manipulation and is easily removed with dialysis. In Germany, thiosulfate is administered along with nitroprusside to avoid toxicity.[63] After administering oxygen and ordering a cyanide toxicity kit for the patient, the physician should call a poison control center for additional specific therapy recommendations.

E. WAR GASES AND PERSONAL PROTECTION SPRAYS

1. Vesicant Agents (Mustard Gas, Lewisite)

The vesicant gases include mustard gas, lewisite, and mustard variants. Mustard gas is presented here because of its current storage and recent use in the Gulf War.

Nitrogen mustard is an oily, yellowish liquid that is vaporized by heat and dispersed by wind currents. Effects are limited to tissue (as opposed to clothing) and blistering may be delayed for hours. The mucosal irritant effects are immediately apparent; respiratory symptoms occur primarily in victims who cannot escape the fumes. No antidote is available, although it is known that the application of warm, moist bandages enhances toxicity.

Sulfur mustard, an alkylating drug, was first synthesized in 1854; however, the vesicant properties were first recognized and employed on a large scale during World War I. Between the world wars, much of the infor-

TABLE 16–5

Agents That Cause Methemoglobinemia

Aminophenones	Nitrobenzene
4-Aminopropiophenone	Occupational hazards
Aniline and derivatives	Aniline
Antimalarials	Chloroaniline
Chloroquine	Dichloroaniline
Primaquine	Dinitrobenzene
Cetrimide	Nitrobenzene
Chlorates	4-Nitrobenzonitrile
Cocaine (adulterated with	Nitrochlorobenzene
benzocaine)	Nitrotoluidine
Copper sulfate	Orthotoluidine
Dapsone	Paratoluidine
4-Dimethylaminophenol	Para-aminosalicylic acid (PAS)
Exhaust fumes (diesel)	Phenacetin
Flutamide	Phenazopyridine
Herbicides (some)	Resorcinol
Hydroxylamine	Smoke inhalation (enclosed-space
Local and topical anesthetics	fires)
Benzocaine	Sodium beta-naphthol disulfonate
Prilocaine	(R salt)
Methylene blue (clinically insignificant)	Sulfonamides
Metoclopramide	
Naphthalene	
Nitrites/nitrates	
Amyl nitrite (inhalation, ingestion)	
Bismuth subnitrate	
Butyl nitrite (inhalation abuse)	
Carrots/spinach (infants)	
Industrial nitrate salts	
Nitroglycerin	
Nitrite/nitrate medications	
Contaminated nitrous oxide	
anesthesia canisters	
Isobutyl nitrite (inhalation abuse)	
Nitrate-contaminated well water	
Nitrite/nitrate meat preservatives	
Silver nitrate (burn therapy)	
Sodium nitrite	

Modified from Hall AH: Systemic asphyxiants. *In* Rippe JM, Irwin RS, Fink MP, Cerra FB (eds): Intensive Care Medicine, ed 3. Boston, Little, Brown, 1996.

mation on nitrogen mustards was classified; however, since then, some of these agents have proved to be effective (yet toxic) chemotherapeutic drugs (see Section VI). Mustard agent dropped on the Kurdish village of Halabja in 1992 killed 5000 unprotected people.[64]

Lewisite is a vesicant that contains arsenic. Pain immediately follows exposure, and even brief contact results in deep ulceration. British antilewisite (BAL or dimercaprol) was developed as an antidote to lewisite exposure when applied as an ointment. Intramuscular BAL has also been used to manage systemic absorption of lewisite.[65] Severe exposure results in hemolysis and hypotension consistent with severe burn injuries. Pulmonary injuries are possible, although the severe pain associ-

ated with exposure provides adequate warning to allow escape from the fumes or donning of mask gear before significant injury occurs. These and other vesicant agents are reviewed further elsewhere.[66]

2. Lacrimators (Tear Gas, Pepper Spray, Mace)

Lacrimators—widely used for crowd control and for personal defense—include such commercial preparations as tear gas, pepper spray, mace, and vomiting gas. There are approximately 60 different chemicals and proprietary compounds in this class, although the three most common ones are chloroacetophenone (CN), chlorobenzylidine malononitrile (CS), and dibenzoxapine (CR).[67] Tear gases are not truly gases at all but rather fine particulates or aerosols that are dispersed via smoke or spray canisters. These agents are noted for their tendency to disperse far enough to cause collateral injury to the deployer. Failing adequate external decontamination of victims, medical personnel may be secondarily overcome by these agents. External decontamination involves cutting away clothing and irrigating affected areas in a well-ventilated area.

Lacrimators are divided into several classes principally according to chemical structure. Their mode of action includes intense chemical irritation of the cornea that typically lasts 30 minutes. Some expulsion vehicles are capable of producing high projection velocities and of embedding the agent in the corneal surface. In these cases, chronic damage with corneal opacification may result. Salivation and throat pain frequently occur. Tachycardia and hypertension may occur in response to pain. Pulmonary symptoms include coughing and chest tightness immediately after exposure. Bronchospasm is common when exposure occurs in a closed space, but responds to usual bronchodilator therapy. Bronchorrhea may be seen. Rarely, pulmonary edema presents between 3 and 24 hours after exposure. Most significant injuries are noted with chloroacetophenone, and there are reports of deaths after exposure to high concentrations. Chlorobenzylidene malononitrile, the agent most often used, has never been associated with a death, even after high-concentration exposures. Occasionally, manufacturers of personal defense products add 1 per cent capsicum oleoresin (chili oil) to the lacrimating agent. Capsicum produces immediate burning on contact with mucous membranes but is not otherwise considered toxic. Tear agents are also sometimes included in pesticide preparations to warn of impending exposure to more toxic substances.[68]

Management begins with application of oxygen, assurance of an airway and adequate ventilation, and establishing a barrier between rescue worker and patient (e.g., gloves, etc.). Next, the patient is decontaminated by removing saturated clothing and irrigating exposed surfaces. Treatment then focuses on bronchodilator therapy and further monitoring of pulmonary status. Contact lenses should be removed and corneas irrigated with sterile pH-balanced saline solution. Immediate ophthalmologic evaluation is imper-

ative. Anesthetic considerations are limited to the management of bronchospasm and other pulmonary sequelae.

3. Nerve Agents

A wide variety of gases and vapors have been used as antipersonnel material, principally during World War I. Phosgene and chlorine gas, which accounted for 80 and 10 per cent of gas-related fatalities, respectively, during World War I, are reviewed in preceding sections. More potent agents subsequently synthesized by the Nazi government before World War II included nerve agents such as tabun (GA), sarin (GB), soman (GD), and VX. All of these agents are currently in production or storage for use. These nerve agents are vapors that have toxic effects similar to those of the organophosphate insecticides but far more potent. These agents have been banned from modern warfare, although, as recently as 1988, traces of nerve agents have been isolated from Kurdish villages in northern Iraq. The potency of these agents is impressive: a single drop of certain agents, properly aerosolized, is capable of killing thousands of people by skin contact alone. The "G" agents have high vapor pressures that facilitate their use as highly toxic and volatile organophosphates, whereas the oily nature of VX makes it a persistent agent that is used much as a mine field is—to deny the enemy use of terrain.

These nerve agents may be absorbed by inhalation or by absorption through the skin; death occurs in minutes to hours. Therapy begins with strict limitation of exposure of health care personnel to the contaminating agent. Supportive care of flaccid paralysis with occult seizures and respiratory arrest must proceed concomitantly with the administration of acetylcholine-blocking agents. Therapy with up to 2000 mg of atropine has been documented.[69] Benzodiazepines may be useful to abort seizures. Oxime agents may be used to unbind acetylcholinesterase from the nerve agent. Oximes are usually effective only over a relatively brief time after exposure, after which the enzyme is irreversibly bound. Pralidoxime is the agent most often used in this context. The toxicity due to acetylcholinesterase inhibition is more fully developed in the section on organophosphate insecticides (the most common civilian source of exposure to this type of drug).

Pretreatment protocols exist that involve the use of carbamates (e.g., pyridostigmine) to bind acetylcholinesterase and thus deny a pool of enzyme to the nerve agent. After the acute exposure to the nerve agent, the enzyme is slowly unbound from the carbamate to permit effective activity. Because nerve agents bind acetylcholinesterase irreversibly, toxic exposures are additive until enzyme is regenerated. Long-term effects not explained solely by the acute effects of these agents include memory loss, concentration deficits, and hallucinations. An excellent review of these agents is available for further study.[70, 71]

F. INHALED DRUGS OF ABUSE

1. Solvents (Gasoline, Cleaning Solvents, Glue, Freon)

A variety of solvents are abused by inhalation in the quest for a quick, inexpensive, euphoric effect. While each of these agents could be considered individually, they are rarely encountered by the anesthesiologist, except in the context of abuse. Industrial accidents and combustion (i.e., smoke inhalation) are the two other common sources of exposure to these agents. As always, when an exposure is suspected, identification of the agent involved is a logical starting point. A certified regional poison control center has the resources to identify specific exposures.

Solvent abuse is limited primarily to the adolescent, predominantly male, population. Substances may be sniffed directly from a tank or container (e.g., gasoline), inhaled from a bag (e.g., adhesives), or insufflated through a cloth held to the nose, also known as "huffing" (e.g., dry cleaning fluid). Commercially available solvents are usually a mixture of several toxic compounds in addition to chemical adulterants. The chemical composition of commonly abused solvents is reviewed in Table 16–6.[72]

The physiologic effects of these agents vary, although a feature of particular interest to anesthesiologists is the potential of the agent to sensitize the myocardium to catecholamines. A classic scenario involves a parent discovering an adolescent son abusing an agent, startling the abuser, followed by the abuser's collapse in sudden cardiac arrest from an acute cardiac dysrhythmia.[73] Myocardial sensitization has been described with gasoline, chlorinated hydrocarbons (includ-

TABLE 16–6

Chemical Composition of Abused Solvents

Inhaled Agent	Toxic Chemical
Aerosol	Fluorocarbons
Dry cleaning fluid	Methylene chloride
	Trichloroethylene
	Carbon tetrachloride
Dyes	Acetone
	Methylene chloride
Gasoline	Petroleum distillates
	Benzene
Glues	Toluene, benzene, xylene
	Acetone
	Trichloroethylene
	Trichloroethane
Lighter fluid	Butane
Liquid typewriter "white-out"	Trichloroethane
Nail polish remover	Acetone, amyl acetate

Modified from Graham DR: Solvent abuse. *In* Haddad LM, Winchester JF (eds): Clinical Management of Poisoning and Drug Overdose, ed 2. Philadelphia, WB Saunders, 1990, pp 1256–1259.

ing carbon tetrachloride, trichloroethylene, and trichloroethane), and freon aerosols. It is not clear how long after sniffing solvents the myocardium remains sensitized, although if the material can be smelled on the patient's breath, in hair, or on clothes, a significant amount may still be present in the body. Means of detection include smelling the agent, looking for a characteristic rash about the nose and mouth ("glue sniffer's rash"), witnessing evidence of acute intoxication (slurred speech, drunken appearance), and detecting the presence of solvent metabolites in the urine (Table 16–7).[74] Anesthetic considerations include limiting the use of agents or circumstances that could further potentiate cardiac dysrhythmias. The patient should be

TABLE 16–7

Detectable Metabolites of Solvents

Solvent	Metabolite
Benzene	Phenol
Toluene	Hippuric acid
Trichloroethylene	Trichloroacetic acid
	Trichloroethanol
Xylene	Methylhippuric acid

Modified from Graham DR: Solvent abuse. *In* Haddad LM, Winchester JF (eds): Clinical Management of Poisoning and Drug Overdose, ed 2. Philadelphia, WB Saunders, 1990, pp 1256–1259.

monitored by ECG throughout the acute course of intoxication. Care should be taken to avoid stimulating or startling the patient. Anesthetic drugs that potentiate myocardial irritability should be avoided, including halothane, cocaine, and ketamine. Hypercarbia, pain, and other indirect sympathetic stimulants should be avoided.

2. Tetrahydrocannabinol

Marijuana is the most prevalent illegal drug in the United States. More than half of all high school seniors who graduated in 1985 had used marijuana. The principal psychoactive ingredient of marijuana and hashish is tetrahydrocannabinol (THC). A marijuana cigarette weighs approximately 0.5 to 1 g and contains between 1 and 3 per cent THC, for a total dose of 5 to 30 mg per cigarette.[75, 76] More concentrated forms of THC such as hash or hash oil can be smoked or baked into cookies, producing larger doses of the drug overall. The effects of marijuana may be divided into low-dose and high-dose effects. Low-dose effects include euphoria, relaxation, and a mild alteration of time and space perception. At higher doses agitation and anxiety seem to predominate. The latter effects are more often noted following oral ingestion of the drug, whereas smoking may be more readily titrated to an overall lower dose level. Side effects of THC include mild tachycardia, increased appetite, a moderate antiemetic effect, bronchodilatation, and conjunctival hyperemia. The use of THC medicinally for bronchodilatation in asthmatics and to decrease ocular hypertension in glaucoma tends to be overshadowed by its psychotropic effects. THC is available commercially as an antiemetic for chemotherapy patients, although specific comparisons of the efficacy of THC versus other antiemetics (e.g., ondansetron) are lacking.

Aside from the psychotropic effects of this agent, chronic pulmonary effects of marijuana smoking are prominent: the toxicity profile is similar to that of cigarette smoking. THC may be combined with other agents, notably PCP ("dipped joints"), alcohol, and various "designer drugs." The use of PCP may produce a profound analgesic and psychotic state. The effects of other combinations have not been fully described. The contamination of marijuana with Paraquat, a potent pesticide, is occurring with less frequency over time but is still described (see section on Paraquat). Overall, anesthetic considerations for the patient exposed to marijuana include assessing the chronic user for chronic lung disease.[77] Acute anxiety reactions may signal a high-dose exposure or mixing of multiple agents. There are no known drug interactions between THC and any anesthetic agent.

3. Cocaine

Cocaine is a drug that has been used and abused since antiquity. Indeed, the Spanish conquistadors discovered that the native Peruvians had developed a vast Incan civilization with many rituals and customs intertwined with the cultivation, harvesting, and chewing of leaves from the plant *Erythroxylon coca*. Chewing the coca leaves was known then, as it is now, to increase stamina and decrease pain. The Inca witch doctors are thought to have used cocaine as an anesthetic by chewing the cocoa leaves and dribbling saliva onto the scalp during trephination. The local anesthetic effects were formally introduced to the medical community for the first time in 1884 by the Viennese ophthalmologist, Carl Koller.

In the 1970s cocaine hydrochloride became available, and in 1982 crack cocaine spawned an epidemic of drug abuse. In 1986, cocaine became the number one cause of emergency room visits for illicit drug abuse. A recent study demonstrated that 57 per cent of violent assault victims and 22 per cent of automobile victims presenting to a Philadelphia trauma center had a urine or blood test positive for cocaine or its metabolites.[78] Currently, in New York City, 18 per cent of motor vehicle accident victims test positive for cocaine.[79]

Cocaine can enter the circulation via inhalation (snorting), intravenously, or inhaled as with crack cocaine. Inhaled crack cocaine is so addicting because it bypasses the liver and travels immediately to the left side of the heart and to the brain following inhalation.

Cocaine has a number of useful clinical effects: it is a local anesthetic, and because of potent vasoconstrictive properties is frequently used by anesthesiologists for topicalization before fiberoptic bronchoscopy. Furthermore, cocaine has more rapid onset and longer action than lidocaine; however, some anesthesiologists refrain from administering cocaine because of its side effects. Cocaine blocks reuptake of catecholamines, both centrally (norepinephrine, dopamine, serotonin) and peripherally (norepinephrine and epinephrine). Cocaine is also an NMDA agonist. Cocaine causes release of the catecholamines norepinephrine and epinephrine and serves as a false neurotransmitter (especially in high concentrations). Cocaine causes direct central nervous system (CNS) stimulation through release of the excitatory amino acids glutamate and aspartate. Additionally, cocaine blocks the sodium channel on CNS neurons and in the cardiac conducting system. These effects are similar to its local anesthetic effects on the sodium channel blockade of peripheral nerves. All of these factors lead to proarrhythmic effects for the drug. Additionally, cocaine can increase platelet aggregation and atherogenesis.

The clinical toxicity of cocaine is related chiefly to CNS hyperactivity and the subsequent seizures, hypertension, tachycardia, and vasospasm. Severe toxicity is seen in almost every organ. In the eyes and brain, manifestations include blindness, infarction, hemorrhage, and seizures. In the chest, pneumothorax and pulmonary infarctions have been reported, as have cardiac dysrhythmias and infarctions, due to both vasospasm and increased myocardial oxygen demand (tachycardia and hypertension). Aortic dissections have also been associated with cocaine intoxication. Additionally, dilated cardiomyopathy, probably secondary to repeated microinfarcts, has been reported, as have ischemic injuries to other organs (including kidneys and liver). The lethality of cocaine is related to the hyperdynamic cardiovascular effects and to the hypermetabolic factors (high fevers, seizures, metabolic acidosis).

The best therapeutic option is treatment with a GABA antagonist drug such as diazepam or midazolam. Beta-adrenergic blockade for hypertension and tachycardia is useful for hemodynamic control; however, beta blockade does not control the propensity for seizures, fever, or metabolic acidosis. Treatment with pancuronium has been shown to diminish fever and the physical manifestations of seizures and acidosis, but death still occurs because very strong electrical seizures can still continue uninterrupted despite absence of overt physical manifestations. Uncontrolled electrical seizures result in brain damage as metabolic activity far exceeds the nutrient supply (especially in oxygen-sensitive neurons). Treatment of cocaine intoxication with benzodiazepine has proven to protect against both seizures and death. The critical element of therapy for cocaine toxicity includes treatment with a GABA antagonist (diazepam or midazolam), control of adrenergic symptoms with additional beta blockade, and active cooling with an ice bath.

Anesthesiologists who care for patients known to have substance abuse problems should be suspicious of patients' administering their own "premedication" via many routes. Indeed, a recent case report in *Anesthesiology* detailed illicit cocaine administration during a spinal anesthetic for a talus fracture.[80] The patient became acutely disruptive and agitated, despite having received 12 mg of midazolam. She required emergent intubation for control of her symptoms. The patient was later found to have placed several "crack rocks" in her nose and mouth before receiving her anesthetic.

When anesthetizing patients with a history of cocaine abuse, anesthesiologists must be vigilant for several intraoperative problems. These patients will have a relatively decreased minimum alveolar concentration (MAC) if they have abstained for a long time preoperatively and an absolutely increased MAC if acutely intoxicated. Other important points about cocaine intoxication and anesthesia are that a history of prolonged succinylcholine effect or a known low dibucaine number is associated with increased susceptibility to the toxicity of cocaine.[81] Because cocaine is hydrolyzed by plasma cholinesterase, patients who have a cholinesterase deficiency are more prone to toxicity from cocaine. Additionally, organophosphates (commonly used in insecticides) can heighten euphoria and prolong cocaine effects.[82] Information from the Flemming article has filtered to the street, as evidenced by a recent report in *Anesthesiology* detailing the use of organophosphate insecticide as an inexpensive way of heightening the "high" of crack cocaine and prolonging its effect.[83] Patients suspected of cocaine intoxication who exhibit concomitant organophosphate symptoms should be treated for the organophosphate intoxication as well as the cocaine. Additionally, patients with a known low dibucaine number or known decreased plasma cholinesterase will have a prolonged succinylcholine effect and increased cocaine toxicity. Furthermore, indirect-acting pressors (such as ephedrine) do not work well in acutely intoxicated or recently intoxicated cocaine addicts.

IV. TOXIC INGESTIONS (POISONING)

A. MEDICATIONS ASSOCIATED WITH OVERDOSE AND TOXICITY (see Table 16–13, p. 625)

1. Acetaminophen

Acetaminophen poisoning is a major source of acute hepatic failure. Although early symptoms may be nonexistent, the delayed manifestations of acetaminophin toxicity are devastating. After a few hours, a patient may complain of anorexia, nausea, vomiting, and diaphoresis. During the first 24 hours, the patient may show no CNS depression unless other drugs were taken concurrently. Because codeine and acetaminophen are frequently packaged together, any patient suspected of codeine overdose should have an acetaminophen level sent immediately. The classic clinical scenario involves a patient who presents to the emergency department comatose, with miotic pupils and shallow respirations and who responds to naloxone (Narcan) and recovers. She wakes up and admits to having taken an overdose of pain pills (codeine). She is discharged to the psychiatric ward and 3 days later returns obtunded and jaundiced because the "pain pills" contained acetaminophen (Tylenol) with codeine. The absence of early toxic symptoms is why acetaminophen overdose may go undiagnosed during the critical early period when N-acetylcysteine therapy is efficacious. Whenever acetaminophen overdose is suspected, a specific drug level should be sent and therapy started.

During the (acute phase of) acetaminophen overdose, blood concentration is elevated and specific therapy with N-acetylcysteine is necessary. In the next 24 to 48 hours plasma acetaminophen levels drop but hepatic necrosis begins. Patients may complain of right upper quadrant pain and become jaundiced on the second or third day following acetaminophen intoxication.

The acute treatment involves removal of any unabsorbed acetaminophen tablets by gastric emptying procedures, including lavage. Additionally, immediately following suspicion of acetaminophen toxicity, N-acetylcysteine therapy should begin by mouth or via nasogastric tube and continued until specific blood levels return. If the measured blood acetaminophen levels are above a specific time-related value (Fig. 16–5), administration of N-acetylcysteine should continue at 4-hour intervals. Enteral dosing of N-acetylcysteine begins with 140 mg/kg, followed by 70 mg/kg every 4 hours for 17 doses. If the first acetaminophen levels are extremely high (greater than 200 mg/dL), hemoperfusion should be instituted to help rid the blood of acetaminophen before seizures occur and to decrease the likelihood of hepatotoxicity.

2. Aspirin

Salicylic acid was first isolated in 1838 from bark of the willow tree *Salix alba*; however it took 60 years for aspirin to be used clinically.[84] Aspirin (salicylate) overdose remains one the most commonly reported poisonings. The classic presenting symptoms of salicylate intoxication include rapid deep respirations, confusion, and coma. With very high salicylate concentrations seizures occur. The skin is diaphoretic, and the patient may have a fever and be dehydrated. The arterial blood gas shows combined metabolic acidosis and respiratory alkalosis that is far greater than respiratory compensation for the metabolic acidosis would dictate. The acidemia of salicylate intoxication is thought to be due to a combination of inhibition of hepatic lactate metabolism and uncoupling of oxidative phosphorylation. The vomiting, sweating, and dehydration lead to electrolyte imbalances.

Treatment. Treatment includes gastric emptying and lavage, fluid replacement with physiologic solutions such as lactated Ringer's, and appropriate electrolyte repletion. Potassium, chloride, and magnesium supplementation is usually required owing to the loss of these electrolytes from vomiting. Alkalinization of the urine is important because salicylic acid (a weak acid) stays in the ionized (nonreabsorbable) state. Alkalinization of urine becomes increasingly important as salicylate levels increase and normal metabolic pathways become saturated. Repeated doses of charcoal further enhance salicylate removal to a greater degree than forced alkaline diuresis alone.[85] Hemodialysis and hemoperfusion are both effective in removing salicylate from the circulation, although hemodialysis has been used more.[86] These invasive treatments are generally reserved for situations where CNS toxicity or cardiovascular collapse are imminent.

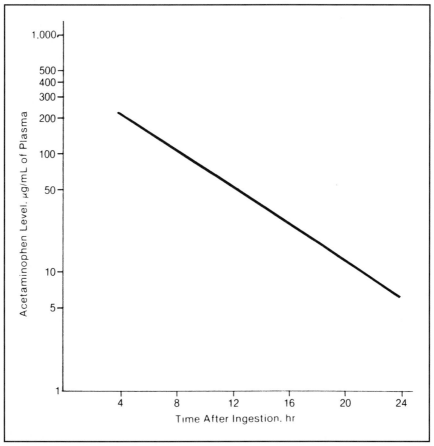

FIGURE 16–5. Semi-logarithmic plot of plasma acetaminophen levels over time. The area above the line indicates probable hepatic toxicity; the area below the line, no hepatic toxicity. (Adapted from Rumack BH, Peterson RC, Coch GG, et al: Acetaminophen overdose: 662 cases with evaluation of oral acetylcysteine. Arch Intern Med 141:380–385, 1981.)

3. Antihistamines

Antihistamines are frequently taken as over-the-counter preparations for colds, pruritus, nasal congestion, or allergic rhinitis. Symptoms of antihistamine overdose include anticholinergic effects (mydriasis, xerostomia, tachycardia, fever) and CNS effects (confusion, hallucinations, delirium, seizures). Treatment begins with gastric emptying and lavage, followed by administration of physostigmine and treatment of associated cardiac dysrhythmias.

4. Digoxin

Symptoms of digoxin intoxication include drowsiness, headache, weakness, tremor, nausea, and vomiting. However, the most important effects are cardiovascular, particularly cardiac dysrhythmias. Bradycardia, various degrees of heart block, and atrioventricular node dissociation are common. Additionally, digoxin has been found to lower the threshold for bupivacaine toxicity in the cardiac and central nervous systems of rats.[87] Thus bupivacaine epidurals are relatively contraindicated for digoxin-intoxicated patients. Because many patients with digoxin toxicity are also taking diuretics, hypokalemia and hypomagnesemia are commonly associated problems. Digoxin toxicity is exacerbated by hypokalemia (premature ventricular contractions, atrial tachydysrhythmias) and hyperkalemia (heart block, asystole). Thus, serum potassium should be repleted to 4.5 mEq/L. Magnesium has rhythm-stabilizing properties (partially involving its role as a cofactor for the sodium-potassium-ATPase pump). Intravenous magnesium, 1 to 2 g, should be administered empirically to all patients with digoxin toxicity, except for those with renal failure or documented hypermagnesemia.[88] Magnesium sulfate is particularly useful for treating ventricular ectopy in the setting of hypokalemia and hypomagnesemia. Magnesium may also be used to treat cardiac dysrhythmia due to digoxin toxicity in the presence of normal or elevated serum magnesium.[89] Specific antidysrhythmia therapy is otherwise focused on the particular dysrhythmia.

Specific therapy to decrease the serum digoxin level begins with gastric emptying followed by activated charcoal; however, most cases of digoxin toxicity seen in the OR occur in patients who have undergone long-term therapy, with or without an acute increase in digoxin level. Digoxin-specific Fab antibody fragments are the definitive treatment for hemodynamically significant cardiac dysrhythmias due to digoxin toxicity.[90] Monitoring of therapeutic response is accomplished by following clinical improvement. This is because the measured serum digoxin level rises following antibody administration (as the assay fails to distinguish between free digoxin and Fab-bound digoxin); however, without clinical improvement, in patients in whom the precise digoxin level is critical, free serum digoxin levels may be obtained via a rapid ultrafiltration assay.[91]

Magnesium is known to suppress early after depolarizations and in supraphysiologic doses may act as an indirect antagonist of digoxin at the sarcolemmal sodium-potassium-ATPase pump. Intravenous magnesium may be used to treat cardiac arrhythmias due to digoxin poisoning when there is likely to be a delay in the availability of digoxin antibodies, even in the presence of elevated serum magnesium.[92]

5. Lithium

Lithium is a common medication for bipolar disorders. It is handled in the body in a manner similar to sodium, but it also competes with other positively charged ions. Lithium displaces these other ions from both intracellular active sites in the following (descending) order: sodium, potassium, magnesium, and calcium.[93] The effects of these ionic interactions in nerve and cardiac tissues are responsible for the toxic complications most important to anesthesiologists.[94]

Lithium-induced neurotoxicity begins with a fine tremor and progresses to spastic dystonia. Mental toxicity ranges from mania to stupor and coma. Unfortunately, some severe cases of intoxication have led to permanent neurologic sequelae.[95] Cardiac manifestations due to lithium include hypotension, dysrhythmias, and circulatory collapse. Dysrhythmias include ST depression, and T-wave inversion in leads V_4 to V_6, premature atrial contractions, and conduction blockade.[96]

Lithium can cause goiter and hypothyroidism.[97] Thus, some patients may be taking Synthroid as well as other drugs that can potentiate the toxicity due to lithium. Combined lithium and tricyclic antidepressant therapy may lead to cardiac toxicity manifested as dysrhythmias.[98]

Lithium is capable of influencing many aspects of hematopoiesis, especially granulocyte formation. The trophic effect of lithium on granulocyte production has led to its use to counteract the granulocyte-suppressing effect of zidovudine (AZT), which is used to suppress virus growth in acquired immunodeficiency syndrome (AIDS).[99]

Because lithium is eliminated from the body almost exclusively via the kidneys, any intervention that alters glomerular filtration rate or electrolyte exchange in the nephrons can affect elimination of lithium. Osmotic and loop diuretics improve lithium clearance and should be used to treat lithium toxicity.[100] In contrast, thiazide diuretics decrease the clearance of lithium and are associated with increased toxicity. Potassium-sparing agents have variable minor effects. Hemodialysis remains the cornerstone of treatment for acute lithium toxicity in patients in renal failure or life-threatening dysrhythmias.[101] Because lithium is removed only slowly from the intracellular compartment, rebound lithium toxicity may follow dialysis. Continuous arteriovenous or venovenous hemodialysis may be superior in this regard.

6. Theophylline

Theophylline and other methylxanthine preparations have a very low therapeutic index. Thus, it is not unusual to see toxicity (including neurologic symptoms and cardiac dysrhythmias) in patients treated with these drugs. Indeed, the first sign of toxicity in adults may be seizures.[102] Symptoms typically begin with nausea and vomiting. The patient may become restless and agitated and eventually obtunded and comatose. Seizures are common with theophylline toxicity. Cardiac dysrhythmias include atrial fibrillation, multifocal PVCs, and ventricular tachycardia. Treatment begins with gastric emptying and saline lavage, followed by activated charcoal. The mainstay of therapy is supportive care. Seizures are controlled with benzodiazepines, and the cardiac effects are attenuated by decreasing sympathetic tone with opiates and beta-adrenergic blockade. For severe toxicity (especially in patients with liver disease or congestive heart failure) hemoperfusion is recommended.

A classic presentation is a teenager with a history of asthma. She denies a drug overdose but is rather uncooperative. She has mild hypertension, significant tachycardia, and rapid breathing. She is tremulous and increasingly restless and soon begins vomiting and has a seizure. She has an elevated glucose value and markedly decreased serum potassium. (Normally, the metabolic acidosis promotes hyperkalemia.)

Tachycardia and seizures, combined with a history of asthma, implicates theophylline toxicity, but when seizures are encountered other possibilities are tricyclic antidepressants, isoniazid, and CNS stimulants like amphetamines and cocaine. Cocaine is the first or second most common drug to cause seizures, depending on the emergency room's location. If the patient lives in or near a farming community, seizures related to organophosphates and other pesticides must be considered.

Hypokalemia, metabolic acidosis, vomiting, tremulousness, tachycardia, and mild hypertension in the setting of an asthma patient with access to theophylline are very characteristic of theophylline overdose, especially with potassium in the very low range (1.8 to 2.0 mEq/L). Intractable seizures occur when the theophylline level is 100 mg/L. Immediate hemoperfusion is necessary to remove the toxic stimulant, but benzodiazepines are also essential for putting the patient's brain to sleep and halting the seizure (as with cocaine intoxication). With slow-release theophylline preparations, the toxic effects can be delayed or can escalate; thus, gastrointestinal washout is important here.

7. Tricyclic Antidepressants

TCAs are one of the more common drugs of overdose. The major toxic manifestations important to anesthesiologists involve the neurologic and cardiovascular systems. The "five Cs" of TCA toxicity can be summarized as abnormalities of conduction, anticholinergic, contractility, convulsions, and coma.

In tricyclic overdose conduction and anticholinergic abnormalities are common. The ECG frequently shows tachycardia due to anticholinergic effects, with a wide QRS complex (conduction blockade). The QRS may continue to widen and develop bundle branch block that may look like ventricular tachycardia.[103] Tricyclics predictably cause significant widening of the QRS complex whenever enough drug is taken to cause coma or seizures. A patient who is thought to have TCAs but does not have a widened QRS probably does not have significant intoxication at that time.

Contractility may be decreased somewhat by TCA overdose due to decreased calcium influx and direct myocardial depression. However, recent studies have deemphasized this aspect. Indeed, alpha-agonist–predominant pressors such as phenylephrine and norepinephrine tend to be most efficacious in supporting the blood pressure for TCA-intoxicated patients.[104]

Some of the newer antidepressant medications like fluoxetine do not have any effect on the ECG but can cause seizures. The newer antidepressant amoxapine (Ascenden) has no effect on the ECG yet is very neurotoxic, causing seizures and coma in the absence of QRS widening. Coloville, amitriptyline, nortriptyline, and doxepin all cause significant QRS widening when there is significant intoxication. In the setting of seizures the physician should always think of TCA overdose and look at the ECG for evidence of QRS widening.

Treatment for TCA overdose begins with airway support for depressed mental status, seizures, or coma. Benzodiazepine or phenytoin and serum alkalinization are used to control seizures. Phentyoin has both antidysrhythmic (specifically improves conduction defects) and anticonvulsant properties, making it an excellent choice for TCA toxicity. Type 1 antidysrhythmics (procainamide, quinidine) are contraindicated in TCA-intoxicated patients, as these drugs cause further conduction abnormalities through a similar mechanism. Despite the refractoriness of the ventricular dysrhythmias associated with TCA overdose, prolonged vigorous resuscitation can have a favorable outcome. Alkalinization of serum pH increases protein binding, reducing the potential for toxicity because less free drug is available, and is an acceptable strategy.[105] Additionally, gastric lavage with charcoal is useful to remove residual TCA tablet residue.

B. NONINFECTIOUS FOOD POISONING

1. Poisonous Plants

The plant kingdom is replete with chemical constituents that are very toxic to humans. Plants have been used both as poisons and medicines since history has been recorded. Some toxins disrupt the oxidative phosphorylation system (e.g., cyanide), inhibit protein synthesis (castor beans, mushrooms), or have antimitotic effects (colchicine). The vast majority of these toxins are derived from alkaloids that have anticholinergic, neuromuscular blocking, neuron transmission blockade, and cardiovascular effects.

a. Anticholinergic Alkaloids

Plants and drugs with anticholinergic properties are ubiquitous in nature. The typical presentation of anticholinergic intoxication includes dilated pupils, dry, flushed skin, tachycardia, mild fever, and CNS symptoms (confusion, ataxia, seizures, coma). A mnemonic for anticholinergic toxicity follows:

Blind as a bat (ciliary muscle paralysis)
Dry as a bone (anhydrosis)
Red as a beet (peripheral vasodilatation)
Fast as a fiddle (tachycardia)
Hot as Hades (hyperthermia)
Mad as a hatter (delirium, coma)

Additional antimuscarinic effects include urine retention, constipation, and decreased bowel sounds. Drugs and plants that cause anticholinergic syndromes are listed in Table 16–8.

Treatment of anticholinergic intoxication is mainly supportive, provided no other toxic drugs or compounds are involved. For example, pancuronium has anticholinergic effects at muscarinic receptors (causing the syndrome described above) but also at nicotinic receptors (leading to neuromuscular blockade). First priority is provision of the ABCs: airway, breathing, and circulation. Next, there is a quick search for the agent that caused the anticholinergic syndrome. Specific antidote therapy involves administration of physostigmine (Antilerium), an anticholinesterase inhibitor, in 1-mg aliquots for adults.

b. Curare and Other Plant-Derived Neuromuscular Blocking Drugs

Curare, the arrow poison used by certain South American tribes, is a powerful neuromuscular blocking drug.[106] The first accounts of curare were written shortly after the voyage of Columbus, by Peter Martyer in his compendium *De Orbo Novo*.[107] Curare is obtained from tropical species of *Strychnos* and *Chondrodendron*. Toxins produced by other plants may produce neuromuscular blockade when ingested, including anatoxin A produced by blue-green algae (*Anabena flos-aquae*) that bloom in farm ponds enriched with fertilizer. Methyllycaconitine, an alkaloid produced by tall larkspur (*Delphinium barbeyi*), has been known to poison livestock in western pastures via a neuromuscular blockade mechanism. Treatment for poisoning with these drugs is supportive, with tracheal intubation and mechanical ventilation for severe toxicity. Neostigmine and physostigmine can be helpful as well.

c. Ergot Poisoning and Lysergic Acid Diethylamide

Ergot poisoning can affect humans and livestock that have ingested rye contaminated by the ergot fungus *Claviceps purpurea*. Poisoning due to this fungus was known in the middle ages as "St. Anthony's fire," owing to the charred and blackened appearance of the victims' extremities. The predominant symptom of acute ergot poisoning is hypertension secondary to the intense vasoconstriction. Later, gangrene of the extremities occurs.[108] Anesthesiologists use ergot alkaloids most often for treating post-partum hemorrhage. Methylergonovine maleate (Methergine) is an ergot amine alkaloid that stimulates uterine and vascular smooth muscle contraction. The usual dose of methylergonovine maleate is 0.2 mg intramuscularly every 2 to 4 hours (not to exceed five doses per 24 hours). Methylergonovine maleate can be administered intravenously, intramuscularly, or by mouth; however, side effects are more frequent and more pronounced when administered IV. The side effects include dizziness, headache, tinnitus, diaphoresis, seizures, hemorrhagic stroke,

TABLE 16–8

Drugs That Cause Anticholinergic Syndrome*

Pharmaceuticals		Plants
Antihistamines **(H¹-blockers)** Brompheniramine Carbinoxamine Chlorpheniramine Clemastine Cyclizine Cyproheptadine Dimenhydrinate Diphenhydramine Hydroxyzine Meclizine Promethazine Pyrilamine Tripelennamine **Anti-Parkinson's** **drugs** Benztropine Biperiden Ethopropazine Procyclidine Trihexyphenidyl **Antipsychotics** Acetophenazine Chlorpromazine Chlorprothixene Fluphenazine Haloperidol Loxapine Molindone Perphenazine Prochlorperazine Thioridazine Thiothixene Trifluoperazine	**Antispasmodics** Anisotropine Clidinium Dicyclomine Isometheptene Methantheline Propantheline Stramonium Tridihexethyl **Belladonna alkaloids and** **related synthetic congeners** Atropine (racemic hyoscyamine) Glycopyrrolate Hyoscine Ipatropium Methscopolamine Scopolamine **Cyclic antidepressants** Amitriptyline Amoxapine Desipiramine Doxepin Imipramine Maprotiline Nortriptyline Protriptyline Trimipramine Zimelidine **Muscle relaxants** Cyclobenzaprine Orphenadrine **Mydriatics** Cyclopentolate Homatropine Tropicamide	Angel's trumpet *Brugmansia arborea* Angel's trumpet *Brugmansia suaveolens* Bittersweet *Solanum dulcamara* Black henbane *Hyoscyamus niger* Black nightshade *Solanum nigrum* Day-blooming jessamine *Cestrum diurnum* Deadly nightshade *Atropa belladonna* Downy thornapple *Datura metel* Fly agaric *Amanita muscaria* Ground cherry *Physalis heterophylla* Jerusalem cherry *Solanum pseudocapsicum* Jimson weed *Datura stramonium* Matrimony vine *Lycium halimifolium* Night-blooming jessamine *Cestrum nocturnum* Nutmeg *Myristica fragrans* Panther mushroom *Amanita pantheria* Potato *Solanum tuberosum* Wild sage *Lantana camara* Wild tomato *Solanum carolinensis* Willow-leaved jessamine *Cestrum parqui*

*Many of these agents have significant toxic effects in addition to their anticholinergic action.
Modified from Ferm RP: Anticholinergic poisoning. *In* Rippe JM, Irwin RS, Fink MP, Cerra FB (eds): Intensive Care Medicine, ed 3. Boston, Little, Brown, 1996.

palpitations, chest pain, dyspnea, hypertension, nausea and vomiting, diarrhea, thrombophlebitis, hematuria, and extremity ischemia (which can lead to gangrene if doses are large enough). Because of the serious cardiovascular effects (chiefly hypertension) ergots should not be administered routinely to hypertensive or preeclamptic patients.

Lysergic acid diethylamide (LSD) is structurally similar to ergonovine and occurs naturally in ergot fungus and in the seeds of the morning glory plant (*Rivea cormbosa*), but most of the LSD consumed as a "recreational drug" is synthesized by reacting lysergic acid with diethylamine. The toxic effects of LSD include hallucinations and centrally mediated autonomic hyperreactivity (hypertension, tachycardia, mild fever, mydriasis, piloerection). The hallucinogenic effects of LSD are mediated by 5-hydroxytryptamine (5-HT) receptor.[109] LSD is rarely lethal, and patients are most often seen by the anesthesiologist after a traumatic event. Treatment of LSD toxicity is mainly supportive, and severe agitation with hallucinations may be controlled with haloperidol.

d. Hemlock (*Conium maculatum*)

Hemlock is a potentially lethal biennial herb of the parsley family that contains many alkaloids (including coniine) that cause anti-cholinergic and neuromuscular blocking effects. Hemlock is a poison that was well-known to the ancient Greeks. Indeed, Socrates was ordered to drink a "cup of hemlock," calculated to be the correct amount. Hemlock poisoning can result from ingestion of wild fowl that have eaten hemlock buds.[110]

Hemlock toxicity includes trembling and weakness of the extremities (nondepolarizing neuromuscular blockade), dilated pupils, and vomiting. Other biphasic nicotinic effects include tachycardia, followed by bradycardia, atrial fibrillation, and death.[111] When death follows hemlock poisoning, it is usually secondary to respiratory failure (largely mediated by neuromuscular blockade).[112] Neuromuscular effects may be accompanied by rhabdomyolysis, myoglobinuria, and acute tubular necrosis (due to myoglobin and actin toxicity at the renal tubule cells). Plasma-exchange transfusions have been found successful in improving the signs of rhabdomyolysis and renal failure following hemlock poisoning.

e. Mescaline

Mescaline is the active phenethylamine alkaloid derived from the peyote cactus. Mescaline use was much a part of the rituals of the native peoples of Mexico and South America.[113] When the Spaniards arrived, they soon began to use the peyote as well. Mescaline was first synthesized in 1918, but native peoples still use the dried peyote buttons, which contain about 6 per cent mescaline (45 mg). Peyote buttons are round tubercles with yellow-white tufts at the apex that grow on the spineless peyote cactus. The buttons are sliced off and, when dried, are hard, brown discs. A mescaline dose of 5 mg/kg (5 to 10 buttons) produces hallucinations in most people. Approximately 30 minutes after ingestion of the buttons, nausea and vomiting occur. Shortly thereafter, diaphoresis, mydriasis, mild tachycardia and hypertension, nystagmus, ataxia, and muscle fasciculations occur. Sensory changes (including visual hallucinations) but a fairly clear sensorium predominate. There is cross-tolerance between most of the hallucinogens, including mescaline, LSD, and psilocybin, which all act at the serotonin (5-HT) receptor. Death is rare, but trauma due to hallucinatory effects is not uncommon. Respiratory depression can accompany massive mescaline overdose, but treatment is generally supportive, and severe agitation with hallucinations may be controlled with haloperidol.

f. Mushrooms

Mushrooms may be one of the most ancient ways of producing inebriation, along with alcohol. Indeed, there is evidence that a sophisticated mushroom cult existed in Guatemala as long as 3500 years ago, and the Spanish conquistadors described mushroom use in Aztec rituals. More than 20 different mushroom varieties were probably used. Several varieties of mushrooms are toxic. Precise identification of poisonous and edible mushrooms is difficult, even for experienced examiners who have detailed knowledge. Typical initial toxic symptoms from mushroom poisoning include nausea, vomiting, and diarrhea. When these symptoms arise more than 6 hours after ingestion, the mushrooms are predictably highly toxic. The specific toxicity of mushroom depends on their group.

i. Cyclopeptide Group

Poisoning with this group occurs from a cyclopeptide α-amanitin toxin and phalloidin toxin. Mushrooms in this group include *Amanita phalloides* (appropriately called "death cap"), *Amanita ocreata* (the equally lethal "death angel"), and others (*Amanita verna* and *Amanita vivosa*). Ingesting one of these mushrooms produces severe diarrhea in the first 6 to 12 hours (mainly because of the phalloidin toxin). Hepatic toxicity and acute fulminant hepatic failure begin in the next 24 to 36 hours, owing to the α-amanitin toxin, which binds to hepatic RNA polymerase II, inhibiting protein synthesis.[114] Initial treatment includes gastric emptying and lavage with activated charcoal, provided diagnosis is made in the first 6 hours after ingestion.

ii. Ibotenic Group

The ibotenic group of mushrooms are those that contain the poison ibotenic acid (an excitatory amino acid). This group includes the mushrooms *A muscaria* (fly agaric, nicknamed for its toxicity to flies) and *A pantharina*. These ibotenics typically produce an inebriated appearance associated with anxiety, hallucinations, seizures, and coma. Patients also manifest anticholinergic symptoms (mydriasis, dry, flushed skin, xerostomia). Anticholinergic symptoms can be treated with physostigmine.

iii. Coprine Group

Coprine mushrooms contain a disulfiram-like chemical. The clinical effects begin within 15 minutes of ingestion and are exacerbated by alcohol.

iv. Muscarine Group

Wild mushroom gathering is so dangerous because (1) many mushrooms look alike and (2) some of the nomenclature is confusing. To wit: muscarine mushrooms are those that contain the alkaloid muscarine. *A. muscaria* contains only trace amounts of muscarine (the chemical for which they were named), and most of its toxicity is due to ibotenic acid.[115] However, mushrooms of the genera *Inocybe* and *Clitocybe* (e.g., *Inocybe sororia* and *Clitocybe dealbata*) contain large quantities of muscarine. Consumption of these mushrooms causes symptoms including salivation, lacrimation, perspiration, diarrhea, bronchospasm. Atropine effectively treats symptoms.

v. Psilocybin Group

Psilocybin mushrooms (*Psilocybe* species) were very popular in the 1960s and early 1970s for their hallucinogenic properties, and they are still used by survivors of the sixties. Psilocybin mushrooms can cause nausea, vomiting, and neurologic symptoms, including hallucinations and seizures. The hallucinogenic effects of psilocybin are due to serotonin-receptor binding (just like those of LSD and mescaline). Benzodiazepines should be used for control of seizures, when present, and Haldol is used for toxic psychotic reactions.

vi. Monomethyl Group

Patients who consume mushrooms of the monomethyl hydrazine group can develop hepatic failure, and occasionally methemoglobinemia. The treatment for mushroom poisoning from this group is pyridoxine.

g. Strychnine

Strychnine, an alcohol derived from the seeds of the Asian tree *Strychnos nux-vomica,* selectively blocks inhibitory neurons in the CNS, resulting in hyperexcitability. It also blocks glycine (an inhibitory neurotransmitter) at the postsynaptic receptors of motor neurons in the spinal cord, causing muscle spasms. Strychnine is frequently mixed with cocaine and heroin by drug dealers to "cut" the drugs and increase their profits. Colorless, and usually odorless, strychnine tastes slightly bitter. Toxicity occurs within 10 to 30 minutes after ingestion, leading to seizures (frequently triggered by minor stimuli such as loud voices or touching). Other manifestations include opisthotonos, risus sardonicus, and severe muscle spasms. Additionally, metabolic acidosis, hypoxia, hyperthermia, rhabdomyolysis, myoglobinuria, and renal failure occur. Treatment is mainly supportive, including airway ventilation and seizure control. Benzodiazepines and barbiturates are used to control seizures and may be given by infusion.

2. Ingested Marine Animal-Derived Toxins: Pelagic Poisoning

Pelagic poisoning is a term coined by Mills and Passamore to describe the toxicity of three agents—fugu (puffer fish), ciguatera, and paralytic shellfish—because these entities cannot be distinguished from one another on the basis of clinical findings.[116] Indeed, the tetrodotoxin (of puffer fish), ciguatoxin (of ciguatera organisms), and saxitoxin (of paralytic shellfish) are produced by the various dinoflagellates that are eaten by the shellfish and by the prey of the puffer fish and carnivorous fish species harboring ciguatera. Furthermore, all three of these toxins affect the sodium channels of nerve tissue (Fig. 16–6).

Toxins formed by microorganisms are transferred from the dinoflagellates to herbivorous species (e.g., fish, invertebrates) and then to carnivorous fish via the marine food chain.[117] Such toxins are distinct from inorganic chemicals or infectious agents that can contaminate seafoods. Clinical manifestations begin with a gastrointestinal prodrome and headache, followed by sensorimotor deficits. Bulbar and cognitive changes are associated with the more lethal tetrodotoxin, saxitoxin,

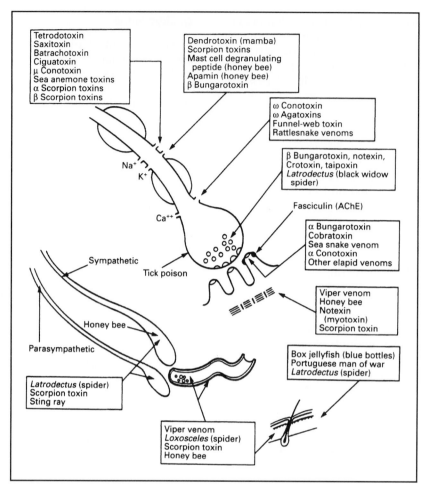

FIGURE 16-6. Principal sites of action of animal toxins. This figure illustrates the site(s) of action for most of the animal-derived toxins detailed in this chapter. The center of the diagram depicts a prejunctional portion of nerve with various ion channels (Na⁺, K⁺, Ca⁺⁺) and continues on to the neuromuscular junction. Both prejunctional and postjunctional components are shown, as well as skeletal muscle. Below the central figure are sympathetic and parasympathetic nerves. A blood vessel is also shown (with cellular elements inside) and a sample of skin. Arrows emanating from the boxed words point to the elements chiefly affected by the various toxins. (From Karalliede L: Animal toxins. Br J Anaesth 74:319–327, 1995. With permission of the British Publishing Group.)

and domoic acid toxin. Tetrodotoxin and saxitoxin block sodium channels; ciguatoxin opens them. Domoic acid stimulates excitatory amino acids at the N-methyl-D-aspartate (NMDA) receptors.[118]

a. Fugu Poisoning

Fugu, also known as blowfish or puffer fish, has been considered a delicacy in Japan for over 2000 years; however, it must be properly cleaned, as the intestines, liver, and ovaries contain tetrodotoxin. Tetrodotoxin causes weakness, paralysis, and death by asphyxiation. On April 29, 1996, three cases of tetrodo-

toxin poisoning occurred among chefs in California who shared contaminated fugu brought from Japan by a coworker as a prepackaged, ready-to-eat product. Although the quantity eaten by each person was minimal, symptoms occurred within 15 minutes. Only one person could still speak when the paramedics arrived (San Diego Union-Tribune, May 5, 1996).[119] Although there is no antitoxin for tetrodotoxin, therapy includes intubation, mechanical ventilation, and supportive care. Additionally, pumping the stomach of patients who eat tetrodotoxin can help diminish toxicity.

Tetrodotoxin is one of the most potent

known nonprotein toxins. Tetrodotoxin blocks the conduction of action potential in nerves without altering the resting membrane potential. Tetrodotoxin displaces thiamine phosphate and occupies its site of action inside the nerve membrane, blocking conduction of action potentials and preventing the increased sodium conduction necessary for depolarization. Cranial nerves are affected first; with larger doses motor nerves are blocked, leading to skeletal muscle weakness and ultimately paralysis and respiratory failure.[120] Tetrodotoxin has local anesthetic potency about 100,000 times that of cocaine.

b. Ciguatera

The word *ciguatera* was probably first used to describe poisoning caused by ingestion of the marine snail *Livona pica* ("cigua"), a staple seafood of the Caribbean. However, the term *ciguatera* is now employed to describe the syndrome of the illness contracted by persons who have eaten tropical and semitropical finfish harboring the ciguatoxin. Ciguatera fish poisoning results from the bioconcentration of a variety of toxins produced by marine dinoflagellates. Signs and symptoms vary much, but the syndrome usually presents as gastrointestinal and neurologic complaints (including paresthesias, paradoxical warm-cold discrimination, weakness, and coma) and bradycardia beginning shortly after ingestion of fish that contain the toxins. Although the degree of neurologic toxicity does not correlate with the amount of toxic fish consumed, the degree of bradycardia does.[121] Because mild symptoms may persist for months or even years, some permanent injury may occur. Poisoning involves ingestion of large carnivorous fish. The first North American epidemic of 25 cases of ciguatera fish poisoning occurred in Southern California with fish caught off the coast of Baja California, Mexico, but even domestic farm-bred fish can harbor the toxin, as can sharks and other species.[122, 123] Indeed, recently more than 500 people (98 of whom died) were poisoned by the flesh of a shark (*Carcharhinus amboinensis*) off the east coast of Madagascar.[124] Although the mechanism is not clear, treatment with mannitol relieves symptoms.[125] Additionally, recent studies show that in rats lidocaine can reverse or block electrophysiologic disturbances due to ciguatoxin.[126]

c. Paralytic Shellfish Poisoning

Paralytic shellfish poisoning (PSP) is caused by a saxitoxin produced by the various dinoflagellates that are filtered out of the water by shellfish. A variety of clams and mussels ingest the dinoflagellates that produce the saxitoxin.[127] During certain summer months in California the mussels that live in the tidal pools become toxic after a bloom of the culprit dinoflagellates (red tide). Some weeks later, the mussels are edible again.

The anesthetic implications for all of these pelagic poisonings are the same: support the airway and cardiovascular system. Most patients with severe poisoning require intubation. Their stomachs should be emptied and charcoal irrigation administered. There is currently no specific antidote.

C. INSECTICIDES

1. Anticholinesterase Drugs

Acetylcholinesterase (AChE) is the enzyme that cleaves the ester bond of acetylcholine (ACh), producing acetate and choline. All synaptic sites that utilize ACh as the neurotransmitter (including all neuromuscular junctions) are richly endowed with the superefficient enzyme AChE. Typically, AChE hydrolyzes ACh in less than a half millisecond. It is critical that ACh be hydrolyzed almost immediately after elaboration, so that rapid repolarization of the postsynaptic membrane occurs.

When AChE is inhibited, ACh has a prolonged effect at all cholinergic sites and, owing to their widespread distribution, produces a massive cholinergic effect. The toxicity of drugs that inhibit AChE prompted the utilization of these drugs as agricultural insecticides and chemical warfare agents (see Section III-E-3). Drugs that inhibit AChE are called *anticholinesterases* (anti-ChE). The first well-known anti-ChE is physostigmine, an alkaloid derived from the calabar bean, a native perennial plant of tropical West Africa. The calabar bean, also called *Esere nut* (thus the alternate name for physostigmine, *eserine*), was used by native tribes as an "ordeal poison" in trials of witchcraft.[128]

a. Organophosphates (Irreversible Anticholinesterases)

Organophosphate poisoning can occur secondary to ingestion of common insecticides, including parathion, malathion, and diazanon. These toxins are absorbed readily through the skin and respiratory and gastrointestinal tracts and can cause severe poisoning. Acute symptoms are related to the accumulation of free ACh at all cholinergic nerve endings owing to the irreversible inhibition of anti-ChE (Table 16–9). Stimulation at muscarinic nerve endings causes salivation, lacrimation, urinary and fecal incontinence, diaphoresis, and miosis. Nicotinic effects include muscle weakness, paralysis and muscle fasciculations, tachycardia, and hypertension (due to sympathetic ganglia stimulation), followed by hypotension. The CNS effects of organophosphates include a combination of muscarinic and nicotinic effects—restlessness, seizures, respiratory depression, and coma.

Treatment of organophosphate toxicity is chiefly supportive care, with gastric emptying and gastric lavage. Muscarinic (cholinergic) symptoms can be treated with atropine. Pralidoxime is a specific additional antidote that can be used to regenerate the AChE that is permanently inhibited by the organophosphate toxicity. When AChE is phosphorylated (as it is with organophosphate toxicity) the enzyme loses its efficacy and regenerates only very slowly. It was discovered that oximes (especially pralidoxime) help regenerate the enzyme.[129] Indications for pralidoxime treatment include muscle weakness, fasciculations, and respiratory failure.

b. Carbamates (Reversible Anticholinesterases)

Carbamates (aldicarb, carbaryl, isocarb, and propoxur) are commonly found in insecticides. Symptoms of carbamate poisoning are cholinergic effects, including constricted pupils, copious salivation and bronchial secretions, vomiting, diarrhea, and sweating. Treatment includes removing unabsorbed carbamate from the stomach using gastric-emptying techniques and lavage. The cholinergic symptoms can be treated with atropine.

The mechanism behind carbamate toxicity is similar to that of organophosphate poisoning. The difference is that carbamates bind

---

TABLE 16–9

Pharmacologic Effects of Cholinesterase Inhibition and Receptor Type

Site	Effects
Muscarinic (increased stimulation)	
Pupils	Miosis (constriction)
Ciliary body	Blurred vision
Exocrine glands	Increased secretions
Lacrimal	Tearing
Salivary	Salivation
Respiratory	Bronchorrhea, rhinorrhea
Heart	Bradycardia
Smooth muscle	Contraction
Bronchial	Bronchoconstriction
Gastrointestinal	Nausea, vomiting, abdominal cramps
Anal sphincter	Relaxation → diarrhea
Bladder muscle	Increased tone (frequency, urgency)
Urinary sphincter	Relaxation → incontinence
Sphincter of Oddi	Contraction → pancreatitis
CNS	Variable
Nicotinic (stimulation, then depression)	
Skeletal muscle	Weakness, cramps, fasciculation, paralysis
Sympathetic ganglia	Tachycardia, hypertension; then hypotension
CNS	Variable symptoms from anxiety and restlessness to confusion, obtundation, coma, and seizures*

CNS = central nervous system.
* Relative contribution of nicotinic and muscarinic receptors to CNS effects unclear. Modified from: Jackson JE, Aaron CK: Cholinergic Agents. In Intensive Care Medicine, ed 3. Edited by James M. Rippe, Richard S. Irwin, Mitchell P. Fink, Frank B. Cerra. Little, Brown and Company, Boston, 1996.

less tightly to cholinesterase and, so, have a shorter duration of action and are slightly less toxic. Carbamates are considered reversible cholinesterase inhibitors. Additionally, carbamates are more selective for insects. Atropine is used for carbamate treatment, and pralidoxime is rarely necessary.

2. Chlorinated Hydrocarbon Insecticides

Chlorinated hydrocarbon insecticides are used in industry and at home and include DDT, lindane, chlordane, aldrin, mirex, and paradichlorobenzene. The toxicity of these compounds varies considerably, but all can be absorbed through the skin and respiratory and gastrointestinal tracts. Symptoms include nausea, vomiting, salivation, and abdominal pain. CNS effects include restlessness, irritability, convulsions, and muscle spasms. If the poison was ingested, gastric emptying and lavage should be performed.

3. Paraquat

Paraquat is an extremely toxic insecticide. Ingestion is followed by burning pain in the mouth and throat, nausea and vomiting, and bloody diarrhea. Later, the patient develops liver failure, renal failure, and severe, irreversible ARDS. Treatment includes gastric emptying and lavage with fuller's earth rather than with activated charcoal (which binds Paraquat poorly). Fluids and electrolytes should be monitored closely, and patients invariably require ventilatory support. Supplemental oxygen should be kept to a minimum as hyperoxia exacerbates pulmonary toxicity (through oxygen-derived free radical mechanisms). Early hemodialysis or hemoperfusion is recommended to prevent the devastating effects of Paraquat poisoning.

D. ORGANIC SOLVENTS AND HYDROCARBONS

1. Alcohols

a. Ethyl Alcohol (Ethanol)

Ethyl alcohol is the intoxicating ingredient in distilled spirits, beer, and wine. Alcohol intoxication is one of the most common forms of drug overdose. Alcohol is frequently encountered in trauma victims and thus is a drug familiar to most anesthesiologists. Any patient who presents to the OR following trauma should have an orogastric or nasogastric tube placed and the stomach emptied. If the patient is profoundly intoxicated before induction, a significant amount of absorption has already occurred, but there could be still more alcohol (or other drugs) in the stomach, and gastric lavage may be warranted. Acute care is mainly supportive, with control of acid-base and electrolyte disturbances.

If the patient is a chronic alcoholic, treatment should also focus on magnesium, potassium, and phosphate replacement and the need for multivitamins, folate, and thiamine. Such patients may have hypoglycemia owing to impaired gluconeogenesis and because of an increased $NADH/NAD^+$ ratio.[130] When chronically starved alcoholics receive glucose for the first time after a long period of subsisting only on hard liquor for calories, several complications can occur. First, they may develop an acute hypophosphate syndrome that can be associated with rhabdomyolysis and neurologic dysfunction. This is because the first step in glucose metabolism involves transformation of glucose to glucose-6-phosphate, thus further depleting the patient's already low phosphate reserves. Second, thiamine is used in the metabolism of glucose and chronic alcoholics typically take in very little. Providing fluids containing glucose to an alcoholic patient without first giving thiamine can trigger Wernicke's encephalopathy. The postoperative focus should be on attenuating symptoms of alcohol withdrawal with prophylactic benzodiazepine administration, avoiding delirium tremens or seizures.

The pathophysiology of ethanol withdrawal is related to stimulation at the GABA receptors. Benzodiazepine is a specific inhibitor of GABA and is thus an excellent treatment, both prophylactically and for delirium tremens. Patients with no history of alcohol withdrawal–related seizures can be treated with benzodiazepines on an individualized "as needed" regimen with efficacy equal to that of a standard fixed schedule.[131]

b. Ethylene Glycol

Ethylene glycol is the active ingredient in antifreeze. Alcoholics have been known to drink large quantities. The lethal dose for a 70-kg adult is around 110 ml of 100 per cent ethylene glycol; however, survivors who drank larger quantities have been documented.[132] Ethylene glycol itself causes little toxicity except "ethanol-like" intoxication, but the metabolic products are very toxic. Ethylene glycol is metabolized via alcohol dehydrogenase to glycoaldehyde, and then by aldehyde dehydrogenase to glycolic acid, and finally by lactate dehydrogenase or glycolic acid dehydrogenase to glyoxylate. Glycoaldehyde and glycolic acid are the most toxic of these metabolites, but most of the damage is done by glyoxylate because it is the only metabolite that accumulates in sufficient concentrations.[133] The anion gap metabolic acidosis seen with ethylene glycol intoxication is due chiefly to glycolic acid and the increased $NADH/NAD^+$ ratio. Pathologic findings include cerebral edema, focal nerve loss, and direct injury to kidneys, lungs, liver, heart, muscles, and retinas.[134]

Treatment, which should commence immediately, consists of airway and circulatory support followed by gastric emptying and lavage and administration of ethyl alcohol (ethanol) to block metabolism of ethylene glycol to the toxic glycolic acid. Hemodialysis should be used for severe toxicity, to remove ethylene glycol and its toxic products.[135]

c. Isopropyl Alcohol (Isopropanol)

Isopropyl alcohol is used as a solvent and disinfectant, in rubbing alcohols, aftershave lotions, and antifreeze. Isopropyl alcohol is two to three times more potent than ethanol as a CNS depressant. Isopropyl alcohol is metabolized chiefly to acetone, which is excreted in the urine. Poisoning symptoms include nausea, vomiting, dizziness, confusion, and occasionally seizures. Very large doses may lead to myocardial depression and hypotension. Treatment includes removal of yet unabsorbed isopropyl alcohol with gastric lavage. Hemodialysis removes isopropyl alcohol and its metabolite acetone and is indicated for very large–dose intoxications.

d. Methyl Alcohol (Methanol)

Several solvents, antifreeze, windshield-washing solutions, and nail polish removers contain methyl alcohol. Methanol is absorbed easily from the gastrointestinal tract. Small amounts may be absorbed through the lungs and skin. Methanol itself is not very toxic, but it is metabolized in the liver by alcohol dehydrogenase to the toxic products of formic acid and formaldehyde. Symptoms of methanol toxicity include nausea, vomiting, abdominal pain, CNS depression, dilated pupils, and optic nerve inflammation (which can lead to blindness). Metabolic acidosis may be severe owing to the formic acid and formaldehyde produced.

Treatment should commence within 2 hours and includes gastric emptying and lavage and administration of ethanol (as for ethylene glycol intoxication) to block metabolism of methanol to its toxic metabolites. Additionally, sodium bicarbonate should be administered to correct existing metabolic acidosis, and hyperventilation is instituted to blow off carbon dioxide. Hemodialysis may be required for severe toxicity, to remove methanol and its toxic products.

2. Alcohol-Free Distilled Hydrocarbons

a. Petroleum-Based Distilled Hydrocarbons

Children are most often poisoned with petroleum-based distilled hydrocarbons (gasoline, kerosene, naphthaline, mineral oils, charcoal lighter fluid). These products are relatively nontoxic while in the gastrointestinal tract, but if aspirated they cause extreme pulmonary toxicity. Therefore, aspiration pneumonia must be avoided if at all possible. Treatment is mainly observation. Removal of the stomach contents is not necessary for small quantities, as long as no other toxic chemical such as a pesticide has been swallowed. If the patient is conscious and cooperative, a nasogastric tube and gastric emptying should precede induction of anesthesia. If toxic chemicals have been ingested gastric emptying is always necessary. If the patient is already comatose or extremely uncooperative, the trachea should be intubated initially with a rapid-sequence technique, after which gastric lavage is performed immediately.

b. Nonpetroleum Distilled Hydrocarbons

Nonpetroleum distilled hydrocarbons (including xylene, toluene, turpentine, benzene) have significant systemic manifestations when ingested in the gastrointestinal tract. Symptoms include nausea, abdominal discomfort, CNS depression, cardiac dysrhythmias, and liver and kidney failure. Treatment includes gastric emptying and lavage to limit systemic absorption, and toxic manifestations of systemic illness are treated by maintaining supportive care. (See also section III-F.)

E. HEAVY METALS

1. Antimony

Antimony is a metalloid that has been used in folk medicine as "tartar emetic" (antimony potassium tartrate). The chemical symbol for antimony, Sb, is derived from *stibium,* the Latin name for stibnite, the name for antimony before the Middle Ages.

Most modern cases of antimony poisoning occur in industrial settings. Antimony is frequently alloyed with lead, providing increased strength and rigidity over lead alone. This application is widely used in the battery industry: inhaling the fumes of overheated batteries can be harmful. Tossing used automobile batteries into hot campfires can yield a toxic smoke containing lead and antimony vapor, which can be lethal. Additionally, antimony is still used in medicinal compounds (i.e., sodium stibogluconate) used to treat parasite infections.[136]

Symptoms of antimony overdose include both acute and chronic cardiac dysfunction. Acutely, the antimony poisoning causes mainly cardiopulmonary dysfunction. ECG demonstrates T-wave changes, QT prolongation, and occasionally sudden death. When antimony exposure occurs via inhalation, upper respiratory symptoms occur. Chronic exposure to antimony can cause cardiomyopathy.[137]

Treatment is mainly supportive, along with removal from toxic exposure, avoidance of other insults that might lead to ventricular fibrillation (i.e., high-catecholamine states), and probably intravenous magnesium, 1 to 2 g, as in other QT prolongation syndromes.

2. Arsenic

Organic arsenic (typically found in the environment) is the least toxic form; however, arsenic of nonorganic sources can be very toxic. Examples include arsenic trioxide found in some pesticides, defoliants, and wood preservatives. Ore-processing and smelting procedures can cause production of arsenic gas (an extremely toxic form of arsenic). Arsenic gas exposure rapidly produces severe hemolysis, anemia, and, subsequently, renal failure. Initially, gastrointestinal symptoms—dysphagia, nausea, diarrhea—occur. Cardiovascular effects include shock, cyanosis, myocardial irritability, and cardiomyopathy. CNS effects include seizures and delirium. Treatment includes removing the patient from the arsenic gas exposure and providing supportive care. Blood-exchange transfusions and hemodialysis for renal failure may eventually be necessary. In the rare case of acute arsenic intoxication from ingestion of a large amount, gastric emptying should be followed by lavage. Fluid replacement is important, and chelation therapy with BAL, followed by D-penicillamine, is useful.

3. Iron

The candylike coatings on ferrous sulfate ($FeSO_4$) tablets have made them a frequent delicacy of children. Toxicity can be seen after 2-g exposure but usually is not severe unless the dose is greater than 10 g.

Iron toxicity begins with vomiting, which may be bloody owing to mucosal erosion. This is followed by metabolic acidosis, coagulopathy, liver dysfunction, and shock. Metabolic acidosis typically commences after depletion of the patient's iron-binding capacity and is multifactorial in origin. Acidosis is produced by the hypovolemia, circulatory shock, and chemical hydration of the ferric ion by water, releasing 3 hydrogen ions ($Fe^{+++} + 3H_2O \rightarrow Fe(OH)_3 + 3H^+$). Hepatic failure results from iron-catalyzed free radical formation and lipid peroxidation of mitochondrial membranes.[138] Renal failure and cirrhosis may follow acute toxicity.

Treatment of acute toxicity is supportive. If measured blood levels are significantly elevated (above 3.5 mg/L), desferroxamine should be administered for chelation therapy. An abdominal radiograph should be obtained, to determine if any iron pills remain in the gastrointestinal tract.[139] Additionally, whole bowel irrigation with GoLYTELY (or another polyethylene glycol solution) helps speed transit of iron concretions through the gastrointestinal tract.

4. Lead

Lead poisoning occurs less frequently today because of strict rules governing manufacture of gasoline and paints and other industrial uses. Lead poisoning has never been a significant source of acute intoxication. For long-term treatment, chelating therapy with EDTA, BAL, or D-penicillamine enhances elimination of lead from the body.

5. Mercury

Mercury intoxication is a rare problem but can follow ingestion of elemental mercury by children when a thermometer breaks in the mouth. Because gastrointestinal absorption of mercury is poor, this method of exposure is usually considered nontoxic, and no specific therapy is required. Inhaled organic or inorganic mercury is, however, very toxic. Chronic inhalation can cause encephalopathy characterized by a tremor and irritability. Acute treatment of mercury intoxication includes gastric lavage, administration of salt-poor albumin (which binds mercury and helps prevent absorption during lavage) and chelating agents such as BAL, followed by D-penicillamine. A recent case report of two patients suggests that, despite treatment as outlined above, relatively high concentrations of mercury remain in the plasma, possibly owing to prolonged release of mercury from red blood cells and tissues after oxidation.[140]

6. Phosphorus

Phosphorus toxicity is manifested in several organ systems, including the cardiovascular, gastrointestinal, hepatic, renal, and nervous systems. Symptoms of burning gastrointestinal and abdominal pain are followed by cardiovascular collapse. The odor of garlic is noted on the patient's breath. The patient's stools and vomitus glow under Wood's lamp. There is no specific antidote, and treatment is mainly supportive. However, gastric emptying and lavage with dilute potassium permanganate is recommended to oxidize any residual phosphorus into the nontoxic oxide.

7. Thallium

Thallium is a rodenticide frequently used in Europe. Like most of the other toxic heavy metals, thallium interferes with metabolism of sulfhydryl groups, especially in the mitochondrial oxidative phosphorylation chain. Thallium also substitutes for potassium, thus depolarizing membranes when present in high concentrations. Thallium toxicity typically occurs 12 to 24 hours after ingestion and has gastrointestinal manifestations of nausea, abdominal pain, diarrhea, and gastroenteritis. An asymptomatic period of perhaps several days is followed by neurologic symptoms, including coma and convulsions. Thallium toxicity, like phosphate and arsenic poisoning, may be associated with a garlicky odor on the patient's breath. Treatment is mainly supportive, and there is no specific antidote. However, absorbed thallium in the gastrointestinal tract can be converted to insoluble forms by a drug such as Prussian blue (potassium ferrocyanide). Dialysis and hemoperfusion are the only therapies for patients who have already absorbed thallium.

F. LYE

Lye ingestion, a toxic exposure with no known effective treatment, frequently results in esophageal injury and risk of acute perforation or tracheoesophageal fistula and healing by stricture formation. Lye-induced tissue injury is liquefaction necrosis resulting from the severe alkalinity, so therapy is logically directed at neutralization with acid. Poisoning patients may be seen by an anesthesiologist for acute airway protection and intubation and for treatment in the ICU. Therapy is predominantly supportive, because the lye may be neutralized before the patient arrives in the OR. A new technique utilizing inhaled carbon dioxide has demonstrated successful results in rabbits, provided it is administered early enough.[141] Inhaled carbon dioxide provides a source of carbonic acid capable of neutralizing tissue and lumen alkalinity. Carbon dioxide inhalation protected anesthetized rabbits' lye-exposed esophaguses against transepithelial necrosis. This approach has the potential to protect the human esophagus against lye injury because it is effective, easy to perform, and relatively safe.

Definitive diagnosis requires endoscopic evaluation. For years, endoscopists were warned to stop at the first evidence of injury to avoid perforating the damaged esophagus, but fiberoptic instruments now allow panendoscopy to be performed safely in almost all cases.[142] Thus, in the future, carbon dioxide might be administered via the suction port of an endoscope during upper endoscopy for lye ingestions.

V. ANIMAL BITES, STINGS, AND ENVENOMATIONS

A. DOMESTICATED ANIMALS AND HUMANS

Animal bites frequently occur on the face and extremities. Patients, especially small children, often present to the OR for débridement and repair of these injuries.[143] Unfortunately, optimal care for these wounds is incompletely understood by many, so an anesthesiologist knowledgeable in this area can facilitate provision of improved medical care. In contrast to most injuries, infections emanating from bites usually reflect the oral flora of the biting animal rather than the skin flora of the host.[144] The most common facultative isolates include *Staphylococcus aureus,* streptococci, *Pasteurella multocida,* and *Eikenella corrodens.* The most common anaerobic organisms include *Peptostreptococcus* and *Bacteroides* species. Penicillin-resistant gram-negative rods are rarely encountered. *E. corrodens,* a common pathogen of bite wounds, is a fastidious gram-negative organism (requiring carbon dioxide to grow in culture). *E. corrodens* is typically sensitive to penicillin and ampicillin but resistant to nafcillin, methicillin, clindamycin, and metronidazole.[145] *P. multocida,* another common cause of infections from animal bites, is quite susceptible to penicillin. Therefore, penicillin is a good choice for empirical coverage because most of the organisms involved with dog, cat, and human bites are sensitive to it. Irrigation of the wound is critical; cat bites are more difficult to irrigate than dog bites because of the puncture wound nature of cat bites. Bites in the hand may enter the bone, joint capsule, or tendon sheaths, which, being avascular, serve as excellent culture media for bacterial growth. These wounds should receive early surgical exploration, copious irrigation and débridement, immobilization of the extremity, and intravenous antibiotic therapy. Antibiotic prophylaxis has not been proven efficacious for dog bites; however, patients with extensive bites or crushed tissue should receive prophylactic antibiotic therapy. Cat bite and human bite victims, on the other hand, should always receive prophylactic antibiotic therapy because the infection rates are higher.

B. VENOMOUS REPTILES, PRINCIPALLY SNAKES

Although the surgical and medical literature teem with interesting articles about animal bites and snake, scorpion, and spider envenomations, very few reports in the anesthesia literature describe the implications of these toxins. In the United States there are approximately 45,000 snake bites per year and 7000 to 8000 of these are venomous, and approximately 10 to 15 bite victims die annually.[146] Worldwide, the number of snake bites is approximately 500,000 per year, and there are 45,000 deaths. The majority of bites occur in Asia, Africa, and South America. Patients are seen by an anesthesiologist when they present to the OR for débridement of snakebite wounds, fasciotomy, or airway support following the development of venom-induced neuromuscular blockade and acute respiratory failure. Figure 16–6 depicts the site of action for most known animal-derived toxins and venoms.

The primary utility of snake venom is to immobilize prey and facilitate its digestion. The lethality of venoms is related principally to their neurotoxic and hematopathologic properties. More than 20 enzymes have been detected in snake venom, and 12 are found in the majority of venoms. Hyaluronidase, present in all snake venoms, facilitates the distribution of venom throughout the tissues of the prey.[147]

Effects of snake venom can be divided into several categories: local tissue reaction, neuromuscular junction effects, hemorrhagic symptoms (including coagulation abnormalities, vascular endothelial injury, intravascular hemolysis), and cardiotoxicity and secondary injuries such as renal failure due to myoglobinemia (from direct injury to the muscle or from compartment syndrome) or stroma-free hemoglobin (following hemolysis).

1. Identification of North American Venomous Snakes

The key to appropriate treatment is accurate identification of the snake that caused the envenomation. Therefore, the snake should be killed at the site and brought into the hospital with the patient. In North America there are only four types of venomous snake: the coral snake (member of the Elapidae family) and three pit vipers, the rattlesnake, the cottonmouth (water moccasin), and the copperhead.

Identification begins with examination of the snake's head. Pit vipers have elliptical pupils, although a dead snake's pupils may become a little less elliptical. Perfectly round pupils, however, occur only in nonvenomous North American snakes (other than the coral snake) and in venomous snakes from foreign soils. The rattlesnake is easy to identify because of its rattle. All pit vipers have heat sensors that they can utilize to home in on a rodent. Pit viper fangs are hinged. A pit viper bite is painful and usually associated with erythema and edema around the puncture marks. If a patient presents with little puncture bites but is not complaining of pain, the bite was not from a pit viper *or* an insignificant amount of pit viper venom was injected. A rattlesnake bite produces pain, swelling, tissue damage, and systemic manifestations (disseminated intravascular coagulation and neurotoxicity).

2. Venom Toxicity

Copperheads are the least lethal of the North American pit vipers. Copperhead envenomations should not be treated with antivenin because the horse serum causes more deaths than copperhead bites. Pygmy rattler bites also are not very fatal. However, Eastern and Western diamondbacks have extremely toxic venom. Diamondbacks account for only 3 per cent of snakebites in the United States, but are responsible for the majority of deaths. The king cobra delivers a lot of venom, but the diamondback has more potent venom and delivers a greater quantity than any other North American snake. The water moccasin and all of the other rattlers fall in between the diamondback, at the potent end of the spectrum, and the copperhead, at the least potent end of the spectrum. Table 16–10 describes the site of action and relative need for antivenin for North American venomous snakebites. Specific issues on the various families of venomous snakes are discussed next.

3. Families of Venomous Snakes (North American Emphasis)

a. Elapidae

Envenomations from elapids account for the majority of deaths worldwide. The family Elapidae includes cobras, kraits, mambas, taipans, tiger snakes, and coral snakes (the only elapid native to the United States). Systemic manifestations of elapid envenomation include ptosis, external ophthalmoplegia, dysphasia, and salivation followed by general paralysis and respiratory failure. Death is due to ventilatory failure secondary to blockade at the neuromuscular junction. Understanding the neuromuscular junction–binding site of α-bungarotoxin (derived from the krait) helped reveal the molecular configuration of the postsynaptic acetylcholine receptors at the neuromuscular junction. Indeed, the 40-kd peptide alpha-subunits of the acetylcholine receptors carry separate binding sites for acetylcholine and α-bungarotoxin.[148, 149] These two alpha subunits, along with three other subunits, are arranged in a ring that forms an ionophore channel for ions.[150]

i. Cobras (Africa, India, Asia)

Cobras, found in Africa, India, and Asia, have a potent neurotoxin that affects the postsynaptic membrane of the neuromuscular junction (Fig. 16–6). The cobra toxin is more easily reversible than α-bungarotoxin (produced by the krait). Cobra venoms also contain potent cardiotoxins.[151] Interestingly, the black-necked cobra (*Naja nigricollis*) discharge their venom by spitting and can injure the eyes, whereas the vast majority of cobras deliver their venom via their fangs. The Indian cobra (*Naja naja*) grows up to 6 feet, whereas the king cobra (*Naja hannah*) grows to 12 feet.

ii. Coral Snakes (North and South America)

Coral snakes have black-tipped heads and alternating red, yellow, and black stripes. In cross-section a coral snake is shaped like a broomstick—perfectly round—whereas most snakes are flatter on the bottom. The bands go all the way around the coral snake. Coral snake venom is the most potent of any snake's in this continent, but the delivery is not as efficient as a rattlesnake's. The coral snake has little, stubby fangs and typically injects little venom. Coral snakes often hang on and chew and contaminate the skin with their extremely potent venom.

Coral snakebite treatment begins by washing the wound with soap and water. A coral snake often stays clamped on for a while after biting. Coral snake venom is almost pure neu-

TABLE 16–10

Site of Venom Action and Relative Need for Antivenin for North American Venomous Snakebites

	Snake			
	Coral Snake	Copperhead	Cottonmouth (water moccasin)	Rattlesnake‡
Identifying features	Red, yellow, black (black-tipped head), round body instead of D-shaped like most snakes. Tends to hang on and bite for a while.	Light to dark tan-copper. Docile nature. Rarely bites unless stepped upon.	Keeps mouth open for a long time whenever provoked.	Rattles, especially if >2 years old; diamondback pattern; sidewinding track.
Site of Action				
Local tissue injury	−*	+ + + +	+ +	+ + + +
Neuromuscular junction	+ + + +	+/−†	+ +	+ + +
Heart	−	−	−	+ +
Blood (DIC)	−	−	−	+ + + +
Kidneys (hemolysis or myoglobinemia causes renal failure)	−	+	+	+ +
Typical quantity of antivenin, for 70 kg adult (when needed)	No antivenin necessary, provided ventilatory support is available. For unstable adult 4–5 vials.	4–5 vials	None	10–20 vials (get coagulation studies first)

*Some Brazilian coral snakebites cause massive tissue injury.
†Of the five subspecies of copperhead, only two have neurotoxic activity: *Agkistrodon contortrix mokasen* and *Agkistrodon contortrix contortrix.*
‡Diamondback and sidewinder rattlesnakes have the most potent venom.

rotoxin. Consequently, there is no tissue damage, no hemotoxin, no significant cardiotoxin, just a neurotoxin that may be slow to develop. The symptoms, which are similar to those of Guillain-Barre syndrome, may take hours to be manifested. Once the symptoms occur, however, the interval between the trivial symptoms and complete paralysis is very short. Thus, the trachea should be intubated early, and health care workers must be prepared to support ventilation. As long as ventilation is ensured, antivenin may be held in reserve.

b. Crotalidae (Pit Vipers)

Vipers are best known for hemorrhagic symptoms resulting from their venom. Russell's viper (India, Sri Lanka), and the saw-scaled (carpet) viper, which species may be responsible for the most deaths worldwide, are the most notorious in this regard. Additionally, Russell's viper has toxins that cause hemolysis leading to renal failure. Interestingly, the Malayan viper produces minimal hemorrhagic symptoms, even though it produces complete anticoagulation in a patient's blood for days. This is due to defibrinogenation without thrombocytopenia or fibrinolysis. Several investigators have studied this phenomenon as an alternative to heparinization during cardiopulmonary bypass.[152]

i. Rattlesnakes

Like other vipers, the rattlesnake (a pit viper) injects venom that has a hemorrhagic effect. Rattlesnake venoms cause defibrinogenation by activating the endogenous fibrinolytic system. Thrombocytopenia and platelet dysfunction are also seen. Additionally, some rattlesnakes produce specific vascular endothelium-disrupting compounds that further accelerate DIC.[153, 154]

Cardiotoxins are found in rattlesnake venom (as in cobras'). In rattlesnake venom the toxins block potassium channels and sodium channels of most excitable membranes, including cardiac muscle. Rattlesnake bites are capable of producing significant local tissue edema. Subsequent tissue injury and hemolysis can lead to renal dysfunction as well. Dickinson and coworkers studied rattlesnake envenomation in 27 horses, demonstrating overall mortality of 25 per cent. The most significant chronic problems were cardiac disease, pneumonia, paralysis, and wound complications.[155]

ii. Cottonmouth (Water Moccasin)

The water moccasin has a tendency to keep its mouth wide open when disturbed and to keep it open for a long time (an unusual behavior for snakes). If you poke a snake with a stick and it does not open its mouth, it is not a water moccasin. Antivenin is reserved for severe cases of cottonmouth envenomation.

iii. Copperhead

Copperheads are very docile snakes. Essentially, they do not bite unless stepped on. Adult copperheads are light to dark copper brown. When copperheads are born, they have a chartreuse-colored tail that is lost when they shed their skin the first time.

Copperhead bites require conservative treatment, as tissue injury is only local. Patients should not be treated with antivenin because the side effects are worse than the snakebite. Wittley reviewed 55 patients treated over a 12-year period, including 12 children who sustained copperhead bites. None was treated with antivenin, and there was no loss of limb or residual disability.[156]

c. Hydrophidae (Venomous Sea Snakes, Indo-Pacific Region)

All sea snakes (the family Hydrophidae) are venomous.[157] The venom of sea snakes contains a neurotoxin that binds to the nicotinic cholinergic receptors on the postsynaptic membrane of the skeletal neuromuscular junction and autonomic ganglia. Some sea snakes have venom that affects the prejunctional membrane at the neuromuscular junction as well. Although sea snake venom is extremely toxic, the amount of venom injected is usually small. Sea snake poisoning also causes direct tissue injury and extreme pain in the envenomated muscles; the result is rhabdomyolysis and myoglobinuria that can promote renal failure.

4. Emergency Treatment of North American Snakebites

Emergency treatment for North American venomous snakebites begins with a quick survey and the ABCs. The physician checks vital signs, draws blood for a type and cross-match and baseline renal panel, hematocrit, platelets, and a disseminated intravascular coagulation panel. This must be done early, since 3 to 4 hours after a rattlesnake bite the patient's serum may no longer be cross-matchable.[158] Blood urea nitrogen and creatinine should be evaluated because nephrotoxicity can occur secondary to venom-induced rhabdomyolysis or after administration of horse serum–derived antivenin. Next, attention should turn to the extremity (checking for swelling) and the type of bite. If there is no swelling by the time the patient arrives at the emergency department or OR, only observation is required for the bite. However, if the snakebite goes directly into a joint or into a fascial plane or directly into a vessel, there may be very little swelling. For instance, if the patient was bitten on the Achilles tendon and directly into some vein, the patient may act very strangely, be confused, and not actually have very much in the way of swelling, but over time swelling will develop. A copperhead bite has almost no systemic symptoms, but the edema is very striking. There is not too much in the way of tissue necrosis, but swelling continues.

Any signs of systemic shock, neurologic alteration, or hemorrhagic symptoms should trigger consideration of antivenin therapy. Crotalid antivenin treats all poisonous North American snakebites except those of coral snakes. The goal is to neutralize the venom, molecule for molecule, before it latches on to a target organ. One vial of antivenin is enough for a copperhead, four or five for a water moccasin or a timber rattler bite, and 15 to 20 vials of antivenin is necessary for an Eastern diamondback bite (Table 16–10).

Like brown recluse spider venom, most snake venoms other than the water moccasin tend to kill bacteria, so primary infections are uncommon. However, secondary infections can occur requiring incision and drainage and antibiotic therapy. These typically occur days after the initial envenomation—and usually well after the most critical phase of venom toxicity has passed. Antibiotics and tetanus prophylaxis should be considered for water moccasin bites, as these snakes harbor *Clostridium* organisms, including *Clostridium tetani*. For other North American snakebites, antibiotic therapy should be reserved for documented secondary infection. Inflammatory conditions not due to infection do not improve with antibiotics. Steroids are of no value except to treat anaphylaxis caused by either the venom or the antivenin. Anaphylaxis should be treated with epinephrine, fluid, antihistamines, and steroid therapy.

Application of tourniquets to the extremities is controversial, as this can lead to increased tissue necrosis from envenomations that cause local tissue injury. A light lymphatic constriction band placed proximal to the site is useful for a snakebite that has prominent neurotoxic effects. However, one must be careful not to release the tourniquet until ventilatory support is available.

Antiserum is life saving in some areas of the world, yet it should not be given to snakebite victims unless there is evidence of systemic manifestations. Some of the systemic manifestations of paralysis can be reversed by administering anticholinesterase drugs such as edrophonium or neostigmine. Some recommend an edrophonium test, alone or with atropine, and if this improves muscle strength the patient can be treated with a neostigmine drip and followed in the intensive care unit. The most important use for antivenin is for bites from vipers, such as the rattlesnake, that cause significant disseminated intravascular coagulation.

5. Helodermatidae (Venomous Lizards)

The Gila monster is a large, relatively slow-moving nocturnal reptile of the deserts of Arizona, Mexico, and surrounding areas. Venom is transferred from glands in the lower jaw via ducts that discharge their contents near the base of the large teeth. The venom is then drawn up along grooves in the teeth by capillary action. The venom of the Gila monster contains serotonin, aminoxidase, phospholipase A, proteolytic compounds, and hyaluronidase. The high hyaluronidase content is responsible for the tissue edema frequently associated with Gila monster bites. There is very little systemic toxicity, except for a slight drop in blood pressure, decreased circulating blood volume, tachycardia, and, occasionally, respiratory distress. Lethal doses are rarely seen but have been associated with decreased ventricular contractility.[159]

C. AMPHIBIAN TOXINS

Amphibians produce poisons in highly developed cutaneous secretory glands. The secretions are excreted continually; however, the secretory rate may be increased at times of stress. The poisons secreted by the skin of amphibians have two protective effects. First they protect against invasion by foreign bacteria and fungi. Second, they serve to discourage predators. Amphibian cutaneous toxins significant to humans include alkaloids and multiple biogenic amines (including epinephrine, norepinephrine, and dopamine).[160] Additionally, a group of bufogenines are secreted by toads. Bufogenines affect smooth muscle and cardiac muscle. Some toads have been found to secrete a tetrodotoxin similar to that produced by the dinoflagellates responsible for pelagic poisoning. Newts and salamanders also have a variety of toxins, including a tetrodotoxin. The presence of toxins and steroid alkaloids in amphibian skin glands provides insight into the reasons that old witches' brew formulas were thought to have magical powers, as they frequently included several of these toxic agents.

More than 100 biologically active alkaloids can be extracted from the skin of Colombian frogs.[161] The skin secretions of the brightly colored Colombian frogs contain a batrachotoxin, which prevents sodium channel inactivation, resulting in a massive influx of sodium and persistent membrane depolarization. Secretory compounds from the skin of Colombian frogs have been used by natives for centuries as arrow and dart poisons.

D. SEA SNAILS

The genus *Conus* includes Pacific and Indian Ocean marine snails that produce beautiful cone-shaped shells. These sea snails also produce a variety of neurotoxins, including alpha, mu, and conotoxins (Fig. 16–6). They can cause death to prey and ventilatory failure in humans.[162] The anesthesiologist might see a patient stung by a snail who develops respiratory failure that requires intubation, mechanical ventilation, and possibly some cardiosupportive therapy.

E. SCORPIONS

Scorpion envenomation (there are more than 650 species worldwide) causes intense local pain and hypesthesia over the envenomated extremity. Local manifestations are followed by systemic symptoms, with alternating cholinergic and adrenergic stimulation. The cholinergic symptoms occur first and are manifested by inability to focus vision, hypersalivation, vomiting, and diarrhea. After the cholinergic symptoms, an adrenergic response is frequently seen, with release of epinephrine and norepinephrine, producing hypertension, tachycardia, and dysrhythmias. Venom of scorpions indigenous to India, North Africa, and the Middle East tends to release catecholamines, causing toxic myocarditis, heart failure, and pulmonary edema.

The bark scorpion *Centruroides exilicauda*, indigenous to Arizona and surrounding states (California, Nevada, New Mexico), is the most important (and lethal) North American scorpion. Bark scorpion venom causes muscle fasciculations, spasms, and respiratory paralysis. *C. exilicauda* venom is the most potent and causes the most diverse manifestations of any scorpion venom. The alpha scorpion toxins delay inactivation of the sodium channel (keeping them open longer) on the presynaptic neuromuscular junction (see Fig. 16–6). The beta scorpion toxins enhance activation of sodium channels (opening them at a membrane potential at which they would normally be closed). The intense local pain may require local or regional nerve blockade for relief. Antivenin also tends to diminish the pain over time and should be administered to any patient with significant symptoms of scorpion envenomation.

Anesthesiologists most frequently care for scorpion-envenomated patients because of respiratory failure (the airway and other tissues swell quickly) or local wound care. These patients should have their trachea intubated immediately following the first symp-

toms of stridor. If intubation is unsuccessful because of periglottic narrowing, transtracheal jet ventilation or cricothyroidotomy should be performed. Emergency drug therapy should include epinephrine, the only antidote known to control the immediate hypersensitivity reactions. If an intravenous line cannot be established quickly, the epinephrine is given through an endotracheal tube. Additionally, epinephrine can be given subcutaneously or into muscle. Additional therapy for anaphylaxis includes an antihistamine and fluid and steroid therapy.

The most important life-sustaining therapy is monitoring of the cardiovascular and pulmonary systems. Occasionally, these patients require intubation and mechanical ventilation to combat the paralysis caused by the California and New Mexico species of scorpions. Treatment of the adrenergic-mediated dysrhythmias and hypertension includes alpha blockers, and calcium channel blockers. Echocardiography has been recommended for management of scorpion envenomation victims because of the myocardial toxicity.[163] Patients should be monitored closely in the ICU until symptoms remit.[164]

F. SPIDERS

Anesthesiologists may be called to see victims of spider bites because of respiratory failure or for intraoperative management of wound care or pain consultation for the misery associated with araneism (spider envenomation). The term *araneism* is derived from *aranea*, which describes the class Arachnida (the spiders). There are two venomous spiders in North America whose bites cause significant disability. These are the black widow (*Latrodectus*) and the brown recluse (*Loxosceles reclusa*), the violin or fiddle-backed spider. Additionally, three important venomous spiders with neurotoxic effects are found outside North America: funnel-web, Joro, and banana.

1. North American Venomous Spiders

a. *Latrodectus* (Black Widow)

Black widows like to live undisturbed in dark areas. The female is a large, jet black spider with a red hourglass on the ventral surface of the abdomen. The adult male is very small and nondescript. Although the black widow is reclusive and not aggressive, a bite may occur when the victim puts on an item of clothing that has been sitting for a long time, like a boot that was in a garage all winter or a coat that hung for a long time in a closet. The black widow is not in the web during the day: she is usually in a crevice or a corner until night, when she returns to her web to wait for food. Black widow webs are made of very strong silk but are very untidy. The web is full of debris and not clean like the web of a garden spider. The venom is a neurotoxin (alpha-latrotoxin) that causes muscle spasms and psychic distress (sometimes referred to as *latrodectism*). The alpha-latrotoxin affects the presynaptic nerve terminals, opening cationic channels and causing massive release of neurotransmitter[165] followed by depletion of synaptic vessels at the neuromuscular junction.[166]

The bite may be as imperceptible as a flea bite or a very mild bee sting. Spasms may "march" up the extremity, entering larger and larger muscle groups. For instance, in the arm the venom progresses to the deltoid group and then to the back and abdominal muscles. The pain from a black widow bite can mimic acute abdomen. There have been bite patients who came to the emergency room with acute abdominal pain and were worked up for exploratory laparotomy. Interestingly, the administration of calcium gluconate can cause the pain to abate and may help diagnostically.[167] Patients with latrodectism have muscle spasms and squirm a lot, which helps distinguish the problem from acute abdomen, where patients lie motionless. There is no abdominal tenderness, but there is abdominal spasm and pain in the back and abdominal muscles. There is a significant elevation in blood pressure, which may be related to the pain and restlessness, but the cause is not clear. Other symptoms include fever, chills, diaphoresis, urine retention, priapism, nausea, and vomiting.

The predominant neurologic symptom is the amazing restlessness of these patients. The restlessness may be partly related to the pain and terror (of having received a black widow bite), but there is also something about the venom that causes this very "hyper," anxious state. There will be very little evidence of injury at the site of the bite (i.e., no swelling, erythema, necrosis, or tissue injury).

Treatment begins with administration of 10 ml of 10 per cent calcium gluconate (diagnos-tic and therapeutic). The specific antidote is black widow antitoxin, which changes the acute state dramatically. The patient may quickly get up and become talkative and happy. For small children or elderly adults, one vial of antivenin is sufficient. A poison control center can provide specific recommendations. For severe cases, general anesthesia with endotracheal intubation and neuromuscular blockade to control the muscle spasms may be necessary until specific antitoxin can be administered).

b. *Loxosceles* (Brown Recluse)

Envenomation from a brown recluse causes significant tissue destruction and coagulation of vessels but has no significant neurotoxic effects. The brown recluse has an inverted violin on its back. The initial bite is seldom detected, but it is usually followed by minor local stinging and pruritus. Some 36 to 48 hours later, a blister with an erythematous base appears at the site of the bite. The blister becomes purple and the base around it develops a faint bluish or ischemic color. Initially, no swelling occurs at the site—just a little depression as the surrounding area shrinks, possibly owing to tissue necrosis; then, a clean ulcer (similar to a syphilis chancre) appears. A scab forms, erythema around the area extends and advances, and then the scab falls off and an even deeper ulcer opens up. This cycle continues without obvious infection, and the rash advances as the ulcer continues to get bigger and bigger.

Dapsone (diaminodiphenylsulfone) has been used, but there is also an antivenin for brown recluse bites (not commercially available, but it has been used in Tennessee[168]). Dapsone is a sulfone used to treat leprosy. It should be started within 1 to 2 days of the bite, with 100 mg administered twice daily for up to 2 weeks. Dapsone causes hemolytic anemia and methemoglobinemia (especially in NADH reductase deficiency states); thus, blood counts should be monitored and methemoglobinemia sought during therapy. Operative therapy is not recommended for the primary injury. However, if the wound becomes secondarily infected, débridement can be life saving, as it is in extremity infections of other causes. When treatment is delayed, surgical excision of necrotic tissue is required. The wound should be treated with wet-to-dry dressings and allowed to heal by secondary intention.

2. Venomous Spiders Not Native to North America

The funnel-web spider (*Atrax*), found in Australia and Tasmania, causes a painful bite followed by nausea, vomiting, abdominal pain, salivation, and dyspnea. The venomous site of action is the calcium channels on the presynaptic portion of the neuromuscular junction. The major cause of the araneism in Brazil and neighboring countries is envenomation from the South American banana spider (*Phoneutria*), which has significant neurotoxic effects. The third non–North American venomous spider of significance is the Joro spider found in Japan and East Asia. The toxin secreted by the Joro spider affects the postsynaptic glutamate receptors, blocking transmission. Envenomation from all of these non–North American spiders can be treated by maintaining supportive care. Neuromuscular blocking drugs should be avoided when anesthetizing these patients.

G. HYMENOPTERA (BEES, WASPS, AND HORNETS)

Hymenoptera (bees, wasps, hornets) are responsible for the majority of deaths due to envenomation in the US. The major symptomatology of Hymenoptera envenomation is IgE-mediated histamine release associated with anaphylactic shock and respiratory failure. *Anaphylaxis* is derived from the Greek word *ana* meaning backward and *phylaxis* meaning protection. Anaphylaxis is currently used to describe rapid, generalized (often unanticipated), immune-mediated events that follow exposure to foreign substances in previously sensitized persons involving an antigen-specific, IgE-mediated mechanism. *Anaphylactoid* reactions are those that may be clinically similar to an anaphylaxis reaction but that are not mediated via the IgE antibody and do not necessarily require prior exposure. The first recorded anaphylactic reaction occurred in an Egyptian Pharoah following a wasp sting and was recorded in hieroglyphics around 2640 BC.[169]

In contrast to snake, spider, and scorpion envenomations, death from Hymenoptera occurs rapidly: 58 per cent within 1 hour.[170] Autopsy reports of 150 sting-induced deaths showed that 70 per cent resulted from airway obstruction. Anaphylactic shock was the next most common cause. The honeybee is the species most frequently responsible for anaphylaxis, followed by the yellowjacket wasp, the white-faced hornet, and the yellow hornet. The most abundant component of Hymenoptera venom is mellitin, which promotes red cell lysis and pigment-induced renal failure. Mast cell degranulation (MCD) peptide leads to mast cell degranulation and histamine release. Apamin is a neurotoxin that blocks potassium channels and may cause CNS hyperreactivity, convulsions, and death.[171] Mellitin and phospholipase A_2 are the allergens most often responsible for the type 1 hypersensitivity that may progress to anaphylactic shock. Hypersensitivity from previous exposure is a critical factor in anaphylactic death from Hymenoptera envenomation.[172] Indeed, only 2 per cent of deaths from Hymenoptera stings in the United States occurred in children younger than 10 years, whereas 50 per cent occurred in persons older than 50.

H. TICK-BORNE PARALYSIS

Tick envenomation can lead to paralysis. Tick paralysis occurs when the tick embeds itself in the victim's skin and produces a toxin while it engorges with the patient's blood. The toxin affects conduction down the motor neuron by blocking acetylcholine release at the neuromuscular junction.[173] Weakness is slow to occur and typically appears 5 days following the attachment of the tick. The toxin can be metabolized and removed completely within 24 hours of tick removal. Tick paralysis has been reported in North America, Australia, and British Columbia.[174] Therapy includes ventilatory support and tick removal.

In summary, most of the animal toxins produce dysfunction at the neuromuscular junction. Acute respiratory care is mainly supportive; however, certain snake, scorpion, and spider venoms may require administration of antivenin to protect against the systemic sequelae, including disseminated intravascular coagulation, rhabdomyolysis, renal failure, and cardiotoxicity.

VI. ANESTHETIC CONSIDERATIONS OF CHEMOTHERAPEUTICS

New and promising antineoplastic agents and combination therapies have produced better therapeutic rates for previously refractory cancers. Experience has led to the recognition of toxicities that may be latent (e.g., progressive cardiac dysfunction following anthracycline therapy). Furthermore, toxicity is frequently seen with combination therapy. This section presents an evaluation of the literature in the evolving area of chemotherapeutic toxicity and the anesthetic considerations for the management of these patients. Any patient with a history of chemotherapy or radiation therapy is at risk for the development of toxicities. Careful preoperative evaluation will help to define the nature of these toxicities and to devise an anesthetic plan to prevent complications.

The goal of this section is to note the effects of chemotherapeutic agents that are expected to have anesthetic considerations. Discussion is limited to effects on the major organ systems that may affect the elimination of medications (e.g., the hepatic and renal systems) or affect the patient's response to medications (e.g., the cardiac and pulmonary systems). Unique effects (e.g., inhibition of pseudocholinesterase activity by cyclophosphamide) are noted when relevant. Other effects, however, such as nausea and vomiting, are not noted unless they are pertinent to a specific clinical scenario (e.g., the effect of instilling mechlorethamine for pleural sclerosing therapy). For a full account of the toxicity of a given agent, the clinician is advised to consult a standard oncology textbook.

A. ALKYLATING AGENTS

Alkylating agents react with nucleophilic substances to form strong covalent linkages. The cellular effects are probably due to alkylating effects on DNA components, with subsequent strand breaks, depurination, inter- or intrastrand linkages, and/or bonding between DNA and various proteins. Interruption of replication and transcription of DNA follows, with cytotoxicity and mutagenesis. There are several different classes of alkylating agents, and, owing to acquired resistance, the effectiveness of agents against various neoplasms, and the synergy of various agents in combination, a patient may receive more than one agent in any given class.

A number of toxic effects are common to alkylating agents, but these do not have specific anesthetic considerations. These include leukemogenesis, amenorrhea, azoospermia, and nausea and vomiting. Of greater concern to the anesthesiologist are the effects of alkyl-

ating agents on cardiac, pulmonary, and hepatic function. For example, cyclophosphamide and dacarbazine exacerbate the effects of anthracycline cardiotoxicity. Busulfan, cyclophosphamide, chlorambucil, and all of the nitrosoureas, but especially carmustine, can produce significant pulmonary injury (Table 16–11). Pulmonary toxicity is frequently exacerbated by exposure to oxygen, and other anesthetic considerations may also apply.

Another form of toxicity common to some alkylating agents is hepatic venoocclusive disease (HVOD), particularly when these agents are given in large doses (i.e., in preparation for bone marrow transplantation). The agents involved include cyclophosphamide, carmustine, lomustine, busulfan, and mitomycin C.[175] The effects of HVOD—jaundice, hepatomegaly with right upper quadrant pain, ascites—may occur in as many as 20 per cent of patients who undergo bone marrow transplant.[176, 177] Evaluation includes the exclusion of other causes of liver disease. HVOD may also be caused by antimetabolite agents (see below). Management involves sodium restriction, spironolactone diuresis, and maintenance of plasma oncotic pressure. HVOD may cause or contribute to death in as many as 30 per cent of bone marrow transplant recipients.[178] Anesthetic considerations for HVOD include careful monitoring for decreased right ventricular filling volume, by invasive means if necessary. Drugs metabolized in the liver may have a diminished rate of elimination and should be avoided.

1. Nitrogen Mustards

Nitrogen mustards are a group of toxic, vesicating, alkylating drugs that are all chemically unstable to some degree. Nitrogen mustards are regarded as analogs of sulfur mustard, which was first synthesized in 1854 and was used during World War I for its vesicant action on the eyes, skin, and lungs.[179] In the interval between World Wars I and II, the nitrogen mustards were studied extensively but secretly. After World War II, much of the data was declassified and efforts toward using these drugs as antineoplastics began.

a. Mechlorethamine

Mechlorethamine, one of the most unstable of the nitrogen mustard alkylating drugs, is favored for treatment of Hodgkin's disease

TABLE 16–11

Pulmonary Toxicity of Antineoplastic Drugs

Drug	Type and Incidence of Injury	Dose Related?/ Dose	Does Oxygen Therapy Worsen Toxicity?	Other Risk Factors
Alkylating Agents				
Cyclophosphamide	1% pulmonary fibrosis†,‡	No	Yes	None
Ifosfamide	Rare interstitial pneumonitis	No	?	None
Chlorambucil	Rare interstitial pneumonitis	2000 mg over 6 months	?	None
Melphalan	Rare interstitial pneumonitis	?	?	None
Busulfan	4% pulmonary fibrosis	? Doses >500 mg	No	Advanced age, rad tx, prolonged tx, combination tx
Nitrosoureas*				
Carmustine	25% pulmonary fibrosis#	Yes; doses >1500 mg/m^2	?Yes	Tobacco use, history of lung disease, cyclophosphamide
Antimetabolites				
Methotrexate	8% incidence of hypersensitivity pneumonitis†	Rare at doses <20 mg/week	No	None
Ara-C	Rare noncardiogenic pulmonary edema	Only w/large doses	No	None
Plant Derivatives				
Vincristine	Rare pulmonary infiltrates with fibrosis	Only with mitomycin	No	Mitomycin coadministration
Antineoplastic Antibiotics				
Bleomycin	5–40% incidence of chronic pulmonary fibrosis†,#	Yes; dose >100 units	Yes	Advanced age, cyclophosphamide, radiation toxicity, tobacco use
Mitomycin	3–12% incidence of interstitial pneumonitis#	No	Yes	Radiation toxicity
Procarbazine	Hypersensitivity pneumonitis	No	No	None

*All nitrosoureas have been associated with pulmonary disease
†Hypersensitivity pneumonitis rarely seen
‡Noncardiogenic pulmonary edema rarely seen
#Acute pulmonary venous vasculitis rarely seen

when used in combination with vincristine, procarbazine, and prednisone (MOPP). This agent may also be used intrapleurally to treat pleural metastases, in which case its toxicity is essentially the same as when it is administered intravenously. Hematologic suppression is dose limiting: leukocyte and platelet counts decline within 1 week of therapy and last 2 to 3 weeks. Nausea and vomiting typically are severe, coming on within 2 hours of the first dose and persisting 24 hours. A possible anesthetic consideration for this agent includes the severe nausea and vomiting that would be expected to follow intraoperative use of this agent as a sclerosing agent and as therapy for carcinomatous pleural or peritoneal involvement. Recent exposure to this agent may be associated with significant suppression in platelet counts and increased risk of hemorrhage.

b. Cyclophosphamide

Cyclophosphamide is a very versatile agent used in the therapy of non-Hodgkin's lymphoma, leukemia, myeloma, sarcomas, and breast and ovarian carcinomas. The most prominent side effect of this agent is hemorrhagic cystitis, although it may also result in pulmonary and cardiac toxicity. Pulmonary toxicity may present in any of three forms and occurs in approximately 1 per cent of those treated (Table 16–11). Cyclophosphamide may provoke an acute, IgE-mediated hypersensitivity reaction similar to that seen with methotrexate, bleomycin, and procarbazine.[180] Rarely, noncardiogenic pulmonary edema may be seen.[181]

The most common form of toxicity, however, is pulmonary fibrosis. In these cases, cyclophosphamide depletes the body's store of antioxidants,[182] and this is thought to contribute to the final common pathway of pulmonary injury secondary to unchallenged oxidant species that participate in oxidation-reduction reactions and fatty acid oxidation, which disrupt cell membranes.[183] No predisposing factors (dose, patient age, previous radiation therapy) appear to be associated with increased risk of pulmonary injury, although exposure to high concentrations of oxygen has been demonstrated in animals to increase the risk of damage.[184] Injury may first appear as early as 3 weeks after therapy starts or as late as 8 years after it ends. Management involves terminating the drug. Recovery occurs in 65 per cent of patients.[185] When suspected, the diagnosis must be aggressively pursued, with bronchoalveolar lavage or lung biopsy, as other studies are nonspecific. The clinical picture is one of pulmonary fibrosis, with decreased compliance and diffusion capacity and a restrictive pattern on pulmonary function tests. Anesthetic considerations for patients with a history of cyclophosphamide exposure include the need for a high index of suspicion for subclinical cases, and the avoidance of high concentrations of oxygen.

Cyclophosphamide may also result in cardiac toxicity (Table 16–12). When administered in large doses (e.g., 120 to 240 mg/kg for induction of bone marrow transplantation), as many as 33 per cent of patients may develop pericarditis and pleural effusion, with possible tamponade.[186] Fewer patients may develop hemorrhagic myocarditis and congestive heart failure.[187] It is hypothesized that cyclophosphamide cardiotoxicity may in-crease the toxic potential of anthracyclines administered concurrently. Unlike anthracyclines, however, cardiotoxicity from cyclophosphamide is not considered to be dose related or cumulative. Many patients develop decreased QRS amplitude and decreased systolic function, but these effects typically resolve over time. Papillary microthrombosis resulting in direct endomyocardial injury is considered to be the cause of cardiac toxicity. Patients with a suggestive history should undergo an echocardiographic evaluation of myocardial function before anesthetic exposure.

Another effect of cyclophosphamide is inhibition of pseudocholinesterase in resulting prolongation of the effects of succinylcholine. This agent may also enhance anticoagulant effects, which may be significant in the setting of acute myelosuppression with thrombocytopenia following chemotherapy. As noted above, this agent may be associated with HVOD. Cyclophosphamide has also been associated with the development of the syndrome of inappropriate antidiuretic hormone secretions (SIADH), which may ultimately result in hyponatremia, coma, and seizures.[188]

Taken in sum, there are many potential toxic sequelae of exposure to cyclophosphamide, including hemorrhagic cystitis, pulmonary fibrosis (which may be exacerbated by high oxygen concentrations), congestive heart failure, sensitivity to succinylcholine, potentiation of anticoagulation, SIADH, and hepatotoxicity.

c. Ifosfamide

Ifosfamide is used to treat testicular cancer, non-Hodgkin's lymphoma, and various sarcomas. Its toxicity profile is expected to be similar to that of cyclophosphamide, including acute noncardiogenic pulmonary edema,[189] and interstitial pneumonitis.[190] As for cyclophosphamide, there does not appear to be any correlation between pulmonary toxicity and dose (see Table 16–11). The most prominent toxic effect of ifosfamide is a 5 to 20 per cent incidence of CNS toxicity, with hallucinations, confusion, and aphasia rapidly progressing to coma, with or without seizures. These symptoms begin within hours of administration and resolve several days after the drug is discontinued. Narcotics and phenothiazine antiemetics are thought to exacerbate this phenomenon.[191] Urothelial protection is necessary with ifosfamide, as it can

TABLE 16–12

Cardiac Toxicity of Antineoplastics

Drug	Toxicity/ Prevalence	Dose Related?/ Dose	Cumulative with Dose?	Exacerbating Drugs	Risk Factors
Cyclophosphamide	Pericarditis 33%, hemorrhagic myocarditis, CHF	120–240 mg/kg	No	None	None
5-FU	Myocardial ischemia 1%	No	No	None	None
Pentastatin	Rare arrhythmias	10 mg/m²/day	No	None	None
Paclitaxel	33% Sinus Bradycardia: also V tach & AV Block	No	No	None	None
Doxorubicin	Cardiomyopathy 7–15%	500 mg/m² total	Yes	Cyclophosphamide, mitomycin, dacarbazine	Extremes of age, history of CHF or MI, hypertension, diabetes
Daunorubicin	Cardiomyopathy 1–2% 12%	550 mg/m² 1000 mg/m²	Yes	Unknown	Pediatric age group
Mitoxantrone	Cardiomyopathy 5%	160 mg/m²	Unknown	Previous anthracycline therapy	Prior disease, radiation therapy
Amsacrine	Ventricular arrhythmias, CHF	Only occurs with rapid infusion	Unknown	Unknown	Hypokalemia
Interferon-alfa	Ischemia, arrhythmias, cardiomyopathy	No	No	No	Prior heart disease
Interleukin 2	Ischemia, arrhythmias, CHF	No	No	No	None

result in hemorrhagic cystitis similar to that produced by cyclophosphamide. Ifosfamide is also expected to have the same drug interactions as cyclophosphamide, including inhibition of pseudocholinesterase with prolongation of succinylcholine, potentiation of anticoagulation, and potentiation of anthracycline toxicity, although none of these effects has been demonstrated in humans. The anesthetic considerations for patients exposed to this agent are not clearly delineated, although prudence suggests an approach similar to that for a patient with a history of exposure to cyclophosphamide but with somewhat lower risk of myelosuppression and a higher risk of urotoxicity and neurotoxicity.

d. Chlorambucil

This agent is employed in the treatment of chronic lymphocytic leukemia, macroglobulinemia, non-Hodgkin's lymphoma, ovarian and breast cancers, and multiple myeloma. It is generally well tolerated; complications are only mild nausea and vomiting and, rarely, hepatotoxicity. There are reports in the literature of pulmonary fibrosis similar to that seen with cyclophosphamide, although this is considered a rare complication. Whether oxygen exposure potentiates pulmonary toxicity is not known (see Table 16–11).[192] In contrast to cyclophosphamide toxicity, toxicity with chlorambucil appears to depend on a total dose of at least 2000 mg and a period of administration of at least 6 months.[193] In the presence of pulmonary fibrosis, it may be prudent to use low inspired oxygen concentrations; there are no other specific anesthetic considerations.

e. Melphalan

Melphalan is used to treat multiple myeloma and carcinomas of the breasts and ovaries. It is also used for isolated limb perfusion for melanomas of the extremities. This procedure is extremely painful and lasts 3 to 4 hours, and, therefore, frequently requires anesthesia. Nausea and vomiting may occur immediately after isolated limb perfusion and may complicate the postanesthetic course. Studies of the cytotoxic potential of melphalan have demonstrated that high tissue oxygen concentrations enhance tumor activity, and this raises the question of whether high concentrations of oxygen may improve the efficacy of melphalan during isolated limb perfusion under general anesthesia.[194] Pulmonary toxicity similar to that seen with cyclophosphamide may be observed, although rarely (see Table 16–11). It is not known whether exposure to high concentrations of oxygen can potentiate lung toxicity. Melphalan may be used for intracavitary treatment of peritoneal metastases, in which case only 1 per cent of the agent concentration of the peritoneal fluid is evident in the bloodstream. Toxicity in this setting is limited.[195] Anesthetic considerations for this agent—mostly limited to the isolated limb perfusion technique—are the potential for postoperative nausea and vomiting.

2. Ethylenimines and Methylmelamines

a. Thiotepa

Thiotepa typically is used in combination with other agents in the treatment of metastatic breast cancer, ovarian cancer, and lymphomas. Its principal use is intracavitary, in the treatment of bladder cancer and of carcinomatous pleural effusions. As with mechlorethamine, the intrapleural or intraperitoneal administration of this agent produces the same toxic effects as parenteral administration, although thiotepa is not as strong a vesicant as mechlorethamine and is associated with less severe nausea and vomiting overall. For these reasons, some practitioners more often use thiotepa. Its most prominent effect is myelosuppression that reaches a nadir in 14 days. It inhibits pseudocholinesterase, and may prolong the effects of succinylcholine. The anesthetic considerations are limited to the effects of this agent after intrapleural therapy, nausea and vomiting, and limitation of the use of succinylcholine.

b. Hexamethylmelamine

Hexamethylmelamine (HMM) is employed principally for the treatment of ovarian cancer. Its most prominent side effects are severe nausea and vomiting and neurotoxicity, which presents both centrally, with lethargy, mood alterations, and hallucinations, and peripherally, with paresthesias and loss of deep tendon reflexes. Neurotoxicity usually resolves with discontinuation of therapy. Patients who take HMM in combination with tricyclic antidepressants or monoamine oxidase inhibitors may suffer orthostatic hypotension. Anesthetic considerations are confined to avoiding drug interactions and titrating centrally acting agents carefully in the presence of central neurotoxicity.

3. Alkyl Sulfonates (Busulfan)

Busulfan is unique in that its pharmacologic action is almost solely myelosuppression. Thus, it is used principally to treat chronic myelocytic leukemia. Its toxicity is pronounced in bone marrow–derived cells: leukocyte and platelet counts start to decrease 10 days after therapy starts and continue to decrease for 2 weeks after therapy finishes. With large doses, seizures and hepatotoxicity may be dose limiting. Ginsberg and Comis report that progressive pulmonary toxicity similar to bleomycin toxicity has been noted. The prevalence of busulfan-induced pulmonary toxicity is 4 per cent, and subclinical fibrosis is apparent at autopsy in 46 per cent of patients. Risk factors for pulmonary toxicity include advanced age and prolonged therapy (i.e., several years). Toxicity has not been reported with doses smaller than 500 mg. Oxygen therapy does not appear to contribute to toxicity, although concurrent administration of other agents or previous radiation treatment may increase the risk of pulmonary toxicity (see Table 16–11).[196] The prognosis after pulmonary fibrosis is poor: survival is less than 5 months. Aside from pulmonary toxicity, busulfan may be associated with HVOD (see Alkylating Agents), hemorrhagic cystitis, and seizures.[197]

4. Nitrosoureas

a. Carmustine

Carmustine, also known as BCNU, is used to treat brain tumors, Hodgkin's disease, and multiple myeloma. Carmustine has multiple—and severe—toxicities. The most predictable is myelosuppression with thrombocytopenia, which starts 4 weeks after the onset of therapy and is prolonged. If cumulative bone marrow toxicity develops, aplastic anemia results. Hepatotoxicity, manifested by elevated liver enzyme values, occurs in 25 per cent of patients but is reversible upon withdrawal of the agent.[198] Nausea and vomiting may be severe.

Anesthesiologists are more likely to be concerned with the pulmonary and renal effects of BCNU. Onset of pulmonary toxicity is heralded by decreased diffusion capacity and is dose related: prevalence is typically 25 per cent and with larger doses (1500 mg/m²) may be as high as 30 to 50 per cent.[199] Preexisting lung disease, concurrent exposure to cyclophosphamide, and tobacco use increase the risk of pulmonary toxicity from BCNU (see Table 16–11).[200, 201] The long-term pulmonary effects of BCNU are particularly striking. O'Driscoll and colleagues report that in children treated for brain tumors with carmustine and radiation, the fatality rate from pulmonary fibrosis was 35 per cent, and that two thirds of these patients died of progressive fibrosis after a symptom-free interval of 7 to 12 years. Fibrosis may be encountered as long as 17 years after cessation of the drug.[202] Owing to the similarity of the pulmonary toxicity associated with carmustine to that associated with bleomycin, some authors recommend avoiding high-concentration oxygen therapy with carmustine, although no available studies have identified oxygen exposure as a risk factor. Rare case reports of carmustine-associated acute pulmonary venous vasculitis (similar to that seen with mitomycin and bleomycin) have been cited.[203]

Nephrotoxicity presents as progressive azotemia, which may not be reversible with withdrawal of therapy. BCNU may be associated with HVOD (see section above on HVOD associated with alkylating agents). Anesthetic considerations for patients with a remote history of exposure to BCNU include the need for a careful preoperative assessment for pulmonary damage and avoidance of oxygen therapy, if possible. Patients exposed recently should be assessed for evidence of renal and hepatic damage and for thrombocytopenia, and therapy should be modified accordingly.

b. Lomustine and Semustine

Lomustine (CCNU) and semustine (methyl-CCNU) are principally used for treatment of lymphomas and brain tumors. The toxicity profiles of these agents are similar to that of carmustine (see above), although the risk of pulmonary and hepatic toxicity is considered to be less. Semustine is remarkable because it carries greater risks of renal toxicity and leukemogenesis, both of which are dose related. Semustine is no longer in commercial development. Lomustine may be associated with HVOD (see above section on HVOD and alkylating agents). The anesthetic considerations for these agents are essentially those for carmustine.

c. Streptozocin

Streptozocin is a naturally occurring nitrosourea antibiotic produced by *Streptomyces acromogenes* fungi that acts as a weak alkylator, as a protein carbamyolator and that affects pyridine nucleopeptide metabolism. It is very specific to pancreatic islet cells and is employed principally in the therapy of islet cell tumors, occasionally in combination with 5-fluorouracil or adriamycin. Toxicities include severe nausea and vomiting after dosing and damage to pancreatic beta cells that is manifested by hypoglycemia and glucose intolerance. Streptozocin can cause nephrotoxicity, but marrow suppression and hepatic toxicity are only mild and transient. Anesthetic management for the acutely exposed patient involves close monitoring of glucose levels; chronically exposed patients should be assessed for glucose metabolism and renal function.

5. Triazenes (Dacarbazine)

A metastatic melanoma drug, dacarbazine is used as a single agent, or in combination with doxorubicin, bleomycin, and vinblastine in the "ABVD" regimen, to treat Hodgkin's disease. The toxicities of dacarbazine include severe nausea and vomiting, myelosuppression with thrombocytopenia, and phototoxicity. Rare cases of hepatic vascular damage, which can be fatal, have been described.[204] Dacarbazine may augment the cardiotoxicity of adriamycin.[205] Anesthetic considerations for this agent include evaluation for thrombocytopenia and for evidence of cardiotoxicity after combination chemotherapy.

B. ANTIMETABOLITES

Antimetabolites are structurally similar to biologically necessary molecules, such as vitamins (e.g., methotrexate, folic acid) or nucleosides (e.g., thioguanine, guanine). By masquerading as essential molecules, antimetabolites substitute for "normal" molecules, creating abnormal products, *or* they compete with normal molecules at important catalytic or enzyme regulatory sites. As a rule, antimetabolites are thought to be less oncogenic than most chemotherapeutic drugs, and rarely are given as single agents. Like the alkylating agents, several of the antimetabolites (6-mercaptopurine, cytosine arabinoside, azathioprine, and 6-thioguanine) have been linked with HVOD. The presentation, prognosis, and management of HVOD are covered in the section on alkylating agents.

1. Folate Analogs (Methotrexate)

Methotrexate is a folic acid analog that acts as an inhibitor of dihydrofolate reductase, the enzyme that converts dihydrofolate to tetrahydrofolate. Decreased tetrahydrofolate limits the synthesis of thymidine and purine, whereas the presence and build-up of methotrexate and dihydrofolate also inhibit synthesis of thymidine and purine. Both thymidine and purine are essential for the synthesis of DNA. Leucovorin (a tetrahydrofolate analog) may be used as rescue therapy from the effects of methotrexate.

Methotrexate is a very versatile agent used to treat both cancer and autoimmune disorders. Aside from the myelosuppression, nausea, and vomiting common with this and other chemotherapeutic agents, methotrexate results in significant pulmonary, neurologic, and hepatic toxicity. Pulmonary toxicity results in desquamative interstitial hypersensitivity pneumonitis in as many as 8 per cent of patients treated with chemotherapeutic doses. This reaction is similar to that noted for procarbazine, cyclophosphamide, and, rarely, bleomycin.[206] There are no known risk factors; oxygen therapy is not thought to increase the risk of pneumonitis. There does not appear to be a dose-response relationship, although toxicity is rare with weekly doses smaller than 20 mg. Management includes cessation of chemotherapy with administration of steroids Mortality is less than 1 per cent.[207] Development of chronic pulmonary fibrosis is

rare.[208] A fulminant noncardiogenic edema with methotrexate has also been described,[209] even when it is administered via the intrathecal route.[210, 211] Possible anesthetic considerations include the need to assess the pulmonary function of symptomatic patients. Anesthesia is often necessary for immobilization of children for intrathecal chemotherapy. Fulminant pulmonary reactions, while rare, can complicate the recovery of these patients.

Methotrexate-induced neurotoxicity involves both the brain and the spinal cord. Brain involvement may be acute, subacute, or chronic.[212] Acute neurotoxicity appears to be limited to large-dose intravenous therapy and results in somnolence and confusion, which rapidly resolves over time.[213] Subacute toxicity presents over weeks, with symptoms of demyelination. This syndrome reverses over a period of weeks and may resolve more quickly with steroids.[214] Chronic toxicity develops months or years after the completion of either intravenous or intrathecal methotrexate therapy. Injury to brain white matter results in progressive loss of cognitive function, onset of focal neurologic symptoms, and dementia. Cranial radiation therapy and the use of combined intravenous and intrathecal chemotherapy increases the risk of chronic neuropathy.[215] There are no reports in the literature about administration of anesthesia to these patients; however, baseline somnolence may exaggerate the response to anesthetics.

Spinal cord toxicity is manifested as progressive myelopathy, occurring weeks or months after intrathecal therapy. These patients may develop a denervation lesion or peripheral weakness.[216] A common side effect of intrathecal treatment with methotrexate is the development, in 60 per cent of patients, of meningeal irritation within hours of therapy.[217] This is manifested by headache, meningismus, nausea, and lethargy. A hyperacute form of the myelopathy described above may also occur in this setting as a paraplegia, which resolves over some months.[218] Significant meningeal symptoms or paraplegia can complicate the postprocedure course of patients receiving intrathecal chemotherapy under anesthesia.

Hepatotoxicity is common after methotrexate therapy: elevated liver function test results typically occur 1 to 2 weeks after therapy.[219] Hepatic fibrosis occurs in 30 per cent of patients. Rarely, these patients develop cirrhosis.[220] Preexisting liver disease appears to prolong recovery of the liver after methotrexate exposure. Anesthetic considerations include limitation of hepatically metabolized agents.

2. Pyrimidine Analogs

a. 5-Fluorouracil

Pyrimidine nucleotides include uracil, cytosine, and thymidine. An analogue of uracil, 5-fluorouracil (5-FU) interferes with RNA processing and function, indirectly interrupting DNA synthesis and repair. 5-FU is used to treat a variety of cancers, including adenocarcinomas of the gastrointestinal tract and squamous cell cancers. It is commonly used in combination with other agents. A major concern with this agent is cardiac and neurotoxicity (the latter does not appear to have any anesthetic implications). In a review of 1000 patients, myocardial ischemia was demonstrated near the time of infusion of 5-FU in 4.5 per cent of those with previously known coronary disease, and in 1 per cent of those without previously known coronary disease.[221] The proposed risk period is from 3 hours to 1 week after administration of 5-FU.[222] The cause of ischemia is not known. Anesthetic implications include the evaluation of patients for this history, including those whose age would otherwise preclude them from developing myocardial ischemia.

b. Fluorodeoxyuridine

Floxuridine (FUdR) is an analog of 5-FU that is used almost solely for intraarterial hepatic infusion for isolated liver metastases. FUdR can be expected to have the same toxicity as 5-FU. No direct anesthetic implications for this agent have been noted in the literature; however, these patients are prone to biliary sclerosis if multiple cycles are used.

c. Cytarabine

Cytarabine (ara-C) is a cytosine analog that inhibits the formation of DNA. It is used in the treatment of acute nonlymphoblastic (myelocytic) leukemia and of chronic myelogenous leukemia. Ara-C may produce neurotoxicity, pulmonary toxicity, and hepatic toxicity. Large doses can result in cerebellar toxicity that presents acutely and usually resolves with withdrawal of ara-C.[223] This syndrome presents as ataxia, dysarthria, and nystagmus; may occur in some 8 to 20 per cent of pa-

tients; and may represent a loss of Purkinje cells in the cerebellum.[224] Patients treated with ara-C can develop encephalopathy and a leukoencephalopathy indistinguishable from that seen after methotrexate therapy.[225] Ara-C can result in myelopathy that presents acutely after intrathecal administration.[226] The anesthetic considerations include the need to alter the dose of anesthetic agents for patients affected with encephalopathy. In addition, acute myelopathy may complicate the immediate postprocedure course in a patient given anesthesia for intrathecal chemotherapy.

Acute, noncardiogenic dose-related pulmonary edema has been described for ara-C, that immediately follows the onset of high-dose systemic chemotherapy.[227] This toxicity is not exacerbated by oxygen therapy and produces no permanent effects. Ara-C results in elevated liver enzymes and has been associated with HVOD (see section on HVOD with alkylating agents).[228]

d. Azacitidine

Azacitidine is an experimental chemotherapeutic that is used in the therapy of nonlymphoblastic leukemia. Nausea, vomiting, and myelosuppression are common side effects. Data on other toxic effects are limited, although both hepatotoxicity and neuromuscular side effects (weakness, lethargy, muscle pain) have been described.

3. Purine Analogs

a. Mercaptopurine

The purine nucleotides include adenine and guanine. Mercaptopurine (6-MP) is a purine analog that interferes with purine synthesis. This agent is used for maintenance therapy of acute leukemias and as an immunosuppressant. The toxic effects of 6-MP include myelosuppression, nausea, vomiting, fever, pancreatitis, and hepatotoxicity. Hepatotoxicity occurs in some 10 to 40 per cent of patients, resulting in cholestasis and parenchymal necrosis.[229] Routine monitoring of hepatic enzymes is elemental to treatment with this agent. As noted above, this agent may be associated with HVOD. Anesthetic considerations include evaluation for hepatic injury and avoidance of hepatic toxins.

b. Thioguanine

Thioguanine (6-TG) is a guanine analog that interferes with purine synthesis. A metabolite of thioguanine is incorporated into DNA, resulting in strand breakage and contributing to cytotoxicity. Thioguanine is used to treat acute, nonlymphoblastic leukemia. Toxicity of this agent is limited to myelosuppression and, occasionally, hepatotoxicity, which is manifested by elevations in liver enzymes and cholestasis. In general, 6-TG manifests less hepatotoxicity and fewer gastrointestinal side effects than 6-MP. This agent may be associated with HVOD. Anesthetic considerations are the same as those for 6-mercaptopurine.

c. Pentostatin and Cladribine

Pentostatin (2'-deoxycoformycin, DCF) is an adenosine analog produced by a *Streptomyces* species. It functions as potent inhibitor of adenosine deaminase and may be a chemical means of producing the clinical effects seen with severe combined immunodeficiency syndrome. It is used principally to treat hairy cell leukemia. Toxicity from this agent is manifested in virtually every system, on a dose-dependent basis. At high doses (e.g., 10 mg/m per day) myelosuppression, immunosuppression, nausea and vomiting, severe renal dysfunction, cardiotoxicity (manifested by arrhythmias, neurotoxicity, and pulmonary toxicity) may occur.[230] At smaller doses (e.g., 4 mg/m^2 per day) that are typically used to treat hairy cell leukemia, toxic effects are mild. Unfortunately, relatively limited and anecdotal data are available on the effects of this agent. At this time, patients with a history of exposure to large doses of this agent should be carefully evaluated for toxicity in every system and appropriate alterations in anesthetic technique should be undertaken. No other specific recommendations are available at this time.

Cladribine is an adenosine analog that interferes with both DNA and RNA synthesis. It is used in the treatment of hairy cell leukemia, non-Hodgkin's lymphoma, and acute and chronic nonlymphocytic leukemias. Except for severe myelosuppression, cladribine has few toxic effects.

d. Fludarabine

Fludarabine is an adenosine analog that inhibits enzymes necessary for DNA synthesis and repair. It has been used in the treatment of chronic lymphocytic leukemia, Hodgkin's and non-Hodgkin's lymphomas. Complications with anesthetic considerations are limited to rare reports of pneumonitis. Data are limited on this issue.

C. PLANT DERIVATIVES

Many of the commonly used antineoplastic agents are plant derivatives. The systematic screening of plant, fungal, bacterial, and marine animal compounds is likely to yield more useful compounds in the future.

1. Vinca Alkaloids

a. Vincristine

Vincristine is a large plant alkaloid that binds to tubulin, interrupting spindle fiber formation and causing mitotic arrest. It is employed in the therapy of acute lymphoblastic leukemia, Hodgkin's and non-Hodgkin's disease, and several of the pediatric tumors. It is often used in combination with cyclophosphamide and dactinomycin. There are several interactions between vincristine and other chemotherapeutic drugs. The only interaction of interest to anesthesiologists is that vincristine may decrease the oral bioavailability of digoxin. The most clinically significant toxicities of vincristine are neurotoxicity and pulmonary toxicity. Neurologic toxicity presents most often as peripheral neuropathy, although the drug can affect the cranial nerves.[231, 232] This effect is correlated with the cumulative dose of drug, and results initially in a loss of deep tendon reflexes, followed by deep sensorimotor polyneuropathy, particularly in the stocking-glove distribution. Autonomic neuropathy, presenting as ileus or orthostatic hypotension, and isolated cranial nerve palsies may also occur. Rare central nervous system toxicity resulting in encephalopathy and coma have been described.[233]

Pulmonary toxicity is rare and is severe only when chemotherapy involves the combination of mitomycin with vincristine. This effect presents with infiltrates and responds to drug withdrawal. Oxygen therapy does not appear to exacerbate this toxicity (see Table 16–11).

b. Vinblastine

Vinblastine is similar to vincristine in its actions and indications. It is commonly given in the "ABVD" combination with doxorubicin, bleomycin, and dacarbazine for Hodgkin's disease, and in the "VPB" combination with cisplatin and bleomycin for nonseminomatous germ cell tumors. The toxicity of vinblastine is essentially the same as for vincristine (see above), although neurotoxicity is generally less severe and myelosuppression is generally greater. Acute bronchospasm has been noted with vinblastine in patients recently exposed to mitomycin C.[234]

c. Other Vinca Alkaloids

Vindesine and navelbine are relatively new agents which are expected to have similar toxicity profiles to vinblastine and vincristine. No specific data on these agents are available at this time.

2. Epipodophyllotoxins

Podophyllotoxin is extracted from the mandrake plant (May apple), *Podophyllum peltatum*, and was used as an herbal remedy by the North American Indians and early colonists. Two podophyllotoxin derivatives, etoposide (VP-16) and teniposide (VM-26), are frequently used as chemotherapeutic drugs today.

Both of these podophyllotoxin derivatives result in DNA strand breakage. They both commonly result in myelosuppression, nausea and vomiting, and occasional anaphylactoid reactions. Peripheral neuropathy is rare and reversible with cessation of these agents. There are rare reports of the administration of teniposide resulting acutely in a noncardiogenic pulmonary edema.[235]

3. Taxol and Its Analogs (Paclitaxel, Taxotere)

Taxol is an antimitotic drug that is isolated from the bark of the western yew tree, *Taxus brevifolia.* Taxol is used against malignant melanoma and carcinoma of the ovary. Toxicity includes myelosuppression and sensory neuropathy.

Paclitaxel is an analog of Taxol, also derived from the western yew tree. Both Taxol and paclitaxel bind to tubulin (at a site distinct from that of the vinca alkaloids) resulting in arrest of cell mitosis. Paclitaxel is a relatively novel agent that has been difficult to derive in sufficient quantities for therapeutic use. Clinical experience is relatively limited, although this agent has shown promise in the treatment of advanced ovarian and breast cancers. Aside from myelosuppression and nausea and vomiting with acute administration, there is some evidence of cardiotoxicity. Both ventricular tachycardia and atrioventricular block have occasionally been described in patients exposed to this agent, whereas one third of patients develop sinus bradycardia alone.[236] The full nature of cardiac effects, including effects on ventricular function, has not been studied. As for all patients exposed to novel agents, anesthesia for these patients should be undertaken with a high index of suspicion for the unusual.

Taxotere is another analog of Taxol with the same proposed mechanism of action. Indications for this agent are still under investigation. There is no known cardiotoxicity for this agent, although a syndrome of peripheral edema and pleural effusions has been described.[237] As with paclitaxel, anesthesia for patients exposed to taxotere should be undertaken with caution.

D. ANTINEOPLASTIC ANTIBIOTICS

The systematic evaluation of the products of various bacteria and fungi has yielded a wide variety of antineoplastic agents. The anthracyclines, known for their potential for cardiotoxicity, are rhodomycins, or colored products, from *Streptomyces* species. Bleomycin, dactinomycin, and mithramycin are similarly products of *Streptomyces* species. All have potency against eukaryotic systems, and are thus toxic to both tumor and normal cell lines. The relative selectivity of toxicity is due to different cell growth rates and minor increased vulnerability of neoplasms to the effects of these agents.

1. Anthracyclines

a. Doxorubicin (Adriamycin)

Doxorubicin is an anthracycline glycoside antibiotic that (1) intercalates between DNA base pairs, resulting in strand breakage, (2) inhibits topoisomerase II, and (3) leads to the formation of free radicals, with resulting disruption of DNA and RNA synthesis. The former two effects are thought to be responsible for the majority of this agent's chemotherapeutic value, whereas the latter effect is thought to be responsible for this agent's cardiotoxicity.[238] Doxorubicin is employed in an exceptionally large number of cancer regimens for treatment of hematologic malignancies, solid organ tumors, sarcomas, and epidermoid carcinomas.

Doxorubicin is a significant cardiotoxin, manifested primarily as congestive heart failure. Toxicity is dose dependent: the prevalence of clinical congestive heart failure is 7 to 15 per cent at doses of 450 to 500 mg/m².[239] Prospective studies involving close observation suggest that the incidence of congestive heart failure at a dose of 450 mg/m² may approach 25 per cent (Fig. 16–7).[240] At doses above 450 to 500 mg/m² the incidence of congestive heart failure rises precipitously. A number of risk factors may predispose to the development of congestive heart failure. These include age over 70, a history of contractile dysfunction, previous myocardial infarction, concomitant treatment with cyclophosphamide, dacarbazine or mitomycin C, radiation therapy to the thorax (greater than 2000 rads), and factors that predispose to the development of organic heart disease, including diabetes and hypertension.[241] Children may be more sensitive than adults to the toxic effects of doxorubicin. Anthracycline may reduce cardiac growth, and produce structural or functional damage which may only become manifest as growth outpaces a fixed cardiac capacity.[242, 243] Factors that increase

cardiac stress, including drug use, pregnancy, and weight lifting, may predispose to the late development of cardiac toxicity.[244] Myocardial toxicity presents in a continuum, cumulative dose being the best predictor of the onset of damage.

The best initial sign of impending congestive heart failure is the onset of resting sinus tachycardia. Other arrhythmias may follow, but they are typically secondary to congestive heart failure. The pathophysiology of anthracycline cardiotoxicity is thought to involve primarily free radical formation, the generation of which is catalyzed by the presence of free ferric ions. This has led to clinical trials involving coadministration of an iron chelator (dexrazoxane or ICRF-187) with doxorubicin, with favorable results. While onset of congestive heart failure usually occurs within several months of anthracycline therapy, in the pediatric population it may present as late as 6 to 10 years after treatment.[245, 246] Once present, congestive heart failure may worsen and progress to death, may remain stable, or may reverse over time.

Given the significant impact of risk factors, the use of chelators, and intersubject variability, it is no longer adequate to assume toxicity or lack of toxicity based solely on a set cumulative dose. To optimize cancer therapy while limiting cardiotoxicity, oncologists monitor the effects on the myocardium of increasing doses of anthracyclines, the goal being to "push the limit," providing as much chemotherapeutic agent as possible. The result of this emerging practice, in terms of the effects on long-term toxicity, has not been established. The best means of assessing myocar-

FIGURE 16–7. Doxorubicin (adriamycin) total dosage versus probability of congestive heart failure. The risk of congestive heart failure increases significantly once a total dose of 450 mg/m² body surface area is administered to a patient. More than 50 per cent of patients have congestive heart failure once a total dose of 1000 mg/m² is administered. (From Von Hoff DD, Layard MW, Basa P, et al: Risk factors for doxorubicin-induced congestive heart failure. Ann Intern Med 9:710–717, 1979.)

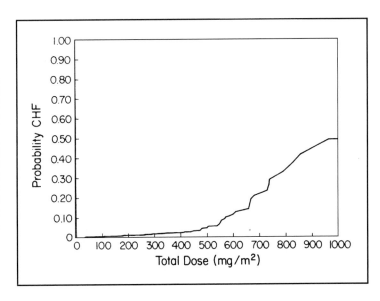

dial damage involves right heart biopsy, which correlates well with clinical examination and is highly specific.[247] Among noninvasive tests, the gated radionuclide scan provides an excellent assessment of ejection fraction, with good longitudinal prognostic value. In the pediatric population, these tests are not as useful and may not be practical. Serial echocardiography is often used instead in the evaluation of children. Decreases in left ventricular ejection fraction of 10 to 20 per cent compared to the initial study triggers discontinuation of therapy. This protocol is based on the assumption that a decrease in left ventricular ejection fraction precedes congestive heart failure, and that stopping therapy before congestive heart failure may limit damage to the myocardium.

Given the variability of risk factors, individual subjects, and dose regimens, as well as the potentially delayed presentation of cardiotoxicity, the anesthesiologist confronted with a patient with a history of exposure to doxorubicin must perform a thorough cardiac evaluation, up to and including the use of echocardiography or gated radionuclide scan.

b. Daunorubicin

An analog of doxorubicin with a similar mechanism of action, daunorubicin is employed in the therapy of acute myelogenous leukemia and acute lymphocytic leukemia. Its cardiotoxicity is similar to doxorubicin, although at a somewhat different dose threshold. Congestive heart failure occurs in 1 per cent to 2 per cent of patients at a dose of up to 550 mg/m^2, increasing to 12 per cent in doses up to 1000 mg/m^2. As for doxorubicin, the pediatric population appears to be more sensitive to the effects of daunorubicin than adults.[248] Anesthetic considerations for this agent are the same as for doxorubicin.

c. Other Anthracyclines

There are a large number of anthracyclines, aside from doxorubicin and daunorubicin, that have been synthesized in an effort to limit cardiac toxicity without decreasing the antitumor effects of the parent compound. Mainly, there are only limited clinical data on the efficacy and toxicity of these agents, although some degree of cardiotoxicity appears to accompany the use of every anthracycline. These agents are idarubicin, epirubicin, esorubicin, carminomycin, marcellomycin, aclarno-

mycin A, and others. Until further clinical data become available, all anthracyclines should be regarded as potentially cardiotoxic, and all patients with a history of exposure to these agents should be evaluated accordingly.

2. Dactinomycin (Actinomycin D)

Dactinomycin (actinomycin D) is a product of *Streptomyces*, which intercalates between cytosine and guanine base pairs in DNA and inhibits RNA synthesis. It is used in the treatment of nephroblastoma, rhabdomyosarcoma, and Ewing's sarcoma, frequently in combination with vincristine, doxorubicin, and/or cyclophosphamide. Hepatic toxicity, particularly after radiation therapy, has been described and is occasionally severe. This agent has been associated with hepatic venoocclusive disease (see the section on HVOD and alkylating agents above). Hepatic toxicity is manifested as elevated liver enzymes, ascites, and hepatomegaly. Anesthetic considerations include making appropriate alterations in the dosing of hepatically metabolized agents.

3. Plicamycin (Mithramycin)

Plicamycin is an antibiotic product of a *Streptomyces* species that forms complexes with DNA, inhibiting RNA synthesis. It has a direct effect on osteoclasts that results in a significant decrease in serum calcium levels and has been employed in the therapy of hypercalcemia when used at less than tumoricidal doses. It is otherwise employed in larger doses for therapy of disseminated, refractory germ cell tumors. Plicamycin is a severely toxic drug, resulting in nausea, vomiting, and myelosuppression. It has a significant effect on the coagulation system owing to its capacity for inducing thrombocytopenia and decreasing the level of clotting factors. It may result in significant hepatic toxicity, with elevations in liver enzymes and renal toxicity. Upon discontinuation of this agent, rebound hypercalcemia may be manifested. Anesthetic management involves the careful monitoring of serum calcium, and the appropriate adjustment of doses in the event of hepatic or renal insufficiency. Coagulation deficits should be assessed and managed with replacement therapy if indicated.

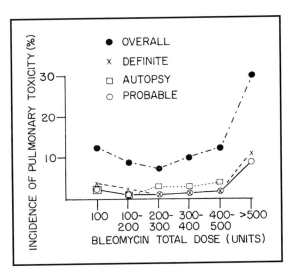

FIGURE 16–8. Risk of pulmonary toxicity and cumulative bleomycin dosage. The risk of pulmonary toxicity increases significantly once a total dose of 400 units is received by the patient. (From Ginsberg SJ, Comis RL: The pulmonary toxicity of antineoplastic agents. Semin Oncol 9(1):34–51, 1982.)

4. Bleomycin

Bleomycin is an antibiotic product of *Streptomyces* species that is a mixture of several sulfur-containing glycopeptides. They function principally by binding to DNA, with resulting strand damage and ultimate inhibition of DNA synthesis. The variable tissue distribution of this agent accounts in part for its efficacy and toxicity. It is mainly distributed to the skin, lungs, kidney, peritoneum, and lymph nodes, but not to the bone marrow. The primary utility of bleomycin is in the therapy of testicular cancers, Hodgkin's disease, diffuse lymphomas, and squamous cell cancers. It is used in some centers for intracavitary treatment of malignant pleural effusions.

The most significant toxicity of bleomycin is pulmonary toxicity (see Table 16–11). Toxicity may occur in one of three forms: as an acute IgE-mediated hypersensitivity reaction, similar to that seen with cyclophosphamide, methotrexate, and procarbazine.[249, 250] Another form of toxicity is an acute pulmonary venous vasculitis with resultant pulmonary hypertension. This toxicity has been demonstrated after carmustine and mitomycin exposure as well. Whether this is a variation on the more common alveolar bleomycin toxicity or occurs through a different mechanism is not known.

A third (and most worrisome) pulmonary toxicity is dose-dependent chronic pneumonitis, with or without progressive fibrosis. The tendency for bleomycin to produce pulmonary toxicity may be due to the distribution of bleomycin to this organ, combined with the relative lack in pulmonary tissue of an inactivating enzyme.[251, 252] Bleomycin results in direct injury to the pulmonary capillary endothelium, followed by injury to the type I and type II pneumocytes. Progressive fibrosis of the alveolar capillary membrane sets in, with a significant decrease in diffusion capacity and the onset of a restrictive lung pattern.[253] Toxicity may be partially caused by free radical formation, which may explain the tendency of oxygen therapy to worsen the effect of bleomycin toxicity.[254] The role of radiation in stimulating free radical formation may explain the potentiating effect of radiotherapy on bleomycin toxicity.[255] The finding of polymorphonuclear blood cells on bronchoalveolar lavage of affected patients has suggested that bleomycin may also act as a chemoattractant for white cells, which may damage the lung by the unconfined elaboration of free radicals.[256]

The likelihood of development of bleomycin pulmonary toxicity is related to several risk factors, the most important being the total cumulative dose of bleomycin. The risk of toxicity is approximately 5 per cent at doses up to 400 units but increases exponentially at higher doses (Fig. 16–8).[257] Toxicity has been noted at doses as low as 100 units, although the presence of other risk factors is considered to have contributed to these cases.[258] Other risk factors include advanced age, combination therapy with other toxins, including cyclophosphamide, chest irradiation (doses larger than 3300 rad), and smoking.[259]

Reports of postoperative complications, including death, among patients exposed to bleomycin first appeared in 1978.[260, 261] The prominent risk factor was initially thought to be oxygen therapy and excessive crystalloid administration, although subsequent studies have implicated only the former.[262–264] Some studies have questioned the role of oxygen therapy in the pathogenesis of bleomycin toxicity, although these studies have been poorly controlled for bleomycin dose and degree of exposure and are considered inconclusive.[265, 266] Given the current information, it is prudent to limit oxygen exposure to patients with a history of exposure to bleomycin. This may be challenging in the case of selective one-lung ventilation (e.g., in the excision of a lung cancer after bleomycin chemotherapy). A useful means of providing precisely controlled oxygen concentrations was described by Hughes and Benumof (Fig. 16–9).[267] The mortality of pulmonary toxicity from bleomycin is 10 per cent; oxygen therapy probably increases the mortality. Pulmonary toxicity may present over 1 year after the last dose of bleomycin. Precautions are therefore indicated for virtually any patient exposed to bleomycin.

As noted, bleomycin may be used as a sclerotic and chemotherapeutic agent for the treatment of malignant pleural effusions. In this scenario, as much as half of the dose may be absorbed systemically and may produce several acute side effects, including allergic reaction. Nausea, vomiting, and myelosuppression are rare with this agent, although desquamation of the skin may be seen. Most of the side effects of bleomycin are reversible, including pulmonary toxicity, although in unusual cases they may be permanent.

5. Mitomycin C

Mitomycin (or mitomycin C) is an antibiotic produced by a *Streptomyces* species that is effectively an alkylating agent. Mitomycin forms covalent bonds with DNA, forming crosslinks and inhibiting DNA synthesis. Part of this drug's effect may derive from the elaboration of oxygen free radicals. The principal activity of this agent is against solid tumors of the stomach, pancreas, colon, breast, lung, and cervix. It may also be used in intravesical therapy of bladder cancer. Significantly, mitomycin appears to significantly increase the degree of cardiotoxicity associated with the anthracyclines when these agents are administered in combination.

There are a number of toxic effects from mitomycin. Unique in its severity is profound myelosuppression with thrombocytopenia, which becomes more severe with cumulative doses. Microangiopathic hemolytic anemia, with renal dysfunction, anemia, and cardiopulmonary collapse is unique to this agent. Renal dysfunction and hepatic dysfunction with coagulopathy, by way of hepatic venoocclusive disease (see HVOD in the section on alkylating agents) have also been described.

Of greatest interest to anesthesiologists is interstitial pneumonitis induced by mitomycin. The mechanism of mitomycin-induced pneumonitis is not fully understood but is thought to be similar to the mechanism responsible for bleomycin-related pulmonary fibrosis (see above).[268] The incidence of pulmonary fibrosis does not appear to be dose related, although oxygen therapy and

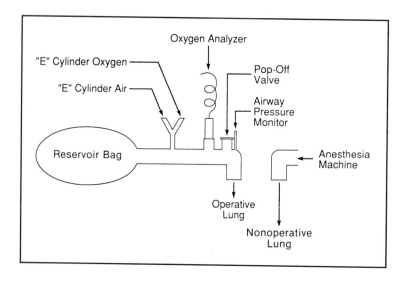

FIGURE 16–9. Schematic of mechanism used to provide a variable FIO$_2$ to the operative lung during continuous positive airway pressure (CPAP) while providing single-lung ventilation. Oxygen and room air tanks are connected by a Y piece leading to an FIO$_2$ analyzer; the FIO$_2$ analyzer is connected in series to a CPAP device consisting of a reservoir bag with pressure-release valve and a pressure manometer. (From Hughes S, Benumof JL: Use of operative CPAP to decrease FIO$_2$ during one-lung ventilation in a bleomycin-treated patient. Anesth Analg 71:92–95, 1990.)

thoracic irradiation are probably contributory.[269, 270] The overall incidence of fibrosis is 3 to 12 per cent with a mortality approaching 50 per cent.[271, 272] Oxygen concentrations are probably best limited for patients with a history of mitomycin exposure. Rare cases of mitomycin-associated pulmonary venous vasculitis have also been noted, similar to that seen with carmustine and bleomycin.[273]

6. Anthraquinones

Mitoxantrone is an anthraquinone (anthracycline analog) that was designed to have less cardiac toxicity than the anthracyclines.[274] Its activity is based primarily upon cross-linking between DNA, and it may also act by interrupting cell division by binding to cell structural proteins. It is used in the therapy of acute nonlymphoblastic leukemia, although with somewhat less activity than the anthracyclines. It is also efficacious in the treatment of breast and ovarian carcinoma. The most profound toxicity of mitoxantrone is myelosuppression, with mild thrombocytopenia.

Of greatest concern to anesthesiologists is the risk of cardiotoxicity with mitoxantrone therapy. Cardiotoxicity may involve relatively minor changes in ejection fraction with decreased voltages on ECG or may present with severe congestive heart failure. At equimyelotoxic doses, mitoxantrone produces less cardiotoxicity than doxorubicin.[275] The incidence of cardiotoxicity is approximately 5 per cent at doses greater than 160 mg/m^2. However, these agents are metabolized to less toxic agents by the liver. Thus, increased toxicity occurs with hepatic dysfunction. A history of cardiac dysfunction, exposure to anthracyclines, or radiation therapy to the thorax increases the risk of cardiotoxicity. Although the pathologic changes seen on endomyocardial biopsy are similar for mitoxantrone and the anthracyclines, the mechanisms are considered to be somewhat different.[276] ICRF-187, an agent that removes free iron from the anthracycline complex, inhibits free radical formation, and somewhat limits anthracycline-induced cardiotoxicity, has no apparent effect on mitoxantrone-related cardiotoxicity.[277] There may be mechanisms common to both agents that result in cardiotoxicity without the elaboration of free radicals. Mitoxantrone therapy, like anthracycline therapy, is generally titrated for maximum effect up to the first evidence of cardiotoxicity. Patients with a history of mitoxantrone therapy should be evaluated with either a multiple gated radionuclide scan or echocardiography for evidence of congestive heart failure before undergoing anesthesia.

E. IMMUNE MODIFIERS

1. Interferon Alfa

Several interferon types are used in the treatment of cancer. Several result in hypotension on infusion, although only interferon alfa has been associated with additional serious cardiac toxicity.[278] Interferon alfa is a glycoprotein derived from leukocytes that is used to treat Kaposi's sarcoma and hairy cell leukemia. The most common symptoms include a flulike illness with malaise, fevers, and chills. It may rarely result in cardiotoxicity with ischemia, arrhythmias, and cardiomyopathy.[279] Cardiotoxicity is not dose or duration dependent. A history of preexisting heart disease may be a risk factor for the development of cardiotoxicity. Relatively little information is available, and the clinician would be prudent to carefully evaluate the cardiac status of any patient with a history of exposure to interferon alfa.

2. Interleukin 2

Administration of interleukin 2 (IL-2) results in minor flulike symptoms in most patients, similar to those associated with interferon alfa. It may also result in a sepsislike picture, with hypotension, arrhythmias, and ischemia. Myocardial suppression may be evidenced by a decreased ejection fraction. These symptoms appear to be reversible by stopping administration of IL-2.[280, 281] Anesthetic considerations are limited to the acute period of administration of IL-2.

F. MISCELLANEOUS CHEMOTHERAPEUTIC DRUGS

1. Cisplatin

Cisplatin is an inorganic planar platinum complex that binds with DNA, altering the conformation of DNA and inhibiting its replication. Cisplatin can affect a large number of cellular functions, including the transport of amino acids, the sodium-potassium exchange pump, and calcium channels. It is among the most widely used agents, effective against testicular and ovarian carcinoma, squamous cell carcinomas, sarcomas, and neuroblastomas.

Renal toxicity is the most prominent side effect of cisplatin: dose-dependent acute impairment of renal function occurs within 3 days after administration as a result of a direct toxicity of the renal tubules and peaks 2 weeks after therapy.[282] Typically, renal function recovers over time, although additional cumulative doses may result in permanent renal damage. As a result of a specific tubular wasting defect, significant hypocalcemia and hypomagnesemia can occur.[283] Optimal management of cisplatin-induced acute tubular necrosis (ATN) involves prevention with hydration and administration of mannitol to maintain tubular flow. Anesthetic considerations include altering the dose of renally eliminated agents, administration of fluids to prevent ATN, and correction of magnesium and calcium deficits. Neuromuscular blockade, which may be prolonged by a decreased serum concentration of calcium and magnesium, may require more careful monitoring.

Cisplatin may be associated with hearing loss, peripheral neuropathy, and central demyelination. Careful attention to administration of neurotoxic agents, such as aminoglycoside antibiotics, is warranted.[284]

2. Carboplatin

Carboplatin is an analog of cisplatin that is 10 times more water soluble than cisplatin. It is used primarily in the treatment of ovarian carcinomas, although it has been used for lung and testicular cancers, pediatric brain tumors, and leukemia. In comparison with cisplatin, it is more myelosuppressive, but less neurotoxic, nephrotoxic, and emetogenic. Thrombocytopenia may be severe: as many as one third of all patients require platelet transfusions.[285] Carboplatin is frequently associated with magnesium wasting and occasionally with potassium, calcium, and sodium wasting. Hepatotoxicity may present as mild elevations in liver function tests. Neurotoxicity is uncommon. Anesthetic considerations include repleting magnesium before anesthesia, to avoid possible complications with prolonged neuromuscular blockade. Renal and hepatic function should be assessed and drug dosages appropriately modified.

3. Asparaginase

Asparaginase is an enzyme produced by bacteria, either *Escherichia coli* or *Erwinia carotovora*, which derives its antitumor efficacy from the absence in some tumor cells of the capacity to synthesize asparagine. Asparaginase is used for induction therapy of acute lymphoblastic leukemia. The toxic effects of asparaginase are related either to an allergic reaction or to inhibition of protein synthesis. Allergic reaction is the most common side effect of asparaginase exposure, occurring in as many as 20 to 30 per cent of patients. This side effect is managed by standard antiallergic therapy, although it may result in anaphylaxis and require a change in agent source from one bacterial preparation to another.[286]

Effects related to inhibition of protein synthesis are manifested in multiple organ systems. The inhibition of synthesis of fibrinogen, antithrombin III, protein C, and protein S may result in clotting or hemorrhagic complications.[287, 288] The decrease in anticoagulant factors precedes the decrease in procoagulants after asparaginase therapy; thrombotic complications are more likely to occur earlier.[289] This may result in thrombotic cerebrovascular events, including sagittal or central venous thrombosis. Neurologic findings include symptoms of elevated intracranial pressure with decreased level of consciousness.[290, 291] Therapy involves heparin, although antithrombin III infusion may be necessary for heparin to have an effect.[292] Decreased levels of asparagine or glutamine in the brain may be responsible for neuropsychiatric symptoms, occasionally as late as 2 weeks after administration, manifested by confusion, lethargy, delusions, and hallucinations.[293] Symptoms are reversible but may require several weeks to resolve.[294] Decreased serum insulin may present with hyperglycemia. Other toxicities include hepatotoxicity with fatty liver infiltration, elevation of liver enzymes, and, occasionally, death. Mild renal dysfunction also occurs occasionally, whereas myelosuppression is uncommon. Anesthetic considerations for patients exposed to this agent include the need for evaluation of neurologic, hepatic, and renal function. Clotting abnormalities should be assessed and resolved.

4. Procarbazine

Procarbazine is a hydrazine derivative that is structurally similar to the hydrazine monoamine oxidase inhibitors phenelzine, isocarboxazid, and iproniazid. Its mechanism of action involves the elaboration of reactive compounds that directly damage DNA. It is used in the MOPP regimen for Hodgkin's disease (with mechlorethamine, vincristine, and prednisone) and in the COPP regimen for non-Hodgkin's lymphoma (with cyclophosphamide, vincristine, and prednisone). Procarbazine is notable for its large number of potential interactions with other drugs. Procarbazine potentiates the effect of other neurologically active drugs, including barbiturates, antihistamines, narcotics, and phenothiazines. As a weak monoamine oxidase inhibitor, this agent may interact with indirect-acting sympathomimetics and tyramine-containing food sources.[295, 296] This agent also produces a disulfiram-like reaction to ethanol.

The toxicity of procarbazine includes neurologic symptoms of paresthesias, lethargy, and neuropathies. Myelosuppression is common, thrombocytopenia being most prominent, occurring up to 6 weeks after therapy. Rarely, administration of procarbazine may be followed within hours to days by an acute pulmonary hypersensitivity reaction manifested by interstitial infiltrates and a pleural effusion. Peripheral eosinophilia is prominent. This reaction is similar to that seen with methotrexate, cyclophosphamide, and, rarely, bleomycin.[297] Management involves discontinuation of procarbazine. There is no evidence that oxygen exposure increases the risk of this toxicity.

Anesthetic considerations for patients exposed to procarbazine center on the many interactions of this agent with other drugs and assessment of neurologic impairment and coagulation function.

5. Amsacrine

Amsacrine (AMSA) is an aminoacridine that intercalates into DNA and inhibits DNA synthesis. It is a relatively new agent, having been introduced in the United States in 1982. This agent is employed in the therapy of acute myelogenous leukemia. It has significant toxicity resulting in myelosuppression, nausea, and vomiting. Although long-term toxicity data are not available for this agent, it appears to have significant cardiotoxic effects. On initial infusion, the rapid administration of this agent has been associated with ventricular arrhythmias, especially in the presence of hypokalemia. Decreased ejection fraction has also been noted after amsacrine therapy; however, since most regimens involve treatment with anthracyclines, the cause of cardiac complications is difficult to establish. Since amsacrine has been associated with prolongation of the QT interval, therapy should be postponed until the potassium value has been confirmed to be normal.[298, 299] Hepatotoxicity and neurotoxicity are unusual but have been reported. Early data permit no conclusions, although anesthetic considerations for patients exposed to this agent include careful cardiac assessment. Since the propensity for prolonged ventricular arrhythmogenesis is not known, it is prudent to maintain a normal serum potassium concentration in patients exposed to potentially arrhythmogenic circumstances (e.g., surgery, sympathetic discharge with exposure with halothane).

6. Mitotane

Mitotane is an analog of the common insecticide DDT. It is a highly specialized agent that blocks adrenal cortical function by inhibiting mitochondrial metabolism and is used in the palliation of adrenal cortical tumors. Mitotane inhibits corticosteroid metabolism; and the development of adrenocortical insufficiency necessitates glucocorticoid and mineralocorticoid replacement. It may also result in neurologic symptoms, with pronounced neurologic depression when administered with other CNS depressants. Principal anesthetic considerations center on the need for corticosteroid replacement therapy, particularly in physiologically stressful circumstances, and the need to titrate CNS depressants carefully to effect.

7. Hydroxyurea

Hydroxyurea is an inhibitor of ribonucleotide reductase, which ultimately results in inhibition of DNA synthesis and repair. It is employed principally in the treatment of chronic myelogenous leukemia and squamous cell carcinomas. The major toxicities of this agent are myelosuppression with leukopenia and thrombocytopenia. Nephrotoxicity

TABLE 16–13

Specific Antidotes for Toxic Substances

Toxin	Antidote	Dose and/or Notes
Acetaminophen	N-Acetylcysteine	140 mg/kg PO followed by 70 mg/kg PO for 17 doses
Anaphylaxis	Epinephrine, antihistamine, fluid, steroids	
Arsenic, mercury, lead	BAL (dimercaprol), D-penicillamine	
Anticholinergic poisoning	Physostigmine	Examples: *Datura stramonium* (thorn apple), belladonna (deadly nightshade), Jimson weed
Benzodiazepines	Flumazenil	Flumazenil may trigger seizures
Cholinergic insecticides, carbamates, and organophosphates	Atropine and pralidoxime	Generally, pralidoxime is necessary only for organophosphates
Coumadin	Vitamin K_1	10 mg IM × 3 days (for hepatic failure FFP is necessary)
Cocaine	GABA antagonist; benzodiazepine, cooling	Avoid succinylcholine, beware concomitant organophosphates
Calcium channel blockers	Calcium chloride, calcium gluconate	AV node action of calcium channel blocker still active despite administration of CaCl
Carbon monoxide	Oxygen, hyperbaric oxygen	Hyperbaric therapy for severe cases
Cyanide	Cyanide antidote kit: Amyl nitrite ampule, sodium nitrite 3% solution, sodium thiosulfate 25% solution	Inhaled 30 seconds of each minute, new ampule every 3 minutes; 0.33 ml/kg IV; 1.7 ml/kg IV
Digoxin	Fab antibody fragments	Magnesium sulfate and potassium repletion for dysrhythmia control
Dystonic reactions	Diphenhydramine	For antipsychotic drugs (i.e., phenothiazines)
Envenomations	Specific antivenin	Skin test prior; be prepared with epinephrine prior to skin test.
Hydrogen sulfide	Oxygen, nitrites	
Iron	Desferrioxamine	
Isoniazid (INH)	Pyridoxine (vitamin B_6), GABA agonists	
Nonethanol alcohols (Ethylene glycol isopropanol, methanol)	Ethanol, 4-methylpyrazole, pyridoxine, folate, thiamine, multivitamins	Ethanol competes with alcohol dehydrogenase, decreasing formic acid production
Methemoglobin	Methylene Blue	Methemoglobin is produced by nitrites, nitrates, anilines, phenacetin, sulfonamides, and prilocaine
Opiates	Naloxone	Titrate to effect, beginning with small doses .01–.04 mg at a time, escalating to 2 mg and continuing larger doses for severe opiate intoxication
Sympathomimetics	Adrenergic blockers	
Strychnine	Benzodiazepines, for seizure control	
Ingested toxins	Activated charcoal	See Table 16–2 to determine utility
Tricyclic antidepressants	Alkalinization Magnesium sulfate (for prolonged Qt)	Magnesium for control of ventricular dysrhythmias

is occasionally seen but is mild. Neurologic complications are rarely seen. There are no major anesthetic considerations for patients exposed to this agent. The major commonly occurring toxic substances and their corresponding antidotes are summarized in Table 16–13.

VII. ANESTHETIC CONSIDERATIONS FOR THE PATIENT WHO HAS UNDERGONE RADIATION THERAPY

Radiation therapy results in injury to many structures. Of primary interest to anesthesiologists are the effects of radiation on the airway and on the pulmonary and cardiac systems.

A. EFFECTS OF RADIATION THERAPY ON THE AIRWAY

Irradiation of the head and neck may substantially affect the ability to secure the airway. The acute response to radiation involves edema of the mucosa with subsequent fibrosis of the involved tissues.[300] Fibrosis may progress over time, become stable, or diminish; a history of easy intubation after or recently associated with radiation therapy is a poor predictor of subsequent intubation conditions. Progressive fibrosis following surgery may compound radiation-induced tissue immobility, markedly worsening the patient's airway. Anesthetic management involves careful assessment of the airway by established techniques, proceeding with anesthesia only after a means of definitively securing the airway has been established.

B. EFFECTS OF RADIATION THERAPY ON THE PULMONARY SYSTEM

The direct effects of radiation therapy are manifested over time in an acute, intermediate, and chronic manner.[301, 302] Acute effects seen almost immediately after therapy starts consist of exudation of proteinaceous material into the alveoli with acute impairment of gas exchange. Inflammatory cells infiltrate alveo-

lar walls, and fibrin is deposited. Over several weeks, intermediate changes are seen, with organization of fibrosis within the alveolar septa and thickening with decreased alveolar oxygen–blood interface. These changes may resolve over weeks, or they may progress to a chronic phase of toxicity. Over several months, progressive fibrosis of alveoli with thickening results in obliteration of gas exchange surfaces. Blood flow to affected regions of the lung becomes markedly diminished, and, depending on the degree of overall ventilation, ventilation-perfusion mismatch may appear.[303] Objective findings on pulmonary function tests include decreased diffusion capacity and oxygenation and a restrictive pattern on dynamic flow studies.

The incidence and severity of radiation pneumonitis have changed markedly with fractionation of total doses into larger numbers of smaller doses and slower administration of radiation during treatment. The overall incidence of pneumonitis varies with previous exposure to chemotherapeutics, total dose, port size, and degree of fractionation.[304, 305] Overall, the incidence of radiation pneumonitis may be as high as 5 to 15 percent for total lung irradiation with a moderate dose. Anesthetic considerations include evaluation of overall lung function via pulmonary function tests. In the event that surgery on the lung is considered, the effect of radiation on the obliteration of the pulmonary vascular bed with increases in pulmonary artery pressure should be considered. It may be necessary to monitor pulmonary artery pressures during excision.

Aside from its direct effects on the pulmonary system, radiation is known to potentiate the toxicity of chemotherapeutics, notably bleomycin, busulfan, and mitomycin.

C. EFFECTS OF RADIATION THERAPY ON THE CARDIOVASCULAR SYSTEM

Radiation therapy involving the heart has undergone significant advances in recent years that are designed to limit the degree of injury to the myocardium. These measures include shielding the cardiac silhouette and applying radiation equally anteriorly and posteriorly.[306] Unfortunately, cardiac shielding is a relatively new technology, and many patients may present for surgery who have not had the benefit of this technology.

Virtually every portion of the heart is affected by radiation. The most severe effects appear to be on the pericardium. In a group of 16 patients who received 3500 rad, all patients had pericardial damage.[307] This is manifested by a pericardial effusion that develops over several days and that over several months may become constrictive. In one study, as many as 15 per cent of patients who received 4000 rad developed constrictive pericarditis.[308] Patients may present with a fixed filling capacity and elevated right heart pressures.

Fibrosis that involves the endomyocardial tissue takes more time to present, at several months after therapy. Fibrosis presents with conduction abnormalities, restrictive cardiomyopathy, and papillary muscle damage with mitral valve dysfunction. Fibrosis may involve the coronary arteries, with the development of occlusive disease. The acute injury to the endothelium of the coronary arteries is plaquelike but lacks the high lipid component of plaques characteristic of atherosclerosis. Coronary vessels are more severely affected proximally with significant loss of the media.

Radiation damage to the heart may present many years after initial therapy. In a study of 81 patients, 11 per cent were symptomatic of constrictive myocardial disease. Six of these patients had constrictive pericarditis, while the other three were considered to have a constrictive myocarditis.[309, 310] The overall incidence of myocardial disease is probably less than was previously seen because of cardioprotective techniques; however, given the delayed and prolonged presentation of many of these patients, anesthetic evaluation of myocardial function and awareness of the incidence of constrictive disease are elemental to their safe management.

REFERENCES

1. Pagel W: Philippus Aureolus Theophrastus Bombastus von Hohenheim-Paracelsus (1493–1541): An Introduction to Philosophical Medicine in the Era of the Renaissance. New York, Karger, 1958.
2. Guyton AC: Textbook of Medical Physiology, ed 8. Philadelphia, W.B. Saunders, 1991.
3. Merigian KS, et al: Prospective evaluation of gastric emptying in self-poisoned patients. Am J Emerg Med 8:479–483, 1990.
4. Goulbourne KB, et al: Small-bowel obstruction secondary to activated charcoal and adhesions. Ann Emerg Med 24:108–109, 1994.
5. Wood JD, Watson WJ: Gamma aminobutyric acid levels in the brain of rats exposed to oxygen at high pressure. Can J Biochem Physiol 41:1907, 1963.
6. Klein J: Normobaric pulmonary oxygen toxicity. Anaesth Analg 70:195–207, 1990.
7. Risberg B, Smith L, Ortenwall P: Oxygen radicals and lung injury. Acta Anaesthesiol Scand 35:106–118, 1991.
8. Fridovich I, Freeman B: Antioxidant defenses in the lung. Ann Rev Physiol 48:693–702, 1986.
9. Heffner JE, Repine JE: Pulmonary strategies of antioxidant defense. Am Rev Respir Dis 140:531–554, 1989.
10. Phan SH, Gannon DE, Varani J, et al: Xanthine oxidase activity in rat pulmonary artery endothelial cells and its alteration by activated neutrophils. Am J Pathol 134:1201–1211, 1989.
11. Lucchesi BR, Werns SW, Fantone JC: The role of the neutrophil and free radicals in ischemic myocardial injury. J Molec Cell Cardiol 21:1241–1251, 1989.
12. Halliwell B, Gutteridge J: Free Radicals in Biology and Medicine. New York, Oxford University Press, 1985.
13. Heffner JE, Repine JE: Antioxidants and the lung. In Crystal RG, West JB (eds): The Lung: Scientific Foundations, Vol. II. New York, Raven Press, 1991, pp. 1811–1820.
14. Sznajder JI, Fraiman A, Hasll JB: Increased hydrogen peroxide in the expired breath of patients with acute hypoxemic respiratory failure. Chest 96:606–612, 1989.
15. Martin WJ II, Gadek JE: Oxidant injury of lung parenchymal cells. J Clin Invest 68:1277–1288, 1981.
16. Ryan SF: Acute alveolar injury: Experimental models. In Gill J (ed): Models of Lung Disease: Microscopy and Structural Methods. New York, Marcel Dekker, 1990, pp. 641–733.
17. Demling R, Lalonde C, Seekamp A, et al: Endotoxin causes hydrogen peroxide–induced lung lipid peroxidation and prostanoid production. Arch Surg 123:1337–1341, 1988.
18. Milligan SA, Hoeffel JM, Goldstein IM: Effect of catalase on endotoxin-induced acute lung injury in unanesthetized sheep. Am Rev Respir Dis 137:420–428, 1988.
19. Warren JS, Johnson KJ, Ward PA: Consequences of oxidant injury. In Crystal RG, West JB (eds): The Lung: Scientific Foundations, vol II. New York, Raven Press, 1991, pp. 1829–1838.
20. Stothert JC Jr, Basadre JO, Herndon D, et al: Conjugated diene production after airway acid aspiration. Prog Clin Biol Med Res 299:69–74, 1989.
21. Clement A, Chandelat K, Masliah J, et al: A controlled study of oxygen metabolite release by alveolar macrophages from children with interstitial lung disease. Am Rev Respir Dis 136:1424–1428, 1987.
22. Kaelin RM, Lapance Y, Tschoop JM: Diffuse interstitial lung disease associated with hydrogen peroxide inhalation in a dairy worker. Am Rev Respir Dis 137:1233–1235, 1988.
23. Allison RC, Kyle J, Adkins KW, et al: Effect of ischemia reperfusion or hypoxia reoxygenation on lung vascular permeability and resistance. J Appl Physiol 69:597–603, 1990.
24. Lynch MJ, Grum CM, Gallagher KP, et al: Xanthine oxidase inhibition attenuates ischemic-reperfusion lung injury. J Surg Res 1988;44:538–544.
25. Klausner JM, Paterson IS, Kobzik L, et al: Oxygen free radicals mediate ischemia-induced lung injury. Surgery 105:192–199, 1989.
26. Detterbeck FC, Keagy BA, Paull DE, et al: Oxygen free radical scavengers decrease reperfusion injury

in lung transplantation. Ann Thorac Surg 50:204–210, 1990.

27. Horgan MJ, Lum H, Malik AB: Pulmonary edema after pulmonary artery occlusion and reperfusion. Am Rev Respir Dis 140:1421–1428, 1989.

28. Kennedy TP, Rao NV, Hopkins C, et al: Role of reactive oxygen species in reperfusion injury of the rabbit lung. J Clin Invest 83:1326–1335, 1989.

29. Klausner JM, Paterson IS, Goldman G, et al: Thromboxane A_2 mediates increased pulmonary microvascular permeability following limb ischemia. Circulation Res 64:1178–1189, 1989.

30. Anner H, Kaufman RP Jr, Kobzik L, et al: Pulmonary leukosequestration induced by hind limb ischemia. Ann Surg 206:162–167, 1987.

31. Klausner JM, Paterson IS, Goldman G, et al: Interleukin-2–induced lung injury is mediated by oxygen free radicals. Surgery 109:169–175, 1991.

32. Grosso MA, Brown JM, Viders DE, et al: Xanthine oxidase–derived oxygen radicals induce pulmonary edema via direct endothelial cell injury. J Surg Res 46:355–360, 1989.

33. Martin WJ II: Neutrophils kill pulmonary endothelial cells by a hydrogen-peroxide–dependent pathway. Am Rev Respir Dis 130:209–213, 1984.

34. Clark JM: Pulmonary limits of oxygen tolerance in man. Exp Lung Res 14:897–910, 1988.

35. Montgomery AB, Luce JM, Murray JF: Retrosternal pain is an early indicator of oxygen toxicity. Am Rev Respir Dis 139:1548–1550, 1989.

36. Merritt JC, Sprague DH, Merritt WE, et al: Retrolental fibroplasia: A multifactorial disease. Anesth Analg 60:109, 1981.

37. Flynn JT: Oxygen and retrolental fibroplasia: Update in challenge. Anesthesiology 60:397, 1984.

38. Dorsch JA, Dorsch SE: Understanding Anesthesia Equipment, ed 3. Baltimore, Williams & Wilkins, 1994, pp. 195–198.

39. Ehrenwerth J, Eisenkraft JB: Anesthesia Equipment: Principles and Practice. St. Louis, Mosby-Year Book, 1993, pp. 97–99.

40. Lauria JI: Soda-lime dust contamination of breathing circuits. Anesthesiology 42:628–629, 1975.

41. Fang ZX, Eger EI 2nd, Laster MJ, et al: Carbon monoxide production from degradation of desflurane, enflurane, isoflurane, halothane, and sevoflurane by soda lime and Baralyme. Anesth Analg 80:1187–1193, 1995.

42. Baum J, Sachs G, von Driesch C, et al: Carbon monoxide generation in carbon dioxide absorbents. Anesth Analg 81:144–146, 1995.

43. Gonsowski CT, Laster MJ, Eger EI 2nd, et al: Toxicity of compound A in rats. Effect of a 3-hour administration. Anesthesiology 80:556–565, 1994.

44. Frink EJ Jr, Malan TP, Morgan SE, et al: Quantification of the degradation products of sevoflurane in two CO_2 absorbants during low-flow anesthesia in surgical patients. Anesthesiology 77:1064–1069, 1992.

45. Brown BR Jr, Frink EJ: The safety of sevoflurane in humans [letter; comment]. Anesthesiology 79:201–202; discussion 202–203, 1993.

46. Fang ZX, Kandel L, Laster MJ, et al: Factors affecting production of Compound A from the interaction of sevoflurane with Baralyme and soda lime. Anesth Analg 82:775–781, 1996.

47. Penny DG: Acute carbon monoxide poisoning: Animal models: A review. Toxicology 62:123–160, 1990.

48. Barker SJ, Tremper KK: The effect of carbon monoxide inhalation on pulse oximetry and transcutaneous PO_2. Anesthesiology 66:677–679, 1987.

49. Gonzalez A, Gomez-Arnau J, Pensado A: Carboxyhemoglobin and pulse oximetry. Anesthesiology 73:573, 1990.

50. Schelble DT: Phosphine and phosgene. In Haddad LM, Winchester JF (eds): Clinical Management of Poisoning and Drug Overdose, ed 2. Philadelphia, W.B. Saunders, 1990, pp. 1235–1240.

51. Lorin HG, Kulling PEJ: The Bhopal Tragedy—What has Swedish disaster medicine planning learned from it? J Emerg Med 4:311–316, 1986.

52. McMullen MJ, Hetrick TJ, Cannon LA: Ammonia, nitrogen, nitrous oxides, and related compounds. In Haddad LM, Winchester JF (eds): Clinical Management of Poisoning and Drug Overdose, ed 2. Philadelphia, W.B. Saunders, 1990, pp. 1270–1279.

53. Horvath EP, doPico GA, Barbee RA, et al: Nitrogen dioxide–induced pulmonary disease. J Occup Med 20:103–110, 1978.

54. Westfelt UN, Lundin S, Stenqvist O: Safety aspects of delivery and monitoring of nitric oxide during mechanical ventilation. Acta Anaesthesiol Scand 40:302–310, 1996.

55. Morrow PE: Toxicology data on NOx: An overview. J Toxicol Environ Health 13:205–227, 1984.

56. Haggerty MA, Soto-Green M, Reichan LB: Caring for victims of toxic gas inhalation. J Crit Illness 2:77–87, 1987.

57. Froner GA, Rutherford GW, Rokeach M: Injection of sodium hypochlorite by intravenous drug users. JAMA 258:325, 1987.

58. Szerlip HM, Singer I: Hyperchloremic metabolic acidosis after chlorine inhalation. Am J Med 77:581–582, 1984.

59. Stair T: Chlorine. In Haddad LM, Winchester JF (eds): Clinical Management of Poisoning and Drug Overdose, ed 2. Philadelphia, W.B. Saunders, 1990.

60. Reisz GR, Gammon RS: Toxic pneumonitis from mixing household cleaners. Chest 89:49–52, 1986.

61. Christel D, Eyer P, Hegemann M, et al: Pharmacokinetics of cyanide poisoning in dogs, and the effects of 4-dimethylaminophenol or thiosulphate. Arch Toxicol 38:177–189, 1977.

62. Isom GE, Way JL: Effects of oxygen on the antagonism of cyanide intoxication: Cytochrome oxidase, in vitro. Toxicol Appl Pharmacol 74:57–62, 1984.

63. Robin ED, McCauley R: Nitroprusside-related cyanide poisoning time (long past due) for urgent, effective interventions. Chest 102:1842–1845, 1992.

64. Mohammed-Ali H: Spatschaden der Giftgaswirkung bei den Überlebenden des irakischen Giftgaskrieges gegen das kurdische Volk. Wien Med Wochschr 142:8–15, 1992.

66. Stewart CE, Sullivan JB: Military munitions and antipersonnel agents. In Sullivan JB, Krieger GR (eds): Hazardous Material Toxicology. Baltimore, Williams & Wilkins, 1992, pp. 986–1014.

67. Graham DR: Tear gas and riot control agents. In Haddad LM, Winchester JF (eds): Clinical Management of Poisoning and Drug Overdose, ed 2. Philadelphia, W.B. Saunders, 1990, pp. 1253–1256.

68. Beswick FW: Chemical agents used in riot control and warfare. Hum Toxicol 2:247–256, 1983.

69. Stewart CE, Sullivan JB: Military munitions and antipersonnel agents. In Sullivan JB, Krieger GR, (eds): Hazardous Material Toxicology. Baltimore, Williams & Wilkins, 1992, pp. 986–1014.

70. Sidell FR: Clinical considerations in nerve agent in-

toxication. In Somani SM (ed): Chemical Warfare Agents. New York, Academic, 1992, pp. 155–194.

71. Somani SM, Solana RP, Dube SN: Toxicodynamics of nerve agents. In Somani SM (ed): Chemical Warfare Agents. New York, Academic Press, 1992, pp. 67–123.

72. Graham DR: Solvent abuse. In Haddad LM, Winchester JF (eds): Clinical Management of Poisoning and Drug Overdose, ed 2. Philadelphia, W.B. Saunders, 1990, pp. 1256–1260.

73. Bass M: Sudden sniffing death. JAMA 212:2075–2079, 1970.

74. Watson JM: Solvent abuse: Presentation and clinical diagnosis. Hum Toxicol 1:249–256, 1982.

75. Szara S: Marijuana. In Haddad LM, Winchester JF (eds): Clinical Management of Poisoning and Drug Overdose, ed 2. Philadelphia, W.B. Saunders, 1990, pp. 737–748.

76. Hollister LE: Health aspects of cannabis. Pharmacol Rev 38:1–20, 1986.

77. Gong H, Fligiel S, Tashkin DP, et al: Tracheobronchial changes in habitual, heavy smokers of marijuana with and without tobacco. Am Rev Respir Dis 136:142–149, 1987.

78. Brookoff D, Campbell E, Shaw L: The underreporting of cocaine-related trauma: Drug abuse warning network versus hospital toxicology test. Am J Pub Health 83:369–371, 1993.

79. Personal communication: Robert S. Hoffman, Director, New York City Poison Control Center. Assistant Professor of Clinical Surgery and Emergency Medicine, New York University School of Medicine, New York, New York.

80. Bernards CM, Teijeiro A: Illicit cocaine ingestion during anesthesia. Anesthesiology 84:218–220, 1996.

81. Jatlow P, Barash PG, VanDyke C, et al: Cocaine and succinylcholine sensitivity: A new caution. Anesth Analg 58:235–238, 1979.

82. Flemming JA, Byck R, Barash PG: Pharmacology and theraputic applications of cocaine. Anesthesiology 73:518–531, 1990.

83. Hershmann Z, Aaron C: Prolongation of cocaine effect. Anesthesiology 74:631–632, 1991.

84. Proudfoot AT: Salicylates and salicylamide. In Haddad LM, Winchester JF (eds): Clinical Management of Poisoning and Drug Overdose, ed 2. Philadelphia, W.B. Saunders, 1990, pp. 909–920.

85. Hillman RJ, Prescott LF: Treatment of salicylate poisoning with repeated oral charcoal. Br Med J 291:1472–1480, 1985.

86. Jacobson D, Wiik-Larson E, Bredesen JE: Haemodialysis or hemoperfusion in severe salicylate poisoning? Hum Toxicol 7:161–171, 1988.

87. De Kock M, Henin D, Gautier M: The endogenous digoxin-like factor enhances bupivacaine toxicity in rats. Reg Anesth 18:369–373, 1993.

88. Cohen L, Kitzes R: Magnesium sulfate and digitalis—toxic arrhythmias. JAMA 249:2808, 1983.

89. Cohen L, Kitzes R: Magnesium sulfate and digoxin—toxic arrhythmias. JAMA 249:2808, 1983.

90. Antman EM, Wenger TL, Butler VP Jr, et al: Treatment of 150 cases of life-threatening digitalis intoxication with digoxin specific Fab antibody fragments: Final report of a multicenter study. Circulation 81:1744, 1990.

91. Ujhelyi MR, Colucci RD, Cummings DM, et al: Monitoring serum digoxin concentrations during digoxin immune Fab therapy. Drug Intell Clin Pharm 25:1047, 1991.

92. Kinlay S, Buckley NA: Magnesium sulfate in the treatment of ventricular arrhythmias due to digoxin toxicity. J Toxicol Clin Toxicol 33:55–59, 1995.

93. Winchester JF: Lithium. In Haddad L, Winchester JF (eds): Clinical Management of Poisoning and Drug Overdose, ed 2. Philadelphia, W.B. Saunders, 1990, pp. 656–665.

94. Groleau G: Lithium toxicity. Emerg Med Clin North Am 12:511–531, 1994.

95. Nagaraja D, Taly AB, Sahu RN, et al: Permanent neurological sequelae due to lithium toxicity. Clin Neurol Neurosurg 89:31, 1987.

96. Salama AA: Complete heart block associated with mesorideazine and lithium combination. J Clin Psychiatry 48:123, 1987.

97. Barclay ML, Brownlie BE, Turner JG, et al: Lithium can cause goitre and hypothyroidism. Lithium associated thyrotoxicosis: A report of 14 cases, with statistical analysis of incidence. Clin Endocrinol 40:759–764, 1994.

98. Dietrich A, Mortensen ME, Wheller J: Cardiac toxicity in an adolescent following chronic lithium and imipramine therapy. J Adolescent Health 14:394–397, 1993.

99. Kazim S, Townsley L, Hughes NK, et al: Lithium and anti-viral drug toxicity: II. Further studies on the ability of lithium to modulate the hematopoietic toxicity associated with the anti-viral drug zidovudine (AZT). Rom J Physiol 30:231–239, 1993.

100. Finley PR, Warner MD, Peabody CA: Clinical relevance of drug interactions with lithium. Clin Pharmacokinet 29:172–191, 1995.

101. Okusa MD, Crystal LJ: Clinical manifestations and management of acute lithium intoxication. Am J Med 97:383–389, 1994.

102. Truwit JD: Toxic effects of bronchodilators. Crit Care Clin 7:639–657, 1991.

103. Marshall JB, Forker AD: Cardiovascular effects of tricyclic antidepressant drugs: Therapeutic usage, overdose, and management of complications. Am Heart J 103:404–414, 1982.

104. Dec WG, Stern TA: Tricyclic antidepressants in the ICU patient. J Intensive Care Med 5:69–78, 1990.

105. Frommer DA, Kulig KW, Marx JA, et al: Tricyclic antidepressant overdose: An overview. JAMA 257:521, 1987.

106. Pelouze M, Bernard C: Recherches sur le curare. C R Acad Sci 533, 1850.

107. McIntyre AR: Historical background, early use and development of muscle relaxants. Anesthesiology 20:410–415, 1959.

108. McKiernan TL, Bock K, Leya F, et al: Ergot induced peripheral vascular insufficiency, noninterventional treatment. Cathet Cardiovasc Diagn 31:211–214, 1994.

109. McKenna DJ, Nazarali AJ, Hoffman AJ, et al: Common receptors for hallucinogens in rat brain: A comparative autoradiographic study using ^{125}I LSD and ^{125}I DOI, a new psychomimetic radioligand. Brain Res 476:45–56, 1989.

110. Scatizzi A, Di Maggio A, Rizzi D, et al: Acute renal failure due to tubular necrosis caused by wildfowl-mediated hemlock poisoning. Renal Fail 15:93–96, 1993.

111. Frank BS, Michelson WB, Panter KE, et al: Ingestion of poison hemlock (*Conium maculatum*). West J Med 163:573–574, 1995.

112. Bowman WC, Sanghvi IS: Pharmacological actions of hemlock (*Conium maculatum*) alkaloids. J Pharm Pharmacol 15:1–25, 1963.

113. SM Shepherd, Jagoda AS: Phencyclidine and the hallucinogens. In Haddad LM, Winchester JF (eds): Clinical Management of Poisoning and Drug Overdose, ed 2. Philadelphia, W.B. Saunders, 1990, pp. 749–780.

114. Jaeger A, Jehl F, Flesch F, et al: Kinetics of amatoxins in human poisoning: Therapeutic implications. Clin Toxicol 31:63–80, 1993.

115. Stollard D, Edes TE: Muscarinic poisoning from medications and mushrooms. Postgrad Med 85:341–345, 1989.

116. Mills AR, Passmore R: Pelagic paralysis. Lancet 1:161–164, 1988.

117. Lewis RJ, Holmes MJ: Origin and transfer of toxins involved in ciguatera. Comp Biochem Physiol C (Engl) 106:615–628, 1993.

118. Watters MR: Organic neurotoxins in seafoods. Clin Neurol Neurosurg 97:119–124, 1995.

119. Tetrodotoxin poisoning associated with eating puffer fish transported from Japan—California, 1996. MMWR 45:389–391, 1996.

120. Russell F: Toxic effects of animal toxins. In Klaassen CD (ed): Casanet and Doul's Toxicology. ed 5. New York, McGraw-Hill, 1996.

121. Katz AR, Terrell-Perica S, Sasaki DM: Ciguatera on Kauai: Investigation of factors associated with severity of illness. Am J Trop Med Hyg 49:448–454, 1993.

122. Barton ED, Tanner P, Turchen SG, et al: Ciguatera fish poisoning. A southern California epidemic. West J Med 163:31–35, 1995.

123. Di Nubile MJ, Hokama Y: The ciguatera poisoning syndrome from farm-raised salmon. Ann Intern Med 122:113–114, 1995.

124. Habermehl GG, Krebs HC, Rasoanaivo P, et al: Severe ciguatera poisoning in Madagascar: A case report. Toxicon (Engl) 32:1539–1542, 1994.

125. Swift AE, Swift TR: Ciguatera. J Toxicol Clin Toxicol 31:1–29, 1993.

126. Cameron J, Flowers AE, Capra MF: Modification of the peripheral nerve disturbance in ciguatera poisoning in rats with lidocaine. Muscle 16:782–786, 1993.

127. Biddard JN, Vijverberg HPM, Frelin C, et al: Ciguatoxin is a novel type of Na⁺ channel toxin. J Biol Chem 259:8353–8357, 1984.

128. Taylor P: Anticholinesterase agents. In Goodman A, Gilman A, Rall T, et al (eds): Goodman and Gilman's The Pharmacological Basis of Therapeutics, ed 8. New York, Pergamon Press, 1990.

129. Wilson IB, Ginsburg S: A powerful reactivator of alkyl phosphate–inhibited acetylcholinesterase. Biochem Biophys Acta 18:168–170, 1955.

130. Lieber CS: Liver adaptation and injury in alcoholism. N Engl J Med 288:356–361, 1973.

131. Saitz R, Mayo-Smith MF, Roberts MS, et al: Individualized treatment for alcohol withdrawal. JAMA 272:519–523, 1994.

132. Linnanvuo-Laitinen M, Huttunen K: Ethylene glycol intoxication. Clin Toxicol 24:167, 1986.

133. Jacobson D, Steinar O, Ostborg J, et al: Glycolate causes the acidosis in ethylene glycol poisoning and is effectively removed by hemodialysis. Acta Med Scand 216:409, 1984.

134. Pons CA, Custer RP: Acute ethylene glycol poisoning: A clinicopathologic report of eighteen fatal cases. Am J Med Sci 211:544, 1946.

135. Gabow PA, Clay K, Sullivan JB, et al: Organic acids in ethylene glycol intoxication. Ann Intern Med 105:16, 1986.

136. Pamplin CL, Desjardins R, Chulay J, et al: Pharmacokinetics of antimony during sodium stibogluconate therapy for cutaneous leishmaniasis. Clin Pharmacol Ther 29:270–271, 1981.

137. Winship KA: Toxicity of antimony and its compounds. Adv Drug Reactions Acute Poison Rev 2:67–90, 1987.

138. Robtham JL, Lietman PS: Acute iron poisoning. Am J Dis Child 134:875, 1980.

139. Tenenbein M: Iron poisoning. In Rippe JM, Irwin RS, Fink MP, et al (eds): Intensive Care Medicine, ed 3. Boston, Little, Brown, 1996.

140. Houeto P, Sandouk P, Baud FJ, et al: Elemental mercury vapour toxicity: treatment and levels in plasma and urine. Hum Exp Toxicol 13:848–852, 1994.

141. Meyers RL, Glenn L, Orlando RC: Protection against alkali injury to rabbit esophagus by CO₂ inhalation. Am J Physiol 264:150–156, 1993.

142. Oakes DD: Reconsidering the diagnosis and treatment of patients following ingestion of liquid lye. J Clin Gastroenterol 21:85–86, 1995.

143. Snyder CC. Animal bite wounds. Hand Clin 5:571–590, 1989.

144. Goldstein EJC, Citron DW, Wield B, et al: Bacteriology of human and animal bite wounds. J Clin Microbiol 8:677, 1978.

145. Tami TA, Parker GS. *Eikenella corrodens*—an emerging pathogen in head and neck infections. Arch Otolaryngol 110:752, 1984.

146. Christopher DG, Rodning CB: Crotalidae envenomation. South Med J 79:159–162, 1986.

147. Karalliede L: Animal toxins. Br J Anaesth 74:319–327, 1995.

148. Dolly JO: Biochemistry of acetylcholine receptors from skeletal muscle. In Tipton KF (ed): International Review of Biochemical, Physiological and Pharmacological Biochemistry 26:257. Baltimore, University Park Press, 1979.

149. Heidmann T, Changeux JP: Structural and functional properties of the acetylcholine receptor protein in its purified and membrane-bound states. Annu Rev Biochem 47:371, 1978.

150. Raftery MA, Hunkapiller MW, Strader CD, et al: Acetylcholine receptor: A complex of homologous subunits. Science 208:1454, 1980.

151. Lee CY, Chang CC, Chin TH: Pharmacological properties of cardiotoxin isolated from Formosan cobra venom. Naunyn-Schmiedebergs Arch Pharmacol 259:360–374, 1968.

152. Viger JR, Glynn MFX. Ancrod (Arvin) as an alternative to heparin anticoagulation for cardiopulmonary bypass. Anesthesiology 71:870–877, 1989.

153. Tiwari I, Johnston WJ. Blood coagulability and viper envenomation. Lancet 1:613–614, 1986.

154. Hasiba U, Rosenbach LM, Rockwell D, et al: DIC-like syndrome after envenomation by the snake *Crotalus horridus horridus*. N Engl J Med 292:505–507, 1975.

155. Dickinson CE, Trub-Dargatz JL, Dargatz DA, et al: Rattle snake venom poisoning in horses: 32 cases 1973–93. J Am Vet Med Assoc 208:1866–1871, 1996.

156. Whitley RE: Conservative treatment of copperhead snake bites without antivenin. J Trauma 41:219–221, 1996.

157. Tu AT: Biotoxicology of sea snake venoms. Ann Emerg Med 16:1023–1028, 1987.

158. Russell FE, Carlson RW, Wainschel J, et al: Snake venom poisoning in the United States: Experiences with 550 cases. JAMA 233:341, 1975.

159. Russell FE, Bogert CM: Gila monster, its biology, venom and bite: A review. Toxicon 19:341, 1981.

160. Daly JW, Garraffo HM, Spande TF: Amphibian alkaloids. Alkaloids 43:186–190, 1993.

161. Daly JW: Biologically active alkaloids from poison frogs (Dendrobatidae). J Toxicol Toxin Rev 1:33–86, 1982.

162. Abogadie FC, Mena EE, Woodward SR, et al: Diversity of conus neuropeptides. Science 249:251–264, 1990.

163. Kumar EB, Soomvo RS, Hamdani A, et al: Scorpion venom cardiomyopathy. Am Heart J 123:725–729, 1992.

164. Gueron M, Ilia R, Sofer S: The cardiovascular system after scorpion envenomation. A review. Clin Toxicol 30:245–258, 1992.

165. Clark AW, Hurlbut WP, Mauro A: Changes in the finite structure of the neuromuscular junction of the frog caused by black widow spider venom. J Cell Biol 52:1–14, 1972.

166. Frontali N, Ceccarelli B, Gorio A, et al: Purification from black widow spider venom of a protein factor causing the depletion of synaptic vesicles at neuromuscular junctions. J Cell Biol 68:462–479, 1976.

167. Verheyden CN: Snakebite and spider bite. Hosp Physician 21–32, 1988.

168. King LE, Rees RS: Dapsone treatment of a brown recluse bite. JAMA 250:648, 1983.

169. Bochner BS, Lichtenstein LM: Anaphylaxis. N Engl J Med 324:1785–1790, 1991.

170. Ennik F: Deaths from bites and stings of venomous animals. West J Med 133:463–468, 1980.

171. Harvey AL, Anderson AJ, Rowman EG: Toxins affecting ion channels. In Harvey AL (ed): Natural and Synthetic Neurotoxins. London, Academic Press, 1993, pp. 129–163.

172. Schmidt JO: Allergy to *Hymenoptera* venoms. In Piek T (ed): Venoms of the Hymenoptera. London, Academic Press, 1986, pp. 509–546.

173. Donat JR, Donat JF: Tick paralysis with persistent weakness and electromyographic abnormalities. Arch Neurol 38:59–61, 1987.

174. Pearn J: Neuromuscular paralysis caused by tick envenomation. J Neurol Sci 34:37–42, 1977.

175. Doll DC, Ringenberg QS, Yarbro JW: Vascular toxicity associated with antineoplastic agents. J Clin Oncol 4:1405–1417, 1986.

176. Shulman HM, McDonald GB, Matthews D, et al: An analysis of hepatic venocclusive disease and centrilobular hepatic degeneration following bone marrow transplantation. Gastroenterology 79:1178–1191, 1980.

177. McDonald GB, Sharma P, Matthews DE, et al: Venoocclusive disease of the liver after bone marrow transplantation: Diagnosis, incidence, and predisposing factors. Hepatology 4:116–122, 1984.

178. D'Cruz CA, Wimmer RS, Harcke HT, et al: Venoocclusive disease of the liver in children following chemotherapy for acute myelocytic leukemia. Cancer 52:1803–1807, 1983.

179. Calabresi P, Chabner BA: Antineoplastic agents. In Goodman A, Gilman A, Rall TW, et al (eds): Goodman and Gilman's The Pharmacological Basis of Therapeutics, ed 8. New York, Pergamon Press, 1990.

180. Weiss RB: Hypersensitivity reaction to cancer chemotherapy. Semin Oncol 9:5–13, 1982.

181. Cooper JA Jr, White DA, Matthay RA: Drug-induced pulmonary disease. Part 1: Cytotoxic drugs. Am Rev Respir Dis 133:321–340, 1986.

182. Smith AC, Boyd MR: Preferential effects of 1,3-bis(2-chloroethyl)-1-nitrosourea (BCNU) on pulmonary glutathione reductase and glutathione/glutathione disulfide ratios: Possible implications for lung toxicity. J Pharmacol Exp Ther 229:658–663, 1984.

183. Freeman BA, Crapo JD: Biology of disease: Free radicals and tissue injury. Lab Invest 47:412–426, 1982.

184. Hakkinen PJ, Whiteley JW, Witschi HR: Hyperoxia, but not thoracic X-irradiation, potentiates bleomycin- and cyclophosphamide-induced lung damage in mice. Am Rev Respir Dis 126:281–285, 1982.

185. Stover DE: Adverse effects of treatment. In Devita VT, Hellman S, Rosenberg SA (eds): Cancer: Principles and Practice of Oncology, ed 3. Philadelphia, J.B. Lippincott, 1989, pp. 2166–2168.

186. Gottdiener JS, Appelbaum FR, Ferrans VJ, et al: Cardiotoxicity associated with high-dose cyclophosphamide therapy. Arch Intern Med 141:758–763, 1981.

187. Cazin B, Gorin NC, Laporte JP, et al: Cardiac complications after bone marrow transplantation. A report on a series of 63 consecutive transplantations. Cancer 57:2061–2069, 1986.

188. DeFronzo RA, Braine H, Colvin M, et al: Water intoxication in man after cyclophosphamide therapy. Time course and relation to drug activation. Ann Intern Med 78:861–869, 1973.

189. Lehne G, Lote K: Pulmonary toxicity of cytotoxic and immunosuppressive agents. A review. Acta Oncol 29(2):113–124, 1990.

190. Baker WJ, Fistel SJ, Jones RV, et al: Interstitial pneumonitis associated with ifosfamide therapy. Cancer 65:2217–2221, 1990.

191. Curtin JP, Koonings PP, Gutierrez M, et al: Ifosfamide-induced neurotoxicity. Gynecol Oncol 42:193–196, 1991.

192. Ginsberg SJ, Comis RL: The pulmonary toxicity of antineoplastic agents. Semin Oncol 9:34–51, 1982.

193. Giles FJ, Smith MP, Goldstone AH: Chlorambucil lung toxicity. Acta Haematol 83:156–158, 1990.

194. Teicher BA, Crawford JM, Holden SA, et al: Effects of various oxygenation conditions on the enhancement by fluosol-DA of melphalan antitumor activity. Cancer Res 47:5036–5041, 1987.

195. Howell SB, Pfeifle CE, Olshen RA: Intraperitoneal chemotherapy with melphalan. Ann Intern Med 101:14–20, 1984.

196. Cooper JA Jr, White DA, Matthay RA: Drug-induced pulmonary disease. Part 1: Cytotoxic drugs. Am Rev Respir Dis 133:321–340, 1986.

197. Peters WP, Henner WD, Grochow LB, et al: Clinical and pharmacologic effects of high dose single agent busulfan with autologous bone marrow support in the treatment of solid tumors. Cancer Res 47:6402–6406, 1987.

198. Perry MC: Hepatotoxicity of chemotherapeutic agents. Semin Oncol 9:65–74, 1982.

199. Weinstein AS, Diener-West M, Nelson DF, et al: Pulmonary toxicity of carmustine in patients treated for malignant glioma. Cancer Treat Rep 70:943–946, 1986.

200. Aronin PA, Mahaley MS Jr, Rudnick SA, et al: Prediction of BCNU pulmonary toxicity in patients with malignant gliomas: An assessment of risk factors. N Engl J Med 303:183–188, 1980.

201. Weiss RB, Muggia FM: Pulmonary effects of carmustine (bischloroethylnitrosourea, BCNU) [letter]. Ann Intern Med 91:131–132, 1979.

202. O'Driscoll BR, Hasleton PS, Taylor PM, et al: Active lung fibrosis up to 17 years after chemotherapy with carmustine (BCNU) in childhood. N Engl J Med 323:378–382, 1990.

203. Doll DC, Ringenberg QS, Yarbro JW: Vascular toxicity associated with antineoplastic agents. J Clin Oncol 4:1405–1417, 1986.

204. Feaux de Lacroix W, Runne U, Hauk H, et al: Acute liver dystrophy with thrombosis of hepatic veins: A fatal complication of dacarbazine treatment. Cancer Treat Rep 67:779–784, 1983.

205. Smith PJ, Ekert H, Waters KD, et al: High incidence of cardiomyopathy in children treated with adriamycin and DTIC in combination chemotherapy. Cancer Treat Rep 61:1736–1738, 1977.

206. Lehne G, Lote K: Pulmonary toxicity of cytotoxic and immunosuppressive agents. A review. Acta Oncol 29:113–124, 1990.

207. Zusman J, Frentz J, Waring W: Rapid resolution of "methotrexate lung" with preoperative steroids. Proc Am Assoc Cancer Res Am Soc Clin Oncol 20:412, 1979.

208. Sostman HD, Matthay RA, Putman CE, et al: Methotrexate-induced pneumonitis. Medicine 55:371–388, 1976.

209. Lascari AD, Strano AJ, Johnson WW, et al: Methotrexate-induced sudden fatal pulmonary reaction. Cancer 40:1393–1397, 1977.

210. Hamous JE, Guffy MM, Aschenbrener CA: Fatal acute respiratory failure following intrathecal methotrexate administration. Cancer Treat Rep 67:1025–1026, 1983.

211. Cooper JA, Zitnik R, Matthay RA: Mechanisms of drug-induced pulmonary disease. Annu Rev Med 39:395–404, 1988.

212. Gilbert M: Neurologic complications. In Abeloff MD, Armitage JO, Lichter AS, et al (eds): Clinical Oncology. New York, Churchill Livingstone, 1995.

213. Walker RW, Allen JC, Rosen G, et al: Transient cerebral dysfunction secondary to high-dose methotrexate. J Clin Oncol 4:1845–1850, 1986.

214. Bleyer WA: Neurologic sequelae of methotrexate and ionizing radiation. A new classification. Cancer Treat Rep 65(Suppl 1):89–98, 1981.

215. Ch'ien LT, Aur RJ, Verzosa MS, et al: Progression of methotrexate-induced leukoencephalopathy in children with leukemia. Med Pediatr Oncol 9:133–141, 1981.

216. Cohen ME, Duffner PK, Terplan KL: Myelopathy with severe structural derangement associated with combined modality therapy. Cancer 52:1590–1596, 1983.

217. Duttera MJ, Bleyer WA, Pomeroy TC, et al: Irradiation, methotrexate toxicity, and the treatment of meningeal leukemia. Lancet 2:703–707, 1973.

218. Gagliano RG, Costanzi JJ: Paraplegia following intrathecal methotrexate: Report of a case and review of the literature. Cancer 37:1663–1668, 1976.

219. Hersh EM, Wong VG, Henderson ES, et al: Hepatotoxic effects of methotrexate. Cancer 19:600–606, 1966.

220. Chabner BA, Donehower RC, Schilsky RL: Clinical pharmacology of methotrexate. Cancer Treat Rep 65(Suppl 1):51–54, 1981.

221. Labianca R, Beretta G, Clerici M, et al: Cardiac toxicity of 5-fluorouracil: A study on 1083 patients. Tumori 68:505–510, 1982.

222. Rinder CS: Cancer chemotherapy and its anesthetic implications. In Barash P, Cullen BF, Stoelting RK (eds): Clinical Anesthesia, ed 2. Philadelphia, JB Lippincott, 1992, pp. 1447–1464.

223. Grossman L, Baker MA, Sutton DM, et al: Central nervous system toxicity of high-dose cytosine arabinoside. Med Pediatr Oncol 11:246–250, 1983.

224. Winkelman MD, Hines JD: Cerebellar degeneration caused by high-dose cytosine arabinoside: A clinicopathological study. Ann Neurol 14:520–527, 1983.

225. Hwang TL, Yung WK, Estey EH, et al: Central nervous system toxicity with high-dose Ara-C. Neurology 35:1475–1479, 1985.

226. Dunton SF, Nitschke R, Spruce WE, et al: Progressive ascending paralysis following administration of intrathecal and intravenous cytosine arabinoside. A Pediatric Oncology Group study. Cancer 57:1083–1088, 1986.

227. Haupt HM, Hutchins GM, Moore GW: Ara-C lung: Noncardiogenic pulmonary edema complicating cytosine arabinoside therapy of leukemia. Am J Med 70:256–261, 1981.

228. Perry MC: Hepatotoxicity of chemotherapeutic agents. Semin Oncol 9:65–74, 1982.

229. Einhorn DI: Hepatotoxicity of 6-mercaptopurine. JAMA 188:802–806, 1964.

230. Chu E, Takamoto CH: Antimetabolites. In DeVita VT, Hellman S, Rosenberg SA (eds): Cancer: Principles and Practice of Oncology, ed 4. Philadelphia, J.B. Lippincott, 1993, pp. 358–374.

231. Gilbert M: Neurologic complications. In Abeloff MD, Armitage JO, Lichter AS, et al (eds): Clinical Oncology. New York, Churchill Livingstone, 1995.

232. Rosenthal S, Kaufman S: Vincristine neurotoxicity. Ann Intern Med 80:733–737, 1974.

233. Scheithauer W, Ludwig H, Maida E: Acute encephalopathy associated with continuous vincristine sulfate combination therapy: Case report. Invest New Drugs 3:315–318, 1985.

234. McDonald S, Missaillidou D, Rubin P: Pulmonary complications. In Abeloff MD, Armitage JO, Lichter AS, et al (eds): Clinical Oncology. New York, Churchill Livingstone, 1995.

235. Cooper JA Jr, White DA, Matthay RA: Drug-induced pulmonary disease. Part 1: Cytotoxic drugs. Am Rev Respir Dis 133:321–340, 1986.

236. Rowinsky EK, McGuire WP, Guarnieri T, et al: Cardiac disturbances during the administration of Taxol. J Clin Oncol 9:1704–1712, 1991.

237. Donehower RC, Rowinsky EK: Anticancer drugs derived from plants. In DeVita VT, Hellman S, Rosenberg SA (eds): Cancer: Principles and Practice of Oncology, ed 4. Philadelphia, J.B. Lippincott, 1993, pp. 358–374.

238. Speyer JL, Freedberg R: Cardiac complications. In Abeloff MD, Armitage JO, Lichter AS, et al (eds): Clinical Oncology. New York, Churchill Livingstone, 1995.

239. Schwartz RG, McKenzie WB, Alexander J, et al: Congestive heart failure and left ventricular dysfunction complicating doxorubicin therapy. Seven-year experience using serial radionuclide angiocardiography. Am J Med 82:1109–1118, 1987.

240. Von Hoff DD, Layard MW, Basa P, et al: Risk factors for doxorubicin-induced congestive heart failure. Ann Intern Med 91:710–717, 1979.

241. Minow RA, Benjamin RS, Lee ET, et al: Adriamycin cardiomyopathy—risk factors. Cancer 39:1397–1402, 1977.

242. Ali MK, Ewer MS: The natural history of anthracycline cardiotoxicity in children. In Muggia FM,

Green MD, Speyer JL (eds): Cancer Treatment and the Heart. Baltimore, Johns Hopkins University Press, 1992, pp. 146–155.

243. Gottdiener JS, Mathisen DJ, Borer JS, et al: Doxorubicin cardiotoxicity: Assessment of late left ventricular dysfunction by radionuclide cineangiography. Ann Intern Med 94 (4 pt 1):430–435, 1981.

244. Steinherz LJ, Graham T, Hurwitz R, et al: Guidelines for cardiac monitoring of children during and after anthracycline therapy: Report of the Cardiology Committee of the Children's Cancer Study Group. Pediatrics 89(5 Pt 1):942–949, 1992.

245. Steinherz LJ, Steinherz PG, Tan CT, et al: Cardiac toxicity 4 to 20 years after completing anthracycline therapy. JAMA 266:1672–1677, 1991.

246. Goorin AM, Chauvenet AR, Perez-Atayde AR, et al: Initial congestive heart failure, six to ten years after doxorubicin chemotherapy for childhood cancer. J Pediatrics 116:144–147, 1990.

247. Ewer MS, Ali MK, Mackay B, et al: A comparison of cardiac biopsy grades and ejection fraction estimations in patients receiving adriamycin. J Clin Oncol 2:112–117, 1984.

248. Speyer JL, Freedberg R: Cardiac complications. In Abeloff MD, Armitage JO, Lichter AS, et al (eds): Clinical Oncology. New York, Churchill Livingstone, 1995.

249. McDonald S, Missaillidou D, Rubin P: Pulmonary complications. In Abeloff MD, Armitage JO, Lichter AS, et al (eds): Clinical Oncology. New York, Churchill Livingstone, 1995.

250. Cooper JA, Zitnik R, Matthay RA: Mechanisms of drug-induced pulmonary disease. Annu Rev Med 39:395–404, 1988.

251. Ishizuka M, Takayama H, Takeuchi T, et al: Activity and toxicity of bleomycin. J Antibiotics 20:15–24, 1967.

252. Ohnuma T, Holland JF, Masuda H, et al: Microbiological assay of bleomycin: Inactivation, tissue distribution, and clearance. Cancer 33:1230–1238, 1974.

253. Cooper JA Jr, White DA, Matthay RA: Drug-induced pulmonary disease. Part 1: Cytotoxic drugs. Am Rev Respir Dis 133:321–340, 1986.

254. Oberley LW, Buettner GR: The production of hydroxyl radical by bleomycin and iron (II). Fed Exp Biol Soc 97:47, 1979.

255. Gross NJ: The pathogenesis of radiation-induced lung damage. Lung 159:115–125, 1981.

256. Wesselius LJ, Catanzaro A, Wasserman SI: Neutrophil chemotactic activity generation by alveolar macrophages after bleomycin injury. Am Rev Respir Dis 129:485–490, 1984.

257. Ginsberg SJ, Comis RL: The pulmonary toxicity of antineoplastic agents. Semin Oncol 9:34–51, 1982.

258. Iacovino JR, Leitner J, Abbas AK, et al: Fatal pulmonary reaction from low doses of bleomycin. An idiosyncratic tissue response. JAMA 235:1253–1255, 1976.

259. Waid-Jones MI, Coursin DB: Perioperative considerations for patients treated with bleomycin. Chest 99:993–999, 1991.

260. Goldiner PL, Carlon GC, Cvitkovic E, et al: Factors influencing postoperative morbidity and mortality in patients treated with bleomycin. Br Med J 1:1664–1667, 1978.

261. Allen SC, Riddell GS, Butchart EG: Bleomycin therapy and anaesthesia. The possible hazards of oxygen administration to patients after treatment with bleomycin. Anaesthesia 36:60–63, 1981.

262. Toledo CH, Ross WE, Hood CT, et al: Potentiation of bleomycin toxicity by oxygen. Cancer Treat Rep 66:359–362, 1982.

263. Tryka AF, Skornik WA, Godleski JJ, et al: Potentiation of bleomycin-induced lung by exposure to 70% oxygen: Morphologic assessment. Am Rev Respir Dis 126:1074–1079, 1982.

264. Tryka AF, Godleski JJ, Brain JD: Differences in effects of immediate and delayed hyperoxia exposure on bleomycin-induced pulmonary injury. Cancer Treat Rep 68:759–764, 1984.

265. Douglas MJ, Coppin CM: Bleomycin and subsequent anaesthesia: A retrospective study at Vancouver General Hospital. Can Anaesth Soc J 27:449–452, 1980.

266. LaMantia KR, Glick JH, Marshall BE: Supplemental oxygen does not cause respiratory failure in bleomycin-treated surgical patients. Anesthesiology 60:65–67, 1984.

267. Hughes SA, Benumof JL. Operative lung continuous positive airway pressure to minimize FIO_2 during one-lung ventilation. Anesth Analg 71:92–95, 1990.

268. McDonald S, Missaillidou D, Rubin P: Pulmonary complications. In Abeloff MD, Armitage JO, Lichter AS, et al (eds): Clinical Oncology. New York, Churchill Livingstone, 1995.

269. Orwoll ES, Kiessling PJ, Patterson JR: Interstitial pneumonia from mitomycin. Ann Intern Med 89:352–355, 1978.

270. Desidero D, Alegesan R, Fischer M, et al: Intraoperative FIO_2 and the development of mitomycin-induced post-operative interstitial pneumonitis. Anesthesiology 73:A1177, 1990.

271. Gunstream SR, Seidenfeld JJ, Sobonya RE, et al: Mitomycin-associated lung disease. Cancer Treat Rep 67:301–304, 1983.

272. Stover DE: Adverse effects of treatment. In DeVita VT, Hellman S, Rosenberg SA (eds): Cancer: Principles and Practice of Oncology, ed 3. Philadelphia, J.B. Lippincott, 1989, pp 2166–2168.

273. Doll DC, Ringenberg QS, Yarbro JW: Vascular toxicity associated with antineoplastic agents. J Clin Oncol 4:1405–1417, 1986.

274. Speyer JL, Freedberg R: Cardiac complications. In Abeloff MD, Armitage JO, Lichter AS, et al (eds): Clinical Oncology. New York, Churchill Livingstone, 1995.

275. Henderson IC, Allegra JC, Woodcock T, et al: Randomized clinical trial comparing mitoxantrone with doxorubicin in previously treated patients with metastatic breast cancer. J Clin Oncol 7:560–571, 1989.

276. Benjamin RS, Chawla SP, Ewer MS, et al: Evaluation of mitoxantrone cardiac toxicity by nuclear angiography and endomyocardial biopsy: An update. Invest New Drugs 3:117–121, 1985.

277. Green MD, Alderton P, Sobol MM, et al: ICRF-187 (ADR-529) cardioprotection against anthracycline-induced cardiotoxicity: Clinical and preclinical studies. Cancer Treat Res 58:101–117, 1991.

278. Speyer JL, Freedberg R: Cardiac complications. In Abeloff MD, Armitage JO, Lichter AS, et al (eds): Clinical Oncology. New York, Churchill Livingstone, 1995.

279. Sonnenblick M, Rosin A: Cardiotoxicity of interferon: A review of 44 cases. Chest 99:557–561, 1991.

280. Speyer JL, Freedberg R: Cardiac complications. In Abeloff MD, Armitage JO, Lichter AS, et al (eds): Clinical Oncology. New York, Churchill Livingstone, 1995.

281. Ognibene FP, Rosenberg SA, Lotze M, et al: Interleukin-2 administration causes reversible hemodynamic changes and left ventricular dysfunction similar to those seen in septic shock. Chest 94:750–754, 1988.

282. Goldstein RS, Mayor GH: Minireview. The nephrotoxicity of cisplatin. Life Sci 32:685–690, 1983.

283. Schilsky RL, Anderson T: Hypomagnesemia and renal magnesium wasting in patients receiving cisplatin. Ann Intern Med 90:929–931, 1979.

284. Gilbert M: Neurologic complications. In Abeloff MD, Armitage JO, Lichter AS, et al (eds): Clinical Oncology. New York, Churchill Livingstone, 1995.

285. Reed E: Platinum analogs. In DeVita VT, Hellman S, Rosenberg SA (eds): Cancer: Principles and Practice of Oncology, ed 4. Philadelphia, J.B. Lippincott, 1993, pp. 390–400.

286. Ohnuma T, Holland JF, Meyer P: *Erwinia carotovora* asparaginase in patients with prior anaphylaxis to asparaginase from *E. coli.* Cancer 30:376–381, 1972.

287. Castaman G, Rodeghiero F, Dini E: Thrombotic complications during L-asparaginase treatment for acute lymphocytic leukemia. Haematologica 75:567–569, 1990.

288. Semeraro N, Montemurro P, Giordano P, et al: Unbalanced coagulation-fibrinolysis potential during L-asparaginase therapy in children with acute lymphoblastic leukaemia. Thromb Haemost 64:38–40, 1990.

289. Chabner B: Miscellaneous agents. In DeVita VT, Hellman S, Rosenberg SA (eds): Cancer: Principles and Practice of Oncology, ed 4. Philadelphia, J.B. Lippincott, 1993, pp. 385–390.

290. Feinberg WM, Swenson MR: Cerebrovascular complications of L-asparaginase therapy. Neurology 38:127–133, 1988.

291. Priest JR, Ramsay NK, Steinherz PG, et al: A syndrome of thrombosis and hemorrhage complicating L-asparaginase therapy for childhood acute lymphoblastic leukemia. J Pediatrics 100:984–989, 1982.

292. Gugliotta L, D'Angelo A, Mattoli-Belmonte M, et al: Hypercoagulability during L-asparaginase treatment: The effect of antithrombin III supplementation in vivo. Br J Haematol 74:465–470, 1990.

293. Gilbert M: Neurologic complications. In Abeloff MD, Armitage JO, Lichter AS, et al (eds): Clinical Oncology. New York, Churchill Livingstone, 1995.

294. Holland J, Fasanello S, Ohnuma T: Psychiatric symptoms associated with L-asparaginase administration. J Psychiatr Res 10:105–113, 1974.

295. Stoelting RK: Chemotherapeutic drugs. In Pharmacology and Physiology in Anesthetic Practice, ed 2. Philadelphia, J.B. Lippincott, 1991, pp. 504–520.

296. Stoelting RK: Drugs used in the treatment of psychiatric disease. In Pharmacology and Physiology in Anesthetic Practice, ed 2. Philadelphia, J.B. Lippincott, 1991, pp. 365–383.

297. Cooper JA, Zitnik R, Matthay RA: Mechanisms of drug-induced pulmonary disease. Annu Rev Med 39:395–404, 1988.

298. Weiss RB, Grillo-Lopez AJ, Marsoni S, et al: Amsacrine-associated cardiotoxicity: An analysis of 82 cases. J Clin Oncol 4:918–928, 1986.

299. Arlin ZA, Feldman EJ, Mittelman A, et al: Amsacrine is safe and effective therapy for patients with myocardial dysfunction and acute leukemia. Cancer 68:1198–1200, 1991.

300. Parsons JT: The effect of radiation on normal tissues of the head and neck. In Million RR, Cassisi NJ (eds): Management of Head and Neck Cancer. A Multidisciplinary Approach. Philadelphia, J.B. Lippincott, 1984, p. 173.

301. McDonald S, Missaillidou D, Rubin P: Pulmonary complications. In Abeloff MD, Armitage JO, Lichter AS, et al (eds): Clinical Oncology. New York, Churchill Livingstone, 1995.

302. Gross NJ: Pulmonary effects of radiation therapy. Ann Intern Med 86:81, 1977.

303. Gross NJ: The pathogenesis of radiation-induced lung damage. Lung 159:115–125, 1981.

304. Siemann DW, Rubin P, Penney DP: Pulmonary toxicity following multifraction radiotherapy. Br J Cancer 53:365–367, 1986.

305. Mah K, Van Dyk J, Keane T, et al: Acute radiation-induced pulmonary damage: A clinical study on the response to fractionated radiation therapy. Int J Radiat Oncol Biol Phys 13:179–188, 1987.

306. Lindower PD, Skorton DJ: Cardiovascular system and anticancer therapy. In Armitage JO, Antman KH (eds): High Dose Cancer Chemotherapy, ed 2. Baltimore, Williams & Wilkins, 1995.

307. Brosius FC, Waller BF, Roberts WC: Radiation heart disease: Analysis of 16 young necropsy patients who received over 3,500 rads to the heart. Am J Med 70:519–530, 1981.

308. Taymor-Luria H, Cohn K, Pasternak RC: Diagnostic challenge: How to identify radiation heart disease. J Cardiovasc Med 8:113–123, 1983.

309. Gottdiener JS, Katin MJ, Borer JS, et al: Late cardiac effects of therapeutic mediastinal irradiation: Assessment by echocardiography and radionuclide angiography. N Engl J Med 308:569–572, 1983.

310. Applefeld MM, Cole JF, Pollock SH, et al. The late appearance of chronic pericardial disease in patients treated by radiotherapy for Hodgkin's disease. Ann Intern Med 94:338–341, 1981.

Index

Note: Page numbers in *italics* refer to figures; page numbers followed by t refer to tables.